Ocular Therapeutics

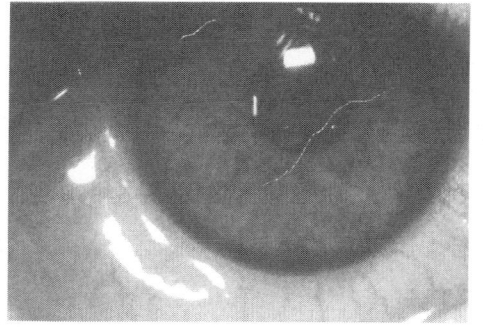

Ocular Therapeutics

Third Edition

Editor-in-Chief

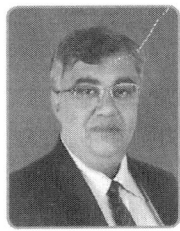

Ashok Garg

MS PhD FIAO(Bel) FRCS FRSM ADM FAIMS FICA
International and National Gold Medalist
Chairman and Medical Director
Garg Eye Institute and Research Center
Hisar, Haryana, India

Foreword

Steve A Arshinoff
Graham Barrett
David J Apple

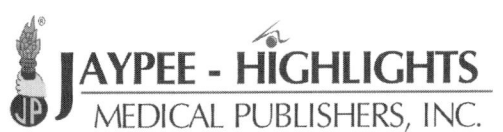

Honorary Editors

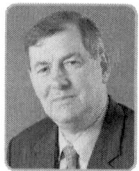

Eric D Donnenfeld MD FCA
Clinical Professor
Ophthalmic Consultants of Long Island
New York, USA

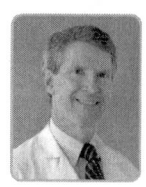

Stephen C Pflugfelder MD
Cullen Eye Institute
Baylor College of Medicine
Houston, Texas, USA

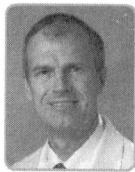

John D Sheppard MD MMSc
Director, Thomas R Lee Center
for Ocular Pharmacology
Professor of Ophthalmology
Eastern Virginia Medical School
Virginia Eye Consultants
Norfolk, Virginia, USA

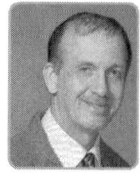

Mitchell Friedlaender MD
Head, Division of Ophthalmology
Director, Laser Vision Center
Scripps Clinic
La Jolla, California
Rockville, USA

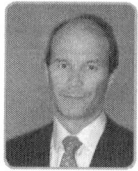

Jose M Ruiz Moreno MD PhD
Professor
Department of Opthalmology
Albacete Medical School
University of Castilla La Mancha
Avenida Almansa, Albacete, Spain

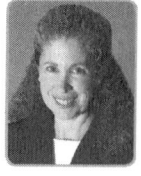

Arbisser Lisa MD
Lisa Brothers Arbisser
Bettendorf, Iowa, USA

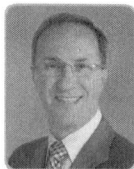

Roberto Bellucci MD
Chief, Ophthalmic Unit
Hospital and Universty of Verona
Via Degli Abeti 17
Salo (BS), Italy

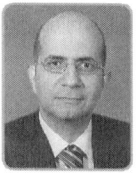

Ahmad K Khalil MD
Professor
Department of Ophthalmology
Research Institute of Ophthalmology
Dokki, Cairo, Egypt

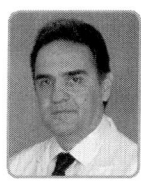

Ashley Behrens MD
Executive Medical Director
Senior Academy Consultant and
KKESH/WEI Professor of International
Ophthalmology
The King Khaled Eye Specialist Hospital
Riyadh, The Kindgom of Saudi Arabia

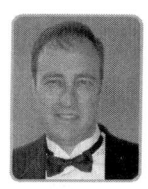

T Mark Johnson MD FRSC
Consultant, Vitreoretinal Surgeon
National Retina Institute
Wisconsin Avenue
Chevy Chase, Maryland, USA

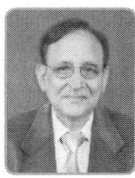

CS Dhull MS PhD FIAO
Director
Postgraduate Institute of
Medical Sciences
Rohtak, Haryana, India

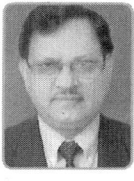

NR Biswas MD DN DNB DSc
Professor
Department of Pharmacology
All India Institute of Medical Sciences
New Delhi, India

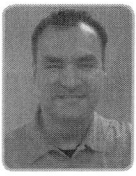

Arturo Perez Arteaga MD
Centro Oftalmologico Tlalnepantla
Dr Perez-Arteaga Vallarta No. 42
Tlalnepantla, Centro Estado de
Mexico

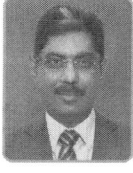

Purendra Bhasin MS
Chairman and Medical Director
Ratan Jyoti Netralaya
Gwalior, Madhya Pradesh, India

Jaypee Brothers Medical Publishers (P) Ltd

Headquarters

Jaypee Brothers Medical Publishers (P) Ltd.
4838/24, Ansari Road, Daryaganj
New Delhi 110 002, India
Phone: +91-11-43574357
Fax: +91-11-43574314
Email: jaypee@jaypeebrothers.com

Overseas Offices

J.P. Medical Ltd.
83, Victoria Street, London
SW1H 0HW (UK)
Phone: +44-2031708910
Fax: +02-03-0086180
Email: info@jpmedpub.com

Jaypee-Highlights Medical Publishers Inc.
City of Knowledge, Bld. 237, Clayton
Panama City, Panama
Phone: +507-301-0496
Fax: +507-301-0499
Email: cservice@jphmedical.com

Jaypee Brothers Medical Publishers Ltd.
The Bourse
111 South Independence Mall East
Suite 835, Philadelphia, PA 19106, USA
Phone: + 267-519-9789
Email: joe.rusko@jaypeebrothers.com

Jaypee Brothers Medical Publishers (P) Ltd.
17/1-B, Babar Road, Block-B, Shaymali
Mohammadpur, Dhaka-1207
Bangladesh
Mobile: +08801912003485
Email: jaypeedhaka@gmail.com

Jaypee Brothers Medical Publishers (P) Ltd.
Shorakhute, Kathmandu
Nepal
Phone: +00977-9841528578
Email: jaypee.nepal@gmail.com

Website: www.jaypeebrothers.com
Website: www.jaypeedigital.com

© 2013, Jaypee Brothers Medical Publishers

All rights reserved. No part of this book may be reproduced in any form or by any means without the prior permission of the publisher.

Inquiries for bulk sales may be solicited at: jaypee@jaypeebrothers.com

This book has been published in good faith that the contents provided by the editors contained herein are original, and is intended for educational purposes only. While every effort is made to ensure accuracy of information, the publisher and the editors specifically disclaim any damage, liability, or loss incurred, directly or indirectly, from the use or application of any of the contents of this work. If not specifically stated, all figures and tables are courtesy of the editors. Where appropriate, the readers should consult with a specialist or contact the manufacturer of the drug or device.

Ocular Therapeutics

First Edition: 2001
Second Edition: 2003
  Revised Reprint: 2006
Third Edition: **2013**

ISBN 978-93-5090-320-9

Printed at Sanat Printers

Dedicated to

My respected Param Pujya Guru Sant Gurmeet Ram Rahim Singh Ji (Insaa) for his blessings and motivation

My respected parents, teachers, my wife Dr Aruna Garg, son Abhishek and daughter Anshul for their constant support and patience during all these days of hard work

My dear friend Dr Amar Agarwal, a leading International Ophthalmologist from India for his continued support and guidance

Ashok Garg
Editor-in-Chief

Contributors

Ahmad K Khalil MD
Professor
Department of Ophthalmology
Research Institute of Ophthalmology
Dokki, Cairo, Egypt

AK Dubey DOMS MD
Assistant Professor
Department of Pharmacology
School of Medical Sciences and
Research, Sharda University
Greater Noida
Uttar Pradesh, India

Alok K Ravi PhD
Department of Ocular Pharmacology
Dr RP Center for Ophthalmic
Sciences
All India Institute of
Medical Sciences
New Delhi, India

Amar Agarwal MS FRCS FRCOph
Consultant
Dr Agarwal's Eye Hospital
Chennai, Tamil Nadu, India

Ammar M Al Mahmood MD FRCS
Consultant
Anterior Segment Division
King Khaled Eye Specialist Hospital
Riyadh, Saudi Arabia

Amit Basia DNB
Consultant, Retina
Vitreous and Uvea
Ratan Jyoti Netralaya
Gwalior, Madhya Pradesh, India

Anand Bagmar MS
Aditya Jyot Eye Hospital Pvt Ltd
Mumbai, Maharashtra, India

Anoop Sivaraman MS
Aditya Jyot Eye Hospital Pvt Ltd
Plot No. 153, Road No. 9
Major Parmeshwaran Road
Opp. SIWS College, Gate No. 3
Wadala, Mumbai
Maharashtra, India

Anthony Vipin Das MS
Clinical Associate
Cornea and Anterior Segment Service
LV Prasad Eye Institute
Hyderabad, Andhra Pradesh, India

Arbisser Lisa MD
Lisa Brothers Arbisser
Bettendorf, Iowa, USA

Arturo Perez Arteaga MD
Centro Oftalmologico Tlalnepantla
Dr Perez-Arteaga Vallarta No. 42
Tlalnepantla, Centro Estado de
Mexico

Ashim K Mitra MD
University of Missouri-Kansas City
School of Pharmacy
Division of Pharmaceutical Sciences
Kansas City, Missouri, USA

Ashley Behrens MD
Executive Medical Director
Senior Academy Consultant and
KKESH/WEI Professor of
International Ophthalmology
The King Khaled Eye Specialist
Hospital, Riyadh
The Kingdom of Saudi Arabia

Ashok Garg MS PhD FIAO(Bel) FRCS
FRSM ADM FAIMS FICA
International and National
Gold Medalist
Chairman and Medical Director
Garg Eye Institute and Research
Center
Hisar, Haryana
India

Ashuma Sachdeva MD
Associate Professor
Department of Biochemistry
Postgraduate Institute of
Medical Sciences
Rohtak
Haryana, India

Ashwin Agarwal
Dr Agarwal's Eye Hospital
Chennai, Tamil Nadu, India

Athiya Agarwal
Dr Agarwal's Eye Hospital
Chennai, Tamil Nadu
India

Carlo Bellucci
Ophthalmic Unit
Hospital and Universty of Verona
Via Degli Abeti 17
Salo (BS), Italy

Cintia S De Paiva MD
Ocular Surface Center
Cullen Eye Institute
Baylor College of Medicine
Houston
Texas, USA

x Ocular Therapeutics

CS Dhull MS PhD FIAO
Director
Postgraduate Institute of
Medical Sciences
Rohtak
Haryana, India

Daphne Bresheaus COA
Division of Ophthalmology
Scripps Clinic
La Jolla
California, USA

De-Quan Li MD PhD
Ocular Surface Center
Cullen Eye Institute
Baylor College of Medicine
Houston
Texas, USA

Douglas W Morck DVM PhD
Department of Ophthalmology
The Eye Care Center
Vancouver, Canada

Eric D Donnenfeld MD FCA
Clinical Professor
Ophthalmic Consultants of
Long Island
New York, USA

Eugenia Sanchis Merino
Department of Opthalmology
Albacete Medical School
University of Castilla La Mancha
Avenida Almansa
Albacete, Spain

Francisco Lugo
Department of Opthalmology
Albacete Medical School
University of Castilla La Mancha
Avenida Almansa
Albacete, Spain

Gagandeep Singh Brar MS
Assistant Professor
Department of Ophthalmology
Postgraduate Institute of Medical
Education and Research
Chandigarh, India

Gina Chavez BSc
Department of Ophthalmology
The Eye Care Center
Vancouver, Canada

GK Das MD
Professor
Department of Ophthalmology
University College of Medical
Sciences and Guru Teg Bahadur
Hospital
New Delhi, India

Harivenkatesh N MD
Senior Resident
Department of Pharmacology
All India Institute of
Medical Sciences
New Delhi, India

Henry D Perry MD FACS
Chief of Cornea Service
Nassau University Medical Center
East Meadow, New York
Rockville Center, New York, USA

Hsi-Kung Kuo MD
Department of Ophthalmology
Chang Gung Memorial Hospital-
Kaohsiung Medical Center
Kaohsiung, Hsien
Taiwan, ROC

Ian Bell MD
Clinical Director
Bell Institute of Ophthalmology
Texas, USA

James M Hill MD
Louisiana State University Eye Center
New Orleans, Louisiana, USA

Javier A Montero MD PhD
Pio del Rio Hortega
University Hospital
Valladolid, Spain

John D Sheppard MD MMSc
Director, Thomas R Lee Center
for Ocular Pharmacology
Professor of Ophthalmology
Eastern Virginia Medical School
Virginia Eye Consultants
Norfolk, Virginia, USA

Jorge Ruiz Medrano MD
St Carlos University Hospital
Madrid, Spain

Jose M Ruiz Moreno MD PhD
Professor
Department of Opthalmology
Albacete Medical School
University of Castilla La Mancha
Avenida Almansa
Albacete, Spain

Kirit Mody MS FRCS FRCO
Consulting Eye Surgeon
Salil Eye Clinic and Contact Lens
Center
Mumbai, Maharashtra, India

KP Biswas
Department of Pharmacology
All India Institute of
Medical Sciences
New Delhi, India

Contributors

Madhurjya Gogoi MD
Department of Pharmacology
Dr RP Center for Ophthalmic Sciences
All India Institute of Medical Sciences
New Delhi, India

Manisha Rathi MD
Professor
Department of Ophthalmology
Regional Institute of Ophthalmology
Postgraduate Institute of Medical Sciences
Rohtak, Haryana, India

Marg E Marquart MD
Department of Ophthalmology
Louisiana State University Health Sciences Center
New Orleans, Louisiana, USA

Mitchell Friedlaender MD
Head, Division of Ophthalmology
Director, Laser Vision Center
Scripps Clinic
La Jolla, California, Rockville
Maryland, USA

Navendu Rai MS
Aditya Jyot Eye Hospital Pvt Ltd
Plot No. 153, Road No. 9
Major Parmeshwaran Road
Opp. SIWS College, Gate No. 3
Wadala, Mumbai
Maharashtra, India

Niranjan Nayak MD
Additional Professor
Department of Ocular Microbiology
Dr RP Center for Ophthalmic Sciences
All India Institute of Medical Sciences
New Delhi, India

NR Biswas MD DN DNB DSc
Professor of Pharmacology
All India Institute of Medical Sciences
New Delhi, India

Pandurang Kulkarni
Aditya Jyot Eye Hospital Pvt Ltd
Plot No. 153, Road No. 9
Major Parmeshwaran Road
Opp. SIWS College, Gate No. 3
Wadala, Mumbai
Maharashtra, India

Pedro Amat Peral
Department of Opthalmology
Albacete Medical School
University of Castilla La Mancha
Avenida Almansa, Albacete, Spain

Pei-Chang Wu MD
Department of Ophthalmology
Chang Gung Memorial Hospital-Kaohsiung Medical Center
Kaohsiung, Hsien
Taiwan, ROC

Prachi Tomar MBBS
Anesthetic
Ratan Jyoti Netralaya
Gwalior, Madhya Pradesh, India

Prateek Gujar MS
Head, Cornea Department
Ratan Jyoti Netralaya
Gwalior, Madhya Pradesh, India

Priyamvada Bhasin MS
Director and Head, Retinal Clinic
Ratan Jyoti Netralaya
Gwalior, Madhya Pradesh, India

Purendra Bhasin MS
Chairman and Medical Director
Ratan Jyoti Netralaya
Gwalior, Madhya Pradesh, India

Rami Pai MS
Senior Research Fellow
Conwest Jain Clinic and Medical Research Society
Mumbai, Maharashtra, India

Reema M Choudhry
Dr Agarwal's Eye Hospital
Chennai
Tamil Nadu, India

Rene-Cano Hidalgo MD
Chairman
Institute of Ophthalmology
Conde de Valenciana
Vitreous and Retina Department
Professor of Ophthalmology
National Institute of Mexico (UNAM)
Mexico

Renee Solomon MD
North Shore University Hospital and Nassau County Medical Center
Rockville Center
New York, USA

Richard Mathias MD FRCP
Department of Ophthalmology
The Eye Care Center
Vancouver, Canada

Rishi Bhardwaj
Aditya Jyot Eye Hospital Pvt Ltd
Plot No. 153, Road No. 9
Major Parmeshwaran Road
Opp. SIWS College, Gate No. 3
Wadala, Mumbai
Maharashtra, India

Robert Latkany MD
Director and Founder
Dry Eye Clinic NY Eye and Ear Infirmary
Dry Eye Center of New York
Manhattan
New York, USA

Roberto Bellucci MD
Chief, Ophthalmic Unit
Hospital and Universty of Verona
Via Degli Abeti 17
Salo (BS), Italy

Saurabh Choudhry
Dr Agarwal's Eye Hospital
Chennai, Tamil Nadu, India

Shachi Desai MS
Aditya Jyot Eye Hospital Pvt Ltd
Plot No. 153, Road No. 9
Major Parmeshwaran Road
Opp. SIWS College, Gate No. 3
Wadala, Mumbai
Maharashtra, India

Simon P Holland MB FRCSC FRCOph
Clinical Professor
Department of Ophthalmology
The Eye Care Center
Vancouver, Canada

S Natarajan MS FRVS
Chairman and Medical Director
Aditya Jyot Eye Hospital Pvt Ltd
Plot No. 153, Road No. 9
Major Parmeshwaran Road
Opp. SIWS College, Gate No. 3
Wadala, Mumbai
Maharashtra, India

SPS Grewal MD
Director
Grewal Eye Institute and Research Center
Chandigarh, India

Srujana Mohanty MD
Dr RP Center for Ophthalmic Sciences
All India Institute of Medical Sciences
New Delhi, India

Stephen C Pflugfelder MD
Cullen Eye Institute
Baylor College of Medicine
Houston
Texas, USA

Sumit Sachdeva MS
Assistant Professor
Regional Institute of Ophthalmology
Postgraduate Institute of Medical Sciences
Rohtak, Haryana, India

Sunita Agarwal MS DO PSVH
Dr Agarwal's Eye Hospital
Chennai, Tamil Nadu
Bangalore
Karnataka, India

T Mark Johnson MD FRSC
Consultant, Vitreoretinal Surgeon
National Retina Institute
Wisconsin Avenue
Chevy Chase, USA

Tracy L Lee BSC MPT
Department of Ophthalmology
The Eye Care Center
Vancouver, Canada

Vinay Prasad MS
Aditya Jyot Eye Hospital Pvt Ltd
Plot No. 153, Road No. 9
Major Parmeshwaran Road
Opp. SIWS College, Gate No. 3
Wadala, Mumbai
Maharashtra, India

Vinay Gupta MD
Assistant Professor
Department of Ophthalmology
Dr RP Center for Ophthalmic Sciences
All India Institute of Medical Sciences
New Delhi, India

Virender Sangwan MS
Associate Director
LV Prasad Eye Institute
Head, Cornea and Anterior Segment
Ocular Immunology and Uveitis Service
Hyderabad
Andhra Pradesh, India

Yumi G Ohashi BSc
Department of Ophthalmology
The Eye Care Center
Vancouver, Canada

Xiadong Zheng MD
Department of Ophthalmology
Ehime University School of Medicine
Ehime, Japan

Foreword to the Third Edition

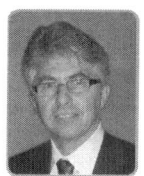

For me, the most difficult course in medical school was therapeutics. It remained the most difficult during my residency in ophthalmology. There were aspects that made obvious sense, like using penicillin to kill streptococci, and things that made a little sense like drugs that seemed to work for rheumatologic conditions that were themselves as yet poorly defined. We were not sure why they worked but somehow they did. We were instructed to simply memorize the lists of agents which had been shown to have some degree of efficacy, as well as second and third choices in the event of allergy to or suboptimal efficacy of the first choice. Therapeutics always seemed like an amalgam of science, may be science, the art of medicine, and placebo tricks. I recall, not too long ago, on one of my lecture trips to India, being asked about the treatment of an unfortunately too common parasitic disorder in India. I looked at the questioner and said, "Do you know where I am from? I have never seen a case of that in my life and never will in Canada. Please ask one of your esteemed local colleagues." The principles of therapeutics are universal, such as how to avoid TASS (the chapter herein is appropriately written by an expert Canadian group), but often the management of a local disease relies upon local knowledge both of the disease and the locally available therapies.

The practice of medicine consists of two steps. The first and perhaps most critical is diagnosis. We all like to believe that we are expert diagnosticians after we have been in practice for a few years. We read journals and textbooks about common and rare disorders to hone our diagnostic skills, and we competed as residents, and still do in various journals to believe we are better than, or at least, just as good, at diagnosis as our peers. We generally leave therapy to be looked up in a recent book, kept in our memory banks, or those of our computers or cell phones, or looked up when needed on the Internet. We believe subconsciously that learning diagnosis creates a permanent addition to our skill set, and can gain us esteem, but that learning therapeutics always seems to only make current trends more easily available transiently.

But textbooks of therapeutics were always the ones that I consulted most frequently after the first 5 years out of my residency. I usually knew what I was looking at, but wanted to see if what I had been taught was still current, and more importantly I wanted to see if some of those nebulous connections between diagnosis and therapy had been enhanced or redirected by new science. Medical and ophthalmic therapeutics only slowly evolves to become more rational and more efficacious. So, we keep reading newer textbooks looking for answers, often in areas that we had not even questioned.

Dr Ashok Garg, along with honoary editors has again assembled a stellar list of editors and authors to try to provide the reader with an updated book for the answers we all seek when confronted by patient problems. The goal of the book, in its 69 chapters, is to provide a quick overview of the therapeutic problem, the ophthalmologist is facing, and to recommend what is currently thought to be the optimum therapy. Hopefully, as you read, along the way each of you will be inspired to see things a bit differently from how you previously viewed the particular issue you are investigating, and perhaps even change a paradigm that may have outlasted its usefulness. After all, we must continually change our paradigms to avoid becoming old and outdated.

The book will hopefully help you, challenge you, make you think, and be well worn in time for the 4th edition, to have served its purpose. Therapeutics is ever changing, and we must eagerly embrace the changes and try to understand them, before we can use them optimally for the benefit of our patients.

Steve A Arshinoff MD FRCSC
Toronto, Ontario, Canada
email: ifix2is@sympatico.ca

Foreword to the Third Edition

There are many textbooks that have been published in the field of Ophthalmology but Dr Ashok Garg with his energy and insights has created a unique publication with this new textbook on *Ocular Therapeutics*.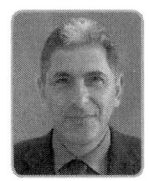

The book contains introductory chapters on basic physiology and drug administration as well as several chapters emphasizing the fundamental role of ocular therapeutics in specific areas of ophthalmology. Dr Ashok Garg is the major contributor to this section and is to be commended for structuring the chapters in a format which is comprehensible and clinically relevant.

The next section focuses on the role of ocular therapeutics in ophthalmic surgery. Together with several international experts, this section of the book is a logical companion to the fundamentals of the previous chapters and highlights the important role of ocular therapeutics in a clinical practice and includes refractive surgery and strategies for the prevention of endophthalmitis. The topics selected cover a broad range of general and subspecialty interests.

The final section on Recent Advances in Ocular Therapeutics addresses conditions such as anti-VEGF treatment and considers the future development of nanotechnology in ophthalmology. The authors who have contributed to this textbook have been selected for their in-depth knowledge and expertise in specific areas and together with Dr Ashok Garg have created an excellent resource on ocular therapeutics for practising Ophthalmologists.

I would like to commend Dr Ashok Garg for his efforts in creating a comprehensive textbook which will be extremely valuable to all Ophthalmologists when selecting appropriate treatment for their patients.

Graham Barrett
Clinical Professor
Department of Ophthalmology
Lions Eye Institute
Head, Department of Ophthalmology
Sir Charles Gairdner Hospital, Nedlands
Western Australia, Australia
President
Asia Pacific Association of Cataract and Refractive Surgeons
e-mail : graham.barrett@uwa.edu.au

Foreword to the Second Edition

It is a distinct pleasure to write Foreword of second edition of the *Textbook of Ocular Therapeutics* edited by Dr Ashok Garg, Garg Eye Institute and Research Center, Hisar, Haryana, India, and my fellow Dr Suresh K Pandey, Center for Research on Ocular Therapeutics and Biodevices, Albert Florens Storm Eye Institute, Medical University of South Carolina, Charleston, South Carolina, USA.

Forty-one chapters, separated in 2 sections, of this book provide a detailed outline for therapy for the basic categories of ocular diseases including infections and inflammations, immune therapy, viscoelastic agents, antioxidants and antiretroviral drugs, antiglaucoma drugs and many others. Detailed and most recent information about the ophthalmic dyes, viscoelastic agents as well as details about the ocular drug toxicity are also addressed in several chapters. An entire new section on applied ocular therapeutics in ophthalmic surgery has been added that includes 11 excellent chapters. A comprehensive text on posterior capsule opacification, cataract surgery in children, ophthalmic dyes for cataract and retinal surgery, photodynamic therapy for age-related macular degeneration as well as indocyanine green angiography and dry eye management are a superb addition to the second edition of this remarkable book. All chapters of the textbook will be very helpful to the practising ophthalmic surgeon in providing clinically useful dosages that are useful in the clinic or field situation. I commend the hard work done by Drs Garg and Pandey to produce this high quality ocular therapeutics textbook.

Chapter 26 on Ocular Drug Toxicity (Complications) of the book is interesting from my perspective. I personally have spent the last 20 years of my professional career describing and evaluating complications of intraocular lenses. Therefore, the topic of complications is in my opinion very important and is a major service provided by this book. Complications of various drugs including toxicity of surgical solutions are covered. This is invaluable to the surgeons who may not have a complete library at hand for consultation on the spot during a clinical practice.

The textbook, for which Drs Garg and Pandey should be congratulated, displays a well-defined view of basic and applied aspect of ocular pharmacology and therapeutics. Each chapter is comprehensive in nature, represents the recent advances in the area of ocular pharmacology and therapeutics. The team of a well-known Indian medical publisher M/s Jaypee Brothers Medical Publishers (P) Ltd, New Delhi, India, provided excellent layout and high quality illustrations for the book. I hope that *Textbook of Ocular Therapeutics* will appear in several more editions with the entry into the new millennium.

David J Apple MD
Fellow, American Ophthalmological Society
Professor, Ophthalmology and Pathology
Pawek-Vallotton Chair of Biomedical Engineering
Director, Ophthalmic Pathology Laboratory and Center for
Research on Ocular Therapeutics and Biodevices
Director, World Health Organization Collaborative Center for
Developing World Ophthalmology
Co-Director, Magill Research Center for Vision Correction
Storm Eye Institute, Medical University of South Carolina
Charleston, South Carolina, USA
e-mail: appledj@musc.edu

Preface to the Third Edition

Ocular Therapeutics have undergone tremendous advances both for anterior and posterior segment diseases in the last one decade. A wide array of new safe, effective drugs with least side effects are available for various ophthalmic surgeries and ocular diseases—new effective FOTE drug therapy based on advanced technology along with invasive and noninvasive ocular drug delivery systems are now available which include the use of nanoparticles, liposomes and dendrimers. Versidoser drug delivery platforms shall revolutionize the FOTE drug delivery system. Genetic, regenerative drugs and stem cell based drug therapy shall make the treatment customized to individual need of ocular disease extent making it more cost-effective and safe.

The third edition of this book has been completely updated with addition of all new ocular drugs and delivery systems in every group of medicine used in ophthalmic disease and surgeries. Sixty-nine chapters of this line have been grouped as preliminary section, Applied Ocular Therapeutics and Recent Advances. In this comprehensive book leading International Ocular Drug Experts have shared their experiences and evidence-based knowledge in the form of chapters.

We are grateful to Shri Jitendar P Vij (Group Chairman), Mr Ankit Vij (Managing Director), Mr Tarun Duneja (Director-Publishing), who took keen interest in this project, and all staff members of M/s Jaypee Brothers Medical Publishers (P) Ltd, New Delhi, India, who worked over time to prepare the book *Ocular Therapeutics,* possible in short time.

We hope the comprehensive book on *Ocular Therapeutics* shall serve as ready reference for all ophthalmologists worldwide who are engaged in eradication of global blindness and make every effort to make eye 6/6 by synergistic combination of ophthalmic drugs and surgery.

Editors

Preface to the Second Edition

We are extremely happy and encouraged to receive the overwhelming response to first edition of *Textbook of Ocular Therapeutics* from all over the world. Keeping in view of this tremendous response, we are presenting the revised and updated second edition of this book within a short period of publication of the first edition.

Research in Ocular Therapeutics is an ongoing continuous process and in last 18-24 months a number of new therapeutic products specially in the field of antiglaucoma, antibiotics, antiallergics, ophthalmic dyes, steroidal and non-steroidal anti-inflammatory drugs have been developed commercially to treat the various ophthalmic diseases in a better way.

The second edition of *Textbook of Ocular Therapeutics* has been written to serve as a comprehensive drug information resource. It was conceived and developed after thorough research of the matter and through a team effort and shall be of great value to both the students and private practitioners. Ophthalmologists shall find the book specially useful in their daily practice.

In the second edition, besides incorporating latest therapeutic drugs, a separate section on Applied Ocular Therapeutics has been added for the benefit of readers to get insight into the role of specific medications in various ophthalmic surgeries.

The text of book is designed in a pharmacotherapeutic format with emphasis on drug entities, commercial product information and specific formulation availability.

We are thankful to contributors, our friends, family members and well wishers who helped us in every possible manner to prepare this edition.

Our sincere thanks are due to M/s Jaypee Brothers Medical Publishers (P) Ltd, New Delhi, India, specially to Shri Jitendar P Vij (Group Chairman) who extended full cooperation to prepare the book and worked hard to publish it expeditiously.

We hope readers shall find the book as a valuable companion in ophthalmic drug product information, selection and use. With God's grace we shall continue the work with future editions. Therefore, your comments and suggestions are always welcome and valuable to us.

Editors

Preface to the First Edition

Textbook of Ocular Therapeutics has been written to provide succinct, reliable, rapid access drug information and facilitate therapeutic decision making.

Due to inspired research in the last decade, a number of new topical drugs are available for better management of different ophthalmic conditions. Significant advancement has taken place in the fields of topical antibiotics, anti-inflammatory (Steroidal and NSAID therapy), third generation antibiotics and NSAIDs are now commercially available for topical use. Tremendous strides have also been made in the field of topical antiglaucoma drugs specially with the advent of Topical Latanoprost, Brimonidine and Acetazolamide eyedrops. A lot of research work is being done on neuroprotective agents. Use of antioxidants in ophthalmology has brought a ray of hope for medical management of Senile cataract and age-related macular degeneration.

Every effort has been made in this book to incorporate the latest advances made in the different branches of ocular therapeutics. The chapters of this textbook has been designed to serve as quick reference to ophthalmologists. In the last chapters of the book Topical and Systemic drugs with common dosages used in ophthalmology has been added to serve as ready reckoner. *Textbook of Ocular Therapeutics* is a comprehensive ophthalmic drug information resource. Detailed information on specific entities as well as many drug combinations has been included.

I am thankful to Dr David J Apple (USA), Dr Suresh K Pandey (USA), Dr Amar Agarwal (Chennai, India), Dr Athiya Agarwal (Chennai, India), Dr Zetterstorm (Germany), Dr Keinkel (Australia) and Dr Patterson (UK), who gave valuable suggestions and tips for preparing the text of the book.

I am grateful to my family members and my wife Dr Aruna Garg who by their tender care and devotion helped me in this formidable task.

It is only appropriate that I thank and acknowledge my gratitude to my staff, Mr Anil Hans (Delhi Type College and Computers, Hisar, Haryana, India), and colleagues who assisted in the writing, editing and production of this text.

My sincere thanks are due to M/s Jaypee Brothers Medical Publishers (P) Ltd, New Delhi, India, specially Shri Jitendar P Vij (Group Chairman) who extended full cooperation to prepare this book and published it expeditiously.

I hope the readers shall find this book as a valuable guide in ophthalmic drug product selection and use. I intend to continue the efforts with future editions, therefore your comments, suggestions are always welcome.

Editor

Contents

SECTION 1: FUNDAMENTALS AND PRELIMINARY CONSIDERATIONS IN OCULAR THERAPEUTICS

1. **Ocular Defense System** 3
   Ashok Garg (India)
   - Physical Protection 3 • Physiological Protection 5

2. **Tear Film Physiology** 9
   Ashok Garg (India)
   - Tear Film Formation Dynamics 14 • Normal Tear Drainage 15 • Tear Composition 16 • Physical Properties of Tears 16 • Chemical Composition of Tear Fluid 18 • Applied Physiology 29 • Hyposecretion of Tears 30 • Hypersecretion of Tears 33

3. **Aqueous Humor Dynamics** 38
   Ashok Garg (India)
   - Blood-Aqueous Barrier 38 • Aqueous Humor Formation 42 • Aqueous Humor Formation Regulation (Control) 44 • Rate of Flow of Movements of Aqueous Humor 45 • Routes of Aqueous Outflow (Escape) 45 • Aqueous Humor Composition 48 • Functions of Aqueous Humor 54

4. **Routes of Administration and Drug Delivery Systems in Ophthalmology** 55
   Ashok Garg (India)
   - Local Application 55 • Systemic Administration 61

5. **Microorganisms and Ocular Diseases** 67
   Ashok Garg (India)
   - Bacteria 67 • Fungi 68 • Viruses 69 • Parasites 69 • Common Microbiological Stains Used in Ophthalmology 69 • Common Ophthalmic Culture Media and Usage 70 • Normal Microbial Flora of the Eye 70

6. **Unique Ocular Drug Delivery Systems** 73
   Xiadong Zheng (Japan), Marg E Marquart, Ashim K Mitra, James M Hill (USA)
   - Unique Ocular Drug Delivery Systems 75 • Other Ocular Drug Delivery Systems 86 • Conclusion and New Perspectives 89

7. **Antibacterial Therapy** 97
*NR Biswas, GK Das, Harivenkatesh N,
Ashok Garg (India)*

• Routes of Antimicrobial Administration in Ophthalmic Practice 97 • Selection of Antimicrobial Agents 98 • Indications for Antimicrobial Therapy 99 • Mechanisms of Resistance to Antibiotics 100 • Steps to be taken to Avoid Antimicrobial Resistance 100 • Antimicrobial Combination Therapy 100 • Microbes Causing Ocular Infections 101 • Classification of Antibacterial Drugs (According to Mechanism of Action) 102 • Drugs that Inhibit Bacterial Cell Wall Synthesis 103 • Beta-Lactam Antibiotics 104 • Glycopeptide Antibiotics 113 • Fosfomycin 115 • Bacitracin 115 • Drugs Attacking Bacterial Cell Membrane 116 • Drugs that Inhibit Bacterial Protein Synthesis 116 • Individual Drugs 120 • Spectinomycin 123 • Tetracyclines 123 • Glycylcycline—Tigecycline 126 • Chloramphenicol 127 • Macrolides 128 • Individual Drugs 131 • Ketolides—Telithromycin 133 • Oxazolidinones—Linezolid 134 • Lincosamides—Clindamycin 135 • Streptogramins—Quinupristin/Dalfopristin 136 • Retapamulin 136 • Fusidic Acid 136 • Drugs Attacking Bacterial DNA 136 • Nitroimidazoles 143 • Drugs Affecting Bacterial Intermediate Metabolism 145 • Cotrimoxazole (Trimethoprim-Sulfamethoxazole) 146 • Mupirocin 147 • Antimicrobial Peptides 147 • Use of Antibiotics in Irrigating Solutions for Intraocular Surgery 149 • Reasons for Failure in Ocular Antibiotic Treatment 152

8. **Anti-inflammatory Therapy** 155
*NR Biswas, AK Dubey, Harivenkatesh N,
Ashok Garg (India)*

• Corticosteroids 155 • Nonsteroidal Anti-inflammatory Drugs 169 • Phenylalkanoic Acids 176 • Indoles 179 • Phenylacetic Acid 180 • Immunosuppressive Agents in Ophthalmology 184

9. **Antiviral Therapy** 193
*NR Biswas, Harivenkatesh N, KP Biswas,
Ashok Garg (India)*

• DNA Viruses 193 • RNA Viruses 193 • Mechanism of Viral Infection/Multiplication 194 • General Mechanisms of Action of Antiviral Agents 195 • Classification of Antiviral Drugs 196 • Antiherpes Agents 198 • Drugs Active Against

Cytomegalovirus 205 • Drugs Active Against Hepatitis Virus 211 • Drugs Used in HIV Infection 214 • Entry Inhibitor (Maraviroc) 221 • Fusion Inhibitor (Enfuvirtide) 221 • Integrase Inhibitor (Raltegravir) 222 • Clinical Use of Antiretroviral Therapy in Ophthalmology 222 • Drugs Active Against Influenza Virus 222

10. **Antifungal Therapy** 225
    NR Biswas, AK Dubey, Harivenkatesh N, Ashok Garg (India)

    • Fungi Causing Ocular Infections 225 • Antifungal Drugs 226 • Polyenes 227 • Antimetabolite (Fluorinated Pyrimidine) 231 • Azole Derivatives 232 • Allylamines 239 • Echinocandins 241 • Silver Compounds 243

11. **Antiglaucoma Therapy** 245
    Ahmad K Khalil (Egypt)

    • Aqueous Solutions 248 • Suspensions 248 • Ointments 248 • Gels 249 • Ocular Inserts 249 • Drug Compliance 249 • Prostaglandins (Hypotensive Lipids; HLS) 254 • Carbonic Anhydrase Inhibitors 258 • A2-Adrenergic Agonists 262 • Cholinergic Drugs 263

12. **Antiallergy Therapy** 280
    NR Biswas, GK Das, Harivenkatesh N, Ashok Garg (India)

    • Type 1 Hypersensitivity Reactions 280 • Antiallergy Medication 281 • Topical Mast Cell Inhibitors 283 • Antihistamines 288 • Oral Antihistamines 293 • NSAIDs (Antiprostaglandin Therapy) 295 • Topical Steroids 295 • Topical Immunosuppressors 296 • Recent Advances in Immunosuppressive Therapy 296

13. **Local Anesthetic Agents** 299
    Ashok Garg (India)

    • Local Anesthetics (Injectables) 299 • Esters 301 • Amides 303 • Local Anesthetics (Topical) 307 • Synopsis of Ophthalmic Uses of Local Anesthetics 313

14. **Ophthalmic Viscosurgical Devices and Other Ocular Surgical Adjuncts** 315
    Ashok Garg (India)

    • Viscoelastic Substances 315 • Criteria for Selection of Viscoelastic Material 315 • Roles of Viscoelastic Substances 316 • Indications for Viscoelastic Substances 316 • Commercially Available Viscoelastic Substances 317 • Future

- Viscoelastics 326 • Irrigating Solutions 326
- Surgical Enzymes 328 • Surgical Adjuncts 330
- Chelating Agents, Collagenase Inhibitors and Mucolytics 335 • Caustic Preparations in Ophthalmology 336 • Cyanoacrylate Tissue Adhesives in Ophthalmology 337

15. Mydriatics and Cycloplegics 340
Ashok Garg (India)

- Mydriatic Adrenergic Agents (Sympathomimetic Agents) 340 • Cholinergic Antagonist as Mydriatic Agents 343 • Cycloplegic Mydriatics 343
- Mydriatic Combinations 348

16. Ophthalmic Dyes 351
Ashok Garg (India)

- Fluorescein Sodium 351 • Fluorexon 356
- Rose Bengal 357 • Lissamine Green 358
- Indocyanine Green 358 • Trypan Blue 360
- Verteporfin (Visudyne) 362

17. Ocular Lubricants and Artificial Tear Solutions 369
Ashok Garg (India)

- Artificial Tear Solutions 370 • Polyvinyl Alcohol Base Solutions 372 • Longer Lasting Mucoadhesive or Increased Viscosity Agents 373 • Polyvinyl Pyrrolidone Polymer Base Tear Solution 373
- Ointments 374 • Ocular Inserts (Solid Devices) 375
- Soft Contact Lens Therapy 376 • Punctal Plugs 376
- Collagen Implants 376 • Miscellaneous Preparations 377 • Recent Advances in New Polymers for Dry Eye Syndrome 377

18. Topical Immune Therapy 380
Ashok Garg (India)

- Ocular Defense System and Immunity 380
- Indications for Topical Immune Therapy 383
- Dosage 384 • Contraindication 385
- Adverse Reactions 385

19. Topical Hyperosmotic Agents 387
Ashok Garg (India)

- Major Causes of Corneal Edema 387 • Various Topical Hyperosmotic Agents Used in Ophthalmology 388

20. Antiretroviral Drug Therapy of Ocular Infections in AIDS 391
Ashok Garg (India)

- HIV-Related Retinopathy 392 • Opportunistic Infections of the Eye 393 • Nonopportunistic

Infections 394 • Tumor Involvement 396
• Neuro-Ophthalmological Manifestations 397
• Cutaneous Hypersensitivity Reactions 397 • HIV
in Ocular Structures 397 • Ocular Manifestations
of HIV Infections in Children 397 • Antiretroviral
Therapy of Ocular Infections in AIDS Patients 398
• Cytomegalovirus Infection 399
• Breakthrough Retinitis 404 • *Toxoplasma*
Infection 405 • Herpes Zoster Ophthalmicus 405
• *Mycobacterium tuberculosis* 406 • *Mycobacterium avium* Intracellulare 406 • Ocular Syphilis 407
• Acute Retinal Necrosis 407 • *Pneumocystis carinii* Choroiditis 407 • Recent Advances in
Antiretroviral Drug Therapy 407

21. **Sterilization, Disinfection and Antiseptics in Ophthalmology** — 410
    Ashok Garg (India)

    • Physical Methods 410 • Chemical Methods 418
    • Soaking in Liquid Chemicals 419 • AIDS and
    Disinfection in Relation to Ophthalmology 426

22. **Miscellaneous Drugs in Ophthalmology** — 430
    Ashok Garg (India)

    • Lid Scrubs 430 • Astringent Ophthalmic
    Solution 431 • Ophthalmic Diagnostic Tear Test
    Strips 431 • Hamameli's Ophthalmic Solution 433
    • Boric Acid 433 • Inactive Ingredients in
    Ophthalmic Products 433 • Viscosurgical
    Devices 436

23. **Ocular Drug Toxicity: Complications** — 438
    Ashok Garg (India)

    • Complications of Topical Antimicrobial Agents 440
    • Complications of Steroids 443 • Systemic Adverse
    Reactions of Glaucoma Medications 452
    • Complications of Topical Ocular Anesthetic
    Agents 457 • Toxicity of Surgical Solutions 460
    • Complications of Contact Lens Solutions 465
    • Complications of Intravenous Fluorescein 466
    • Classification of Adverse Reactions 467 • Drug-induced Ocular Cicatrization 469 • Systemic Drugs
    Causing Ocular Toxicity 472

24. **Topical and Systemic Ophthalmic Drugs with Common Dosages** — 492
    Ashok Garg (India)

    • Antibiotic Therapy 492 • Topical Anti-inflammatory Therapy 494 • Antiviral Therapy 496
    • Antifungal Therapy 498 • Antiglaucoma Therapy 499
    • Antiallergy Therapy 502 • Local Anesthetic

Agents 504 • Mydriatics and Cycloplegics 505
• Artificial Tears and Lubricants 506 • Ophthalmic
Viscosurgical Devices 508 • Irrigating Solutions 508
• Surgical Enzymes 509 • Surgical Adjuncts 509
• Topical Immune Therapy 510 • Topical
Hyperosmotic Agent 510 • Anticataract Therapy 511
• Medical Therapy for Armd (Age-related Macular
Degeneration) 512 • Medical Therapy for Diabetic
Retinopathy 512 • Ophthalmic Dyes 512 • Contact
Lens Care Products 514 • Recent Multipurpose
Soft Lens Care Systems 515 • Antiretroviral Drugs
in Ophthalmic Infections 516 • Ocular Therapeutics
in Refractive Surgery 520

25. **Ocular Manifestations of Systemic Diseases** 523
    Ashok Garg (India)
    • Various Systemic Diseases 523

26. **Quick Look Tabulated Ocular Therapeutics
    Information** 541
    Ashok Garg (India)
    • Antibacterials 541 • Combination Antibiotics 542
    • Anti-inflammatory Drugs 543 • Topical Steroid-
    antibiotic Combinations 544 • Antiviral Therapy 545
    • Antifungal Therapy 546 • Anti-allergy Therapy 547
    • Antiglaucoma Therapy 548 • Local Anesthetic
    Agents 551 • Local Anesthetic Combinations 552
    • Mydriatics and Cycloplegics 552 • Ophthalmic
    Viscosurgical Devices (OVD) and Surgical
    Adjuncts 552 • Ophthalmic Dyes 555 • Lubricants
    and Artificial Tear Solutions 556 • Topical Immune
    Therapy 559 • Topical Hyperosmotic Agents 559
    • Contact Lens Care Products 559 • Rewetting
    Solutions (Soft Lenses) 566 • Nonsurgical
    Adjuncts 566

SECTION 2: APPLIED OCULAR THERAPEUTICS IN OPHTHALMIC SURGERY

27. **Comprehensive Review of Topical Ophthalmic
    Antibacterial Agents: Their Mechanisms of Action
    and Adverse Effects Including Long-Standing
    Drugs and the Most Recent Preparations** 573
    Renée Solomon, Eric Donnenfeld (USA)
    • Bacterial Conjunctivitis 573 • Bacterial Keratitis 574
    • Properties of Topical Ophthalmic Antibacterial
    Agents 575 • Extemporaneously Compounded
    Fortified Antibiotics 582 • Aminoglycosides 582
    • Bacitracin 584 • Beta-Lactam Antibiotics 585
    • Chloramphenicol 587 • Macrolides 588

- Erythromycin 588 • Azithromycin 589
- Polymyxin and Combination Products 591
- Sulfacetamide 592 • Tetracyclines 593
- Vancomycin 594 • Selecting the Optimal Ophthalmic Antibiotic 595 • Clinical Judgment in Choosing an Ophthalmic Antibiotic 595
- Bacterial Conjunctivitis 596 • Bacterial Keratitis 596
- Norfloxacin 0.3 Percent Solution 597

28. **Preoperative and Postoperative Antibiotic Prophylaxis in Cataract Surgery** 606
    NR Biswas, Srujana Mohanty, GK Das, Madhurjya Gogoi (India)
    - Antibiotic Prophylaxis 607 • Chloramphenicol 609
    - Topical Fluoroquinolones 610 • Lomefloxacin 610
    - Fourth Generation Fluoroquinolones 611
    - Intracameral Antibiotics 612

29. **Management of Iatrogenic Inflammation of the Eye** 615
    NR Biswas, GK Das, Vinay Gupta (India)
    - Topical Application 615 • Use of Nonsteroidal Anti-inflammatory Drugs in Inflammation 619

30. **Management of Postrefractive Keratitis** 625
    Eric D Donnenfeld (USA)

31. **Ocular Pharmacotherapeutics in Corneal Refractive Surgery** 631
    Ashok Garg (India)
    - Preprocedure Therapeutic Medications 631
    - Postprocedure Therapeutic Medications 632

32. **Antioxidants and Their Role in Ophthalmology** 635
    CS Dhull, Sumit Sachdeva, Manisha Rathi, Ashuma Sachdeva (India)
    - Classification of Antioxidants 637

33. **Tetracyclins for Ocular Surface Diseases** 647
    Robert Latkany (USA)

34. **Clinical Applications of Antimycotic Agents in the Eye** 651
    Niranjan Nayak (India)
    - Keratomycosis 651 • Orbital Cellulitis 655
    - Dacryocystitis 656 • Endophthalmitis 656

35. **Recommended Antibiotic Dosages for Various Clinical Conditions of the Eye** 662
    Ashok Garg (India)

xxxii Ocular Therapeutics

36. **Endophthalmitis Prevention Strategies**   670
   John D Sheppard (USA)
   - New Concepts in Endophthalmitis Treatment 670
   - Existing Literature 671 • Practical Clinical Practice 671 • Microbial Antibiotic Resistance 672

37. **Management of Myopic Choroidal Neovascularization**   674
   Jose M Ruiz Moreno, Javier A Montero (Spain)
   - Photodynamic Therapy 674
   - Intravitreal Anti-VEGF Drug Injection 676

38. **Treatment of Central Serous Choroidopathy**   685
   Pedro Amat Peral, Francisco Lugo, Jose M Ruiz Moreno (Spain)
   - Differential Diagnosis 689 • Treatment 689
   - Pathogenesis 693 • Case Report 694

39. **Treatment of Retinal Angiomatous Proliferation**   702
   Javier A Montero, Jose M Ruiz-Moreno, Jorge Ruiz-Medrano (Spain)
   - Natural History 704

40. **Conjunctival Allergen Challenge for Evaluating Anti-inflammatory Therapy**   716
   Mitchell Friedlaender, Daphne Bresheaus (USA)
   - Abstract 716 • Methods 717 • Results 719

41. **Steroid Therapy for Allergic Ocular Disease**   725
   John D Sheppard (USA)
   - New Concepts in Topical Steroid Therapy 725
   - The Nature of Allergic Disease 727 • Combined Surface Diseases Present Diagnostic Challenges 728
   - Innovative Strategies for Ocular Surface Diseases 730
   - Blepharitis Exacerbates Dry Eyes and Allergy 735
   - Steroids for Contact Lens Wearers and Refractive Surgery Patients 740

42. **Optimizing Visual Outcomes with NSAIDs Therapy in Cataract and Refractive Surgeries**   744
   Eric D Donnenfeld, Henry D Perry (USA)
   - Rationale for Treating Ocular Inflammation 745
   - Pharmacologic Therapy for Ocular Inflammation 746

43. **Immunosuppressive Drugs in Ophthalmology**   756
   Ashok Garg (India)
   - Selection of Patients 756 • Alkylating Agents 756
   - Antimetabolites 757 • Antibiotic Cyclosporin A 758

Contents **xxxiii**

- Ocular Drug Toxicity of Immunosuppressive Agents used in Ophthalmic Conditions 759 • Recent Advances in Immunosuppressive Therapy 759

44. **Management of Cystoid Macular Edema** 762
    Arturo Perez Arteaga, Rene-Cano Hidalgo (Mexico)
    - Definition 762 • Etiology 762 • Histopathology 765
    - Clinical Findings 765 • Paraclinical Approach 766
    - Treatment 767

45. **Blepharitis** 775
    Mitchell Friedlaender (USA)
    - Classification 775 • Genetics 775 • Infection 776
    - Allergy 777 • Corneal Manifestations 778
    - Chemistry 779 • Treatment 779

46. **Trypan Blue in the Management of Mature Cataract** 782
    Amar Agarwal, Athiya Agarwal, Sunita Agarwal (India)
    - Rhexis in Mature Cataracts 782 • Trypan Blue 782
    - Technique 783 • Adverse Effects 790
    - Sterilization 790 • Indocyanine Green Dye 790

47. **Trypan Blue Assisted Epiretinal Membrane Removal** 791
    Amar Agarwal, Athiya Agarwal, Sunita Agarwal, Saurabh Choudhry, Reena M Choudhry (India)
    - Patients and Technique 791 • Results 793

48. **Perfluorocarbon Liquids in Vitreoretinal Surgery** 795
    Amar Agarwal (India)
    - Types 795 • Physical Properties 795
    - Indications 802 • Miscellaneous 807
    - Other Medical Applications 808
    - Complications 808

49. **Use of Tissue Adhesives in Ophthalmology** 810
    Prateek Gujar, Purendra Bhasin, Priyamvada Bhasin (India)
    - Cyanoacrylate Tissue Adhesives 811
    - Human Fibrin Glues 812 • Recent Advances in Tissue Adhesives in Ophthalmology 813

50. **Photodynamic Therapy (Verteporfin) in Age-related Macular Degeneration** 816
    S Natarajan, Anand Bagmar (India)
    - Technique 817 • Preparation of the Patient for PDT 818 • Calculation of the Treatment Spot Size Required Covering the CNV 819

51. Indocyanine Green Angiography 822
    S Natarajan, Anand Bagmar (India)
    - Advantages of ICG 822 • History 822
    - Pharmacology 823 • Toxicity 823 • Technique 823
    - Various Phases of ICG Angiography 823 • ICG in Age Related Macular Degeneration 824

52. Management of Dry Eye—Current Trends and Recent Advances 833
    Anthony Vipin Das, Virender Sangwan (India)
    - Medical Management 833 • Ongoing Clinical Trials 841

53. Management of Endophthalmitis: Antibiotic Schedule and Dosages 847
    Pei-Chang Wu, Hsi-Kung Kuo (Taiwan)
    - Acute Postoperative Endophthalmitis 847

54. Surgical Techniques of Glued IOL 860
    Ashvin Agarwal, Amar Agarwal (India)
    - Scleral Fixated IOL 860 • Fibrin Glue 860
    - Surgical Technique 860 • Discussion 861

55. Intraocular Gases 870
    S Natarajan, Pandurang Kulkarni, Navendu Rai, Shachi Desai, Vinay Prasad, Rishi Bhardwaj, Anoop Sivaraman (India)
    - Physical Properties of Gases 870 • Intraocular Gas Geometry 871 • Intraocular Gas Kinetics 871
    - Effect of Anesthetic Gases and Atmospheric Depressurization 873 • Clinical Considerations 873
    - Choice of Gas 873 • Nonexpansile Concentration 876 • Techniques of Fluid-Air Exchange and Intraocular Gas Injection 876
    - Clinical Uses 878 • Postoperative Management 879
    - Toxicity and Complications 880

56. Pharmacology of Anti-VEGF Therapy 883
    T Mark Johnson (USA)
    - Vascular Endothelial Growth Factor and Angiogenesis 883 • Administration of Anti-VEGF Therapy 885 • Side Effects of Anti-VEGF Therapy 885

SECTION 3: RECENT ADVANCES IN OCULAR THERAPEUTICS

57. Toxic Anterior Segment Syndrome 891
    Simon P Holland, Douglas W Morck, Richard Mathias, Tracy L Lee, Gina Chavez, Yumi G Ohashi (Canada)

Contents

58. Anesthesia Trends in Ophthalmology — 899
Arbisser Lisa
- History 899 • Perioperative Workup 899
- Trends in Topical Anesthesia 900 • Trends in Regional Anesthesia 900 • Author's Technique 901

59. Azithromycin in Ophthalmology: A New Therapy — 905
Eric Donnenfeld, Mitchell Friedlaender (USA)
- Topical Azithromycin Eyedrop (Azasite) 905
- Chemical Structures of Azithromycin and Erythromycin 906 • Modeled Bioavailability of Azithromycin from Azasite 907

60. Use of Beta-adrenergic Blockers in Ocular Vascular Diseases — 911
Javier A Montero, Jose M Ruiz-Moreno, Eugenia Sanchis-Merino (Spain)

61. Clinical Applications of Anti-inflammatory and Anti-protease Effects of Tetracyclines in Ocular Surface Disease — 924
Stephen C Pflugfelder, Cintia S De Paiva, De-Quan Li (USA)

62. Optimized NSAIDs and Antibacterial Regimen is Key to Ocular Surgical Prophylaxis — 935
Ashok Garg (India), Ian Bell (USA)
- Postoperative Schedule for Cataract Patients 936
- Measuring Potency 937 • Penetration Tracking 938
- Safety Evaluation 938

63. Ophthalmic Medications in Pediatric Age Group — 940
Rami Pai, Kirit Mody (India)
- Precautions 940 • Mydriatic Agents 941
- Glaucoma Medications 944 • Anti-inflammatory Drugs 950 • Anti-allergy Medications 953
- Antibiotics 956 • Sulfonamides 960
- Aminoglycosides 961 • Macrolides 962
- Tetracyclines 962 • Chloramphenicol 963
- Fluoroquinolones 964 • Antivirals 964
- Antifungals 967

64. Management of Uveitis in Children — 971
Gagandeep Singh Brar, SPS Grewal (India)
- Juvenile Idiopathic Arthritis Associated Uveitis 972
- Fuchs Heterochromic Uveitis 974
- Intermediate Uveitis 975 • Behçet's Disease 976
- Toxoplasmosis 977 • Toxocariasis 979

65. **Management of Anticoagulation Therapy in Elective Ophthalmic Procedures** 982
Purendra Bhasin, Prateek Gujar, Priyamvada Bhasin, Prachi Tomar (India)

• Identifying the Patients at Risk 982 • Risk of Bleeding Complications 983 • Modifying Antithrombotic Therapy During Ophthalmic Surgery 984 • Intraoperative Considerations to Reduce Bleeding in Patients Using Anticoagulation Therapy 985

66. **Ocular Pharmacology of Intravitreal Dexamethasone Sustained Release Implant** 988
Priyamvada Bhasin, Amit Basia, Purendra Bhasin (India)

• Mechanism of Action 988 • Chemical Formula 989
• Technique 990 • Pharmacokinetics 990
• Indications 991 • Contraindications 994
• Adverse Effects 994

67. **Nanotechnology in Ophthalmology** 996
NR Biswas, Harivenkatesh N, KP Biswas, Alok K Ravi, Madhurjya Gogoi (India)

• Medicine and Nanotechnology 996
• Nanotechnology in Ophthalmology 1000
• Ocular Distribution of Nanoparticles 1004
• Future of Nanotechnology 1005

68. **Photochemical Therapy for Corneal Infections** 1007
Ammar M Al Mahmood, Ashley Behrens (Saudi Arabia)

• Antimicrobial Effects of PCTCI 1007
• Microbial Keratitis Following CXL 1012
• Microbial Keratitis Following Other PDT Approaches 1014 • Antimicrobial Effect of Other PDT Approaches 1014

69. **Recent and Future Drugs in Ophthalmology** 1020
Roberto Bellucci, Carlo Bellucci (Italy)

• Recent and Emerging Drugs 1020
• New Drug Delivery in Ophthalmology 1023
• Biological Transporters and Prodrugs 1024
• Colloidal Carriers and Nanoparticles 1025

Index *1035*

Section 1

Fundamentals and Preliminary Considerations in Ocular Therapeutics

1

Ocular Defense System

Ashok Garg (India)

Eye like the other parts of the body has natural defence mechanism.

Eye is one of the highly specialized sensory organs of the body. Nature has provided eye with bony and anatomical protection and physiological reflexes. Eyes are protected from radiational hazards. Immunological process, Biochemical and enzymatic systems protect the eyes from ocular inflammation.

Ocular defence system is broadly classified in two categories:
a. Physical protection.
b. Physiological protection.

PHYSICAL PROTECTION

Eyeballs are well-protected in the bony orbit. The eye lies in the front half of the orbit surrounded by fat and connective tissue and is supported by a fascial hammock. The eyeball lies in a quadrilateral pyramid or pear-shaped bony cavity situated on the either side of the root of the nose called orbit. Orbit stalk is the optic canal. The orbit lies behind the orbital septum and has a roof, a floor; a medial wall and a lateral wall. The protective orbit is made up of seven bones namely maxilla, frontal, zygomatic, lacrimal, ethmoid, sphenoid and palatine. The bones of the anterior margin of the orbit are thick and strong but most of the walls are thin. Its two medial walls are parallel and two lateral walls form a 90° angle with each other. Each eyeball is suspended by extraocular muscles and their facial sheath. The anterior part of eyeball and center of cornea are just at the level of line joining the upper and lower bony orbital margins so that eyeball is protected from any kind of damage as a result of fall on the face side or when a large object hits the orbits. The eyeball is also protected by orbital fat to absorb any shock or vibrations specially in condition of concussion and free fall injury and provides a protective cushion. However, in counter coup injury the medial walls of the bony orbit give way as these are the weakest part of the orbits (Figs 1.1 and 1.2).

Lattice arrangement of collagen fibers adds to the strength of the cornea. Descemet membrane elasticity reduces the risk of corneal perforation. Criss-cross pattern of zonular fibers hold the lens in place.

Condensed part of the peripheral vitreous supports the retina.

The special physical protection in term of anatomical safeguards is provided by extra-length of the optic nerve between scleral entry and optic canal so that even if the eye is temporarily

4 Fundamentals and Preliminary Considerations in Ocular Therapeutics

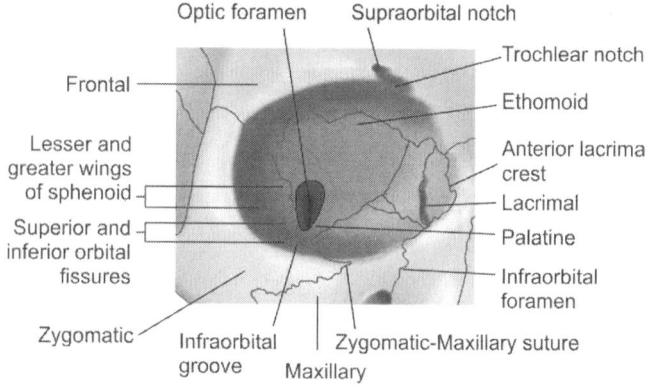

Fig. 1.1: Anatomy of the orbital cavity (Physical defense system of the eye). *Courtesy:* Kanski Clinical Ophthalmology, Butterworths International Edition

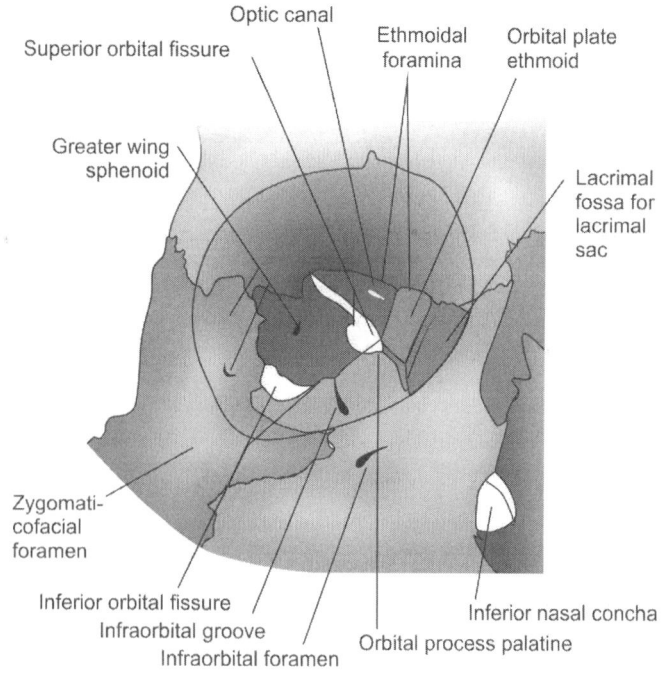

Fig. 1.2: Walls of the orbit

expulsed, the optic nerve cannot detach itself away from the eyeball. The firm attachment of optic nerve to the bony optic canal through its dural covering also ensures that optic nerve cannot be pulled out of intracranial cavity. The intraorbital portion of optic nerve is much longer (25 mm) than the distance between the back of globe to the optic foramen (18 mm). This allows for significant forward displacement of globe without causing excessive stretching of the optic nerve.

PHYSIOLOGICAL PROTECTION

A number of physiological factors provide protection to the eye.

The blinking reflex of the eye protects and helps to moisten and lubricate the exposed part of the eyeball. The eyelashes acts as antennae to warn against any foreign body coming near to eyeball and reflexly stimulate the closure of eyelids. Eyelashes also produce physical obstruction against flying particles, dust and dirt, etc. The Bell's phenomenon protects the cornea from exposure and injury. The pupil regulates the entry of light into the eyes. Iris diaphragm makes the posterior segment, a dark-room.

The pigment epithelium of the retina adsorbs the light after it passes through the anterior layers of retina. Cilioretinal arteries also acts as nutrition of the macula in CRA occlusion cases.

The cornea absorbs most of the infrared rays of the sunlight. The lens by its biochemical mechanism absorbs most of the UV rays of the sunlight so that retina is protected from the harmful effects of the sunrays. Intact corneal epithelium acts as a strong barrier against invasion by most of the microorganisms and also acts as selective permeable membrane. Micropolysaccharides in the corneal stroma prevent swelling of the cornea. Descemet membrane acts as a strong barrier against invading organisms. Due to absence of blood vessels in the cornea and lens, these two structures do not suffer from primary inflammation and also from neoplastic pathology. The optical integrity and normal function of the eye depend on an adequate supply of fluid covering its surface. The exposed part of the globe—the cornea and the bulbar conjunctiva—is covered by a thin fluid film referred to as preocular tear film. Tears refer to fluid film known as preocular tear film, and the conjunctival sac.

The volume of the tear fluid is about 5–10 microliter and about 95 percent of it, is produced by the goblet cells and the accessory lacrimal glands of the conjunctiva, in healthy individuals.

Tear film is a complete trilaminar structure which is directly in contact with the environment and is critically important for protecting the eye from external influences.

The precorneal tear film consists of three layers each of which has separate functions (Figs 1.3 and 1.4).

Outer Lipid Layer

It is secreted by meibomian glands and has three main functions:
  i. To retard the evaporation of the aqueous layer of the tear film.
 ii. To increase surface tension and assist in the vertical stability of the tear film so that tears do not overflow the lower lid margin.
iii. To lubricate the eyelids as they pass over the surface of the globe.

Middle Aqueous Layer

This is secreted by main lacrimal gland and the accessory lacrimal glands and has four main functions:

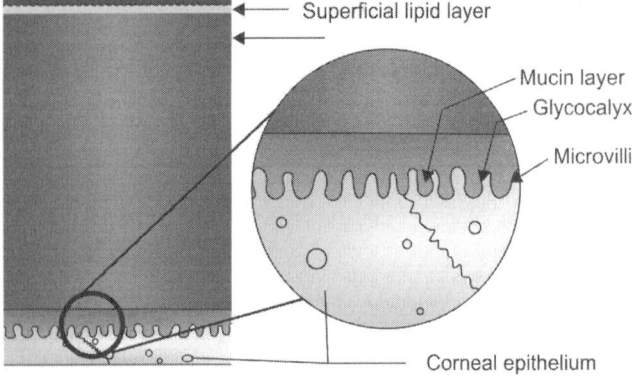

Fig. 1.3: Tear film layers (Physiological protection of the eye). *Courtesy:* Allergan India Limited

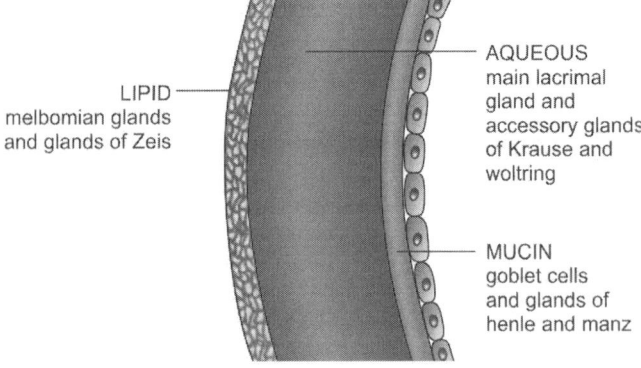

Fig. 1.4: Three layers of precorneal tear film. *Courtesy:* Kanski Clinical Ophthalmology, Butterworths International Edition

i. It supplies atmospheric oxygen to the corneal epithelium.
ii. It has antibacterial substances like lactoferrin and lysozyme.
iii. It provides a smooth optical surface by abolishing any minute irregularities of the cornea.
iv. It washes away debris from the conjunctiva and cornea.

Inner Mucin Layer

This is very thin and is secreted by the goblet cells in the conjunctiva and also by the crypts of Henle and glands of Manz. The main function of this layer is to convert the corneal epithelium from a hydrophobic to the hydrophilic surface. An aqueous solution form a smooth and even layer when dropped on to a hydrophilic surface. This layer enables the corneal epithelium to be adequately wetted.

In addition to adequate amounts of aqueous tears and mucin, three other factors are necessary for effective resurfacing of the cornea by the precorneal tear film.
1. A normal blink reflex which ensures that the mucin is brought from the inferior conjunctiva and rubbed into the corneal epithelium.
2. Congruity between the external ocular surface and the eyelids ensures that the precorneal tear film spread evenly over the entire cornea.
3. Normal epithelium is necessary for the adsorption of mucin on to its surface cells.

The chemical composition of human tear is quite complex containing proteins, lipids, metabolites, enzymes, electrolytes and other elements which play an important role in the defence of the outer eye.

The tear protein fraction forms the first line of defence against external influences.

In normal human tears, three types of immunoglobulins, namely IgA, IgG and IgM are present.

In normal tears secretory IgA and IgG form the first line of ocular defence and may act to modulate the normal flora of ocular adnexa allowing saprophytic growth which prevents pathological flora colonizing the ocular surface.

These globulins also prevent adherence of bacteria to the mucosal surface and neutralize viruses and toxins.

Tears transport metabolic products and provide a pathway for WBC in cases of injury.

Avascularity of the cornea is an important factor for antigenicity.

HDA in the peripheral cornea allows tissue immune reaction only when the blood vessels invade the corneal tissue.

In short, the eye is physically well-protected and the physiological mechanisms retain the transparency of media and visuosensory character of the retina. Cornea and lens are immunologically well-protected.

The ocular defence system during physical or pathological attacks is too strong to break the defence barrier.

BIBLIOGRAPHY

1. Adler. Physiology of the Eye; CV Mosby, 1992.
2. Agarwal A. Textbook of Ophthalmology, 1st edn. New Delhi: Jaypee Brothers Medical Publishers, 2002.
3. Bartlett JD. Clinical Ocular Pharmacology, 4th edn. Boston: Butterworth-Heinemann, 2001.
4. Bartlett JD. Ophthalmic Drug Facts: Lippincott-William and Wilkins, 2001.
5. Chong. Clinical Ocular Physiology: Lippincott-William- Wilkins, 1997.
6. Crick RP, Trimble RB. Textbook of Clinical Ophthalmology; Hodder and Stoughton, 1986.
7. Duane TD. Clinical Ophthalmology, 4th edn. Butterworth-Heinemann, 1999.

8. Duvall. Ophthalmic Medications and Pharmacology: Slack Inc, 1998.
9. Ellis PP. Ocular Therapeutics and Pharmacology, 7th edn. CV Mosby, 1985.
10. Fechner. Ocular Therapeutics: Slack Inc., 1998.
11. Fraunfelder. Current Ocular Therapy, 5th edn. WB Saunders, 2000.
12. Garg Ashok. Current Trends in Ophthalmology, 1st edn. New Delhi: Jaypee Brothers Medical Publishers, 1997.
13. Garg Ashok. Manual of Ocular Therapeutics, 1st edn. New Delhi: Jaypee Brothers Medical Publishers, 1996.
14. Garg Ashok. Ready Reckoner of Ocular Therapeutics, 1st edn. New Delhi, 2002.
15. Goodman LS, Gilman A. Pharmacological Basis of Therapeutics, 7th edn. New York: Macmillan, 1985.
16. Havener's, Ocular Pharmacology, 6th edn. CV Mosby, 1994.
17. Kanski. Clinical Ophthalmology, 4th edn. Butterworth-Heineman, 1999.
18. Kershner. Ophthalmic Medications and Pharmacology: Slack. Inc., 1994.
19. Korb. The Tear Film: Butterworth – Heinemann, 2001.
20. Lens, Ocular Anatomy and Physiology, Lippincott – William and Wilkins, 1999.
21. Olin BR, et al. Drugs Facts and Comparisons: Facts and Comparisons, St Louis, 1997.
22. Onofrey. The Ocular Therapeutics; Lippincott-William and Wilkins, 1997.
23. Rhee. The Wills Eye Drug Guide: Lippincott – William and Wilkins, 1998.
24. Saude. Ocular Anatomy and Physiology: Blackwell Science, 1993.
25. Snell. Clinical Anatomy of the Eye: Blackwell Science, 1998.
26. Steven Podos. Textbook of Ophthalmology, New Delhi: Jaypee Brothers Medical Publishers, 2001.
27. Zide. Surgical Anatomy of the Orbit: Lippincott – William and Wilkins, 1985.
28. Zimmerman. Textbook of Ocular Pharmacology: Lippincott and William and Wilkins, 1997.

Tear Film Physiology

Ashok Garg (India)

INTRODUCTION

The exposed part of the ocular globe—the cornea and the bulbar conjunctiva is covered by a thin fluid film known as preocular tear film. Tear film is that surface of the eye, which remains most directly in contact with the environment. It is critically important for protecting the eye from external influences and for maintaining the health of the underlying cornea and conjunctiva. The optical stability and normal function of the eye depend on an adequate supply of fluid covering its surface.

The tear film is a highly specialized and well-organized moist film which covers the bulbar and palpebral conjunctiva and cornea. It is formed and maintained by an elaborate system—the lacrimal apparatus consisting of secretory, distributive and excretory parts. The secretory part includes the lacrimal gland, accessory lacrimal gland tissue, sebaceous glands of the eyelids, goblet cells and other mucin-secreting elements of the conjunctiva (Fig. 2.1). The elimination of the lacrimal secretions is based on the movement of tears across the eye aided by the act of blinking and a drainage system consisting of lacrimal puncta, canaliculi, sac and nasolacrimal duct (Figs 2.2A to C).

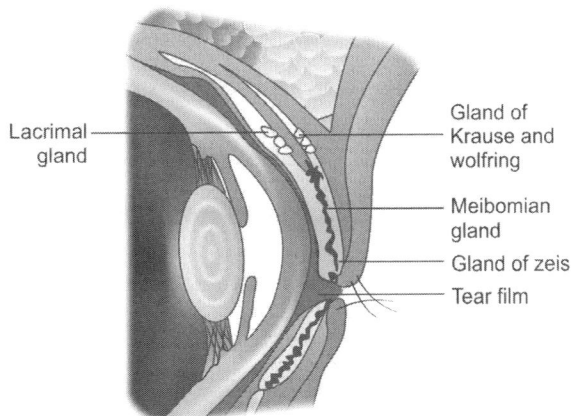

Fig. 2.1: Cross-section of eye showing tear film (blue) in its natural distribution along with tear producing glands (*Courtesy:* Allergan India Limited)

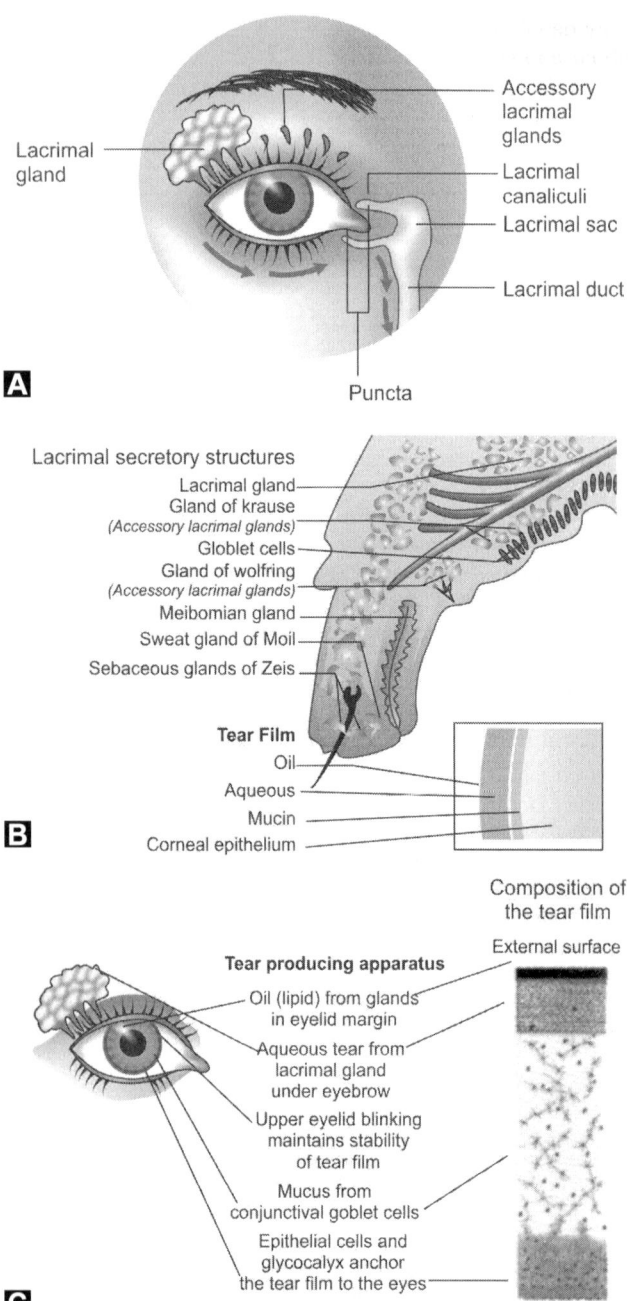

Figs 2.2A to C: (A) Tear drainage system (*Courtesy:* Allergan India Limited) (B) Tear film and lacrimal secretory structures (C) Composition of tear film and tear producing apparatus (*Courtesy:* FDC Limited)

By definition, a film is a thin layer that can stand vertically without appreciable gravitational flow and the tear film meets this criterion very well. The presence of continuous tear film over the exposed ocular surface is imperative for good visual acuity and wellbeing of the epithelium and facilitates blinking. Tear film serves:
- An optical function by maintaining an optically uniform corneal surface
- A mechanical function by flushing cellular debris, foreign matter from the cornea and conjunctival sac and by lubricating the surface
- A corneal nutritional function
- An antibacterial function.

The composition of the tear film must be kept within rather narrow quantitative and qualitative limits in order to maintain the wellbeing and proper functioning of the visual system. Abnormalities of the tear film affecting its constituents or volume lead to serious dysfunction of the eyelids and the conjunctiva with the concomitant loss of corneal transparency. A thin tear film is uniformly spread over the cornea by blinking and ocular movements. The tear film can be arbitrarily divided into four main parts:
- The marginal tear film along the moist portions of the eyelid which lie posterior to the lipid strip secreted by the tarsal glands
- Portion covering the palpebral conjunctiva
- Portion covering the bulbar conjunctiva
- Precorneal tear film which covers the cornea.

The marginal, palpebral and conjunctival portions are regarded as making the preocular tear film.

Tears refers to the fluid present as the precorneal film and in the conjunctival sac. The volume of tear fluid is about 5–10 ml with normal rate of secretion about 1–2 ml/minute. About 95 percent of it is produced by the lacrimal gland and lesser amounts are produced by goblet cells and the accessory lacrimal glands of the conjunctiva. The total mass of the latter is about one-tenth of the mass of the main lacrimal gland.

The secretory part of the lacrimal apparatus provides the aqueous tear, lipids and mucus all the important components of the tear film and its boundary.

The tear film is composed of three layers (Fig. 2.3).

Superficial Lipid Layer

The superficial layer at the air-tear interface is formed over the aqueous part of the tear film from the oily secretions of meibomian glands and the accessory sebaceous glands of Zeiss and Moll. The meibomian gland openings are distributed along the eyelid margin immediately behind the lash follicles.

The chemical nature of the lipid layer is essentially waxy and consists of cholesterol esters and some polar lipids. The thickness of this layer varies with the width of the palpebral fissure and is between 0.1 and 0.2 mm. Being oily in nature it forms a barrier

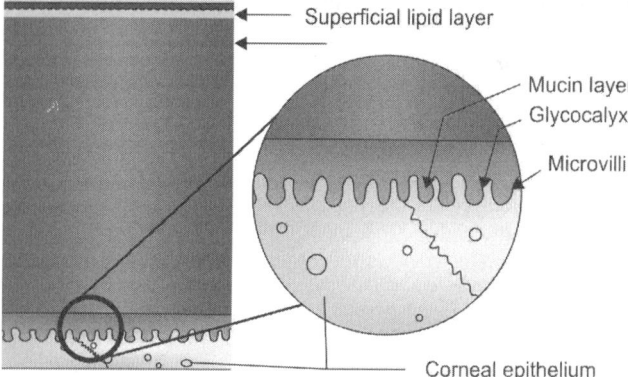

Fig. 2.3: Tear film layers (*Courtesy:* Allergan India Limited)

along the lid margins that retains the lid margin tear strip and prevents its overflow on to skin. This layer is so thin that there are no interference color patterns such as one normally sees on an oily surface. However, if one squints, the oily layer thickness and distinct interference colors may be seen.

While the bulk of tarsal gland secretions are nonpolar lipid compounds which do not spread over an aqueous surface alone, many surface active components are also present. It appears that the tarsal gland secretions which are transported to the cornea in the tear film are massaged into the outermost layer of corneal epithelial cells by eyelid action and then possibly are changed by local metabolic processes in the epithelium combining with conjunctival mucus to form a stable hydrophilic base for the precorneal tear film.

This outer lipid layer has the following main functions:
- It reduces the rate of evaporations of the underlying aqueous tear layer
- It increases surface tension and assists in the vertical stability of the tear film so that tears do not overflow the lower lid margin
- It lubricates the eyelids as they pass over the surface of the globe.

Middle Aqueous Layer

The intermediate layer of tear film is the aqueous phase which is secreted by the main lacrimal gland and the accessory glands of Krause and Wolfring.

This layer constitutes almost the total thickness of the tear film 2.5 to 10 mm, many times thicker than the fine superficial oily layer. This layer contains two phases—a more concentrated and a highly dilute one. The interfacial tension at the adsorbed mucin-aqueous layer is apt to be rather small due to the intensive hydrogen bond formation across the interface. This layer contains inorganic salts, water proteins, enzymes, glucose, urea, metabolites, electrolytes, glycoproteins and surface active biopolymers. Uptake of oxygen

through the tear film is essential to normal corneal metabolism. This layer has four main functions:
- Most importantly it supplies atmospheric oxygen to the corneal epithelium
- It has antibacterial substances like lactoferrin and lysozyme. Therefore, dry eye patients are more susceptible to infection than a normal eye
- It provides smooth optical surface by removing any minute irregularities of the cornea
- It washes away debris from the cornea and conjunctiva.

Posterior Mucin Layer

The innermost layer of tear film is a thin mucoid layer elaborated by goblet cells of the conjunctiva and also by the crypts of Henle and glands of Manz. It is the deepest stratum of the precorneal tear film. This layer is even thinner than the lipid layer and is 0.02 to 0.04 mm thick. This adsorbs on the epithelial surface of the cornea and conjunctiva rendering them hydrophilic. It assumes the ridged appearance of the microvilli of superficial epithelial cells which it covers. The preocular tear film is dependent upon a constant supply of mucus which must be of proper chemical and physical nature to maintain corneal and conjunctival surfaces in the proper state of hydration. The mucous threads present in the tear film provides lubrication allowing the eyelid margin and palpebral conjunctiva to slide smoothly over one another with minimal energy lost as friction during blinking and ocular rotation movements. They also cover foreign bodies with a slippery coating thereby protecting the cornea and conjunctiva against the abrasive effects of such particles as they are moved about by the constant blinking movements of eyelids. The mucus contributes stability to the preocular tear film as well as furnishing an attachment for the tear film to the conjunctiva but not to the corneal surface. The corneal surface is covered with a myriad of fine microvilli which provides some support for the tear film. The mucus dissolved in the aqueous phase facilitates spreading of the tear film by smoothening the film over the corneal surface to form a perfect, regular refracting surface.

So the mucin layer which is a glycoprotein converts a hydrophobic surface into a hydrophilic surface and enables the corneal epithelium to be adequately wetted.

In addition to sufficient amounts of aqueous tears and mucin three other important factors are necessary for effective resurfacing of the cornea by the precorneal tear film:
- A normal blink reflex is essential to ensure that the mucin is brought from the inferior conjunctiva and rubbed into the corneal epithelium. Patients suffering from facial palsy and lagophthalmos therefore develop corneal drying
- Congruity between external ocular surface and the eyelids ensures that the precorneal tear film shall spread evenly over the entire cornea. Patients suffering from limbal lesions like dermoids face the problem of apposition of the eyelids to the globe leading to local selective areas of drying

- Normal epithelium is necessary for the adsorption of mucin on to its surface cells. Patients suffering from corneal scars and keratinizations have problem of interference with the corneal wetting.

The tear film is not visible apparently on the surface of the eye but at the upper and lower lid margins a 1 mm strip of tear fluid with concave outer surface can be seen. It is here that the oily surface prevents spillage of the tear fluid over the lid margin. Tears forming the upper tear strip are conducted nasally from the upper temporal fornix. At the lateral canthus the tears fall by gravity to form the lower strip, spreading medially the upper and lower strips reach the plica and caruncle where they join together. The tear fluid does not flow over the eye by gravity but a thin film is spread over the cornea by blinking and eye movements.

TEAR FILM FORMATION DYNAMICS

It is interesting to know the tear film formation. Generally during the closure of the eyelids the superficial lipid layer of the tear film is compressed by the eyelid edges because it is energetically unfavorable for the lipid to penetrate under the lids into the fornix. The thickness of lipid layer therefore increases by a factor of 1000 resulting in thickness of 0.1 mm which is easily contained between the adjacent eyelid edges. The aqueous tear layer remains uniform under the lids and acts as a lubricant between the eyelids and the globe. In a complete blink phenomenon, the two tear minisci join and most of their bulk is held at their junction to fill the slight bridge formed by the meeting eyelids and at the canthus.

When the eyelids open, first they form an aqueous tear surface on which the compressed lipid rapidly spread. Monomolecular lipid layer is the first to spread at speeds limited only by the moving eyelid. Following the spread of lipid monolayer, the excess lipid and associated macromolecules shall distribute themselves over the tear film surface at a lower speed, usually the lipid layer ceases within 1 second after the opening of the eye.

Under normal conditions a person blinks on an average 15 times per minute. Some of these blinks may not be complete (the upper eyelid descends only half way towards the lower eyelid). Normally the tear film break-up time (BUT) is longer than the interval between blinks and no corneal drying occurs.

A deficiency in the conjunctival secretions can lead to dry eye symptoms even in the presence of an adequate aqueous tear component (Fig. 2.4).

Break-up time is generally determined after the instillation of a drop of fluorescein solution in the eye or after staining the tear miniscus and the tear film by a wetted paper strip containing fluorescein. Normal BUT value ranges from 10–40 seconds for normal eyes (Fig. 2.5), when the BUT is determined by a noninvasive method (e.g. by the toposcope). BUT values of as long as 3–5 minutes can be recorded.

If the BUT is shorter than the average time interval between two consecutive blinks, tear film rupture can cause pathological changes in the underlying epithelium. The tear film breaks

Tear Film Physiology

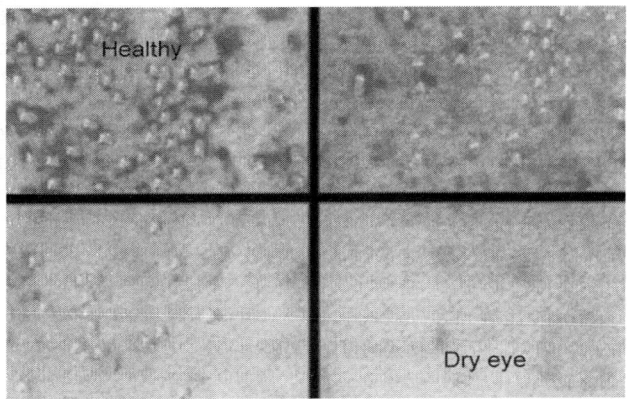

Fig. 2.4: Impression cytology mapping
(*Courtesy:* Allergan India Limited)

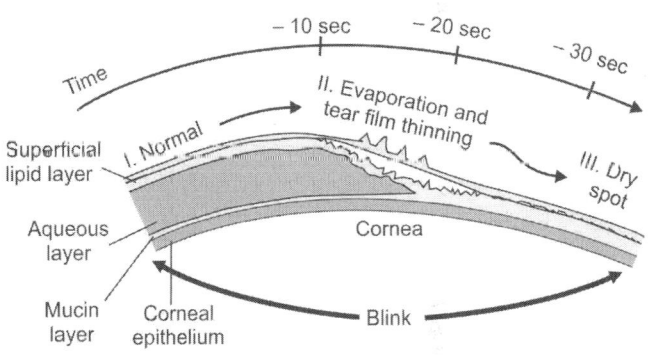

Fig. 2.5: Mechanism of tear film break-up
(*Courtesy:* Allergan India Limited)

up prematurely over the damaged epithelial surface thereby exacerbating the injury.

Generally, there is balance between the secretion and excretion of tears and the rate of tear drainage increases with increased tear volume.

NORMAL TEAR DRAINAGE

In the normal tear film between 10 and 25 percent of the total tears secreted are lost by evaporation. Evaporation rate is low because of the protective oily surface.

In the absence of the protective oily layer the rate of evaporation is increased 10 to 20 times. Normally tear flows along the upper and lower marginal strips and enters the upper and lower canaliculi by capillarity and possibly by suction also. About 70 percent of tear drainage is via the lower canaliculus and the remaining through the upper canaliculus. With each blink the superficial and deep heads of pretarsal orbicularis muscle compress the ampullae, shorten the horizontal canaliculi and move the puncta medially. Simultaneously the deep heads of preseptal orbicularis muscle which are attached to the fascia of the lacrimal sac contract and expand the sac. This creates a negative pressure which sucks the tears from the canaliculi into the sac. When the eyes are opened the muscles relax, the sac collapses and a positive pressure is created which forces the tear down the duct into the nose. Gravity also plays an important role in the sac emptying. The puncta move laterally, the canaliculi lengthen and become filled with tears.

TEAR COMPOSITION

Tears contain 98.2 percent water and 1.8 percent solids. The high percentage of water in tears is a natural consequence of the need for lubrication of the conjunctiva and corneal surface (Tables 2.1 and 2.2). The evaporation of water between blinks may influence the concentration of the tear film. The evaporation rate of water from the intact precorneal tear film through the superficial lipid layer has been shown to be 8×10^{-7} cm^{-2} sec^{-1}. In a time interval of 10 seconds (between two consecutive blinks) the thickness of the tear film decreases about 0.1 mm resulting in nearly 1–2 percent decrease in water concentration. The solute concentration however increases about 20 percent.

PHYSICAL PROPERTIES OF TEARS

Tear pH

The pH of unstimulated tears is about 7.4 and it approximates that of blood plasma. Although wide variations are found in normal individuals (between 5.0 and 8.35) the usual range is from 7.3 to 7.7. A more acidic pH of about 7.25 is found following prolonged lid closure possibly due to carbon dioxide produced by the cornea and trapped in the tear pool under the eyelids. Tear pH is characteristic for each individual and the normal buffering mechanism maintain the pH at a relatively constant level during waking hours. The permeability of the corneal epithelium does not seem to be affected by wide variations in the pH of tear fluid.

TABLE 2.1: Relative water contents of tears and other body fluids	
Fluid	Percentage water
Tear	98.2
Aqueous humor	98.9
Vitreous humor	99.0
Blood	79.5
Serum	91.0
Urine	96.5

Osmotic Pressure

The osmotic pressure in tears mainly caused by the presence of electrolytes is about 305 mOsm/kg equivalent to 0.95 percent sodium chloride. Individual values over the waking day may range from 0.90 to 1.02 percent NaCl equivalents. A decrease to an average of 285 mOsm/kg equivalent to 0.89 percent NaCl has been reported following prolonged lid closure which accounts for the reduced evaporation. When the aqueous component of tears decreases, the tears become markedly hypertonic (0.97% NaCl solution or more) and corneal dehydration results. When the eyes are closed, there is no evaporation of tears and the precorneal tear film is in osmotic equilibrium with the cornea. When the eyes are open evaporation takes place, increasing the tonicity of the tear film and producing an osmotic gradient from the aqueous through the cornea to the tear film. This direction of flow will continue as long as evaporation maintains the hypertonicity of the tear film. Osmotic pressure is sensitive to changes in tear flow. Reflex stimulation of tears in early adaptation to contact lenses results in a decrease in electrolytes and in total protein leading to hypotonicity. This relative hypotonicity may account for the corneal edema often seen in early stages of contact lens wearing.

Other Physical Properties of Tear (Table 2.2)

- Refractive index—1.357
- Tear volume—0.50–0.67 g/16 hr (waking).

TABLE 2.2: Composition of human tears and plasma

Composition	Tears	Plasma
Physical properties		
pH	7.4 (7.2–7.7)	7.39
Osmotic pressure	305 mOsm/kg Equiv. 0.95% NaCl	6.64 atm
Refractive index	1.357	1.35
Volume	0.50–0.67 g/16 hour (waking)	
Chemical properties		
1. General tear composition		
Water	98.2 g/100 ml	98 g/100 ml
Solids (total)	1.8 g/100 ml	8.6 g/100 ml
Ash	1.05 g/100 ml	0.6–1.0 g/100 ml
2. Electrolytes		
Sodium	120–170 mmol/l	140 mmol/l
Potassium	26–42 mmol/l	4.5 mmol/l
Calcium	0.3–2.0 mmol/l	2.5 mmol/l

Contd...

Contd...

	Composition	Tears	Plasma
	Magnesium	0.5–1.1 mmol/l	0.9 mmol/l
	Chloride	120–135 mmol/l	100 mmol/l
	Bicarbonate	26 mmol/l	30 mmol/l
3.	Antiproteinasis		
	α_1-Anti trypsin (a1-at)	0.1–3.0 mg%	280 mg%
	α_1-Anti chymotriypsin	1.4 mg%	24 mg%
	Inter-α trypsin inhibitor	0.5 mg%	20 mg%
	α_2 Macroglobulin	3-6 mg%	—
4.	Nitrogenous substances		
	Total protein	0.668-0.800 g/ 100 ml	6.7 g/100 ml
	Albumin	0.392 g/100 ml	4.0–4.8 g/100 ml
	Globulin	0.2758 g/100 ml	2.3 g/100 ml
	Ammonia	0.005 g/100 ml	0.047 g/100 ml
	Uric acid		
	Urea	0.04 mg/100 ml	26.8 mg/100 ml
	Total nitrogen	158 mg/100 ml	1140 mg/100 ml
	Nonprotein nitrogen	51 mg/100 ml	15–42 mg/100 ml
5.	Carbohydrates		
	Glucose	2.5 (0–5.0) mg/ 100 ml	80–90 mg/100 ml
6.	Sterols		
	Cholesterol and cholesterol esters	8–32 mg/100 ml	200–300 mg/100 ml
7.	Miscellaneous		
	Citric acid	0.6 mg/100 ml	2.2–2.8 mg/100 ml
	Ascorbic acid	0.14 mg/100 ml	0.1–0.7 mg/100 ml
	Lysozyme	1–2 mg/ml	—
	Amino acid	7.58 mg/100 ml	—
	Lactate	1–5 mmol/l	0.5–0.8 mmol/l
	Prostaglandin	75 pg PF/ml 300 pg PF/ml	80–90 pg PF/ml
	Catecholamine	0.5–1.5 mg/ml	
	Complement	1:4 dilution (Hemolytic assay)	1.32 dilution (Hemolytic assay)

CHEMICAL COMPOSITION OF TEAR FLUID

The chemical composition (Table 2.2) of tear fluid is quite complex. The first chemical analysis of tears was studied in 1791 by Fourcroy and Van Que Lin Fleming (1922) and Ridley (1934) demonstrated the detailed chemical composition of normal tears.

Immunoelectrophoretic studies have shown that tears contain lipids, proteins, enzymes, metabolites, electrolytes and hydrogen ions, etc.

Lipids

Lipids are present in small amount in tears as they are contained only in the very thin superficial lipid layer of the tear film. Chromatographic studies of meibomian lipids reveal the presence of all possible lipid classes mainly waxy esters, hydrocarbons, triglycerides, cholesterol esters and in lesser amount diglycerides, monoglycerides, free fatty acids, free cholesterol and phospholipid. However, great individual variations occur in lipid composition.

Cholesterol

Cholesterol has been reported to be present in tear fluid in concentrations of about 200 mg percent which is same as in the blood. Like all lipids in biological fluids cholesterol has to be transported by α and β lipoproteins. In normal tears the very low protein content and the absence of lipoproteins is incompatible with a cholesterol concentration of 20 mg percent.

Proteins

About 60 components to tear protein fraction have been reported which form the first line of defense against an external infection and seen to be more effective than systemically produced antibodies. The protein content of tears differ from that of blood plasma in several respects. Proteins can be divided in two groups.

Group A: Proteins which are similar to serum proteins with a low concentration representing less than 15 percent of all tear proteins. Some of them are always present in tears (Table 2.3) namely albumin, IgG, α-L antitrypsin, transferrin, α-L antichymotrypsin and β-2 microglobulin others which appears sporadically are ceruloplasmin, haptoglobin and Zinc α-2 glycoprotein.

Group B: Specific proteins synthesized by tear gland are RMP (rapid migration protein) and some other proteins (Tables 2.4 and 2.5) which are also present in other external secretions (lysozyme, lactoferrin and IgA).

Tear Albumin

Albumin represents about 60 percent of the total protein in tears as it does in plasma. Tear albumin is a unique protein fraction. It is electrophoretically a prealbumin and migrates to a position similar to serum prealbumin. Genetic polymorphism has been reported of the tear albumin.

Electrophoresis of tears shows several peaks of migration. These peaks are main which correspond to proteins synthesized by the lacrimal gland—rapid migrant proteins and lactoferrin migrating to the anode and lysozyme migrating to the cathode.

The total tear proteins content strongly depends upon the method of collection of tears. Small unstimulated tears show levels of about 20 mg/ml while stimulated tears show much lower values in the range of 3–7 mg/ml reflecting the level of lacrimal gland fluid.

TABLE 2.3: Amino acid composition of human tear lysozyme

Amino acids	Residues (gm/100 g protein)
Aspartic acid	13.23
Arginine	13.05
Glutamic acid	8.55
Tryptophane	6.89
Alanine	6.36
Leucine	6.11
Trypsin	5.65
Glycine	4.94
Lysine	4.92
Valine	4.62
Serine	4.02
Half-cysteine	4.01
Threonine	3.67
Isoleucine	3.59
Phenylalanine	1.97
Proline	1.72
Methionine	1.50
Histidine	1.01

TABLE 2.4: Relative quantity of various protein fractions in tears

Fractions	Normal tears (Percentage)	Stimulated flow (Tears) Percentage
Albumin	58.2	20.2
Globulin	23.9	56.9
Lysozyme	17.9	22.9

Lysozyme

Fleming first discovered an antibacterial substance and showed that this substance is an enzyme which he named lysozyme because of its capacity to lyze bacteria. In normal tears concentration of lysozyme is much higher than in any other body fluid. The normal level for human tear lysozyme (HTL) is 1–2 mg/ml. The enzymic activity of lysozyme is optimal at pH 5.2 and decreases above and below this pH value.

Lysozyme is a long chain, high molecular weight proteolytic enzyme produced by lysosomes—a known cellular ultrastructure. Lysozyme acts upon certain bacteria and dissolves them by

TABLE 2.5: Origin of various tear protein fractions

Protein fraction	Lacrimal gland proper	Accessory lacrimal gland	Goblet cells
Lysozyme	+	—	—
Component-I	—	+	±
Component-II	+	±	±
Component-III	+	±	±
Serum albumin	—	—	+
Tear albumin	+	—	—
Mucin	—	—	+

+ means fraction is present
— means fraction is absent
± Means fraction is indifferently present

cleaning the polysaccharide component of their cell walls. As the function of cell wall in bacteria is to confer mechanical support a bacterium devoid of its cell wall usually bursts because of the high osmotic pressure inside the cell.

Lysozyme level in tears can be measured with a diffusion method or with a spectrophotometric assay.

In addition to lysozyme, presence of other antibacterial factors in human tears have been shown. The nonlysozymal bactericidal protein beta lysin has been reported to be derived chiefly from platelets but it exists in higher concentration in tears than in blood plasma. The lysozyme and beta lysin protein fractions can be separated by filtering the tears. The antibacterial activity of the filtrate results from lysozyme but in whole tears beta lysin is responsible for three-fourth of the bactericidal effect. Beta lysin acts primarily on cellular membrane while lysozyme dissolves bacterial cell walls.

The action of lysozyme depends on the pH. The optimum pH for lysis varies with the solubility of the bacterial proteins but in general it ranges between 6.0 and 7.4. Low salt concentrations favor lysis by increasing solubility.

Human tear lysozyme (HTL) levels have been shown to be greatly decreased in tears of patients suffering from Sjogren's syndrome and ocular toxicity from long-term use of practolol therapy thus making it a useful diagnostic aid. Other disease states where HTL level is lowered include herpes simplex virus infection and malnutrition in children.

Lactoferrin

It is an iron carrying protein and appears to be a major tear protein in the intermediate fraction. Its property of iron binding (Fe III) is 300 times stronger than the other iron binding protein (transferrin). This is probably significant for its bacteriostatic activity in tears making essential metal ions unavailable for microbial metabolism.

Transferrin

Transferrin has been shown to be present in tears. Transferrin along with serum albumin and IgG can be detected only after mild trauma to the mucosal surface of the conjunctiva or in tears.

Ceruloplasmin

Ceruloplasmin, a copper carrying protein is regularly found in tears. In electrophoresis the migration rate of tear ceruloplasmin varies from its serum counter part.

Immunoglobulins

Tiselius (1939) for the first time separated the plasma proteins by electrophoresis and isolated three types of globulins—alpha, beta and gamma. Antibody property of the immune serum resides in the gamma globulin fraction. Immunoglobulins are elaborated by plasma cells following transformation of antigen stimulated B-lymphocytes. This elaboration constitutes the humoral immune system.

Five major classes of immunoglobulins have been recognized (Table 2.6). These are:

    Immunoglobulin A   (IgA)
    Immunoglobulin G   (IgG)
    Immunoglobulin M   (IgM)
    Immunoglobulin E   (IgE)
    Immunoglobulin D   (IgD)

Immunoglobulin A (IgA): It is the major immunoglobulin present in tears, saliva and colostrum. Almost all of the IgA have a secretory component attached to them when they occur in external secretions. It participates in the functioning of IgA as antibody in the external environment. The possible functions of secretory IgA include prevention of viral and bacterial infections that may have an access to the external secretions, e.g. tears and participate as opsonins in the phagocytosis process.

The average levels of IgA—the predominant immunoglobulin in normal human tear is 14 mg/dl.

In the human lacrimal gland, IgA appears to be synthesized by interstitial plasma cells and after entry into the intercellular spaces it is coupled to SC and secreted as secretory IgA (IgA-SC) through the blood-tear barrier involving intracellular transport by acinar

TABLE 2.6: Immunoglobulin levels in tear and serum

Ig Class	Tears	Serum
Total proteins	800 mg/100 ml	6500 mg/100 ml
IgA	14–24 mg/100 ml	170–200 mg/100 ml
IgG	17 mg/100 ml	1000 mg/100 ml
IgM	5–7 mg/100 ml	100 mg/100 ml
IgE	26–250 mg/ml	2000 mg/ml

epithelial cells into the lumens. In the conjunctiva IgA and plasma cells are located in the substantia propria. Only in the acinar epithelium of the accessory lacrimal glands can SC material be present indicating that these are the sites of synthesis of secretory IgA of the conjunctival secretions. Depending upon the method of tear collection IgA values can vary from 10 to 100 mg percent.

Immunoglobulin G (IgG): It is present in very low concentrations in normal tears. However, after mild trauma to the mucosal surface of the conjunctiva it can be easily detected.

IgG is the most prominent circulating (serum) immunoglobulin present in concentrations five times that of IgA. The average level of IgG in normal human tears range from 17 to 20 mg/100 ml.

The serum level of IgG is about 1000 mg/dl. IgG molecule has a molecular weight of about 150,000. Each molecule of IgG consists of 2 L chains and 2 H chains linked by 20-25-S-S bonds. The antigenic analysis of IgG myelomas show four subclasses now termed as IgG_1, IgG_2, IgG_3, and IgG_4. IgG_1 is the predominant variant and together with IgG_3 possesses the ability to combine with complement to bind to macrophages and to cross the placenta. IgG synthesis in humans is about 35 mg/kg/d and its half-life is about 23 days. IgG molecules are Y-shaped with a hinge region near the middle of the heavy chain connecting the 2 Fab segments to the Fc segment.

During the secondary response, IgG is the major immunoglobulin to be synthesized probably because of its small size, IgG diffuses more readily than other immunoglobulins into the tears, therefore as the predominating immunoglobulin it carries the major burden of neutralizing bacterial toxins and of binding to microorganisms (specially streptococci, pneumococci and staphylococci) to enhance their phagocytosis. IgG is most efficient in killing and stopping the progress of microorganism's invasion.

Immunoglobulin M (IgM): It is present in very low concentrations in normal tears. The average level of IgM in normal tears range from 5 to 7 mg percent. Barnett (1968) reported first the presence of IgM in normal tears.

The serum level of IgM is about 100 mg/dl. The IgM molecule with a molecular weight 900,000 is the largest of the immunoglobulins. Often referred to as macroglobulin because of its size, the IgM molecule are pentamers with a high valency or anticombining capacity. Due to its high valency IgM is extremely efficient agglutinating and cytolytic agent and is the first type of antibody which is formed after the initial encounter with antigen. It appears early in response to infection and is confined mainly to the blood stream.

Even minimum trauma to conjunctiva would cause serum proteins to leak into the tears. There is increased concentrations of IgA, IgG and IgE in tears. Either these immunoglobulins are selectively excreted into the tears or they are locally synthesized. Increased concentrations of IgA, IgG and IgM are reported in cases of blepharoconjunctivitis, herpes keratitis, vernal conjunctivitis, acute follicular conjunctivitis, phlyctenular conjunctivitis, keratomalacia, corneal ulcer and acute endogenous uveitis.

Immunoglobulin E (IgE): It is mostly extravascular in distribution. IgE values ranges from 26 to 144 mg/ml in normal tears. Normal serum contains only traces of IgE but greatly elevated levels are seen in atopic conditions.

Immunoglobulin D (IgD): IgD levels are quite low in tears as well as in serum. It is mostly intravascular.

Complement

Complement in tears has been shown in hemolytic assays up to dilution of 1.4 whereas serum is active in this system up to 1:32.

Glycoproteins

Glycoproteins are present in the mucoid layer as well as in the tear fluid since they are highly soluble in water. Glycoproteins contribute significantly to the stickiness of the material forming the mucoid layer. N-acetylneuraminic acid (a sialic acid) has been indentified in normal tears. Glycoproteins may play a critical role in the lubrication of the corneal surface by rendering its hydrophobic surface more hydrophilic permitting spreading and stabilization of the tear film. The mucus is secreted by the conjunctival goblet cells as a solution of glycoproteins (mucoids) and this sticky mixture adheres to the surface of the epithelium even though the glycoproteins are water soluble.

The glycoproteins are carbohydrate-protein complexes characterized by the presence of hexosamines, hexoses and sialic acid. In normal tears relative hexosamine content of the protein which is used as indicator for glycoproteins varies from 0.5 to 17 percent, the hexosamine concentration from 0.05 to 3 g/l. Sialic acid concentration of human tears has been reported to be 114 mmol/100 ml.

Antiproteinases

Antiproteinases, inhibitors of proteinases are present in tears at levels much lower than in plasma (Table 2.7).

TABLE 2.7: Antiproteinases concentration in tears and plasma		
Antiproteinases	mg percentage	
	Plasma	Tears
α_1-antitrypsin ($\alpha_1$at)	280	0.1-0.4
α_1-antichymotrypsin		1.5
		3.0
α_1-antichymotrypsin	24	1.4
Inter-α-trypsin inhibitor	20	0.5
α_2-macroglobulin		3
		6

These includes α_1-antitrypsin, α_1-antichymotrypsin, intratrypsin inhibitor and α_2-macroglobulin. The source of-α_1 antitrypsin is the lacrimal gland while other antiproteinases originate from corneal and conjunctival surfaces. In various inflammatory conditions of the eye the levels of α_1-at and α_2-m in tear fluid are increased.

In bacterial and viral infections of the eye (Table 2.8) and in corneal ulceration the levels of α_1-at and α_2-m in tear fluids are increased. Using albumin as a marker protein there is evidence suggesting that these two collagenase inhibitors are derived either from plasma by a general increase in vascular permeability to proteins or they are produced locally.

Metabolites

A number of metabolites have been reported to be present in normal human tears. These include organic constituents of low molecular weight like glucose, urea, amino acids and other metabolites like lactate, histamine, prostaglandins and catecholamines.

Glucose

Glucose is present in minimal amounts of about 0.2 mmol/liter in tear fluids of normal glycemic persons. This low concentration of glucose appear to be insufficient for corneal nutrition. There is no definitive evidence that cornea metabolizes glucose emanating from the tears.

It has been shown that some glucose in tears originates from the goblet cells of the conjunctiva. There is corresponding rise in tear glucose level with elevation of plasma glucose level above 100 mg percent. However, there is no significant rise in tear glucose levels in diabetics with blood glucose level of more than 20 mmol/liter

TABLE 2.8: Antimicrobial factors in tears

Compound	Evidence
Lysozyme	+
IgA	+
IgG	±
IgE	+
IgM	±
Complement	+
Lactoferrin	+
Transferrin	±
Betalysin	+
Antibiotic producing Commensal organism	+

+ present in normal tears.
± Present in tears after stimulation (mild trauma to the conjunctiva)

which demonstrates the barrier function of the corneal and conjunctival epithelium against loss of glucose from the tissues into the tear fluid. It is the tissue fluid which contributes to the tear glucose after mechanically stimulated methods of tear collection.

Urea

Urea concentration in tear fluid and plasma has been found to be equivalent suggesting an unrestricted passage through the blood-tear barrier in the lacrimal gland. Urea concentration in tears decreases with increasing secretion rate.

Amino Acids

Free amino acid concentration in tears is reported to be 7.58 mg/100 ml. This value is 3-4 times higher than the free amino acid concentration in serum.

Lactate

Lactate levels of 1-5 mmol/l in tears are far higher than the normal blood levels of 0.5-0.8 mmol/l. Pyruvate from 0.05 to 0.35 mmol/l is about the same as is normal for blood (0.1-0.2 mmol/l). These levels do not show significant alterations after mechanical irritation. The epithelium does not possess a barrier function for lactate and pyruvate.

Histamine

Histamine is present in normal tears collected from the conjunctival sac at a level of about 10 mg/ml. In vernal conjunctivitis specifically a variable increase up to 125 mg/ml has been observed.

Prostaglandins

Prostaglandins are present in normal tears at the level of 75 pg prostaglandin F/ml and it is little lower than in serum. In inflammatory conditions of the eye significant higher values are found up to 300 pg/ml of tears.

Catecholamines, Dopamine, Noradrenaline and Dopa

Catecholamines, dopamine, noradrenaline and dopa have been found in the tear fluid. Their levels vary from 0.5 to 1.5 mg/ml. Dopamine has values as high as 280 mg/ml.

In glaucoma patients lower values have been reported for these compounds which reflect the diminished activity of the sympathetic innervation of the eye. The determination of catecholamines in tears has been advocated as a test in glaucoma diagnosis.

TABLE 2.9: Human tear electrolytes						
Concentration in mmol/l						
	Na^+	K^+	Ca^{++}	Mg^{++}	Cl^-	HCO_3^-
Tears	120–170	6–26	0.5–1.1	0.3–0.6	118–138	26
	145	24	0.4–1.1	0.5–1.1	106–130	
	134–170	26–42	0.3–2.0		120–135	
Serum	140	4.5	2.5	0.9	100	30

Electrolytes and Hydrogen Ions

The predominant positively charged electrolytes (cation) in tears are mainly sodium and potassium while the negative ions (anions) are chloride and bicarbonate (Table 2.9).

Sodium

Sodium concentration in tears 120–170 mmol/liter is about equal to that in plasma suggesting a passive secretion into the tears. While potassium with an average value of about 20 mmol/l is much higher than the corresponding plasma concentration of about 5 mmol/l. This indicates an active secretion of potassium into the tears. It is interesting to observe that while the main cationic constituent of the aqueous and vitreous humor is sodium while cornea (mainly corneal epithelium) contains a much higher concentration of potassium than sodium. These two cations play an essential role in the osmotic regulation of the extracellular and intracellular spaces and in general changes in sodium level are the reverse of changes in potassium level.

Calcium

Calcium is independent of the tear production and is lower than the free fraction of plasma. In cystic fibrosis patients have much higher calcium values. An average of 2.5 mmol/l have been shown only at slow rates concomitant with lower tear sodium values.

Magnesium

Magnesium in tears is little lower than corresponding serum value possibly reflecting the free fraction of magnesium. Both calcium and magnesium play a role in controlling membrane permeability.

Chloride

Chloride, an anion essential to all tissues also plays an important role in osmotic regulation much like sodium and potassium. The chloride concentration is slightly higher in tears than in serum.

Bicarbonate

The bicarbonate together with the carbonate ions in tears may be involved in the regulation of pH. This buffer system maintains the near neutral pH of the tear film, the surface of which is exposed to atmospheric changes.

Enzymes

Enzymes of Energy Producing Metabolisms

Glycolytic enzymes and enzymes of tricarboxylic acid cycle can be detected in high values only in human tear samples. These enzymes form a blood-tear barrier against penetration from the blood. The source of these enzymes is in the conjunctiva where they are secreted in small amounts. The lacrimal gland apparently does not secrete these enzymes. These enzymes can be obtained during mechanical irritation.

Lactate Dehydrogenase

Lactate dehydrogenase (LDH) is the enzyme in the highest concentration in tears. It can be separated electrophoretically into its five isoenzymes showing a pattern with more of the slower migrating muscle type isoenzymes. This is closely related to the distribution pattern of corneal tissue in contrast to serum LDH where the faster migrating heart type isoenzymes prevail.

These findings indicate that tear LDH originates from the corneal epithelium. Therefore, in patients suffering from corneal disease, the distribution of LDH isoenzymes in tears differs from those found in healthy individuals. LDH isoenzymes bound to immunoglobulin have been found in blood and it is probable that here an analogous binding takes place in tears.

Lysosomal Enzymes

Lysosomal enzymes include a number of lysosomal acid hydrolases, which are present in tears in concentration of 2 to 10 times than those in serum. The lacrimal gland is the main source of the lysosomal enzymes but conjunctiva may act as a second source for lysosomal enzymes after mild trauma. The relative high values are found in tear fluid collection where the epithelial cells of conjunctiva remain intact and contain very low levels of lactate dehydrogenase or other cytoplasmic enzymes. Lysosomal enzyme activities in tears are used for diagnosis and identification of carriers of several inborn errors of metabolism.

The concentration of β-hexosaminidase in tears collected on filter paper strips is an index for the development and prognosis of diabetic retinopathy. The tears would reflect the decreased enzyme activity of β-hexosaminidase and of other lysosomal glycosidases in the retina showing a negative correlation with the increased plasma levels of these enzymes.

Amylase

Amylase is the enzyme present in tear fluid in relatively moderate levels. The origin of this enzyme is in lacrimal gland. The reported presence of amylase in the cornea might be due to contamination by tear fluid.

Peroxidase

Peroxidase (POD) is present in human tears originating from the lacrimal gland and not from the conjunctiva. The level of tear POD in human tears is 103 m/l. POD activity found in the conjunctiva is probably derived from the tears.

Plasminogen Activator

Plasminogen activator has been demonstrated in tear fluid and corneal epithelium is suggested to be the source of this urokinase-like fibrinolytic activity.

Collagenase

Collagenase has been shown to be present in tear fluid in the presence of corneal ulceration, due to infection, chemical burn, trauma and desiccation. Corneal collagenase is present as an inactive precursor "latent collagenase" which can be activated with trypsin and *in-vivo* possibly by plasmin resulting from plasminogen activator activity in tears.

Drugs Excreted in Tears

Tears represent a potentially more stable body fluid of low protein content and with modest variations of pH. Passage of drugs from the plasma to the tears apparently takes place by diffusion of the non-protein bound fraction. However, presence of tight junctions between the acinar epithelial cells in the lacrimal gland forming a blood-tear barrier, the lipid solubility is expected to play a major role. The blood-tear barrier shows the same characteristics as that of cell membrane. Phenobarbital and carbamazepine are excreted in tears in about 0.5 percent of corresponding plasma concentration.

Methotrexate, an antimetabolite reaches tear levels of 5 percent of the corresponding plasma concentrations and is in equilibrium with the unbound fraction in plasma. Ampicillin is present in tears in concentration of about 0.02 of the corresponding serum level.

APPLIED PHYSIOLOGY

Basic secretion of tear fluid is made up of the secretions of the lacrimal gland and accessory lacrimal gland tissue together with the secretions of meibomian glands and the mucous glands of the conjunctiva. Reflex secretions of tears is hundreds time greater than basal or resting secretion. The stimulus to reflex secretions appears to be derived from the superficial corneal and conjunctival sensory stimulation as a result of tear break up and dry spot formation. The secretory stimulus to the lacrimal glands is parasympathetic with reflex secretions occurring in both eyes following superficial stimulation of one eye. The whole mass of lacrimal tissue responds as one unit to reflex tearing. Reflex secretion is reduced by topical corneal and conjunctival anesthesia.

HYPOSECRETION OF TEARS

Hyposecretion means decreased formation of tears.

Lacrimal hyposecretion may be congenital although not very common. Acquired lacrimal hyposecretion may be due to:
- Atrophy and fibrosis of lacrimal tissue due to a destructive infiltration by mononuclear cells as in keratoconjunctivitis sicca and Sjogren's syndrome
- Local inflammatory diseases of the conjunctiva commonly conjunctival scarring secondary to bacterial or viral infection
- Chronic inflammatory disease of the salivary and lacrimal glands (Mikulicz's syndrome)
- Damage or destruction of lacrimal tissue by granulomatous (sarcoidisis), pseudotumor or neoplastic lesions
- Absence of lacrimal gland
- Blockage of excretory ducts of the lacrimal gland
- Neurogenic lesions
- Meibomian gland dysfunction.

Diagnostic Tests for Tear Hyposecretions (Table 2.10)

Tear Film Break-up Time (BUT)

The tear film break-up time is a simple physiological test to assess the stability of the precorneal tear film. This test is performed by instilling fluorescein into the lower fornix, taking precaution not

TABLE 2.10: Diagnostic tests and drug assays in tears		
Compound	*Diagnosis*	*Usefulness*
Lysozyme	Sjögren's disease	+
	Practolol induced toxicity	+
	Traumatic inflammation of eye	+
Lysosomal enzymes	Lysosomal storage disease	+
Collagenase	Corneal ulceration	+
α_1-Antitrypsin	Bacterial infections	±
Glucose	Diabetes mellitus	±
Tear albumin	Genetic marker	+
Immunoglobulins (IgA, IgG and IgM)	Iatrogenic inflammation of anterior-segment	+
+ Useful		
± Comparatively useful		

to touch cornea. The patient is asked to blink several times and then to refrain from blinking. The tear film is scanned with a broad beam and cobalt blue filter. After an interval of time black spots or line indicating dry spots appear in the tear film. BUT is the interval between the last blink and appearance of the first randomly distributed dry spot. Ideally average of three measurements is taken. A normal BUT is more than 10 seconds and a BUT of less than 10 seconds is considered abnormal. This test may also be abnormal in eyes with mucin or lipid deficiency.

Schirmer's Test

The rate of tear formation is estimated by measuring the amount of wetting on a special filter paper which is 5 mm wide and 35 mm long (Fig. 2.6).

Previously Schirmer's test 1 and 2 were used in diagnostic practice but nowadays modified Schirmer-I test is employed. This test is performed as follows:

Schirmer strips are prepared by cutting out Whatman filter paper No. 41 into the strips of 5 mm × 35 mm dimensions. A 5 mm tab is folded over at one end. Before use, these strips are autoclaved.

The bent end is placed into lower conjunctival sac at the junction of lateral one-third and medial two-third of the lower eyelid so that a 5 mm bent end rests on the palpebral conjunctiva and the folding crease lies over the eyelid margin. This test is usually performed in sitting posture in dim light.

The patient is asked to keep the eyelid open and look slightly upwards at a fixation point. Blinking is allowed while the patient gazes at the fixation point.

After one minute, the strips are carefully removed and moistening of the exposed portion of the strip is measured in millimeters with the help of a millimeter ruler.

The measurements are made from the notch at the bend of the Schirmer strip to the distal end of the wetting on the strip (excluding the folded over tab). The amount of wetting of the Schirmer strip in one minute is multiplied by three to correspond roughly to the amount of wetting that would have occurred in five minutes (Jones, 1972). It is a measure of the rate of tear secretion in a five-minute period.

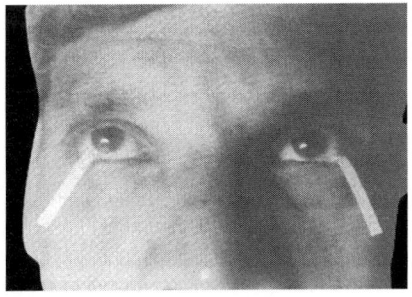

Fig. 2.6: Modified Schirmer test

A normal eye will wet between 10 mm and 25 mm during that period. Measurements between 5 mm and 10 mm are considered borderline and values less than 5 mm is indicative of impaired secretion.

Vital Dye Staining

- Rose Bengal 1 percent has an affinity for devitalized epithelial cells and mucus in contrast to fluorescein which remains extracellular and is more useful in showing up epithelial defects. Rose Bengal is very useful in detecting even mild cases of keratoconjunctivitis sicca (KCS) by staining the interpalpebral conjunctiva in the form of two triangles with their base at the limbus.

    The only disadvantage with Rose Bengal staining is that it may cause ocular irritation specially in eyes with severe KCS. In order to reduce that amount of irritation only a small drop should be instilled into the eye. A topical anesthetic should not be used prior to the instillation of Rose Bengal as it may produce a false-positive result.
- Alcian blue has similar properties as Rose Bengal and is less irritant but it is not generally available.

Lysozyme Assay

Lysozyme assay is based on the fact that in hyposecretion of tears, there may be reduction in the concentration of lysozyme. This test is performed by placing the wetted filter strip into an agar plate containing specific bacteria. The plate is then incubated for 24 hours and the zone of the lysis is measured. The zone will be reduced if the concentration of lysozyme in the tears is decreased.

Tear Globulin Assay

Tear IgA levels are measured in this test. This test is also based on the principle that decreased tear formation will lead to decreased IgA (immunoglobulin A) levels in tears. This test is performed on a specific tripartigan immunodiffusion plates containing specific agar gel in wells (Figs 2.7 and 2.8). Twenty ml of tear samples is put into these wells and plates are incubated for 48 hours. The diffusion of rings around wells are measured to the nearest 0.1 mm with a partigen ruler. The ring will be reduced if the concentration of IgA in tears is decreased. This is a reliable test for measuring tear globulins.

Tear Osmolarity

Tear osmolarity is increased in cases of hyposecretion.

Biopsy of the Conjunctiva

Biopsy of the conjunctiva and an estimation of the number of goblet cells are other tests which can be done. In mucin deficiency states the number of goblet cells shall be decreased.

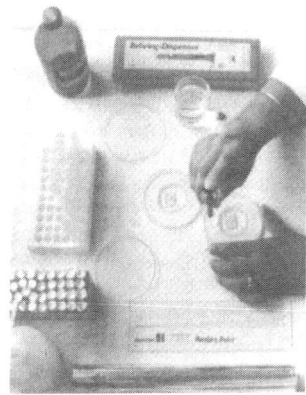

Fig. 2.7: Tear globulin assay (diagnostic test)

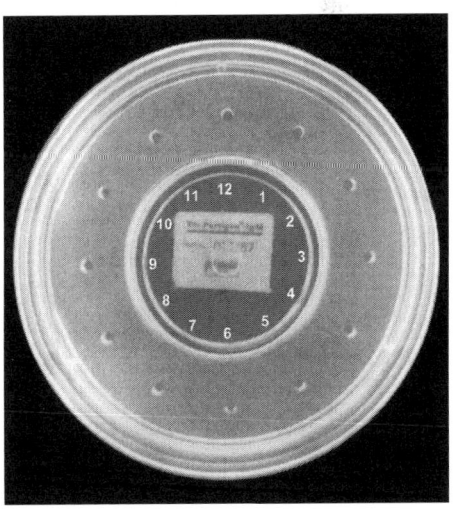

Fig. 2.8: Tripartigen immunodiffusion plates (diffusion of rings around agar wells is measured up to 0.1 mm)

HYPERSECRETION OF TEARS

In practice when patient complains of a wet eye there are two possibilities of excessive watering of the eye.
- Lacrimation from reflex hypersecretion due to irritation of cornea and conjunctiva.
- Obstructive epiphora as a result of failure of tear drainage or evacuation system. The main causes are lacrimal pump failure due to lower lid laxity or weakness of the orbicularis muscle and more commonly due to mechanical obstructions of the drainage system.

If the wet eye is caused by hypersecretion the Schirmer test values (technique already mentioned) will be increased and the Jones Fluorescein dye test will reveal normal outflow function.

Physiological Diagnostic Test for Hypersecretions

Jones I (Primary) Test

This is a physiological test which differentiates an excessive watering due to a partial obstruction of the lacrimal passages from primary hypersecretion of tears (Fig. 2.9).

In this test 1 drop of 2 percent fluorescein solution is instilled into the conjunctival sac. After about 5 minutes a cotton-tipped bud or applicator (moistened in coccaine 4% or proparacaine 0.75%) is inserted under the inferior turbinate at the nasolacrimal duct opening. This is situated about 3 cm from the external nares.

The results are interpreted as follows:
- If the fluorescein is recovered from the nose on the applicator and aqueous solution passes from the conjunctival sac to the nose in 1 minute then the excretory system is patent and cause of watering is primary hypersecretion. No further tests are required then and the test is inferred as positive

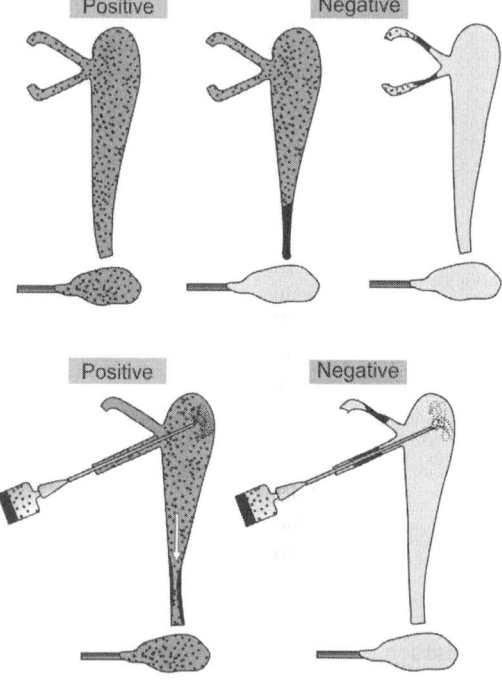

Fig. 2.9: Dye testing: Jones primary test (top) and Jones secondary test (bottom) (*Courtesy:* Kanski Clinical Ophthalmology Butterworth International Edition)

- If no dye is recovered from the nose a partial obstruction is present or there is failure of the lacrimal pump mechanism. In this situation secondary dye test or Jones II test is required.

Jones II (Secondary Irrigation) Test

This test helps to identify the probable site of partial obstruction.

In this procedure topical anesthesia (4% Xylocaine or 0.5% proparacaine) is instilled into the conjunctival sac and any residual fluorescein is washed out. The nasolacrimal system is then irrigated with normal saline. The patient is positioned with his or her head down by about 45° so that the saline runs out of the nose into white paper tissues and not into the pharynx.

This test is interpreted as follows:
- Positive—if fluorescein-stained saline is recovered from the nose, the dye must have reached the lacrimal sac during the primary dye test but was stopped from entering the nose by a partial obstruction in the nasolacrimal duct. However, syringing of the lacrimal system had pushed the dye past the obstruction into the nose. A positive secondary dye test indicates a partial obstruction to the nasolacrimal duct which can be treated by a dacryocystorhinostomy (DCR) procedure.
- Negative—if unstained saline is recovered from the nose it means that no dye has entered the lacrimal sac during the primary dye test. This means a partial obstruction in the upper drainage system (punctum, canaliculi or common canaliculus) or a defective lacrimal pump mechanism. In such a situation DCR would fail and some other operative procedure will be required.

Fluorescein Dye Disappearance Test

An accurate status of the excretory capability of the lacrimal system can be obtained by observing the behavior of a single drop of 2 percent fluorescein solution instilled into the inferior conjunctival cul-de-sac. The color intensity after 5 minutes is measured and graded on a scale of 0 to 4+. The normal excretion of the retained fluorescein shall be 0 to 1+. Any greater residual then is indicative of impaired outflow. However, by this test one cannot distinguish between impairment of the upper and lower segments of the system, but it may complement the Jones tests.
- Nasal examination should be performed in order to determine the position of normal nasal structures specially the position of the anterior end of the middle turbinate when surgery is contemplated. It will also detect the presence of polyps or tumors, etc.

Special Tests

Intubation Dacryocystography

The conventional method of dacryocystography consists of injecting contrast medium into one of the canaliculi followed by the taking of posteroanterior (PA) and lateral views, radiographs. However, far superior status of the canalicular system can be obtained by using a technique that combines injection of lipoidol ultrafluid through a cathetar with macrography. In common canalicular lesions, subtraction macrodacryocystography may provide more sophisticated details.

These specific investigations are not only extremely valuable in depicting the exact location of the obstruction but they are also of help in the diagnosis of diverticula, fistulae, filling defects due to tumors, stones and infections by *streptothrix* species.

Scintillography (Radionuclide Testing)

This test involves the labeling of tears with gamma-emitting substances such as technetium-99m and monitoring their progress through the drainage system. This is a sophisticated and reliable test for better understanding of excretory physiology.

Color Doppler Scanography

Color Doppler scanography is the latest technique for evaluating the status of the drainage system. It is a recently introduced test with accurate results.

BIBLIOGRAPHY

1. Agarwal A. Textbook of Ophthalmology, 1st edn. New Delhi: Jaypee Brothers Medical Publishers, 2002.
2. Bartlett JD. Clinical Ocular Pharmacology, 4th edn. Boston: Butterworth-Heinemann, 2001.
3. Bartlett JD. Ophthalmic Drug facts: Lippincott—William and Wilkins, 2001.
4. Crick RP, Trimble RB. Textbook of Clinical Ophthalmology: Hodder and Stoughton, 1986.
5. Duane TD. Clinical Ophthalmology, 4th edn. Butterworth – Heinemann, 1999.
6. Duvall. Ophthalmic Medications and Pharmacology: Slack Inc, 1998.
7. Ellis PP. Ocular Therapeutics and Pharmacology, 7th edn. CV Mosby, 1985.
8. Fechner. Ocular Therapeutics: Slack Inc, 1998.
9. Fraunfelder. Current Ocular Therapy, 5th edn. WB Saunders, 2000.
10. Garg A. Current Trends in Ophthalmology, 1st edn. New Delhi: Jaypee Brothers Medical Publishers, 1997.
11. Garg A. Manual of Ocular Therapeutics, 1st edn. New Delhi: Jaypee Brothers Medical Publishers, 1996.
12. Garg A. Ready Reckoner of Ocular Therapeutics, 1st edn. New Delhi, 2002.
13. Goodman LS, Gilman A. Pharmacological Basis of Therapeutics, 7th edn. New York: Macmillan, 1985.
14. Havener's. Ocular Pharmacology, 6th edn. C.V. Mosby, 1994.
15. Kanski. Clinical Ophthalmology, 4th edn. Butterworth – Heineman, 1999.

16. Kershner. Ophthalmic Medications and Pharmacology: Slack. Inc, 1994.
17. Olin BR, et al. Drugs Facts and Comparisons: Facts and Comparisons, St Louis, 1997.
18. Onofrey. The Ocular Therapeutics; Lippincott-William & Wilkins, 1997.
19. Rhee. The Wills Eye Drug Guide: Lippincott – William & Wilkins, 1998.
20. Steven Podos. Textbook of Ophthalmology, New Delhi: Jaypee Brothers Medical Publishers, 2001.
21. Zimmerman. Textbook of Ocular Pharmacology: Lippincott & William & Wilkins, 1997.

3

Aqueous Humor Dynamics

Ashok Garg (India)

INTRODUCTION

Aqueous humor is a clear slightly alkaline watery fluid occupying both the anterior and posterior chambers of the eye. It is not a stagnant fluid but continuously secreted and passed over the lens through the pupil into the anterior chamber and then drained into the vascular system—the anterior ciliary veins.

Aqueous humor has a density slightly higher than water. The volume of aqueous in the anterior chamber is about 0.25 cc whereas that in the posterior chamber is about 0.06 cc.

BLOOD-AQUEOUS BARRIER

The system of semipermeable membranes separating the blood from the ocular cavity is known as the blood-aqueous barrier. The tight junctions between the nonpigmented epithelial cells (NPE) together with the nonfenestrated iris vessels represent the morphological contribution to the blood-aqueous barrier.

It is formed in the posterior segment of the globe by the walls of the retinal capillaries which like those of the central nervous system (CNS) are very impermeable, and by Bruch's membrane and retinal pigment epithelium (RPE). In the ciliary region, it is formed by the two-layered ciliary epithelium through which fluid has to pass before reaching the posterior chamber (Figs 3.1 and 3.2). The junctions between the ciliary epithelial cells have been described by the Freeze-fracture technique. These consist of a network of anastomosing strands that firmly unite adjacent cells. In the iris blood-aqueous, barrier is formed by the walls of the capillaries in this tissue which are openly exposed to the anterior chamber through the crypts and spongy stroma.

The specific impermeability of the retinal capillaries and of the Bruch's membrane pigment epithelial barrier prevents the ready passage of large-sized molecules of any kind into the eye. However, substances with high lipid solubility easily traverse the barrier much more readily (e.g. chloramphenicol, sulfonamides, etc.).

The extracellular space between the apices of pigmented and nonpigmental epithelial cells is bordered by gap junctions, not by tight junctions through which tracer material passes freely. After the injection of horseradish peroxidase (mol. wt. 40,000) and microperoxidase (mol. wt. 1900), the electron dense tracer enters

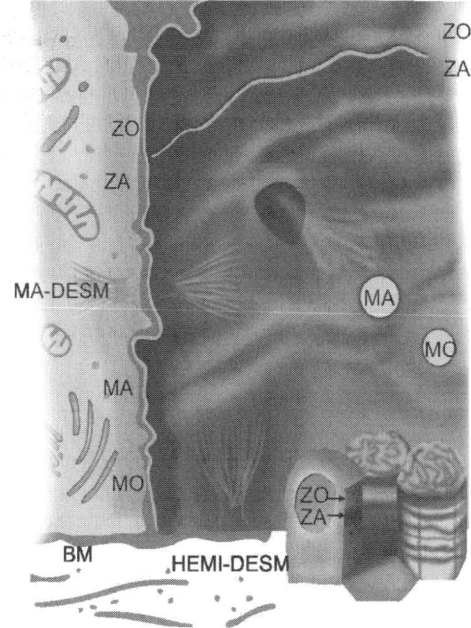

Fig. 3.1: View of the intercellular junctions of ciliary epithelium. (ZO—the zonula occludens forms the tight junctions by completely obliterating the intercellular space—the blood-aqueous barrier resides here)

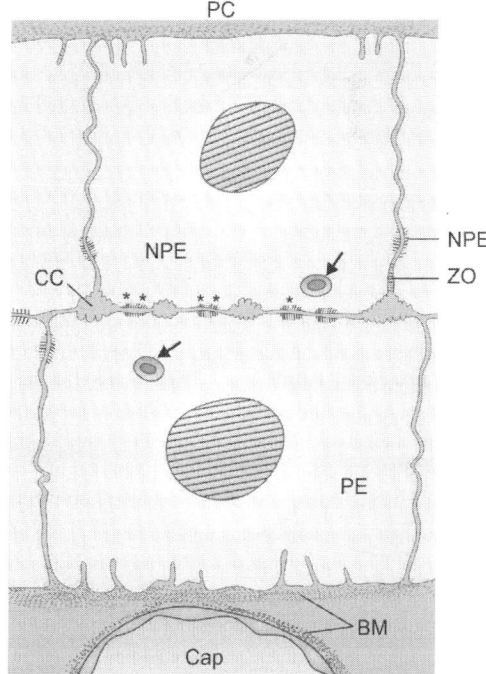

Fig. 3.2: Normal ciliary epithelium (the blood-aqueous barrier resides in the tight junctions marked ZO at the apex of NPE cells of ciliary epithelium)

the space between the two layers of epithelial cells through the gap junctions and into the ciliary channels where it is stopped by the tight junctions. The effectiveness of the blood-aqueous barrier is proved by its impermeability to a small track such as microperoxidase. However, it is important to note that no single anatomic structure can explain all the transport characteristics of the ciliary epithelium and that other metabolic or transport functions also come into play.

The blood-aqueous barrier is permeable to fluorescein, a water-soluble molecule that penetrates into the posterior chamber probably through the anterior part of the ciliary processes. Some of the fluorescein diffuses into the anterior chamber through the iris vessels.

The blood-aqueous barrier is highly permeable to water but less to salts. Consequently, abrupt increase in the osmotic pressure of plasma occurs after intravenous injections of hyperosmotic agents used to treat acute attack of congestive angle-closure glaucoma (ACG). It will cause the rapid removal of water from the eye followed by a drop in intraocular pressure (IOP). The permeability of blood-aqueous barrier to water is also the basis of the water drinking test in open-angle glaucoma (OAG). In this case, penetration of water into the eye from the diluted plasma results in increased aqueous formation.

Most of the cells of the nonpigmented epithelium show deep infoldings which are U-shaped and reach almost to the nucleus. In the basal or inner third of the nonpigmented cells there is accumulation of the enzyme ATPase. This enzyme plays an important role in the active transfer of sodium across the cell membrane during the process of aqueous formation.

Breakdown of Blood-Aqueous Barrier

Under normal conditions, the blood-aqueous barrier remains stable and this stability contributes to the normal dynamics of aqueous resulting in a steady state of normal IOP. The stability of the blood-aqueous barrier may be disturbed by inflammatory conditions of the eye specially those involving the ciliary body. It may also be disturbed under the effects of certain medications.

The destabilization of the blood-aqueous barrier with leakage of plasma proteins into the anterior chamber has significant clinical implications. Fragmentation of tight junctions specially in the anterior parts plicata region of the ciliary body occurs after paracentesis with subsequent leakage of plasma proteins into the aqueous humor. This inflow of plasma like or "plasmoid" aqueous (or secondary aqueous) into the anterior chamber is responsible in part for increase in IOP.

If the permeability of the capillaries is increased, large molecules shall be able to pass through their walls so that a turbid fluid rich in protein is formed. This increase in permeability may be brought about by the vasodilator drugs in inflammatory conditions such as iridocyclitis or choroiditis and also happens when the capillary walls are mechanically stretched.

A variety of noxious stimuli can lead to the incompetence of blood-aqueous barrier. Following trauma to the eye, a substance from irides named irin is released into the aqueous in response to trauma. It contains both E and F prostaglandins. Prostaglandins implicated in the irritative response after mechanical trauma to the eye result in miosis, vasodilation, increased protein levels in the aqueous and increased IOP. Prostaglandins applied topically to the eye result in breakdown of the tight junctions of NPE and increased protein into the aqueous humor with highest levels in the posterior chamber. Alteration of blood-aqueous barrier can also be induced by intracarotid infusion of hyperosmotic agents which causes separation of the pigment epithelium (PE) and nonpigment epithelial layers, opening of the blood-aqueous barrier and severe permanent damage of the PE cells. Significant disruption of the blood-aqueous barrier has been recently reported in literature in the contralateral eyes of patients undergoing cataract extraction and lens implantation surgery and in the eye of patients undergoing argon laser trabeculoplasty for OAG.

The anatomic basis for the breakdown of the barrier is found in the formation of cysts containing protein rich fluid and edema of the ciliary processes due to increased permeability of capillaries to the proteins (Fig. 3.3). The increased pressure within the ciliary processes stretches the epithelial cells and separates them causing leakage of proteins including fibrinogen into the posterior chamber.

Such a two-way transference of fluid across the capillary wall would tend to stagnation. To it is added a secretory process conducted by the metabolic activity of the cells of the ciliary epithelium, it is probable that this accounts for about 95 percent of total quantity of aqueous.

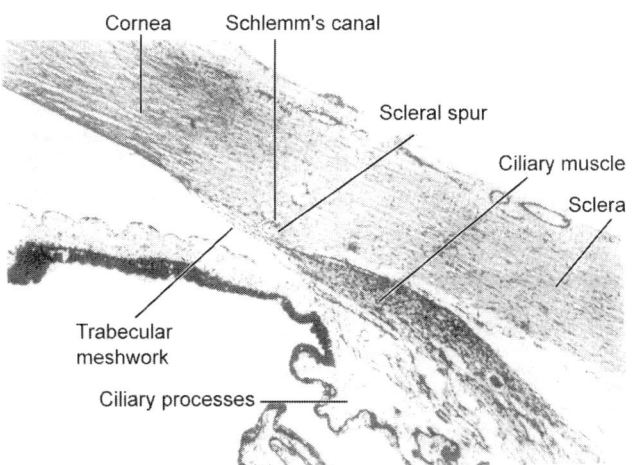

Fig. 3.3: Photomicrograph of ciliary body in human eye and its relationships

AQUEOUS HUMOR FORMATION

Production or formation of aqueous humor occurs in the secretory ciliary epithelium by three basic mechanisms: (i) diffusion, (ii) active secretion, and (iii) ultrafiltration.

Diffusion

Diffusion of solutes across cell membrane occurs from the side of greater concentration to the side of lesser concentration. Lipid-soluble substances that easily penetrate cell membranes readily move in this fashion. Ultrafiltration occurs when the flux of substance across a membrane is increased by a hydrostatic driving force (i.e. transport is increased under the effect of increased hydrostatic pressure). The process of active transport or secretion requires the input of cellular energy (in form of adenosine triphosphate) to secrete material against a concentration gradient.

Although all the three processes may contribute to the formation of aqueous humor, the maximum contribution likely comes from active transport of the solute followed by the osmotic flow of water into the posterior chamber (Fig. 3.4).

Active Secretion

Secretion or active pumping of substances into the posterior chamber is the primary means of aqueous production. Secretion is the result of an active metabolic process and is independent of the level of IOP.

It is now well-accepted that active transport of certain solutes by the ciliary epithelium is the most important in aqueous humor formation. The rate of aqueous formation depends on the rate of active solute transport by ciliary epithelium. The membrane-

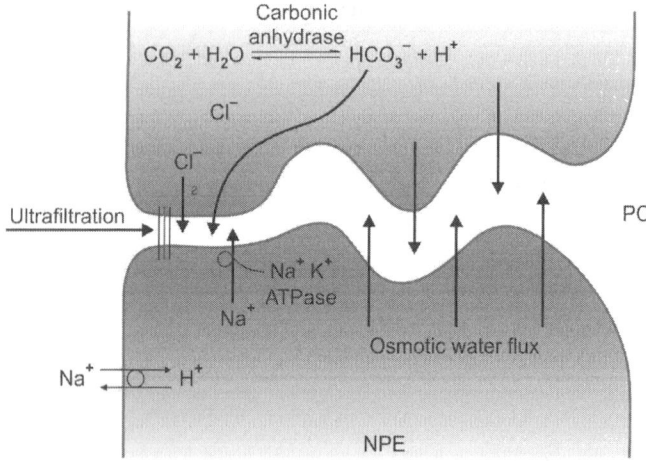

Fig. 3.4: Osmotic flow model of aqueous production

bound enzyme system known as sodium-potassium adenosine triphosphatase (Na^+/K^+ ATPase) is an active energy-dependent transport system present in the nonpigmented epithelium (NPE) and is present in maximum concentration along the lateral cellular interdigitations. Usually Na^+ is the actively transported ion with Cl^- or HCO_3^- following to maintain electroneutrality. Measurements of electric potential across the ciliary epithelium shows that aqueous is positive with respect to ciliary body stroma. Active transport of Cl^- may also occur but magnitude of this transport is very small as compared to that of Na^+.

The relationship concerning ciliary metabolism and the actual site of ion transport is complex because of the unique arrangement of the ciliary epithelial cells.

On biochemical assay a number of enzyme systems have been shown to be present in the NPE layer. It includes Nucleotide phosphotases (specially ATPase), adenylate cyclase and carbonic anhydrase. There is greater development of intracellular organelles and a higher metabolic rate in NPE as compared to PE layer. These findings indicate that the NPE probably plays the dominant role in the aqueous humor formation.

The mechanism of aqueous humor formation by the transporting epithelium (NPE cells) is best described by the standing gradient osmotic flow model.

A steady state standing osmotic gradient is maintained in the lateral intercellular channel with the maximal concentration of solute occurring proximally in the channel adjacent to the tight junction. This hypertonic fluid in the proximal region of the channel pushes an osmotic flux of water into channel. The solute concentration decreases from the proximal to the distal end of the channel as water enters. Slightly hypertonic fluid flows into the posterior chamber as nascent aqueous.

Ultrafiltration

The rate of ultrafiltration is influenced by the level of blood pressure in the ciliary capillaries, the plasma oncotic pressure and the level of IOP. The process of ultrafiltration of fluid from the plasma into the posterior chamber is responsible for as much as 75 percent of aqueous humor formation.

Hydrostatic and oncotic forces across the ciliary epithelium favor reabsorption of the aqueous humor into the ciliary process (Fig. 3.5). The stroma of ciliary processes has a certain oncotic pressure (approx 14 mm Hg) as a result of protein leakage through its fenestrated capillaries. Ciliary body stroma is a potential site of extravascular diffusion of fluid and solutes from ciliary capillaries. The concentration of proteins in the ciliary body stroma is approximately 75 percent of the intravascular level. This significant concentration of extravascular protein produces a high oncotic pressure attracting fluid to this location from areas with fluids of less oncotic pressure. Smooth muscle cells of the ciliary muscle and fibroblasts of the connective tissue layer in the ciliary body may also alter this fluid biochemically although degree of alteration from these cells appears to be minimal.

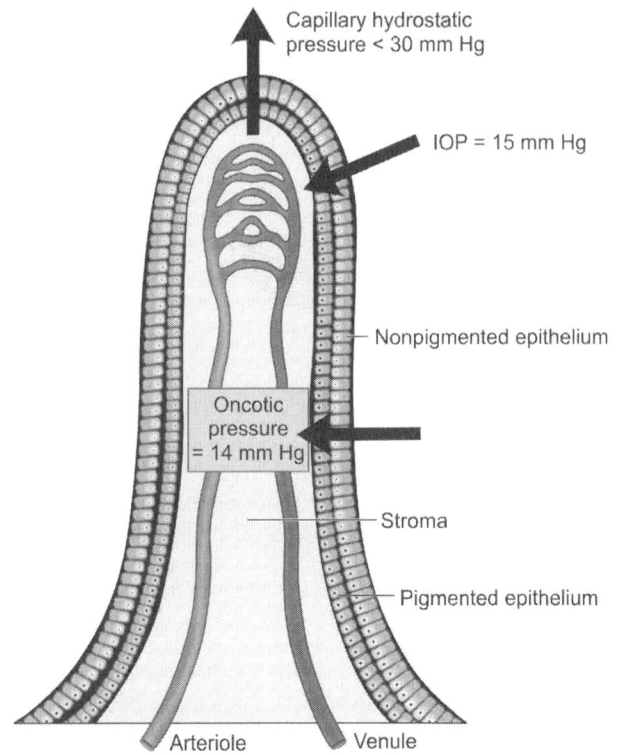

Fig. 3.5: Hydrostatic forces involved in aqueous humor production

It has been shown that capillary hydrostatic pressure in excess of 29 mm Hg shall be required for the formation of an ultrafiltrate. The capillary hydrostatic pressure in ciliary process has been estimated to be 27 to 32 mm Hg.

AQUEOUS HUMOR FORMATION REGULATION (CONTROL)

Clinical data suggest that humoral or neurohumoral pathways influence the steady state level of IOP by altering the rate of aqueous formation. The ciliary epithelia contain an enzyme receptor complex (adenylate cyclase) which is responsible for formation of cyclic AMP, an intracellular second messenger. Stimulation of this enzyme complex in ciliary epithelia can cause a decrease in the net rate of aqueous humor inflow. Adenylate cyclase can be activated by catecholamines, glycoprotein hormones, organic fluorides, etc. Topical application of Forsokolin a diterpene significantly decreases IOP by reducing net aqueous humor inflow. The production of cyclic AMP by ciliary adenylate cyclase may represent a final common pathway in IOP regulation with the possibility of modulation of this receptor complex by a number of humoral, neurohumoral and pharmacological agents.

RATE OF FLOW OF MOVEMENTS OF AQUEOUS HUMOR

Depending upon the technique employed the rate of flow of the aqueous homor has been shown to vary from 1 to 5 cumm/minute. Movement of aqueous humor takes place by two ways.

Thermal Circulation

Normally, there is a difference of temperature between the cornea which is cooled by air and the vascularized iris which is warmed up by the blood. This difference of temperature is about 3–5°C. As a result of this temperature difference, a convection current is in the aqueous of the anterior chamber causing a constant flow of the aqueous upwards in the region of the iris and downwards in the region of the cornea. This movement is known as thermal circulation.

Bulk Flow

This type of circulation of aqueous occurs in the following pattern. Aqueous humor originated by ciliary body—posterior chamber—through pupil into anterior chamber—through spaces of Fontanna in the trabecula at the angle of anterior chamber to the afferent channels of the canal of Schlemm—canal of Schlemm—efferent channels (aqueous veins)—intrascleral and episcleral plexus of veins.

ROUTES OF AQUEOUS OUTFLOW (ESCAPE)

There are two paths by which aqueous escapes from the eye. One is pressure dependent while the other is pressure independent.

Trabecular Meshwork Outflow (Conventional Outflow)

Approximately 80 percent of total outflow of aqueous is through the trabecular meshwork into Schlemm's canal and then into venous circulation by way of the aqueous veins (Figs 3.6A and B).

The pressure-dependent pathway is through the many progressively smaller pores of the trabecular meshwork into Schlemm's canal, to the few collector channels and into the episcleral veins (Fig. 3.7).

Mechanism of aqueous flow across the Schlemm's canal is partially understood, however, various possibilities are as follows:

Vacuolation Theory

According to this, transcellular spaces exist in the endothelial cells forming inner wall of the canal of Schlemm. These spaces open as a system of vacuoles and pores primarily in response to pressure and transport the aqueous from the juxtacanalicular connective tissue to the canal of Schlemm.

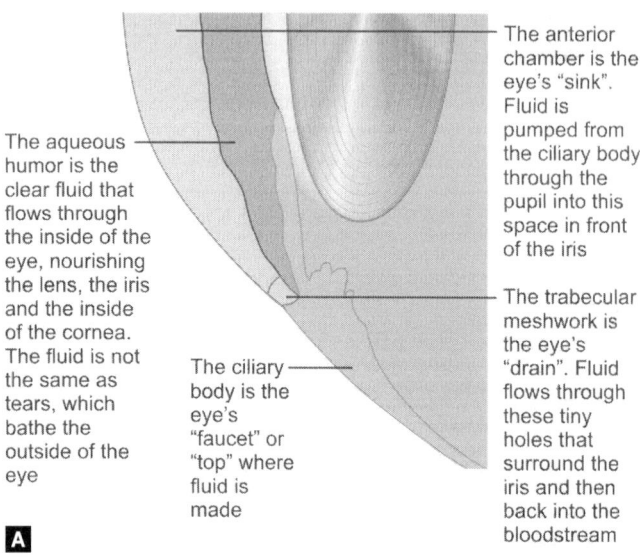

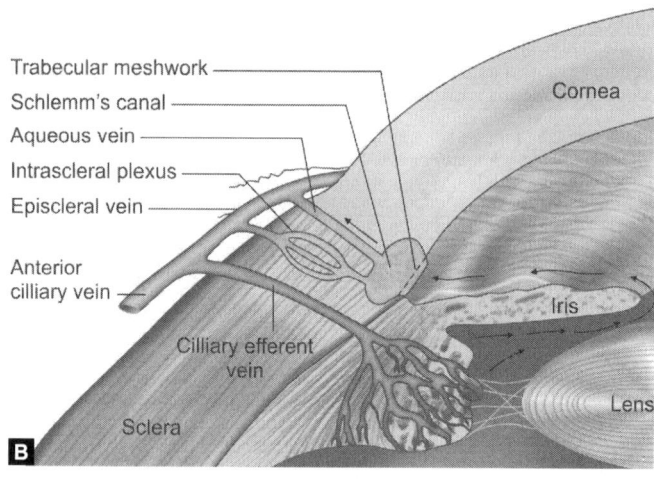

Figs 3.6A and B: The aqueous outflow system

Leakage of endothelial cell junctions may allow aqueous drainage.

Transcellular channels might be present in endothelial cells.

From Schlemm's canal the aqueous is transported via 20 to 30 external collector channels into the episcleral veins by direct and indirect systems. A pressure gradient between IOP and intrascleral venous pressure (about 10 mm Hg) is responsible for unidirectional flow of aqueous.

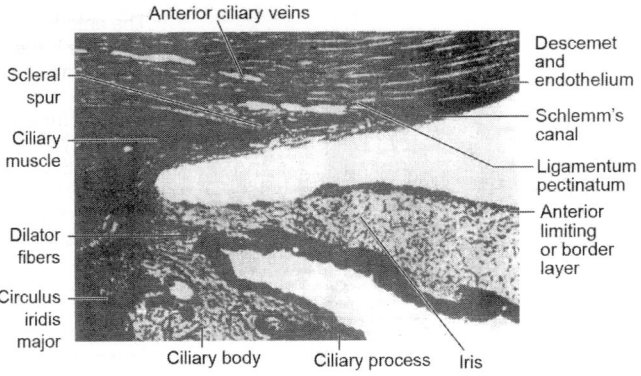

Fig. 3.7: Anterior chamber angle in cross-section

The facility of the total pathway is usually designated as Ctrab. The high pressure end of flow path is IOP or P1, the low pressure end is episcleral venous pressure Pe. The rate of flow through the trabecular meshwork system is Ftrab = (P1-Pe)Ctrab.

However, several authors have shown that this simple pressure flow relation of the trabecular outflow system is not accurate. Brubaker formulated the trabecular system outflow resistance changes as—

$$Rtrab. = Ro + (Pi-Pe) RoQ$$

Here, Ro = Resistance when outflow pressure head, Pi-Pe = O and Q is the obstruction coefficient (demension mm Hg-1).

The mechanism of the increased outflow resistance (decreased facility) as Pi increases appears to be apposition of the walls of Schlemm's canal by the increased IOP with resulting decreased filtering area and increased resistance to flow in the canal.

Uveoscleral Outflow Pathways

Uveoscleral outflow pathways account for the remaining 20 percent of the aqueous outflow. Here, the aqueous flows through the ciliary body into the suprachoroidal space to be drained by the venous circulation in the ciliary body, choroid and sclera (Fig. 3.8).

In this pathway, aqueous seeps into the face of the ciliary body which forms part of the chamber angle between the root of the iris and the scleral spur. Aqueous percolates far back into the ciliary body and choroid partly to be absorbed into blood vessels and partly to leak through the sclera into the orbital tissues. The rate of aqueous outflow through this uveoscleral pathway is not affected by the pressure. Uveoscleral outflow (U) works like a constant rate pump. The lack of effect of IOP on the U rate is possibly due to compression of the soft uveal tissue against the sclera thus valving the flow in proportion to IOP.

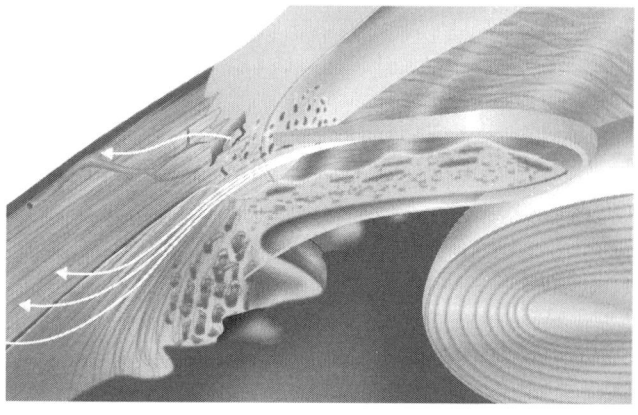

Fig. 3.8: Uveoscleral aqueous outflow pathway
(*Courtesy:* Pharmacia and Upjohn India Pvt Ltd)

AQUEOUS HUMOR COMPOSITION

Physical Properties

pH	—	7.1-7.3 (Alkaline)
Specific gravity	—	1.002-1.004
Viscosity	—	1.029
Refractive index	—	1.34
Composition-water	—	98.69%
Solids	—	1.31%

The composition of the aqueous humor depends on the nature of the freshly secreted fluid, the subsequent passive and active solute exchange across adjacent tissues and the rate of exit from the eye. The metabolic requirements to tissues such as the cornea, lens and trabecular meshwork are met by the continuous flow of aqueous through the posterior and anterior chambers. Diffusional and metabolic alterations of the aqueous occur constantly.

Osmolarity

The aqueous humor is slightly hyperosmotic to the plasma. No significant difference in osmolarity between samples of anterior and posterior chamber aqueous have been shown.

Exchange of Substances between Aqueous Humor and Surrounding Tissues

As we know that vitreous humor is a gel containing a network of collagan fibers bound together by hyaluronic acid. About 98 percent of this gel is water. The diffusion of solutes from the posterior aqueous into the vitreous contributes significantly to the concentration gradients of low molecular weight substances in the vitreous.

Solute exchanges between the aqueous and the cornea are necessary for normal corneal metabolism (except atmospheric oxygen). Although the peripheral cornea is supplied by the limbal vasculature yet the central cornea must derive its nutrition from the aqueous.

The flux of glucose into the cornea and lactic acid out of cornea contribute significantly to the lower concentration of glucose and higher concentration of lactic acid present in the anterior aqueous as compared to posterior aqueous.

Amino acids are also supplied to the cornea by the aqueous by a diffusion process. The corneal endothelium serves as a fluid pump to keep the cornea in a clear deturgescent state. About 10 ml/hour of fluid is pumped back into the anterior aqueous by the corneal endothelium. The normal measured flow rates of aqueous humor through the anterior chamber is about 150 ml/hour.

The crystalline lens takes up amino acids from the aqueous under normal conditions and may release accumulated amino acids into the aqueous when aqueous amino acids concentrations are low. Active transport of potassium occurs across the anterior surface of the lens. In short, the crystalline lens alters the aqueous by using glucose, amino acids and other solutes, releases metabolic products such as lactic acid and may act as homeostatic reservoir for amino acids.

The anterior border of the iris does not consist of continuous cell layer therefore the extracellular space of iris tissue is in continuity with the aqueous humor. Although diffusional exchange across the iris vessels is likely, there are no clinical research data to indicate active transport of any material across these vessels.

Chemical Composition of Aqueous Humor

Proteins

The most common difference in chemical composition of aqueous humor and blood plasma is found in the protein contents of two fluids. In the plasma, it has the order of 6.0 to 7.0 gm/100 ml whereas in the aqueous humor it is only 5.0 to 15.0 mg/100 ml. The blood-aqueous barrier normally limits the total protein content of the aqueous humor to less than one nintieth of the plasma concentration.

The protein composition of aqueous humor differs substantially from that of blood plasma. Normal aqueous humor consists of lower molecular weight proteins like albumin and beta-globulins while heavy molecular weight proteins such as beta-lipoproteins and immunoglobulins are present in traces. The albumin-globulin ratio is several times higher in aqueous as compared to that of plasma due to exclusion of heavy globulins from the aqueous by the blood-aqueous barrier.

In inflammatory conditions of the eye, the aqueous humor protein levels become higher than 1 g/100 ml as there is total breakdown of the selectivity of blood-aqueous barrier and aqueous humor protein fractions become qualitatively similar to those of plasma.

Immunoglobulins

Normally immunoglobulin G (IgG) is present in aqueous humor in a concentration of about 3 mg/100 ml. IgA, IgM and IgD are not present commonly in detectable amounts. However in inflammatory conditions of the anterior segment of the eye, IgG levels increases and IgM and IgA also become detectable.

Regarding complement activity, normal human aqueous contains only functional C2, C6 and C7 fractions. In inflamed conditions of the eye complement components are also found in increased amounts and increased levels are proportional to elevated IgG levels. Aqueous immue complexes are present in patients with Fuch's heterochromic iridocyclitis, sympathetic ophthalmitis and endogenous uveitis.

Coagulation and Cell Growth Inhibitors

The normal aqueous humor contains only the traces of the components of coagulation and fibrinolytic systems except plasminogen and plasminogen proactivator which are present in significant concentration in normal aqueous humor.

The presence of plasminogen and plasminogen proactivator and absence of inhibitors of these fibrinolytic protein serve as a physiological function in keeping the outflow pathways free of fibrin.

Secondary aqueous contains significant amounts of all the chief components of coagulation and fibrinolysis. Research studies have shown that aqueous humor promotes coagulation by shortening the prothrombin and partial thromboplastin times. These unique characteristics of the aqueous humor are responsible for the difference in evolution of intracameral clots as compared to intravascular clots.

Recent studies have shown that aqueous humor from patients with senile cataract inhibit the growth of subconjunctival fibroblasts. After glaucoma filtering surgery, the aqueous humor supports the growth of fibroblasts the effect lasting as long as 10 weeks after surgery. It supports that fibroblast proliferation inhibitor is present in normal aqueous humor while that is not present in secondary aqueous.

Crystalline Lens Proteins

The alpha- and gamma-crystallines are normally present in smaller amounts in aqueous humor of the eye with clear lenses. The concentration (levels) of these lens crystalline increases in eyes with senile cataract supporting the view that these proteins leak from the lens.

In patients suffering from phacolytic glaucoma, the aqueous contains heavy molecular weight soluble proteins. These proteins having molecular weight greater than 150×10^6 daltons are responsible for increase in IOP by obstructing the aqueous outflow channels.

TABLE 3.1: Electrolyte concentrations in normal aqueous humor

Substance	Anterior aqueous	Posterior aqueous	Plasma
Sodium(Na⁺) (mmol/ml)	146	143.5	146
Potassium K⁺ (mmol/ml)	5.25	5.4	5.50
Ca⁺⁺ (mmol/ml)	1.70	1.76	2.60
Mg⁺⁺ (mmol/ml)	0.8	0.78	1.00
Chloride (Cl⁻) (mmol/ml)	109.5	109.00	108.00
Bicarbonate HCO_3^- (mmol/ml)	33.6	34.1	27.40
Hydrogen ion (pH)	7.60	7.57	7.40
Oxygen (mm/Hg)	55	—	100-150
Phosphate (mmol/ml)	0.62	0.57	1.11

Lipids

Research studies have shown that normal aqueous contains less than 1 mg/100 ml of lipoprotein and phospholipids. Lysophosphatidyl choline, sphingomyelin and phosphatidylcholine constitute the main fractions of phospholipids in aqueous humor. A significant blood-aqueous barrier exists for phospholipids with their concentration ranging between 1-30th to one-half of the corresponding plasma concentrations.

Noncolloidal Composition

The crystalloidal composition of the aqueous humor is near similar to that of plasma. The detailed constituents of aqueous humor and plasma are given in Table 3.1.

Electrolytes: From Table 3.1 data Na⁺ concentration in aqueous and plasma are to be very similar. Despite equimolar concentrations of Na⁺ in aqueous and plasma a slightly higher effective osmotic pressure caused by Na⁺ is present in the aqueous humor. It is the concentration of electrolytes near to NPE cells specially in intercellular channels is important.

Regarding K⁺ and Ca⁺⁺ and Mg⁺⁺ concentrations in aqueous, they are near similar to that present in plasma except for calcium which is present in a slightly lower concentration in normal aqueous humor. Regarding anions Cl⁻ is present in apparent excess and HCO_3^- in deficit in relation to plasma concentrations. The apparent difference in the aqueous or plasma distribution of Cl⁻ may depend on the relative concentrations of Na⁺ and Cl⁻ actively transported into the posterior chamber.

Glucose and lactate: Glucose concentration in aqueous is about 80 percent of that in the plasma (Table 3.2). Glucose enters the aqueous by simple diffusion from the plasma. Transport of glucose across the ciliary body is due to increase in the permeability of the ciliary epithelium and has been reported in diabetic patients.

TABLE 3.2: Organic solutes concentrations in aqueous humor

Substance	Aqueous humor	Plasma
Ascorbate (mmol/ml)	0.96	0.02
Citrate (mmol/ml)	0.38-0.48	
Glucose (mmol/ml)	4.9-6.9	5.9-8.30
Lactate (mmol/ml)	7.40	4.30
Creatinine (mmol/ml)	0.18	0.18
Pyruvate (mmol/ml)	0.66	0.22
Hyaluronate (mmol/ml)	4.0	4.1
Protein (mg/100 ml)	13.5	—
Urea (mmol/ml)	6.3	7.3

Corneal uptake of glucose also occurs by diffusion. Its concentration in corneal endothelium and the extracellular stromal space is about 50 percent of the aqueous concentration. Similarly lactic acid is present in aqueous humor in much higher levels than in the plasma. Lactate enters the posterior chamber readily across the ciliary epithelium but does not get accumulated in the posterior chamber appreciably above the plasma level. Immunoelectrophoretic studies have shown that glucose metabolism by the ciliary epithelium, retina, lens and cornea contributes significantly to the lactate content of the aqueous.

Oxygen: Normal oxygen tension in aqueous humor range between 13 and 80 mm Hg depending upon the estimation method used. Polymethylmethacrylate (PMMA) corneal contact lenses produce outer corneal hypoxia by restricting the access of atmospheric oxygen to the cornea. Under such situations, an increase in the flux of oxygen from the anterior chamber into the cornea occurs and a decrease in the partial pressure of oxygen in the aqueous humor occurs.

Ascorbate: Aqueous humor has higher concentration of ascorbic acid. The amount of ascorbic acid secreted into the aqueous may be dependent directly on the quantity reaching the site of secretion. Ascorbic acid in aqueous increases to certain limiting level (about 50 mg/100 ml) with increasing concentration in the blood. With higher blood levels no further increase in aqueous concentration of ascorbic acid occurs even though the blood concentration is more than twice that of aqueous. Ascorbic acid is secreted actively by a specific transport mechanism that can be saturated. Ascorbate in aqueous may act as an antioxidant regulating the solution-gel balance of mucopolysaccharides in the trabecular meshwork. It also serves to partially absorb cataractogenic ultraviolet radiation.

Amino acids: The cocentrations of amino acids in normal aqueous is given in Table 3.3.

Most of the amino acids are secreted into the aqueous via an active process. Kinsey postulated at least three transport systems for amino acids: one each for the basic, acidic and neutral groups.

TABLE 3.3: Amino acids concentrations in aqueous humor and aqueous/plasma ratio

Amino acids (mmol/kg H$_2$O)	Aqueous conc	Aqueous/plasma ratio
Alanine	306	0.94
Arginine	105	1.50
Glutamate	9	0.19
Glycine	24	0.11
Histidine	67	0.85
Isoleucine	65	1.30
Leucine	139	1.42
Lysine	159	0.64
Methionine	44	2.54
Phenylalanine	93	2.01
Proline	44	0.19
Taurine	66	1.02
Threonine	128	1.17
Tyrosine	91	1.84
Valine	285	1.35

Research studies have shown that there exist six transport systems in the ciliary epithelium—three independent mechanisms for neutral amino acids and independent mechanisms for basic amino acids, acidic amino acids and urea. Amino acids enter the posterior chamber across the ciliary epithelium by an active process, the exact nature of transport is still not very defined.

Tapetoretinal degenerations have been reported to cause specific abnormalities in the concentration of certain amino acids of the aqueous.

Lactic Dehydrogenase

The enzyme lactic dehydrogenase (LDH) has been reported to be present in small quantities in the normal aqueous humor where isoenzyme 3, 4 and 5 predominates. The aqueous/plasma ratio of LDH is greater than 1.50 in patients with retinoblastoma and less than 0.60 in a variety of other ocular conditions. The source of LDH in the aqueous of patients suffering from intraocular malignancy is the release of cytosol enzymes into the surrounding medium. A high degree of necrosis as in retinoblastoma allow more free enzyme to reach the aqueous.

Miscellaneous Substances

Other substances such as hyaluronic acid, sialic acid, trivalent chromium ions, vitamin B$_{12}$, monoamine metabolites are also present in normal aqueous humor in varying concentrations.

FUNCTIONS OF AQUEOUS HUMOR

- Aqueous humor maintains the nutrition of the avascular structures like the cornea, lens and also carries away their waste products. So, it plays an important metabolic role by providing substrates and removing metabolites from the avascular cornea and lens
- The clear aqueous in anterior chamber play a role in the refraction of the light rays
- The most important function of aqueous is its role in maintaining a proper and constant IOP. The rate of aqueous formation and aqueous outflow are vital for maintaining normal IOP.

BIBLIOGRAPHY

1. Agarwal A. Textbook of Ophthalmology, 1st edn. New Delhi: Jaypee Brothers Medical Publishers, 2002.
2. Bartlett JD. Clinical Ocular Pharmacology, 4th edn. Boston: Butterworth-Heinemann, 2001.
3. Bartlett JD. Ophthalmic Drug Facts: Lippincott – William and Wilkins, 2001.
4. Crick RP, Trimble RB. Textbook of Clinical Ophthalmology: Hodder and Stoughton, 1986.
5. Duane TD. Clinical Ophthalmology, 4th edn. Butterworth – Heinemann, 1999.
6. Duvall. Ophthalmic Medications and Pharmacology: Slack Inc, 1998.
7. Ellis PP. Ocular Therapeutics and Pharmacology, 7th edn. CV Mosby, 1985.
8. Fechner. Ocular Therapeutics: Slack Inc., 1998.
9. Fraunfelder. Current Ocular Therapy, 5th edn. WB Saunders, 2000.
10. Garg A. Current Trends in ophthalmology, 1st edn. New Delhi: Jaypee Brothers Medical Publishers, 1997.
11. Garg A. Manual of Ocular Therapeutics, 1st edn. New Delhi: Jaypee Brothers Medical Publishers, 1996.
12. Garg A. Ready Reckoner of Ocular Therapeutics, 1st edn. New Delhi: 2002.
13. Goodman LS, Gilman A. Pharmacological Basis of Therapeutics, 7th edn. New York: Macmillan, 1985.
14. Havener's. Ocular Pharmacology, 6th edn. CV Mosby, 1994.
15. Kanski. Clinical ophthalmology, 4th edn. Butterworth – Heineman, 1999.
16. Kershner. Ophthalmic Medications and Pharmacology: Slack. Inc., 1994.
17. Olin BR, et al. Drugs Facts and Comparisons: Facts and Comparisons, St. Louis, 1997.
18. Onofrey. The Ocular Therapeutics; Lippincott-William and Wilkins, 1997.
19. Rhee. The Wills Eye drug Guide: Lippincott – William and Wilkins, 1998.
20. Steven Podos. Textbook of Ophthalmology, New Delhi: Jaypee Brothers Medical Publishers, 2001.
21. Zimmerman. Textbook of Ocular Pharmacology: Lippincott and William and Wilkins, 1997.

4

Routes of Administration and Drug Delivery Systems in Ophthalmology

Ashok Garg (India)

For ocular drugs to be effective an ideal drug delivery system (DDS) should deliver the drug at the receptor site in ocular tissues in relatively high concentration to elicit the desired pharmacological response. Most of the ophthalmic drugs are applied topically in the form of eyedrops. The time course of drug deliver from an eyedrop follows a first order kinetics. It is well known that about 1 percent or less of an applied dose is absorbed across the cornea topically to reach the anterior segment of eye.

The major problem in the drug treatment (topical) of ocular diseases is the difficulty of achieving a sufficient quantity of drug at the desired site of action. The tight junctions of iris capillaries and retina act as a barrier to the diffusion of drugs from the blood into the aqueous and vitreous and the cornea acts as a barrier to drugs applied locally. Another factor quite important is the rate of removal from the eye of any drug that does actually penetrate into the aqueous or vitreous because although inflammation may reduce the barrier to penetration of the drug into the eye, the associated hyperemia will also speed the removal of the drug from the eye.

During the last decade research is going on in ophthalmic field for a suitable mode of ocular therapy to provide higher and sustained penetration of the drugs into the ocular tissues and anterior chamber promptly and effectively.

Most important factor which modify drug penetration is slow release of the drug thereby increasing the contact time of the drug to the ocular structures. The duration of drug action in the eye can be extended by:
- Reducing drainage through the use of viscosity enhancing agents.
- Improving corneal drug penetration. An ideal drug delivery system should have:
  - Spatial placement.
  - Controlled drug delivery.

The routes of administration are local and systemic for ocular diseases.

LOCAL APPLICATION

Local application of drugs for the treatment of superficial eye diseases is a very satisfactory route. When the desired site of action of the drug is inside the eye then the problem of ocular barrier arises.

Corneal Barrier

For practical purposes cornea can be considered to consist of three layers. The outer and inner layers (The epithelium and the endothelium) prevent water soluble agents, e.g. ionized molecules passing into the eye, but permit the passage of lipid soluble agents whereas the corneal stroma resists the passage of lipid soluble agents but freely allows the passage of water soluble agents. Drugs with dual capability are usually capable of changing from lipid solubility to water solubility of ionization. The effectiveness of corneal barrier may be considerably reduced by damage to the corneal epithelium.

Scleral Barrier

The sclera unlike cornea does not act as a differential solubility barrier and is relatively porous. However, there is unidirectional flow across the sclera from the inside to the outside of the eye. The intraocular pressure may be partially responsible for this.

Methods of Local Application of Drugs

- Application to corneal surface.
- Subconjunctival route.
- Retrobulbar route.
- Direct injection into the aqueous or vitreous.

Application to the Corneal Surface

The drug through this route must fulfill the necessary criteria for passing the corneal barrier to penetrate into the eye.

Formally, the drug delivery kinetics passing through this route can be divided in two parts:

1. *First order kinetics:* In this concentration of drug available for penetration falls off exponentially as the medication is diluted and washed away by the tear film and drug concentration achieved in posterior segment of the eye is very less. This type of drug delivery is provided by aqueous or high viscosity solutions, ointments or hydrogel drug delivery system.
2. *Zero order kinetics:* In this system drug is held in reservoir and is released into the tear film at the constant rate to provide constant drug concentration in the cornea or aqueous.

This drug delivery system is provided by ocuserts, soluble ophthalmic drug inserts (SODI) and the osmotic pumps, and liposomal drug delivery system, cotton pledgets and filter paper strips.

Application to the corneal surface may be in form of topical drops, ointments, gels, viscous preparations, constant release membranes and soft lenses. Topical drops route is commonly used to treat various ocular infections, inflammation and as topical anesthesia in modern cataract surgery, phacoemulsification and lasik surgery.

The passage of the drug is aided by damage to the corneal epithelium and on the amount of drug in contact with cornea and duration of contact.

When topical drops are used, much is lost because it is washed away by the tears.

Viscous and ointment preparations of drugs including oil suspensions and methyl cellulose solutions prolong contact time. This reduces the total quantity of drug given to the patients as well as reducing the unwanted frequency of medication giving better patient compliance.

Membrane Bound Devices

Ocusert System

This system was the first ophthalmic drug delivery system approved by US FDA for use in human beings.

Ocuserts provide zero order kinetics drug release.

The ocuserts is a device with a two membrane sandwich with a pilocarpine reservoir in the center. The copolymeric membrane is ethyline vinylacetate also encased between the membranes is a white titanium dioxide ring that aids in visualizing and handling the inserts.

Ocuserts not only provides zero order delivery of the drug but also the total amount of drug needed for therapeutic effect is much less than what used as drops or suspension.

Ocuserts are soft and extremely flexible and can be placed either under the upper or lower lid.

The problems with ocuserts can be cost factor, foreign body sensation or incidental loss of ocusert from the cul-de-sac. Other type of ocuserts are diffusible units osmotic units and erodible units. Drugs that can be delivered through ocuserts are pilocarpine, antibiotics, steroids, carbachol or a combination.

Drug Impregnated Inserts

Soluble ophthalmic drug inserts (SODI) were first introduced in seventies and are made of polymers of acrylamide, ethlacrylate and vinyl pyrrolidone. SODI dissolve in the cul-de-sac and is capable to provide detectable drugs levels in the cornea up to 48 hours.

Wafers were introduced in eighties. Wafers are soluble ophthalmic inserts made of succinylated collagen. These wafers are 6 x 12 mm in size and are inserted into the inferior cul-de-sac. Antibiotics can be delivered through this route.

Hydrogel Contact Lens Delivery

The hydrogel contact lenses (soft lenses) by virtue of their high water content and large intermolecular pore size, absorb water soluble drugs and release them initially in a high pulse and then release gradually. Hydrogel lenses can be used to deliver water soluble drugs like dexamethasone, antibiotics and pilocarpine. These lenses can be an excellent route of administration. The lens is inserted into the eye after being presoaked in the drug solution. This device is often used in the management of dry eye disorders.

Osmotic Pumps

Osmotic pump recently introduced is the drug delivery system of future to treat various ocular diseases commonly. Osmotic pumps, contain salt enclosed in one compartment and drug enclosed in an adjacent compartment. Both compartments have flexible walls.

This type of device can deliver any type of medication into the eye regardless of its solubility or molecular weight. The development of new polymeric membranes for use as drug inserts envelops, has recently begun.

Research work is going on suitable new site specific drugs delivery system, one side coated hydroxypropyl cellulose inserts, sub-Tenon administration of drug through collagen sponges connected with silicon tube work is going on Margan Therapeutic Lens as continuous corneal perfusion system and on colloidal suspension capsules with an oily core in which drugs is dissolved (nano capsules).

Periocular Administration

When higher concentrations of drugs are required they can be injected locally into the periocular tissues. Periocular drug administration include injection under bulbar conjunctiva, under Tenon capsule (sub-Tenon's) (Fig. 4.1) and behind globe itself and peribulbar route. Drugs most often delivered in this manner include steroids and antibiotics. Local anesthetics are commonly injected through peribulbar route prior to cataract extraction and other intraocular surgical procedures.

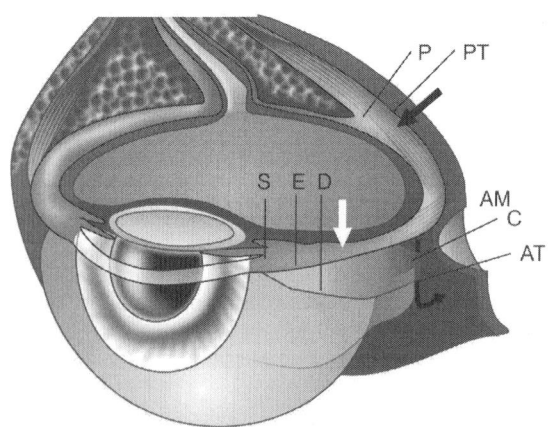

Fig. 4.1: Sub-Tenon's plane relationship (cross-section view)

Subconjunctival Route

This route including injection under the bulbar conjunctiva used to achieve high concentrations of drug in the anterior chamber. Antibiotics, steroids, mydriatics can be given by this route.

Subconjunctival injections are painful so this route is used only in severe cases of ocular inflammation or infection of the anterior segment.

Retrobulbar Route

Drugs can be delivered to the back of the orbit by retrobulbar injections. This is the route for local anesthesia in ocular surgery. Steroids may also be injected by this route to reduce optic nerve or posterior segment inflammation (Fig. 4.2).

Intracameral Administration

Intracameral administration involves placing drug directly into the anterior chamber of the eye. This is most commonly associated with cataract extraction, IOL implantation and phacoemulsification during which a viscoelastic substance is injected into the anterior chamber to protect the corneal endothelium. Antibiotics are not routinely injected into the anterior chamber as there is significant risk of complications as well as drug toxicity.

Intravitreal Administration

The intravitreal injection is primarily reserved as a last effort to save eye with severe acute infection or intraocular inflammation. Intravitreal antibiotics is the treatment of choice for endophthalmitis. Intravitreal liquid silicone is used for the treatment of complicated retinal detachment. Recently intravitreal ganciclovir has been used with success in treating cytomegaloretinitis in patient with AIDS.

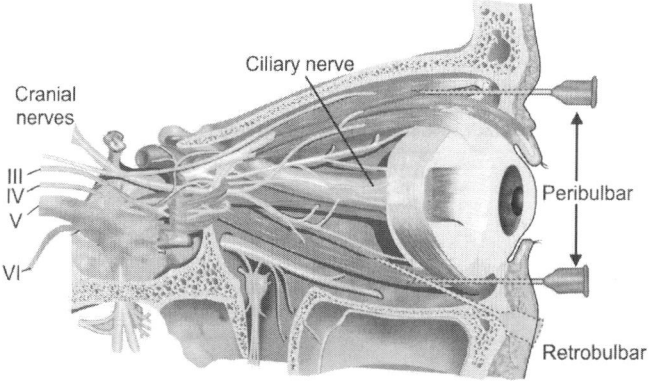

Fig. 4.2: Retrobulbar and peribulbar anesthesia (needle positions)

Parabulbar (Flush) Administration

This is new administration route for local anesthesia which is highly useful, safe, effective and technically easier. In this method consisting of a limbal sub-Tenon administration of retrobulbar anesthesia using a blunt irrigating cannula. This technique can be used involving anterior and posterior segment surgery (Figs 4.3 and 4.4).

Peribulbar Administration

Peribulbar administration is mainly used for giving local anesthesia for modern intraocular surgery. Since the exit of retrobulbar route peribulbar is safe and effective route of administrating local anesthesia. Peribulbar route is safe because here local injection is given out of muscle cone and complications like intraconal hemorrhage or damage to optic nerve are ruled out.

In this method a cocktail of lignocaine and bupivacaine is injected at the junction of lateral 1/3rd and medial 2/3rd of inferior orbital rim by 26 gauge 1" long needle which is directed

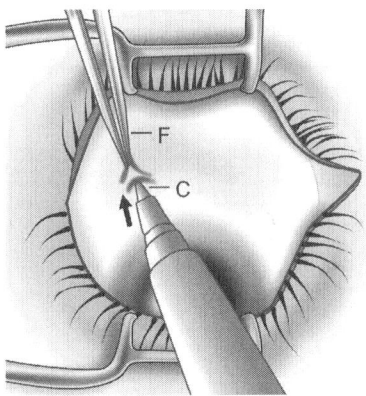

Fig. 4.3: Parabulbar (flush) local anesthesia (surgeon's view)

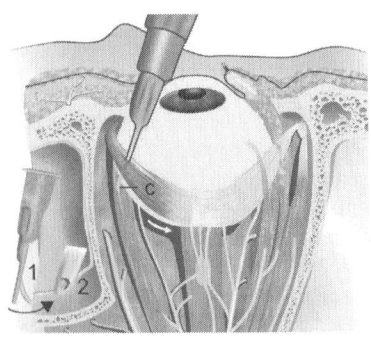

Fig. 4.4: Parabulbar (flush) local anesthesia (cross-section view)

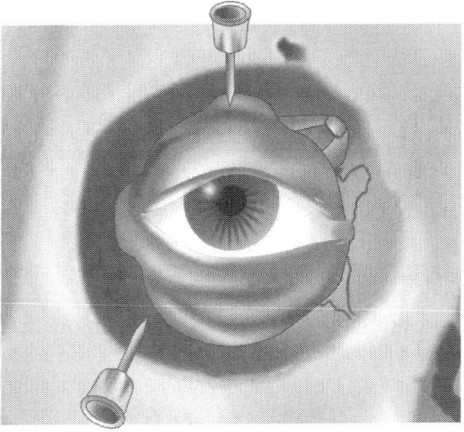

Fig. 4.5: Needle positions for retrobulbar or peribulbar anesthesia (frontal view)

backward and medially to its whole length. At present after topical anesthesia, peribulbar anesthesia is most commonly used method of giving local anesthesia worldwide (Fig. 4.5).

Direct Injection into the Globe

Drugs are often introduced into the eye during ocular surgery. Care is taken that the concentration of drug the vehicle and the type of preservative is suitable. Antibiotics may be injected directly into the aqueous and vitreous in cases of endophthalmitis.

SYSTEMIC ADMINISTRATION

General rules for system drug administration apply but there is an effective blood aqueous and blood vitreous barrier so that intraocular levels of systemically administered drugs are usually lower than the serum.

Most drugs will cross the aqueous and vitreous in cases of ocular inflammatory diseases which increases permeability. In systemic administration drugs can be given orally or by intramuscular intravenous injections. Although most ocular diseases respond to topical therapy but certain ocular disorders require systemic drug administration. Oral administration of certain drugs may be most effective route of drug delivery. Carbonic anhydrase inhibitors for treatment of glaucoma, steroids for optic neuritis, uveitis, analgesics for the management of pain associated with ocular trauma, antibiotic therapy for ocular infections and antihistaminic therapy for acute ocular allergy are few examples of oral administration.

Parental administration includes intramuscular (IM) and intravenous (IV) injections. Hydroxycobalamin (Vitamin B_{12}) and certain antibiotics are given through IM route. Continuous IV infusion of various antibiotics may be required for treatment of endophthalmitis and other severe ocular infections.

The futuristic considerations in ocular drug delivery system is to make drug delivery in therapeutic concentration in the posterior segment of the globe. The new modifications in ocular DDS design must not only work on the corneal route for drug absorption but also of other routes like scleral route. There is also need of sophisticated technology to monitor the pharmacokinetics.

Medications Forms Used in Ophthalmology

Solutions and Suspensions

This is one of the most common forms of drug delivery system being used in ophthalmology today. Most of the topical ocular preparations are commercially available as solutions or suspensions which are applied directly to the eye from the bottle via sterile eyedropper provided alongwith.

Patient should be cautioned about touching the dropper tip to the eye as it can lead to contamination of the medication beside causing ocular injury. Patient should not also touch tip of the dropper with hand to avoid contamination of preparation. Suspension forms should be shaken before use to provide an accurate dosage of drug.

Ointments

This is second most common form of drug delivery system used in ophthalmology. The main purpose for an ophthalmic ointment vehicle is to prolong drug contact time with the eye. Ointments are specially useful for treating children who may not cooperate for topically applied solutions. Ointments are specially useful for medicating ocular injuries such as corneal abrasions where the eye needs to be patched. Always administer solutions before ointments as ointments preclude entry of subsequent drops. In general put 0.25-0.50 inch ribbon of ointment with a sweeping motion inside the lower lid by squeezing the tube gently and slowly release the eyelid. Ask the patient to close the eye for 1-2 minutes and remove excessive ointment around the eye. Patients should be cautioned about temporary blurring of vision due to ointment. Patients should avoid activities requiring visual acuity until blurring clears.

Gels

In modern ophthalmic drug delivery systems gels are fast gaining importance. Ophthalmic gels are similar in viscosity and clinical usage to ophthalmic ointments. Gels provide prolonged contact time for medication within the precorneal tear film.

Sprays

Some ophthalmic medications like mydriatics and cycloplegics alone or in combination can be administered as spray to the eye to dilate pupil or cycloplegic examination. This form is specially used for pediatric patients and solution is administered using a sterile perfume atomizer or plastic spray bottle.

Lid Scrubs

Certain commercial ophthalmic preparations (eyelid cleansers, antibiotic solutions or ointments) can be applied directly to eyelid margin for the treatment of non-infectious blepharitis. This is ideally achieved by applying the medication to the end of the special cotton tipped applicator and then scrubbing the eyelid margins several times daily. Gauze pads supplied with commercially available eyelid cleansers are also suitable.

Medication Devices Used in Ophthalmology

Contact Lenses

Therapeutic soft contact lenses with high water content are of great benefit in treating several ophthalmic diseases. Soft contact lenses can absorb water soluble drugs and release them into the eye over a prolonged duration. These lenses are specially useful in promoting sustained release of solutions or suspensions that normally would be removed quickly from the external ocular tissues. Therapeutic soft contact lenses are used commonly as drug delivery devices in the management of dry eye disorders. Sometimes these lenses are also used for the treatment of ocular infections specially bacterial corneal ulcers.

Corneal Shields

Porcine or bovine scleral collagen shields are commercially available which are usually non-cross linked and homogenized. Corneal shields are generally placed as a bandage on the cornea following surgery or injury to protect and lubricate the cornea. For treating bacterial corneal ulcers corneal shields are used in conjunction with topical antibiotics with good results.

Cotton Pledgets

Small cotton pieces can be soaked with topical ophthalmic solutions and placed in conjunctival sac. Such devices certainly allow a prolonged ocular contact time with solutions that are normally instilled topically into the eye. Generally cotton pledgets are used for the administration of mydriatic solutions. This drug delivery device promotes maximum mydriasis in an effort to break posterior synechiae or to dilate sluggish pupils.

Filter Paper Strips

Fluorescein strips are commercially available as drug impregnated filter paper strips (Sodium fluorescein, Rose bengal or Flurexon). These filter strips help to ensure sterility of sodium fluorescein which can be easily contaminated with *Pseudomonas aeruginosa* when prepared in solution. These test strips are used diagnostically to identify corneal injuries and infections. Schirmer tear test strips are also available commercially for diagnosing dry eye disorders.

Artificial Tear Inserts

A specially designed rod-shaped pellet of hydroxy propyl cellulose without preservative is commercially available to be inserted into the inferior conjunctival sac with a special applicator. Following insertion, these devices absorbs fluid, swells and then releases the non-medicated polymer to the eye for a duration of 24 hours. Ocuserts are specially used in the treatment of dry eye disorders.

Membrane Bound Inserts

Ocuserts are membrane controlled drug delivery system which deliver a constant quantity of medication to the eye for a week continuously. Pilocarpine ocuserts are commonly used in the treatment of glaucoma. These ocuserts are placed on to bulbar conjunctiva under the upper or lower eyelid. Pilocarpine ocusert is a useful substitute for pilocarpine drops or gel in glaucoma patients who have poor compliance with more frequent drug instillation.

Practical Tips for Use of Various Ophthalmic Medications

Proper administration of ophthalmic drugs is absolutely essential to achieve optimal therapeutic results. Here I shall describe several common practical points which should be informed to the patients before starting any ophthalmic formulation.

- Never instill more than one properly placed drop of ophthalmic solution or suspension into the affected eye. Normal eye retains 10 mcl of fluid on an average. Generally eyedropper delivers 25–50 mcl/drop of fluid.

    For proper placement of drop into the eye ask the patient to tilt head backward or lie down in supine position with gaze upward. Gently grasp lower eyelid below eyelashes and pull the eyelid away from the eye to form a pouch. Put dropper directly over eye. Avoid contact of dropper with the eye. Keep the dropper tip about one inch away from the eye. Look upward before instilling the drop. Release the lid slowly and close eye gently for 2–3 minutes.

- Systemic absorption of ophthalmic solution or suspension can be minimized by compressing the canaliculus and lacrimal sac for 3–5 minutes after instillation. This compressing certainly retards the passage of drops via nasolacrimal duct into the areas of potential absorption like nasal and pharyngeal mucosa.

- When multisolution therapy is indicated ideally instill the drops separately at 5 minutes interval. This ensures that first solution drop is not flushed away by the second or second is not diluted by first one.

- Certain ophthalmic factors may increase absorption from ophthalmic dose forms like lax eyelids specially in elderly patients and diseased eyes which forms a great pool for retention of topical solution or suspension.
- Discourage the use of eye cup in cases of eye lotions due to risk of contamination and spreading disease.
- Ophthalmic suspensions generally mix with tears poorly and remain in the lower cul-de-sac longer than solutions.
- Ophthalmic ointments are helpful in maintaining contact between ocular tissues and drug by decreasing the rate as slow as 0.5 percent per minute. Ophthalmic ointments provide maximum contact between drug and ocular tissues.
- Ophthalmic ointments should be instilled preferably at bedtime as it may impede delivery of other ophthalmic drugs to the affected eye by acting as a barrier to contact.
- Ointments may blur vision during waking hours so bedtime use is generally recommended.
- Monitor expiration dates of ophthalmic medications. Do not use outdated drugs.
- Ophthalmic solutions and ointments are generally misused. Patient use these medications on their own without counseling ophthalmologists. Appropriate patient education and counseling with prescribing and dispensing of ophthalmic medicines is essential.

BIBLIOGRAPHY

1. Agarwal A. Textbook of Ophthalmology, 1st edn. New Delhi: Jaypee Brothers Medical Publishers, 2002.
2. Bartlett JD. Clinical Ocular Pharmacology, 4th edn. Boston: Butterworth-Heinemann, 2001.
3. Bartlett JD. Ophthalmic Drug Facts: Lippincott – William and Wilkins, 2001.
4. Crick RP, Trimble RB. Textbook of Clinical Ophthalmology: Hodder and Stoughton, 1986.
5. Duane TD. Clinical Ophthalmology, 4th edn. Butterworth – Heinemann, 1999.
6. Duvall. Ophthalmic Medications and Pharmacology: Slack Inc, 1998.
7. Ellis PP. Ocular Therapeutics and Pharmacology, 7th edn. CV Mosby, 1985.
8. Fechner. Ocular Therapeutics: Slack Inc., 1998.
9. Feibel RM. Current Concepts in Retrobulbar Anaesthesia: Surv. Ophthalmol 1985;30:102.
10. Fraunfelder. Current Ocular Therapy, 5th edn. WB Saunders, 2000.
11. Fraunfelder FT. Ophthalmic Drug Delivery Systems: Surv. Ophthalmol 1974;18:292.
12. Garg A. Current Trends in Ophthalmology, 1st edn. New Delhi: Jaypee Brothers Medical Publishers, 1997.
13. Garg A. Manual of Ocular Therapeutics, 1st edn. New Delhi: Jaypee Brothers Medical Publishers, 1996.
14. Garg A. Ready Reckoner of Ocular Therapeutics, 1st edn. New Delhi, 2002.

15. Goodman LS, Gilman A. Pharmacological Basis of Therapeutics, 7th edn. New York: Macmillan, 1985.
16. Halberg GP. Drug Delivery Systems for Topical Ophthalmic Medication, Ann. Ophthalmol 1975;7:1199.
17. Havener's. Ocular Pharmacology, 6th edn. CV Mosby, 1994.
18. Kanski. Clinical Ophthalmology, 4th edn. Butterworth – Heineman, 1999.
19. Kershner. Ophthalmic Medications and Pharmacology: Slack. Inc., 1994.
20. Olin BR, et al. Drugs Facts and Comparisons: Facts and Comparisons, St Louis, 1997.
21. Onofrey. The Ocular Therapeutics; Lippincott-William and Wilkins, 1997.
22. Rhee. The Wills Eye drug Guide: Lippincott – William and Wilkins, 1998.
23. Robin JS. Ophthalmic ointments; Surv. Ophthalmol 1978;22:335.
24. Steven Podos. Textbook of Ophthalmology. New Delhi: Jaypee Brothers Medical Publishers, 2001.
25. Zimmerman TJ. Therapeutic Index of Topically Applied Ocular Drugs, Arch. Ophthalmol 1984;102:551.
26. Zimmerman. Textbook of Ocular Pharmacology: Lippincott and William and Wilkins, 1997.

5
Microorganisms and Ocular Diseases

Ashok Garg (India)

INTRODUCTION

About every known pathogenic microorganism can cause ocular infection, some pathogens have specific affinity for special ocular structures, e.g. *Gonococcus* causes conjunctivitis but does not involve lacrimal apparatus. For the purpose of discussion, organisms affecting the eye may be classified as follows.

BACTERIA

On the basis of gram reaction and shape they are divided into:
- Gram-positive rods ⎤
- Gram-negative rods ⎥ Aerobic and
- Gram-positive cocci ⎥ anaerobic
- Gram-negative cocci ⎦

1. Most pathogenic cocci are gram-positive. These are:
   - *Staphylococcus aureus*
   - *Staphylococcus epidermidis*
   - *Staphylococcus saprophyticus*
   - *Streptococcus pyogenes*
   - *Streptococcus pneumoniae*
   - *Pneumococcus* (*Diplococcus pneumoniae* and *Streptococcus pneumoniae*)
   - Anaerobic *Streptococcus* (*Peptostreptococcus*)
   - α and β hemolytic *Streptococcus*.

2. Gram-negative cocci are
   - *Meningococcus*
   - *Gonococcus* ⎤ *Pharyngis flavescens*
   - *Neisseria* ⎦ *Mucosa sicca*
   - *Branhamella*

3. Most pathogenic rods are gram-negative. These are:
   - *Pseudomonas aeruginosa*
   - *Pseudomonas cepacia*
   - *Haemophilus influenzae and aegyptius*
   - *Moraxella* ⎤ *M. lacunata*
     ⎥ *M. nonliquefaciens*
     ⎦ *M. bovis*
   - *Acinetobacter*
   - *Klebsiella* ⎤ *K. pneumoniae*
     ⎦ *K. oxytoca*

- *E. coli*
- *Shigella* — *S. sonnei*, *S. flexneri*
- *Brucella* — *B. abortus*, *B. suis*, *B. melitensis*
- *Serratia* — *S. marcescens*, *S. flexneri*
- *Proteus* — *P. mirabilis*, *P. vulgaris*

4. Gram-positive rods are:
   - *Bacillus subtilis*
   - *Bacillus anthracis*
   - *Bacillus cereus*
   - *Clostridia (welchii)*
   - *Clostridia tetani*
   - *Corynebacteria* — *C. diphtheriae*, *C. xerosis*, *C. pseudodiphtheriticum*, *C. hemolyticus*
   - *Listeria monocytogenes*

5. Mycobacteria (acid-fast bacilli)
   - *Mycobacterium tuberculosis*
   - Atypical *mycobacteria*
   - *Mycobacterium leprae*

6. Higher bacteria (*Actinomycetales*)
   - *Actinomyces israelii*
   - *Nocardia* species — *N. asteroides*, *N. caviae*, *N. brasiliensis*
   - *Streptothrix*

7. Spirochaetes
   - *Treponema pallidum*

8. *Chlamydia* (Between bacteria and virus)
   - *Chlamydia trachomatis*
   - *Chlamydia psittaci*

FUNGI

1. Yeast and yeast-like fungi:
   - *Cryptococcus*
   - *Candida* (*albicans, parapsilosis* and *tropicalis* species)
2. Filamentous fungi
   a. Aseptate fungi:
      - Mucor
      - Rhizopus
   b. Septate fungi:
      - Aspergillus — *A. fumigatus*, *A. flavus*, *A. niger*, *A. terreus*
      - Fusarium (*F. solani, oxysporum, episphaeria* and *monilformae* species)

Microorganisms and Ocular Diseases

- *Dematiaceous fungi*
- *Drechslera* species
- *Curvularia lunare*
- *Cladosporium* species
- *Alternaria*
- *Penicillum* species
- *Cephalosporium* (*Acremonium* species)
c. Dimorphic (*Histoplasma capsulatum*)
d. *Rhinosporidium seeberi.*

VIRUSES

DNA Viruses

1. Herpes group
   - Herpes simplex (HSV_1 and HSV_2 types)
   - Varicella zoster
   - Cytomegalovirus
2. Adenoviruses (8 and 19, 3 and 7 type)
3. Variola and vaccinia
4. *Molluscum contagiosum*
5. Human papovavirus.

RNA Viruses

- Picorna viruses
  - Enterovirus type 70
  - Coxsackie A 24
- Measles
- Mumps
- Rubella.

PARASITES

- *Taenia solium*
- *Cysticerus cellulosae*
- *Echinococcus granulosus*
- *Toxoplasma gondii*
- *Toxocara canis*
- *Loa loa*
- *Wuchereria bancrofti*
- *Onchocerca volvulus*
- *Acanthamoeba* (*Castellanii, Culberisono* and *Polyphaga* species)
- *Demodex organisms* (*folliculorum* and *brevis*)
- *Phthirus pubis.*

COMMON MICROBIOLOGICAL STAINS USED IN OPHTHALMOLOGY

Diff quick stain: Used to differentiate white blood cell types in eye disease like:
- Bacterial—neutrophils
- Viral—lymphocytes

- Allergic—eosinophils and basophils
- Vernal—mast cells/lymphocytes

Gram stain: To differentiate gram +ve (blue) and gram –ve (red) organisms.

Giemsa stain: To identify cellular inclusion bodies in chlamydial infection.

Wright stain: To reveal the condition and character of epithelial cells and inflammatory cells.

Calcofluor stain: For identification of *Acanthamoeba*.

Ziehl-Neelsen's stain: For differential staining of acid-fast bacilli.

Kinyoun's method: For identifying *Nocardia* species.

Lactophenol cotton blue mount: For filamentous fungal culture.

Hansel stain: For rapid identification of any eosinophilic response.

COMMON OPHTHALMIC CULTURE MEDIA AND USAGE (TABLE 5.1)

TABLE 5.1: Different culture media and their usage

	Media	Composition	Usage
1.	Blood agar	Defibrinated sheep's blood	To detect hemolytic activity
2.	Chocolate agar	Heat denaturalized sheep's blood and nutrients	Best medium for *Haemophilus* and *Neisseria*
3.	Sabouroud's medium	Glucose/peptone and antibiotics	Fungal culture media
4.	Thioglycolate broth	Sodium thioglycolate	General culture media
5.	Brain-heart infusion broth	Beef brain and heart/protease/dextrose/neopeptone/antibiotic	Fungal growth media
6.	Page's medium	*E. coli* plates	For *Acanthamoeba*
7.	Thayer-Martin medium	Modified chocolate agar with nutrients and selected antibiotics	Best for *Neisseria*
8.	Löwenstein-Jensen media		For mycobacteria
9.	Viral carrier medium	Contain Hank's BSS to human cell tissue culture	For herpes simplex, zoster and adenovirus

NORMAL MICROBIAL FLORA OF THE EYE

The conjunctival sac and eyelid margins harbor a variety of microorganisms. The inner structures are sterile. The normally present flora can be divided into two groups: the resident flora and transient flora.

Resident Flora

It consists of fixed type of microorganisms regularly found in the eye. The predominant of these microorganisms are *Staphylococcus epidermedis* and *Corynebacterium xerosis*.

Transient Flora

It consists of nonpathogenic or potentially pathogenic microorganisms that inhabit the eye for short duration. They may be derived from the environment (exogenous) or from other parts of the body (endogenous). Members of transient flora are generally of little clinical significance as long as the normal resident flora and host resistance remain intact. However, under favorable pathological conditions, these transient mircoorganisms may colonize, proliferate and produce clinical ocular diseases. The various organisms that may be encountered as transient flora are:

Gram-positive Bacteria

- Diphtheroids (*Corynebacterium* species)
- *Staphylococcus aureus* and other species
- Haemolytic and non-haemolytic streptococci
- Aerobic spore beares (*Bacillus* species).

Gram-negative Bacteria

- *Haemophilus* species
- *Moraxella* species
- *Neisseria* species.

Enteric Bacilli

- *E. coli*
- *K. pneumoniae*
- *Enterobacter* species.

Fungi

Due to omnipresence of fungal spores in air, they are some times present in the conjunctival sac. The common fungi are *Aspergillus fumigatus, Aspergillus flavus, Mucor* species, *Dematiaceous fungi* (*Alternaria, Curvularia, Helminthosporium*, etc.), *Penicillium* species, etc.

The microbial flora of the conjunctiva is normally held in check by the following factors:
- Flushing mechanism provided by tears
- Bactericidal action of lysozyme present in tears
- Phagocytosis by epithelial cells and inflammatory cells

- Mechanical barrier of intact mucous membrane
- Blinking action of lids.

BIBLIOGRAPHY

1. Apple. Ocular Pathology, 5th edn. CV Mosby, 1998.
2. Agarwal A. Textbook of ophthalmology, 1st edn. New Delhi: Jaypee Brothers Medical Publishers, 2002.
3. Bartlett JD. Clinical Ocular Pharmacology, 4th edn. Boston: Butterworth-Heinemann, 2001
4. Bartlett JD. Ophthalmic Drug facts: Lippincott–William and Wilkins, 2001.
5. Crick RP, Trimble RB. Textbook of Clinical Ophthalmology: Hodder and Stoughton, 1986.
6. Duane TD. Clinical Ophthalmology, 4th edn. Butterworth–Heinemann, 1999.
7. Duvall. Ophthalmic Medications and Pharmacology; Slack Inc., 1998.
8. Ellis PP. Ocular Therapeutics and Pharmacology, 7th edn. CV Mosby, 1985.
9. Fechner. Ocular Therapeutics: Slack Inc., 1998.
10. Fraunfelder. Current Ocular Therapy, 5th edn. WB Saunders, 2000.
11. Garg A. Current Trends in Ophthalmology, 1st edn. New Delhi: Jaypee Brothers Medical Publishers, 1997.
12. Garg A. Manual of Ocular Therapeutics, 1st edn. New Delhi: Jaypee Brothers Medical Publishers, 1996.
13. Garg A. Ready Reckoner of Ocular Therapeutics, 1st edn. New Delhi, 2002.
14. Goodman LS, Gilman A. Pharmacological Basis of Therapeutics, 7th edn. New York: Macmillan, 1985.
15. Harry. Clinical Ocular Pathology: Butterworth–Heinemann, 1993.
16. Havener's. Ocular Pharmacology, 6th edn. CV Mosby, 1994.
17. Kanski. Clinical Ophthalmology, 4th edn. Butterworth-Heineman, 1999.
18. Kershner. Ophthalmic Medications and Pharmacology; Slack. Inc., 1994.
19. Olin BR, et al. Drugs Facts and Comparisons: Facts and Comparisons, St Louis, 1997.
20. Onofrey. The Ocular Therapeutics; Lippincott-William and Wilkins, 1997.
21. Rhee. The Wills Eye drug Guide; Lippincott – William and Wilkins, 1998.
22. Steven Podos. Textbook of Ophthalmology; New Delhi: Jaypee Brothers Medical Publishers, 2001.
23. Zimmerman. Text book of Ocular Pharmacology; Lippincott–William and Wilkins, 1997.

6

Unique Ocular Drug Delivery Systems

Xiadong Zheng (Japan), Marg E Marquart, Ashim K Mitra, James M Hill* (USA)

INTRODUCTION

Drug delivery, as it pertains to ocular tissues, is defined as an approach to controlling and ultimately optimizing delivery of the drug to its target tissue in the eye or its adnexal tissues.[1] Ocular drug delivery is one of the most interesting and challenging endeavors facing ophthalmologists and pharmaceutical scientists. The anatomy, physiology, and biochemistry of the eye render this organ exquisitely impervious to foreign substances. However, the eye is vulnerable to endogenous inflammation and exogenous infectious agents, such as bacteria and viruses. Effective ocular drug delivery depends on numerous factors, such as concentration of the drug, the contact time at the corneal surface, the route of drug delivery, and the physical chemical properties of the compound. An optimal topical drug delivery system would be one that can be administered in eyedrop form with no blurred vision or irritation and that would need no more than one instillation each day to maintain therapeutic effect. The benefits to patients are simplicity, higher efficacy, lower toxicity, and minimal side effects.

Conventional ocular drug delivery systems, such as topical administration of ophthalmic suspensions, solutions, or ointment, account for 90 percent of the currently accessible marketed formulations. One of the major problems encountered with the conventional topical delivery of ophthalmic drugs is the rapid and extensive precorneal loss caused by drainage and high tear fluid turnover. After instillation of an eyedrop, in most cases only 10 percent of applied dose is absorbed.[2] Most of the applied drug is immediately diluted in the tear film and rapidly drained from the conjunctival sac to the nasolacrimal duct (tear turnover). The drainage rate becomes even higher when the formulation is irritating. Also, overflow of eyedrops onto lids and evaporation of tear film contribute to loss and waste of the drug. The ocular disposition of ophthalmic formulations is diagrammed in Figure 6.1.

Behind the tear film, the corneal epithelial layer is the second barrier for drug penetration. The epithelium facing the tear film is a lipophilic layer. This layer retards the diffusion of water-soluble (hydrophilic) substances through both the apical superficial cell membranes and the paracellular pathways between cells, which are

---

*Recipient of award for the Research to prevent Blindness, "Senior Scientific Award"

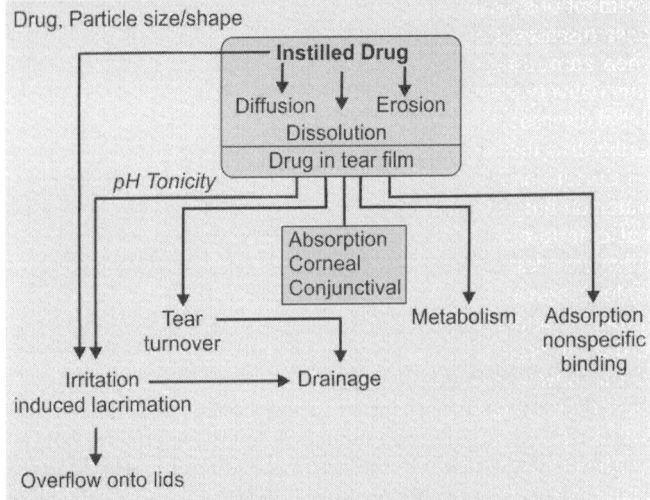

Fig. 6.1: The ocular disposition of ophthalmic formulations. About 10 percent of the applied drug is actually absorbed by the cornea. The majority of the drug is lost by drainage (Reprinted with permission from Mitra AK (Ed): Ophthalmic Drug Delivery Systems, Marcel Dekker: New York, 178, 1993)

filled with a continuous band of tight junctions. The stromal layer allows for relatively free diffusion of drugs because of its aqueous environment. Although lipid-soluble (hydrophobic) substances permeate cell membranes with ease, they are immiscible in the aqueous phase of the tear film. Therefore, biphasic compounds that possess both lipid and water solubility are necessary components of topical drugs for adequate penetration of the corneal barrier.[3]

All factors considered, the challenge to the formulator is to circumvent the protective barriers of the eye without causing permanent tissue damage. The specific aim of designing a drug delivery system is to achieve a sustained therapeutic concentration of medication to the targeted site(s) while bypassing healthy tissue and lowering nonproductive loss for the appropriate duration, thereby improving the ratio of effectiveness to toxicity. To date, scientists have attempted to improve the bioavailability of topical ocular drugs by extending the drug contact time, using techniques such as subconjunctival injection, application of nanoparticles, liposomes, gels, inserts, latex systems, and mucoadhesives. Others have attempted to increase specific drug penetration by using prodrugs generated by modification of the drug's chemical structure. Attempts have also been made to improve the corneal permeability of drugs by iontophoresis or transiently modifying the integrity of the corneal epithelium through chelating agents and surfactants. However, effective ocular drug delivery has never been fully achieved and drug toxicity has been an obstacle for physicians and pharmaceutical scientists. In addition, with the emergence of virulent uveitis and retinopathies that patients develop after potent immunosuppressant therapy or with acquired immunodeficiency syndrome, the traditional ophthalmic solutions, suspensions, and ointment dosage forms are clearly no longer sufficient to combat these diseases. Poor penetration, lack of specificity, and toxicity when administered in high concentrations render conventional drug delivery systems of limited use in the treatment of posterior global diseases. Therefore, the need to develop even more efficient ocular drug delivery systems is becoming urgent.

Current research in ophthalmology has greatly increased our understanding of the physiological and biochemical constraints that determine the relatively low ocular bioavailability of many drugs. Progress in the chemical and pharmaceutical industry has explored a great number of new chemical entities and novel devices for ocular delivery in experimental eye research and clinical trials. In this chapter, we introduce some representative achievements in the development of unique ocular drug delivery systems, specifically, corneal collagen shields, iontophoresis, liposomes, and dendrimers. We will also review some of the alternative ophthalmologic drug delivery systems including those that have been tested, are being refined, or are still in the developmental stages.

UNIQUE OCULAR DRUG DELIVERY SYSTEMS

Corneal Collagen Shield

Development of Collagen Shield

The development of the corneal collagen shield as an ocular drug delivery system stems from two innovative approaches in ophthalmology. The first is to use bandage shields to protect eyes from ocular insults, such as postoperative recovery from corneal transplantation, refractive surgery, and recovery from recurrent epithelial erosions after ocular infection. The second approach is to use the soft contact lens to deliver drugs across the cornea. In this procedure, the hydrophilic lens is placed on the cornea and the drug is administered topically onto the surface of the lens. The contact lens is thought to act as a drug depot, binding the drug and releasing it slowly, thereby increasing retention of the therapeutic agent in the tear film. Although these soft lenses can enhance healing and deliver drugs for an extended period while allowing the eye to remain open, their cost is relatively high. Also, the contact lens must be fitted accurately and usually needs to be inserted and removed only in the ophthalmologist's office. Furthermore, soft contact lenses could harbor ocular pathogens, which can cause secondary infection of the treated eye. In addition, the drug releasing time has been found to be relatively shorter than expected. Ocular drug delivery by soft contact lenses, therefore, is not an ideal approach to effective, safe ocular disease treatment.

Over nearly two decades, interest in the use of the collagen shield as a unique ocular drug delivery system has been intensively pursued in numerous animal experiments and clinical trials[4-33] of the drug delivery systems described in this chapter, only collagen shields have been used in routine clinical practice.

Principle and Properties

The corneal collagen shield is fabricated from porcine or bovine scleral tissue, which bears a collagen composition similar to that of the human cornea. Therefore, the collagen shield displays characteristics of high biocompatibility and low immunogenicity. The collagen shield is shaped like a contact lens. Multiple base curves are not necessary because the shield can easily conform to the shape of the cornea. The mechanical properties of the shield are to protect the corneal epithelium from the action of the eyelids and the collagen acts as a drug reservoir for long-term release.

The collagen shield is packaged in a dehydrated form to be rehydrated before application. Typically, the drug is loaded into the collagen shield simply by soaking the shield in the intended drug solution prior to application. The hydrated shield forms a clear, pliable, thin film approximately 0.1 mm in thickness, with a diameter of 14.5 mm and base curve of 9 mm that conforms to the corneal surface. Drug delivery by collagen shields is dependent on absorption and subsequent release of the medication by the shield. When a water-soluble drug is used for rehydration, the drug becomes trapped in the interstices of the collagen matrix. Some drugs undergo reversible binding to collagen. The shield is designed to dissolve slowly within 12, 24, or 72 hours, thereby releasing the drug. For water-insoluble drugs such as cyclosporine, the drugs need to be incorporated into the shield at the time of manufacturing.

In the manufacture of collagen shields, the ability to control the amount of crosslinking in the collagen subunits by exposure to ultraviolet (UV) light is an important physiochemical property, because the amount of crosslinking is related to the dissolution time of the shield on the corneal surface. Some of the properties of commercially available corneal collagen shields, such as Medilens and Bio-Cor 24 have been described elsewhere.[34]

The collagen shield offers the advantage of being entirely soluble so that it does not need to be removed from its site of application. Other advantages of collagen shields include prevention of delay in treatment and maintenance of high concentrations of a variety of drugs in the eye. Collagen shields avoid some of the disadvantages of bandage soft contact lenses, such as the "suck-on syndrome" and the risk of infection; neovascularization can also be prevented, as the shield seems to increase oxygen absorption as it dissolves. In addition, collagen shields have shown to cause no systemic side effects and minimal corneal surface irritation in comparison to common preservatives in conventional ophthalmic antibiotics.[35]

Therapeutic Approach in Ophthalmology

A number of studies have described the ocular pharmacokinetics of dyes such as fluorescein[4] and other drugs by collagen shields, as well as the use of collagen shields in the chemotherapy of various disorders. The drugs that have been investigated include antibiotics, such as tobramycin,[5-13] gentamicin,[6,14-19] vancomycin,[19] and ofloxacin,[20,21] antifungal agents, such as amphotericin B,[22,23] antiviral agents, such as trifluorothymidine,[24,25] anti-inflammatory agents, such as dexamethasone,[5,6,14,15,26] prednisolone,[27] anticoagulants, such as heparin,[28] and immunosuppressive agents, such as cyclosporin A.[29-32] In the majority of instances in experimental studies, there is moderate to marked improvement in ocular drug absorption. The ability of the shield to deliver a drug to the cornea adds benefit to its usual purpose of promoting wound healing.

However, some recent clinical studies have shown that the use of corneal collagen shields to prevent ocular infection is not warranted. Taravella et al,[5] for example, conducted a prospective, randomized study of 32 patients undergoing cataract surgery. Compared with the conventional eyedrop group, eyes preoperatively treated with collagen shields did not show any difference in the delivery of tobramycin-dexamethasone combination into aqueous humor. Studies by the same group also showed that collagen shields did not enhance delivery of trifluorothymidine to the corneas with intact epithelium before penetrating keratoplasty.[24] Callizo et al found that there were no differences in the time course of the healing process between control and collagen shield treated eyes after keratectomy. There was an important polymorphonuclear infiltration in shield treated eyes, indicating a subacute inflammatory immunological reaction.[33]

In addition, there are a number of difficulties related to the design and use of collagen shields. Hydrated shields are difficult to handle and need to be inserted by ophthalmologists, often producing some discomfort, and interfering with vision. Shields are not individually tailor-made to fit each patient, and therefore, expulsion of the shield may occur.[34,36]

Conclusion

The collagen shield has provided a means of delivery of a variety of medications to ocular tissues. There are many indications that the shields deliver drugs as well as, if not better, than topical drops. Because of their biological inertness, structural stability, good biocompatibility and low cost of production, collagen shields could become promising carriers for ocular drugs. However, some problems exist and the collagen shield, in its present form, is not the most ideal sustained ocular drug delivery system. Collagen shields are not indicated for most patients with conditions requiring chronic rather than acute therapy. For it to be useful in sustained drug delivery, the existing biomaterials in the collagen shield must be modified or new biomaterials must be used. Also more clinical trials are needed to further determine its clinical efficacy and safety.

Iontophoresis

Principle and Properties

Ion transfer (Greek: iontophoresis) is a procedure whereby ions are driven across a barrier by an electric current. The mechanism of iontophoresis is based on the following physical principle like charged ions repel and oppositely charged ions attract.

In ocular drug delivery, iontophoresis transiently modifies the integrity of the corneal epithelium or sclera, by physical means, hence facilitating the penetration of ionized drugs across or into the targeted tissues. For best delivery, the solution of medication to be iontophoresed should have a minimum of extraneous ions. The molecule to be delivered by iontophoresis should have a strong net charge: anions (negative ions) or cations (positive ions). In general, the concentration of the ionized drug in solution can range from 0.01 to 5.0 percent. Other physicochemical characteristics, such as pH, conductivity, and ionic strength of the solution, often need to be taken into consideration for the specific drug to be iontophoresed.

One major advantage of iontophoresis for drug delivery is the elimination of systemic toxicity. This procedure can deliver a high concentration of drug to the targeted tissue where it can achieve the maximum benefit with little waste or systemic absorption. This physical approach can be precisely controlled by using the directly applied current. Another advantage is the very rapid delivery with improved consistency in the drug penetration to a specific ocular site.

Device and Procedure

The iontophoretic equipment consists of a device to deliver direct current with a current meter, a rheostat to control the amount of current flowing through the system, and two electrodes. Platinum is the best material for the electrode, since it releases almost no ions, undergoes degradation at a very slow rate, and is nontoxic.

Iontophoresis can be used in ophthalmology to deliver drugs by two approaches. Corneal iontophoresis delivers high concentrations of a drug to the anterior segment of the eye (cornea, aqueous humor, ciliary body and lens). In phakic eyes, the lens-iris-diaphragm limits penetration of a drug into the posterior tissues of the eye such as the posterior vitreous and retina. This barrier can be overcome by applying the current through the pars plana (transscleral iontophoresis), which can produce significantly high and sustained drug concentration in vitreous and retina.

Transcorneal iontophoresis: In this procedure, an eyecup, which is filled with medication, is placed over the cornea. A platinum electrode is positioned in contact with the top of the solution. To drive electropositive drugs (cations) from the eyecup solution into the cornea, the positive pole of the circuit (anode) is connected to the eyecup electrode. The negative pole (cathode) is attached to the neck, hand or ear of the subject. Figure 6.2 shows a diagram of transcorneal iontophoresis of a positively charged drug (e.g. gentamicin, epinephrine) in a rabbit eye model.

Transscleral iontophoresis: For transscleral iontophoresis, the drug solution is contained in a narrow tube within an eyecup held to the conjunctiva by suction. The tube is placed over the pars plana to avoid current damage to the retina. This technique circumvents

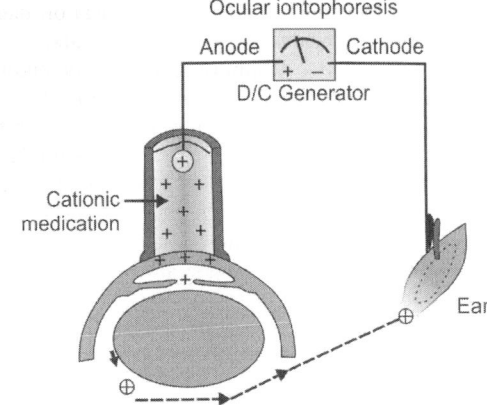

Fig. 6.2: Transcorneal iontophoresis in the rabbit. A positively-charged drug is passed through the cornea by means of a direct electric current [Reprinted with permission from AK Mitra, (Ed): Ophthalmic Drug Delivery Systems, Marcel Dekker: New York, 332, 1993]

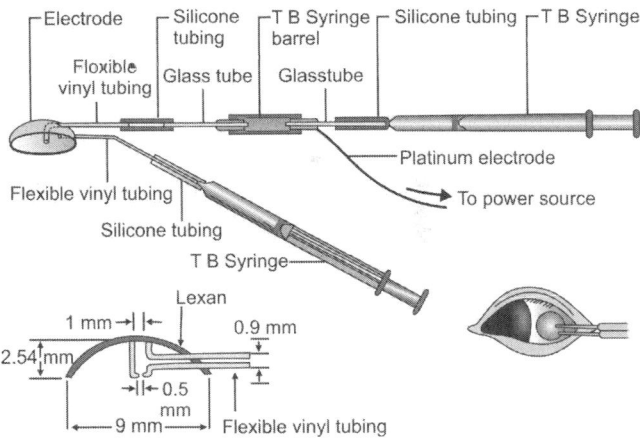

Fig. 6.3: Apparatus used for transscleral iontophoresis. Drug is delivered to the vitreous or retina by passing the drug through the conjunctiva. A syringe delivers the drug to a small eyecup that is suctioned to the conjunctiva [Reprinted with permission from AK Mitra (Ed): Ophthalmic Drug Delivery Systems, Marcel Dekker: New York, 341, 1993]

the lens-iris barrier and delivers drugs into the vitreous or retina. Figure 6.3 shows a diagram of transscleral iontophoresis.

Therapeutic Approaches in Ophthalmology

Iontophoresis was employed in ophthalmology as early as 1908 by Wirtz who passed an electric current through electrolyte-saturated cotton sponges placed over the eye for the treatment of conditions such as corneal ulcers, keratitis, and episcleritis.[37] During the first half of the twentieth century iontophoresis was used all over the world and studied extensively in the field of ophthalmology. Hill et al in the 1993 edition of the book of Ophthalmic Drug Delivery Systems, reviewed the use of iontophoresis in ophthalmology.[38] In general, iontophoresis has been used as a noninvasive, effective drug delivery system to deliver high concentrations of dyes, antibiotics, antifungal agents, anesthetic agents, and adrenergic agonists and antagonists. Ocular iontophoresis offers a fast, painless, safe, reliable and sustained concentration of drug delivery. Experimentally, iontophoresis has proven extremely useful as a reliable system for inducing reactivation of herpes virus in various models of this ocular disease.[39-44] Clinically, studies have found that this unique drug delivery system is promising in the delivery of dyes and drugs for a variety of ocular diseases. Within the past 10 years, in addition to the review chapter mentioned above, a number of authors have reviewed the application of iontophoresis in therapeutic approaches in ophthalmology with its advantages and disadvantages, such as Pillai et al,[45] Sasaki et al,[46] Sarraf and Lee,[47] Callegan et al.[48] In the following paragraphs, we review some of recent studies in animal models and human approaches utilizing iontophoresis as a unique ocular drug delivery system.

Studies by Frucht-Pery et al[49] showed that although higher current intensity did not significantly enhance drug concentration in the cornea, adequate bactericidal concentrations of gentamicin could be obtained in iontophoresis-treated corneas. In an animal study, Yoshizumi et al[50] found that transscleral iontophoresis of foscarnet represents a noninvasive drug delivery system for the local treatment of cytomegalovirus (CMV) retinopathy.

Frucht-Pery et al[51] also studied the distribution of gentamicin in the rabbit cornea following transcorneal iontophoresis. The highest concentration of the drug remained in the central cornea while the midperipheral cornea had higher levels than the peripheral cornea. Rieger et al[52] investigated iodine distribution in a porcine eye model following iontophoresis and found that the rank of iodine content in the ocular tissues in descending order was cornea> retina> vitreous> anterior chamber fluid> lens. This result provided evidence for the possible approach to protective, antioxidative treatment of ocular tissues by iontophoresis.

Behar-Cohen et al investigated the efficacy of the iontophoretic system in the delivery of dexamethasone for the treatment of rat endotoxin-induced uveitis. They found that iontophoretic administration of dexamethasone exerted a therapeutic effect on the posterior as well as anterior segment of the eye, and there was no clinical and histological damage caused by this technique, indicating that this system presents a safe, viable alternative to systemic administration of glucocorticoids in severe ocular inflammations.[53]

Yoshizumi et al are the first to study the ocular toxicity in multiple applications of foscarnet iontophoresis. They applied foscarnet to rabbit eyes by transscleral iontophoresis for a total of 7 regimens over a period of 21 days. Therapeutic concentrations of foscarnet in the vitreous capable of treating CMV retinitis was achieved. Electroretinography (ERG) and slit-lamp biomicroscopy revealed no evidence of ocular toxicity, indicating multiple applications of transscleral iontophoresis can safely deliver high concentrations of the drug into vitreous.[54]

Another potential application of iontophoresis worth mentioning is the delivery of dyes for gonioscopic pulsed dye laser sclerostomy. Studies have been reported in which dyes were delivered to the sclera by transscleral iontophoresis. Grossman et al[55] delivered methylene blue into rabbit eyes, Melamed et al[56] delivered methylene blue into the sclera of glaucoma patients, and Sarraf et al[57] delivered reactive black 5 dye into rabbit eyes. These three studies reported the delivery of a pulsed dye laser beam to the stained area through a goniolens to treat glaucoma. Iontophoresis was used to effectively deliver dyes into sclera. This system is technically feasible and could be a viable adjunct to pulsed dye laser sclerostomy procedures in ophthalmology.

Conclusion

Iontophoresis offers a unique ocular drug delivery system that is fast, painless, safe, and in most cases, results in the delivery of a high concentration of the drug to a specific target tissue. In glaucoma studies, iontophoresis applications include fluorescein to study aqueous humor dynamics,[58-60] adrenergic agents for treatment of glaucoma,[61,64] and 5-fluorouracil for control of cellular proliferation after glaucoma surgery.[65] In ocular anesthesia, iontophoresis can be used before ocular surgery.[66,67] In the treatment of ocular infections, antibiotics and antifungal agents can be delivered transcorneally or transsclerally according to the site of infection.[68-72] In the treatment of ocular inflammation, steroids can be delivered efficiently to animal or human eyes.[53,73,74] In the treatment and study of ocular herpes simplex virus infection, antivirals and adrenergic agents have been tested in various animal models.[39-44] In addition, alternative substrates have been tested for the diagnosis and/or treatment of ocular disorders.[75,76] However, this procedure is not a panacea for all eye disorders, but has importance for those substances that are not amenable to topical delivery and require repeated administration over an extended period of time. The role of iontophoresis in the field of clinical ophthalmology is currently being redefined. With this renewed interest, more and more clinical approaches utilizing this unique ocular drug delivery system need to be tested before it becomes a routine clinical procedure to treat patients.

Liposomes

Principle and Property

Liposomes are microscopic vesicles formed when certain phospholipid molecules interact to form a lipid bilayer in an aqueous environment. According to their size, liposomes are known as either small unilamellar vesicles (SUV; 10-100 nm) or

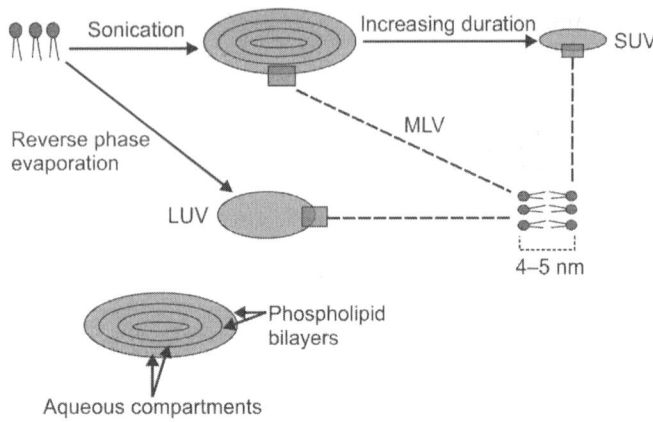

Fig. 6.4: Liposome preparation. Liposomes are made by constructing phospholipid bilayers into spherical structures containing hydrophilic molecules in an inner aqueous compartment, or hydrophobic molecules within the lipid bilayer. Sonication produces multilamellar vesicles (MLV) or small unilamellar vesicles (SUV). Reverse phase evaporation produces large unilamellar vesicles (LUV) [Reprinted with permission from AK Mitra, (Ed): Ophthalmic Drug Delivery Systems, Marcel Dekker: New York, 290, 1993]

large unilamellar vesicles (LUV; >100-3000 nm). If more bilayers are present, they are referred to as multilamellar vesicles (MLV). All the vesicles share the property of a liquid crystalline bilayer, similar to an outer cell membrane. Depending on the composition, liposomes can have a positive, negative, or neutral surface charge.[77]

Figure 6.4 depicts two commonly used methods for liposome preparation, sonication and reverse phase evaporation. Since liposomes are composed of lipids similar to those present in biological membranes, they are expected to be biocompatible and biodegradable. If the liposomes are formed in the presence of a drug, the drug will be incorporated into either the aqueous compartment or the lipid layer depending on its solubility. Thus, liposomes can accommodate both hydrophilic and lipophilic compounds.

A drug can be incorporated into a liposome in several ways depending on its chemical properties. In general, a water-soluble drug is dissolved in the aqueous phase in the interior compartment, whereas a more hydrophobic drug may be incorporated into the lipid bilayer itself, forming part of the vesicle membrane. The oil/water partition coefficient of the drug determines the stability of the drug in the liposome.

Probable mechanisms by which liposomes interact with cells include: (i) intermembrane transfer; (ii) contact release; (iii) adsorption of the liposome to the cell surface via nonspecific means or specific ligands such as antibodies, hormones, and lectins; (iv) fusion of the liposomes with the cell membranes and (v) endocytosis of the liposomes by the cell (Fig. 6.5).

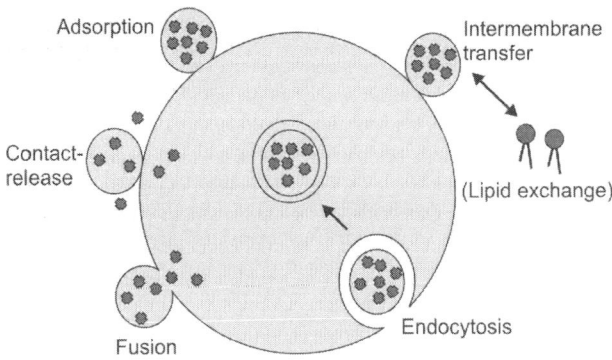

Fig. 6.5: Possible liposome-cell interactions [Reprinted with permission from AK Mitra, (Ed): Ophthalmic Drug Delivery Systems, Marcel Dekker: New York, 293, 1993]

Therapeutic Approaches in Ophthalmology

Liposomes have been widely studied for nearly two decades with the objective of increasing the specificity of action of drugs towards specific targets, to facilitate the bioavailability of drugs through biological membranes, or to protect a drug against enzyme inactivation. Their use in topical administration and especially in ocular administration has not received as much attention as other routes of administration.[77]

Although there is no commercially available product for repeated application in the eye, this colloidal system has been intensively studied as a means to improve and facilitate corneal drug transport. A great number of drugs and even some types of genes have been tested in this unique drug delivery system by experimental research or clinical trials.[35,77-81]

Three approaches have attempted utilizing liposomes as drug delivery systems: (i) topical application;[82-85] (ii) subconjunctival and intravitreal injection,[86-91] and (iii) targeting liposomal drug release with antibody,[92,93] laser,[94-96] and microwave radiation.[97,98] Most of the results have indicated that liposomes as drug carriers provide the possibility of controlled selective drug delivery and improved bioavailability. However, their usefulness is hindered by short shelf-life, limited drug loading capacity, and difficulty in sterilizing the drug preparations.[35,77,81]

In addition, these studies have also revealed that the potential of liposomes in ocular drug delivery appears to be greater for lipophilic than hydrophilic compounds. Liposome encapsulation has been found to alter ocular drug disposition depending on the type of liposomes and the physicochemical properties of the encapsulated drug.[99,100] Positively charged liposomes are preferentially captured at the negatively charged corneal surface as compared with neutral or negatively charged liposomes.[101]

Conclusion

Liposomal drug delivery system appears to have potential for ocular applications on the basis of studies in animal models. Liposomes can be easily prepared from nontoxic lipid materials, which are nonirritant and do not obscure vision. Although the potential of liposomes in ocular drug delivery appears greater for lipophilic than hydrophilic compounds, liposomes as drug carriers provide the possibility of controlled and selective drug delivery and improved bioavailability. Further research is needed to refine the procedures for use in humans and to elucidate the various parameters, which may influence the liposome as a means of ocular drug delivery.

Dendrimers

Property and Principle

In the past decade, a new macromolecular architecture has been developed. This new architecture mimics the dendritic branching of trees and is referred to as dendrimers, dendrons or dendrigrafts.[102-105] Dendrimers are different from all other classical synthetic polymers both by their unprecedented structure control, as well as by the fact that they are solvent-soluble, covalently fixed, three-dimensional megamolecules.[102] This unique macromolecular structure has been referred to as the fourth inventive architectural class of polymer that chemists have developed this century.

Dendrimers can be designed to mimic proteins and also be made in very robust forms to withstand both severe thermal and hydrolytic conditions. They are indeed reminiscent of biological cells, displaying three major architectural components: a core, an interior and a surface (Fig. 6.6).

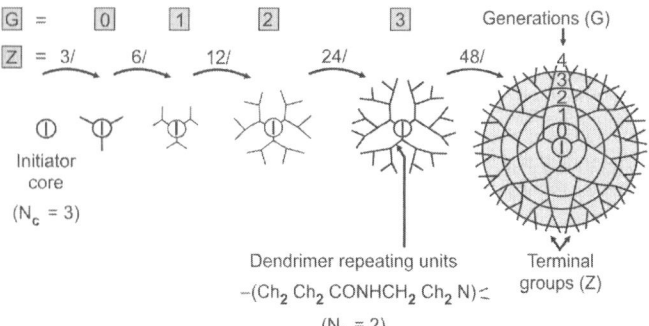

Fig. 6.6: Dendrimer formation. Through successive generations (G), terminal chemical groups (Z) are added to a starting structure, the initiator core. The initiator core depicted is one that allows three terminal groups to be added onto it in the first generation, G_0. Each generation allows two more terminal groups to be added to each terminal group from the preceding generation. By the fourth generation (G_3), there are 48 terminal groups. (Kindly provided by Donald A Tomalia, Michigan Molecular Institute, Ann Arbor, Michigan)

One of the most remarkable features of dendrimers is that these molecules are nanoscale in size and shape. The compounds closely match the sizes and contours of many important proteins and bioassemblies. For example, insulin ($\cong$30A), cytochrome C ($\cong$40A) and hemoglobin ($\cong$55A) are roughly the same size and shape, respectively, as generations 3, 4 and 5 of ammonia core, PAMAM (polyamidoamines) dendrimers.[102-105]

Another important asset of dendrimers is their ability to present functional groups or be transformed into a wide variety of nanoscaled chemical surfaces. Nanoscopic reagents such as DNA, antibodies or proteins have been combined with dendrimers to produce new gene delivery vectors.[106-110] This architectural function of the dendrimer is related to its guest-host, containment property, known as the "dendrimer box". There are now numerous examples demonstrating the cargo space that can be found in various dendrimer families. For example, the PAMAM dendrimers can host as much as three times the weight of aspirin or agricultural chemicals compared with dendrimer weight very recent research has shown that this space has unique shape-specific recognition properties for guest molecules that will undoubtedly offer exciting options for "smart drug delivery" systems.[102,105]

Potential Application of a Unique Drug Delivery System

One practical use of dendrimers in medicine is in gene therapy. Dendrimers can be made into the size and shape of histones, the proteins that carry DNA in cells. In an *in vitro* experiment, Tomalia et al has combined histone-like dendrimers and the luciferase gene with close to 30 different types of cells from various species, including humans. In nearly all cases, the dendrimers successfully transported genetic material into the cells and luciferase protein was expressed as a reporter. Although the exact mechanisms of how this dendrimer-DNA unit delivers the DNA of interest into cells has not been completely determined, this research shows the promising avenue of new gene therapy.[105] The profound advantages of this unique system include great capacity of delivery, nontoxicity, and non-immunogenicity, unlike conventional modified viral vectors.

Recently, many research teams are developing techniques for transporting other classes of drug molecules to selected targets in the body including ocular tissues. The dissolution of water insoluble ibuprofen in dendrimer host molecules clearly demonstrates the exciting potential in this area. Esfand et al have shown that the aqueous solubility of ibuprofen increases significantly in the presence of dendrimers.[111] Other related researches include the study of biodistribution of lipidic peptide dendrimer carrier after oral administration in rats,[112] an *in vitro* study of the interaction of synthetic oligonucleotide with mycobacteria after treatment of fourth generation dendrimers,[113] and a study of antisense pharmacology in the potential treatment of cancer.[106] For the practicing ophthalmologist, drug-releasing dendrimers are an emerging area of intense research activity and not an available technology.

Conclusion

Dendrimers are one of the most important and exciting contributions in synthetic chemical and pharmaceutical areas preceding the 21st century. The application of this unique macromolecular structure as means of gene and drug delivery is promising. Following optimization, these supermolecules whose properties can be made to order and easy and rapid to perform could launch a significant new industry in medicine. We look forward to an extensive exploration of the study of this unique drug delivery system.

OTHER OCULAR DRUG DELIVERY SYSTEMS

Pumps

Pumps are small devices that deliver drugs to the eye via a tube for extended periods of time. These devices are usually designed small enough to be implanted in the subcutaneous space and do not need an external power source or battery. The tube is passed from the pump to the eye through a subcutaneous tunnel. The distal end of the tube can be located in the conjunctival sac, corneal stroma, anterior chamber, or vitreous.

Various types of pumps have been tested or are being invented. Pumps can be made to fit different tissue structures and for different durations of drug delivery. The following are a few examples.

Two-chamber Pump

One chamber contains the drug in aqueous solution and the other a charging solution. The charging fluid is in liquid-gas equilibrium that expands at body temperature driving the drug at a constant flow rate. An example is Infusaid pump (Metal Bellows Corporation, Sharon, MA).

Osmotic Pump

Such a pump is driven by osmotic imbibition of extracellular water. This pump can deliver fluid for up to 7 days. An example is Alzet osmotic minipump (Alza Corporation, Palo Alto, CA).

Adjustable Pump

Adjustable pump contains a miniaturized pump and a port for transcutaneous refilling. One unique feature of this pump is that if used in the clinic, the patient can release a preset quantity of intended drug by finger pressure on the modular miniature plunger as required. An example is TI-DDS (totally implantable drug delivery system, Micro Infusions Systeme GmbH, Bruhlstr, Germany).

Although a variety of pumps have been studied in animal models for their possible applications in ocular drug delivery systems, and some promising results have been obtained (i.e.

sustained, high concentrations of drugs in targeted tissues),[114-119] pumps have not gained wide acceptance in practical clinical ophthalmology. The surgical procedure required for their insertion and potential problems with infection and extrusion limit their usefulness.

Ocular Inserts

Ocular inserts are unique devices made for extended duration of drug delivery and maintenance of an effective drug concentration in the target tissues.[120] Usually, they are small enough to be inserted into the cul-de-sac of the conjunctiva or vitreous. Corneal collagen shields that have been described earlier in this chapter are considered to be ocular inserts. The ocular pump may be considered as a form of ocular insert. The general characteristics of ocular inserts are listed and some specific types of inserts are described.

Criteria for Successful Ocular Inserts

- Comfort and noninterference with vision
- Sufficient oxygen permeability
- Biocompatibility and stability
- Reproducibility of release kinetics
- Applicability to a variety of drugs
- Ease of sterility and nontoxicity
- Ease of handling (insertion and removal)
- Ease of manufacture and low cost.

Although most of the above features are not unique to ocular drug delivery systems, a few of them are required by all controlled-release devices.[120]

In general, ocular inserts can be made erodible or nonerodible. Compared to erodible ocular inserts, the advantages of nonerodible ocular inserts are: (i) better release kinetics of drug; (ii) ease of detection when they are expelled, and (iii) greater reliability. The disadvantage is that the nonerodible insert has to be removed after the intended drug delivery period.

Some marketed nonerodible ocular inserts include contact lenses and the ocusert®. Erodible ocular inserts include the Lacrisert®, the SODI (soluble ocular drug insert) and collagen shield. These devices are currently being used in ophthalmic clinics and they are reviewed in a variety of articles.[120-122]

Another development of ocular inserts is the minidisk, which is made like a miniature contact lens. The diameter of the minidisk is between 4 and 5 mm, which allows the device to be easily placed behind the lower or upper eyelid without compromising comfort, vision, or oxygen permeability. Minidisks can also be prepared from erodible or nonerodible polymers, and the nonerodible minidisk has hydrophilic and hydrophobic types.

In summary, ocular inserts have shown some efficacy for prolonged-release ocular drug delivery. However, some of the devices are not accepted universally by all patients due to discomfort and high dosing frequencies. To completely meet the criteria of successful ocular inserts, there are still many experimental and clinical studies that need to be done. The physical and chemical design of the ocular inserts have to be refined in order to optimize the device and eliminate current problems.

Particulate Polymers

Particulate polymeric drug delivery system refers to nano- (< 1 μm) and microparticles (> 1 μm), which are designed to be used to reduce the precorneal elimination rate from the eye and hence increase the extent of ocular absorption.[123-126] The upper size limit for microparticles for ophthalmic administration is about 5 to 10 mm. Above this size, a scratching feeling will occur after topical application, which causes the microparticles not to be suitable for ophthalmic use.

Nanoparticles are produced by emulsion polymerization. Polyalkylcyanoacrylates are the most frequently used ophthalmologic nanoparticles.[123] The binding of drugs depends on the physicochemical properties of the drugs as well as of the nano- or microparticle polymer and also on the manufacturing process for these vehicles. In most experimental studies, the drug absorption in the eye is enhanced significantly in comparison with conventional eyedrops owing to the much slower ocular elimination rates of the particles from the cul-de-sac. For instance, several antiglaucoma drugs have been successfully loaded onto nanoparticles for testing the drug delivery efficacy.[77,123-129]

Because smaller particles are better tolerated by patients, nanoparticles may become very comfortable ophthalmic prolonged-action drug delivery systems. However, more clinical trials of a variety of drugs need to be done for optimization of this unique ocular drug delivery system.

Mucoadhesive Polymers

Mucoadhesive (bioadhesive) ocular drug delivery system refers to applying natural or synthesized polymers to the corneal surface, where the dosage form adheres to the precorneal mucus and resides in the eye until the polymer dissolves or the mucin replaces itself. One obvious advantage of the mucoadhesive device is prolongation of drug release for ocular tissues, hence increasing the drug bioavailability.

A number of studies have been done regarding the issues of chemical structure and biophysical properties of mucoadhesive polymers relevant to their ocular drug delivery ability. Some representative mucoadhesives with good mucoadhesive performance include carboxymethylcellulose, carbopol, polymethylmethacrylate, acrylic acid, polycarbophil and sodium alginate. So far, mucoadhesives have shown some promising and beneficial properties as a unique ocular drug delivery system.[77,130,131]

Since the potential of a mucoadhesive agent is determined by a number of parameters, such as chain length, configuration, and molecular weight and electronic charges, the research on mucoadhesives is still in its early stages and further advances in understanding and manipulation of the dosage form are necessary to translate this unique drug delivery system into practical application in controlled drug delivery.

Penetration Enhances

One of the principal problems in ocular drug delivery is relatively low permeability of a drug across the ocular surface. Enhancement of drug penetration through intercellular junctions or the cell membrane is one solution.

Substances used to enhance corneal penetration of ophthalmic drugs include surfactants, bile acids, fatty acid, preservatives, and chelating agents. The mechanisms of action of enhancers include: (i) cytoskeletal modulation of corneal permeability; (ii) alteration of tight cellular junctions by promoting glucose or amino acid with sodium cotransport; and (iii) change of drug charge type or charge density for enhanced absorption, etc.[40,132]

Penetration enhancers have not been extensively studied to date. Since the eye is very sensitive to most penetration enhancers and these compounds are required to be pharmacologically inert, chemically stable, specific and nonsensitizing, more research is needed to develop new penetration enhancers with a high specificity of action and minimal local and systemic toxicity.

CONCLUSION AND NEW PERSPECTIVES

For over a century ophthalmologists and pharmacologists have been searching for the best ocular drug delivery system that can provide a sustained therapeutic concentration of a drug at targeted tissue in a safe and highly efficient way. Although only very few ophthalmic drug delivery systems have been commercialized and are currently available in clinic, research on new drug delivery systems has definitely provided an important dynamism as never before, with the promise of new and exciting directions. With further research on the understanding of the physiological and biochemical constraints that determine the relatively low ocular bioavailability of many drugs, we look forward to the development of new, unique ocular drug delivery systems that can eventually be widely used in clinic to benefit patients.

REFERENCES

1. Schoenwald RD. Ocular drug delivery. Clin Pharmacokinet 1990;18:255-69.
2. Mitra AK. Ophthalmic Drug Delivery Systems. Marcel Dekker: New York, 1993.
3. Klyce SD, Beuerman RW. Structure and function of the cornea. In Kaufman HE, Barron BM, McDonald MB (Eds): The Cornea (2nd edn) Butterworth-Heinemann: Boston; 1998.pp.3-50.
4. Reidy JJ, Limberg M, Kaufman HE. Delivery of fluorescein to the anterior chamber using the corneal collagen shield. Ophthalmology 1990;97:1201-3.

5. Taravella M, Stepp P, Young D. Collagen shield delivery of tobramycin to the human eye. CLAO J 1998;24:166-8.
6. Mahlberg K, Krootila K, Uusitalo R. Compatibility of corticosteroids and antibiotics in combination. J Cataract Refract Surg 1997;23:878-82.
7. Chen CC, Takruri H, Duzman E. Enhancement of the ocular bioavailability of topical tobramycin with use of a collagen shield. J Cataract Refract Surg 1993;19:242-5.
8. Clinch TE, Hobden JA, Hill JM, et al. Collagen shields containing tobramycin for sustained therapy (24 hours) of experimental Pseudomonas keratitis. CLAO J 1992;18:245-7.
9. Assil KK, Zarnegar SR, Fouraker BD, et al. Efficacy of tobramycin-soaked collagen shields vs. tobramycin eyedrop loading dose for sustained treatment of experimental Pseudomonas aeruginosa-induced keratitis in rabbits. Am J Ophthalmol 1992;113:418-23.
10. Unterman SR, Rootman DS, Hill JM, et al. Collagen shield drug delivery: Therapeutic concentrations of tobramycin in the rabbit cornea and aqueous humor. J Cataract Refract Surg 1988;14:500-4.
11. Poland DE, Kaufman HE. Clinical uses of collagen shields. J Cataract Refract Surg 1988;14:489-91.
12. Sawusch MR, O'Brien TP, Dick JD, et al. Use of collagen corneal shields in the treatment of bacterial keratitis. Am J Ophthalmol 1988;106:279-81.
13. O'Brien TP, Sawusch MR, Dick JD, et al. Use of collagen corneal shields versus soft contact lenses to enhance penetration of topical tobramycin. J Cataract Refract Surg 1988;14:505-7.
14. Milani JK, Verbukh I, Pleyer U, et al. Collagen shields impregnated with gentamicin-dexamethasone as a potential drug delivery device. Am J Ophthalmol 1993;116:622-7.
15. Renard G, Bennani N, Lutaj P, et al. Comparative study of a collagen corneal shield and a subconjunctival injection at the end of cataract surgery. J Cataract Refract Surg 1993;19:48-51.
16. Silbiger J, Stern GA. Evaluation of corneal collagen shields as a drug delivery device for the treatment of experimental Pseudomonas keratitis. Ophthalmology 1992;99:889-92.
17. Liang FQ, Viola RS, del Cerro M, et al. Noncross-linked collagen discs and cross-linked collagen shields in the delivery of gentamicin to rabbit eyes. Invest Ophthalmol Vis Sci 1992;33:2194-8.
18. Baziuk N, Gremillion CM Jr, Peyman GA, et al. Colagen shields and intraocular drug delivery: Concentration of gentamicin in the aqueous and vitreous of a rabbit eye after lensectomy and vitrectomy. Int Ophthalmol 1992;16:101-7.
19. Phinney RB, Schwartz SD, Lee DA, et al. Collagen-shield delivery of gentamicin and vancomycin. Arch Ophthalmol 1988;106:1599-604.
20. Taravella MJ, Balentine J, Young DA, et al. Collagen shield delivery of ofloxacin to the human eye. J Cataract Refract Surg 1999;25:562-5.
21. Kuwano M, Horibe Y, Kawashima Y. Effect of collagen cross-linking in collagen corneal shields on ocular drug delivery. J Ocul Pharmacol Ther 1997;13:31-40.
22. Pleyer U, Legmann A, Mondino BJ, et al. Use of collagen shields containing amphotericin B in the treatment of experimental Candida albicans-induced keratomycosis in rabbits. Am J Ophthalmol 1992;113:303-8.

23. Schwartz SD, Harrison SA, Engstrom RE Jr, et al. Collagen shield delivery of amphotericin B. Am J Ophthalmol 1990;109:701-4.
24. Kuster P, Taravella M, Gelinas M, et al. Delivery of trifluridine to human cornea and aqueous humor using collagen shields. CLAO J 1998;24:122-4.
25. Gussler JR, Ashton P, van Meter WS, et al. Collagen shield delivery of trifluorothymidine. J Cataract Refract Surg 1990;16:719-22.
26. Hwang DG, Stern WH, Hwang PH, et al. Collagen shield enhancement of topical dexamethasone penetration. Arch Ophthalmol 1989;107:1375-80.
27. Sawusch MR, O'Brien TP, Updegraff SA. Collagen corneal shields enhance penetration of topical prednisolone acetate. J Cataract Refract Surg 1989;15:625-8.
28. Murray TG, Stern WH, Chin DH, et al. Collagen shield heparin delivery for prevention of postoperative fibrin. Arch Ophthalmol 1990;108:104-6.
29. Kanpolat A, Batioglu F, Yilmaz M, et al. Penetration of cyclosporin A into the rabbit cornea and aqueous humor after topical drop and collagen shield administration. CLAO J 1994;20:119-22.
30. Kaufman HE. New approaches in topical drug administration and treatment of the dry eye. Klinische Monatsblatter fur Augenheilkunde 1993;202:195-8.
31. Reidy JJ, Gebhardt BM, Kaufman HE. The collagen shield. A new vehicle for delivery of cyclosporin A to the eye. Cornea 1990;9:196-9.
32. Chen YF, Gebhardt BM, Reidy JJ, et al. Cyclosporine-containing collagen shields suppress corneal allograft rejection. Am J Ophthalmol 1990;109:132-7.
33. Callizo J, Cervello I, Mayayo E, et al. Inefficacy of collagen shield in the rabbit corneal wound-healing process. Cornea 1996;15(258):262.
34. Hill JM, O'Callaghan RJ, Hobden JA, et al. Corneal collagen shields for ocular delivery. In Mitra AK (Ed). Ophthalmic Drug Delivery Systems. Marcel Dekker: New York; 1993.pp.261-73.
35. Shofner RS, Kaufman HE, Hill JM. New horizons in ocular drug delivery. Ophthalmol Clin North Am 1989;2:15-24.
36. Kaufman HE, Steinemann TL, Thompson HW, et al. Collagen-based drug delivery and artificial tear. J Ocul Pharmacol 1994;10:17-27.
37. Wirtz R. Die ionentherapie in der augenheilkunde. Klin Monatsbl Augenheilkd 1908;46:543-79.
38. Hill JM, O'Callaghan RJ, Hobden JA. Ocular iontophoresis. In Mitra AK (Ed): Ophthalmic Drug Delivery Systems. Marcel Dekker: New York; 1993.pp.331-54.
39. Zheng X, Marquart ME, Loutsch JM, et al. HSV-1 migration in latently infected and naive rabbits after penetrating keratoplasty. Invest Ophthalmol Vis Sci 1999;40:2490-7.
40. Gangarosa LP Sr, Ozawa A, Ohkido M, et al. Iontophoresis for enhancing penetration of dermatologic and antiviral drugs. J Dermatol 1995;22:865-75.
41. Rootman DS, Haruta Y, Hill JM. Reactivation of HSV-1 in primates by transcorneal iontophoresis of adrenergic agents. Invest Ophthalmol Vis Sci 1990;31:597-600.
42. Hill JM, Haruta Y, Rootman DS. Adrenergically induced recurrent HSV-1 corneal epithelial lesions. Curr Eye Res 1987;6:1065-71.

43. Hill JM, Rayfield MA, Haruta Y. Strain specificity of spontaneous and adrenergically induced HSV-1 ocular reactivation in latently infected rabbits. Curr Eye Res 1987;6:91-7.
44. Willey DE, Trousdale MD, Newburn AB. Reactivation of murine latent HSV infection by epinephrine iontophoresis. Invest Ophthalmol Vis Sci 1984;25:945-50.
45. Pillai O, Nair V, Poduri R, et al. Transdermal iontophoresis. Part II: Peptide and protein delivery. Methods Find.Exp.Clin Pharmacol 1999;21(3):229-40.
46. Sasaki H, Yamamura K, Mukai T, et al. Enhancement of ocular drug penetration. Crit Rev Ther Drug Carrier Syst 1999;16:85-146.
47. Sarraf D, Lee DA. The role of iontophoresis in ocular drug delivery. J Ocular Pharm 1994;10:69-81.
48. Callegan MC, O'Callaghan RJ, Hill JM. Pharmacokinetic considerations in the treatment of bacterial keratitis. Clin Pharmacokinet 1994;27:129-49.
49. Frucht-Pery J, Solomon A, Doron R, Ever-Hadani P, et al. Efficacy of iontophoresis in the rat cornea. Graefe's Arch Clin Exp Ophthalmol 1996;234:765-9.
50. Yoshizumi MO, Lee DA, Sarraf DA, et al. Ocular toxicity of iontophoretic foscarnet in rabbits. J Ocul Pharmacol Ther 1995;11:183-9.
51. Frucht-Pery J, Goren D, Solomon A, et al. The distribution of gentamicin in the rabbit cornea following iontophoresis to the central cornea. J Ocular Pharm Therapeut 1999;15(3):251-6.
52. Rieger G, Winkler R, Buchberger W, et al. Iodine distribution in a porcine eye model following iontophoresis. Ophthalmologica 1995;209:84-7.
53. Behar-Cohen FF, Parel JM, Pouliquen Y, et al. Iontophoresis of dexamethasone in the treatment of endotoxin-induced-uveitis in rats. Exp Eye Res 1997;65:533-45.
54. Yoshizumi MO, Dessouki A, Lee DA, et al. Determination of ocular toxicity in multiple applications of Foscarnet iontophoresis. J Ocular Pharmcol Therapeut 1997;13(6):529-36.
55. Grossman RE, Sarraf D, Lee DA. Iontophoresis of methylene blue for gonioscopic pulsed dye laser sclerostomy. J Ocul Pharmacol 1993;9:277-85.
56. Melamed S, Solomon A, Neumann D, et al. Internal sclerostomy using laser ablation of dyed sclera in glaucoma patients: A pilot study. Br J Ophthalmol 1993;77:139-44.
57. Sarraf D, Lee DA. Iontophoresis of reactive black 5 for pulsed dye laser sclerostomy. J Ocul Pharmacol Ther 1993;9:25-33.
58. Jones RF, Maurice DM. New methods of measuring the rate of aqueous flow in man with fluorescein. Exp Eye Res 1966;5:208-20.
59. Starr PAJ. Changes in aqueous flow determined by fluorophotometry. Tans Ophthalmol Soc UK 1966;86:639-46.
60. Holm O. A photogrammetric method for estimation of the pupillary aqueous flow from the living human eye. Acta Ophthalmol 1968;46:254-77.
61. Kitazawa Y, Horie T. Denervation supersensitivity induced by chemical sympathectomy with 6-hydroxydopamine. Jpn J Ophthalmol 1974;18:109-18.
62. Kitazawa Y, Nose H, Horie T. Chemical sympathectomy with 6-hydroxydopamine in the treatment of primary open-angle glaucoma. Am J Ophthalmol 1975;79:98-103.

63. Watanabe H, Levene RZ, Bernstein MR. 6-hydroxydopamine therapy in glaucoma. Trans Am Acad Ophthalmol Otolaryngol 1977;83:69-77.
64. Colasanti BK, Trotter RR. Enhanced ocular penetration of the methyl ester of alpha-methyl-para-tyrosine after iontophoresis. Arch Int Pharmacodyn Ther 1977;228:171-6.
65. Kondo M, Araie M. Iontophoresis of 5-fluorouracil into the conjunctiva and sclera. Invest Ophthalmol Vis Sci 1989;30:583-5.
66. Sisler HA. Iontophoretic local anesthesia for conjunctival surgery. Ann Ophthalmol 1978;10:597-8.
67. Meyer DR, Lindberg JV, Vasquez RJ. Iontophoresis for eyelid anesthesia. Ophthalmic Surg 1990;21:845-8.
68. Rootman DS, Jantzen JA, Gonzalez JR, et al. Pharmacokinetics and safety of transcorneal iontophoresis of tobramycin in the rabbit. Invest Ophthalmol Vis Sci 1988;29:1397-1401.
69. Hodben JA, Reidy JJ, O'Callaghan RJ, et al. Ciprofloxacin iontophoresis for aminoglycoside-resistant *Pseudomonas* keratitis. Invest Ophthalmol Vis Sci accepted, 1990.
70. Choi TB, Lee DA. Transscleral and transcorneal iontophoresis of vancomycin in rabbit eyes. J Ocular Pharmacol 1988;4:153-64.
71. Barza MM, Peckman C, Baum J. Transcleral iontophoresis of gentamicin in monkeys. Invest Ophthalmol Vis Sci 1987;28:1033-6.
72. Church AL, Barza M, Baum J. An improved apparatus for transcleral iontophoresis of gentamicin. Invest Ophthalmol Vis Sci 1992;33:3543-5.
73. Lachaud JP. Considerations on the use of corticosteroids by ionization in certain ocular diseases. Bull des Societies D'Ophthalmologie de France 1965;65:84-9.
74. Lam TT, Edward DP, Zhu X, et al. Transcleral iontophoresis of dexamethasone. Arch Ophthalmol 1989;107:1368-71.
75. Asahara T, Shinomiya K, Naito T, et al. Induction of genes into the rabbit eye by iontophoresis. Acta Soc Ophthalmol Jpn 1999;103:178-85.
76. Shimomura Y. Iontophoresis for postherpetic neuralgia. Folia Ophthalmol Jpn 1987;38:175-82.
77. Bourlais CL, Liliane A, Hosein Z, et al. Ophthalmic drug delivery system—recent advances. Prog Retin Eye Res 1998;17:33-58.
78. Reimer K, Fleischer W, Brogmann B, et al. Povidone-iodine liposomes—an overview. Dermatology 1997;195(Suppl 2):93-9.
79. Desmettre T, Mordon S, Soulie S, et al. Liposome in ophthalmology. Review of the literature. J Francais d Ophthalmol 1996;19:716-31.
80. Niesman MR. The use of liposomes as drug carriers in ophthalmology. Crit Rev Ther Drug Carrier Syst 1992;9:1-38.
81. Langer R. New methods of drug delivery. Science 1990;249:1527-33.
82. Pleyer U, Elkins B, Ruckert D, et al. Ocular absorption of cyclosporine A from liposomes incorporated into collagen shields. Curr Eye Res 1994;13:177-81.
83. Velpandian T, Gupta SK, Gupta YK, et al. Ocular drug targeting by liposomes and their corneal interactions. J Microencapsulation 1999;16(2):243-50.
84. Whitcup SM, Pleyer U, Lai JC, et al. Topical liposome-encapsulated FK506 for the treatment of endotoxin-induced uveitis. Ocul Immunol Inflamm 1998;6:51-6.

85. Milani JK, Pleyer U, Dukes A, et al. Prolongation of corneal allograft survival with liposome-encapsulated cyclosporine in the rat eye. Ophthalmology 1993;100:890-6.
86. Van der Veen G, Broersma L, Dijkstra CD, et al. Prevention of corneal allograft rejection in rats treated with subconjunctival injections of liposomes containing dichloromethylene diphosphonate. Invest Ophthalmol Vis Sci 1994;35:305-15.
87. Assil KK, Frucht-Perry J, Ziegler E, et al. Tobramycin liposomes. Single subconjunctival therapy of pseudomonal keratitis. Invest Ophthalmol Vis Sci 1991;32:3216-20.
88. Wiechens B, Grammer JB, Johannsen U, et al. Experimental intravitreal application of ciprofloxacin in rabbits. Ophthalmologica 1999;213:120-8.
89. Garcia-Arumi J, Pascual R, Fonseca MJ, et al. Pharmacokinetics and retinal toxicity of intravitreal liposome-encapsulated 5-fluorouridine. Ophthalmologica 1997;211: 344-50.
90. Akula SK, Ma PE, Peyman GA, et al. Treatment of cytomegalovirus retinitis with intravitreal injection of liposome encapsulated ganciclovir in a patient with AIDS. Br J Ophthalmol 1994;78:677-80.
91. Salah-Eldin M, Peyman GA, el-Aswad M, et al. Evaluation of toxicity and efficacy of a combination of antineoplastic agents in the prevention of PVR. Int Ophthalmol 1994;18:53-60.
92. Norley SG, Sendele D, Huang L, et al. Inhibition of herpes simplex virus replication in the mouse cornea by drug containing immunoliposomes. Invest Ophthalmol Vis Sci 1987;28:591-5.
93. Norley SG, Huang L, Rouse BT. Targeting of drug loaded immunoliposomes to herpes simples virus infected corneal cells: An effective means of inhibiting virus replication *in vitro*. J Immunol 1986;136:681-5.
94. Desmettre TJ, Soulie-Begu S, Devoisselle JM, et al. Diode laser-induced thermal damage evaluation on the retina with a liposome dye system. Lasers Surg Med 1999;24:61-8.
95. Guran T, Zeimer RC, Shahidi M, et al. Quantitative analysis of retinal hemodynamics using targeted dye delivery. Invest Ophthalmol Vis Sci 1990;31:2300-6.
96. Zeimer RC, Khoobehi B, Niesman MR, et al. A potential method for local drug and dye delivery in the ocular vasculature. Invest Ophthalmol Vis Sci 1988;29:1179-83.
97. Khoobehi B, Peyman GA, Niesman MR, et al. Hyperthermia and temperature-sensitive liposomes: Selective delivery of drugs into the eye. Jpn J Ophthalmol 1989;33:405-12.
98. Khoobehi B, Peyman GA, McTurnan WG, et al. Externally triggered release of dye and drugs from liposomes into the eye. An *in vitro* and *in vivo* study. Ophthalmology 1988;95:950-5.
99. Singh K, Mezei M. Liposomal ophthalmic drug delivery system. I. Triamcinolone acetonide. Int J Pharm 1983;16:339-44.
100. Singh K, Mezei M. Liposomal ophthalmic drug delivery system. II. Dihydrostreptomycin sulfate. Int J Pharm 1984;16:263-9.
101. Lee VHL. Application of liposomes in ocular drug delivery. In Pleyer D, Schmidt K, Tiel HJ, (Eds): Liposomes in Ophthalmology and Dermatology. Hippokrates: Stuttart; 1993.pp.53-9.
102. Tomalia DA, Esfand R. Dendrons, dendrimers, and dendrigrafts. Chemistry and Industry; 1997.pp.416-20.
103. Veprek P, Jezek J. Peptide and glycopeptide dendrimers. Part II. J Pept Sci 1999;5:203-20.

104. Tomalia DA, Naylor AM, Goddard WAI. Starburst dendrimers: molecular-level control of size, shape, surface chemistry, topology, and flexibility from atoms to macroscopic matter. Angew Chem Int Ed Engl 1990;29:138-75.
105. Tomalia DA. Dendrimer molecules. Scientific Am; 1995.pp.42-6.
106. Bielinska A, Kukowska-Latallo JF, Johnson J, et al. Regulation of in vitro gene expression using antisense oligonucleotides or antisense expression plasmids transfected using starburst PAMAM dendrimers. Nucleic Acids Res 1996;24(11):2176-82.
107. Hudde T, Rayner SA, Comer RM, et al. Activated polyamidoamine dendrimers, a non-viral vector for gene transfer to the corneal endothelium. Gene Therapy 1999;6:939-43.
108. Qin L, Pahud DR, Ding Y, et al. Efficient transfer of genes into murine cardiac grafts by Starburst polyamidoamine dendrimers. Hum Gene Ther 1998;9:553-60.
109. Kukowska-Latallo JF, Bielinska AU, Johnson J, et al. Efficient transfer of genetic material into mammalian cells using Starburst polyamidoamine dendrimers. Proc Natl Acad Sci USA 1996;93: 4897-902.
110. Tang MX, Redemann CT, Szoka FC Jr. *In vitro* gene delivery by degraded polyamidoamine dendrimers. Bioconjug Chem 1996;7: 703-14.
111. Esfand R, Beezer AE, Mitchell JC. An investigation of synthesis and potential application of tetradirectional cascade dendrimers as drug delivery systems. 96 AD; London, 1996.
112. Sakthivel T, Toth I, Florence AT. Distribution of a lipidic 2.5 nm diameter dendrimer carrier after oral administration. Int J Pharm 1999;183:51-5.
113. Attia SA, Shepherd VE, Rosenblatt MN, et al. Interaction of oligodeoxynucleotides with mycobacteria: Implications for new therapeutic strategies. Antisense Nucleic Acid Drug Dev 1998;8: 207-14.
114. Reidy JJ, Mondino BJ, Brown SI, et al. A long-term implantable aqueous delivery system for the external rabbit eye. Invest Ophthalmol Vis Sci 1980;19:428-30.
115. Michelson JB, Nozik RA. Experimental endophthalmitis treated with an implantable osmotic minipump. Arch Ophthalmol 1979;97:1345-6.
116. Roussel TJ, Osato MS, Wilhelmus KR. Cyclosporine and experimental corneal transplantation. Transplant Proc 2000;15: 3081-3.
117. Eliason JA, Maurice DM. An ocular perfusion system. Invest Ophthalmol Vis Sci 1980;19:102-5.
118. Ishibashi T, Miki K, Patterson R, et al. An intravitreal cannula system: Long-term follow-up study. Int Ophthalmol 1986;9:5-9.
119. Miki K, Patterson R, Ryan SJ. An indwelling cannula system for the primate eye. J Neurosci Methods 1985;13: 267-79.
120. Bawa R. Ocular inserts. In Mitra AK (Ed): Ophthalmic Drug Delivery Systems. Marcel Dekker: New York; 1993.pp.223-60.
121. Lee VH, Robinson JR. Topical ocular drug delivery: Recent developments and future challenges. J Ocul Pharmacol 1986;2:67-108.
122. Sieradzki E. Bioavailability of drugs applied to the eye externally. Klinika Oczna 1991;93:34-6.
123. Calvo P, Vila-Jato JL, Alonso MJ. Comparative *in vitro* evaluation of several colloidal systems, nanoparticles, nanocapsules, and

nanoemulsions, as ocular drug carriers. J Pharm Sci 1996;85: 530-6.
124. Das SK, Tucker IG, Hill DJ, et al. Evaluation of poly (isobutylcyanoacrylate) nanoparticles for mucoadhesive ocular drug delivery. I. Effect of formulation variables on physiochemical characteristics of nanoparticles. Pharm Res 1995;12:534-40.
125. Joshi A. Microparticulates for ophthalmic drug delivery. J Ocul Pharmacol 1994;10:29-45.
126. Kreuter J. Particulates (nanoparticles and microparticles). In Mitra AK (Ed): Ophthalmic Drug Delivery Systems. Marcel Dekker; New York; 1993.pp.275-87.
127. Calvo P, Alonso MJ, Vila-Jato JL, et al. Improved ocular bioavailability of indomethacin by novel ocular drug carriers. J Pharm Pharmacol 1996;48:1147-52.
128. Zimmer A, Mutschler E, Lambrecht G, et al. Pharmacokinetic and pharmacodynamic aspects of an ophthalmic pilocarpine nanoparticle-delivery system. Pharm Res 1994;11:1435-42.
129. Harmia T, Speiser P, Kreuter J. A solid colloidal drug delivery system for the eye: Encapsulation of pilocarpine in nanoparticles. J Microencapsul 1986;3:3-12.
130. Krishnamoorthy R, Mitra AK. Mucoadhesive polymers in ocular drug delivery. In Mitra AK (Ed): Ophthalmic Drug Delivery Systems. Marcel Dekker: New York; 1993.pp.199-221.
131. Robinson JR, Longer MA, Veillard M. Bioadhesive polymers for controlled drug delivery. Ann NY Acad Sci 1987;507:307-14.
132. Liaw J, Robinson JR. Ocular penetration enhancers. In Mitra AK, (Ed): Ophthalmic Drug Delivery Systems. Marcel Dekker: New York; 1993.pp.369-81.

Antibacterial Therapy

NR Biswas, GK Das, Harivenkatesh N, Ashok Garg (India)

INTRODUCTION

Principles in antibiotic therapy remain the same in all medical specialties. The rational selection of antimicrobial drugs depends upon the diagnosis, sensitivity and assay of bactericidal activity. In most infections the relationship between causative agent and clinical picture is not constant. It is, therefore, important to obtain proper specimens from diseased ocular tissue for bacteriological identification of causative agent. Ideally the antibacterial agent should be started based on sensitivity of the organisms.

The eye is particularly suitable for local application of antibiotics. The use of systemic antibiotics is limited by relatively poor penetration of antibiotics into the eye through the blood-eye barrier. However, during infection, the impermeability of the barrier reduces thereby allowing drugs and other molecules to pass through it.

The general principles of management of infection in any part of the body also apply to the ocular infection. An accurate diagnosis confirmed by the culture and sensitivity from the samples (corneal scraping in corneal ulcers, conjunctival swab in conjunctivitis and vitreous tap in endophthalmitis, etc.) is necessary before selecting the most effective antibiotic.

ROUTES OF ANTIMICROBIAL ADMINISTRATION IN OPHTHALMIC PRACTICE

- Topical
- Subconjunctival/subtenon/retrobulbar injections
- Intracameral injections
- Intravitreal injections/implants
- Systemic

External ocular infections can be treated with topical antibiotics. If used at proper concentration most of the commercially available antibiotics are safe. However, higher concentrations and more number of applications than the prescribed limit may cause toxic effects like corneal epithelial defect and tear film instability. The goal of achieving high antibiotic concentration in anterior segment can be achieved by frequent instillation of antibiotic drops into the conjunctival sac. Ophthalmic ointments have better retention time and hence better corneal penetration.

Subconjunctival antibiotic injection produces a constant and prolonged depot of medication supplying effective drug concentration in the anterior segment. Intracameral injections directly deliver the drug into the anterior chamber. The vitreous cavity is the most difficult area to be penetrated by topical and subconjunctival routes. Therefore, direct intravitreal injection of antibiotic is recommended in desperate situation like endophthalmitis. Recently intravitreal implants (e.g. ganciclovir implant) are available for treatment of retinitis.

Topical antibiotics are also used prophylactically before surgery. Organisms that are otherwise considered normal flora such as *Staphylococcus epidermidis* are potential pathogens to the eye. *Staphylococcus epidermidis*, the commensal organism in the conjunctival sac is the most common cause of postoperative endophthalmitis. The use of preoperative antibiotics decrease or eliminate bacterial flora from the conjunctiva and prevent intraoperative contamination of wound and anterior chamber.

SELECTION OF ANTIMICROBIAL AGENTS

Antibiotics are chemical substances produced by microorganisms that have the capacity to inhibit growth of or even destroy bacteria and other microorganisms in dilute solution. The chemical structures of most therapeutics have been identified.

The best prerequisite for the correct choice of an antimicrobial which at the same time will be fully active, safe and well-tolerated is an exact clinical and bacteriological diagnosis.

The choice of an antimicrobial is not only influenced by the type and susceptibility of the infecting organism but also by mode of action and pharmacokinetics of the antibiotic, the severity and localization of infection, age, hepatic and renal functions of the patient.

When more than one antibiotic is used, apart from the spectrum of the individual antibiotic, synergism and antagonism must be kept in mind, since these antibiotics may have variable mechanism of action.

The antibiotics exert their action by various means which is described in the subsequent sections. Antibiotics may be either bactericidal (those which kill organisms) or bacteriostatic (which inhibit bacterial multiplication). Some bacteriostatic drugs become bactericidal when used in higher concentration as may occur with topical ophthalmic applications.

Similarly the antibacterial activity of the given drug may be concentration dependent or time dependent. For example, the bactericidal activity of amino glycosides increases with the increasing drug concentrations (concentration dependent killing). Such drugs show antibacterial activity even after their plasma levels become undetectable (postantibiotic effect). On the other hand, the bactericidal activity of penicillin increases with the increasing amount of time the blood levels remain above the minimum bactericidal concentration (time dependent killing).

During antibiotic selection, the pharmacokinetics of the antibiotics must be taken into consideration. Absorption, tissue diffusion and distribution, intraocular penetration, protein binding, metabolism and excretion differ for each antimicrobial agent.

The 'suitable drug' for a causative organism is based on the following:
- The site of infection.
- Antimicrobial spectrum of the drug.
- Age, hepatic and renal functions of the patient.
- Previous history of drug allergies.
- The place where the infection was acquired and local susceptibility pattern.
- Mechanical predisposing factors.
- Predisposing host facts.

Because of tear flow, topically instilled antibiotics have a limited life span in the conjunctival sac and only a fraction of their volume penetrates the eyeball across the cornea. Drug penetration may be improved by frequent instillation, increasing the viscosity of the drug, by employing the vehicle, by altering the PH of the drug or by the use of fortified drops.

Topical antibiotics should be selected depending upon the severity of infection and the suspected ocular pathogen. Preferably use less potent antibiotics in common ocular infection and reserve broad spectrum and more potent antibiotics for more severe or fulminant infections.

INDICATIONS FOR ANTIMICROBIAL THERAPY

- Bacteriologically and clinically proven infection of the eye.
- Topical antibiotics are more useful in external ocular infections like conjunctivitis, keratitis, keratoconjunctivitis, dacryocystitis, stye and chalazion.
- As prophylaxis to
  - Prevent secondary bacterial infection in patients who are ill with other diseases
  - To protect healthy persons from the acquisition or invasion by specific infection to which they are exposed
- Confirmation of suspected diagnosis of significant bacterial infection by observing clinical response.

The commercially available antibiotic drops and ointments are marketed in various strengths from 0.3 to 1 percent. However, in severe infections of the eye in addition to systemic therapy, high potency fortified drops are freshly prepared and used. But these fortified eyedrops have a very short life span.

But at the same time, indiscriminate use of antibiotics should be checked as it leads to:
- Widespread sensitization resulting in hypersensitivity/anaphylaxis.
- Change in normal flora of the tears resulting in super infection.
- Direct drug toxicity due to prolonged use.
- Masking serious infections without eradicating it.
- Development of drug resistance.

MECHANISMS OF RESISTANCE TO ANTIBIOTICS

Bacteria develop various strategies to resist the action of antibiotics and to safeguard themselves, some of which are given below:
- Production of enzymes that inactivate the drug
  - β-lactamase inactivates penicillins and cephalosporins, acetyltransferase inactivates chloramphenicol, aminoglycoside inactivating enzymes inactivate aminoglycosides.
- Alteration of drug binding sites
  - Methicillin resistance in *Staphylococcus* is due to altered penicillin binding protein. Resistance to aminoglycosides, erythromycin and fluoroquinolones may occur by similar fashion.
- Decreased drug uptake by the bacteria
  - Intracellular concentration of tetracycline and aminoglycosides are very low in the resistant bacteria.
- Active efflux of the drug by the bacteria
  - Resistance to erythromycin and tetracyclines occur by development of efflux pumps.
- Alteration of metabolic enzymes and development of alternative metabolic pathway
  - Sulfonamide resistant bacteria develop alternative pathway to synthesize folic acid.
- Combination of the above

Once the bacteria develop resistance then it can be transferred to other bacteria by gene transfer through conjugation, transduction or transformation.

STEPS TO BE TAKEN TO AVOID ANTIMICROBIAL RESISTANCE

In order to avoid resistance to topical antibiotics the following principles might be followed:
- Limit antibiotic use when it is definitely required. It is unnecessary to use broad spectrum antibiotics in condition like viral conjunctivitis.
- Avoid chronic use of antibiotics. Ask the patient to follow the ophthalmologist advice strictly regarding the duration of antibiotics use.
- Use newer antibiotics only when necessary for treatment of resistant infections.
- Completely treat all clinical infections and consider using a second therapeutic agent to prevent emergence of resistant organisms.

ANTIMICROBIAL COMBINATION THERAPY

Sometimes combinations of antimicrobial agents are used in the treatment of ocular infections, if necessary.

Indications of Combination Therapy
- To give prompt treatment to the patient.

- To delay the emergence of microbial mutants resistant to one drug on chronic use.
- To treat mixed infections.
- To achieve bactericidal synergism.

Disadvantages of Antimicrobial Combination

- The more the drugs are used, the greater the chances for drug reaction to occur.
- The cost is unnecessarily high.
- Relax in attitude of clinician in the effort to establish a specific diagnosis.
- Antimicrobial combinations may accomplish no more than an effective single drug.
- Increased incidence of adverse effects.
- High chances of super-infections.

MICROBES CAUSING OCULAR INFECTIONS

Most common pathogens seen in ocular infective conditions are:
a. Gram-positive cocci:
   - *Staphylococcus aureus*
   - *Staphylococcus epidermidis*
   - *Streptococcus pneumoniae*
   - *Streptococcus faecalis*
   - α and β hemolytic streptococci
b. Gram-negative cocci:
   - *Neisseria gonorrhoeae*
   - *Neisseria meningitides*
   - *Neisseria sicca, mucosa* and *flavescens*
c. Gram-negative rods:
   - *Haemophilus species* (*influenzae* and *aegyptius*)
   - *Escherichia coli*
   - *Pseudomonas aeruginosa*
   - *Klebsiella* species (*pneumonia* and *oxytoca*)
   - *Moraxella* species (*lacunata, bovis, catarrhalis* and non-liquefaciens)
   - *Serratia marcescens*
   - *Acinetobacter* species
   - *Enterobacter* species
   - *Shigella* species (*sonnei* and *flexneri*)
   - *Proteus* (*mirabilis* and *vulgaris* species)
   - *Brucella* species (*abortus, suis* and *melitensis*)
d. Gram-positive rods:
   - *Clostridium* species (*tetani* and *welchii*)
   - *Corynebacterium* species (*diphtheria* and *xerosis*)
   - *Bacillus* species (*anthracis, cereus* and *subtilis*)
   - *Listeria monocytogenes*
e. Miscellaneous:
   - *Chlamydia trachomatis*
   - *Nocardia* species

The broad-spectrum antibiotics are variably effective against Gram +ve and –ve organisms.

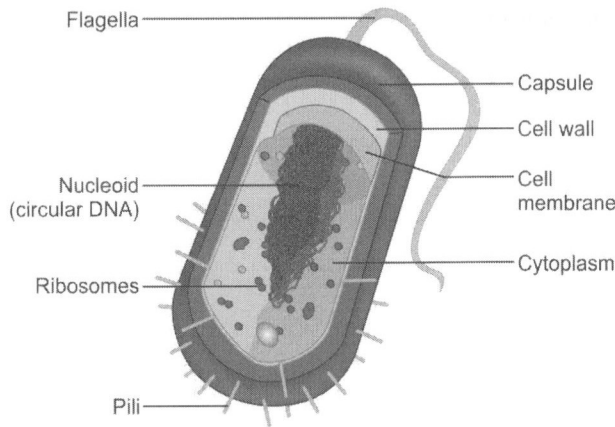

Fig. 7.1: Structure of bacteria

CLASSIFICATION OF ANTIBACTERIAL DRUGS (ACCORDING TO MECHANISM OF ACTION)

1. Drugs inhibiting bacterial cell wall synthesis
   a. Beta-Lactam antibiotics
      - Penicillins
      - Cephalosporins (including Cephamycins)
      - Monobactams
      - Carbapenems
   b. Glycopeptide antibiotics
      - Vancomycin
      - Teicoplanin
      - Dalbavancin
      - Telavancin
   c. Fosfomycin
   d. Bacitracin
   e. Cycloserine
2. Drugs attacking bacterial cell membrane
   a. Daptomycin
   b. Polypeptide antibiotics (except bacitracin)
      - Polymyxin B
      - Colistin
      - Tyrothricin
3. Drugs inhibiting bacterial protein synthesis
   a. Tetracyclines
   b. Glycylcyclines
      - Tigecycline
   c. Chloramphenicol
   d. Macrolides
      - Erythromycin
      - Roxithromycin
      - Clarithromycin
      - Azithromycin
   e. Ketolides
      - Telithromycin
   f. Streptogramins
      - Quinupristin-Dalfopristin

g. Oxazolidinones
   - Linezolid
h. Lincosamide
   - Clindamycin
i. Aminoglycosides
j. Spectinomycin
k. Retapamulin
l. Fusidic acid
4. Drugs attacking bacterial DNA
   a. Fluoroquinolones
   b. Nitroimidazoles
   c. Nitrofurantoin
5. Drugs affecting bacterial intermediate metabolism
   a. Sulfonamides
   b. Trimethoprim
   c. Pyrimethamine
   d. Cotrimoxazole (Sulfamethoxazole-Trimethoprim)
6. Miscellaneous drugs
   a. Mupirocin
   b. Antimicrobial peptides

DRUGS THAT INHIBIT BACTERIAL CELL WALL SYNTHESIS

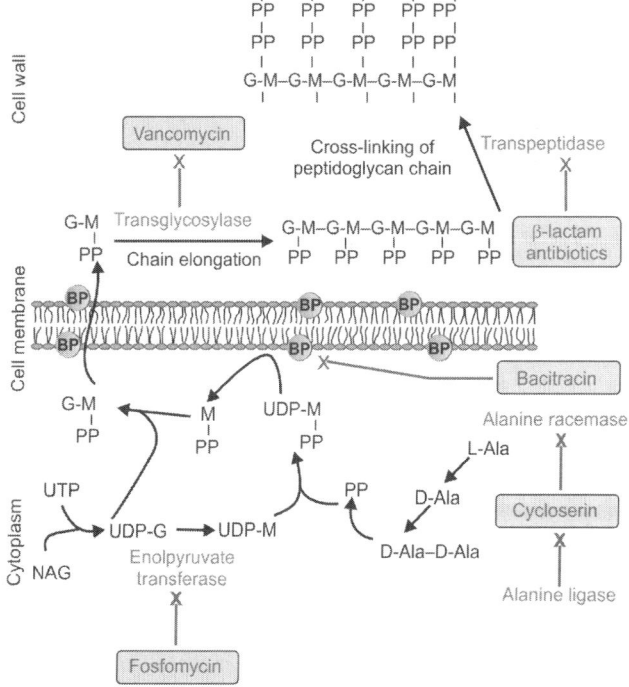

Fig. 7.2: Steps in bacterial cell wall synthesis and various drugs interfering in the pathway. *Note:* Enzymes are shown in green and drugs are shown in red; G: N-Acetylglucosamine (NAG); M: N-Acetylmuramic acid; Ala: Alanine; PP: Pentapeptide; BP: Bactroprenol; UDP: Uridine diphosphate

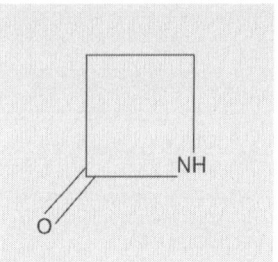

Fig. 7.3: Structure of β-lactam ring

BETA-LACTAM ANTIBIOTICS

These are so called because they contain β-lactam ring in their structure (Fig. 7.3). They are bactericidal drugs and include penicillins, cephalosporins, monobactams and carbapenems.

Mechanism of Action

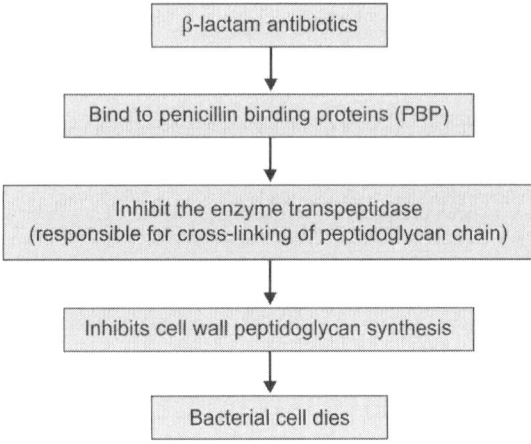

Mode of Resistance

Bacteria develop resistance to Penicillins and other β-lactam antibiotics by the following modes:
- Production of β-lactamases that destroy the β-lactam antibiotics
- Altered penicillin binding proteins (Methicillin resistance to *Staphylococcus aureus*)
- Decreased entry or active efflux of the antibiotic.

Penicillins

Penicillins are derivatives of 6-aminopenicillanic acid (Fig. 7.4).

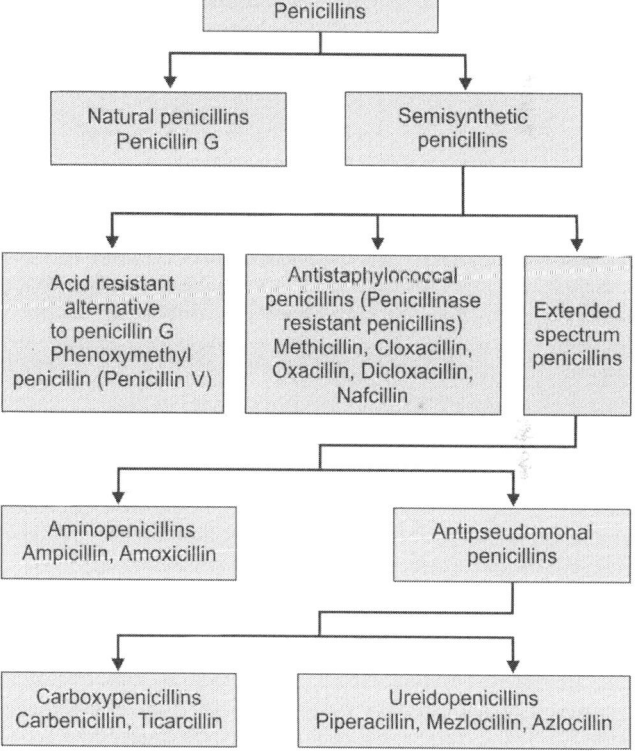

Fig. 7.4: Structure of 6-aminopenicillanic acid

Penicillins are further classified into the following groups:

- **Penicillins**
  - **Natural penicillins** — Penicillin G
  - **Semisynthetic penicillins**
    - **Acid resistant alternative to penicillin G** — Phenoxymethyl penicillin (Penicillin V)
    - **Antistaphylococcal penicillins (Penicillinase resistant penicillins)** — Methicillin, Cloxacillin, Oxacillin, Dicloxacillin, Nafcillin
    - **Extended spectrum penicillins**
      - **Aminopenicillins** — Ampicillin, Amoxicillin
      - **Antipseudomonal penicillins**
        - **Carboxypenicillins** — Carbenicillin, Ticarcillin
        - **Ureidopenicillins** — Piperacillin, Mezlocillin, Azlocillin

Penicillin G (Benzyl Penicillin/Crystalline Penicillin)

Penicillin G is the first antibiotic isolated from a fungus (*Penicillium notatum*). It is destroyed by gastric acid and hence not effective orally. It is short acting and is excreted intact by the kidneys by tubular secretion. Probenecid inhibits tubular secretion and prolongs duration of action of Penicillin.

It has narrow antimicrobial spectrum covering Gram +ve organisms (cocci and rods) and some Gram –ve cocci and anaerobes except *Bacteroides fragilis*. *Treponema pallidum* and *Borrelia burgdorferi* are extremely sensitive while *Leptospira* and *Actinomyces* are moderately sensitive to Penicillin G. *Staph. aureus* and Gonococci have become resistant to Penicillin G.

Penicillin G is the drug of choice for treatment of syphilis, streptococcal infections, actinomycosis, rheumatic fever, meningococcal infections, tetanus, gas gangrene and rat bite fever. Penicillin G can be made long acting by adding either procaine group (Procaine penicillin) or benzathine group (Benzathine penicillin) to it.

Benzathine penicillin G 1.2 million units given intramuscularly once a month is the drug of choice for secondary prophylaxis of rheumatic fever.

Penicillin V (Phenoxymethyl Penicillin)

It is an acid stable analog of Penicillin G and can be given orally. Antimicrobial spectrum is same as Penicillin G but it is less effective against *Neisseria sp*. Penicillin V 250 mg twice daily is an alternative to benzathine penicillin for prophylaxis of rheumatic fever.

Penicillinase Resistant Penicillins (Methicillin, Cloxacillin, Oxacillin, Dicloxacillin, Nafcillin)

They are highly effective against *Staphylococcus sp.* that produce penicillinase. They are used in the treatment of Staphylococcal infections. Methicillin is no longer used due to interstitial nephritis. Methicillin Resistant *Staph. aureus* (MRSA) have emerged and Vancomycin is used to treat MRSA infections.

Aminopenicillins (Ampicillin, Amoxycillin)

They have extended spectrum of activity which includes *Listeria monocytogenes, H. influenzae, E. coli, Salmonella, Shigella,* penicillin resistant pneumococci. However, they are susceptible to β-Lactamase and are not effective against *Pseudomonas, Klebsiella* and *Enterobacter* infections.

Ampicillin is partly excreted in bile and undergoes enterohepatic circulation. Amoxicillin is better absorbed than ampicillin. Aminopenicillins are used in the treatment of respiratory and urinary tract infections and enteric fever. Ampicillin is the drug of choice for meningitis caused by *Listeria monocytogenes*.

Carboxypenicillins (Carbenicillin, Ticarcillin)

They have good activity against *Pseudomonas* and *Proteus sp*. But they are not active against *Klebsiella sp*. Carbenicillin is not used currently due to bleeding tendencies but its indanyl ester salt is used orally in the treatment of urinary tract infections.

Ureidopenicillins (Piperacillin, Mezlocillin, Azlocillin)

In addition to *Pseudomonas* and *Proteus sp.* they are also active against *Klebsiella sp*. They are frequently combined with aminoglycosides for serious infections caused by Gram –ve organisms and in neutropenic patients with sepsis.

Dose of commonly used penicillins is given below.

Drug	Dose	Fortified preparations
Penicillin G	IV/IM : 2-24 million Units/day in 4-6 divided doses	Topical fortified drops: 1 Lakh Units/ml (Shelf life- 4 days*) Subconjunctival : 1 million Units
Penicillin V	PO : 1-2 g/day in 4 divided doses	---
Methicillin Cloxacillin Dicloxacillin Nafcillin Oxacillin	Cloxacillin and Dicloxacillin PO : 250-500 mg 6th hourly Nafcillin and Oxacillin IV : 1-2 g 4th – 6th hourly	Methicillin: Topical fortified drops: 50 mg/ml (Shelf life- 4 days*) Subconjunctival: 100 mg
Ampicillin Amoxicillin	PO: 250-500 mg 6th hourly (ampicillin) and 8th hourly (amoxicillin). IV/IM: Dose varies with indication	Ampicillin: Topical fortified drops: 50 mg/ml (Shelf life- 1 day*) Subconjunctival: 100 mg
Carbenicillin Ticarcillin	Ticarcillin: IV. 3g 4th – 6th hourly	Carbenicillin: Topical fortified drops: 4-6 mg/ml (Shelf life- 3 days*) Subconjunctival: 100 mg Intravitreal: 2 mg Ticarcillin: Fortified drops: 6-20 mg/ml Subconjunctival: 100 mg
Piperacillin Mezlocillin Azlocillin	Piperacillin: IV: 3-4 g 4th-6th hourly	Piperacillin: Topical fortified drops: 6-8 mg/ml (Shelf life- 3 days*) Subconjunctival: 100 mg
PO—Per Oral; IV—Intravenous; IM—Intramuscular * Shelf life if refrigerated proper		

Adverse Effects of Penicillins

- Hypersensitivity reactions (Minor rash to Anaphylaxis)
- Jarisch-Herxheimer reaction (when penicillin G is given to patient with syphilis)
- Pain on injection site
- Interstitial nephritis with methicillin
- Diarrhea with ampicillin
- Bleeding tendencies with carbenicillin
- Cross-sensitivity with other β-lactam antibiotics except Aztreonam. Aztreonam is the only β-lactam antibiotic which can be safely given to a patient allergic to penicillin.

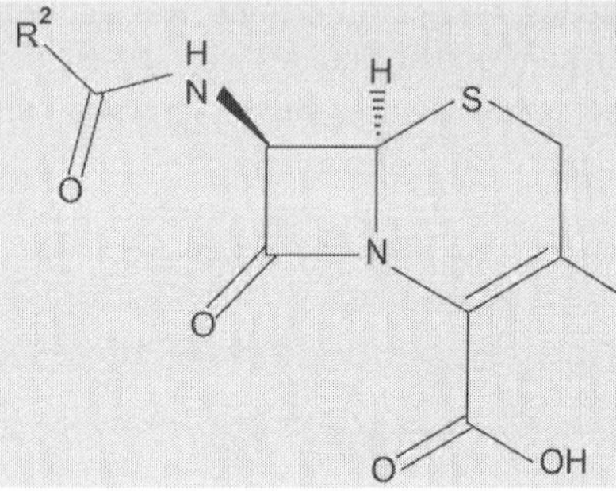

Fig. 7.5: Molecular structure of cephalosporins

β-Lactamase Inhibitors

β-Lactamase is an enzyme produced by the resistant bacteria that degrades β-lactam antibiotics. β-Lactamase inhibitors prevent the destruction of the antibiotic and thereby restores the antibacterial activity of these drugs. Three β-Lactamase inhibitors used clinically are:
1. Clavulanic acid
2. Sulbactam
3. Tazobactam

Clavulanic acid is frequently combined with Amoxicillin (Co-Amoxyclav), while sulbactam is combined with ampicillin and tazobactam is combined with piperacillin. Avibactam is a novel β-Lactamase inhibitor currently in phase 3 clinical trials.

Cephalosporins

Cephalosporins are obtained from a fungus *Cephalosporium*. These are derivatives of cephalosporin C produced by fungus *Cephalosporium acremonium*. Molecular structure (Fig. 7.5) is closely related to that of penicillins. Mode of action is similar to penicillins since both group posses β-lactam ring.

Cephalosporins are classified in to five generations based on antimicrobial activity and pharmacological properties:

Classification of cephalosporins				
1st generation cephalosporins	2nd generation cephalosporins	3rd generation cephalosporins	4th generation cephalosporins	5th generation cephalosporins*
Cephalexin	Cefuroxime	Cefotaxime	Cefepime	Ceftaroline
Cefadroxil	Cefoxitin	Ceftriaxone	Cefpirome	Ceftobiprole
Cefazolin	Cefotetan	Ceftizoxime		
Cephaloridine	Cefaclor	Ceftazidime		
		Cefoperazone		
		Cefixime		
		Cefpodoxime		
		Cefdinir		
		Ceftibuten		
		Moxalactam		

* Not available in India

None of the cephalosporins (except 5th generation) are active against MRSA.

First Generation Cephalosporins

They have good activity against gram +ve bacteria and relatively modest activity against Gram –ve microorganisms. Most gram +ve cocci except enterococci are susceptible.

Drug	Dose	Fortified preparations
Cefazolin	IV/IM : 1-6 g/day in 3-4 divided doses	Topical fortified drops: 50 mg/ml (Shelf life- 7 days*) Subconjunctival : 100 mg Intravitreal : 2 mg
Cephalexin	PO : 1-4 g/day in 4 divided doses	----
Cefadroxil	PO : 1-2 g/day in 2-4 divided doses	----
Cephradine	PO : 1-4 g/day in 4 divided doses	----
Cephalothin	Not used systemically	Subconjunctival : 50-100 mg
Cephaloridine	Not used systemically	Subconjunctival : 100 mg
PO—Per Oral; IV—Intravenous; IM—Intramuscular * Shelf life if refrigerated properly		

All these drugs are excreted by kidneys and hence dose reduction is mandated in renal impairment patients. They are used in treatment of staphylococcal and streptococcal infections. Cefazolin is used as a prophylactic antibiotic for surgical procedures due to its good tissue penetration.

Second Generation Cephalosporins

They have excellent activity against gram +ve organisms — *Staphylococcus* and *Streptococcus* except *Streptococcus faecalis* and are more active than 1st generation cephalosporins against gram –ve bacteria like *E. coli, Klebsiella, H. influenzae* but are inactive against *Pseudomonas*.

Drug	Dose	Fortified preparations
Cefuroxime	IV/IM : 0.75-1.5 g 8th hourly PO (Cefuroxime axetil) : 250-500 mg 12th hourly	----
Cefaclor	PO : 250-500 mg 8th hourly	----
Cefoxitin	IV/IM : 1-2 g 6th – 8th hourly	----
Cefotetan	IV/IM : 1-2 g 12th hourly	----
Cefmetazole	IV/IM : 1-4 g/day in 2-4 divided doses	----
PO—Per Oral; IV—Intravenous; IM—Intramuscular * Shelf life if refrigerated properly		

They are used in treatment of sinusitis, otitis media and lower respiratory tract infections. Cefoxitin, cefmetazole and cefotetan belong to cephamycins and are active against anaerobes like *Bacteroides fragilis*.

Third Generation Cephalosporins

These agents are mainly effective against gram –ve organisms and to some extent gram +ve organisms but not against staphylococci. Ceftazidime and cefoperazone are active against *Pseudomonas aeruginosa* while ceftizoxime and moxalactam are active against *Bacteroides fragilis*. Ceftriaxone and Cefotaxime can cross blood-brain barrier and attain therapeutic levels in CSF. Ceftriaxone and cefotaxime are active against penicillin resistant pneumococci. Ceftriaxone and cefoperazone are mainly excreted in bile and are safe in patients with renal impairment.

Drug	Dose	Fortified preparations
Cefotaxime	IV/IM : 1-2 g 6th – 12th hourly	Topical fortified drops: 50 mg/ml (Shelf life- 7 days*)
Ceftriaxone	IV/IM : 1-4 g/day in 1-2 divided doses	Topical fortified drops: 50 mg/ml (Shelf life- 7 days*)
Ceftizoxime	IV/IM: 1-2 g 8th – 12th hourly	Subconjunctival: 100 mg
Ceftazidime	IV/IM : 0.5-2 g 8th – 12th hourly	Topical fortified drops: 50 mg/ml (Shelf life- 7 days*) Intravitreal: 2.25 mg
Cefoperazone	IV/IM: 2-4 g/day in 2 divided doses	---
Cefixime	PO : 200-400 mg/day	---
Cefpodoxime	PO: 100-400 mg 12th hourly	---
Cefdinir	PO: 300 mg 12th hourly	---
Ceftibuten	PO: 400 mg/day	---
Moxalactam	IV/IM: 2-6 g/day in 2-3 divided doses	---
PO—Per Oral; IV—Intravenous; IM—Intramuscular; * Shelf life if refrigerated properly		

Ceftriaxone and cefotaxime are useful in treatment of meningitis. Ceftriaxone is preferred in treatment of gonorrhea and enteric fever. Ceftazidime has excellent activity against *Pseudomonas* and is frequently combined with aminoglycosides for treating *Pseudomonas* infections and in febrile neutropenic patients.

Fourth Generation Cephalosporins

They are highly active against gram –ve bacteria (including *Pseudomonas*) that are resistant to other cephalosporins especially enterobacteriaceae. They are also active against methicillin sensitive *Staphylococcus aureus* and penicillin resistant streptococci but not against MRSA.

Drug	Dose	Fortified preparations
Cefepime	IV: 0.5-2 g 8th – 12th hourly	----
Cefpirome	IV: 1-2 g 12th hourly	----

Fifth Generation Cephalosporins

They are active against methicillin resistant *Staphylococcus aureus* (MRSA) and penicillin resistant pneumococci. Ceftobiprole is also active against *Pseudomonas*.

Drug	Dose	Fortified preparations
Ceftaroline	IV: 600 mg 12th hourly	----
Ceftobiprole	IV: 500 mg 8th – 12th hourly	----

They are used in treatment of acute bacterial skin and skin structure infections and community acquired bacterial pneumonia.

Adverse Effects of Cephalosporins

- Hypersensitivity reactions (Minor rash to Anaphylaxis)
- Cross-reactivity with other β-Lactam antibiotics
- Diarrhea
- Pseudomembranous enterocolitis due to *C. difficile*
- Hypoprothrombinemia and bleeding (with cefoperazone, cefmetazole and cefotetan)
- Disulfiram like reactions with alcohol (with cefoperazone, cefmetazole and cefotetan)
- Pain on injection site
- Nephrotoxicity with cephaloridine and cephalothin.

Ocular Uses of Cephalosporins

Subconjunctival cephalosporins are used as adjuncts to aminoglycosides to enhance surgical prophylaxis. Intravitreal cephalosporins provide excellent adjunct to aminoglycosides in treatment of endophthalmitis. Ceftazidime with vancomycin or cefazolin with amikacin provide broad spectrum coverage on intravitreal administration.

After IV administration, vitreous levels of ceftriaxone achieved concentrations which exceed MIC for 90 percent of gram –ve rods and sensitive *Staphylococus aureus* except *Pseudomonas* and *Staphylococcus epidermidis*. Other cephalosporins do not achieve vitreous levels in bactericidal range. Hence systemic cephalosporins play a limited role in treatment of endophthalmitis. Aqueous and vitreous levels achieved with some cephalosporins are given in the below table.

Drug	Dose	Aqueous levels (µg/ml)	Vitreous levels (µg/ml)
Cephalexin	2 g (Oral)	1.2	-
Cefoxitin	2 g (IV)	3.1	-
Ceftazidime	2 g (IV)	3.39	-
Cefuroxime	1.5 g (Oral/IV)	2.7-6.2	-
Moxalactam	2 g (IV)	2.4-9.6	-
Ceftizoxime	2 g (IV)		7.8
Cefpirome	1 g (IV)	-	1.29-1.33
	2 g (IV)	-	1.6-2.39
Ceftriaxone	1 g (IV)	-	0.93
	2 g (IV)	-	2.47

Topical cephalosporins are useful in treatment of severe bacterial conjunctivitis and keratitis and give excellent results when combined with topical aminoglycosides. Topical cefazolin alternating with topical aminoglycosides every 30 minutes round the clock is the most commonly used preparation for severe bacterial corneal ulcer.

Monobactams—Aztreonam

Aztreonam is the only monobactam in clinical use. It is active against aerobic gram-negative bacteria including *Pseudomonas*. It is not active against anaerobes and gram +ve bacteria. Its antimicrobial spectrum resembles that of aminoglycosides. The structure of aztreonam is shown in Figure 7.6.

It is used in treatment of infections caused by gram –ve bacteria in a dose of 1-2 g 6th-8th hourly. The characteristic feature of aztreonam is that it is safe in patients allergic to penicillins and cephalosporins (except ceftazidime).

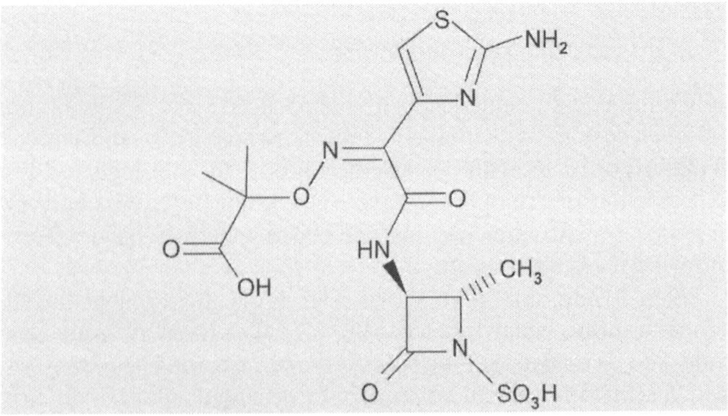

Fig. 7.6: Molecular structure of aztreonam

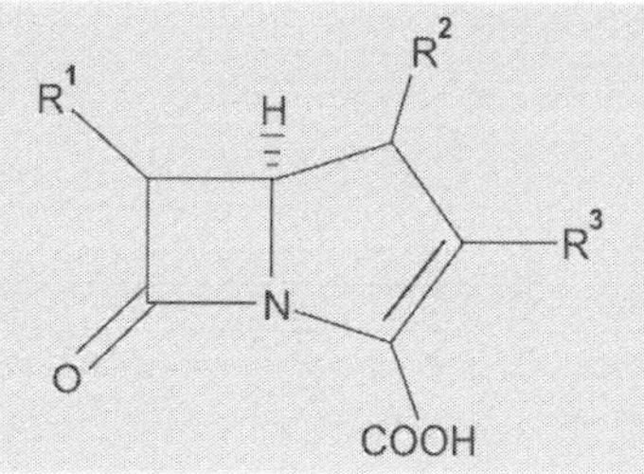

Fig. 7.7: Molecular structure of carbapenems

Carbapenems

They have wide antimicrobial spectrum that includes gram -ve bacteria (including *Pseudomonas*), gram +ve bacteria and anaerobes. They are resistant to hydrolysis by most β-lactamases including extended spectrum β-lactamase (ESBL) but are susceptible to metallo-β-lactamase.

The dose of clinically used carbapenems is given below:

Drug	Dose	Comments
Imipenem	IV: 0.25-1 g 6th – 8th hourly	Degraded by renal dehydropeptidase enzyme; hence combined with cilastatin which inhibits the enzyme
Ertapenem	IV/IM: 1 g/day	No need to combine with cilastatin. Ertapenem has long t½ and given once daily
Doripenem	IV: 500 mg 8th hourly	
Meropenem	IV: 1 g 8th hourly	

Carbapenems are used in treatment of mixed aerobic and anaerobic infections and in resistant infections. They are used in treatment of febrile neutropenic patients (±aminoglycosides).

Adverse Effects of Carbapenems

- Nausea, vomiting, diarrhea
- High dose imipenem can cause seizures in renal failure patients
- Cross-reactivity with other β-lactam antibiotics.

GLYCOPEPTIDE ANTIBIOTICS

The glycopeptide antibiotics in clinical use are vancomycin, teicoplanin and telavancin. Dalbavancin and oritavancin are newer drugs under clinical trials. All of them are bactericidal agents.

Mechanism of Action

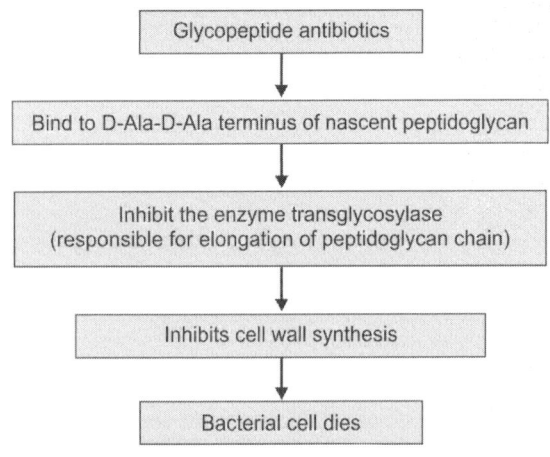

Mode of Resistance

Bacterial resistance to vancomycin is due to alteration of binding site D-Ala–D-Ala to either D-Ala–D-lactate or D-Ala–D-serine.

Antimicrobial Spectrum

Have excellent activity against gram +ve bacteria including MRSA and enterococci. However, they are inactive against gram –ve bacteria and mycobacteria. Vancomycin exhibits synergistic bactericidal activity with aminoglycosides against enterococci.

Drug	Dose	Fortified preparations	Comments
Vancomycin	IV: 2 g/day in 2-4 divided doses	Topical fortified drops: 25-50 mg/ml (Shelf life- 4 days*) Subconjunctival: 25 mg Intravitreal: 1-2 mg	Oral vancomycin 0.5-2 g/day in 2-4 divided doses is used in treatment of pseudomembranous enterocolitis
Teicoplanin	IV: 200-400 mg/day	----	Long t½; used once daily
Telavancin	IV: 10 mg/kg/day	----	In addition to inhibition of transglycosylase, it also disrupts membrane potential

Vancomycin is the drug of choice for MRSA infections. It is also used in treatment of enterococcal endocarditis and in meningitis caused by *Streptococcus pneumoniae*. Oral vancomycin is used

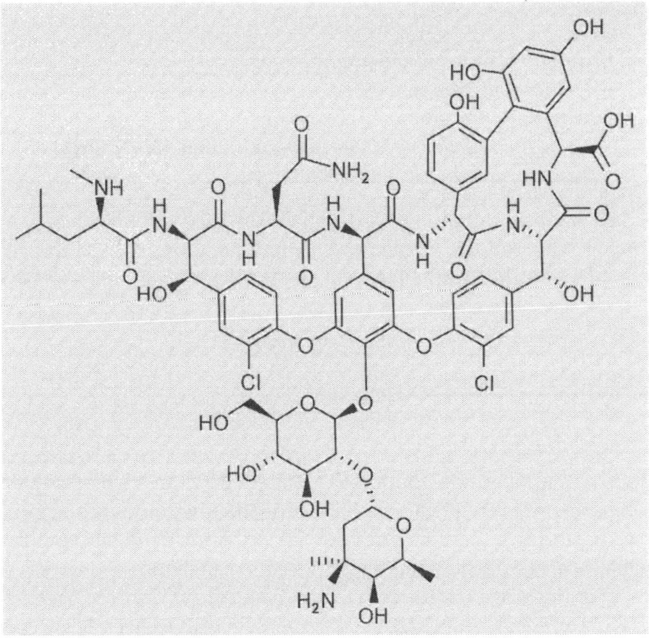

Fig. 7.8: Chemical structure of vancomycin

in treatment of pseudomembranous enterocolitis. Intravitreal vancomycin with an aminoglycoside has been recommended as initial empiric therapy for bacterial endophthalmitis. A dose of 1 mg in 0.1 ml intravitreally establishes intraocular levels significantly higher than MIC for most gram-posititve organisms.

Adverse Effects

- Red man syndrome due to histamine release (with vancomycin)
- Chills and fever
- Ototoxicity and nephrotoxicity at high doses.

FOSFOMYCIN

It inhibits the enzyme enolpyruvate transferase and thereby inhibiting cell wall synthesis. Antimicrobial spectrum includes both gram +ve and –ve bacteria. It is used in the treatment of uncomplicated urinary tract infections.

BACITRACIN

It is a polypeptide antibiotic obtained from *Bacillus subtilis*. It is mainly active against gram +ve bacteria. It interferes with dephosphorylation of bactoprenol which transfers the peptidoglycan unit to growing cell wall and thus inhibits bacterial cell wall synthesis. Due to nephrotoxicity it is used only topically.

Dosage

- Commercially available preparations
  - *Ointment:* 500 units/g
- Fortified preparations
  - *Fortified eyedrops:* 10000 units/ml (Shelf life—7 days)
  - *Subconjunctival:* 5000-10000 units

It is often combined with polymyxin-B or neomycin in the topical preparations. Ocular uses include treatment of superficial eye infections like staphylococcal blepharitis.

DRUGS ATTACKING BACTERIAL CELL MEMBRANE

Daptomycin

It is a lipopeptide antibiotic obtained from *Streptomyces roseosporus*. It is highly bactericidal drug that mainly acts on gram +ve bacteria. It depolarizes the cell membrane of susceptible bacteria and leads to potassium efflux and cell death.

It is active against vancomycin resistant *Staphylococcus aureus* (VRSA) and vancomycin resistant enterococci. It is given in a dose of 6 mg/kg for treatment of skin and soft tissue infections and bacteremia caused by gram +ve organisms. Adverse effects include myopathy and diarrhea.

Polymixin-B, Colistin and Tyrothricin

These agents are polypeptide antibiotics that attack the bacterial cell membrane by their detergent like action. They are bactericidal drugs but are not used systemically due to nephrotoxicity and neurotoxicity. Polymixin B is mainly effective against gram –ve bacteria. They are used topically in treatment of skin diseases and superficial eye infections.

Dosage of Polymixin-B

- Commercially available preparations
  - *Ointment:* 10000 units/g
- Fortified preparations
  - *Fortified eyedrops:* 50000 units/ml (Shelf life—3 days)
  - *Subconjunctival:* 100000 units

DRUGS THAT INHIBIT BACTERIAL PROTEIN SYNTHESIS

Aminoglycosides

They are bactericidal drugs obtained from soil actinomycetes. They contain two or more amino sugars glycosidally linked to hexose

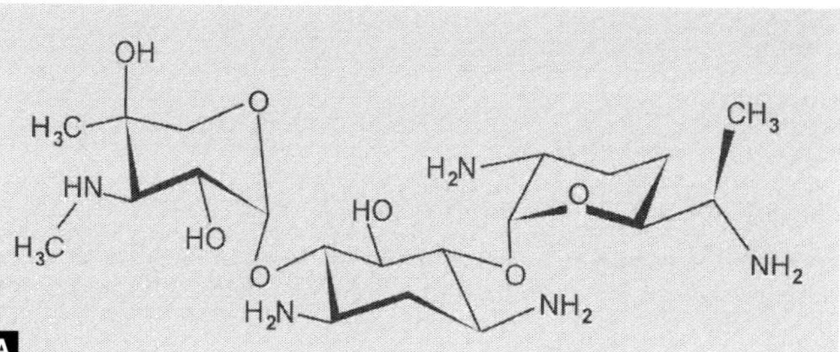

A

Gentamicin

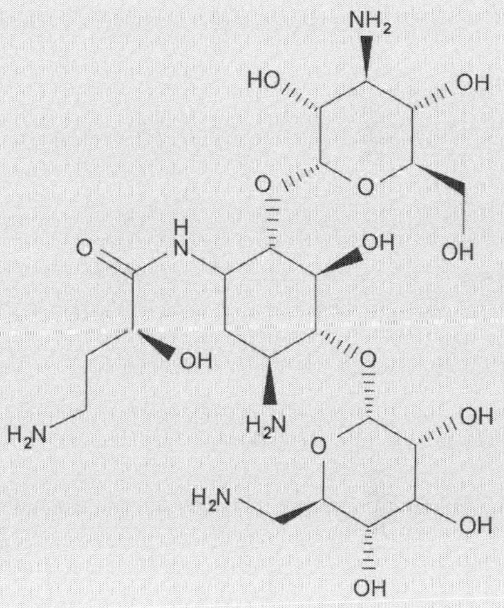

B

Amikacin

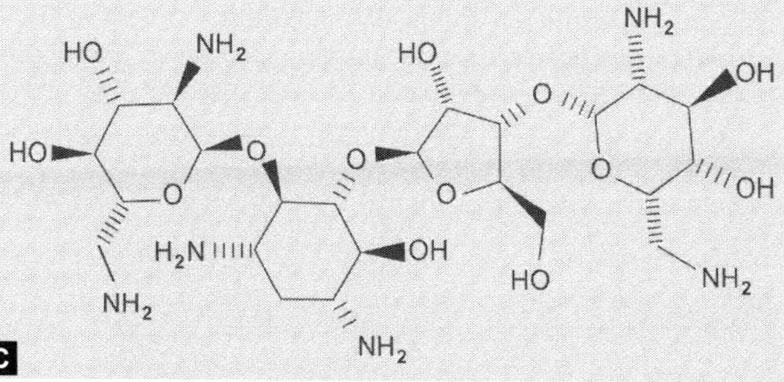

C

Neomycin

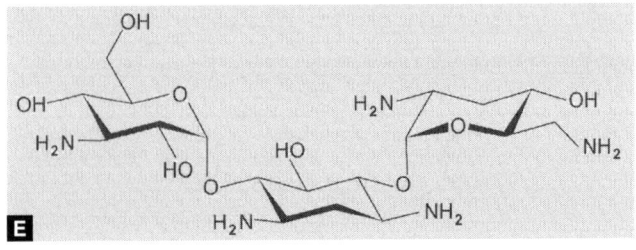

Figs 7.9A to E: Chemical structures of aminoglycosides

or aminocyclitol. They are poorly absorbed orally and hence usually given parenterally or topically. They exhibit concentration dependent killing as mentioned previously and have a narrow therapeutic margin. Hence therapeutic drug monitoring plays a key role in optimizing the dosage of these drugs.

Aminoglycosides are one among the most commonly used antibiotics in ophthalmic practice. Clinically useful aminoglycosides include streptomycin, gentamicin, neomycin, kanamycin, amikacin, tobramycin, sisomicin and netilmicin. Molecular structures of some of them are shown below in Figures 7.9A to E.

Mechanism of Action

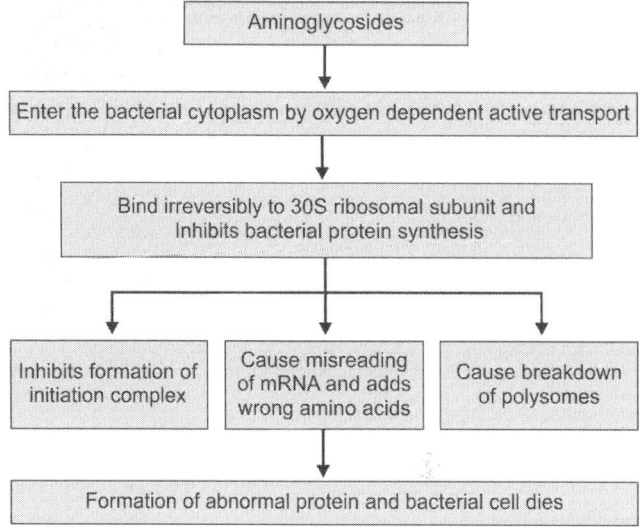

Antimicrobial Spectrum

They are mainly active against aerobic gram –ve bacteria including *Pseudomonas*. They are inactive against anaerobes. Aminoglycosides exhibit synergistic bactericidal effects when used along with cell wall inhibitors like penicillins or vancomycin.

Mode of Resistance

- Production of enzymes that inactive aminoglycosides
- Impaired entry of the drug into the bacterial cell
- Alteration of binding site in 30S ribosomal subunit.

Amikacin and netilmicin are least susceptible to enzymatic destruction and hence are active against the bacteria that are resistant to other aminoglycosides.

Systemic Uses

These agents are used in treatment of gram negative infections, urinary tract infections, pneumonia, meningitis, peritonitis, *Pseudomonas* infection in burns patients and sepsis usually in combination with penicillins or cephalosporins.

Orally administered neomycin is useful in treatment of hepatic encephalopathy. It acts by suppressing the gut flora which acts as the main source for ammonia production in the intestinal tract.

Streptomycin is a commonly used first line antitubercular drug while amikacin and kanamycin are used as second line agents in treatment of resistant tuberculosis.

Adverse Effects

- Ototoxicity (cochlear and vestibular toxicity)
- Nephrotoxicity
- Neuromuscular blockade
- Rarely hypersensitivity reactions
- Teratogenicity.

Amikacin, neomycin and kanamycin produce cochlear toxicity while streptomycin and gentamicin produce vestibular toxicity. Netilmicin is the least ototoxic aminoglycoside.

Neomycin, tobramycin and gentamicin are highly nephrotoxic while streptomycin is least nephrotoxic. Hence dose reduction is mandatory in patients with renal impairment.

Neomycin and streptomycin produce maximum neuromuscular blockade while tobramycin produces least neuromuscular toxicity.

INDIVIDUAL DRUGS

Gentamicin

It is a commonly used aminoglycoside in ophthalmic practice. It is obtained from *Micromonospora purpurea*. It is active against aerobic gram –ve bacteria like *E. coli*, *Klebsiella*, *Pseudomonas*, *Enterobacter* and *Proteus*.

Dosage

- *Parenteral (IV/IM):* 3 mg/kg/day
- Commercially available ophthalmic preparations
  - *Drops:* 0.3 percent
  - *Ointment:* 0.3 percent
- Fortified preparations
  - *Fortified eyedrops:* 16-20 mg/ml (Shelf life—30 days)
  - *Subconjunctival:* 10-20 mg
  - *Intravitreal:* 200-400 µg

Ocular Uses

Topically it is used in the treatment of superficial eye infections like bacterial conjunctivitis. Topical drops achieve concentrations sufficient to treat ocular surface infections while fortified eyedrops are required to achieve therapeutic levels consistently in the anterior chamber. Fortified gentamicin eyedrops in combination with cephalosporins or vancomycin is frequently used as initial empiric treatment of bacterial corneal ulcer.

Systemically administered gentamicin is useful in treatment of ocular injuries with retained foreign bodies while intravitreal injection of 200–400 µg is used in case of endophthalmitis. Gentamicin is more toxic to retina than amikacin.

Subconjunctival gentamicin produces local toxicity which manifests as papillary mydriasis, conjunctival paresthesias and delay in corneal wound healing.

Tobramycin

It is obtained from cultures of *Streptomyces tenebrarius*. Its antimicrobial spectrum and pharmacokinetics are similar to gentamicin. It is highly effective against *Pseudomonas* when compared to gentamicin.

Dosage

- *Parenteral (IV/IM):* 3-5 mg/kg/day
- *Nebulization/Inhalation:* 300 mg 12th hourly
- Commercially available ophthalmic preparations
  - *Drops:* 0.3 percent
  - *Ointment:* 0.3 percent
- Fortified preparations
  - *Fortified eyedrops:* 16-20 mg/ml (Shelf life—30 days)
  - *Subconjunctival:* 10-20 mg
  - *Intravitreal:* 200-400 µg

Uses

Inhaled tobramycin is used in treatment of respiratory infections due to pseudomonas in cystic fibrosis patients. Other uses of tobramycin are similar to gentamicin.

Amikacin

It is a semisynthetic aminoglycoside that is derived from kanamycin, due to which it is resistant to enzymatic destruction. It is active against many gram –ve bacteria that are resistant to gentamicin. Among the aminoglycosides, amikacin has the lowest frequency of resistant strains so far reported.

Dosage

- *Parenteral (IV/IM):* 15 mg/kg/day
- Commercially available ophthalmic preparations
  - *Drops:* 0.5-1 percent
- Fortified preparations
  - *Fortified eyedrops:* 20 mg/ml (Shelf life—30 days)
  - *Subconjunctival:* 125 mg
  - *Intravitreal:* 400 µg

Ocular Uses

Intravitreal injection of amikacin in combination with vancomycin or cephalosporins is used in the treatment of bacterial endophthalmitis. Intravitreal amikacin in concentration of 400 µg in 0.1 ml is nontoxic to the retina. Retinal toxicity with intravitreal amikacin occurs only in dose 1500 µg compared with 400 µg of gentamicin or 800 µg of tobramycin. Hence in sight threatening endophthalmitis, amikacin offers a broader spectrum with less toxicity.

Topical use of amikacin in the treatment of bacterial keratitis should be restricted to culture proven organisms that are resistant to gentamicin and tobramycin. Subconjunctival injection gives adequate bactericidal concentration in the anterior chamber without systemic toxicity.

Neomycin

It is obtained from *Streptomyces fradiae*. It is usually used in combination with polymixin-B, gramicidin or bacitracin for a broad spectrum antibiotic coverage.

Dosage

- *Parenteral (IV/IM):* 15 mg/kg/day
- Commercially available ophthalmic preparations
  - *Drops:* 0.3 percent
  - *Ointment:* 0.3 percent
- Fortified preparations
  - *Fortified eyedrops:* 30-40 mg/ml (Shelf life—3-7 days)
  - *Subconjunctival:* 100 mg

Various combinations available commercially:
- Neomycin/Polymixin B/Bacitracin combination:
  Topical ophthalmic oint: 5000 units/g Polymixin B, 500 units/g Bacitracin and 5 mg/gm neomycin.
- Neomycin/Polymixin B combination:
  Topical ophthalmic oint: 6000 units/g Polymixin B and 5 mg/g Neomycin.
- Neomycin/Polymixin B/Gramicidin combination:
  Topical ophthalmic solution: 1.75 mg neomycin, 10000 units of Polymixin B and 0.025 mg gramicidin/ml.
  Neomycin is also used in the treatment of acanthamoeba keratitis in combination of other antiacanthamoeba drugs.

Sisomycin

It has antibacterial activity similar to gentamicin. It is effective in gentamicin and tobramycin resistant strains.

Dosage

- Commercially available ophthalmic preparations
  - *Drops:* 0.3 percent
  - *Ointment:* 0.3 percent
- Fortified preparations
  - *Fortified eyedrops:* 20 mg/ml (Shelf life—30 days)
  - *Subconjunctival:* 20-80 mg

Netilmicin

It is N-ethyl derivative of sisomycin and has antibacterial activity similar to that of tobramycin.

Dosage

- *Parenteral (IV/IM):* 4-6 mg/kg/day
- Fortified preparations
  - *Subconjunctival:* 20-40 mg

Kanamycin

It is obtained from *Streptomyces kanamyceticus*. It is used for streptomycin resistant gram –ve bacillary infections and resistant tuberculosis. It is not active against *Pseudomonas*.

Dosage

- *Parenteral (IV/IM):* 15 mg/kg/day
- Fortified preparations
  - *Fortified eyedrops:* 10 mg/ml

Framycetin

Its antibacterial activity is similar to that of neomycin.
- Commercially available ophthalmic preparations
  - *Drops:* 0.5 percent
  - *Ointment:* 0.5-1 percent

Streptomycin

It is obtained from *Streptomyces griseus*. It is antimicrobial activity is similar to that of other aminoglycosides. It is commonly used in the treatment of tuberculosis as a first line drug. Other uses include tularemia, plague and brucellosis. It is not commonly used in ophthalmic practice.

SPECTINOMYCIN

It is an aminocyclitol antibiotic closely related to aminoglycosides but it lacks the sugar moiety. It shares the same mechanism of action with aminoglycosides. It is used as 2 g single dose intramuscular injection for treatment of gonorrheal urethritis, cervicitis and proctitis in penicillin allergic and drug resistant patients.

TETRACYCLINES

They are broad spectrum bacteriostatic antibiotics which inhibit bacterial protein synthesis. Oral bioavailability varies with individual drugs and absorption of tetracyclines is impaired by the presence of food, antacids, calcium and iron salts. The structure of tetracycline is shown in Figure 7.10.

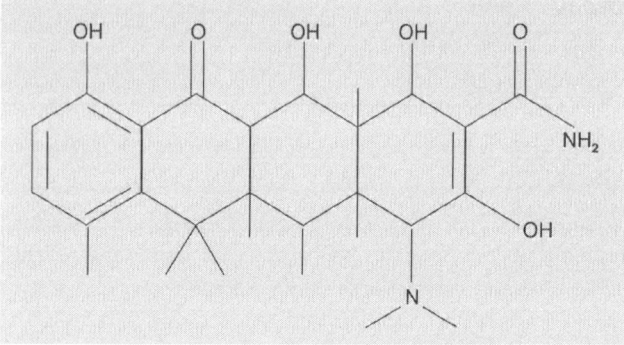

Fig. 7.10: Chemical structure of tetracyclines

Classification

Tetracyclines are classified into three groups based on duration of action as given here:

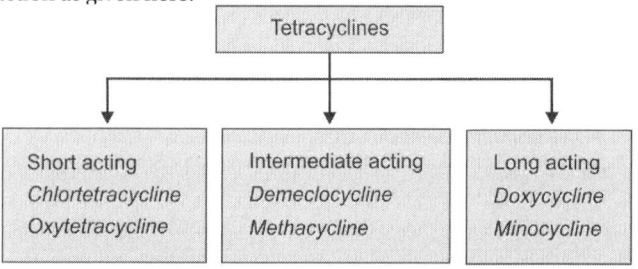

Mechanism of Action

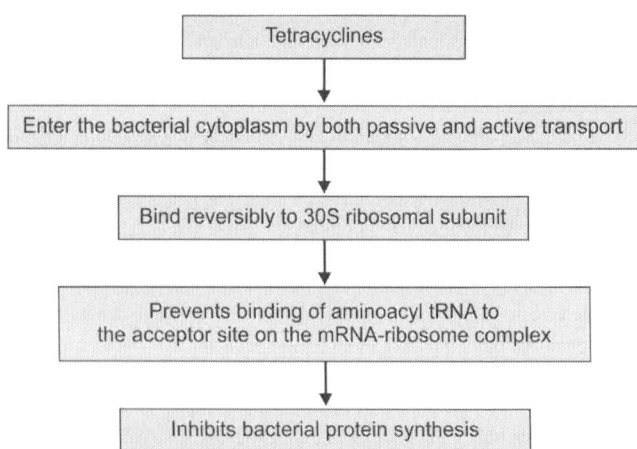

Antimicrobial Spectrum

They have broad antimicrobial spectrum that includes gram +ve and gram –ve bacteria, anaerobes, rickettsiae, chlamydiae, mycoplasma and some protozoa. But they are not active against proteus, serratia and *Pseudomonas*.

Mode of Resistance

- Impaired entry into the cell or increased efflux from the cell through efflux pump
- Ribosomal protection due to synthesis of some proteins that hamper the binding of the drug to 30S ribosomal subunit
- Inactivation of the drug by enzymes.

Adverse Effects

- GI disturbance—Nausea, vomiting, diarrhea
- Occurrence of superinfections due to suppression of normal bacterial flora
- Photosensitivity reactions and rash
- Fanconi syndrome with out-dated tetracyclines
- Teratogenicity
- Discoloration of teeth and bony deformity in children.

All tetracyclines are contraindicated in renal failure except doxycycline because doxycycline is excreted in bile and is safe in renal impairment.

Dosage

Drug	Systemic dose	Ophthalmic preparations
Tetracycline	PO: 1-2 g/day in 2-4 divided doses	1 percent ophthalmic drops 1 percent ophthalmic ointment
Oxytetracycline	PO : 500 mg 6th hourly	1 percent ointment commercially available
Chlortetracycline	----	1 percent ointment commercially available
Demeclocycline	PO: 150 mg 6th hourly or 300 mg 12th hourly	
Doxycycline	PO: 100-200 mg 12th hourly	----
Minocycline	PO: 50-200 mg 12th hourly IV: 100-200 mg/day	----

Systemic Uses of Tetracyclines

Tetracyclines are the drug of choice for treatment of infections caused by chlamydiae, rickettsiae and *Mycoplasma pneumoniae*. Tetracyclines are commonly employed in combination therapy for eradication of *H. pylori* infection implicated in peptic ulcer disease. Doxycycline is used in treatment of cholera, acne vulgaris, leptospirosis and malaria. Tetracycline combined with aminoglycosides is preferred in treatment of plague, tularemia and brucellosis. Minocycline is useful in eradication of meningococcal carrier state. Demeclocycline is the drug of choice for treatment of SIADH (Syndrome of inappropriate secretion of antidiuretic hormone).

Ocular Uses of Tetracyclines

Surface ocular infections caused by susceptible microorganisms respond well to topical tetracycline despite poor intraocular penetration. Large oral dosage (6-8 gm/day) produces demonstrable aqueous concentration and may be advised for the treatment of intraocular infections.

- Chlamydial disease: Systemic tetracycline is used in treatment of adult inclusion conjunctivitis acquired from genital contact. A three-week course of tetracycline or minocycline is recommended and effective.
- Topical tetracycline is used in prophylaxis for ophthalmia neonatorum in newborn.
- Acute trachoma may be cured by topical and systemic tetracycline. Treatment should be continued for 2-4 weeks.
- Phlyctenular keratoconjuctivitis: It is considered to be a nonspecific hypersensitive reaction to bacterial proteins and responds well to systemic tetracycline.
- Toxoplasmosis: Combination of minocycline and sulfadiazine is useful for treatment of active toxoplasmic retinochoroiditis.
- Ocular rosacea: Tetracycline 1 g/day for 4-6 weeks followed by a slow taper to 250 mg every 1-2 days is useful in treatment of ocular rosacea. The clinical improvement results from reduced lipase production by staphylococci as well as reduction in microflora.
- Spirochetal infection: Tetracycline or doxycycline is recommended for the treatment of Lyme disease. Tetracycline is an acceptable alternative in treatment of syphilis.
- Persistent epithelial defects: Persistent epithelial defects are caused by tissue and leukocytic collagenases. Tetracyclines have anticollagenolytic effect independent of their antimicrobial properties. Systemic tetracyclines have been useful in healing persistent epithelial defects.
- Identification of neoplasms: Oxytetracycline is preferentially concentrated in rapidly growing neoplastic tissues. The presence of oxytetracycline in tissue can be detected at the time of surgery by examination under UV light which causes a brilliant yellow fluorescence. This method of tumor detection is applicable to surgery of orbital neoplasms. The dose of oxytetracycline for the fluorescent detection of neoplasm is 15 mg/kg/day for three days.

GLYCYLCYCLINE—TIGECYCLINE

Tigecycline is a newer antibacterial agent that belongs to glycylcyline group. It is a bacteriostatic agent and derived from minocycline. It has a very broad antimicrobial spectrum that includes both gram +ve and gram –ve bacteria, anaerobes and

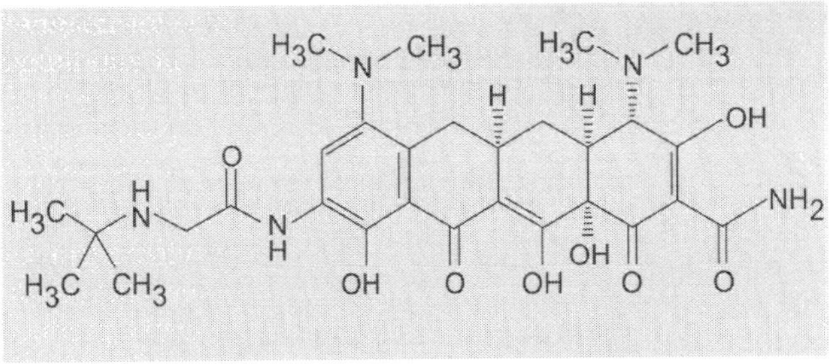

Fig. 7.11: Chemical structure of tigecycline

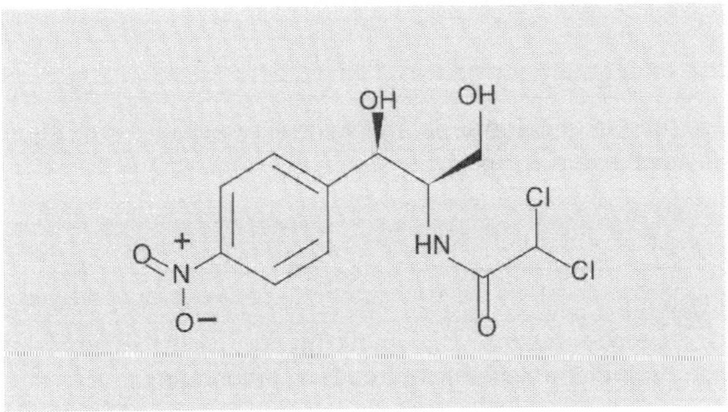

Fig. 7.12: Chemical structure of chloramphenicol

atypical agents. It is active against MRSA, VRSA, coagulase negative *Staphylococcus aureus*, vancomycin resistant enterococci and other multidrug resistant strains including tetracycline resistant strains but not against *Pseudomonas* and proteus. It is eliminated in bile and hence no dose reduction is needed in renal insufficiency.

Dosage: 100 mg IV stat followed by 50 mg 12th hourly.

Uses: It is used in treatment of complicated skin and skin structure infections, community acquired pneumonia and intra-abdominal infections.

CHLORAMPHENICOL

It is a broad-spectrum bacteriostatic antibiotic obtained from *Streptomyces venezuelae*. It is ideally suited for topical use in eye as it has least tendency to produce allergic reactions and has good corneal and intraocular penetration due to its high lipid solubility.

Antimicrobial Spectrum

It is broad spectrum antibiotic effective against a wide range of gram +ve and –ve bacteria including anaerobes but is not active against *Pseudomonas*.

Mechanism of Action

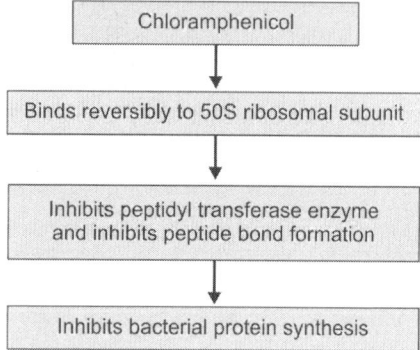

Mode of Resistance

By production of chloramphenicol acetyl transferase enzyme that inactivates the drug.

Dosage

- Systemic
  - *Oral/Parenteral (IV):* 50-100 mg/kg/day in 4 divided doses
- Commercially available ophthalmic preparations
  - *Drops:* 0.5-1 percent
  - *Ointment:* 0.5-1 percent
- Fortified preparations
  - *Fortified eyedrops:* 5-10 mg/ml
  - *Subconjunctival:* 50-100 mg
  - *Intravitreal:* 1-2 mg

Ocular Uses

It was used as a topical antibiotic in treatment of bacterial conjunctivitis but currently it has very limited use due to occurrence of aplastic anemia even with topical applications.

Adverse Effects

- Reversible bone marrow depression
- Aplastic anemia (idiosyncratic reaction)
- Superinfections
- Gray baby syndrome in infants.

MACROLIDES

They are bacteriostatic drugs that contain a lactone ring attached to deoxy sugar. Macrolides in clinical use are erythromycin, roxithromycin, clarithromycin and azithromycin. Erythromycin is obtained from *Streptomyces erythreus*. Clarithromycin and azithromycin are derived from erythromycin. The chemical structures of macrolides are shown in Figures 7.13A to D.

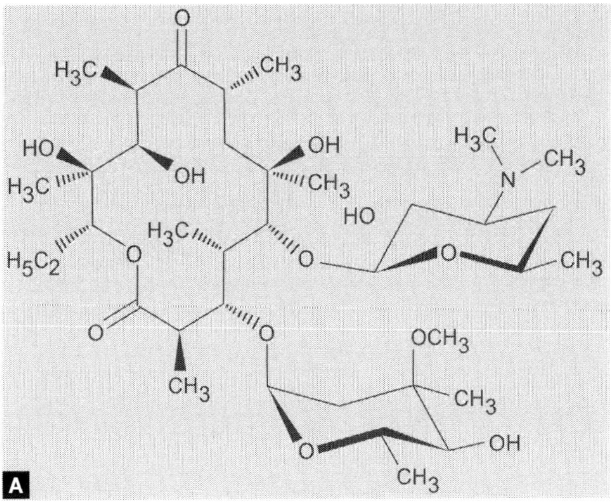

A Erythromycin

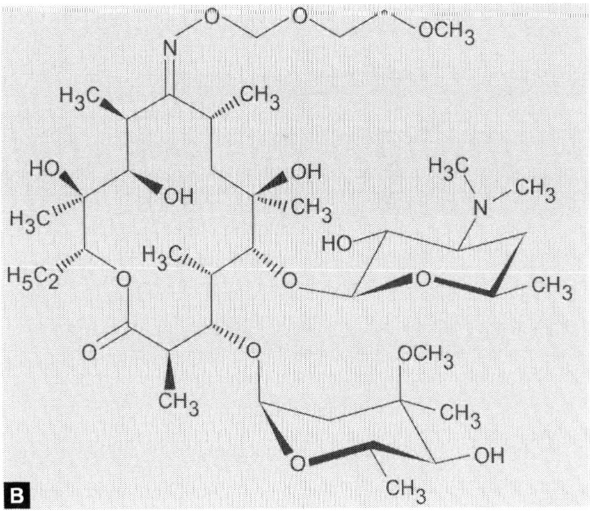

B Roxithromycin

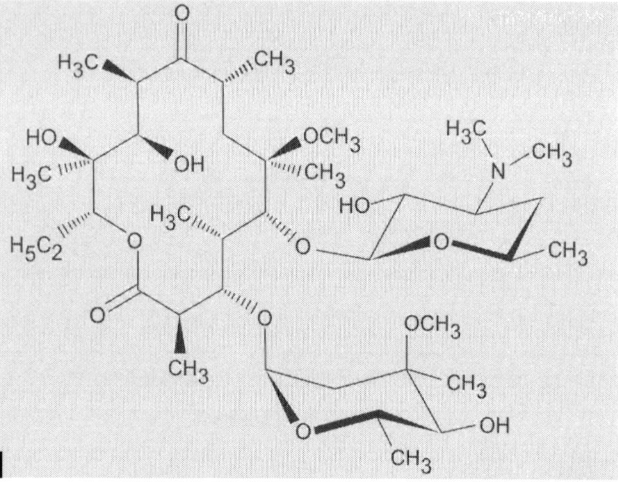

Clarithromycin

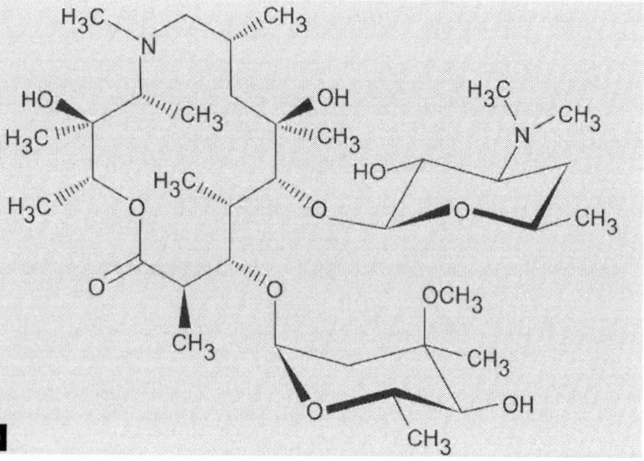

Azithromycin

Figs 7.13A to D: Molecular structure of macrolides (A) Erythromycin; (B) Roxithromycin; (C) Clarithromycin and (D) Azithromycin

Mechanism of Action

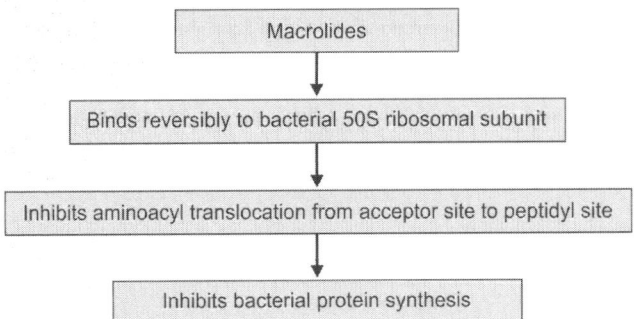

Mode of Resistance

- Increased efflux of the drug by active efflux pump
- Production of enzymes (esterases) that inactivate the drug
- Ribosomal protection due to synthesis of some proteins that hamper the binding of the drug to 50S ribosomal subunit.

INDIVIDUAL DRUGS

Erythromycin

Erythromycin is a bacteriostatic drug but becomes bactericidal in high concentrations. It is active against gram +ve bacteria like staphylococci, streptococci, pneumococci and cornybacteria, mycoplasma, legionella, chlamydia, gram –ve bacteria like *Neisseria, Bordetella, Campylobacter, H. influenzae* and some *Rickettsia*. It is also effective against certain mycobacterial species. It is mainly excreted in bile.

Dosage

- Systemic dose
  - *Oral:* 1-4 g/day in 4 divided doses
  - *Parenteral (IV):* 1-2 g/day in 2-4 divided doses
- *Topical gel/ cream for acne vulgaris:* 2 percent
- Commercially available ophthalmic preparations
  - *Ointment:* 0.5 percent
- Fortified preparations
  - *Fortified eyedrops:* 25 mg/ml
  - *Subconjunctival:* 50-100 mg
  - *Intravitreal:* 500 µg

Adverse Effects

- GI intolerance—Nausea, vomiting, diarrhea
- Cholestatic hepatitis
- Erythromycin is a CYP450 enzyme inhibitor and hence involved in many drug interactions.

Roxithromycin

It is a semisynthetic macrolide which has similar antimicrobial spectrum to that of erythromycin. It has low affinity for CYP450 enzymes and has less drug interactions when compared to erythromycin. It is better absorbed in empty stomach and is given at a dose of 150 mg twice daily for treatment of susceptible infections. The main adverse effect is gastrointestinal intolerance.

Clarithromycin

It is a semisynthetic derivative of erythromycin and has better bioavailability following oral administration. Antimicrobial spectrum is similar to that of erythromycin but it is more active against *Mycobacterium avium* complex (MAC) than any other macrolide. It is also active against *Mycobacterium leprae* and *Toxoplasma gondii*.

Dosage: 250-500 mg 12th hourly orally.

Adverse Effects

It is a potent CYP450 enzyme inhibitor and hence involved in many drug interactions. However, it produces less GI intolerance when compared to erythromycin.

Azithromycin

It is also a semisynthetic derivative of erythromycin. Absorption is better in empty stomach. It has long half life which makes it suitable for once daily administration. It has excellent tissue penetration. Antimicrobial spectrum is similar to that of clarithromycin. It is more active against *H. influenzae* and *Chlamydia* but less effective against gram +ve bacteria when compared to erythromycin. In ophthalmic use, azithromycin is the preferred drug in the management of trachoma.

Dosage

- Systemic dose
    - Oral: 0.5-1g once daily
    - Parenteral (IV): 500 mg/day
- Commercially available ophthalmic preparations
    - Drops: 1 percent.

Adverse Effect

It does not inhibit CYP450 enzymes and hence is free of drug interactions.

Spiramycin

It is a macrolide antibiotic obtained from *Streptomyces ambofaciens*. It is used in the treatment of acute toxoplasmosis in pregnancy and in congenital toxoplasmosis.

Uses of Macrolides

Macrolides are the drug of choice for treatment of respiratory tract infections, community acquired pneumonia, diphtheria, erythrasma, pertussis, chancroid due to *Haemophilus ducreyi* and infections caused by *Mycoplasma, Chlamydia, Legionella* and *Campylobacter jejuni*.

Clarithromycin is used in combination therapy for eradication of *H. pylori* infection that causes peptic ulcer and in treatment of leprosy along with minocycline.

Azithromycin is preferred for treatment of chlamydial infections and repiratory tract infections especially those caused by *H. influenzae*.

Clarithromycin and azithromycin are used in prophylaxis as well as treatment of MAC infection in HIV patients.

Erythromycin is an alternative drug for prophylaxis of rheumatic fever in penicillin allergic patients.

Topical azithromycin is used in the treatment of bacterial conjunctivitis. Erythromycin ointment is used in prophylaxis of neonatal gonococcal and chlamydial conjunctivitis in the newborns.

KETOLIDES—TELITHROMYCIN

They are semisynthetic macrolides that have a 3-keto group in its structure. Telithromycin is the only antibiotic in this group. It is less susceptible to the efflux pumps and hence it is active against macrolide resistant strains. Antimicrobial spectrum is similar to that of macrolides. Molecular structure of telithromycin is shown in Figure 7.14.

Telithromycin is used in the treatment of respiratory tract infections including community acquired pneumonia caused by multidrug resistant pneumocooci, *Moraxella catarrhalis, Chlamydophila pneumoniae, Haemophilus influenzae* and *Mycoplasma pneumoniae*, bronchitis, sinusitis and streptococcal pharyngitis.

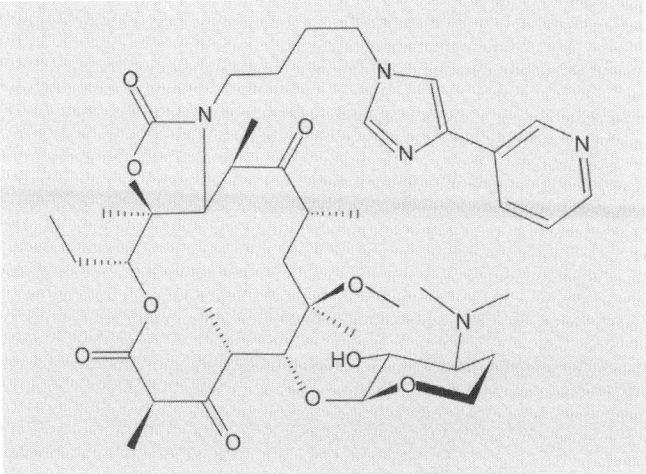

Fig. 7.14: Chemical structure of telithromycin

Dosage

800 mg once daily orally.

Adverse Effects

Hepatotoxicity, drug interaction due to CYP450 enzyme inhibition.

OXAZOLIDINONES—LINEZOLID

Linezolid is a synthetic agent and the only member of this group currently in clinical use. Other oxazolidinones in clinical trials are Torezolid, Posizolid and Radezolid. Systemically administered linezolid has good intraocular penetration. The chemical structure of linezolid is given in Figure 7.15.

Antimicrobial Spectrum

It is highly active against gram +ve bacteria (both aerobic and anaerobic) including staphylococci (including MRSA), streptococci, enterococci (including vancomycin resistant enterococci), corynebacteria and *Listeria monocytogenes*. It is a bacteriostatic agent but it is cidal for streptococci. It has some activity against *Mycobacterium tuberculosis*. But it is not active against gram –ve organisms.

Mechanism of Action

It binds to bacterial 50S ribosomal subunit and inhibits protein synthesis by preventing the formation of ribosomal complex that initiates protein synthesis.

Dosage

- *Oral:* 400-600 mg 12th hourly
- *IV:* 600 mg 12th hourly.

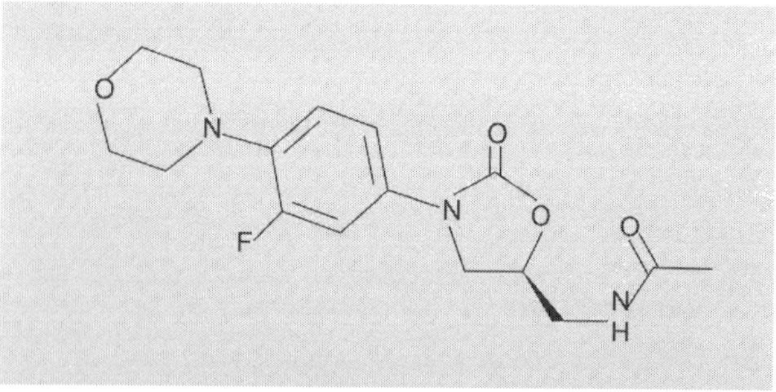

Fig. 7.15: Chemical structure of linezolid

Adverse Effects

- Thrombocytopenia, anemia and neutropenia
- Lactic acidosis
- Serotonin syndrome if given with serotonergic drugs.

Uses

It is used in treatment of vancomycin resistant enterococci infections, nosocomial pneumonia, community acquired pneumonia, skin and skin structure infections.

LINCOSAMIDES—CLINDAMYCIN

Clindamycin is a lincosamide antibiotic derived from lincomycin. It is highly active against *Bacteroides sp.* and other anaerobes (both gram +ve and –ve). Antimicrobial spectrum also includes streptococci, staphylococci and pneumococci. It is also active against *Pneumocystis jiroveci* and *T. gondii*. However, it is not active against MRSA, enterococci and aerobic gram –ve bacteria.

Clindamycin binds to bacterial 50S ribosomal subunit and inhibits protein synthesis. It is a bacteriostatic drug. It penetrates well in to the tissues and abscess cavity.

Dosage

- Systemic dose:
  - *Oral:* 150-450 mg 6th hourly
  - *Parenteral (IV/IM):* 600-1200 mg/day in 2-4 divided doses
- *Topical gel/lotion/solution for acne vulgaris:* 1 percent
- Fortified ophthalmic preparations:
  - *Fortified eyedrops:* 50 mg/ml
  - *Subconjunctival:* 25-50 mg
  - *Intravitreal:* 1000 µg or 1 mg

Adverse Effect

Diarrhea including pseudomembranous enterocolitis by *Clostridium difficile* and skin rashes.

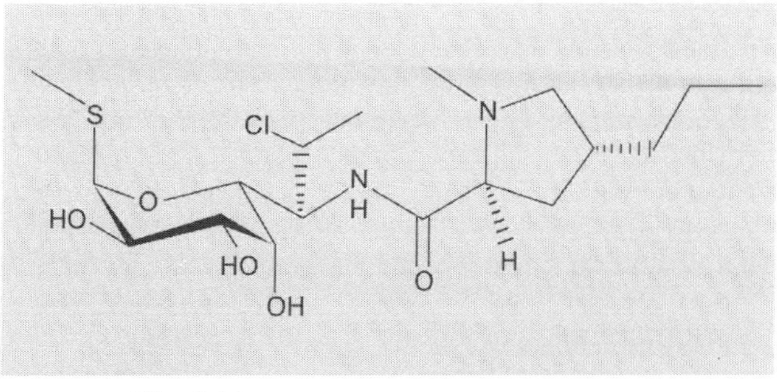

Fig. 7.16: Chemical structure of clindamycin

Uses

Clindamycin is used in the treatment of anaerobic infections, skin and soft tissue infections due to staphylococci and streptococci, lower respiratory tract infections including pneumonia caused by pneumococci, gynecological infections, intra-abdominal infections, septicemia, bone and joint infections and treatment of bacterial vaginosis.

Clindamycin in combination with primaquine is an alternative treatment for *Pneumocystis jiroveci* pneumonia. Clindamycin-pyrimethamine combination is used in toxoplasmosis of brain in HIV patients. Topically clindamycin is useful in the treatment of acne vulgaris.

STREPTOGRAMINS— QUINUPRISTIN/ DALFOPRISTIN

Quinupristin/Dalfopristin is a synergistic combination of streptogramin B (quinupristin) and streptogramin A (dalfopristin) in 30:70 ratio. It is a bactericidal drug and inhibits bacterial protein synthesis by binding to bacterial 50S ribosomes.

It is active against gram +ve cooci including MRSA, multidrug resistant streptococci, pneumococci and *Enterococcus faecium*. But it is not active against *Enterococcus faecalis* and gram –ve bacteria.

It is primarily excreted in bile and no dosage adjustment is required in renal impairment. It is given intravenously in dose of 7.5 mg/kg 8th–12th hourly in treatment of serious infections caused by vancomycin resistant *Enterococcus faecium* and in complicated skin and skin structure infections caused by drug resistant staphylococci.

RETAPAMULIN

It is a newer topical antibiotic that belong to pleuromutilin group. It binds with bacterial 50S ribosomes and inhibits protein synthesis.

It is effective against streptococci and staphylococci. It is used as 1 percent ointment in topical treatment of impetigo caused by *Staphylococcus aureus* or *Streptococcus pyogenes*.

FUSIDIC ACID

It is a bacteriostatic drug that acts by inhibiting bacterial protein synthesis. It is obtained from the fungus *Fusidium coccineum*. It is active against gram +ve bacteria especially streptococci and staphylococci. It is used topically as 2 percent sodium fusidate cream or ointment.

DRUGS ATTACKING BACTERIAL DNA

Fluoroquinolones

Nalidixic acid is the first quinolone antibiotic to be used clinically. It is mainly active against gram –ve bacteria and was used for treatment of urinary tract infections.

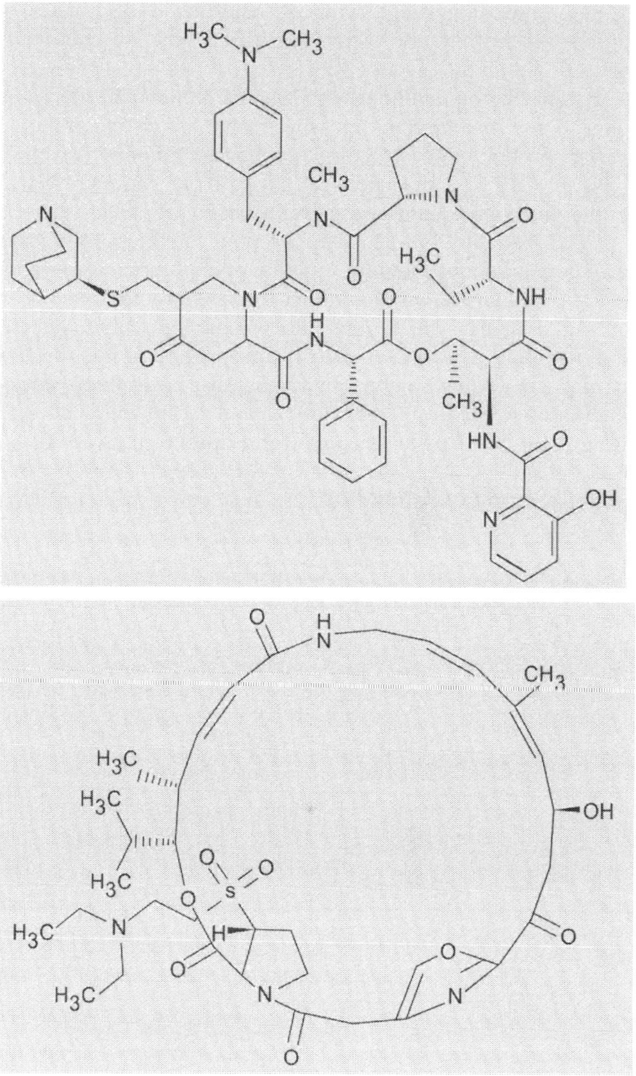

Antibacterial Therapy

Fig. 7.17: Chemical structure of Quinupristin/Dalfopristin

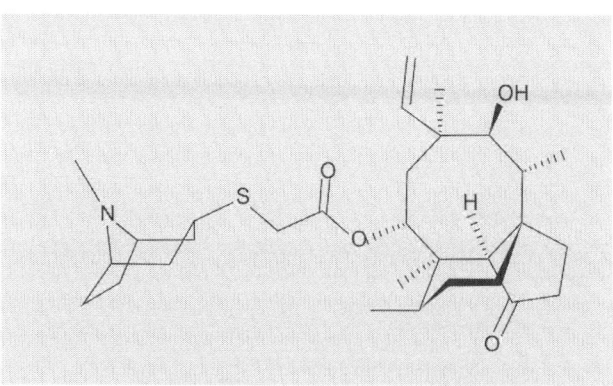

Fig. 7.18: Structure of retapamulin

Fluoroquinolones are synthetic fluorinated derivatives of nalidixic acid. They are bactericidal drugs and are commonly used in ophthalmic practice with excellent response. The newer generation fluoroquinolones have broad antimicrobial spectrum, better tissue penetration and lower rate of development of resistance. The basic structure of fluoroquinolones is shown in Figure 7.19 and the chemical structure of commonly used ophthalmic fluoroquinolones are shown in Figure 7.20.

Good aqueous humor concentrations of fluoroquinolones have been demonstrated in uninflamed human eyes after systemic administration in addition to topical route. It has been shown that ocular penetration of fluoroquinolones after systemic administration is related to their relative degree of lipophilicity. Sparfloxacin being highly lipophilic had excellent ocular penetration (55%) comparing vitreous and serum levels followed by ofloxacin (30%), pefloxacin (10%) and ciprofloxacin (5.5%).

Classification of Quinolones

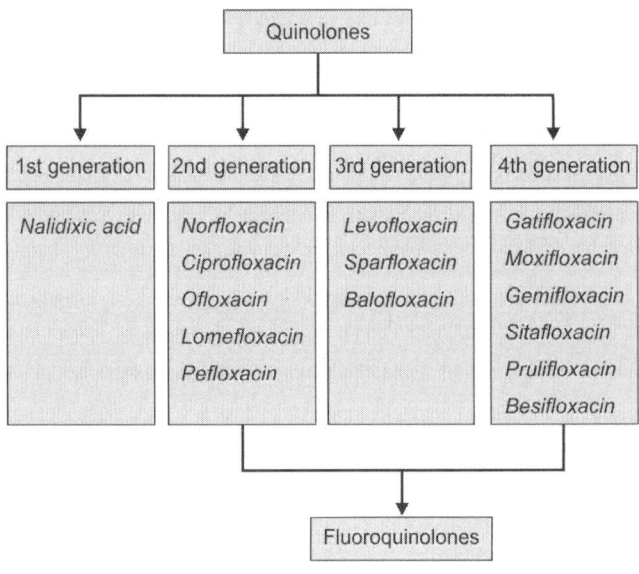

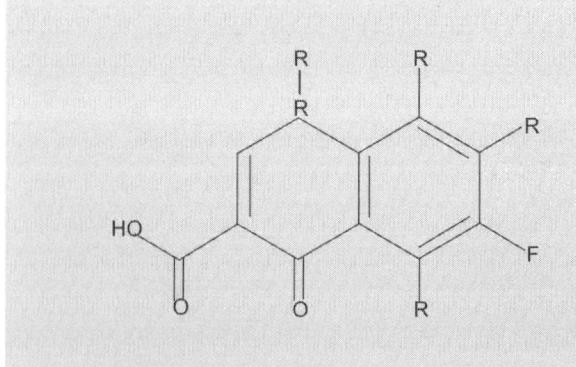

Fig. 7.19: Basic structure of fluoroquinolones

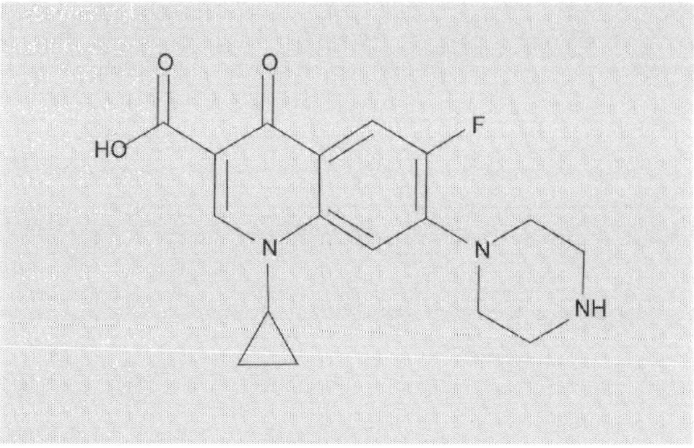

Antibacterial Therapy

Ciprofloxacin

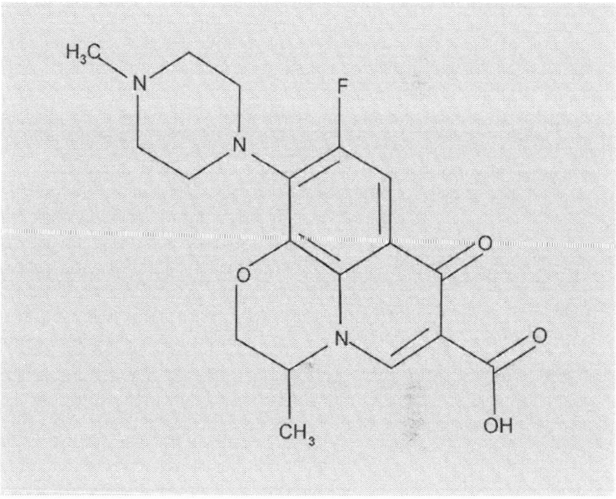

Ofloxacin

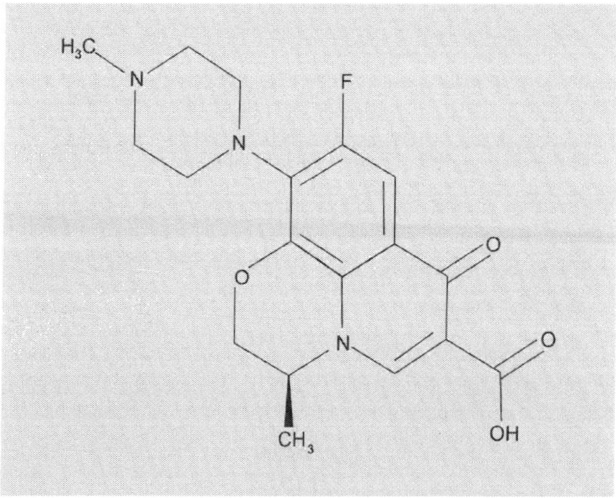

Levofloxacin

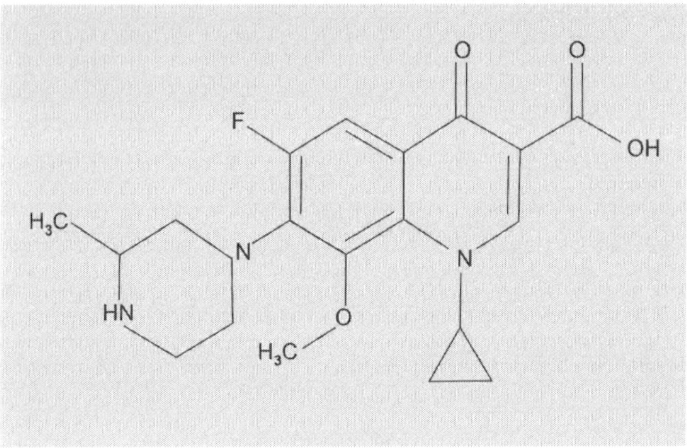

Gatifloxacin

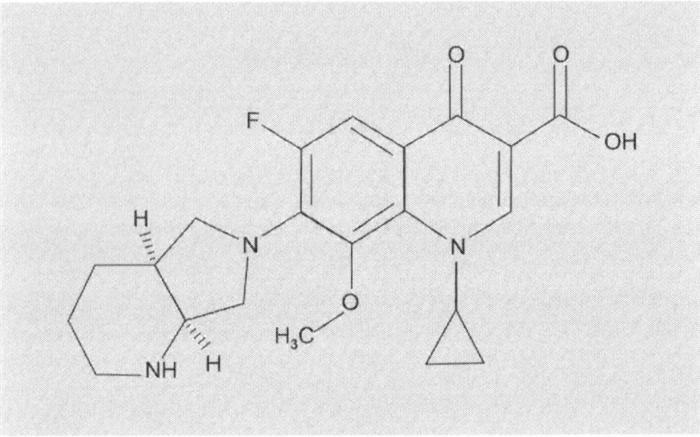

Moxifloxacin

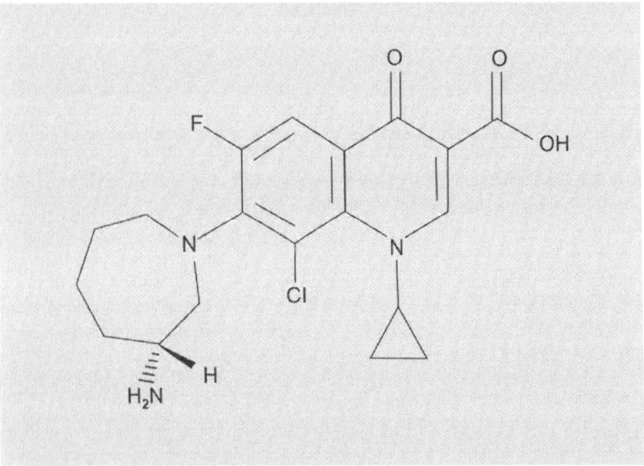

Besifloxacin

Fig. 7.20: Chemical structure of commonly used fluoroquinolones in ophthalmic practice

Mechanism of Action

Quinolones inhibit the enzyme DNA gyrase in gram –ve organisms and Topoisomerase-IV in gram +ve organisms.

During DNA replication, positive supercoils are introduced into the DNA strand. DNA gyrase is the enzyme present in gram –ve bacteria which nicks the DNA strand and introduces negative supercoils into the DNA and reseals it. The corresponding function in gram +ve bacteria is carried out by Topoisomerase IV. Quinolones inhibit this process thereby resulting in excessive positive super coiling which inhibits DNA replication and leads to cell death.

Antimicrobial Spectrum

Fluoroquinolones are bactericidal drugs that are highly active against gram –ve bacteria including *E. coli, Salmonella, Shigella, Pseudomonas, H. influenzae, Neisseria sp.* and *Campylobacter*. Newer generation fluoroquinolones also have good activity against gram +ve organisms like *Streptococcus* and Staphylococci but are not active against MRSA. Antimicrobial spectrum of fluoroquinolones also includes intracellular organisms like *Chlamydia, Mycoplasma* and *Legionella*. Newer drugs like garenoxacin, gemifloxacin and moxifloxacin are also active against anaerobes. However, fluoroquinolones are not active against *Treponema pallidum*.

Among the fluoroquinolones, ciprofloxacin has maximum activity against *Pseudomonas*. Levofloxacin, gatifloxacin, moxifloxacin and gemifloxacin have good activity against Streptococci especially *Streptococcus pneumoniae*. Ciprofloxacin, ofloxacin and pefloxacin are also active against mycobacterial species including *M. tuberculosis* and *Mycobacterium avium* Complex while ofloxacin and pefloxacin have some activity against leprosy.

Mode of Resistance

- Alteration of quinolone binding region in the target enzymes due to point mutations
- Active efflux of the drug by the bacteria.

Dosage

The dose of commonly used fluoroquinolones is given in the below table:

Drug	Systemic dose	Ophthalmic preparations
Norfloxacin	PO: 400 mg 12th hourly	Ophthalmic drops: 0.3% Ophthalmic ointment: 0.3%
Ciprofloxacin	PO: 1000-1500 mg/day in 2 divided doses IV: 200-400 mg 8th–12th hourly	Ophthalmic drops: 0.3% Ophthalmic ointment: 0.3%
Ofloxacin	PO/IV: 200-400 mg 12th hourly	Ophthalmic drops: 0.3% Ophthalmic ointment: 0.3%
Pefloxacin	PO: 400 mg 12th hourly	Ophthalmic drops: 0.3%
Lomefloxacin	PO: 400 mg once daily	Ophthalmic drops: 0.3%
Levofloxacin	PO/IV: 250-750 mg once daily	Ophthalmic drops: 0.5% and 1.5%
Sparfloxacin	PO: 400 mg on day 1 and 200 mg on following days	Ophthalmic drops: 0.3%
Balofloxacin	PO: 100 mg 12th hourly	----
Gatifloxacin	----	Ophthalmic drops: 0.3% Ophthalmic ointment: 0.3%
Moxifloxacin	PO: 400 mg once daily	Ophthalmic drops: 0.5% Ophthalmic ointment: 0.5%
Gemifloxacin	PO: 320 mg once daily	----
Prulifloxacin	PO: 600 mg once daily	----
Besifloxacin	----	Ophthalmic drops: 0.6%

Systemic Uses of Fluoroquinolones

Fluoroquinolones are used in treatment of urinary tract infections (UTI), prostatitis, gastrointestinal infections like enteric fever, shigellosis and gastroenteritis, respiratory tract infections, bone, skin and soft tissue infections and pelvic inflammatory disease.

In treatment of UTI, ciprofloxacin, norfloxacin and prulifloxacin are preferred while levofloxacin, sparfloxacin, moxifloxacin and gemifloxacin are indicated for respiratory tract infections. Ciprofloxacin is effective in treatment of *Pseudomonas* infections and in treatment of anthrax. Ciprofloxacin, moxifloxacin and levofloxacin are used as second line drugs in treatment of drug resistant tuberculosis. Ofloxacin is a second line drug for leprosy. Nadifloxacin is a topical fluoroquinolone used in topical treatment of acne vulgaris.

Ocular Uses of Fluoroquinolones

Topical fluoroquinolones are effective in various infective conditions of the eye. They have good intraocular penetration and achieve adequate concentrations in aqueous humor. In fact systemically administered fluoroquinolones attain good intraocular concentrations and hence they are rarely used intravitreally.

Topical fluoroquinolones are commonly used in treatment of bacterial conjunctivitis, keratitis, keratoconjunctivitis, blepharitis and dacryocystitis. Systemic fluoroquinolones are used in the treatment of bacterial endophthalmitis. Topical fluoroquinolones are well-tolerated when compared to topical aminoglycosides which are toxic to corneal and conjunctival epithelium.

Adverse Effects of Systemic Fluoroquinolones

- *GI disturbances:* Nausea, vomiting and diarrhea
- Headache, dizziness and sleep disturbances
- Skin rashes
- Photosensitivity (especially with lomefloxacin, pefloxacin and sparfloxacin)
- Tendinitis and achilles tendon rupture
- Arthropathy in children
- Teratogenicity
- QT interval prolongation with sparfloxacin, gatifloxacin and moxifloxacin.

Fluoroquinolones withdrawn from the market due to adverse effects:
- Gatifloxacin due to increased incidence of hypoglycemia in diabetic patients taking oral hypoglycemic agents. However, it can cause both hypo- and hyperglycemia
- Trovafloxacin due to hepatotoxicity
- Clinafloxacin due to phototoxicity
- Grepafloxacin due to cardiotoxicity (QT interval prolongation).

Adverse Effects of Topical Fluoroquinolones

Topical fluoroquinolones are well-tolerated and safe. Topical ciprofloxacin can cause following adverse effects:
- Local burning, itching and discomfort
- Conjunctival hyperemia
- Photophobia
- White precipitates in corneal surface if used frequently for treatment of corneal ulcer.

NITROIMIDAZOLES

Nitroimidazoles are commonly used drugs for the treatment of anaerobic and protozoal infections. Nitroimidazoles in clinical use include metronidazole, tinidazole, secnidazole and ornidazole.

Mechanism of Action

Nitroimidazoles enter the cell by passive diffusion. The nitro group is reduced inside the anaerobic bacteria and certain protozoa thereby producing highly active nitro radicals that damage the DNA of organism leading to cell death.

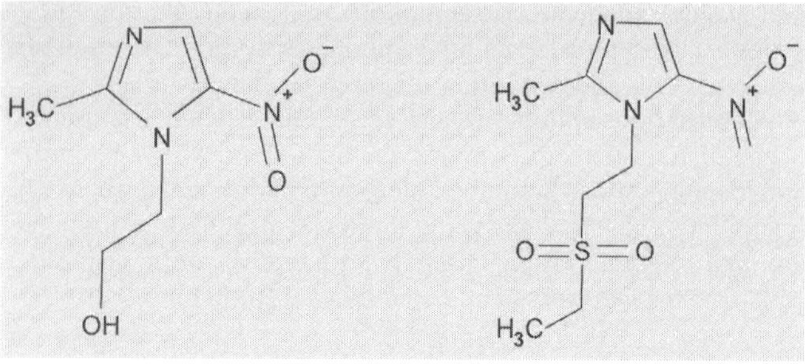

Fig. 7.21: Chemical structures of metronidazole (left) and tinidazole (right)

Antimicrobial Spectrum

Nitroimidazoles are active against anaerobic bacteria like *Bacteroides, Clostridium, H. pylori, Campylobacter, Fusobacterium* and anaerobic streptococci; and protozoa like Entamoeba histolytica, *Trichomonas vaginalis* and *Giardia lamblia*, Although metronidazole does not directly affect the guinea worm (*Dracunculus medinensis*), it helps in extraction of the worm from the skin of infected patients.

Dosage

The dosage of nitroimidazoles is given below. No ophthalmic preparations are available commercially.

Drug	Oral dose	Parenteral (IV) dose
Metronidazole	PO: 200-800 mg 8th hourly	IV: 500 mg 8th hourly
Tinidazole	PO: 0.5-2 g once daily	IV: 800 mg/day in 1-2 divided doses
Secnidazole	PO: 1.5-2 g/day	----
Ornidazole	PO: 0.5-1.5 mg/day	IV: 0.5-1 g/day

Adverse Effects

- *GI effects:* Nausea, metallic taste, dry mouth
- *CNS effects:* Headache, dizziness, vertigo, paresthesias
- Metronidazole can cause disulfiram like reactions with alcohol.

Uses

Metronidazole is the preferred drug for treatment of protozoal infections like amebiasis, trichomoniasis and giardiasis. It is used in treatment of anaerobic bacterial infections like pseudomembranous enterocolitis due to *Clostridium difficile, H. pylori* infection, bacterial vaginosis, acute necrotizing ulcerative gingivitis (trench mouth/ vincent's angina) and intra-abdominal infections.

DRUGS AFFECTING BACTERIAL INTERMEDIATE METABOLISM

Sulfonamides

Sulfonamides are structural analogs of p-amino benzoic acid (PABA) and they are the first group of antibiotics to be used clinically. They are bacteriostatic drugs and their role in medical practice has been superseded by the other newer antimicrobial agents.

Classification

1. Orally absorbed sulfonamides:
   Short acting   : Sulfisoxazole, Sulfamethizole, Sulfacytine
   Intermediate acting: Sulfadiazine, Sulfamethoxazole
   Long acting   : Sulfadoxine
2. Orally nonabsorbed but active in bowel lumen: Sulfasalazine
3. Topical sulfonamides: Sulfacetamide, Silver sulfadiazine, Mafenide

Mechanism of Action

Sulfonamides competitively inhibit the enzyme dihydropteroate synthase that produces dihydropteroic acid (precursor of dihydrofolic acid) from PABA. As a result of this inhibition bacteria cannot synthesize folic acid.

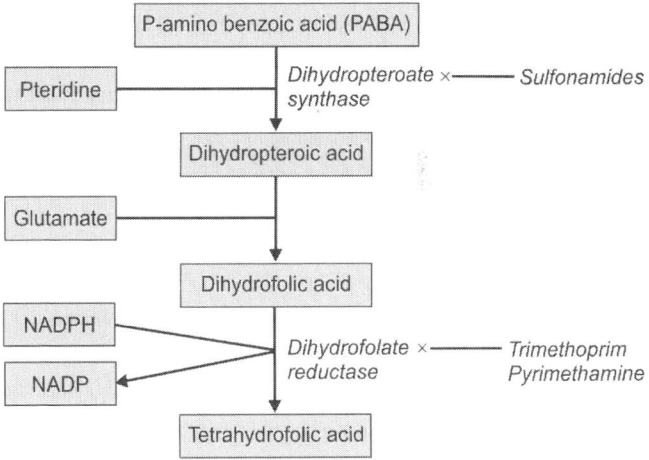

Antimicrobial Spectrum

Sulfonamides inhibit gram +ve and –ve bacteria, *Nocardia, Chlamydia trachomatis* and some protozoa like *Toxoplasma gondii*. But many of these organisms have become resistant to sulfonamides thereby limiting the role of sulfonamides in clinical practice.

Mode of Resistance

- Decreased affinity of the enzyme dihydropteroate synthase
- Increased production of PABA
- Alternative metabolic pathway to produce folic acid.

COTRIMOXAZOLE (TRIMETHOPRIM-SULFAMETHOXAZOLE)

It is a synergistic fixed dose combination of trimethoprim and sulfamethoxazole in a dose ratio of 1:5. The combination is bactericidal to many organisms like streptococci, staphylococci including MRSA, *E. coli*, *Salmonella*, *Shigella*, *Proteus*, *Klebsiella*, *Nocardia*, *Toxoplasma* and *Pneumocystis jiroveci*.

Trimethoprim and pyrimethamine are inhibitors of the enzyme dihydrofolate reductase. Cotrimoxazole produces a sequential inhibition in the bacterial folic acid synthesis pathway thereby acting as a bactericidal agent. However, many organisms have developed resistance to cotrimoxazole.

Topical preparations of sulfonamides available in market:
- Sulfacetamide ocular drops: 10 percent, 20 percent, 30 percent
- Silver sulfadiazine 1 percent topical ointment/ cream.

Dosage of Cotrimoxazole

- For infections other than *Pneumocystis jiroveci* pneumonia
  - *Oral:* 1 double strength tablet (Trimethoprim 160 mg and Sulfamethoxazole 800 mg) twice daily
  - *IV treatment:* 8-10 mg/kg/day in 2-4 divided doses

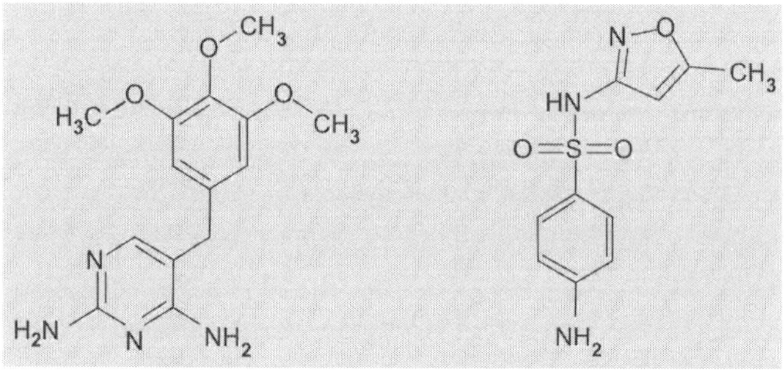

Trimethoprim Sulfamethoxazole

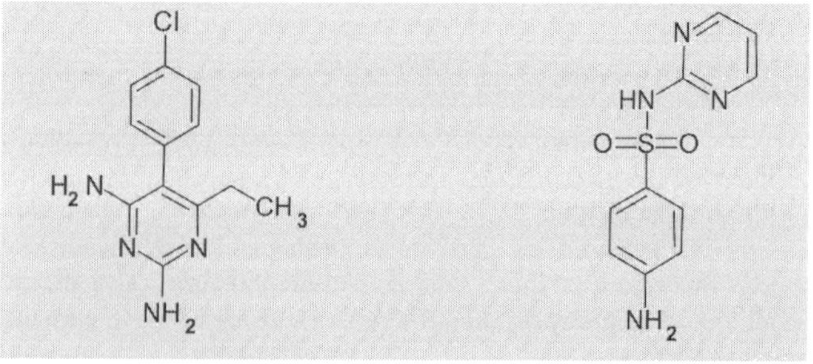

Pyrimethamine Sulfadiazine

Fig. 7.22: Chemical structures of trimethoprim (top left), sulfamethoxazole (top right), pyrimethamine (bottom left) and sulfadiazine (bottom right)

- For *Pneumocystis jiroveci* pneumonia
  - *Oral prophylaxis:* 1 double strength tablet once daily or thrice weekly
  - *Oral treatment:* Trimethoprim 15–20 mg/kg and sulfamethoxazole 75–100 mg/kg/day in 3-4 divided doses
  - *IV treatment:* 15–20 mg/kg/day (based on trimethoprim) in 3-4 divided doses
- Fortified eyedrops
  - Trimethoprim 16 mg/ml and Sulfamethoxazole 80 mg/ml.

Adverse Effects of Sulfonamides and Cotrimoxazole

- Fever
- Hypersensitivity reactions: Skin rashes, exfoliative dermatitis, photosensitivity reactions
- Crystalluria, hematuria
- Bone marrow suppression: Anemia, granulocytopenia, thrombocytopenia
- Hemolysis in G6PD deficient individuals
- Kernicterus in newborns.

Clinical Uses of Sulfonamides and Cotrimoxazole

Sulfacetamide eyedrops are used in treatment of superficial bacterial eye infections, conjunctivitis and trachoma. Silver sulfadiazine is used topically to prevent infection of burn wounds. Sulfasalazine is used in treatment of inflammatory bowel diseases like ulcerative colitis. Sulfadiazine—pyrimethamine combination is used in the treatment of toxoplasmosis, leishmaniasis and falciparum malaria. Cotrimoxazole is used in the treatment of *Pneumocystis jiroveci* pneumonia, urinary tract infections, prostatitis and nocardiosis. Fortified cotrimoxazole drops are used in the treatment of corneal ulcer caused by *Nocardia* species.

MISCELLANEOUS AGENTS

MUPIROCIN

It is a topical antibiotic obtained from *Pseudomonas fluorescens*. It is mainly active against gram +ve bacteria including streptococci and staphylococci (methicillin sensitive and resistant). It is bacteriostatic at low concentrations and bactericidal at high concentrations.

It binds to bacterial isoleucyl-tRNA synthetase and inhibits bacterial protein and RNA synthesis. It is used as 2 percent topical cream in treatment of skin infections including impetigo caused by *Staphylococcus aureus* and *Streptococcus pyogenes* and in eradication of nasal colonization of MRSA.

ANTIMICROBIAL PEPTIDES

Antimicrobial peptides are small molecular weight proteins isolated from the immune defense system of organisms such as insects, amphibians and mammals including humans. They have

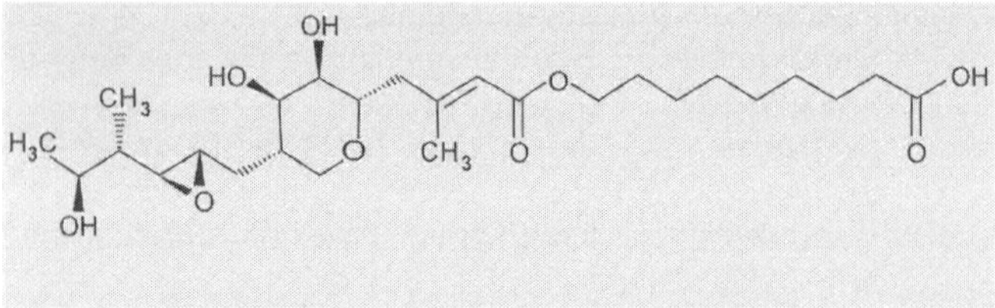

Fig. 7.23: Chemical structure of mupirocin

broad-spectrum of antimicrobial activity. The antimicrobials of this group are:

Defensins

Defensins are a group of antimicrobial and cytotoxic peptides with three distinct peptide families – α, β and θ defensins determined both by source and chemical structure. The alpha and beta defensins are derived mainly from mammalian source.

These are active against a number of organisms including gram-negative and gram-positive bacteria, mycobacteria, fungi and viruses. Insect defensins are active predominantly against gram-positive bacteria. Classic and beta defensins are highly active against human isolates from ulcerative keratitis. Organisms tested include alpha hemolytic *Streptococcus sp. S. pneumoniae, P. aeruginosa* and *Morganella*. At a concentration of 10 ug/ml there was a marked bactericidal effect.

Classic and beta defensins have a possible application as a microbicide in corneal storage media. A concentration of 200 ug/ml successfully killed 99.9 percent of three main organisms namely *S. aureus, S. pneumoniae* and *P. aeruginosa* within 30 minutes at all three temperatures (4°C, 23°C and 37°C). This bactericidal effect is impressive especially when the rapidity and low temperatures are considered. Conventional antibiotics do not have significant effect on lower temperatures.

Cecropins

These antimicrobial peptides are produced by giant silk moth (*Hyalophora cecropia*) in response to bacterial challenge. The antimicrobial properties are similar to defensins.

Synthetic cecropin analog D5C and natural antimicrobial peptides have potential bactericidal effect at concentration of 100 μg/ml at 4°C and 27°C. The cecropin D5C has also been investigated as a possible antimicrobial additive for contact lens disinfecting solutions. The addition of D5C to leading disinfecting solutions did enhance the bactericidal effect for certain organisms.

Magainins

Magainins were isolated from the skin of frog *Xenopus laevis*. They have broad spectrum activities like the above mentioned peptides. Initial investigations into the antimicrobial activity into ocular infections are promising.

Another antimicrobial peptide discovered in rabbit aqueous humor is under investigation for bactericidal activity.

Other antimicrobial peptides under investigation are indolicidins, dermicidin, protegrins and dermaseptin.

USE OF ANTIBIOTICS IN IRRIGATING SOLUTIONS FOR INTRAOCULAR SURGERY

Irrigation solutions supplemented with antibiotics are used widely for intraocular surgeries. Gentamicin (8 µg/ml), vancomycin (20 µg/ml) or gentamicin and vancomycin combination are the most common antibacterial agents investigated in this manner. It has been reported that incidence of endophthalmitis reduces drastically when gentamicin or vancomycin is added to the cataract infusion solution and then filtered. The antibiotic supplementation in the infusion solution kills bacteria and prevents endophthalmitis. On examination of anterior chamber aspiration after cataract surgery in which gentamicin was used in the irrigating solution, no organisms were isolated. These results are encouraging and research is being done on *in vitro* model to evaluate the potential antimicrobial effects of piperacillin (512 µg/ml) and tazobactam (64 µg/ml) combination used in irrigating solution. Other antibiotic agents examined to determine their utility in intraocular infusions include fluoroquinolones like ofloxacin and sparfloxacin.

TABLE 7.1: Recommended nontoxic doses of antimicrobial infusion fluids for vitrectomy	
Agent	Dose (mg/ml)
Amikacin	0.01
Ceftazidime	0.04
Chloramphenicol	0.01
Ciprofloxacin	0.01
Clindamycin	0.009
Dicloxacillin	0.01
Gentamicin	0.008
Imipenem	0.01
Lincomycin	0.01
Lomefloxacin	0.01
Methicillin	0.02
Ofloxacin	0.01
Oxacillin	0.01
Pefloxacin	0.01
Penicillin G	0.01
Sparfloxacin	0.01
Tobramycin	0.01
Vancomycin	0.03

TABLE 7.2: Recommended doses of intravitreal antimicrobial agents

Agent	Dose (mg/ 0.1ml)
Amikacin	0.04
Ampicillin	5.0
Carbenicillin	2.0
Cefazolin	2-2.25
Ceftazidime	2.0
Chloramphenicol	2.0
Ciprofloxacin	0.1
Clarithromycin	0.5
Clindamycin	0.45-1.0
Gentamicin	0.02
Imipenem	0.5
Kanamycin	0.04
Lincomycin	1.5
Lomefloxacin	0.08
Methicillin	2.0
Netilmicin	0.01
Norfloxacin	0.1
Ofloxacin	0.1
Oxacillin	0.5
Pefloxacin	0.1
Sparfloxacin	0.08
Tobramycin	0.02
Vancomycin	1.0

TABLE 7.3: Preparation of intravitreal antibiotic injections

Agent	Commercial availability	Initial diluent (ml)	Initail conc. (mg/ml)	Aliquot (ml)	Final diluent (ml)	Final conc. (mg/ml)	Final intravitreal dose (in 0.1 ml)
Amikacin	500 mg/2 ml	---	250	0.1	6.15	4	400 µg
Ampicillin	1 g	4	250	0.3	1.2	50	5 mg
Cefazolin	500 mg	2	225	0.1	0.9	22.5	2.25 mg
Chloramphenicol	1 g	10	100	0.1	0.4	20	2 mg
Clindamycin	300 mg/2 ml	---	150	0.1	1.4	10	1 mg
Gentamicin	80 mg/2 ml	---	40	0.1	1.9	2	200 µg
Kanamycin	500 mg/2 ml	---	250	0.1	6.15	4	400 µg
Tobramycin	80 mg/2 ml	---	40	0.1	1.9	2	200 µg
Vancomycin	500 mg	10	50	0.2	0.8	10	1 mg

TABLE 7.4: Various topical antibiotic preparations (Commercial and Fortified)

Agent	Commercial drops	Fortified drops	Shelf life	Subconjunctival dose
Amikacin	0.5 – 1%	20 mg/ml	30 days	125 mg
Ampicillin	---	50 mg/ml	1 day	100 mg
Azithromycin	1%	---	---	---
Bacitracin	---	10000 units/ml	7 days	5000-10000 units
Besifloxacin	0.6%	---	---	---
Carbenicillin	---	4-6 mg/ml	3 days	100 mg
Cefazolin	---	50 mg/ml	4 days	100 mg
Cefoperazone	---	50 mg/ml	7 days	100 mg
Cefotaxime	---	50 mg/ml	7 days	100 mg
Ceftazidime	---	50 mg/ml	7 days	100 mg
Ceftriaxone	---	50 mg/ml	7 days	100 mg
Chloramphenicol	0.5 – 1%	5-10 mg/ml	15 days	50-100 mg
Ciprofloxacin	0.3%	---	---	---
Clarithromycin	---	10 mg/ml	14 days	---
Clindamycin	---	50 mg/ml	7 days	25-50 mg
Erythromycin	---	25 mg/ml	14 days	50-100 mg
Framycetin	0.5%	---	---	---
Gatifloxacin	0.3%	---	---	---
Gentamicin	0.3%	16-20 mg/ml	30 days	10-20 mg
Kanamycin	---	10 mg/ml	7 days	---
Levofloxacin	0.5 – 1.5%	---	---	---
Lomefloxacin	0.3%	---	---	---
Methicillin	---	50 mg/ml	4 days	100 mg
Moxifloxacin	0.5%	---	---	---
Neomycin	0.3%	30-40 mg/ml	7 days	100 mg
Netilmicin	---	20-40 mg/ml	7 days	---
Norfloxacin	0.3%	---	---	---
Ofloxacin	0.3%	---	---	---
Pefloxacin	0.3%	---	---	---
Penicillin G	---	1 lakh units/ml	4 days	1 million units
Piperacillin	---	12 mg/ml	3 days	100 mg
Polymyxin-B	10000 units/ml	50000 units/ml	7 days	100000 units
Sisomicin	0.3%	20 mg/ml	30 days	20-80 mg
Sparfloxacin	0.3%	---	---	---
Tetracycline	1%	---	---	---
Ticarcillin	---	6-20 mg/ml	3 days	100 mg
Tobramycin	0.3%	16-20 mg/ml	30 days	10-20 mg
Vancomycin	---	25-50 mg/ml	4 days	25 mg

TABLE 7.5: Initial topical antibiotic of choice for external ocular infections based on Gram stain findings

Type of bacteria	First line drug	Alternative drug
Gram-positive cocci	Cefazolin Vancomycin	Penicillin G, Bacitracin, Fluoroquinolones
Gram-positive bacilli	Penicillin G	Vancomycin, Bacitracin
Gram-negative cocci	Ceftriaxone	Ceftazidime, Fluoroquinolones
Gram-negative bacilli	Tobramycin, Gentamicin, Amikacin	Ticarcillin, Ceftazidime, Fluoroquinolones
Bacteria suspected (No organism seen)	Cefazolin plus Tobramycin	Fluoroquinolones

TABLE 7.6: Topical antibiotic therapy for culture specific bacterial ulcers

Organism	Topical (Fortified/Nonfortified)	Subconjunctival
Pseudomonas	Tobramycin plus Ticarcillin/ Piperacillin Ciprofloxacin	Tobramycin/ Amikacin plus Piperacillin/ Ticarcillin
Staphylococcus	Penicillin G (if sensitive) Methicillin/ Cefazolin (if sensitive) Vancomycin (for MRSA) Bacitracin	Cefazolin, Vancomycin
Enterobacter E.coli Klebsiella Proteus	Aminoglycosides Fluoroquinolones	Tobramycin, Amikacin
Bacillus	Vancomycin Plus Gentamicin/ Tobramycin Fluoroquinolones	Vancomycin, Gentamicin
Nocardia	Cotrimoxazole Amikacin Sulfacetamide	Amikacin

REASONS FOR FAILURE IN OCULAR ANTIBIOTIC TREATMENT

1. Inaccurate diagnosis: Antibiotics are effective only against bacterial infections. However, many times for common ocular inflammation like viral keratitis and allergic conjunctivitis antibiotics has no role though prescribed more often as the first line of treatment. So proper diagnosis should be made and antibiotics should be used whenever it is required.
2. Development of drug resistance: Indiscriminate use of antibiotics has resulted in more and more drug resistance to commonly available antibiotics. So it is recommended that the sensitivity of the organisms causing infections should be

TABLE 7.7: Specific antibiotic therapy for treatment of bacterial endophthalmitis

Organism	Intravitreal	Systemic	Topical/sub-conjunctival
Staphylococcus	Cefazolin Vancomycin (MRSA)	Vancomycin Linezolid	Cefazolin
Streptococcus	Vancomycin	Ceftriaxone, Cefotaxime	Levofloxacin, Moxifloxacin
Haemophillus	Chloramphenicol	Fluoroquinolones	Fluoroquinolones
Pseudomonas	Amikacin Ceftazidime	Ceftazidime plus gentamicin Fluoroquinolones	Fluoroquinolones Aminoglycosides
Bacillus	Clindamycin Vancomycin Amikacin	Clindamycin Vancomycin Fluoroquinolones	Clindamycin Fluoroquinolones
Moraxella	Ceftazidime	Ceftriaxone Cefotaxime	Moxifloxacin Levofloxacin
Enterococcus	Vancomycin	Vancomycin	Aminoglycosides
E. coli	Amikacin	Amikacin Fluoroquinolones	Amikacin Fluoroquinolones
Proteus	Amikacin Cefazolin	Amikacin Fluoroquinolones	Amikacin Fluoroquinolones
Corynebacterium	Vancomycin Cefazolin	Cefazolin	Cefazolin

known before starting antibiotics or at least the newer and stronger should be avoided for mild ocular infections.
3. Patient noncompliance.
4. Inadequate dose.
5. Inadequate immune system of the patient.

CONCLUSION

In ophthalmic practice, the mode of administration of antibiotics is highly significant as the intraocular penetration of drugs differ considerably. Intravitreal administration of antibiotics has the advantage of achieving high concentration in vitreous cavity without systemic exposure and hence preferred in the treatment of endophthalmitis. Shelf life of the drugs should be kept in mind to optimize the therapeutic effect during topical, subconjunctival and intraocular therapy. Emerging antimicrobial resistance is a global problem. Rational use of these antibiotics will prevent the development of resistance of these valuable drugs.

BIBLIOGRAPHY

1. American Academy of Ophthalmology Retina Panel. Preferred Practice Pattern® Guidelines. Bacterial Keratitis - Limited Revision. San Francisco, CA: American Academy of Ophthalmology; 2011 [updated 2011; cited]; Available from: www.aao.org/ppp.

2. American Academy of Ophthalmology Retina Panel. Preferred Practice Pattern® Guidelines. Conjunctivitis - Limited Revision. San Francisco, CA: American Academy of Ophthalmology; 2011 [updated 2011; cited]; Available from: www.aao.org/ppp.
3. Agarwal A. Textbook of Ophthalmology. 1st edn. New Delhi: Jaypee Brothers Medical Publishers (P) Ltd.; 2002.
4. Albert DM. Albert and Jakobiec's Principles and Practice of Ophthalmology. 3rd edn. Saunders, Elsevier; 2008.
5. Bartlett JD. Ophthalmic Drug Facts. 23rd edn. Wolters Kluwer Health; 2011.
6. Bartlett JD, Jaanus SD. Clinical Ocular Pharmacology. 5th edn. Butterworth-Heinemann, an imprint of Elsevier Inc.; 2008.
7. Bertino JS, Jr. Impact of antibiotic resistance in the management of ocular infections: the role of current and future antibiotics. Clin Ophthalmol 2009;3:507-21.
8. Brunton LL. Goodman and Gilman's. The Pharmacological Basis of Therapeutics. 12th edn. New York: The McGraw-Hill Companies, Inc.; 2011.
9. Garg A. Advances in Ophthalmology. 1st edn. New Delhi: Jaypee Brothers Medical Publishers (P) Ltd.; 2005.
10. Garg A. Clinical Applications of Antibiotics and Anti-inflammatory Drugs in Ophthalmology. 1st edn. New Delhi: Jaypee Brothers Medical Publishers (P) Ltd.; 2007.
11. Gordon YJ, Romanowski EG, McDermott AM. A review of antimicrobial peptides and their therapeutic potential as anti-infective drugs. Curr Eye Res 2005;30(7):505-15.
12. Hancock RE, Sahl HG. Antimicrobial and host-defense peptides as new anti-infective therapeutic strategies. Nat Biotechnol 2006;24(12):1551-7.
13. Karpecki P, Paterno MR, Comstock TL. Limitations of current antibiotics for the treatment of bacterial conjunctivitis. Optom Vis Sci 2010;87(11):908-19.
14. Katzung BG. Basic and Clinical Pharmacology. 12th edn. New York: The McGraw-Hill Companies, Inc; 2012.
15. Lopez-Cabezas C, Muner DS, Massa MR, Mensa Pueyo JM. Antibiotics in endophthalmitis: microbiological and pharmacokinetic considerations. Curr Clin Pharmacol 2010;5(1):47-54.
16. McDonald M, Blondeau JM. Emerging antibiotic resistance in ocular infections and the role of fluoroquinolones. J Cataract Refract Surg 2010;36(9):1588-98.
17. Onofrey BE. Ocular Therapeutics Handbook: A Clinical Manual. 3rd edn. Philadelphia: Lippincott Williams and Wilkins; 2011.
18. Scoper SV. Review of third- and fourth-generation fluoroquinolones in ophthalmology: *in vitro* and *in vivo* efficacy. Adv Ther 2008;25(10):979-94.
19. Sharma S. Antibiotic resistance in ocular bacterial pathogens. Indian J Med Microbiol 2011;29(3):218-22.
20. Smith A, Pennefather PM, Kaye SB, Hart CA. Fluoroquinolones: place in ocular therapy. Drugs 2001;61(6):747-61.
21. Tasman W, Jaeger EA. Duane's Ophthalmology on DVD-ROM. 2011 ed: Lippincott Williams and Wilkins; 2011.
22. Yount NY, Yeaman MR. Emerging themes and therapeutic prospects for anti-infective peptides. Annu Rev Pharmacol Toxicol 2012;52:337-60.

8

Anti-inflammatory Therapy

NR Biswas, AK Dubey, Harivenkatesh N, Ashok Garg (India)

Inflammation is the manifestation of vascular and cellular response of the tissue to an injury. Ocular inflammation can be due to iatrogenic or accidental injury and sometimes due to endogenous injury to eye. Response to the injury is marked by the production and release of many inflammatory mediators. Various anti-inflammatory drugs developed so far have been directed against different cellular and chemical mediators of inflammation, e.g. mast cells, lymphocyctes, leukocytes, complement, histamine, plasma kinins, proteolytic enzymes and derivates of arachidonic acid. Anti-inflammatory drugs can broadly be classified as:
1. Corticosteriods
2. Nonsteroidal anti-inflammatory drugs (NSAIDs)
3. Immunosuppressive agents.

CORTICOSTEROIDS

Since their introduction into ocular therapy, corticosteroids have been useful to control inflammatory and immunological diseases of the eye. The anti-inflammatory effects of corticosteroids are nonspecific and they inhibit inflammation without regard to cause. Topical corticosteroids exert an anti-inflammatory action. Aspects of the inflammatory process such as hyperemia, cellular infiltration, vascularization and fibroblastic proliferation are suppressed. Steroids cause inhibition of inflammatory response to inciting agents of mechanical, chemical or immunological nature. Topical corticosteroids are effective in acute inflammatory conditions of conjunctiva, sclera, cornea, lids, iris, ciliary body and anterior segment of the globe. They are effective in ocular allergic conditions. In the treatment of ocular diseases, the route depends on the site and extent of the disorder.

The mechanism of the anti-inflammatory action is shown to be potentiation of epinephrine, vasoconstriction, stabilization of lysosomal membranes, retardation of macrophage movement, prevention of kinin release, inhibition of lymphocyte and neutrophil function, inhibition of prostaglandin synthesis and in prolonged use decrease of antibody production. By inhibition of fibroblastic profileration, symblepharon formation in chemical and thermal burns may be prevented. Decreased scarring with clearer corneas following topical corticosteroid therapy is the result of inhibiting fibroblastic proliferation and vascularization.

The central mechanism of all these inflammation inhibitory processes is probably the induction of lipocortin production by the corticosteroids. These lipocortins inhibit phospholipase A2, which plays a key role in the production of inflammatory mediators such as prostaglandins and leukotrienes at the site of tissue injury. The use of corticosteroids in ocular diseases remains largely empirical but some general principles should be kept in mind.

After topical application some systemic absorption does take place but that is not significant enough to produce any untoward effect.

1. Type and location of inflammation determines which route of administration is appropriate.
2. A particular preparation is selected over others based on the potency of the steroid.
3. Dosage is largely determined by clinical experience and should be reassessed at frequent intervals during the course of therapy.
4. Treatment in most of the mild-to-moderate external inflammatory conditions of the eye should not generally be extended for more than three to four weeks.
5. Therapy should be reduced gradually, not discontinued abruptly.
6. The minimum effective dose should be used for the shortest time necessary.
7. Individualize dose.
8. Maintain close follow-up to assess the effects of therapy on the disease and possible adverse effects to be patient.
9. Patient compliance watch with the drug regimen is important in resolution of the inflammation.

Clinical use experience indicates that corticosteroids differ in their ability to suppress inflammation. They fall into three categories:

1. Glucocorticoids
2. Mineralocorticoids
3. Sex hormones.

Only the glucocorticoids have role in ophthalmic practice. They have powerful anti-inflammatory action and it is this property that has made them such an important agent in the treatment of many ocular diseases. However, they have a number of adverse effects.

Steroids may be administered locally in the form of eyedrops, ointments, injections (Subconjuctival, sub-Tenon, retroequatorial, retrobulbar, intracameral, intravitreal and intralesional) and systemically in the form of tablets or injections.

Indications

Topical corticosteroids are used for the treatment of steroid responsive inflammatory conditions of the palpebral and bulbar conjunctiva, lid, cornea and anterior segment of the globe. Indications for topical use include various allergic and hypersensitivity conditions of the eye like.

- Postoperative phase of Excimer Laser and Lasik surgery.
- Iatrogenic inflammation of the eye.

- Contact dermatitis of eyelids
- Pseudophakic inflammation and after phacoemulsification
- Nonspecific superficial keratitis
- Allergic conjunctivitis and blepharitis
- Vernal conjunctivitis
- Phlyctenular keratoconjuctivitis
- Herpes zoster keratitis
- Disciform and interstitial keratitis
- Corneal graft reactions
- Anterior and panuveitis
- Episcleritis and scleritis
- Chlazion, iritis, cyclitis
- Hemangioma
- Postkeratoplasty phase
- Superficial punctuate keratitis
- Traumatic inflammation of eye.
- Corneal injury from chemical, radiation or thermal burns.

Use higher strengths for moderate-to-severe inflammations. In difficult cases of anterior segment eye disease, systemic therapy may also be required in addition.

Contraindications

Topical corticosteroids should not be used in acute superficial herpes simplex keratitis, fungal diseases of ocular structures, vaccinia, varicella and other viral diseases of cornea and conjunctiva, ocular tuberculosis, hypersensitivity and after uncomplicated removal of superficial corneal foreign body.

Topical steroids are not effective in Sjögrens keratoconjunctivitis. Acute purulent untreated eye infections may be masked or activity enhanced by topical steroids. Stromal herpes simplex keratitis treatment with steroid medication requires great caution.

Usage of topical steroids in pregnancy and lactation: Safety of intensive or protracted use is not fully substantiated. Use with caution, when clearly needed and when potential benefits outweigh potential hazards.

Administration and Dosage

Topical steroid treated duration varies with the type of lesion and may extend from few days to several weeks depending on therapeutic response. Relapse may occur if therapy reduced too rapidly.

Taper over several days. Relapse more common in chronic active lesions usually respond to retreatment.

Topical solutions: Instill 1 to 2 drops into the conjunctival sac every hour during the day and every 2 hours during the night in acute inflammatory conditions of the eye in mild-to-moderate inflammation use dosage of 1 drops every 4-6 hours.

Ointments: Apply a thin coating in lower conjunctival sac 3-4 times a day in severe inflammation. In mild to moderate cases, one application at bed time may be sufficient to control symptoms. Ointments are specially convenient when eye pad is used and may be preparation of choice when prolonged contact of drug with ocular tissues is needed.

Many of the steroid preparations are formulated as suspensions because of their inability to dissolve in a solution. Various topical steroidal agents used in ophthalmology are:

Hydrocortisone

1. Acetate suspension—0.5 to 2.5 percent
2. Acetate solution—0.2 percent
3. Acetate ointment—1.5 percent.

Prednisolone

1. Acetate suspension—0.12 percent, 0.25 percent and 1.0 percent
2. Sodium phosphate soln—0.12 percent, 0.5 and 1.0 percent
3. Phosphate soln—0.5 percent
4. Phosphate ointment—0.25 percent.

Dexamethasone

1. Sodium phosphate soln—0.1 percent, 0.05 percent, 0.01 percent
2. Suspension—0.1 percent
3. Sodium phosphate oint—0.05 percent.

Betamethasone

1. Sodium phosphate solution—0.1 percent
2. Sodium phosphate oint—0.1 percent.

Triamcinolone

1. Triamcinolone acetonide suspension—0.1 percent
2. Triamcinolone acetonide ointment—0.1 percent
3. Can also be given as periocular injection.

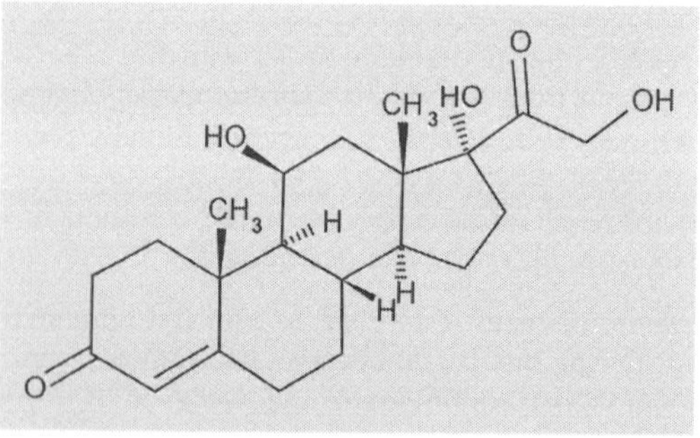

Fig. 8.1: Chemical structure of hydrocortisone

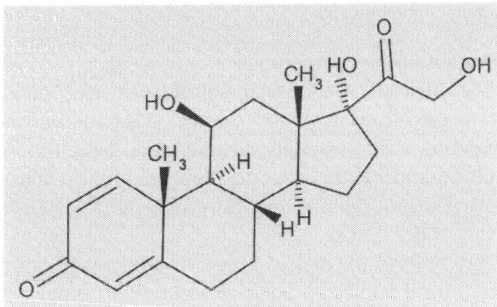

Fig. 8.2: Chemical structure of prednisolone

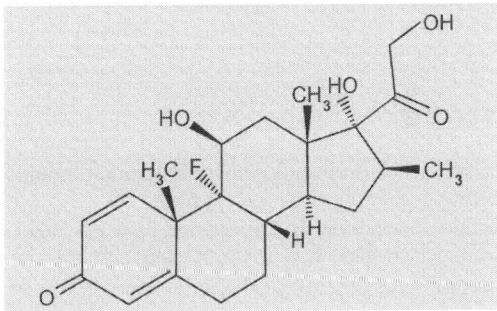

Fig. 8.3: Chemical structure of betamethasone

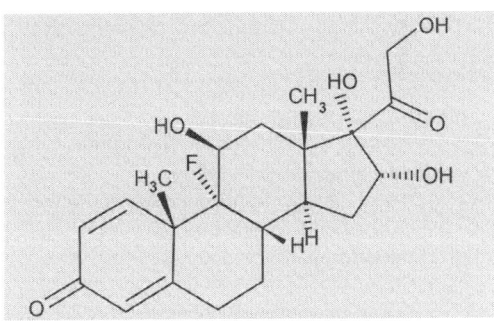

Fig. 8.4: Chemical structure of triamcinolone

Progesterone Like Agents

1. Medrysone suspension – 1 percent
2. Fluorometholone suspension – 0.1 percent (FML), 0.25 percent (FML Forte) and ointment (0.1%)
3. Fluorometholone acetate suspension 0.1 percent.

Rimexolone

Ophthalmic suspension- 1 percent.

Loteprednol Etabonate

Ophthalmic solution- 1 percent.

Some groups of the topical steroids (drops) have better intraocular penetration than others. Dexamethasone and betamethasone have better intraocular penetration than triamcinolone and hydrocortisone. New generation steroids like rimexolone, flurometholone are powerfrul corticosteroids with very low risk of IOP spikes.

Medrysone (Hydroxymethyl progesterone) has poor intraocular penetration. It is more related structurally to progesterone as compared to other steroids. It has less anti-inflammatory potency as compared to 0.1 percent dexamethasone, but the propensity to cause the rise in IOP is also less as compared to dexamethasone or betamethasone. Medrysone is usually recommended for minor reaction involving lids and conjunctiva. Its efficacy has not been demonstrated in iritis or uveitis.

Full strength topical corticosteroids are indicated in severe allergic or immunological responses, severe uveitis with hypopyon but without corneal epithelial break and microbial infective element, iatrogenic and pseudophakic inflammation and in Post Excimer PRK Laser and Lasik surgery phases.

In certain ophthalmic inflammatory diseases however, full strength topical steroids are not indicated and diluted steroid regime should be used. Topical dexamethasone phosphate (0.01 diluted solution) is commonly prescribed by the ophthalmologists. The diluted corticosteroids (1:10) have clear advantages in the therapy of ophthalmic disorders. These are as follows:

1. Enhance resistance to infection.
2. Possess effective anti-inflammatory response even in 1:20 dilutions.
3. Do not enhance microbial fungal flora of their lesions.
4. Do not produce ocular hypertension.
5. Do not delay healing when used in 1:10 dilution.
6. Do not enhance collagenase release.
7. Effective control of allergic conditions of conjunctiva.
8. Stabilize the corneal endothelial function.
9. Do not produce keratopathy.
10. Do not cause dry eye.

Thus advantages of diluted corticosteroids are non-promotion of organism growth, non-interference in healing processes without compromising their therapeutic effects. Strict precaution should be taken, topical steroids are never stopped suddenly to avoid high chances of recurrence of disease and adverse effects owing to tissue addiction. The therapy must be tapered gradually in dose and frequency over a period of time. The diluted corticosteroid regime should be continued for a period of one week after the clinical cure.

Since the advent of new generation topical corticosteroid like rimexolone and flurometholone topical steroid therapy has revolutionized. Unlike topical dexamethazone, betamethasone, prednisolone and hydrocortisone ophthalmic solutions, these new generation steroids have low incidence of adverse effects specially rise of IOP spikes leading to steroid induced glaucoma. A brief description of the new generation topical steroids is given below.

Rimexolone

Rimexolone (Vexol) 1 percent ophthalmic suspension is the first new ocular steroid with classic steroid power in 20 years. With this unique new design rimexolone displays a strong affinity for human glucocorticoid receptor and high *in vitro* activity. It has powerful anti-inflammatory effect like other steroids but significantly with low risk of IOP spikes similar to FML (0.1% soln).

Indications

Topical rimexolone (1%) is:
- Highly effective in reducing postoperative inflammation of eye (Intraocular surgery). In postsurgery inflammation following Excimer Laser PRK and Lasik Surgery.
- In pseudophakic inflammation of the eye.
- Highly effective in treating anterior uveitis
- Treating allergic conjunctivitis, keratoconjuctivitis.

Contraindications

It should not be used in the below conditions:
- Dendritic keratitis
- Vaccinia varicella
- Mycobacterial infection of the eye
- Fungal disease of the eye
- Acute purulent untreated infections which may be masked or enhanced by the presence of steroid
- Persons with hypersensitivity to any component
- Pregnancy, lactating mothers and in children.

Dosage

One percent ophthalmic sterile multidose suspension (5 ml and 10 ml vials). Patient is advised to put one drop in the affected eye

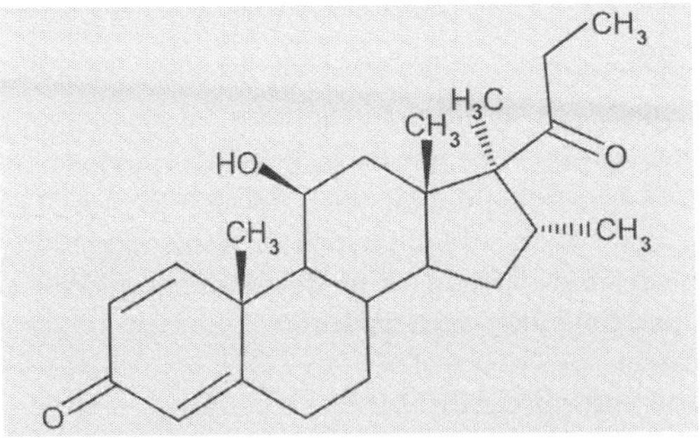

Fig. 8.5: Chemical structure of rimexolone

3-4 times a day. Dosage can be increased depending upon severity of the condition. Rimexolone provides well tolerated, comfortable and ease to use therapy.

Adverse Reactions

In addition to standard adverse effects of topical steroids being discussed separately in details. Topical rimexolone can cause blurred vision, discharge, discomfort, ocular pain, foreign body sensation, hyperemia, increased fibrin, dry eye, conjunctival edema, corneal staining, photophobia,, non-ocular adverse effect although very low can be headache, hypotension, rhinitis, taste perversion and pharyngitis.

Fluorometholone

Fluorometholone (FML) is a topical corticosteroid being prescribed commonly by ophthalmologists worldwide. It is powerful anti-inflammatory agent of steroidal group. Chemically it is 9-fluor-11β, 17-dihydroxy-6α-methyl pregna-1,4-diene-3,20-dione 17-acetate.

In topical suspension (0.1% and 0.25% FML forte), it is available with liquifilm (polyvinyl alcohol). It is well tolerated in ocular tissue and is distributed throughout the ocular tissues rapidly.

Mechanism of Action

Topical flurometholone acts by inhibiting the inflammatory response to a variety of inciting agents. They inhibit the edema, fibrin deposition, capillary dilation, leukocyte migration, phago-cytic activity. Capillary proliferation, fibroblast proliferation, deposition of collagen and scar formation associated with inflammation. It inhibits the synthesis of histamine within mast cells. The FML also decreases prostaglandin synthesis and retards epithelial regeneration. The special character of topical FML is that it has powerful anti-inflammatory property similar to topical dexamethasone, betamethasone and prednisolone (diluted and undiluted) but has a significant lower propensity to increase intraocular pressure which leads to steroid induced glaucoma.

Indications

For steroid responsive inflammation of the palpebral and bulbar conjunctiva, cornea and anterior segment of the globe.
- In iatrogenic inflammation specially after Excimer Laser PRK and Lasik Surgery, Pseudophakic inflammation.
- In Phaco emulsification (Postsurgical inflammation)
- Disciform and interstitial keratitis
- Panuveitis
- Scleritis and episcleritis
- Traumatic inflammation of the eye.

Anti-inflammatory Therapy

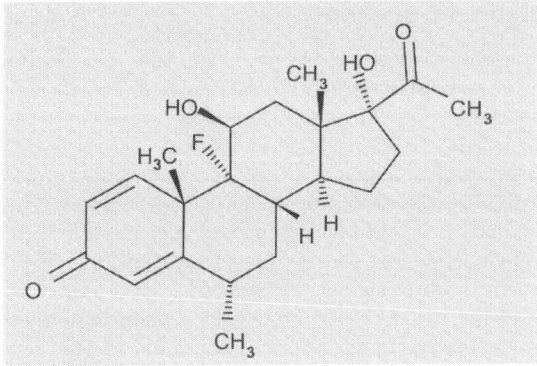

Fig. 8.6: Chemical structure of fluorometholone

Contraindications

Contraindications are similar to standard topical steroid therapy already mentioned.

Precautions should be taken while prescribing topical FML medication for herpes simplex keratitis involving stroma, as it requires greater and frequent slit-lamp microscopy for adverse effects. Topical FML should not be used for injection.

Dosage and Administration

Fluorometholone is available as sterile suspension in 5 ml vials in strength of 0.1 percent and 0.25 percent (FML forte). Besides it, FML is also available as ophthalmic ointment (0.1%) and as acetate suspension (0.1%).

Patients should be advised to instill one drop of topical FML into conjunctival sac 2-4 times daily. During the initial 24-48 hours the dosage may be safely increased two drops every hour depending upon severity of the condition. Care should be taken not to discontinue therapy prematurely and abruptly.

Unique features of topical FML suspension are:
- Its efficacy on ocular surface well established all over the world.
- It is safer than currently available low dose preparations which are up to 10 times diluted
- It is micro fine suspension which ensures uniform particle distribution, longer residence time and rapid absorption.
- Its liquifilm advantage soothes, cools, enhances patient comfort and micro fine suspension minimizes mechanical irritation.
- It has less risk to raise IOP spikes established worldwide through clinical trials.

Due to these special features topical FML suspension is widely and frequently prescribed by ophthalmologists worldwide specially to control iatrogenic inflammation in modern high-tech ophthalmic surgery of PRK, lasik and phacoemulsification.

Loteprednol Etabonate

Loteprednol etabonate (0.5% Ophthalmic soln) is a site reactive corticosteroid with powerful anti-inflammatory activity similar to dexamethasone and FML with marked low propensity to increase IOP spike.

Loteprednol etabonate (0.5%) is a unique ester-based corticosteroid and is a soft drug. Soft drug is a biological compound with predictable inactivation to nontoxic moieties after achieving its therapeutic role thus causing less adverse reactions. The design of this drug (retrometabolic drug design) incorporates a "Soft spot" into the structure that undergoes a predictable metabolic inactivation leading to lower toxicity and more specific action on target organ.

It has high lipophilicity with good intraocular penetration and its predictable degradation is depicted to provide an improved safety profile. That is the reason it causes less increase in intraocular pressure than dexamethasone.

Predictable intraocular conversion of the drug to an inactive compound reduces the amount of active corticosteroid in the trabecular meshwork. Loteprednol etabonate (0.5%) is indicated in steroid responsible inflammatory conditions of the eye, iatrogenic and pseudophakic inflammation of the eye and in anterior uveitis. It is effective in post PRK and Lasik surgery inflammation. Loteprednol 0.2 percent has been approved for seasonal allergic conjunctivitis.

It is available as 0.2 percent and 0.5 percent ophthalmic suspension in 2.5, 5 and 10 ml vials.

Difluprednate

This is a relatively newly developed topical anti-inflammatory steroid with high efficacy and is available as 0.05 percent ophthalmic emulsion. The stable oil-in-water emulsion formulation has an advantage of producing dosage consistency as

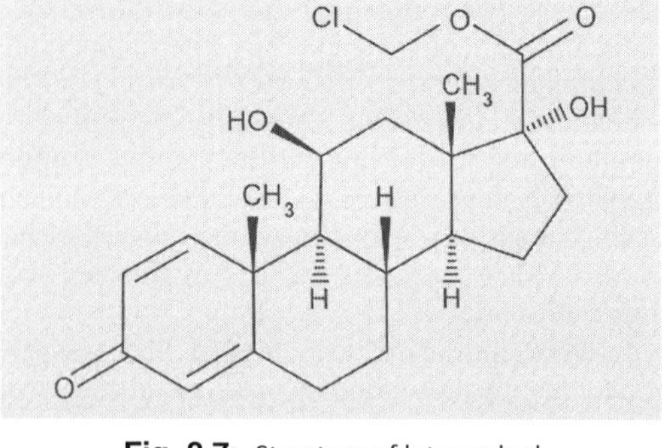

Fig. 8.7: Structure of loteprednol

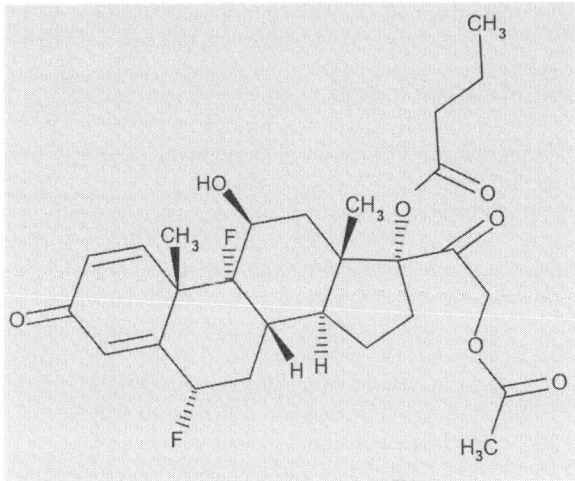

Fig. 8.8: Chemical structure of difluprednate

the other formulations in suspension are needed to be shaken by the patient before instilling the drop for homogeneity of dosage. It has good tissue penetration and better bioavailability, along with fast local metabolism.

It is mainly recommended to treat pain and inflammation associated with ocular surgery and can be used in other ocular inflammatory conditions. One drop four times daily is to be instilled in the conjunctival sac beginning 24 hours postoperatively for two weeks followed by one drop two times daily for one week and then tapered depending on the response. Because of enhanced penetration it may also be used in managing posterior segment inflammation.

As with other moderate to strongly potent steroids, difluprednate also carries an associated risk of increased intraocular pressure, and other adverse effects, but the increased potency, less frequent dosing and the emulsion formulation are some of the advantages of this drug over the others.

Corticosteroids drops are used either in solo or in combination of topical antibiotics to produce maximal benefit to the patient.

Topical Steroid Antibiotic Combinations

Various topical steroid-antibiotic combinations used in ophthalmic field are:
1. Dexamethasone (0.1%) with neomycin (0.5%) in solution form.
2. Dexamethasone (0.1%) with neomycin (0,35%) and polymyxin B (10000 units/ml) suspension or ointment.
3. Dexamethasone (0.1%) with chloramphenicol (0.5 to 1%) soln.
4. Dexamethasone (0.1%) with framycetin (0.3%) suspension.
5. Dexamethasone (0.1%) and tobramycin (0.3%) suspension.
6. Dexamethasone (0.1%) with chloramphenicol (1%) and polymyxin B 5000 I.U. soln and oint.
7. Dexamethasone (0.1%) with gentamicin (0.3%)-soln.

8. Dexamethasone (0.1%) with ciprofloxacin (0.3%)
9. Dexamethasone (0.1%) with ofloxacin (0.3%)
10. Dexamethasone (0.1%) with lomefloxacin (0.3%)
11. Dexamethasone (0.1%) with sparfloxacin (0.3%)
12. Betamethasone (0.1%) with neomycin (0.5%) soln
13. Betamethasone (1%) with chloramphenicol (0.5%) in soln. and oint form.
14. Betamethasone (0.1%) with gentamicin (0.3%) in soln.
15. Hydrocortisone (0.5%) with neomycin (0.5%) oints and soln.
16. Hydrocortisone (0.5%) with neomycin (0.5%) oint and soln.
17. Hydrocortisone (1.5%) and neomycin (0.5%) ointment.
18. Hydrocortisone 10 mg/gm, polymyxin B 0.5 mg/gm ointment.
19. Hydrocortisone (1%) with gentamycin (0.3%)- Suspension.
20. Hydrocortisone (0.5%) with chloramphenicol (1%)- ointment.
21. Prednisolone (0.5%) neomycin -0.35 percent and Polymyxin B 10000 units/ml suspension.
22. Prednisolone (1%) with gentamicin (0.3%) suspension.
23. Prednisolone (0.2%) with sulphacetamide (10%) and phenylephrine (0.12%)-soln.
24. Fluorometholone (0.1%) with neomycin (0./35%) in solution.
25. Fluorometholone (0.1%) with gentamicin (0.9%) in soln.
26. Fluorometholone (0.1%) with tobramycin (0.3%) in soln.

Indications of topical antibiotic steroid combinations:
- In treatment of anterior segment inflammatory disorders which may be threatened with or complicated by bacteria sensitivity to antibiotics.
- In pre-and postoperative phase of intraocular surgery where the possibility of infection with susceptible organisms exists.
- In chronic anterior uveitis and corneal injury from chemical, radiation or thermal burns.

Contraindications of antibiotic-steroid combination:
- In acute untreated purulent ocular infections caused by microorganisms not sensititve to antibiotics in steroid combination
- Acute superficial herpes simplex (dendritic keratitis)
- Vaccinia, varicella and other viral diseases of the conjunctiva and cornea
- Fungal diseases
- Ocular tuberculosis
- Hypersensitivity of drug
- In diseases due to microorganisms resistant to associated antibiotic with concerned steroid combination, infection may be masked, enhanced or activated by the steroid
- Prolonged use may result in overgrowth of non-susceptible organisms.

The advantage of topical steroid-antibiotic combination is that when decision is taken to administer such drugs combination, there is greater patient compliance and convenience with the added assurance that the appropriate dosage of both the drugs is administered. When both the drugs are in the same formulation, compatibility of ingredients is assured and the correct volume of drug is delivered and retained. In antibiotic steroid topical combination, steroids provided powerful anti-inflammatory effect while associated antibiotic provide broad spectrum bactericidal effect. Even pus, exudates and bacterial growth products cannot inactivate the antibiotics in such combinations.

Dosage and Administration

Patient is advised to put 1-2 drops in the conjunctival sac 2-4 times daily. Care should be taken not to discontinue the treatment prematurely and abruptly.

Adverse Reactions

In addition to topical steroid complications already mentioned in this chapter, the most frequent reactions reported are ocular discomfort, irritation upon instillation of the medication and punctuate keratitis. These reactions resolve with the discontinuation of the medication.

In present day ophthalmic practice topical fluorometholone neomycin (FML-neo), dexamethasone-tobramycin and dexamethasone-neomycin-polymixin B combinations are commonly prescribed as effective treatment when infection and inflammation or injection and allergy coexist.

Modes of Corticosteroid Delivery

The various modes of corticosteroid drug delivery systems have their limitations in the form of their questionable reach in desired concentration at the target site, and the associated unwanted ocular and systemic adverse effects.

In severe forms of anterior uveitis or iatrogenic inflammation, topical steroid therapy may require supplementation with periocular injection of systemic steroids. Periocular steroids help in delivering a higher dose and sustained delivery to the posterior segment and thus are effective for intermediate uveitis, uveitic macular edema, and posterior uveitis. Generally, 40 mg triamcinolone is administered through the posterior sub-Tenon or orbital floor or 40 mg methylprednisolone through the orbital floor. Periocular triamcinolone has been used due to its lesser tendency to cause scar formation and extraocular muscle fibrosis. Compared to other steroids, triamcinolone has no mineralocorticoid activity. The clinical improvement is apparent after 2-3 days. Periocular injections are contraindicated in toxoplasmosis and necrotising scleritis. Injections can be repeated after 2-4 weeks.

Triamcinolone has also been tried as intravitreal implant. Intravitreal triamcinolone injection of 1-4 mg in 0.1 ml can be given in some specific cases. But the therapeutic effects on intravitreal injections are normally not sustained for long because of the short half lives of the drugs in vitreous. The intravitreal injections also carry an increased risk of elevated intraocular pressure, cataract, and endophthalmitis.

There have been efforts to device new ways to deliver steroids to ocular tissues to overcome the shortcomings of conventional routes, such as the variable bioavailability and numerous side effects of the systemic steroids, and the need for repeated injections or eyedrop instillation with the local steroidal therapy. So formulations in the form of sustained-release intraocular corticosteroid implants have been developed. The fluocinolone acetonide implant was developed to deliver corticosteroid for up to 30 months in chronic non-infectious posterior uveitis. The dexamethasone drug delivery system is another such biodegradable intravitreal implant approved by the FDA for the treatment of macular edema and noninfectious posterior uveitis. It can be implanted intravitreally by an injector as compared to the fluocinolone implant which needs surgical placement. These implants also carry the risk of increased IOP, cataract formation, conjunctival hemorrhage and the other traumatic complications.

Systemic Corticosteroids

Systemic steroids are the mainstay of treatment of inflammation of the posterior segment and orbit. They are used as supplement to topical steroids in severe inflammation of the anterior segment of the eye.

Anti-inflammatory effect of dexamethasone is 30–50 times more than that of cortisone; prednisolone is 5 times more potent than cortisone as an anti-inflammatory agent.

Indications for systemic steroids:
- Posterior uveitis
- Sympathetic ophthalmia
- Papillitis and retrobulbar neuritis
- Anterior ischemic optic neuropathy
- Scleritis
- Severe anterior uveitis
- Malignant exophthalmos
- Orbital pseudotumor
- Herpez zoster ophthalmicus
- IOL implantation
- Refractive keratotomy
- Vogt-Koyanagi-Harada syndrome
- Macular edema.

Dosage, duration and type of systemic steroids use depends upon the severity and type of ocular diseases in which it is required.

Ocular complications of topical steroid use:
Complications of topical steroids are due to their intraocular penetration, collagenolytic and immune-suppressive prosperities. Topical steroids must be used with caution in herpetic keratitis properties. Some common complications of topical steroid therapy are mentioned below.
- Reduced resistance of viral, bacterial and fungal infection
- Cataract (Posterior subcapsular cataract type)
- Raised intraocular pressure in susceptible patients (Glaucoma-open angle type) with optic nerve damage defects in visual field and acuity

- Secondary ocular infections from fungi and viruses liberated from ocular tissues
- Delayed wound healing
- Dry eye
- Ptosis
- Mydriasis
- Perforation of globe when used in conditions where there is thinning of cornea and sclera.

Ocular complications of systemic steroid use:
Systemic corticosteroids produce several ocular side effects on extensive use. These are:
- Posterior subcapsular cataract
- Activation of infections
- Glaucoma, exophthalmos, papilledema.

The undesirable effects of steroids led to the development of nonsteroidal anti-inflammatory agents which are relatively free of serious side effects.

NONSTEROIDAL ANTI-INFLAMMATORY DRUGS

In the treatment of ocular inflammation, need of nonsteroidal anti-inflammatory drugs (NSAIDs) was felt due to the complications associated with the more established corticosteroid therapy such as elevation of intraocular pressure, progression of cataracts, increased risk of infection, worsening of stromal melting, etc. Although an overlap between the mechanisms of action of both NSAIDs and steroids exists, yet the use of NSAIDs in ophthalmology is safer than the use of corticosteroids as NSAIDs are relatively free of potential adverse effects of steroids.

The history of NSAIDs use in ophthalmology dates back to 1971 when Vane and Smith established the connection between the clinical effect of acetylsalicylates and inhibition of prostaglandin synthesis.

Since the detection of presence of prostaglandins in rabbit iris tissue on 1955, this substance has been established in elevated levels in the anterior chamber that have been associated with inflammation triggered by trauma, uveitis, cataract, IOL surgery and laser iridotomy. Topical NSAIDs are now widely used in iatrogenic and other inflammatory conditions of the eye.

Classification and Structure of NSAIDs

Nonsteroidal anti-inflammatory drugs are chemically heterogeneous groups that can be grouped into various classes as given below:
- Salicylates
- Fenamates
- Indoles
- Phenylalkanoic acids
- Pyrazolones
- Phenylacetates
- Para-aminophenols.

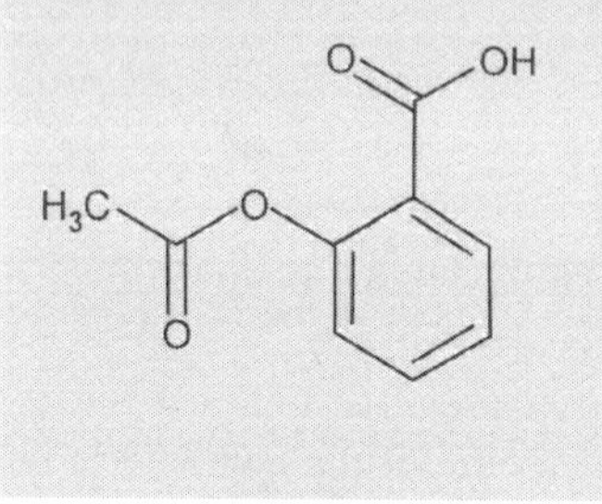

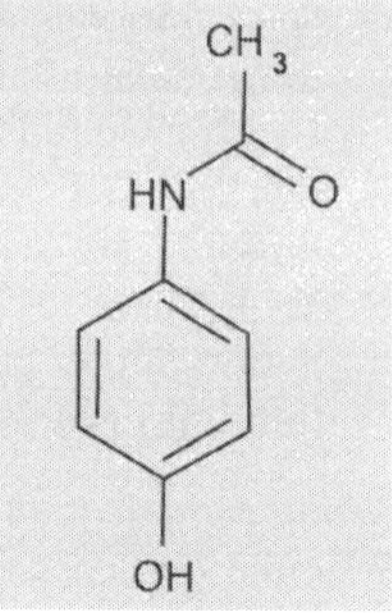

Acetylsalicylic acid

Acetaminophen

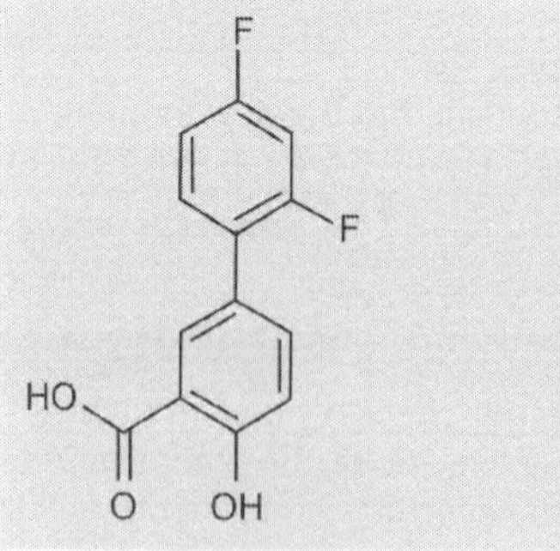

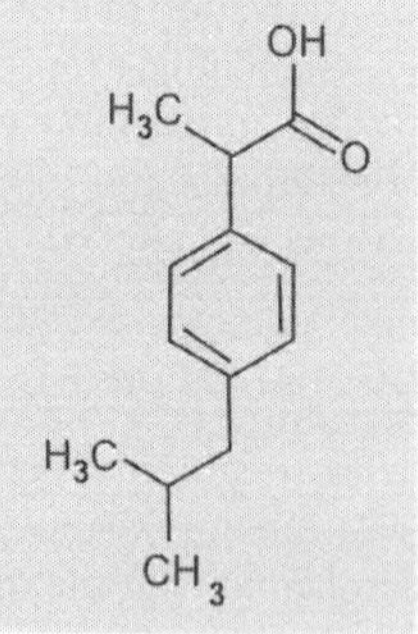

Diflunisal

Ibuprufen

Fig. 8.9: Chemical structures of some systemically used NSAIDs

The chemical feature shared by all these classes is the absence of cholesterol derived steroid nucleus hence the term non-steroidal. The pharmaceutical emphasis has been on the indoles, phenylacetates and phenylalkanoic acids because of instability in solution and hence high ocular toxicity of salicylates, fenamates and pyrazolone derivatives. Specific drugs belonging to each class are listed in Tables 8.1 and 8.2.

Mechanism of Action

Nonsteroidal anti-inflammatory drugs provide symptomatic relief by helping in suppressing the inflammation but they do not modify the inflammatory etiology. Nonsteroidal anti-inflammatory drugs act mainly as anti-inflammatory agents by inhibiting cyclo-oxygenase and lipo-oxygenase enzymes which lead to inhibition of products like prostaglandins, thromboxane and leukotrienes which induce inflammation. The synthesis of prostaglandins is dependent upon the activity of enzyme cyclo-oxygenase, while formation of leukotrienes is dependent upon the activity of lipo-oxygenase. Prostaglandins in eye cause miosis, increased vascular permeability, breakdown of blood-aqueous barrier, conjunctival hyperemia and changes in intraocular pressure. Prostaglandins have also been implicated in allergic reactions. Most of the NSAIDs

TABLE 8.1: Systemic nonsteroidal anti-inflammatory agent

Drug class	Drug name	How supplied (mg) (Commercially)	Typical adult Daily dose (mg)
Salicylates	Aspirin	325-650	650-975 mg q4h
	Diflunisal	250,500	250 qid
	Choline magnesium Trisalicylate	250,500	1000-1500 mg bid
	Sodium salicylate	325-650	325-650 mg q3-4h
Fenamates	Mefenamate	250	250 qid
	Meclofemate	50,100	50-100 qid
Indoles	Indomethacin	25,50,75 (slow release)	25,50 tid-qid, 75 bid
	Sulindac	150,200	150-200 bid
	Tolmetin	200,400,600	400 tid
Phenyl acetic acid	Diclofenac	25,50,75	50-75 bid
Phenyl alkanoic acids	Fenoprofen	200,300,600	300-600 tid
	Ketoprofen	25,50,75	75 tid-50 qid
	Piroxicam	10,20	10 bid, 20 daily
	Flurbiprofen	50,100	100 tid
	Ketorolac	10	10 qid
	Naproxen	250,375,500	250-500 bid
	Naproxen Na	275,550	275-550 bid
	Ibuprofen	200,300,400, 600,800	400-800 tid
	Nabumetone	250,300	1 g q night
Pyrazolones	Phenylbutazone	100	100 tid-qid
Para-aminophenols	Acetaminophen	80,325,500,650	650 q 4th hourly

inhibit enzyme cyclo-oxygenase where as some of them inhibit both cyclo-oxygenase and lipo-oxygenase.

Apart from the inhibition of COX, NSAIDs produce anti-inflammatory effect by other mechanisms such as suppression of polymorphonuclear (PMN) chemotaxis as well as decreased expression of inflammatory cytokines and mast cell degranulation. The NSAIDs also have free radical scavenging activity during inflammation and thus help in the prevention of tissue damage.

Depending on the step at which action is exerted they have been categorized in two types.

Type I Inhibitors

These inhibit cyclo-oxygenase and therefore also the cyclic endoperoxidase activity. Hence PG G_2 and PG H_2 are not formed,

TABLE 8.2: Topical nonsteroidal anti-inflammatory agents

Drug name	How supplied commercial	Typical dose
Flurbiprofen	0.03% solution	1 drop every 30 minutes, 2 hours preoperatively (total dose-4 drops)
Suprofen	1.0%	2 drops at 1, 2 and 3 hours preoperatively or every 4 hours while awake on the day of surgery
Diclofenac	0.1% solution	-qid
Ketorolac	0.5% solution	-tid
Indomethacin	• 0.5-1.0% suspension	
	• 0.1% ophthalmic solution	-qid
Bromfenac	0.09% solution	- bid
Nepafenac	0.1% suspension	- tid
Freshly prepared topical NSAIDs		
Asprin	1.0%	-qid
Acetyl salicylic acid	0.03% solution	-qid
Diflunisal	0.03% solution	-qid
Ointment		
Oxyphenbutazone	10% ointment	HS - bid
Phenylbutazone	10% ointmernt	HS - bid

thus the whole range of PG, thromboxane A_2 and PGI_2 cannot be synthesized. Examples of type I inhibitors include salicylates, the fenamates, propionic acid derivatives and indomethacin.

Type II Inhibitors

These inhibit isomerases and reductases, i.e. the step from cyclic endoperoxide to PGE_2 PGF_2, e.g. pyrazolones.

Arachidonic Acid Metabolites and Inflammation

A variety of phenomena in the inflammatory response are mediated by three interrelated plasma derived factors the complement, kinin and clotting system.

The products derived from metabolism of arachidonic acid (AA) affect a variety of biological processes including inflammation and hemostasis. Arachiodonic acid metabolism proceeds along one of the two major pathways: Lipo-oxygenase or cyclo-oxygenase. The cyclo-oxygenase (COX) enzymes exists in two forms COX-1 and COX-2. COX-1 is the constitutive enzyme found in most cells. It is thought that the prostanoids produced by them are involved in normal homeostasis. COX-2 is induced in inflammatory cells by an inflammatory stimulus. Thus, COX-2 has relevance for the mechanisms of action of the NSAIDs.

Pharmacokinetics

Nonsteroidal anti-inflammatory drugs are well-absorbed after oral administration and have measurable ocular penetration. The NSAIDs are 90 to 99 percent protein bound and therefore are easily recovered from ocular tissues. However topical NSAIDs appear to penetrate the eye better than oral administration. Topical instillation of these drugs provides adequate levels of agents in ocular tissue and aqueous humour for inhibition of prostaglandin synthesis. However, topical NSAIDs can gain access to the systemic circulation via mucosal absorption. Therefore, even local administration of NSAIDs can be accompanied by systemic toxicity if nasolacrimal occlusion and eyelid closure are not employed following eyedrop instillation.

The NSAIDs have three type of effects:
- Anti-inflammatory effect
- Analgesic effect
- Antipyretic effect.

In ophthalmology these drugs are used primarily for their anti-inflammatory effects and when required for the analgesic effect.

The NSAIDs are inhibitors of both isoenzymes COX-1 and COX-2 though they vary in degree of inhibition of each.

The anti-inflammatory action is mediated by their inhibition of COX-2. Drugs with selective action on COX-2 could bring in a major advancement. The anti-inflammatory effect of NSAIDs varies. Drug such as indomethacin and piroxicam are strongly anti-inflammatory some such as naproxen, ibuprofen and nabumetone are moderately anti-inflammatory while drugs like paracetamol have essentially no anti-inflammatory activity.

In ophthalmic topical preparations flurbiprofen (0.03 percent), diclofenac (0.1%), ketorolac (9.5%), indomethacin (1%), suprofen (1%), bromfenac (0.09%), and nepafenac (0.1%) are commonly used.

Topical NSAIDs when used stabilize the blood-ocular barriers and are as effective in reducing iatrogenic inflammation as topical corticosteroids. NSAIDs like steroids are also used systemically specially when their action needs to be combined with anti-inflammatory effects or when higher intraocular levels are desirable such as in CME or diffuse retinitis.

Topical NSAIDs like indomethacin (Indole derivative) is commercially available as 1 percent aqueous suspension. A 0.1 percent indomethacin ophthalmic solution has recently been commercially launched. The phenyl alkanoic acids are water soluble and are formulated as ophthalmic solutions. Flurbiprofen (0.03%) and suprofen (1%) are approved by FDA (USA) for intraoperative use to inhibit miosis during cataract surgery. Ketorolac tromethamine (0.5%) has been approved for the treatment of seasonal allergic conjunctivitis. While topical diclofenac (1%) is a phenylacetic acid derivative that is approved by FDA for use to minimize postoperative inflammation after cataract surgery.

Ocular Indications for use of NSAIDs

Maintenance of Intraoperative Mydriasis

Adequate pupillary dilation specially its maintenance during intraocular surgery undergoing ECCE and in posterior segment procedures (Vitreo-retinal surgery). Endogenous factors other than prostaglandins and surgical techniques have been responsible for this condition. NSAIDs use can cause pharmacological effect on the pupil lessening intraoperative miosis. NSAIDs that are commonly used for this purpose include topical flurbiprofen 0.3 percent. Suprofen 1 percent and indometacin 1 percent suspension. Clinical data have shown that topical indomethacin 1 percent Suspension or 0.1 percent ophthalmic solution maintain pupillary dilation in statistically significant higher number of patients undergoing cataract surgery. Topical flurbiprofen and suprofen solutions are commonly sued by ophthalmologists to inhibit intraoperative miosis. This pharmacological activity of NSAIDs is of potential clinical benefit because decreasing pupil size is a well established risk factors for vitreous loss and zonular breaks during ECCE with IOL implantation.

Reduction of Postoperative Inflammation

Surgical injury to the eye leads to breach of the blood aqueous barrier and subsequent cellular infiltration leading to intraocular inflammation. Topical NSAIDs drops are potentially useful in managing postoperative inflammation following intraocular surgery. Flurophotometric analysis offers a quantitative means of studying anterior chamber inflammation.

Several clinical studies have shown the efficacy of NSAIDs specially indomethacin 1 percent, flurbiprofen 0.03 percent, ketorolac 0.5 percent and diclofenac 0.1 percent. On postoperative inflammation NSAIDs positive effect has been reported both in intracapsular and extracapsular cataract surgery. Fluorophotometry studies have shown that topical NSAIDs achieve better inflammation control than the corticosteroids in double masked randomized studies. Topical NSAIDs treatment has been shown to be more effective in re-establishing the disrupted blood-aqueous barrier as compared to the topical steroids. Topical diclofenac 0.1 percent and indomethacin 1 percent suspension or 0.1 ophthalmic solution have been proved to be better in controlling inflammation after cataract surgery. Studies have advocated the use of topical diclofenac 0.1 percent four times daily starting 24 hours after cataract surgery to control postoperative inflammation. It is possible practically to prescribe a topical NSAIDs for a topical corticosteroid to control iatrogenic inflammation specially in eyes with significant steroid responsive glaucoma.

Prevention and Treatment of Aphakic and Pseudophakic Cystoid Macular Edema

Cystoid macular edema (CME) is the most common cause of visual decline following cataract surgery. Angiographically proven CME after cataract surgery occurs in 50-70 percent of patients undergoing ICCE and in 20-30 percent patients who undergo ECCE. The common denominator of all the CME is believed to be mainly prostaglandin mediated breach of blood-retina barrier. Clinical studies have shown that oral and topical NSAIDs are effective in the prophylaxis of angiographic pseudophakic and aphakic CME.

In Summary

a. Topical NSAIDs are effective in preventing postsurgical angiographic CME when topical or sub-Tenon corticosteroid is given concurrently.
b. Prophylactic treatment with topical NSAIDs has a beneficial effect on visual function.
c. Topical NSAIDs are also effective in the treatment of angiographically documented subclinical CME and this can turn into improved visual function.
d. Topical NSAIDs are also effective in treating chronic symptomatic established CME (of 6 months or greater duration). One percent topical fenoprofen and oral indomethacin has been shown to be quite effective in such condition. In the treatment of CME, standard recommendation is to use combination of a topical corticosteroid and topical NSAIDs and then tapering of corticosteroid as the clinical situation improves.

Uveitis

In contrast to postsurgical inflammation, many forms of uveitis require prolonged steroid therapy to control inflammation. Of course, the risk of iatrogenic glaucoma and cataract becomes substantial in these situations. Therefore, NSAIDs are gaining a more secure position in the treatment of certain uveitis.

Systemic NSAIDs have shown to prevent attacks of juvenile rheumatoid arthritis associated iridocyclitis, acute non-granulomatous anterior uveitis and chronic iridocyclitis.

In cases of posterior uveitis and secondary vasculitis, oral NSAIDs are shown to be effective in eliminating macular edema and preventing recurrence. Standard recommend regime is combination of topical corticosteroid and an oral NSAIDs (specially diclofenac 75 mg bd daily) as initial therapy.

Scleritis and Episcleritis

Systemic NSAIDs are agents of choice in the treatment of non-necrotising, simple diffuse and nodular scleritis. Furthermore, when a steroid is needed, the duration and dose of the steroid may be reduced with the adjunctive use of an NSAIDs.

Allergic and Giant Papillary Conjunctivitis

Vernal keratoconjunctivitis most commonly occurs in children and young adults. It shares with contact lens-associated giant papillary conjunctivitis (GPC), the common finding of giant papillae. Ketorolac 0.5 percent ophthalmic solution is effective in reducing eye itching often associated with allergic conjunctivitis. It can also be useful in cases of steroid induced open angle glaucoma and also to prevent cataract formation. One percent topical suprofen has been shown to effective in the treatment of contact lens related GPC.

Recent studies have shown that 1 percent acetyl salicylate and 1 percent piroxicam solutions are effective in treating seasonal allergic conjunctivitis.

Reduction of Discomfort after Refractive Surgery

Topical kerotolac 0.5 percent has been reported to be effective in the management of certain corneal conditions. Well known analgesic effect of topical ketorolac has been shown to reduce corneal pain following Excimer Laser PRK surgery.

Combination of topical diclofenac 1 percent and topical steroid (FML) has been shown to be statistically superior to corticosteroid alone in controlling post PRK myopic regression.

Topical NSAIDs have been used to lessen pain and inflammation after Nd: Yag and photocoagulating lasers.

The use of topical indomethacin 1 percent has been found to be effective to treat symptoms associated with corneal scars, edema, infiltrates and erosions.

VARIOUS TOPICAL NSAIDS USED COMMONLY IN OPHTHALMIC PRACTICE WORLDWIDE

PHENYLALKANOIC ACIDS

Flurbiprofen

It is one of the most potent NSAIDs of the group which is found to be very effective in various ocular conditions. Topical flurbiprofen is available as 0.03 percent in ophthalmic solution (5 ml pack). It is indicated for the inhibition of intraoperative miosis. It is also indicated for treatment of postoperative (iatrogenic) and post-laser trabeculoplasty, inflammation of anterior segment of the eye. It has no significant effect on IOP.

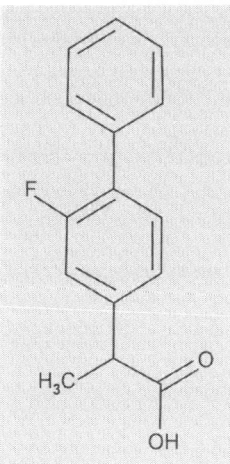

Fig. 8.10: Chemical structure of flurbiprofen

Dosage

For inhibition of intraoperative miosis, a total of four drops of topical flurbiprofen should be administered in the eye by instilling one drop every half hour beginning two hours before surgery.

One drop should be instilled into the conjunctival sac every four hours for one week following laser trabeculoplasty or 2-3 weeks after other surgical procedures.

Topical flurbiprofen is contraindicated in dendritic keratitis and in individuals who are hypersensitive to the drug. Precaution should be taken as there exists the potential for cross-sensitivity to acetylsalicyclic acid and other NSAIDs. Use of flurbiprofen sodium with an anti-infective drug in the presence of ocular infections should be monitored closely.

Adverse Reactions

The most frequent adverse reactions reported with the use of topical flurbiprofen solution are transient burning and stinging upon instillation and other minor symptoms of ocular irritation. It may cause an increased bleeding tendency of ocular tissues in conjunction with surgery.

Ketorolac Tromethamine

It is an alpha substituted aryl acetic acid NSAID. It has both analgesic and anti-inflammatory properties. It is highly soluble in water.

As it is non-narcotic, nonsteroidal agent, its mechanism of action is by its ability to inhibit prostaglandin biosynthesis. Ocular administration of ketorolac reduces prostaglandin biosynthesis. Ocular administration of ketorolac reduces prostaglandin E_2 levels in aqueous humor. Clinical studies have shown that the mean concentration of PGE_2 was 90 pg/ml in aqueous humor prior to the start of topical ketorolac treatment which was reduced drastically to 28 pg/ml in the eye receiving ketorolac ophthalmic solution. It has no significant effect upon intraocular pressure.

Ketorolac ophthalmic solution has following salient features.
- It can be safely administered in conjunction with other ophthalmic medications such as antibiotics, beta blockers, carbonic anhydrase inhibitors, cycloplegic and mydriatics.
- Inhibits leukocyte accumulation even better than dexamethasone.
- Microfine suspension helps in uniform distribution and rapid absorption.
- Lesser propensity to raise IOP than low dose and comparable dose dexamethasone.
- Proven safety in children.

Indications and Usage

- Indication for relief of ocular itching due to seasonal allergic conjunctivitis. It significantly reduces conjunctival inflammation, lid edema, foreign body sensation and photophobia
- Post-Excimer PRK surgery pain management
- Chronic conjunctivitis
- Iatrogenic inflammation of the eye
- Treating aphakic and pseudophakic CME
- For treating episcleritis, patients with corneal edema or erosions
- For prophylaxis associated with retinal detachment surgery.

Dosage and Administration

- Topical ketorolac tromethamine ophthalmic solution is available in strength of 0.5 percent. The recommended dose is one drop four times a day in seasonal allergic conjunctivitis, post PRK pain management and in iatrogenic inflammation of the eye. On topical use it is distributed throughout ocular tissues.

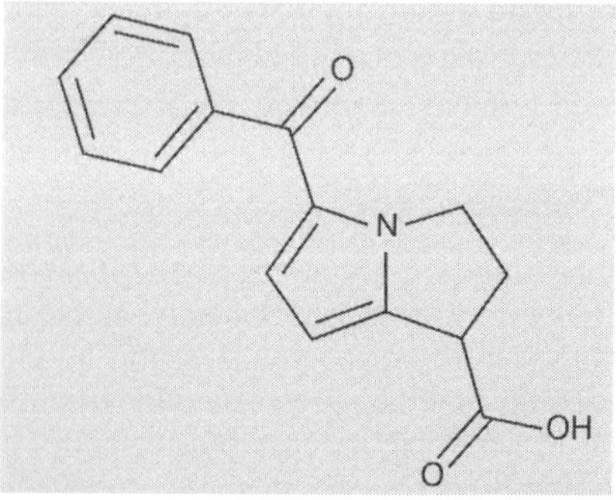

Fig. 8.11: Chemical structure of ketorolac

- Systemic 10 mg tablets (one tablet 3-4 times daily depending upon the severity of pain).
- Injection 1 ml ampule containing 4.35 mg of ketorolac.
- Precautions should be taken regarding its potential for cross-sensitivity to acetylsalicylic acid, phenyl acetic acid derivatives and other NSAIDs.
- There is report that it may cause increase bleeding of ocular tissues including hyphema in conjunction with ocular surgery as it has potential for increased bleeding time due to interference with thrombocyte aggregation.

Adverse Reactions

On topical use ketorolac is well tolerated except for transient stinging and burning sensation on instillation. Other ocular adverse effect reported are ocular irritation, allergic reactions, superficial ocular infections and superficial keratitis. On systemic use it can cause GIT disturbances like nausea, vomiting, constipation, anorexia, pain and ulceration, dermatological and hypersensitivity reactions, CNS effects like headache, dizziness, depressions, confusion and insomnia.

Suprofen

It is available as 1 percent topical ophthalmic solution. Following topical application it achieves significant intraocular levels and inhibit the release of prostaglandin E_2 and $F_{2\alpha}$ and thromboxane B_2 from the inflamed cornea more effectively.

It is good NSAIDs in treating giant papillary conjunctivitis, iatrogenic inflammation of eye and in preventing intraoperative miosis.

Dosage

It is available as 5 ml pack in 1 percent concentration. Patient is advised to put 2 drops at 1, 2, 3 hours preoperatively and four times a day postoperatively and in other ocular inflammatory conditions. Besides these NSAIDs, the other phenylalkanoic acid derivative used in topical forms are:
- Fenoprofen (0.3%)
- Ibuprofen (0.5%)
- Ketoprofen (1.0%)
- Naproxen (0.5%)
- Piroxicam (1%).

INDOLES

Indomethacin

Topical indomethacin is used in the form of 1 percent aqueous suspension and recently introduced 0.1 percent ophthalmic solution.

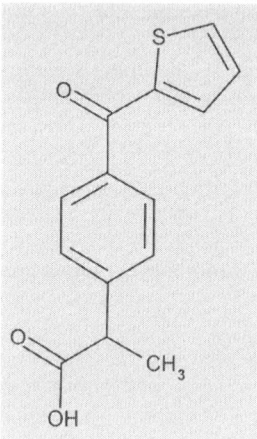

Fig. 8.12: Structure of suprofen

- It is an excellent NSAIDs to treat aphakic and pseudophakic CME following cataract surgery and retinal detachment surgery.
- It has an excellent anti-inflammatory property in treating iatrogenic inflammation, episcleritis and patients of corneal edema and erosions. It has good intraocular penetration. Its mechanism of action and adverse reactions are similar to other NSAIDs mentioned earlier in this chapter.

Other indole NSAIDs used topically are:
- Tolmetin (5% Ophthalmic solution)
- Sulindac (1%).

PHENYLACETIC ACID

Diclofenac Sodium

Diclofenac sodium is a potent nonsteroidal anti-inflammatory drug with analgesic activity which inhibits prostaglandin synthesis. Sodium salt of diclofenac is commercially used. It is one of the most widely prescribed NSAIDs (Either topical or systemic) in ophthalmology. It is most commonly used for its marked anti-inflammatory and analgesic activities in ophthalmology.

Indications

1. In topical form, it is most commonly prescribed in iatrogenic inflammation, pseudophakic inflammation of the eye following cataract and IOL surgery.
2. In aphakic, pseudophakic CME following intraocular surgery.
3. In reduction of post excimer laser PRK surgery pain in the patients.
4. Inhibition of surgically induced miosis during intraocular surgery.

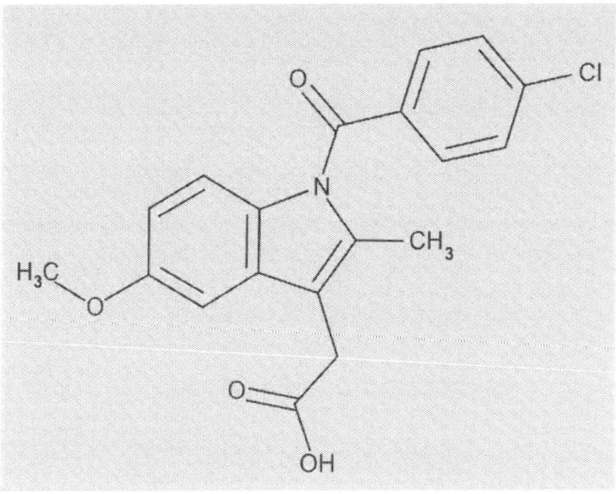

Fig. 8.13: Structure of indomethacin

Dosage and Administration

- In topical form, it is used as ophthalmic solution in strength varying from 0.1 to 1 percent. It has good intraocular penetration. Patient is advised to put one drop 4 times a day postoperatively till the complete clinical cure is achieved. For preoperative use 1 drop of topical diclofenac 0.1 percent solution may be instilled in the affected eye 5 times during 3 hours (prior to surgery).
- In systemic form, it is available as tablet in the strength of 25, 50 and 75 mg. Patient is given oral dose in certain ocular condition where systemic administration is warranted in addition to topical use.
- It is also available in injection form as 75 mg/3 ml ampule. In certain cases of severe postoperative pain 1-2 deep intramuscular injection is indicated following cataract surgery for analgesic effect.

Topical diclofenac does not cause rise in intraocular pressure. It is contraindicated in patients allergic or sensitive to aspirin or other NSAIDs. Patients with blurred vision should not drive or operate machinery and soft contact lenses should not be worn during the treatment period.

Role of Ocular Diclofenac in Therapy

As the world population ages, cataract becomes an even more common problem facing clinicians and surgeons. Identification of effective pharmacological method of treating or preventing acute inflammatory processes associated with surgical extraction of cataract constitute an important goal of pre-and postoperative management.

Topical diclofenac, a potent NSAID has shown equivalent efficacy (when formulated as 0.1% solution) to dexamethasone 0.1 percent solution in attenuating signs of ocular inflammation. The

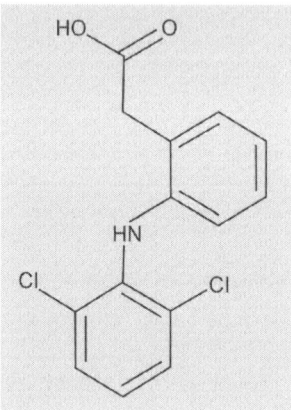

Fig. 8.14A: Chemical structure of diclofenac

drug is similar to indomethacin 0.1 percent in preventing elevation of IOP following cataract surgery. The occurrence and severity of cystoids macular edema is lessened with prophylactic instillation of topical diclofenac and drug appears to prevent surgically induced miosis to greater degree.

Adverse Reactions

Topical diclofenac solution is well tolerated except for a transient localized burning and tingling sensation as reported by some patients.

On systemic use it causes GIT disturbances, headache, dizziness, rash, pruritis, peripheral edema, GI bleeding and peptic ulcer, etc.

Bromfenac

Bromfenac is a lately introduced nonsteroidal anti-inflammatory drug for topical ophthalmic use. It blocks prostaglandin synthesis by inhibiting cyclo-oxygenase 1 and 2, thus producing its anti-inflammatory action.

Clinical Indications

Bromfenac is mainly recommended for the treatment of postoperative inflammation in patients who have undergone cataract extraction.

Dosage

It is available as 0.09% solution. One drop of bromfenac solution is instilled in the affected eye(s) two times daily beginning 24 hours after cataract surgery and is to be continued for two weeks.

Adverse Reactions

- Burning/stinging sensation
- Pain
- Itching
- Redness
- Iritis/keratitis
- Increased risk of bleeding
- Delayed healing (with concomitant use of topical steroids).

Nepafenac

Nepafenac is also a relatively newer anti-inflammatory drug developed for topical ophthalmic use. Unlike majority of topical anti-inflammatory drugs which are formulated as solutions, nepafenac is available as suspension. Nepafenac is also not a free acid as other NSAIDs. Nepafenac is the first prodrug NSAID and gets converted into Amfenac after penetrating the cornea upon topical application. Amfenac is the active moiety which has nonsteroidal anti-inflammatory action. It inhibits the synthesis of prostaglandins, which are responsible for pain and inflammation, by inhibiting the enzyme cyclo-oxygenase (prostaglandin synthase).

Dosage

It is available as 0.1 percent solution. One drop is instilled in the affected eye(s) three-times-daily beginning one day before and then continued for 2 weeks postoperatively.

Indications

It is mainly indicated for the treatment of pain and inflammation associated with cataract surgery and can be used for similar iatrogenic inflammatory conditions.

Adverse Reactions

- Capsular opacity
- Blurring
- Foreign body sensation
- Increased intraocular pressure
- Sticky sensation

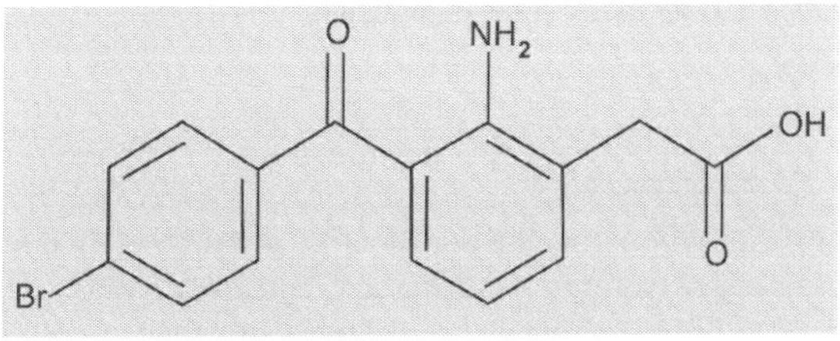

Fig. 8.14B: Structure of bromfenac

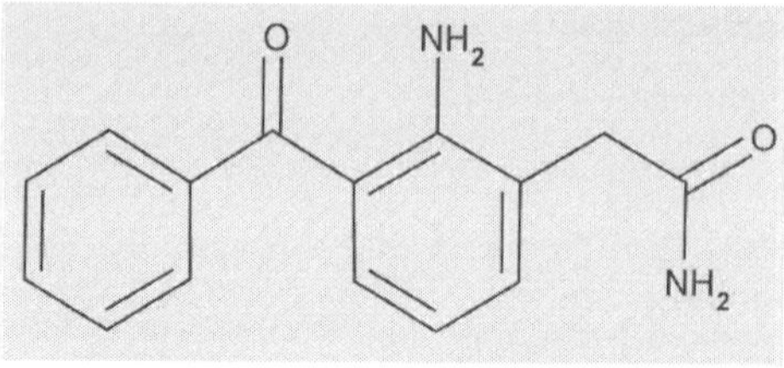

Fig. 8.15: Structure of nepafenac

- Increased bleeding time
- Keratitis.

Hypersensitivity to any of the ingredients in the formulation or to other NSAIDs is a contraindication for use.

General Local and Systemic Toxicities of NSAIDs

The most common adverse reactions after topical instillation as already described in individual NSAIDs are transient blurring, stinging and hyperemia of the conjunctiva.

Manufacturers have used various new formulation methods to minimize this potential discomfort. Indomethacin solution in sesame seed oil was abandoned in favor of aqueous suspension or ophthalmic solution. Suprofen is prepared with 1 percent caffeine because it is less irritating in this form. Ketorolac is formulated as tromethamine salt as its moiety enhances the aqueous solubility and results in solution which is less irritating to the eye.

Generally all the topical NSAIDs have the potential of delaying wound healing. The risk is further enhanced with the concomitant use of topical steroids. Keratitis, epithelial breakdown, corneal thinning, corneal erosion, corneal ulceration or corneal perforation may occur in susceptible patients on the prolonged use of any of the topical NSAIDs. So, one should be watchful for these adverse effects in patients with complicated ocular surgeries, ocular surface diseases, corneal denervation and corneal epithelial defects. In addition allergic and hypersensitive reactions have been reported with topical NSAIDs. Systemic administration of NSAIDs can be accompanied by serious side effects such as gastrointestinal, central nervous system, hematological, renal, liver, dermatological and metabolic changes. These adverse effects are minimized by topical administration.

Therefore, NSAIDs use must be carefully monitored for adverse events as with any other class of drug use.

IMMUNOSUPPRESSIVE AGENTS IN OPHTHALMOLOGY

Many of the actions of glucocorticoids, apart from being anti-inflammatory, are immunosuppressive. Glucocorticoids and their popular established rationale for use have already been discussed earlier. Here, drugs which are especially immunosuppressive in nature, are being discussed. The immunosuppressant drugs should be prescribed by ophthalmologists with caution and preferably in concert with an oncologist.

Till date, there appears to have been very low incidence of severe complications from the combined regimen of corticosteroids and immunosuppressive agents probably because of lower dosage use and better general health of ophthalmic patients receiving them. Patients should be fully informed as to potential risk and benefits.

Selection of Patients

- Selection involves those patients who have progressive, usually bilateral vision-threatening disease.
- Failed to respond to conventional corticosteroid therapy or have unacceptable side effects from them.
- Have Wegener's granulomatosis, polyarteritis nodosa or Behçet's disease (Drugs of first choice).
- Can be adequately followed up
- Good compliance about following instructions.
- Are ready to undergo therapy voluntarily with knowledge of potential side effects.
- May benefit certainly from the use of the drugs.
- Have no primary contraindication like active tuberculosis, toxoplasmosis or other infectious process.

Classification of Immunosuppressive Agents Used in Ophthalmology

Immunosuppressive agents used in ocular inflammatory diseases are classified as under:
a. Corticosteroids (Already discussed separately)
b. Antimetabolities (Cytotoxic agents)
   - Alkylating agents: Cyclophosphamide, chlorambucil,
   - Azathioprine, methotrexate
c. Calcineurin inhibitors: Cyclosporin A
d. Antibodies: Infliximab, vascular endothelial growth factors (VEGF), inhibiting monoclonal antibodies (Bevacizumab, Ranibizumab) and Pegaptanib.

Alkylating Agents

Common Alkylating agents used in ophthalmic conditions are cyclophosphamide and chlorambucil. Both are structurally related to nitrogen mustard but are less toxic to the hematopoietic system as compared to nitrogen mustard. These agents work by suppressing the B cell lymphocytes (humoral immunity) and the T cells lymphocytes (cell mediated immunity).

Clinical Indications

Behçet's disease, sympathetic ophthalmia, rheumatoid arthritis, polyarteritis nodosa, Wegener's granulomatosis, relapsing polychondritis, bulluous pemphigoid and malignancy.

Dosage

Cyclophosphamide: In adult patients start at 1–2 mg/kg/day, to be taken in empty stomach. A white blood count (WBC) is taken at day 1 and after every 2–3 days until about 7 days. At this point dosage is reduced by 25–50 mg if needed, to stabilize the WBC between 2500 and 5000/mm^3. The WBC and CBC with differential are then followed weekly and fortnightly once stabilized.

Chlorambucil: In adult patients start at 0.1–0.2 mg/kg/day and increase every 3–4 day if there is no idiosyncratic reaction. The WBC and CBC with DLC are followed as for cyclophosphamide.

Adverse reactions:
- Thrombocytopenia
- Anemia and opportunistic infections
- GIT disturbances
- Alopecia (common with cyclophosphamide)
- Jaundice
- Pulmonary interstitial fibrosis
- Renal toxicity and testicular atrophy
- Hemorrhagic cystitis is an indication for discontinuing cyclophosphamide. There is report of increased incidence of myeloproliferative and lymphoproliferative malignancy in patients on these drugs.

Antimetabolites

The antimetabolites used in ophthalmology are:
1. Azathioprine—interferes with purine metabolism.
2. Methotrexate—interferes with folate action by inhibiting the enzyme dihydrofolate reductase.

Both functions are essential for nucleic acid synthesis and cellular proliferation.

Clinical Indications

- In rheumatoid arthritis, pemphigoid and regional ileitis.
- Sympathetic ophthalmia and VKH syndrome.

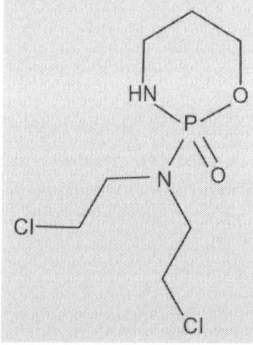

Fig. 8.16: Chemical structure of cyclophosphamide

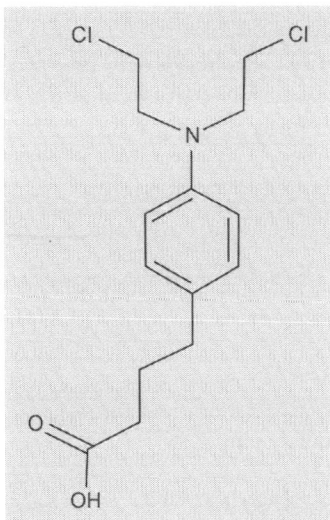

Fig. 8.17: Structure of chlorambucil

- Pars planitis and Behçet's disease.
- Recalcitrant cases of intermediate uveitis.

Dosage

Azathioprine dosage starts at 1–2 mg/kg/day, gradually increasing to 2.5 mg/kg/day. The usual dose range is 100–200 mg/day in one or divided doses. Patient's WBC, CBC with differential are taken at regular intervals.

Methotrexate dosage is variable due to high drug toxicity. Generally for 1–4 weeks oral, IM or IV dose of 2.5–15 mg is given over 36–48 hours until a therapeutic response is noted and then maintained as per hematologic (weekly) and renal and hepatic (monthly) monitoring.

Adverse Effects of Azathioprine

Nausea, vomiting, leukopenia, and bone marrow depression.

Adverse Effects of Methotrexate

- Leukopenia and thrombocytopenia
- Hepatic and renal toxicity
- GIT disturbances, stomatits, hemorrhagic enteritis
- Interstitial pneumonitis
- CNS toxicity and sterility

Hematological monitoring (WBC, CBC with differential) is similar to that of cyclophosphamide.

Cyclosporin A

It interferes with T cell lymphocyte activation and blocks the gene transcription of interleukins (IL-2, IL-3), IFN-γ and other factors stimulated by T-cells.

Clinical Indications for Cyclosporin A

- Behçet's disease (for which corticosteroids are contraindicated)
- Birdshot chorioretinopathy
- Sarcoid, VKH and sympathetic ophthalmia

Relative Indications

- All noninfectious cases of uveitis unresponsive to maximum tolerated steroid therapy.
- Eales' disease
- Retinal vasculitis (non infectious)
- Serpiginous choroiditis

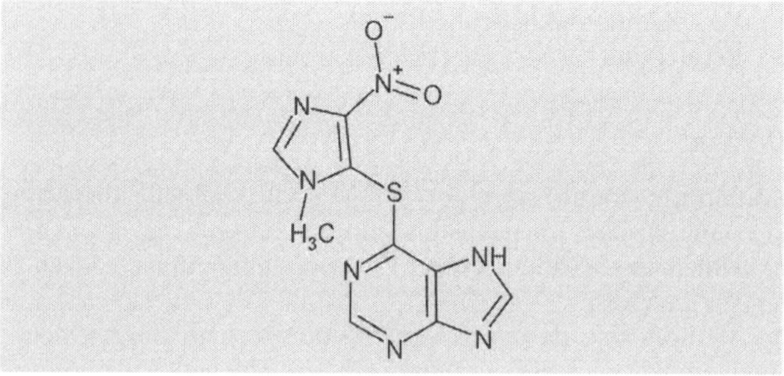

Azathioprine

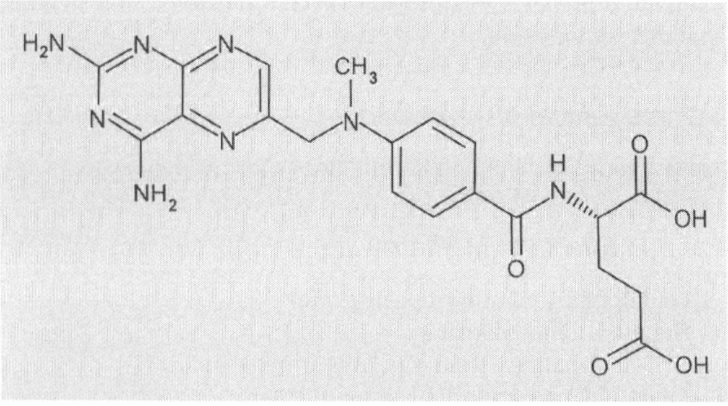

Methotrexate

Fig. 8.18: Chemical structure of azathioprine and methotrexate

Anterior segment diseases include pemphigoid, Mooren's ulcer, high risk corneal transplant rejection and cataract surgery in uveitis patients.

Dosage

Around 2.5–5 mg/kg/day given orally in an olive oil ethanol solution with milk or juice. Maximum dose is 10 mg/kg/day.

Adverse Effects

- Systemic hypertension
- Partially reversible renal toxicity
- Opportunistic infections
- Hyperuricemia
- Hepatotoxicity.

Monthly and if required weekly blood tests (CBC with differential and WBC) should monitor these effects.

- A combination of steroid and cyclosporin A therapy augment each other such that addition of prednisolone (10–20 mg/day) or short-term 1 mg/kg/day may allow a lowering of the cyclosporin A dosage (4–6 mg/kg/day) with no loss of therapeutic efficacy).
- Chlorambucil or cyclophosphamide and steroid management module:

    It involves initial treatment with prednisolone 1 mg/kg/day along with cytotoxic drug at an appropriate dose. This treatment should be continued for 4 weeks until the disease is suppressed, then steroids are tapered and stopped over 2 months. The cytotoxic drug dose is adjusted to keep the

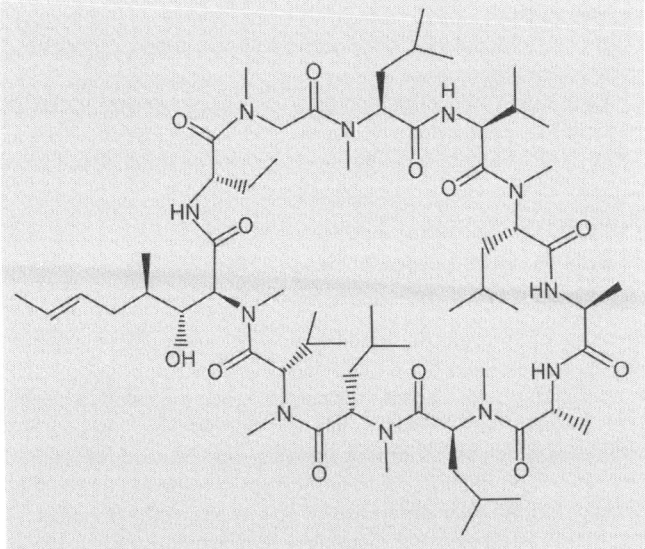

Fig. 8.19: Chemical structure of cyclosporin A

WBC at 3000–4000/ul and continued for one year to induce remission before being stopped. Monitor the CBC and urine analysis weekly until stable, then at every 2 weeks.

Infliximab

Infliximab is an anti-TNF-alpha monoclonal antibody. It has been approved for the treatment of many extraocular inflammatory conditions and has also been tried successfully in various ocular conditions.

Clinical Indications in Ophthalmology

- Behçet's disease
- Noninfectious scleritis
- Severe ocular rheumatoid disease
- Scleromalacia perforans
- Neovascular age-related macular degeneration
- Vogt-Koyanagi-Harada disease
- Retinal vascular tumors
- Refractory retinal vasculitis due to sarcoidosis
- Diffuse subretinal fibrosis syndrome
- Idiopathic sclerosing orbital inflammation (myositis)
- Sight threatening thyroid associated ophthalmopathy.

Dosage

5 to 10 mg/kg is administered by IV infusion at 6–8 weeks intervals.

Adverse Effects

- Infusion related reactions
- Hepatitis
- Increased incidence of opportunistic infections, reactivation of latent tuberculosis
- Lymphoma and other malignancies have been reported in children and adolescent patients treated with TNF blockers, so such rare but fatal adverse effects have to be watched out for.

Vascular Endothelial Growth Factors Inhibitors: Ranibizumab, Bevacizumab, Pegaptanib Sodium

These agents prevent the binding of VEGF, an angiogenic factor, with its receptors on the endothelial cells thus inhibiting cellular proliferation, new vessel formation and vascular leakage. Ranibizumab and Bevacizumab are humanized monoclonal antibodies which act as antiangiogenic drugs. Most of the studies have shown ranibizumab and bevacizumab to be of comparable efficacy, with no clear superiority of one over the other in efficacy. Pegaptanib is a pegylated oligonucleotide which binds to VEGF (not the receptors) and produces the antiangiogenic effects.

Clinical Indications

- Neovascular (wet) form of age-related macular degeneration (AMD)
- Choroidal neovascularization
- Proliferative diabetic retinopathy with macular edema
- Neovascular glaucoma
- Retinopathy of prematurity
- Macular edema secondary to retinal vein occlusions.

Dosage

Ranibizumab

Intravitreal ranibizumab 0.5 mg (0.05 ml) can be given once a month. It has been administered once every three months also when the monthly injection is not feasible, but this is supposed to reduce the efficacy. It is available as 10 mg/ml solution in a single-use vial for intravitreal injection. Ranibizumab intravitreal or intracameral injection is generally given in the dose range of 1.25–2.5 mg (0.05 ml).

Pegaptanib

0.3 mg is administered once every six weeks by intravitreous injection into the affected eye.

Adverse Effects

Conjunctival hemorrhage, blurred vision, anterior chamber inflammation, pain, vitreous floaters, increased intraocular pressure, anterior chamber inflammation, blurred vision, punctate keratitis, and opacities may occur. One has to be cautious for the inherent risks of ocular injections such as endophthalmitis, retinal detachment, cataract and thromboembolic events. These drugs should be avoided in the presence of ocular or periocular infections and hypersensitivity to any of the ingredients in the formulation.

Ocular Drug Toxicity of Immunosuppressive Agents used in Ophthalmic Conditions

- Decrease in vision
- Visual hallucinations
- Lids or conjunctival redness, conjunctivitis, subconjunctival hemorrhage and hypertrichosis
- Loss of eyelashes or eye brow
- Retinal hemorrhages
- Retinal pigment epithelium disturbances
- Cortical blindness (cyclosporin).

BIBLIOGRAPHY

1. Agarwal A. Textbook of Ophthalmology, 1st edn. New Delhi: Jaypee Brothers Medical Publishers, 2002.

2. Albert DM. Albert and Jakobiec's Principles and Practice of Ophthalmology, 3rd edn. Saunders, Elsevier, 2008.
3. Bartlett JD. Ophthalmic Drug Facts, 23rd edn. Wolters Kluwer Health, 2011.
4. Bartlett JD, Jaanus SD. Clinical Ocular Pharmacology. 5th edn. Butterworth-Heinemann, an imprint of Elsevier Inc, 2008.
5. Brunton LL. Goodman and Gilman's The Pharmacological Basis of Therapeutics, 12th edn. New York: The McGraw-Hill Companies, 2011.
6. Duvall. Ophthalmic Medications and Pharmacology. Slack Inc, 2006.
7. Ellis PP. Ocular Therapeutics and Pharmacology, 7th edn. CV Mosby, 1985.
8. Fechner. Ocular Therapeutics. Slack Inc, 1998.
9. Flach AJ. Nonsteroidal Anti-inflammatory Drug in Ophthalmology. Int. ophthalmol. Clinic 1993;33:1.
10. Franzie JP. Steroids. Int. Ophthalmol. Clinic, 1993;33:9.
11. Garg A. Advances in Ophthalmology, 1st edn. New Delhi: Jaypee Brothers Medical Publishers, 2005.
12. Garg A. Clinical Applications of Antibiotics and Anti-inflammatory Drugs in Ophthalmology, 1st edn. New Delhi: Jaypee Brothers Medical Publishers, 2007.
13. Garg A. Current Trends in Ophthalmology, 1st edn. New Delhi: Jaypee Brothers Medical Publishers, 1997.
14. Garg A. Manual of Ocular Therapeutics, 1st edn. New Delhi: Jaypee Brothers Medical Publishers, 1996.
15. Garg A. Ready Reckoner of Ocular Therapeutics, 1st edn. New Delhi, 2002.
16. Havener's Ocular Pharmacology, 6th edn. CV Mosby, 1994.
17. Kanski. Clinical Ophthalmoloy, 7th edn. Expert Consult, 2011.
18. Katzung BG. Basic and Clinical Pharmacology, 12th edn. New York: The McGraw-Hill Companies, 2012.
19. Leibowitz HM. Anti-inflammatory Medications. Int Ophthalmol Clinic, 1980;20:117.
20. Olin BR. Drugs Facts and Comparisons. St. Louis, 1997.
21. Onofrey BE. Ocular Therapeutics Handbook: A Clinical Manual, 3rd edn. Philadelphia: Lippincott Williams and Wilkins, 2011.
22. Rhee. The Wills Eye Drug Guide. Lippincott–William and Wilkins, 2001.
23. Roy and Fraunfelder's Current Ocular Therapy, 6th edn. WB Saunders, 2007.
24. Tasman W, Jaeger EA. Duane's Ophthalmology on DVD-ROM, 2011 edn. Lippincott Williams and Wilkins, 2011.
25. Zimmerman. Textbook of Ocular Pharmacology. Lippincott William and Wilkins, 1999.

9

Antiviral Therapy

NR Biswas, Harivenkatesh N, KP Biswas, Ashok Garg (India)

INTRODUCTION

During the last decade, incidence of ocular viral infections has increased manifold. Ocular viral infections have become a major cause of corneal blindness in the developed as well as developing countries. Its management poses a great challenge because of the nature of the disease and its profound consequences. Among the infectious organisms, viruses are the smallest in size. The major viruses that have been reported to cause ocular diseases include:

DNA VIRUSES

- Herpes group
  - Herpes simplex virus (HSV1 and HSV2 type)
  - Varicella zoster virus (VZV)
  - Cytomegalovirus (CMV)
  - Epstein-Barr virus (EBV)
- Adenovirus (3, 7, 8, 19 and 37 types)
- Variola and vacinnia virus.

RNA VIRUSES

- Picorna virus
- Enterovirus type 70
- Coxsackie A 24
- Measles
- Mumps
- Rubella
- Human immunodeficiency virus.

Viruses are the smallest living units which do not possess a cellular organization. Viruses are the ultimate expression of parasitism; they not only take nutrition from the host cell but also direct its metabolic machinery to synthesize new virus particles. Viral chemotherapy is therefore difficult as it would require interference with cellular metabolism in the host. However, virus directed enzymes have been identified in the infected cell and these may have higher affinities than the regular cellular enzymes. Another difficulty is that in majority of acute infections, viral replication is already at its peak when symptoms appear. Therefore, therapy has to be started in the incubation period as a prophylactic measure.

Development of antiviral drugs has lagged behind due to above mentioned problems unlike the rapid development of antibacterial antibiotics.

It is difficult to block the viral activity in the cell without adversely affecting the host cell metabolic activity since virus replicate using host cell machinery. Most of the antiviral drugs available today mainly inhibit viral nucleic acid synthesis without unduly harming the host cells. There are a few drugs which inhibit viral entry into the cell or block viral protein synthesis. Other peculiar problem includes the nature of viral illness and latency of viruses. Diagnosis is difficult during incubation period and laboratory diagnosis of viral infections is often delayed.

Albeit antiviral drugs exert their action on actively replicating viruses, they have failed to act on the latent forms of viruses like herpes simplex virus (HSV) and varicella zoster virus (VZV).

Clinical importance of viruses lies in their ability to cause huge number of human diseases. Viral infections of the eye ranges from benign to malignant; from a transient keratitis of mononucleosis to progressive sarcoma associated with AIDS. More than 100 viruses are known to be pathogenic to man.

MECHANISM OF VIRAL INFECTION/MULTIPLICATION

Viral replication involves a series of events. DNA virus particle or virion consists of DNA core surrounded by protein capsid coat and lipid envelope. The first step in viral replication is the attachment of the virus to the host cell followed by penetration of the host cell membrane resulting in the entry of virus inside the host cell. On entry into the host cell the virus loses its lipid and protein coats and passes into the host cell nucleus.

Viral DNA gets integrates with host DNA and starts replicating. With the transcription of viral mRNA, virus specific proteins are synthesized. Then the viral particles are assembled after gaining further proteins and lipid coats from host cell. Multiple virions are then released from the host cell. Various stages of viral replication are shown schematically in Figure 9.2 and the antiviral drugs acting on various sites are summarized in Table 9.1.

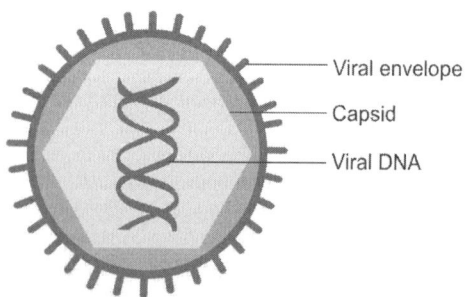

Fig. 9.1: Structure of virus

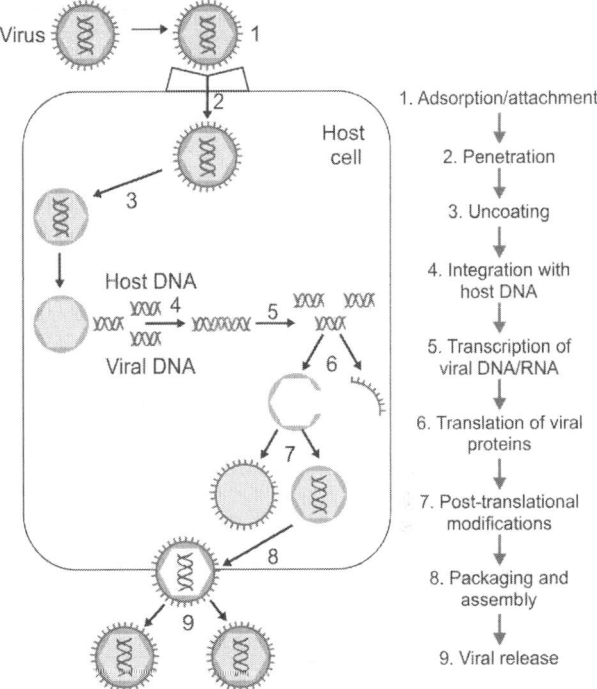

Fig. 9.2: Multiplication of virus—Schematic representation

GENERAL MECHANISMS OF ACTION OF ANTIVIRAL AGENTS

The chemotherapy of intracellular DNA viral infection is based primarily on the disruption of viral DNA synthesis. The site of viral infection is also critical to the success of antiviral agents. With the transcription of viral mRNA, viral specific proteins including thymidine kinase and DNA polymerase are synthesized. Purine and pyrimidine bases (nucleic acid of viruses) are phosphorylated to triphosphorylated purine and pyrimidine bases with the help of thymidine kinase. This triphosphorylated purine and pyrimidine base get incorporated into DNA virus with the help of DNA polymerase and lead to the formation of new DNA which synthesize late proteins that are responsible for the formation of daughter virion capsids hence forming the daughter virion. Most of the known antiviral compounds are virustatic and their antiviral activity is based on the inhibition of virus replication in the presence of drug.

In spite of extensive research for new antiviral agents, only selected compounds are commercially available for clinical use. The reason for this as already mentioned is inability to find substances which selectively influences the viral replication without causing toxic effects on the cells. Moreover, cell damage caused by viral infection is extensive at the stage when first clinical symptom appears.

TABLE 9.1: Drugs acting on various stages of viral replication

Stage of viral replication	Antiviral drugs acting on this stage
Virus attachment	*Entry inhibitors:* Maraviroc (HIV) Palivizumab (RSV) Docosanol (HSV)
Fusion of virus with host cell membrane	*Fusion inhibitors:* Enfuvirtide (HIV)
Penetration of the virus	Interferons (HBV, HCV)
Uncoating	Amantadine (Influenza) Rimantadine (Influenza)
Integration of viral genome and host genome	Integrase inhibitors: Raltegravir (HIV)
Viral DNA/RNA synthesis	Acyclovir, Valacyclovir (HSV, VZV) Ganciclovir, Foscarnet (CMV) Adefovir, Entecavir (HBV) NRTIs- Zidovudine and others (HIV) NNRTIs- Nevirapine, Efavirenz (HIV)
Viral protein synthesis	Interferons (HBV, HCV) Fomivirsen (CMV)
Post-translational modification and maturation	Protease inhibitors: Ritonavir, Indinavir and others (HIV)
Viral assembly	Interferons (HBV, HCV)
Virus release	Neuraminidase inhibitors: Oseltamivir (Influenza) Zanamivir (Influenza)

HIV- Human Immunodeficiency Virus; HBV- Hepatitis B Virus; HCV- Hepatitis C Virus; HSV- Herpes Simplex Virus; CMV- Cytomegalovirus; VZV- Varicella Zoster Virus; RSV- Respiratory Syncytial Virus; NRTIs- Nucleoside Reverse Transcriptase Inhibitors; NNRTIs- Non-nucleoside Reverse Transcriptase Inhibitors

CLASSIFICATION OF ANTIVIRAL DRUGS

Most of the antiviral drugs available today are analogs of nucleosides. Antiviral drugs may be classified according to their activity against particular viruses.

Drugs Active Against Herpes Simplex Virus and Herpes Zoster Virus

- Vidarabine
- Idoxuridine
- Acyclovir
- Valacyclovir
- Famciclovir
- Penciclovir
- Docosanol

- Trifluridine
- Foscarnet.

Drugs Active Against Cytomegalovirus

- Ganciclovir
- Valganciclovir
- Foscarnet
- Cidofovir
- Fomivirsen (Anti-sense oligonucleotide).

Drugs Active Against Influenza Virus

- Active only against Influenza A:
  - Amantadine
  - Rimantadine
- Active against both Influenza A and B:
  - Neuraminidase inhibitors
    - Oseltamivir
    - Zanamivir.

Drugs Active Against Hepatitis Virus

- Active against Hepatitis B Virus (HBV):
  - Nucleotide analogs
    - Adefovir
    - Tenofovir
  - Nucleoside analogs
    - Lamivudine
    - Entecavir
    - Telbivudine
  - Interferons
- Active against Hepatitis C Virus (HCV):
  - Nucleoside analog
    - Ribavirin
  - Protease inhibitors (NS3/4A protease)
    - Telaprevir
    - Boceprevir
  - Interferons.

Drugs Active Against Respiratory Syncytial Virus

- Palivizumab (monoclonal antibody)
- Ribavirin (aerosolized).

Drugs Active Against Human Immunodeficiency Virus

- Nucleoside Reverse Transcriptase Inhibitors (NRTIs)
  - Zidovudine
  - Stavudine
  - Lamivudine

- Abacavir
- Zalcitabine
- Didanosine
- Emtricitabine
- Nucleotide Reverse Transcriptase Inhibitors
  - Tenofovir
- Non-Nucleoside Reverse Transcriptase Inhibitors
  - Efavirenz
  - Nevirapine
  - Delavirdine
  - Etravirine
- Protease inhibitors
  - Ritonavir
  - Indinavir
  - Nelfinavir
  - Saquinavir
  - Amprenavir
  - Fosamprenavir
  - Lopinavir
  - Atazanavir
  - Darunavir
  - Tipranavir
- Entry inhibitor
  - Maraviroc (CCR5 antagonist)
- Fusion inhibitor
  - Enfuvirtide
- Integrase inhibitor
  - Raltegravir.

Details of individual antiviral agents are given below:

ANTIHERPES AGENTS

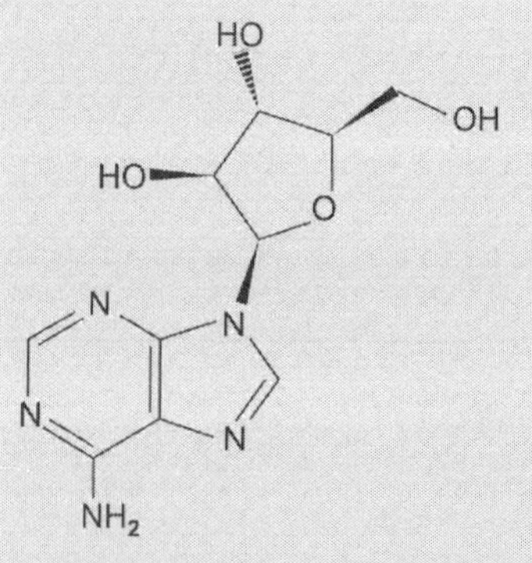

Vidarabine

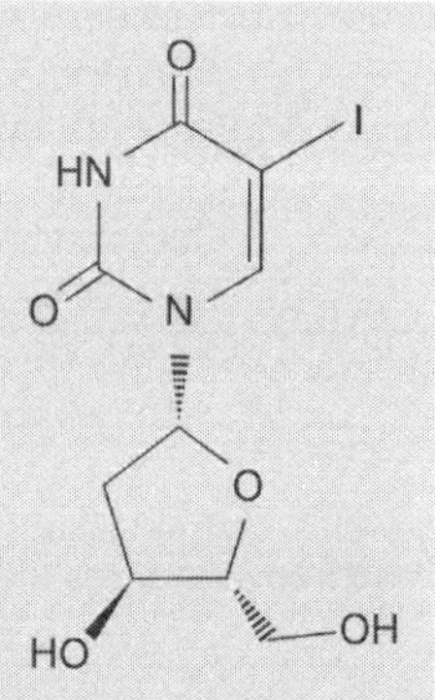

Idoxuridine

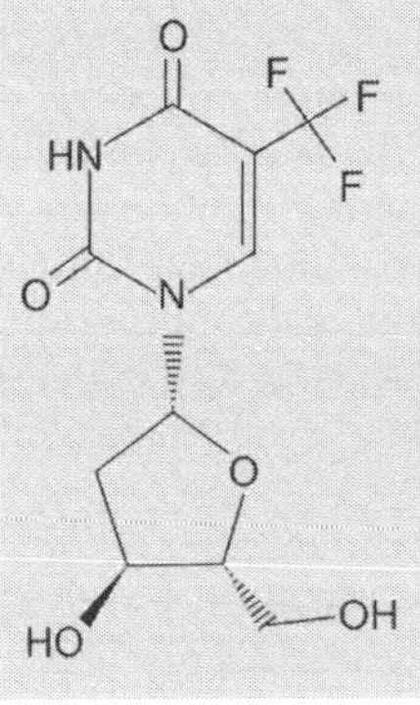

Antiviral Therapy

Trifluridine

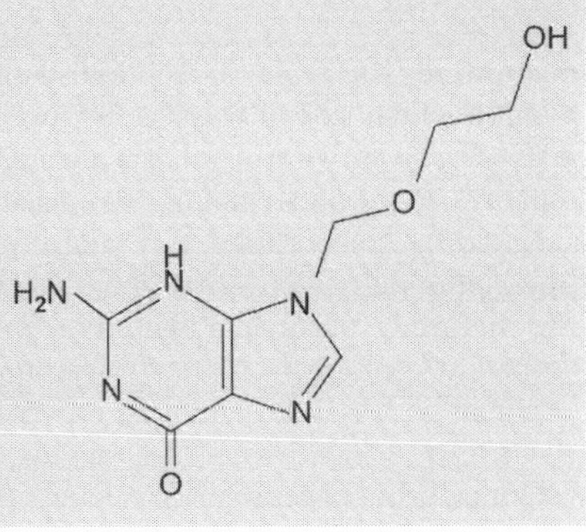

Acyclovir

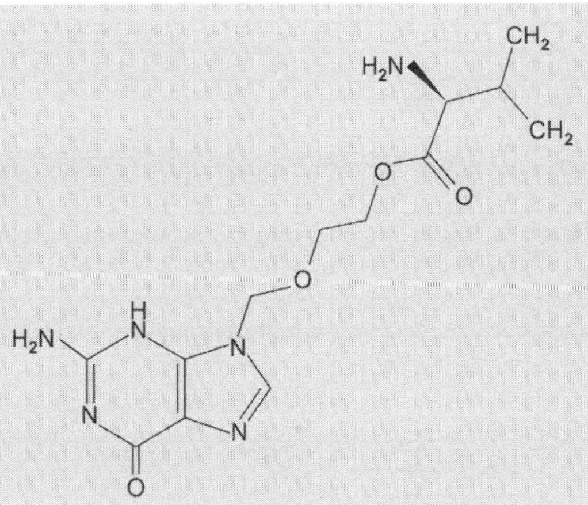

Valacyclovir

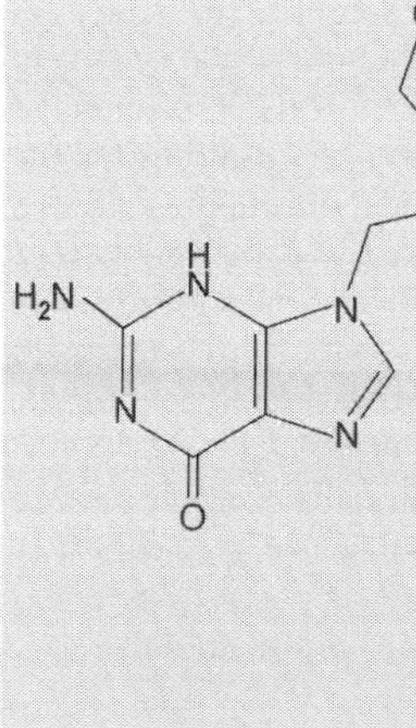

Famciclovir

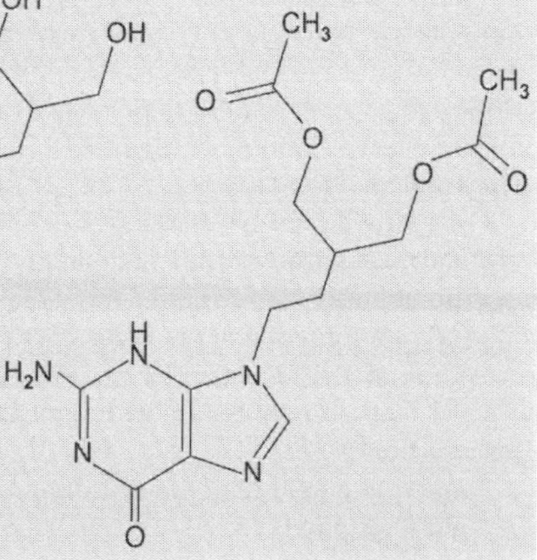

Penciclovir

Fig. 9.3: Structure of commonly used antiherpes drugs

Idoxuridine

Idoxuridine (IDU) is a 5-iodo-2-deoxy uridine which is a thymidine analogue. It was the first pyrimidine antimetabolite to be used as an antiviral agent. It is a halogenated pyrimidine where 5-methyl group of thymidine is replaced by iodine. The drug is activated by both cellular and viral thymidine kinase to form a triphosphorylated derivative. The phosphorylated drug competes with naturally occurring thymidine in DNA chain elongation ultimately resulting in chain termination.

Since both cellular and viral enzymes activate the drug, side effects also include severe host cell toxicity. Initially, it was used systemically but because of associated toxicity and lack of efficacy, its systemic use has been abandoned. It is now used only in topical form for treatment of viral keratitis.

It inhibits, the viral replication in the cornea. IDU is rapidly degraded into an inactive idouracil in the tissue. Its intraocular penetration is poor. It is effective against DNA viruses. Viral selectivity of IDU is low.

It is effective in treatment of HSV keratitis especially superficial epithelial infections. Herpes simplex virus readily develops resistance to it. Initial attacks and dendritic corneal ulcers respond well but poorer results are obtained in recurrent attacks or when corneal stroma is involved or HSV type 2 infection occurs. It is contraindicated during first few weeks of keratoplasty and penetrating corneal ulcer as it inhibits corneal stromal healing.

Dosage

- 0.1 percent eyedrops
- 0.5 percent eye ointment

Topical IDU given for 2 weeks continuously cures 75 percent of superficial HSV Keratitis. Treatment should not be prolonged beyond 3 weeks since it may lead to corneal toxicity. It is used both for primary as well as recurrent HSV keratitis. The drug does not penetrate cornea and is water insoluble hence little activity in stromal keratitis. In HSV epithelial keratitis topical IDU 0.1 percent solution is given to patient to put one drop every hour during the day and every 2-3 hours at night. IDU (0.5%) ointment is advised to be applied 6 times a day.

Once the fluorescein staining of cornea becomes negative, the frequency of topical solution instillation is reduced to 4-6 times a day. The treatment is continued for at least 3 weeks to counter the rebound phenomenon of the virus reactivation.

Although IDU is effective in HSV epithelial keratitis, yet in some cases treatment failure with topical IDU has been reported. This may be due to:

- Inadequate treatment due to infrequent administration
- Viral resistance
- Insufficient potency
- Improper diagnosis
- Toxicity or allergy.

Adverse Effects

Short-term reversible toxic effects resulting from disruption of normal cellular DNA synthesis like toxicity to cornea, conjunctiva and lids are seen. On prolonged use of IDU, it causes:
- Blepharitis
- Papillary conjunctivitis
- Punctal occlusion
- Superficial punctate keratopathy
- Delayed epithelial healing
- Ghost dendrites and scarring
- Corneal clouding
- Photophobia
- Lid edema
- Ptosis.

If no healing is seen within two weeks most probably the virus is resistant to IDU and an alternative drug should be used.

Vidarabine (Ara-A)

Vidarabine is an adenosine analog. It is converted into phosphorylated drug by cellular and viral kinases. Phosphorylated drug is a potent inhibitor of viral (HSV) DNA polymerase. It was the first drug to be used intravenously for life threatening HSV infection and is an alternative to acyclovir. Unlike IDU, Ara-A can achieve viricidal concentration in aqueous humor after 2 hours of topical administration due to improved corneal penetration. It is effective for the treatment of HSV type 1 and type 2 infections including stromal keratitis, iritis and cases resistant to IDU therapy. Currently, it is available only for topical use. Systemic use of this drug has been discontinued due to availability of better and safe drugs.

Dosage

It is available as 3 percent ophthalmic ointment and the ointment is to be applied 5 times a day for 14–21 days. After epithelization, dose is reduced to 1–2 times/day for 4–5 days.

The drug is rapidly deaminated in tissues including the cornea. It is generally given not for more than 3 weeks due to fear of toxicity.

Adverse Effects

- Superficial punctate keratitis
- Photophobia
- Lacrimation
- Allergic reactions.

Trifluridine

Trifluridine (TFT) is a halogenated pyrimidine analog (trifluoro-thymidine). It is more soluble than IDU and is effective against IDU resistant strains. It is phosphorylated to active drug inside the cell. The active drug trifluridine triphosphate is a potent inhibitor of both viral and host DNA synthesis. It competes with thymidine triphosphate for incorporation into DNA strand and thus inhibits DNA synthesis. Due to toxicity, it is not used systemically and is only available for topical use.

Dosage

It is available as topical 1 percent solution. For HSV epithelial keratitis, patient is advised to instill the eyedrops 6–9 times/day for 14 days. After epithelization dose is reduced to 1 drop 4 times/ day for a week.

TFT does not penetrate the intact cornea but in the diseased eye, it attains antiviral concentration in the aqueous humor.

Adverse Effects

Adverse effects of trifluridine are much less when compared to vidarabine or IDU. Prolonged use of TFT causes:
- Irritation and burning sensation
- Delayed epithelial healing
- Conjunctival keratinization and scarring
- Corneal stromal edema
- Contact blepharodermatitis
- Raised IOP
- Dry eyes
- Epithelial keratopathy.

Ocular Uses

Topical trifluridine is used in the treatment of:
- Primary and recurrent HSV epithelial keratitis, vaccinia and adeno virus keratitis
- IDU and vidarabine resistant cases
- Deeper infections/ stromal involvement
- Thygeson's superficial punctate keratitis
- Dendritic and geographical HSV keratitis.

Bromovinyl Deoxyuridine

It is thymidine analog like IDU and TFT. It is more effective against varicella-zoster virus (VZV).

Bromovinyl Deoxyuridine (BVDU) is more potent than IDU in healing epithelial HSV keratitis and better to TFT in the treatment of stromal keratitis and iritis. It penetrates easily the intact cornea to attain viricidal concentration in the aqueous humor.

Dosage

It is available as 0.1 percent ophthalmic solution. Patient is advised to put 1–2 drops 8–9 times a day. All ulcers heal within 8–10 days. BVDU has good effect in dendritic ulcer and stromal keratitis.

Adverse Effects

Local hypersensitivity reactions to eyedrops.

Acyclovir

Acyclovir is a purine analog of guanosine. It is converted to active triphosphate form by the viral and host cell enzymes and this active triphosphate form inhibits DNA synthesis and viral replication. Acyclovir is selectively activated in virus infested cells only resulting in minimum toxicity to uninfected normal host cells. Acyclovir has a low toxicity for host cell and has 100 fold chemotherapeutic indexes.

Even in the presence of intact epithelium, it achieves sufficient antiviral concentration in the aqueous humor. It is a broad spectrum drug that is active against HSV 1 and 2 subtypes and VZV.

The high degree of selectivity of acyclovir is related to its unique mechanism of action. Acyclovir is phosphorylated to acyclovir monophosphate in the virus infected cells by viral thymidine kinase enzyme. In uninfected cell, little phosphorylation occurs and hence the drug is concentrated mainly in virus infected cells. Acyclovir monophosphate is subsequently converted by host cell kinases to a triphosphate form which is a potent inhibitor of virus induced DNA polymerase with relatively little effect on host cell DNA polymerase.

Acyclovir triphosphate is also incorporated into the elongating viral DNA resulting in DNA chain termination. Thus, normal cellular function is unaffected while the virus replication is inhibited in the virus infected cells. This highly selective property makes acyclovir a potent antiherpetic drug with minimal side effects.

Dosage

The dose of acyclovir for various indications is summarized in the table below:

Ophthalmic preparations	Oral preparations	IV dose	Topical (For dermatological use)
Available as 3% ophthalmic ointment	Available as 200, 400 and 800 mg tablets	Available as 250 mg, 500 mg and 1 g injection	Available as 5% ointment/ cream
3% ophthalmic ointment to be applied 5 times a day for 2 weeks then gradual tapering to maintenance dose of 1–2 times per day	200-800 mg 4–5 times/day depending on the infection	5–10 mg/kg slow IV infusion over 1 hour thrice daily	5% dermal cream/ ointment applied 5 times a day to the affected areas

Intravitreal Dosage

In acute retinal necrosis syndrome intravitreal acyclovir has been used in dose of 5 µg in 0.1 ml given weekly.

Uses

- Primary HSV keratits, dendritic ulcers
- Infectious epithelial keratitis
- HSV iritis and blepharitis
- Patients at risk for recurrent disease more than twice annually
- Patients in whom keratoplasty has been performed for active HSV keratitis
- Herpes zoster infection
- Varicella zoster infection (Chicken pox)
- In acute retinal necrosis syndrome
- Immunosuppressed patients such as AIDS and organ transplant recipients.

  In patients of HSV epithelial keratitis, stromal keratitis, and iritis, in addition to topical acyclovir, oral acyclovir is given in dose of 200–800 mg 5 times daily and in case of immunocompromised patients IV acyclovir is given in additional to topical therapy.

  For treatment of HSV stromal keratits, combination of acyclovir and steroids is more effective.

  In HSV blepharitis and orofacial lesions, 5 percent dermal cream/ ointment is to be applied 5 times a day to the affected areas.

Resistance to Acyclovir

In AIDS patients, development of resistance and clinical failure has been reported with chronic or intermittent administration of acyclovir. The most common mechanism of resistance is a deficiency of the virus induced thymidine kinase enzyme. These patients with resistance to acyclovir frequently respond to foscarnet.

Adverse Effects

Generally acyclovir is well tolerated. Adverse effects reported with acyclovir are given below:
- Topical use
  - Superficial punctate epithelial keratopathy
  - Topical burning sensation
- Systemic use
  - GIT disturbance, dizziness, anorexia, fatigue, edema, rashes, lymphadenopathy
  - Renal dysfunction especially with rapid IV administration
  - Reversible neurological manifestation.

Valacyclovir

This prodrug is the L-valyl ester form of acyclovir. It is converted to acyclovir rapidly after oral administration. Valacyclovir has better oral bioavailability than acyclovir. It is available only for oral use.

Famciclovir

Famciclovir is a prodrug for penciclovir with similar actions like acyclovir. It also inhibits viral DNA polymerase. It has good bioavailability when compared to acyclovir and thus has the advantage of requiring, smaller doses.

Dosage and Indication

It is mainly used for Herpes Zoster ophthalmicus. Oral dosage is 500–700 mg three times a day for 7 days (equal to acyclovir in acute disease and better in reducing late neuralgia).

Penciclovir

It is the active form of famciclovir and is only available for topical use as 1 percent cream. It is used in treatment of recurrent herpes labialis.

DRUGS ACTIVE AGAINST CYTOMEGALOVIRUS

Ganciclovir

Ganciclovir is a synthetic guanosine derivative and has activity against all types of herpes viruses both *in vivo* and *in vitro* but the difference in chemical structure makes it 10–25 times more potent against cytomegalovirus (CMV).

Ganciclovir gets converted to its active triphosphate form which inhibits CMV DNA polymerase and gets incorporated into CMV DNA resulting in eventual termination of DNA chain elongation. The initial conversion to monophosphate form is catalyzed by viral thymidine kinase enzyme in HSV infected cells and by viral phosphotransferase enzyme in CMV infected cells. Cellular kinases in CMV infected cells subsequently phosphorylate ganciclovir monophosphate to diphosphate and active triphosphate moieties. Ganciclovir triphosphate once formed appears quite stable and persists for days in the CMV infected cell. Oral bioavailability of ganciclovir is poor.

Indications

- Intravenous ganciclovir
    - Treatment of CMV retinitis in immunocompromised patients including AIDS patients
    - Prevention of CMV disease in transplant recipients at risk

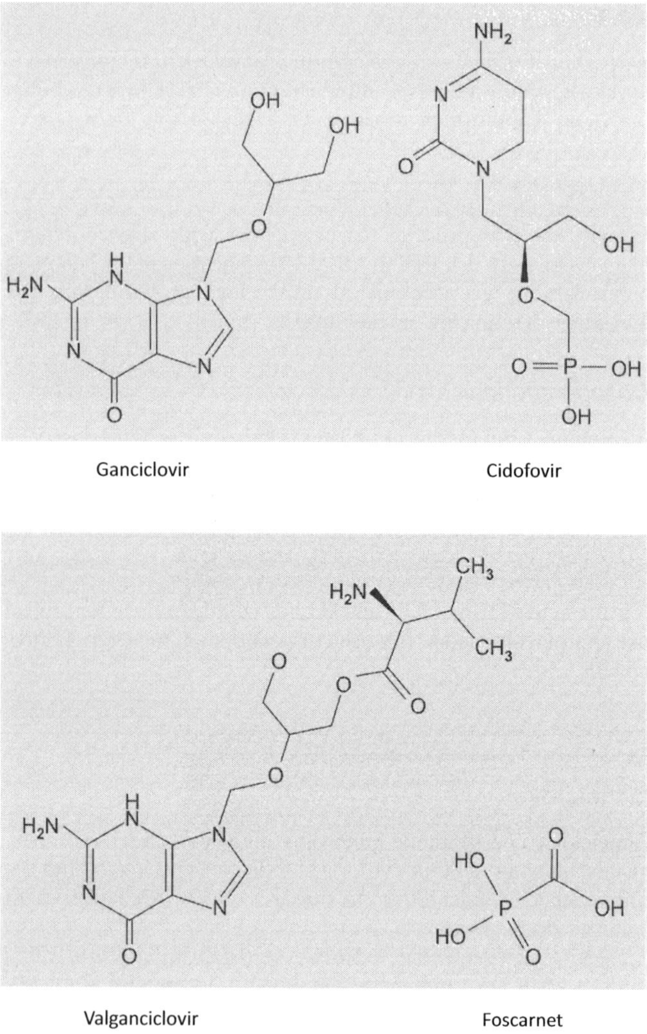

Fig. 9.4: Chemical structure of commonly used antiviral agents for cytomegalovirus infections

- Oral ganciclovir:
  - Alternative to IV formulation for maintenance treatment of CMV retinitis in AIDS patients after appropriate IV induction therapy
  - CMV prophylaxis for patients at risk
- Ophthalmic gel:
  - Treatment of active herpetic keratitis (dendritic ulcer)
- Intravitreal implant:
  - Treatment of CMV retinitis.

Dosage and Adverse Effects

	Ophthalmic preparations	Oral preparations	IV dose	Intravitreal implant
Marketed preparations	Available as 0.15% ophthalmic gel	Available as 250 and 500 mg capsules	Available as 500 mg injection	Available as 4.5 mg intravitreal implant
Dosage	0.15% ophthalmic gel to be applied 5 times a day till corneal ulcer heals followed by thrice daily for 7 days	1000 mg thrice daily OR 500 mg 4th hourly	5 mg/kg slow IV infusion over 1 hour twice daily	4.5 mg intravitreal implant releases the drug for 5-8 months
Uses	In topical treatment of acute herpetic keratitis (dendritic ulcer)	Maintanance treatment of CMV retinitis, CMV prophylaxis in transplant and HIV patients	Induction treatment of CMV retinitis, CMV prophylaxis in transplant patients	Treatment of CMV retinitis
Adverse effects	Blurred vision, eye irritation, punctate keratitis, conjunctival hyperemia	GI disturbance like diarrhea, anorexia, vomiting; CNS effects like neuropathy, headache; myelosuppression	-do-	Retinal detachment, visual acuity loss, vitreous hemorrhage

Combination of ganciclovir and foscarnet has been found to be more effective in delaying progression of CMV retinitis than administration of individual drugs alone.

Additive myelosuppression may occur when ganciclovir is used with zidovudine or Azathioprine. Hence, concomitant administration of these drugs with ganciclovir requires careful monitoring.

Ganciclovir Intravitreal Implant

Ganciclovir intravitreal implants are commercially available for the treatment of CMV retinitis in patients with AIDS. Each implant contains 4.5 mg of ganciclovir and is designed to release the drug over a period of 5–8 months. Following depletion of ganciclovir from the implant, the implant may be removed and replaced.

Implants should be stored at room temperature 15–30°C. Exercise caution in handling the implant in order to avoid damage to the polymer coating on the implant which may result in the increased rate of drug release from the implant. The implant should be handled by the suture tab only.

Valganciclovir

It is L-valyl ester prodrug of ganciclovir that gets rapidly converted to ganciclovir after oral administration. Oral bioavailability of valganciclovir is much better than ganciclovir. It is available only for oral use. Indications and adverse effects are same as that of ganciclovir.

Foscarnet Sodium (Phosphonoformic Acid)

Foscarnet is an analog of inorganic pyrophosphate which is a potent inhibitor of replication of all known herpes viruses including cytomegalovirus (CMV). Foscarnet exhibits its antiviral activity by a selective inhibition at the pyrophosphate binding site on virus specific DNA polymerases and reverse transcriptases at doses that do not interfere with host cell DNS polymerase.

Foscarnet does not require activation (phosphorylation) to exert its antiviral activity. Foscarnet is active against acyclovir resistant herpes virus and ganciclovir resistant CMV.

Indications

- Treatment of CMV retinitis in AIDS patients
- Treatment of acyclovir- resistant HSV infections
- Treatment of Ganciclovir and Cidofovir resistant CMV retinitis
- Combination therapy with ganciclovir in patients who have relapsed after monotherapy with either drug.

Dosage

Commercially foscarnet is available as IV infusion bottle that contains 24 mg/ml.
- For CMV retinitis:
  - 60 mg/kg slow IV infusion over 1 hour thrice daily for 2–3 weeks followed by maintenance dose of 90 mg/kg/day IV infusion over 2 hours.
- For resistant HSV keratitis:
  - 40 mg/kg slow IV infusion over 1 hour twice or thrice daily for 2–3 weeks or until ulcer heals followed by maintenance dose of 90 mg/kg/day IV infusion over 2 hours.

Adverse Effects

The most common adverse effects reported are fever, nausea, anemia, diarrhea, abnormal renal functions including acute renal failure, increased serum creatinine, hypocalcemia, hypokalemia, hypophosphatemia, vomiting, headache, seizure, bone marrow suppression. Infusion of normal saline before foscarnet administration helps to reduce nephrotoxicity. Concomitant use of other nephrotoxic drugs like aminoglycosides, amphotericin B should be avoided.

Cidofovir

Cidofovir is a cytosine nucleotide derivative with broad spectrum of antiviral activity against CMV, HSV-1 and 2, VZV, EBV and other herpes group of viruses, adeno virus and pox virus. Conversion of cidofovir to active form cidofovir diphosphate does not require the presence of viral enzymes. Cidofovir diphosphate inhibits CMV DNA polymerase and thus DNA synthesis.

Indications

Cidofovir is indicated for the treatment of CMV retinitis in AIDS patients.

Contraindications

Hypersensitivity to cidofovir, renal insufficiency, patients receiving other nephrotoxic agents.

Dosage

Cidofovir is commercially available as 75 mg/ml injection in 5 ml ampoules. Cidofovir must be diluted in 100 ml 0.9 percent saline solution prior to the administration. To minimize potential nephrotoxicity, oral probenecid and IV saline preloading must be given before starting cidofovir infusion.

Recommended dose of cidofovir for 5 mg/kg once weekly as slow IV infusion over 1 hour for 2 consecutive weeks followed by maintenance dose of 5 mg/kg IV infusion once in every 2 weeks.

Probenecid should be administered orally with each cidofovir dose. 2 gm 3 hours prior to the cidofovir dose and 1g again at 2 and 8 hours after completion of cidofovir infusion. Patients should receive 1 liter of normal saline IV infusion over 1-2 hour period immediately before the cidofovir infusion.

Adverse Effects

Adverse effects reported are renal toxicity, proteinuria, serum creatinine elevation, metabolic acidosis, nausea, vomiting, diarrhea, anorexia, abdominal pain, allergic reactions and elevated liver enzymes. Concomitant use of other nephrotoxic drugs like aminoglycosides, amphotericin B should be avoided.

Fomivirsen

Fomivirsen is chemically a phosphorothioate oligonucleotide that inhibits cytomegalovirus (CMV) replication through an antisense mechanism. The nucleotide sequence of fomivirsen is complementary to a sequence in mRNA transcripts of the immediate early region 2 (IE_2) of CMV. Binding of fomivirsen to the target mRNA results in the inhibition of IE_2 protein synthesis, subsequently inhibiting replication of CMV.

Since the action of fomivirsen is unique than that of other antiviral drugs, it is active against the CMV isolates resistant to ganciclovir, foscarnet or cidofovir.

Indication

Fomivirsen is indicated for the treatment of CMV retinitis in AIDS patients who:
- Are intolerant to other drugs
- Have a contraindication to use of other antiviral drugs
- Fail to respond adequately to other drugs.

Dosage and Administration

Fomivirsen is commercially available as injection for intravitreal use. The recommended induction dose, i.e. 330 µg (0.05 ml) as a single intravitreal injection every alternate week for 2 doses followed by maintenance doses of 330 µg (0.05 ml) once a month. If the disease progresses during fomivirsen maintenance phase, reinduction at the same dose may control the disease progression.

Fomivirsen's ocular concentrations are reported to be greatest in the iris and retina. It is detectable in the retina within hours after injection and concentration increase over a period of 3–5 days.

Fomivirsen is administered by intravitreal injection into the affected eye using 30 G needle on a low volume syringe, after application of topical local anesthetic and antimicrobial.

Instructions for Intravitreal Injection

- Disinfect rubber stopper with 70 percent ethyl alcohol or acetone.
- Attach a 5 micron filter needle to the injection syringe for solution withdrawal and 0.15 ml solution should be withdrawn through the filter needle.
- Remove filter needle and put a 30 G needle to syringe containing fomivirsen. Inject excess volume and air from the syringe.
- Stabilize globe with cotton tip applicator and insert needle fully through an area 3–4 mm posterior to the limbus aiming towards the center of globe. Keep the fingers off the plunger until the needle has been completely inserted.
- Deliver the injection volume (0.05 ml) by slow injection. Roll cotton tip applicator over injection site as the needle is withdrawn to reduce the loss of eye fluid.
- Monitor light perception and optic nerve head perfusion. If not completely perfused by 10 minutes, perform anterior chamber paracentesis with a 30 G needle on a plungerless tuberculin syringe at the slit lamp.

Adverse Effects

Adverse effects reported are ocular inflammation (uveitis), iritis, vitritis, abnormal vision, anterior chamber inflammation, cataract, conjunctival hemorrhage, floaters, increased IOP, photophobia, retinal detachment and retinal edema.

DRUGS ACTIVE AGAINST HEPATITIS VIRUS

Interferons

Interferons are proteins produced by host cell in response to viral infection and some other inducers. These interferons belong to cytokine family and possess broad antiviral, immune modulating and anti-proliferative properties.

Interferons are of three types – α, β and γ interferons. Among these, only α-interferons are used in ophthalmic practice. Pegylated interferons are obtained by addition of polyethylene glycol to interferons (pegylation). Pegylation increases the half-life of interferons thereby decreasing the frequency of administration.

Mechanism of Action of α-interferons

Interferons bind to specific receptors and active JAK-STAT signal transduction pathway leading to various effects like:
- Inhibition of viral penetration
- Inhibition of transcription
- Inhibition of translation
- Inhibition of post-translational processing
- Inhibition of viral maturation and release.

Antiviral activities of interferons are mainly due to inhibition of viral protein synthesis.

Indications

- Treatment of Hairy cell leukemia
- AIDS related Kaposi sarcoma
- Chronic myelogenous leukemia
- Chronic hepatitis B infection
- Acute and chronic hepatitis C infection
- Treatment of drug resistant HSV keratitis

Interferons given in combination with other antiviral drugs markedly reduce the duration of treatment.

Dosage

Interferons are generally given by subcutaneous or intramuscular route. Dose of interferons varies according to different indications.

Interferons are also given topically for treatment of HSV keratitis.

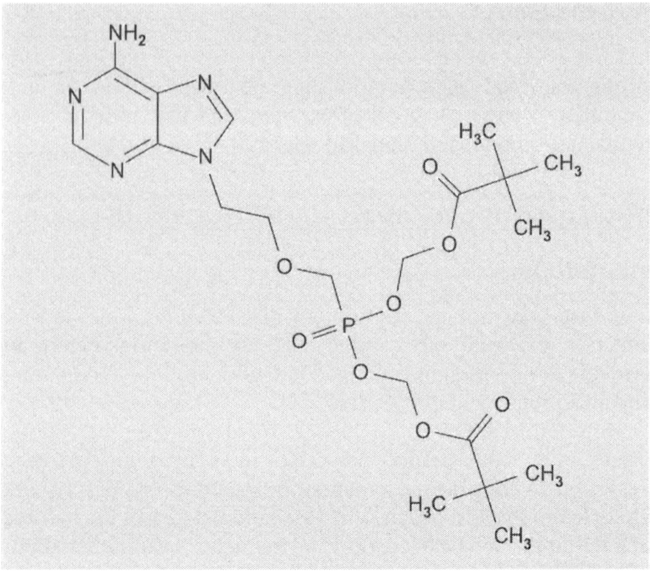

Adefovir

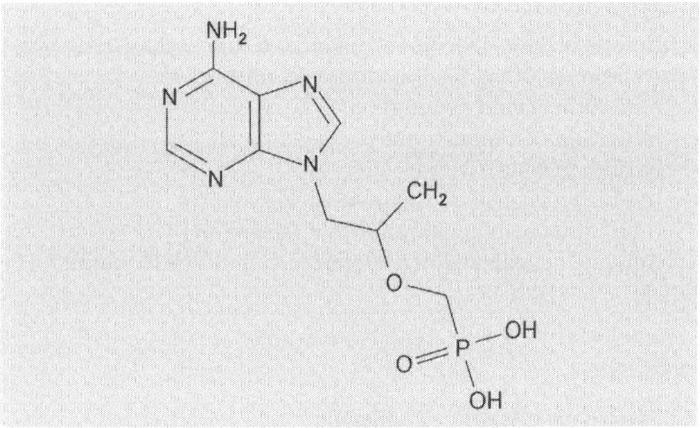

Tenofovir

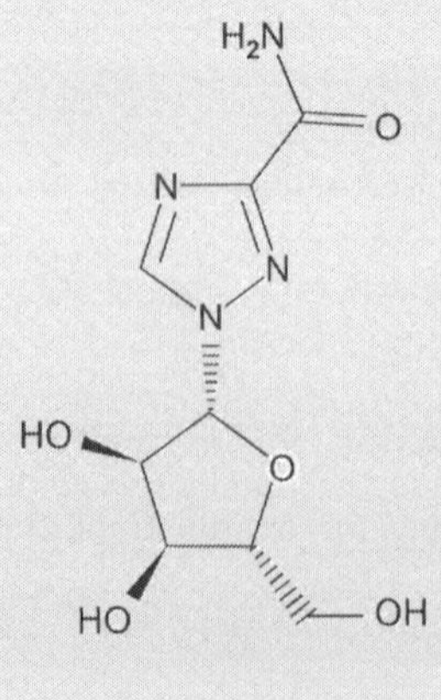

Ribavirin

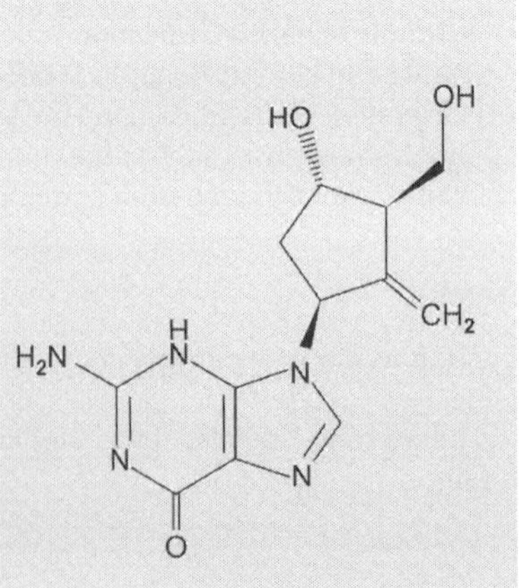

Entecavir

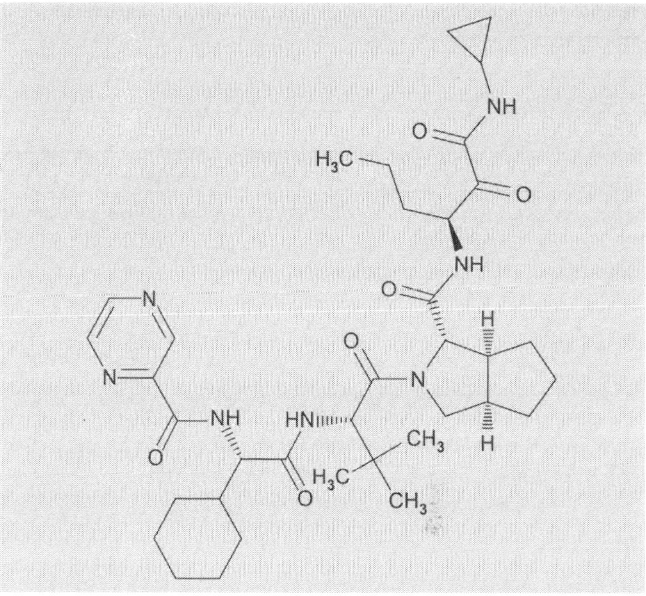

Telaprevir

Fig. 9.5: Chemical structure of commonly used drugs in hepatitis

Adverse Effects

Adverse effects commonly encountered with interferon therapy are given below:
- Fever, chills, myalgia and fatigue
- Bone marrow depression
- Neurotoxicity
- Hypersensitivity reactions.

Adefovir

Adefovir is adenine nucleotide analog that was originally developed for treatment of HIV infection. In less toxic doses, it was found to be effective in treatment of hepatitis B infection and has gained approval for treatment of HBV infection. It is marketed as the prodrug adefovir dipivoxil.

The active diphosphate form inhibits HBV DNA polymerase, causes DNA chain termination and hence inhibits HBV DNA synthesis. It is used as 10 mg tablet once daily in treatment of chronic HBV infection. Adverse effects include nephrotoxicity, headache, diarrhea, abdominal pain, hepatic steatosis and lactic acidosis.

Tenofovir

This adenosine nucleotide analog previously used in treatment of HIV infection, has recently been approved for treatment of chronic HBV infection including those resistant to lamivudine and entecavir.

Lamivudine

This nucleoside analog is an antiretroviral drug that belongs to nucleoside reverse transcriptase inhibitors (NRTIs). It has also been approved for treatment of chronic HBV infection in dose of 100 mg once daily orally. The efficacy in HBV infection is due to inhibition of HBV DNA polymerase.

Entecavir

It is a guanosine analog that is highly active against HBV. The active phosphorylated form inhibits HBV DNA polymerase. It is used orally in a dose of 0.5–1 mg daily for treatment of chronic active HBV infection.

Ribavirin

It is a guanosine analog used in treatment of chronic HCV. It is active against HCV, influenza virus A and B, Respiratory syncytial virus (RSV) and HIV-1. The active form of the drug is ribavirin triphosphate. It is used orally in a dose of 400–600 mg twice daily in combination with pegylated α-interferon for treatment of chronic HCV infection. The main adverse effects of ribavirin include dose dependent hemolytic anemia and teratogenicity.

Boceprevir and Telaprevir

These newer agents act by inhibiting NS3/4A serine protease enzyme of HCV. This enzyme is essential for proteolytic cleavage of HCV-encoded polyprotein into mature form that is necessary for replication of the virus. By inhibiting the enzyme, these drugs inhibit HCV viral replication. They are used orally in combination with pegylated interferon-α and ribavirin in treatment of chronic HCV infection including resistant cases.

DRUGS USED IN HIV INFECTION

Nucleoside Reverse Transcriptase Inhibitors

These agents are nucleoside analogs that act as competitive inhibitors of HIV-1 reverse transcriptase. NRTIs used clinically for treatment of HIV infection include Zidovudine, Stavudine, Lamivudine, Abacavir, Zalcitabine, Didanosine and Emtricitabine. Tenofovir is a nucleotide reverse transcriptase inhibitor used in HIV infection.

Zidovudine is the first antiretroviral drug approved for treatment of HIV infection. The chemical structures of some of these drugs are shown in Figure 9.6.

Antiviral Therapy

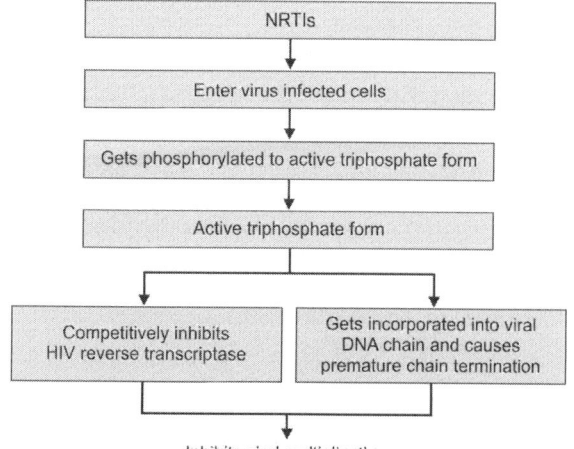

Fig. 9.6: Chemical structure of some commonly used Nucleoside Reverse Transcriptase Inhibitors

Mechanism of Action

Tenofovir being a nucleotide analog only requires two phosphorylations and the active form is tenofovir diphosphate.

These drugs inhibit both HIV 1 and 2 and some drugs like lamivudine, tenofovir and emtricitabine are also effective against HBV.

Adverse Effects

These drugs selectively inhibit HIV reverse transcriptase without affecting host cell DNA polymerase. Despite their low affinity for human DNA polymerase, some of these drugs also inhibit human DNA polymerase resulting in toxicities like anemia, granulocytopenia, myopathy, peripheral neuropathy, pancreatitis and lactic acidosis.

Peripheral neuropathy is more common with stavudine, zalcitabine and zidovudine. Pancreatitis is commonly associated with didanosine, stavudine and zalcitabine. Anemia is more common with zidovudine. Stavudine and zidovudine can cause lipodystrophy. Abacavir can cause hypersensitivity reactions (more common in patients with HLA-B*5701 allele) and can increase the risk of myocardial infarction.

Dosage

Drug	Dosage when used in combination with other drugs
Zidovudine	400–600 mg/day in 2 divided doses
Lamivudine	300 mg/day in 2 divided doses
Stavudine	60–80 mg/day in 2 divided doses
Abacavir	600 mg/day in 2 divided doses
Zalcitabine	2.25 mg/day in 3 divided doses
Didanosine	250–400 mg/day in 1–2 divided doses
Emtricitabine	200 mg/day (once daily)
Tenofovir	300 mg/day (once daily)

Emtricitabine is fluorinated analog of lamivudine with long half-life and hence used once daily.

Non-nucleoside Reverse Transcriptase Inhibitors

These drugs noncompetitively inhibit HIV reverse transcriptase. They do not require phosphorylation for activation and directly bind to HIV reverse transcriptase enzyme and inhibit it. Non-nucleoside reverse transcriptase inhibitors (NNRTIs) in clinical use include nevirapine, efavirenz, delavirdine and etravirine. NNRTIs are only active against HIV-1 and are inactive against HIV-2.

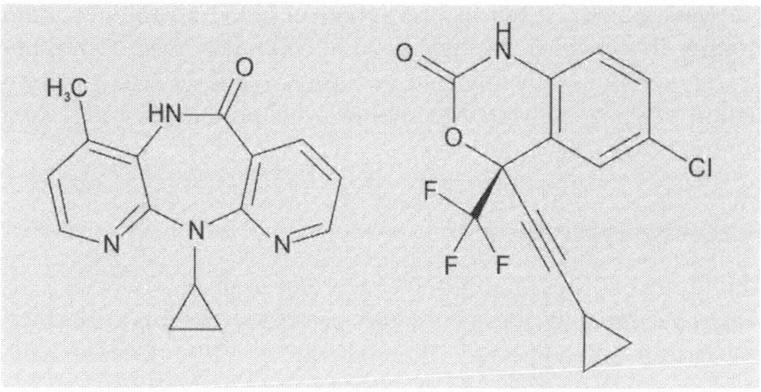

Antiviral Therapy

Fig. 9.7: Structure of Non-nucleoside reverse transcriptase inhibitors Nevirapine (left), Efavirenz (center) and Etravirine (right)

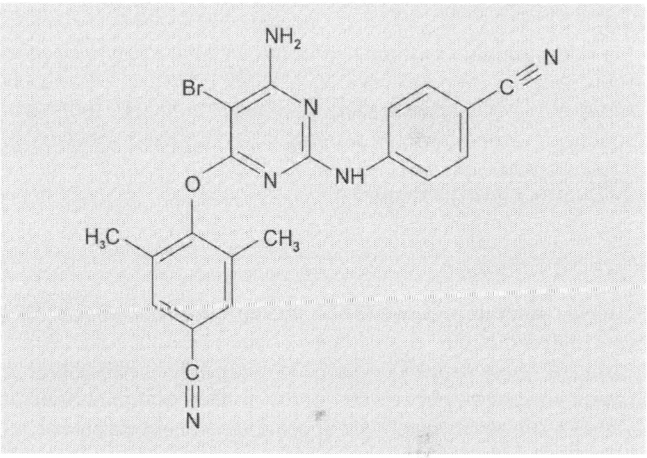

Adverse Effects

Non-nucleoside reverse transcriptase inhibitors (NNRTIs) can produce skin rash, nausea, head ache and diarrhea. Efavirenz can cause psychiatric symptoms like depression and mania. Delavirdine and efavirenz are teratogenic and should be avoided in pregnancy.

Dosage

Drug	Dosage when used in combination with other drugs
Nevirapine	400 mg/day in 2 divided doses
Efavirenz	600 mg/day (once daily)
Delavirdine	1200 mg/day in 3 divided doses
Etravirine	400 mg/day in 2 divided doses

Nevirapine is used in prevention of HIV transmission from mother to newborn. A single dose of 200 mg is given to mother at the onset of labor followed by 2 mg/kg oral dose to newborn within 3 days of delivery. Nevirapine is not teratogenic and is used commonly for this indication.

Protease Inhibitors

This group of drugs inhibits the viral protease enzyme. During later stages of viral replication, immature precursor proteins are formed due to translation of Gag-Pol gene products. HIV protease enzyme is responsible for cleavage of precursor proteins to final mature structural protein of the virus. Protease inhibitors (PIs) inhibit this process and result in formation of immature and nonfunctional virions.

Protease inhibitors do not require intracellular phosphorylation to get activated. They are active against both HIV 1 and 2. Clinically used drugs in this class include Ritonavir, Indinavir, Nelfinavir, Saquinavir, Amprenavir, Fosamprenavir, Lopinavir, Atazanavir, Darunavir and Tipranavir. Chemical structure of some protease inhibitors is shown in Figure 9.8.

Adverse Effects

Protease inhibitors can cause metabolic side effects like hypertriglyceridemia, dyslipidemia, hyperglycemia and insulin resistance. These drugs alter body fat and produce redistribution of body fat resulting in central obesity, buffalo hump, peripheral wasting resulting in cushingoid appearance. Except atazanavir, all other PIs can produce the above metabolic side effects. Protease inhibitors cause many drug interactions due to their interaction with CYP450 enzymes (inhibition or induction).

Dosage

Drug	Dosage when used in combination with other drugs
Ritonavir	1200 mg/day in 2 divided doses
Indinavir	2400 mg/day in 3 divided doses
Nelfinavir	2250–2500 mg/day in 2–3 divided doses
Saquinavir	2000 mg/day in 2 divided doses (with ritonavir boosting)
Fosamprenavir	2800 mg/day in 2 divided doses OR 1400 mg/day with ritonavir boosting
Lopinavir	800 mg/day in 1–2 divided doses (with ritonavir boosting)
Atazanavir	300 mg/day (with ritonavir boosting)
Darunavir	800 mg/day (with ritonavir boosting)
Tipranavir	100 mg/day in 2 divided doses (with ritonavir boosting)

Ritonavir is a potent CYP3A4 inhibitor and is used to increase the blood levels of other PIs. Hence, ritonavir is known as

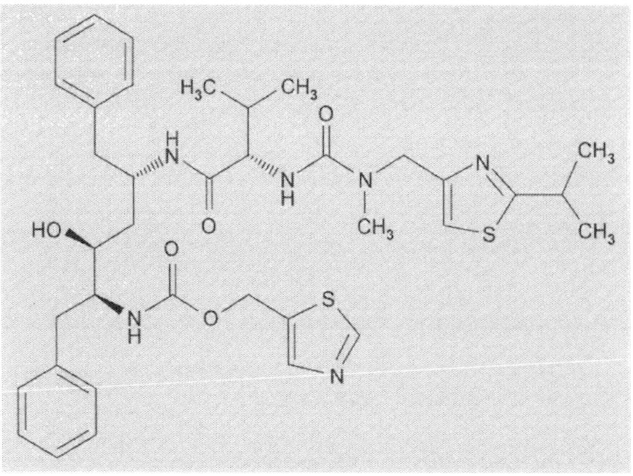

Ritonavir

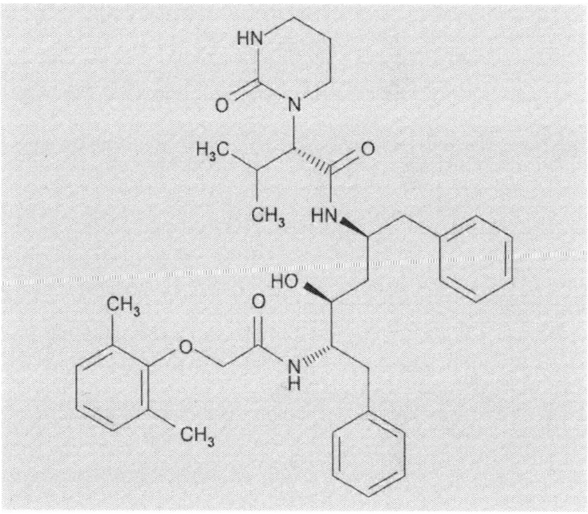

Lopinavir

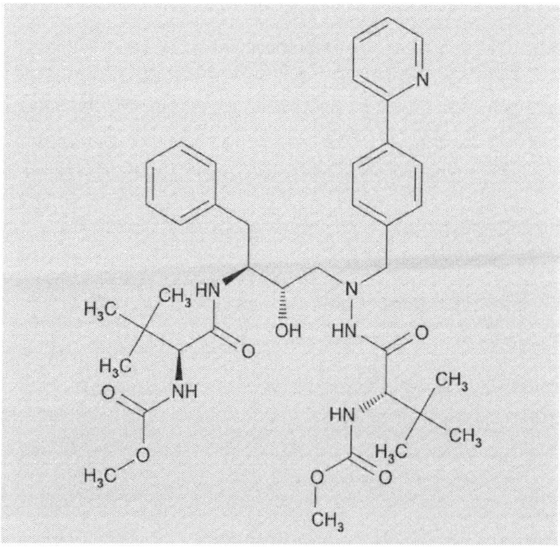

Atazanavir

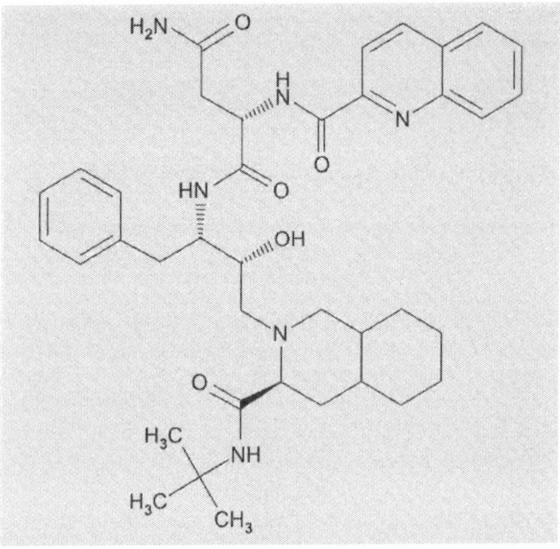

Saquinavir

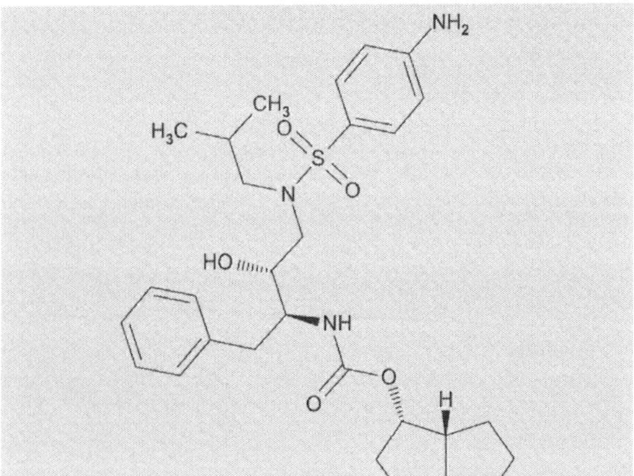

Darunavir

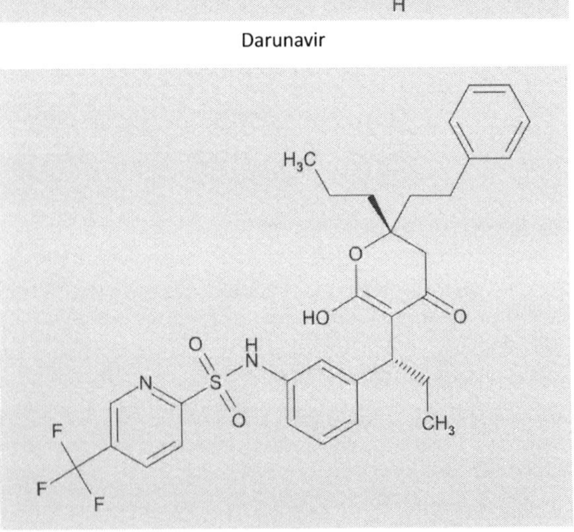

Tipranavir

Fig. 9.8: Chemical structure of some protease inhibitors

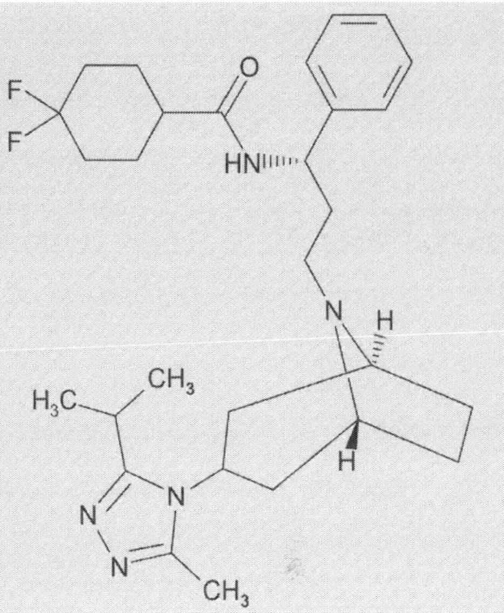

Fig. 9.9: Chemical structure of maraviroc

"pharmacokinetic enhancer". Darunavir and tipranavir are active against HIV-1 resistant to other protease inhibitors.

ENTRY INHIBITOR (MARAVIROC)

Maraviroc is a chemokine receptor (CCR5) antagonist that prevents the entry of HIV inside the host cell. It is effective only against HIV-1 virus that has affinity for CCR5 receptor. It is neither effective against CXCR4 tropic HIV nor HIV-2.

Maraviroc is used orally in a dose of 300 mg twice daily in the treatment of CCR-5 tropic HIV-1 infection including those with resistance to other antiretroviral drugs. Since maraviroc is a substrate for CYP3A4, dosage adjustment must be done in patients receiving CYP3A4 inducers or inhibitors. Adverse effects include cough, upper respiratory tract infections and elevated liver enzymes.

FUSION INHIBITOR (ENFUVIRTIDE)

Enfuvirtide is a synthetic peptide that binds to gp41 subunit of the viral envelope glycoprotein and prevents the fusion of viral and host cell membrane. It is active only against HIV-1 infection and not against HIV-2. It is given by subcutaneous injection in dose of 90 mg twice daily. Common side effects include local reactions in the injection site and eosinophilia.

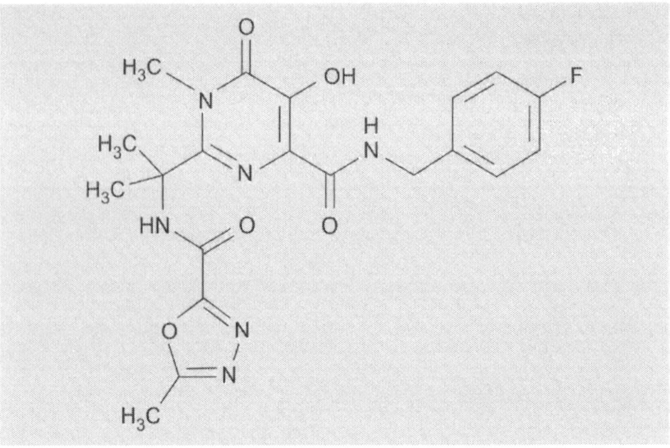

Fig. 9.10: Chemical structure of raltegravir

INTEGRASE INHIBITOR (RALTEGRAVIR)

Raltegravir inhibits the viral enzyme integrase, thereby preventing the integration of reverse transcribed HIV DNA with the host cell DNA. Hence, replication of HIV is halted. It is active against both HIV 1 and 2.

It is used orally in dose of 400 mg twice daily for treatment of drug resistant HIV infection. Adverse effects include diarrhea, nausea, insomnia, dizziness and headache.

CLINICAL USE OF ANTIRETROVIRAL THERAPY IN OPHTHALMOLOGY

Ocular complications occur in more than 50 percent of AIDS patients with advanced disease. These include retinal microvasculopathy, Kaposi's sarcoma, opportunistic infection like cytomegalovirus (CMV) retinitis, zoster ophthalmicus, toxoplasma retinochoroiditis, H. simplex infection and pneumocystis jerovicii choroiditis, HIV induced iridocyclitis and anterior uveitis.

By decreasing the viral load and by increasing the CD4 count, the antiretroviral drugs retard the progression of the disease and prevent the occurrence of these ocular complications.

DRUGS ACTIVE AGAINST INFLUENZA VIRUS

See Figure 9.11.

Amantadine and Rimantadine

These drugs inhibit uncoating of virus particle. They exert their antiviral effect by inhibiting the function of M2 protein that acts as ion channel in the virus particle and hence preventing viral replication. These agents are active only against influenza A. Rimantadine is α-methyl derivative of amantadine and is more

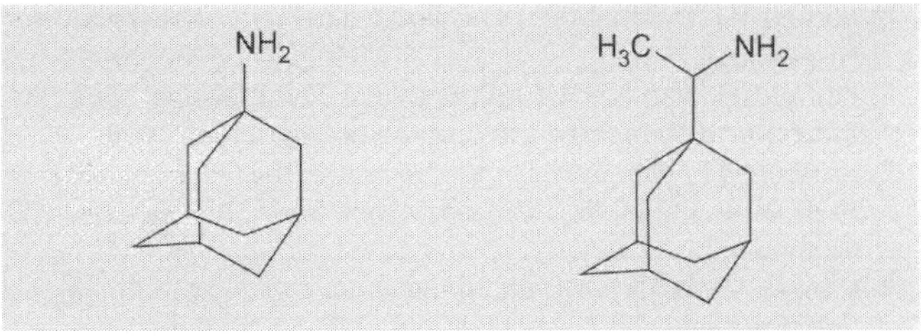

Amantadine Rimantadine

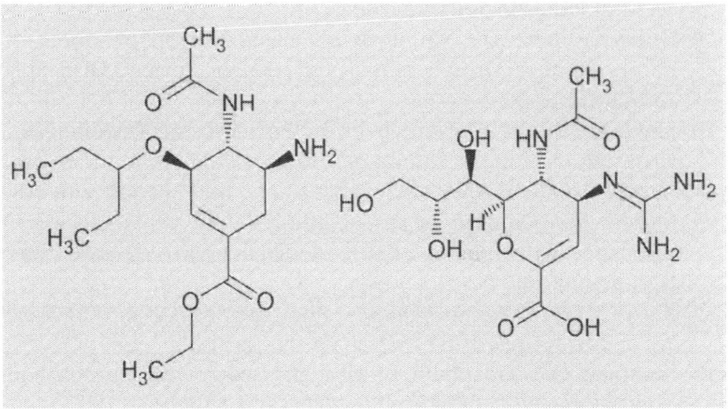

Oseltamivir Zanamavir

Fig. 9.11: Structure of drugs used in treatment of influenza

active than amantadine. These drugs are used in prophylaxis and treatment of influenza A viral infection. Amantadine (but not rimantadine) is also used in treatment of Parkinson's disease.

Oseltamivir and Zanamivir

These agents are active against both influenza A and B. They inhibit the viral enzyme neuraminidase thereby interfering with the release of virus from the infected cells. Oseltamivir is used orally (75 mg twice daily for 5 days) and zanamivir by inhalation (10 mg twice daily for 5 days) in treatment of both influenza A and B viral infections. These drugs were widely used during the recent epidemic of H1N1 infection (swine flu).

BIBLIOGRAPHY

1. Agarwal A. Textbook of Ophthalmology. 1st edn. New Delhi: Jaypee Brothers Medical Publishers (P) Ltd.; 2002.
2. Albert DM. Albert and Jakobiec's Principles and Practice of Ophthalmology. 3rd edn: Saunders, Elsevier, 2008.
3. Al-Dujaili LJ, Clerkin PP, Clement C, McFerrin HE, Bhattacharjee PS, Varnell ED, et al. Ocular herpes simplex virus: how are latency, reactivation, recurrent disease and therapy interrelated? Future Microbiol 2011;6(8):877-907.

4. Bartlett JD. Ophthalmic Drug Facts. 23rd edn. Wolters Kluwer Health 2011.
5. Bartlett JD, Jaanus SD. Clinical Ocular Pharmacology. 5th edn. Butterworth-Heinemann, an imprint of Elsevier Inc. 2008.
6. Brunton LL. Goodman and Gilman's The Pharmacological Basis of Therapeutics. 12th edn. New York: The McGraw-Hill Companies, Inc. 2011.
7. Garg A. Advances in Ophthalmology. 1st edn. New Delhi: Jaypee Brothers Medical Publishers (P) Ltd. 2005.
8. Garg A. Clinical Applications of Antibiotics and Anti-inflammatory Drugs in Ophthalmology. 1st edn. New Delhi: Jaypee Brothers Medical Publishers (P) Ltd. 2007.
9. Guess S, Stone DU, Chodosh J. Evidence-based treatment of herpes simplex virus keratitis: a systematic review. Ocul Surf 2007;5(3):240-50.
10. Jabs DA, Griffiths PD. Fomivirsen for the treatment of cytomegalovirus retinitis. Am J Ophthalmol 2002;133(4):552-6.
11. Jeng BH, Holland GN, Lowder CY, Deegan WF, 3rd, Raizman MB, Meisler DM. Anterior segment and external ocular disorders associated with human immunodeficiency virus disease. Surv Ophthalmol 2007;52(4):329-68.
12. Katzung BG. Basic and Clinical Pharmacology. 12th edn. New York: The McGraw-Hill Companies, Inc, 2012.
13. Kaufman HE. Treatment of viral diseases of the cornea and external eye. Prog Retin Eye Res 2000;19(1):69-85.
14. Marangon FB, Miller D, Alfonso E. Laboratory results in ocular viral diseases: implications in clinical-laboratory correlation. Arq Bras Oftalmol 2007;70(2):189-94.
15. Onofrey BE. Ocular Therapeutics Handbook: A Clinical Manual. 3rd edn. Philadelphia: Lippincott Williams and Wilkins, 2011.
16. Razonable RR. Antiviral drugs for viruses other than human immunodeficiency virus. Mayo Clin Proc 2011;86(10):1009-26.
17. Romanowski EG, Gordon YJ. Update on antiviral treatment of adenoviral ocular infections. Am J Ophthalmol 2008;146(5): 635-7.
18. Tasman W, Jaeger EA. Duane's Ophthalmology on DVD-ROM 2011 edn: Lippincott Williams and Wilkins, 2011.
19. Wilhelmus KR. The treatment of herpes simplex virus epithelial keratitis. Trans Am ophthalmol Soc 2000;98:505-32.
20. Wilhelmus KR. Therapeutic interventions for herpes simplex virus epithelial keratitis. Cochrane Database Syst Rev 2007(1): CD002898.

Antifungal Therapy

NR Biswas, AK Dubey, Harivenkatesh N, Ashok Garg (India)

INTRODUCTION

Fungal keratitis results from invasion of cornea by a fungal organism. Unfortunately because of difficulty in diagnosing and treating these infections they often result in devastating ocular consequences. The incidence of fungal keratitis has risen sharply in last few decades probably due to increased use of topical corticosteroids and broad spectrum antibiotics, better diagnostic techniques and due to increased prevalence of immunocompromised patients. Fungi do not invade the cornea easily and seems to require trauma, contact lens wear or immunological compromise for infection. In the rural areas, trauma with vegetative material is a common cause while contact lens wear is a common in the urban areas.

Fungal endophthalmitis, albeit less common than fungal keratitis, is also seen in ophthalmic practice. It could be due to exogenous infection, as with penetrating trauma, or endogenous hematological spread.

The fungi can be broadly divided into two types namely yeasts and molds (filamentous fungi).

FUNGI CAUSING OCULAR INFECTIONS

The most common organisms responsible for fungal keratitis worldwide are given below:

Yeast Fungi

Candida species are common offenders in this group. *Candida* ulcer commonly occurs in eyes with predisposing alterations in host defense like chronic use of corticosteroids, exposure keratitis, keratitis sicca, herpes simplex keratitis and prior keratoplasty. *Candida* ulcers produce a relatively indolent stromal infiltration with smaller satellite lesions.

Filamentous Fungi

Fusarium, Aspergillus, Curvularia and *Cephalosporium* are the most common filamentous fungi. These organisms usually infect normal eyes following mild abrasive trauma especially after injury from vegetable matter. The organisms are ubiquitous and can be isolated readily from soil, air and organic waste. In contact lens wearers, filamentous fungi are commonly associated with cosmetic or aphakic lens wear and yeasts with therapeutic lenses.

Management of keratomycosis is often difficult because the disease process is often advanced at the time of first examination. The infecting fungi cause hypopyon by infiltrating the stroma without perforating the cornea. Because of favorable climate for fungal development keratomycosis is frequent in tropical countries.

ANTIFUNGAL DRUGS

Despite the availability of many antifungal drugs in the market, ocular uses of antifungals are limited by their poor intraocular penetration, narrow spectrum and side effects. Often debridement has to be done to facilitate the drug entry and prolonged aggressive treatment is needed. There is no single broad spectrum antifungal drug which could be used effectively to treat all the fungal infections and hence the treatment is usually initiated empirically till the offending organism is confirmed.

Systemically administered amphotericin B attains poor concentration in the vitreous while fluconazole, flucytosine and voriconazole have shown to achieve high concentrations. Intravitreal injections of amphotericin B or voriconazole are being used increasingly to quickly achieve the therapeutic antifungal activity in the posterior segment of the eye in severe cases like fungal endophthalmitis.

An ideal ocular antifungal drug must be long-acting, non-irritating, possess good intraocular penetration and should be highly effective.

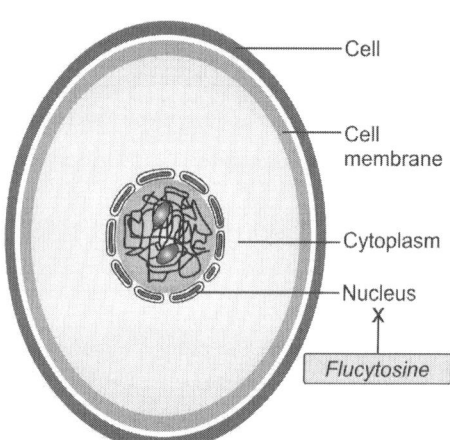

Fig. 10.1: Schematic structure of a fungal cell. Flucytosine (X) inhibit fungal nucleic acid synthesis

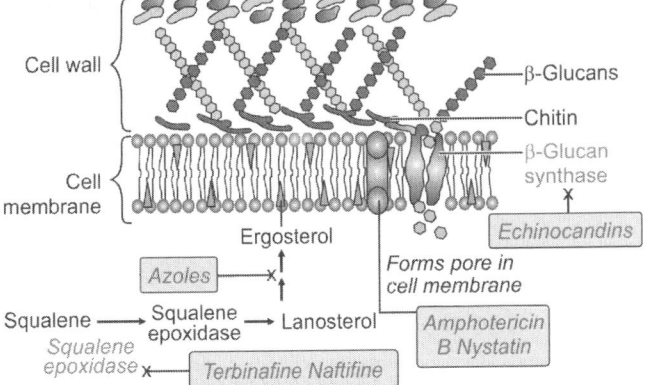

Fig. 10.2: Schematic representation of fungal cell wall and cell membrane and various drugs acting on it. Drugs are shown in red and enzymes are shown in green

Classification

Various antifungal agents used for the management of keratomycosis can be classified on the basis of their chemical structures.

- Polyene antibiotics
  - Amphotericin-B, nystatin, hamycin, natamycin
- Anti-metabolite
  - flucytosine
- Azoles
  - Imidazoles
    - Ketoconazole, miconazole, econazole, clotrimazole, oxiconazole, butoconazole
  - Triazoles
    - Itraconazole, fluconazole, voriconazole, posaconazole, isavuconazole
- Allylamines
  - Terbinafine, naftifine
- Echinocandins
  - Caspofungin, micafungin, anidulafungin
- Others
  - Griseofulvin, ciclopirox olamine, haloprogin, tolnaftate, butenafine
- Miscellaneous drugs
  - Undecylenic acid, benzoic acid, salicylic acid, silver compounds

The polyenes and azoles are commonly used for the treatment of ocular fungal infections.

POLYENES

The first effective antifungal agents used were polyenes (Fig. 10.3). These compounds share a common molecular structure consisting of a conjugated double bond system of variable size linked to

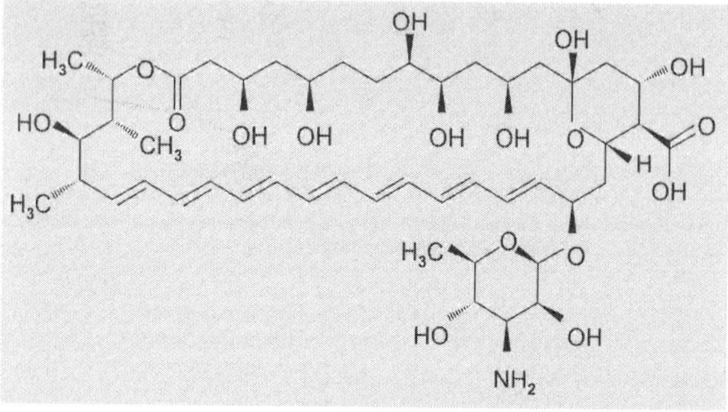

Amphotericin B

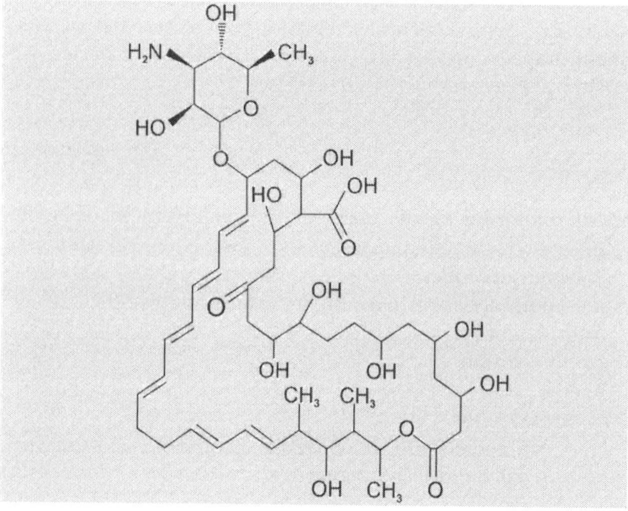

Nystatin

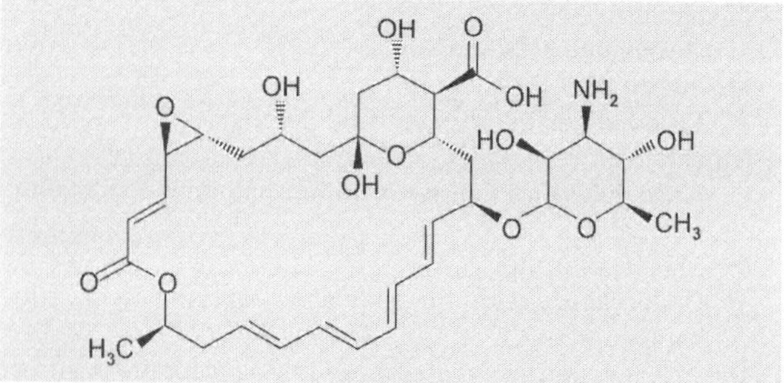

Natamycin

Fig. 10.3: Chemical structure of polyenes—amphotericin B (top left), nystatin (top right) and natamycin (bottom) mycosamine, an amino acid sugar. The various members of this group are classified according to number of double bond present. Clinically used polyenes include amphotericin B, nystatin, hamycin and natamycin.

Mechanism of Action

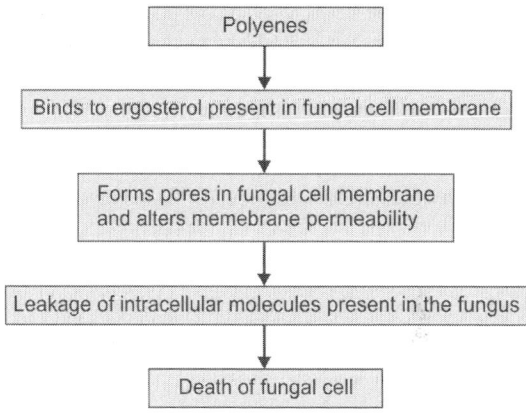

Amphotericin B

Amphotericin B, a heptaene polyene (7 double bonds) is produced from *Streptomyces nodosus*. Amphotericin B is insoluble in water, unstable at 37°C and degrades rapidly if exposed to light. However, solubility is improved by the addition of deoxycholate. It is the most effective topical antifungal for candida keratitis but penetration through intact cornea is poor as compared to natamycin.

Antifungal Spectrum

Amphotericin B is fungicidal drug and has a broad antifungal spectrum that includes *Candida, Aspergillus, Cryptococcus, Coccidioides, Sporothrix, Blastomyces, Histoplasma* and *Mucor* species.

Dosage

For treatment of keratomycosis, amphotericin B can be given by topical, subconjuctival, intracameral and intravenous routes. Since adequate intravitreal levels of amphotericin B are not attained by systemic route, intravitreal injections are required in the management of severe fungal endophthalmitis.

- As topical fortified ophthalmic eye drops, it is used for treatment of fungal keratitis in concentration of 0.075–0.3 percent (usually 0.15%) at hourly interval and then gradually tapered over several weeks (Topical amphotericin B is superior to 5 percent natamycin or 1% miconazole and ketoconazole regarding efficacy).
- Dosage of sub-conjunctival injection is 0.8–1.0 mg for 1–2 doses (24–48 hours interval).

- Dose of intravitreal injection is 5–10 µg/0.1 ml
- Systemic (intravenous): Given in dose of 0.5–1 mg/kg/day as slow IV infusion (in 5% dextrose solution) over 4 hours.

The insolubility of this drug limits its penetration into the eye when given topically or systemically.

Adverse Effects

The toxicity of systemic amphotericin B include infusion related reactions and cumulative toxicity. Anaphylaxis, fever, chills, headache, nausea and vomiting are infusion related adverse reactions and can be minimized by starting with a low dose and by pretreatment with hydrocortisone or antihistamines. Nephrotoxicity is the dose limiting adverse effect of amphotericin B.

Newer formulations of amphotericin B like liposomal amphotericin B and lipoidal amphotericin B produce fewer incidences of adverse effects like nephrotoxicity when compared to conventional amphotericin B, but they are highly expensive.

Nystatin

Nystatin was the first polyene antibiotic to be identified by Hazen and Brown in 1950. It is derived from *Streptomyces noursei*. It is effective against *Candida* infections.

Dosage

It is available in topical ointment/cream that contains 100000 units/g. Patient is advised to apply 4–5 times a day till the ulcer heals. Nystatin is used orally in treatment of oropharyngeal and intestinal candidiasis and topically for treatment of vaginal candidiasis.

Adverse reactions include allergic hypersensitivity reactions.

Natamycin

Natamycin is a tetraene antifungal drug and is the only antifungal agent of this group commercially available as topical ophthalmic solution.

It is derived from *Streptomyces natalenses*. It is most effective against filamentous fungi and has been of special use in the treatment of *Fusarium* and *Aspergillus* infections, the commonest cause of fungal keratitis around the world. It is also effective against *Candida*, *Histoplasma* and *Cladosporium*.

Dosage

It is available as 5 percent ophthalmic suspension. Patient is advised to put 1–2 drops 4–6 times a day till the ulcer heals (maximum for 2 weeks). Natamycin is gradually tapered over weeks. Topical suspension should be shaken well before use. Natamycin often adheres to areas of corneal ulceration, perhaps increasing the duration of drug contact time. This drug cannot be given systemically. The relatively high total corneal drug concentration ensures that adequate amount of bioactive drug is available on topical use.

Adverse Effects

In general, topical natamycin is well tolerated. Adverse effects include irritation, burning sensation, punctate keratitis and allergic reactions in the eye.

ANTIMETABOLITE (FLUORINATED PYRIMIDINE)

Flucytosine

It is a fluorinated pyrimidine (5-flurocytosine). The antifungal properties of this compound were first reported in 1963. It is effective against *Candida, Cryptococcus, Aspergillus, Cladosporium* and *Penicillium* species.

Mechanism of Action

```
┌─────────────────┐
│   Flucytosine   │
└────────┬────────┘
         ↓
┌─────────────────────────────────────────────┐
│ Transported across fungal cell membrane by  │
│         cytosine permease enzyme            │
└────────┬────────────────────────────────────┘
         ↓
┌─────────────────────────────────────────────┐
│ Converted intracellularly to 5-fluorouracil │
│ and then to 5-deoxyuridine monophosphate    │
│     and 5-fluoridine triphosphate           │
└────────┬────────────────────────────────────┘
         ↓
┌─────────────────────────────────────────────┐
│     Inhibits fungal RNA and DNA synthesis   │
└─────────────────────────────────────────────┘
```

It has synergistic antifungal action with amphotericin B.

Dosage

- Oral: 50–150 mg/kg/day in four divided doses.
- Topically it is used as one percent ophthalmic drops. Patient is advised to instill one drop hourly and then gradually tapered to 4 times a day over 3 weeks duration.

The effectiveness of this drug is limited due to poor cell wall penetration in certain fungal species. For this reason, it is not

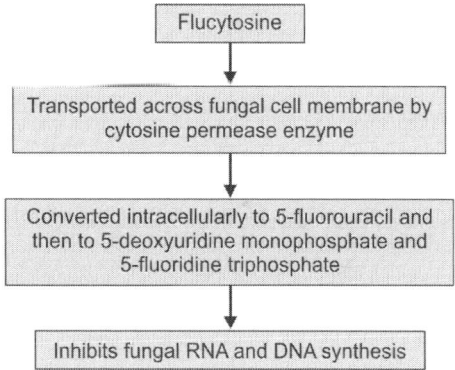

Fig. 10.4: Chemical structure of flucytosine

administered alone in the treatment of keratomycosis. Its use is as an adjunctive therapy in the treatment of *Candida keratomycosis*.

Adverse Effects

Topically it can cause ocular irritation, itching and transient burning sensation. On systemic use adverse effects include nausea, vomiting and diarrhea.

AZOLE DERIVATIVES

The antifungal activity of the azole group of compounds was first recognized more than 30 years ago. Since the initial introduction of clotrimazole, a number of antifungals in this group have become available today.

Currently there are two major types of azoles. The imidazoles, first to be developed are five member ring structures containing two nitrogen atoms. The other group is triazoles that contain three nitrogen atoms in the five membered ring (Figure 10.4).

Triazoles by their improved pharmacokinetics profile and antifungal activity have replaced imidazoles in ophthalmic practice. Many newer drugs in the azole group have come up in the recent years.

Mechanism of Action

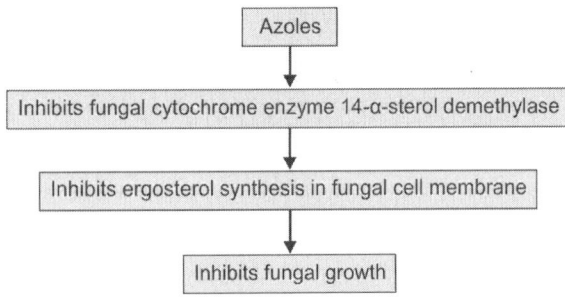

The affinity for fungal and human cytochrome P-450 enzymes varies with different azoles. Newer triazoles like flucanozole, itraconazole and posaconazole have high affinity specifically for

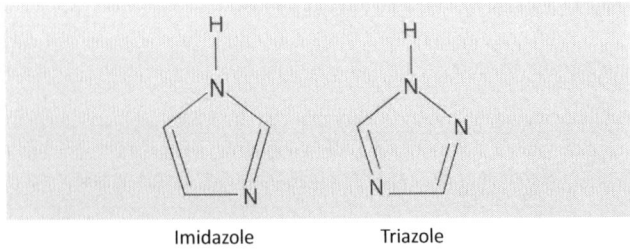

Fig. 10.5: Chemical structure of azoles: Imidazoles (left) and triazoles (right)

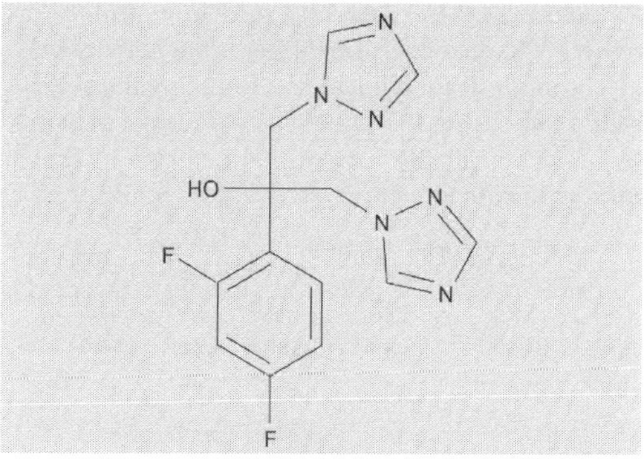

Fluconazole

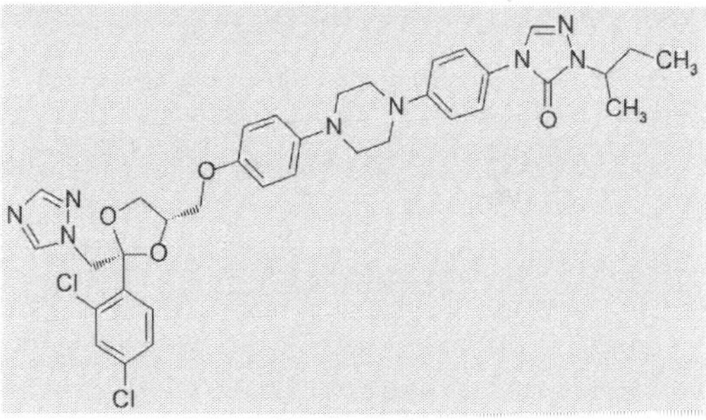

Itraconazole

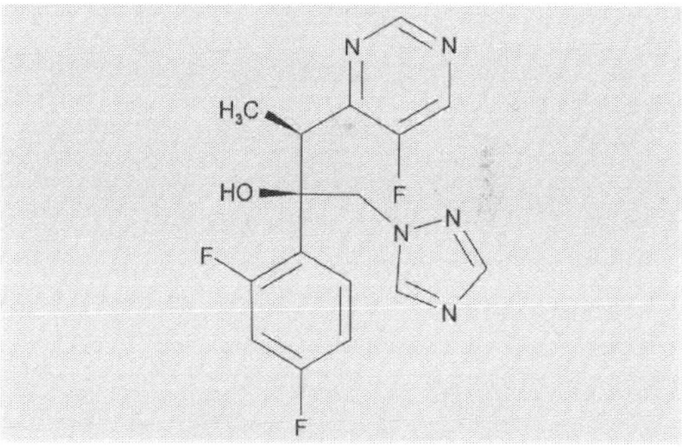

Voriconazole

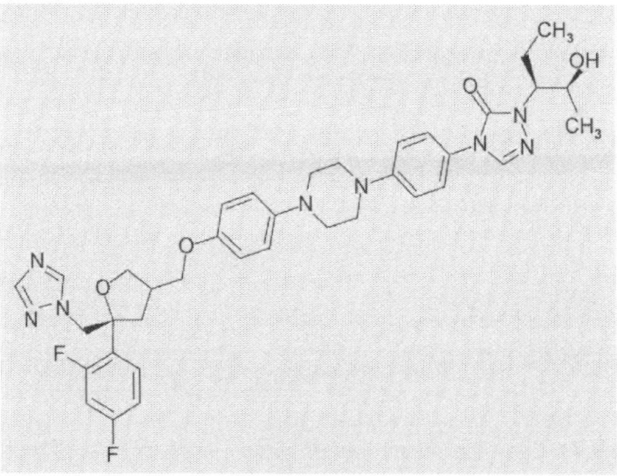

Posaconazole

Fig. 10.6: Chemical structures of some commonly used triazoles

fungal cytochrome P-450 enzymes and low affinity for human cytochrome P-450 enzymes. This differential activity makes them attractive compounds for clinical use, reducing the severity of side effects while increasing the effective anti-fungal activity. Various azole derivatives available for commercial use in fungal ocular infections are discussed below:

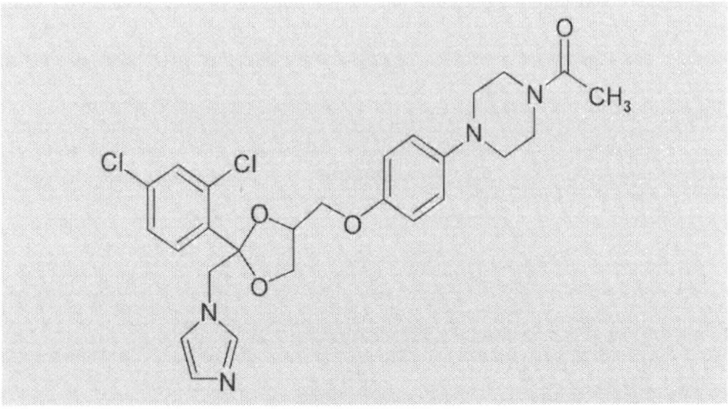

Ketoconazole

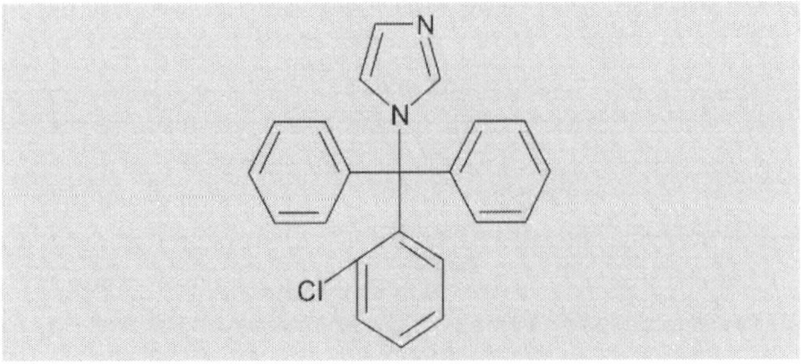

Clotrimazole

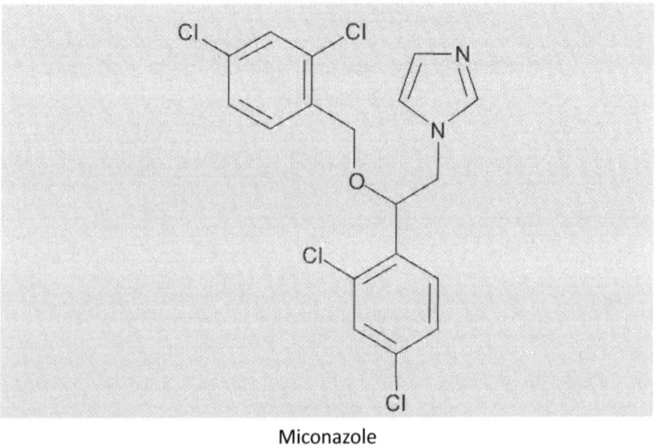

Miconazole

Fig. 10.7: Chemical structures of some commonly used imidazoles

Clotrimazole

It is a chlorinated trityl imidazole, first synthesized in 1967. Clotrimazole is available only for topical use and is used in the treatment of superficial fungal infections like tinea infections. It is also effective in treatment of corneal ulcers due to *Aspergillus*. It is also active against *Candida, Fusarium, Penicillium, Alternaria, Cladosporium* and *Actinomyces*.

Dosage

It is available as 1 percent topical solution and was used in the past for treatment of fungal keratitis. One drop of this solution to be instilled on hourly basis over the days till the ulcer heals and then tapering (3-4 times a day) over several weeks.

A dermatological cream containing 1 percent clotrimazole is well tolerated when applied to eye also. Clotrimazole is poorly soluble in water and cannot be given parenterally.

Adverse Reactions

On topical instillation, ocular irritation and punctuate keratopathy have been reported. On systemic admistration hepatotoxicity, nausea and diarrhea are some of the adverse effects seen.

Miconazole

Miconazole is a phenethyl imidazole, first synthesized in 1969. It is available only for topical use and is effective against yeast and filamentous fungi (*Candida, Fusarium, Aspergillus, Penicillium, Alternaria, Histoplasma, Cladosporium, Coccidioides* and *Actinomyces*).

Dosage

It is available as 1 percent ophthalmic solution and applicaps. The initial dosage in fungal keratitis is one drop of miconazole at hourly interval, which may be gradually reduced with the response. Sub-conjunctival injection dose is 5-10 mg every 48 hourly for 2-3 doses. The corneal epithelium appears to be a potent barrier following topical administration.

Adverse Effects

Conjunctival chemosis, punctuate epithelial corneal erosions, pruritus are seen in some individuals.

Econazole

Econazole, a di-chlorimidazole, is a phenyl imidazole with broad spectrum of activity and low toxicity. It is available only for topical use and is effective against *Candida, Aspergillus* and other fungal species. The action against filamentous fungi is greater than against yeasts.

Dosage

It is available as (1%) ointment and topical ophthalmic preparation (1%) can be freshly prepared and well tolerated. Patient is advised to instill topical preparation 4-6 times a day. Because of poor intraocular penetration, it is effective only in superficial infections of the eye.

Ketoconazole

This imidazole derivative is highly effective in the treatment of keratomycosis. The increased water solubility and enhanced absorption are valuable properties of this drug that set it apart from earlier imidazoles. Despite availability for systemic use, it is not routine used systemically due to high incidence of adverse effects and drug interactions.

Ketoconazole is effective against *Candida*, *Aspergillus*, *Fusarium* and *Curvularia* species in particular.

Dosage

- *Topical preparations:* Concentration ranging from 1–5 percent. Also available as 2 percent shampoo for treatment of seborrheic dermatitis.
- *Oral:* Available as 200 mg tablets. Dose is 200–400 mg/day.

Adverse Effects

Systemic use of ketoconazole has reduced now with the advent of better and safe drugs. Ketoconazole also inhibits human cytochrome P450 enzymes and hence results in many adverse effects and drug interactions. Adverse effects seen are GIT disturbances, abnormal liver function tests and hypersensitive reaction. The hepatotoxicity of systemic ketoconazole is usually reversible with cessation of drug although recovery may be slow.

Topical preparations of ketoconazole are well tolerated. One percent ketoconazole did not retard the closure of epithelial defects.

Fluconazole

Fluconazole is a triazole derivative (bis-triazole) used for ocular fungal infections. It has a good pharmacokinetic profile and relative low side effects. Fluconazole is highly water soluble and exhibits low protein binding. It is highly specific for fungal cytochrome enzymes and usually does not interfere with human cytochrome enzymes. Among the azole group of antifungals, fluconazole has the least activity towards human cytochrome P450 enzymes and hence does not produce drug interactions. It is available for both systemic and topical use.

Fluconazole is most effective against *Candia albicans* and *Cryptococcus* species. It is also active against *Histoplasma capsulatum, Blastomyces dermatidis* and *Coccidiodes*. Fluconazole has no activity against *Aspergillus* and other filamentous fungi.

Fluconazole is the agent of choice for treatment of cryptococcal meningitis. The most common ophthalmic use of systemic fluconazole is in the treatment of *Candida endophthalmitis* in combination with amphotericin B.

Dosage

It is available as oral tablet, intravenous injection and topical solution.

- Topically it is available as (0.3%) ophthalmic solution. Patient is advised to instill one drop in the conjunctival sac every 4 hours. Tapering is done (1 drop 4 times a day) and therapy is generally continued for 14–21 days until there is resolution of active ulcer/keratitis.
- Systemic dose of fluconazole (Oral/ IV):
    - 200-600 mg/day for 10–12 weeks for cryptococcal meningitis and for 3–5 weeks for disseminated candida infections.
    - 150 mg single dose for treatment of vaginal candidiasis

Ophthalmic use of fluconazole has the following advantages:
- Topically it has faster and deeper penetration which ensures 100 percent cure in 21–24 days therapy
- Highly effective in topical treatment of fungal keratitis with deep abscess and corneal ulcers because of deep corneal penetration
- Broad spectrum coverage with faster and complete eradication
- It is very well tolerated and has wide therapeutic index
- Presurgical use ensures maximum prophylaxis against fungal infections
- Fluconazole can also be given intravitreally in dose of 100 µg/ 0.1 ml in treatment of fungal endophthalmitis due to *Candida*. This dose is not toxic to the retina.

Adverse Effects

On topical application fluconazole is well tolerated. Adverse effects like irritation and transient burning sensation of the eye can occur. When used systemically, it can cause nausea, headache and skin rash.

Itraconazole

Itraconazole is a triazole antifungal compound. Although it is less attractive agent than fluconazole because of its poor water solubility, yet its spectrum of activity is in some respects broader than fluconazole. It is highly effective in treatment of infections caused by dimorphic fungi like *Histoplasma, Blastomyces* and *Sporothrix*. Despite the apparent indifferent pharmacokinetic profile, it is well distributed in lipid rich tissues. It is given orally, intravenously and topically. Effective oral absorption depends upon presence of food in the stomach and low pH.

Currently, itraconazole is prescribed for treatment of fungal infections caused primarily by *Aspergillus*, histoplasmosis, blastomycosis, onychomycosis and dematiceous fungi. It has moderate efficacy against *Candida* and *Fusarium* infections.

Dosage

- Oral: 100–200 mg once or twice daily depending upon the severity of infections.
- IV: 200 mg slow IV infusion over 1 hour given twice daily for severe systemic fungal infections.
- Topical: Topical ophthalmic drops are not commercially available and hence it has to be prepared freshly for such use.
- Sub-conjunctival injection provides adequate therapeutic levels in the cornea.

Adverse Effects

On systemic administration adverse reactions reported are GIT disturbances and hypersensitive reactions.

Voriconazole

This newer antifungal agent has excellent activity against *Aspergillus* species and *Candida*. It is also active against *Fusarium* and *Scedosporium* species. It is also effective against drug resistant *Candida* infections.

Voriconazole has replaced amphotericin B as the antifungal agent of choice for the treatment of invasive aspergillosis due to better safety profile. It is used in topical treatment of fungal corneal ulcer especially in serious infections when aggressive treatment and broad spectrum of activity is required. It is less toxic than amphotericin B and has good corneal penetration.

Dosage

- Oral: 200 mg twice daily for treatment of invasive aspergillosis and candidemia.
- IV (Slow infusion): Loading dose of 6 mg/kg 12th hourly on day 1 followed by maintenance dose of 4 mg/kg 12th hourly on consecutive days.
- Intravitreal injections have been tried for severe fungal endophthalmitis.

Adverse Effects

Visual disturbance, blurring of vision and disturbed color vision are the common adverse effects reported with voriconazole. However, these visual disturbances are transient and resolve within an hour. Other adverse effects reported include rashes, photosensitivity, dermatitis and drug interactions due to microsomal CYP450 enzyme inhibition.

Posaconazole

This newer antifungal agent belongs to triazole group. Among the azole group of antifungal agents, posaconazole has the broadest antifungal spectrum. Currently it is the only member in the azole family that is highly active in treatment of zygomycosis and mucormycosis. It is active against *Candida* and *Aspergillus* species.

It is available only for oral administration. Oral absorption is better if taken with fatty food. Ocular penetration of posaconazole is poor and hence it is not used in initial treatment of fungal endophthalmitis. However, it may be considered when other antifungal drugs failed to produce a therapeutic response.

Dosage (Oral)

- 100–200 mg twice or thrice daily
- 400 mg twice daily for treatment of refractory and drug resistant infections.

Adverse Effects

Diarrhea, nausea, vomiting and headache are the common adverse effects reported with posaconazole. Other adverse effects include hypertension, rash, elevated liver enzymes, thrombocytopenia and anemia.

ALLYLAMINES

Terbinafine

This antifungal agent belongs to synthetic allylamine group. It is available for both systemic and topical use. It is highly effective against a broad range of dermatophytes, the pathogens responsible for the majority of superficial fungal infections.

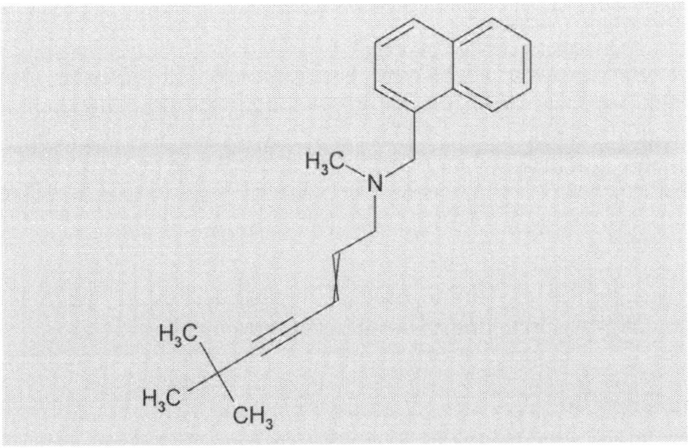

Fig. 10.8: Chemical structure of terbinafine

Mechanism of Action

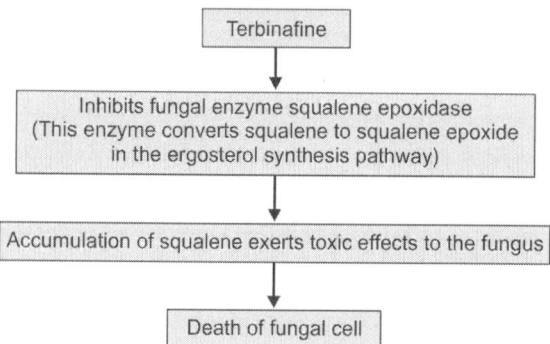

Terbinafine differs from previous groups of antifungal agents in three main ways.
- Fungicidal action
  - Unlike azoles, terbinafine has primary fungicidal activity causing fungal cell death at very low concentrations. It interferes with the fungal ergosterol synthesis by inhibiting the fungal enzyme squalene epoxidase.
- Selectivity
  - It is highly selective for fungal enzymes and unlike azoles, it does not affect the cytochrome P-450 system.
- Lipophilicity
  - It is highly lipophilic and diffuses well through the infected tissues.

Due to its primary fungicidal activity, mycological cure is achieved before clinical cure. This offers an advantage over topical azole antifungal therapy where symptomatic relief is often achieved before mycological cure.

Dosage

- Oral: 125–250 mg once daily
- Topical: One percent cream

Adverse Effects

Systemic adverse effects are gastrointestinal symptoms, skin reactions, taste disturbances, hepatobiliary dysfunction, hematological disorders. On topical use it may cause redness, itching, stinging and dryness.

Naftifine

It is a topical allylamine used as 1 percent topical cream for dermatophyte infections. It is not used systemically.

Butenafine

It is synthetic benzylamine used as 1 percent topical cream for dermatophyte infections. It is not available for systemic use.

ECHINOCANDINS

These newer agents are the latest addition in antifungal drug therapy. They are peptide molecules that are linked to fatty acids. Echinocandins approved for clinical use include caspofungin, micafungin and anidulafungin. The chemical structures of echinocandins are shown in Figure 10.9.

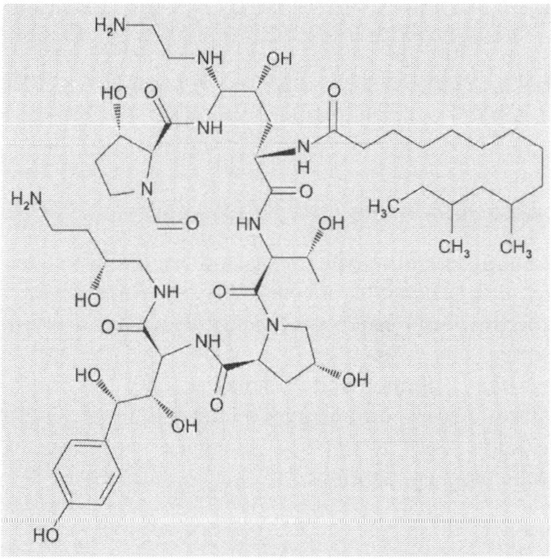

Caspofungin

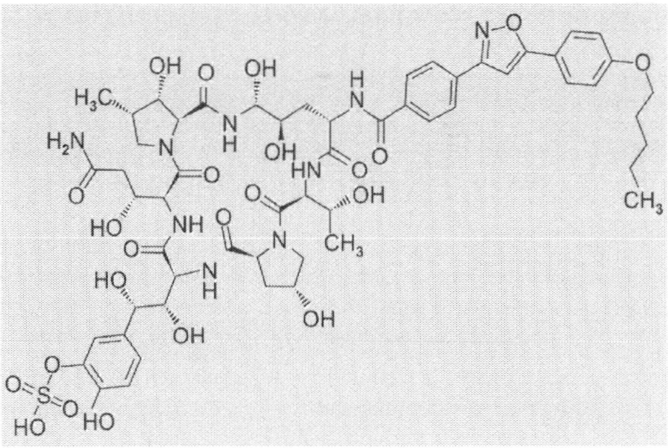

Micafungin

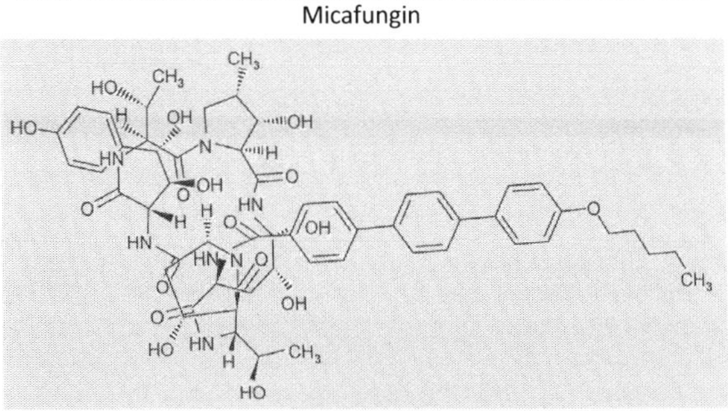

Anidulafungin

Fig. 10.9: Chemical structure of echinocandins—Caspofungin, Micafungin and Anidulafungin

Mechanism of Action

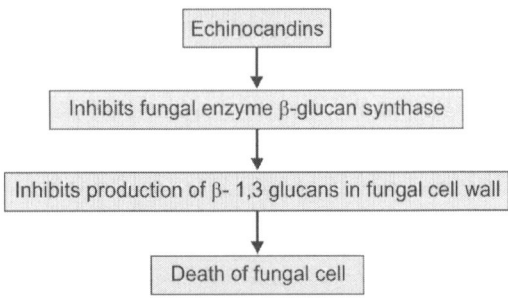

Antifungal Spectrum

Echinocandins are fungicidal drugs and are highly active against *Candida* and *Aspergillus* species. They are not active against *Cryptococcus* species and causative agents of *Mucor* mycosis and zygomycosis.

They are commercially available only as intravenous formulations. The intraocular penetration of intravenous echinocandins is not satisfactory. Hence it is not routinely used in ophthalmic practice currently.

Individual Drugs

A brief description of individual drugs is given in the below table.

Drug name	*Dosage*	*Adverse effects*
Caspofungin	IV (slow infusion): 70 mg loading dose followed by 50 mg daily for 14 days	Infusion related reactions, rash, elevated liver enzymes, electrolyte imbalance
Micafungin	IV (slow infusion): 100–150 mg daily for treatment and 50 mg daily for prophylaxis of systemic candidiasis	Nausea, vomiting, diarrhea, electrolyte imbalance, hypersensitivity reactions, elevated liver enzymes, drug interactions with cyclosporine and sirolimus
Anidulafungin	IV (slow infusion): 200 mg loading dose followed by 100 mg daily for 2 weeks for treatment of candidemia. 100 mg loading dose followed by 50 mg daily for 2 weeks for treatment of esophageal candidiasis	Hypersensitivity reactions

Uses of Echinocandins

Echinocandins are used in the treatment of systemic invasive candidiasis, candidemia, and mucocutaneous candidiasis. They can also be used as salvage therapy in treatment of invasive aspergillosis that failed to respond to amphotericin B.

SILVER COMPOUNDS

The combination of silver with sulfonamides significantly increases the activity against bacterial and fungal infections. This combination probably functions as an organic base-heavy metal release system, and the release of silver ions is said to be responsible for its antimicrobial action.

Silver Sulfadiazine

It is highly effective against *Candida*, *Aspergillus* and *Fusarium* species. Topically it is well tolerated. It is broad spectrum fungistatic agent and is effective in both superficial and deep ocular fungal infections.

Dosage

It is available as 1 percent ophthalmic drops and in aplicaps. Patient is advised to put one drop at hourly interval initially, then tapering to 4 times a day over a period of 14–21 days.

Adverse Effects

Adverse effects include local irritation, foreign body sensation and itching.

BIBLIOGRAPHY

1. Agarwal A. Textbook of Ophthalmology, 1st edn. New Delhi: Jaypee Brothers Medical Publishers (P) Ltd, 2002.
2. Albert DM. Albert and Jakobiec's Principles and Practice of Ophthalmology, 3rd edn. Saunders, Elsevier, 2008.
3. Bartlett JD. Ophthalmic Drug Facts, 23rd edn. Wolters Kluwer Health, 2011.
4. Bartlett JD, Jaanus SD. Clinical Ocular Pharmacology, 5th edn. Butterworth-Heinemann, an imprint of Elsevier Inc, 2008.
5. Brunton LL. Goodman and Gilman's the Pharmacological Basis of Therapeutics, 12th edn. New York: The McGraw-Hill Companies, Inc, 2011.
6. Chowdhary A, Singh K. Spectrum of fungal keratitis in North India. Cornea 2005(1):8-15.
7. Garg A. Advances in Ophthalmology, 1st edn. New Delhi: Jaypee Brothers Medical Publishers (P) Ltd, 2005.
8. Garg A. Clinical Applications of Antibiotics and Anti-inflammatory Drugs in Ophthalmology, 1st edn. New Delhi: Jaypee Brothers Medical Publishers (P) Ltd, 2007.

9. Jurkunas U, Behlau I, Colby K. Fungal keratitis: changing pathogens and risk factors. Cornea 2009;28(6):638-43.
10. Kalkanci A, Ozdek S. Ocular fungal infections. Curr Eye Res 2011;36(3):179-89.
11. Katzung BG. Basic and Clinical Pharmacology, 12th edn. New York: The McGraw-Hill Companies, Inc, 2012.
12. Klotz SA, Penn CC, Negvesky GJ, Butrus SI. Fungal and parasitic infections of the eye. Clin Microbiol Rev 2000;13(4):662-85.
13. Manzouri B, Vafidis GC, Wyse RK. Pharmacotherapy of fungal eye infections. Expert Opin Pharmacother 2001;2(11):1849-57.
14. Nayak N. Fungal infections of the eye–laboratory diagnosis and treatment. Nepal Med Coll J 2008;10(1):48-63.
15. Onofrey BE. Ocular Therapeutics Handbook: A Clinical Manual. 3rd edn. Philadelphia: Lippincott Williams and Wilkins, 2011.
16. Saha R, Das S. Mycological profile of infectious Keratitis from Delhi. Indian J Med Res 2006;123(2):159-64.
17. Tasman W, Jaeger EA. Duane's Ophthalmology on DVD-ROM. 2011 edn. Lippincott Williams and Wilkins, 2011.
18. Thomas PA. Current perspectives on ophthalmic mycoses. Clin Microbiol Rev 2003;16(4):730-97.
19. Vanzzini Zago V, Alcantara Castro M, Naranjo Tackman R. Support of the laboratory in the diagnosis of fungal ocular infections. Int J Inflam 2012;2012:643104.

Antiglaucoma Therapy

Ahmad K Khalil (Egypt)

Ocular medications have an important role in the treatment of glaucoma. Medications are usually considered the first line of treatment for glaucoma, and in many instances, medications alone can control the disease. All lines of treatment of glaucoma aim at o preserve the patient's vision during his/her lifetime to meet their functional needs. The only way currently proven to slow or stop damage from progressing is to reduce intraocular pressure (IOP) below the level that will cause continued damage to the optic nerve.

Medical therapy for glaucoma has been very well used for the past decades. With an ever increasing armamentarium of new drugs being introduced, and its proven success in achieving IOP lowering with various degrees, it has become the mainstay of initial glaucoma treatment. Most patients respond to a simple regimen with a desirable reduction in IOP. Side effects are usually few and tolerable, and are often reversible by stopping the medication. Even with cases who are deemed for surgical treatment, many expect a trial of medical therapy first and are likely to be somewhat suspicious of a too rapid suggestion for surgery. On the other hand, several prospective studies have pointed to medical therapy as less effective in lowering IOP and perhaps in preventing further visual field loss than filtering surgery.[1,2] These studies were however carried out in the 1980s, 90s, when many of the currently available potent medications were not there. The Collaborative Glaucoma Initial Therapy Trial at the end of 5 years showed no difference in the progression of visual field loss with either medication as initial therapy in glaucoma or trabeculectomy.[3]

The attempt to stabilize or at least minimize the damage to both structure and function involves these therapeutic approaches:
1. The reduction of intraocular pressure to or below a presumed "safe" target pressure that arrests the disease process or slows it sufficiently that patients will have the preservation of visual acuity and visual field consistent with their activities of daily living and their expected life span. Different optic nerves demand different intraocular pressures in order not to sustain progression. The same pressure does not suit every optic nerve.
2. Maintaining and theoretically increasing ocular perfusion pressure to the optic nerve and retina. Vascular factors play a significant role in maintaining the health of the optic nerve. Protecting the optic nerve head and retinal ganglion cells from

chemical mediators and other damaging agents that may result from intraocular pressure, vascular insult, or other unknown factors. Thus, neuroprotection is the final goal of all glaucoma therapies, although the term itself considers treatment approaches separate from directly lowering intraocular pressure or raising ocular perfusion pressure.

Currently, the only way proven to slow or stop damage from glaucomatous progression is to reduce intraocular pressure (IOP) below the level that will cause continued damage to the optic nerve.

In treating the patient, the ophthalmologist needs to take into account new understandings of risk factors as well as new concepts of the disease process and evolving therapies.

Despite challenging the concept that lowering IOP really helps glaucoma patients, and prevent damage progression by some authors,[4] the general consensus of the majority of studies in this context point out that IOP lowering if indeed beneficial for the control of glaucoma.[5] Most studies clearly point to IOP as an important risk factor, if not a causal factor in the pathogenic process of glaucoma. These studies strongly suggest that the lower the IOP, the less likely optic nerve damage is to develop or progress.

There are, of course, many other non-IOP factors that influence the choice of medical. The decision really rests upon the clinician's accounting of risk factors for an individual patient. In addition to the ability of medications to lower intraocular pressure, we must also consider the natural course of the disease and the age of the patient, topical and systemic side effects of medications, preservative toxicities, dosing intervals, adherence to medical regimens and, of course, the possibility of no treatment at all for select patients.

Before beginning medical therapy, the physician should set a "target-IOP" for the patient. The target-IOP is the clinician's best estimate of the maximum intraocular pressure the specific glaucoma patient can tolerate without further damage to their optic nerves and visual fields.[6] This target pressure is only a clinical estimate and must be updated periodically if progression is noted. Rather than a single numerical value for an initial target pressure, most glaucoma specialists set a preliminary goal for target IOP as a range of percentage reduction from the initial presenting IOP in the office setting.[7,8] The less the initial pretreatment IOP, the more advanced the optic nerve damage, and the older the patient, the lower the target pressure should be set. The presence of diabetes or arteriosclerotic cardiovascular disease should also lower the target pressure. A cup-to-disc ratio of 0.9, and advanced visual field loss may require a target pressure of 15 mm Hg or lower. Expert panel recommendations for initial target pressure range from 25 percent reduction for patients with mild glaucoma to more than 35 percent initial reduction for patients with severe damage[9]

While naturally available substances provided the earliest glaucoma medications, new drugs are now developed through computational and synthetic chemical techniques

An ideal drug would have no side effects, would be effortless to administer, would cost nothing, and would be 100 percent effective in controlling or eliminating the problem. Currently, the ideal drug for glaucoma does not exist.

Drug Delivery

Glaucoma drugs come in many preparations. Topical medications for glaucoma are available as aqueous solutions, suspensions, ointments, inserts placed within the fornices of the eye, and gels. Systemic medications used to treat glaucoma also have several routes of administration

Instilling Drops into the Conjunctival Cul-de-sac

The precorneal tear film normally contains 7 to 10 µl.[10] After instillation of an eyedrop, the tear film can momentarily hold up to 30 µl before the patient blinks. Blinking causes the majority of the drop to spill out onto the cheek while the remaining portion is pumped into the lacrimal system and becomes available for systemic absorption The average size of a commercial eyedrop is 39.0 µl.[11] Only 1 to 7 percent of an instilled dose penetrates the cornea.[12]

Most eyedrops preparations enter the eye by passing through the cornea. The movement of drugs across the conjunctiva and sclera accounts for less than 2 percent of the intraocular concentration.[13] The multilayered cornea is not easily penetrated by drugs. The corneal structure may be described as a lipid-water-lipid Sandwich. Three layers of the cornea act as barriers to drug permeability: the epithelium, the stroma, and the endothelium. The lipid-rich epithelium is the strongest barrier. Thus, molecules with high lipid solubility will have better corneal penetration. The stroma is 78 percent water and is passed most easily by hydrophilic drugs. Because the lipophilic endothelium is only one cell layer thick, it is a much weaker barrier than the epithelium. This dual nature of the corneal barriers causes drugs possessing both lipid and water solubility to penetrate the cornea more readily.

Under normal circumstances the turnover rate of the tear film is 15 percent per minute[10]. The instillation of eyedrops stimulates tearing and increases the turnover rate to 30 percent per minute. Furthermore, blinking and squeezing propels tears toward the lacrimal drainage system. Applying pressure on the canaliculi and closing the eyelids gently after administering eyedrops can reduce the flow of tears and medication into the lacrimal system and prolong drug-cornea contact.[14] Drugs that pass into the nasolacrimal system can be absorbed rapidly by the heavily vascularized mucosa of the nasopharynx and oropharynx. Drugs absorbed in this manner do not pass through the gastrointestinal tract and the liver and are not metabolized by these tissues.[14] It is estimated that as much as 80 percent of an eyedrop volume drains through the nasolacrimal system, where it is available for systemic absorption.[15] Again, a minute of eyelid closure following an eyedrop is a very practical, effective, and inexpensive way to reduce systemic drug absorption.

Ocular drug delivery systems are designed to increase ocular absorption in a convenient manner while minimizing local and systemic side effects. The large variety of drug forms points to the difficulty of achieving these goals. Topical glaucoma medications can be formulated as aqueous solutions, suspensions, ointments, inserts, emulsions, and gels. Each formulation also contains inactive ingredients (excipients) that adjust pH, tonicity, and viscosity. In addition, all dosage forms designed for multidose administration must reduce the risk of contamination, through either preservatives or special containers.

The pH of an eyedrop affects comfort, corneal penetration, and, ultimately, ocular absorption. Changes in pH can increase ocular penetration of topical carbonic anhydrase inhibitors five- to six-fold.[16]

Preservatives, of which benzalkonium chloride is the most common, are added to all multidose formulations to minimize microbial contamination. In addition to their antimicrobial activity, preservatives may also increase ocular absorption by enhancing corneal penetration and can contribute significantly to ocular allergies. In 2001, a chloro-oxy compound, Purite, was introduced in place of benzalkonium cloride in a new formulation of brimonidine (Alphagan-P) to help diminish allergic side effects.[17]

VARIOUS FORMS OF OCULAR DRUG ADMINISTRATION

AQUEOUS SOLUTIONS

Most topical glaucoma medications are formulated as aqueous solutions. This is probably the least expensive and easiest to apply, and generally does not cause blurred vision. However, aqueous solutions drain rapidly into the lacrimal system, which limits corneal contact time and ocular penetration.

SUSPENSIONS

Drugs with limited water solubility can be suspended as solid particles in a liquid vehicle and applied as an eyedrop. Prednisolone acetate and other topical corticosteroids are some of the most commonly used suspensions.

OINTMENTS

Ointment formulations are commonly used for antibiotics and corticosteroids, and they improve ocular absorption through prolonged retention of drug in the cul-de-sac. Blurred vision generally limits patient acceptance of ointments for chronic glaucoma therapy

GELS

Gels that form after contact with the ocular surface constitute *in situ*, gel-forming systems. When these medications are given as an aqueous solution, factors in the conjunctival cul-de-sac, such as temperature, pH, or the ionic milieu, trigger formation of the gel. Gels have proved useful in prolonging the duration of action of pilocarpine.[18] Timolol has now been formulated in Gelrite, a polysaccharide gellan gum in which gel formation is triggered by the presence of sodium ions in the tears. In chronic treatment, once-daily use of timolol in this gel product is equivalent to twice-daily use of timolol in solution.[19,20]

OCULAR INSERTS

Numerous devices have been developed to enhance delivery of ocular medications. The ocusert (no longer commercially available), was a membrane ring applied underneath a patient's eyelid to provide a continuous delivery of pilocarpine. The zero-order kinetics was said to allow a much smaller total dose of pilocarpine to achieve IOP reduction equivalent to that of conventional pilocarpine eyedrops.[21] Other devices, such as ophthalmic rods and paper strips, have been investigated for glaucoma treatment, but did not become commercially available.[22,23]

DRUG COMPLIANCE

Eliciting compliance is the key to successful glaucoma therapy. Selection of medications should be based on scientific concepts such as receptor binding, duration of action, and consideration of preservatives. Obviously, not every medication is good for every patient and what is a good first medication is not always a good second one. Future developments in glaucoma therapy will get us away from medications needed even just "once-a-day" and thereby increase compliance.

Drugs for Medical Therapy of Glaucoma

The rationale for treatment of glaucoma is based on the assumption that lowering intraocular pressure currently is the most important thing we can do for the patient. At the present time, benefits such as improved blood flow or direct neuroprotection of retinal ganglion cells are secondary considerations when choosing primary therapy for patients with ocular hypertension or open angle glaucoma.

Medications for the treatment of glaucoma may be divided into six classes:
- Beta-adrenergic antagonists
- Prostaglandins
- Carbonic anhydrase inhibitors, topical, oral
- Sympathomimetic agonists, non-selective, selective
- Parasympathomimetic agents, miotics
- Hyperosmotic agents.

Beta-Adrenergic Antagonists

In 1967 Phillips and coworkers reported that an intravenous injection of propranolol, a β-adrenergic antagonist, lowered intraocular pressure (IOP) in humans.[24] In following years, a number of other β-adrenergic antagonists were also found to be effective ocular hypotensive agents.[25,26] A paper by Katz et al in 1976 demonstrated that topical timolol reduced IOP in normal volunteers.[27] From the late 1970s through the beginning of the twenty-first century, beta-adrenergic antagonists (beta-blockers) became the mainstay of initial clinical treatment for lowering intraocular pressure in glaucoma patients. Timolol and its pharmacologic cousins replaced both miotics and epinephrine analogues. The adrenergic antagonists were prescribed commonly because they are both effective in most types of glaucoma and relatively free of the annoying ocular side effects (e.g. miosis, myopic shift in refraction, conjunctival hyperemia) produced by other classes of drugs. As will be noted, however, these agents may have profound although sometimes subtle systemic side effects; it is this latter problem that has seen them take second place to the Hypotensive lipids.

Beta-blockers reduce IOP by about 20–25 percent by suppression of aqueous humor formation. These drops inhibit cyclic adenosine monophosphate (cAMP) in ciliary epithelium.[28,29] Most investigators find little or no change in outflow facility after administration of various topical beta-blockers.[30-32]

Aqueous humor production is reduced greatly during sleep and that little additional reduction occurs with the administration of timolol either just before or during sleeping hours. This suggests that circulating catecholamines stimulate the ciliary processes to produce aqueous humor. During sleep, the level of circulating catecholamines falls and aqueous humor production diminishes. Timolol could act by antagonizing the catecholamine-induced stimulation of aqueous humor production during waking hours. Thus, it would have little effect during sleep when catecholamine levels are low.[33] Topical administration of timolol and the other β-adrenergic antagonists to one eye reduces IOP in the contralateral eye.[34,35] The fact that IOP in the contralateral eye is reduced less than in the ipsilateral eye suggests a local effect in the eye rather than an effect mediated by the central nervous system or by a reduction of blood pressure. Substantial levels of timolol are found in the contralateral eye after unilateral topical administration in rabbits, and small but clinically significant levels are found in humans.[36]

Timolol is available in either 0.25 or 0.5 percent strengths. Although, both concentrations produce the same peak IOP-lowering effect,[37,38] their trough effect may differ, depending on the ocular pigmentation. It seems that melanin readily binds timolol and may become a slow release depot for the drug. Thus patients with dark irides may need a higher concentration of timolol than those with less pigment to achieve the same response.

Many investigators have debated the necessity of using any of the beta-blockers more frequently than once a day.[39] Most product monographs recommend and declare FDA approval for twice-daily administration. Clinical trials have shown that an anionic heteropolysaccharide gellan gum, which prolongs the residence time of the drug in the tear film, given once a day, has an efficacy equivalent to twice-a-day timolol maleate.[40,41] However, several clinical studies demonstrate that timolol maleate solutions (0.25 or 0.5%) used once every 24 hours are as efficacious as when used twice daily.[42] Even though the serum half-life of absorbed topical beta-blockers may only be several hours (betaxolol is the longest at 12 to 20 hours), the ocular availablity of the drug is prolonged due to the melanin binding previously noted. This depot storage phenomenon may, in part, explain the observation that at least 2 weeks is needed to entirely "wash out" the effects of timolol maleate after the drug is stopped.[43]

Side Effects

Applied topically, beta-blocker agents are generally well tolerated. In particular, local ocular side effects of beta-blockers are relatively uncommon. As the systemic absorption of topically applied beta-blockers can be substantial, however, systemic side effects, some potentially life-threatening, can occasionally lead to discontinuance of these drugs.

Ocular Side Effects

Compared with their predecessors, topical beta-blockers have a very favorable ocular tolerability. However, some users do not transient stinging and burning, most commonly with betaxolol hydrochloride 0.5 percent solution. This has led to the development of the better-tolerated 0.25 percent suspension, Betoptic S.[44] Metipranolol hydrochloride (Optipranolol) has also caused more burning and stinging than other beta-blockers.[45] Carteolol hydrochloride (Occupress) may be the most comfortable beta-blocker following instillation.

It was speculated that chronic beta-blocker application might cause changes in the conjunctiva that increase the tendency for scarring following subsequent filtering surgery. Histopathologic evidence later supported this contention by demonstrating that chronic topical glaucoma medications are associated with an increased cellularity (fibroblasts and lymphocytes) in the conjunctiva.[46]

Systemic Side Effects

Many patients cannot use topical beta-blockers because of systemic side effects. Approximately 80 percent of an eyedrop (volume 30 to 80 µl) passes through the proximal nasolacrimal ducts to the nasal mucosa and its microvasculature, and is equivalent to an intravenous injection. Eighty percent of one 50 µl drop of a 0.5 percent solution contains 200 of active ingredient. For an infant weighing 3 or 4 kg, or a full-sized adult with labile asthma, this amount of beta-blocker could be seriously compromising. Because drops are usually instilled in both eyes twice a day, and patients often squeeze more than one drop with each application, it is essential to limit systemic absorption as much as possible. Simple digital nasolacrimal occlusion, or eyelid closure, for 5 minutes can markedly reduce serum concentrations of drugs.[14]

The nonselective beta-blockers (timolol, levobunolol, metipranolol, and carteolol) are particularly contraindicated in people with a history of reactive airway diseases, such as asthma, emphysema, and chronic bronchitis. Betaxolol is relatively specific for beta1-receptors and may be a safe alternative for very mild asthma, but several reports indicate that this drug can compromise breathing in patients with preexisting lung disease.[47]

Beta1-receptor blockade also reduces heart rate and contractile force. This decreases cardiac output, which partially explains why these drugs lower blood pressure. Patients with compromised myocardial function can suffer congestive heart failure, heart block, or bradyarrhythmias, and exacerbation of sinus bradycardia.

In addition to decreasing cardiac output, blockade of beta2-receptors can theoretically induce vasospasm by leaving alpha-receptors, which mediate vasoconstriction, free to bind circulating norepinephrine. Blood flow to organs other than the brain is reduced with propranolol.[48] This has generated considerable discussion about the possible effects of beta-blockade on optic nerve head perfusion[49]

Lastly, Beta-blockers may cause depression caused by down-regulation of neurotransmitter pathways in the central nervous system,[50] or exacerbate preexisting depression.[51] Although depression occurs more frequently with oral beta-blockers than with eyedrops, the latter gain access to the CNS by their lipophilic nature and ready transport across the blood–brain barrier.

Beta-blockers in Clinical Ophthalmic Use

Beta-blockers are available in solutions, gel forming solutions, and suspensions.

Generic/brand names
- *Nonselective* (B1–B2 blockade)—timolol maleate (Timoptic, Timoptic XE, Timoptic Ocudose, Timolol GFS, Istalol); timolol hemihydrate (Betimol), levobunolol (Betagan); metipranolol (Optipranolol 0.3%), carteolol HCl (Ocupress 1%)
- *Selective* (B2 blockade)—Betoptic-S.25%

The nonselective agents (all but betaxolol) appear clinically more alike than different, although there are some differences that may be important in selected patients, In the following timolol will be discussed as the prime example of nonselective and betaxolol as the selective agent

Timolol

This lipophilic, nonselective beta-blocker solution is available as the maleate salt and the hemihydrate salt; it is also available in various gel formulations (gellan gum (Gelrite), a surface-activated gel, to prolong ocular contact and improve penetration and enhance its transit into the anterior segment) which has the same IOP-lowering efficacy as twice-daily timolol solution.[41] Timolol maleate (Timoptic™, Merck, West Point, Penn and generics) is a nonselective β1- and β2-adrenergic antagonist that lacks substantial intrinsic sympathomimetic activity and membrane-stabilizing properties. Timolol reduces IOP in normal and glaucomatous eyes without changing visual acuity, accommodation, or pupil size.[27,34] On average, timolol lowers IOP by about 5 mm Hg over a 6–12 month period.[52] Timolol penetrates the eye rapidly; following topical administration, IOP begins to fall in 30–60 minutes, reaches a low in 2 hours, and returns to baseline in 24–48 hours.[27] Some residual effect of timolol on IOP may be detected for as long as 2–3 weeks, and beta-blockade can be detected up to 1 month after discontinuation of the drug.[53] Timolol and other beta-blockers flatten the diurnal IOP curve, they are generally less effective during the night-time hours, possibly because the secretion of aqueous is lowest during the night.[54]

Timolol has become the 'gold' standard against which all newer glaucoma hypotensive agents are compared. It is less potent than the major prostaglandin analogs and equivalent to unoprostone, brimonidine, and the topical carbonic anhydrase inhibitors.[55-57] The ocular hypotensive effect of timolol is additive to that of the miotics[58-60] and the carbonic anhydrase inhibitors (CAIs).[61,62] Timolol adds well to the topical carbonic anhydrase inhibitors with a decrease in aqueous humor formation and IOP with the two drugs greater than either alone.[63] Additivity of brimonidine's effect to timolol both in reducing aqueous formation and IOP has been recorded.[64]

Finally, Topical beta-blockers used to treat glaucoma are less effective at lowering IOP in patients already taking oral beta-blockers.[65]

Betaxolol

Betaxolol (Betoptic, Alcon Laboratories, Fort Worth, TX) is a relatively selective β1-adrenergic antagonist that lacks intrinsic sympathomimetic activity and membrane-stabilizing properties. Patients with ocular hypertension and glaucoma experienced 20 to 30 percent lowering of IOP with Betoptic.[66,67] The drug reduces IOP by decreasing aqueous humor formation,[68,69] but appears to lower IOP as much as timolol,[66] with most studies showing about a 2 mm Hg difference. Despite this, some published evidence shows a better preservation, and even improvement, of visual fields with betaxolol as compared with timolol[70] which some investigators attribute to a beneficial effect on optic disc blood flow.

Evidence suggests that betaxolol may be more 'neuroprotective' than its nonselective cousins despite a weaker effect on IOP lowering. It seems to reduce the progression of visual field defects compared with timolol.[70] and may even increase retinal sensitivity.[71] topical betaxolol seems to increase retinal blood flow.[72] This appears to be particularly true in patients with normal-pressure glaucoma.[73]

PROSTAGLANDINS (HYPOTENSIVE LIPIDS; HLS)

The prostaglandins have become one of the mainstays of glaucoma treatment around the world. Although their ocular effects have been known for some time, investigators have only recently succeeded in separating their ability to lower intraocular pressure (IOP) from their other, less desirable, side effects. The resulting PG formulations constitute our most potent glaucoma drugs. Prostaglandins for treating OAG fall into three subcategories. The prostaglandin analogues (PGAs) include latanoprost (Xalatan 0.005%) and travoprost (Travatan and Travatan Z, both 0.004%); there is one prostamide – bimatoprost (Lumigan 0.03%); and the deconsanoid class is represented by unoprostone isopropyl (Rescula 0.15%). They function as prodrugs. Latanoprost, travoprost, and unoprostone are esterified derivatives of prostaglandin F2a, while bimatoprost contains an amide group in the same position as the isopropyl ester of the other molecules.

Acting as local hormones, PGs are quickly inactivated systemically. Because of this, and their low therapeutic concentrations, these agents have relatively few systemic side effects. However, as relative newcomers to the glaucoma armamentarium, their long-term side effects remain to be explored.

Early drugs developed to control glaucoma either decreased aqueous production (beta-blockers) or increased conventional, trabecular-meshwork-mediated outflow (miotics). The major innovation of the PGs medications is their ability to increase uveoscleral outflow. They also increase trabecular meshwork outflow to a lesser extent. Most of the increased outflow facility can be attributed to their effects on the pressure-independent uveoscleral outflow pathway.[74-76] PGs IOP lowering is less affected by circadian variations in aqueous production than the beta-blockers.[77,78] The increased uveoscleral outflow was confirmed with the use of tracer substances in primate eyes.[79] Studies in humans are confirmatory.[80] Prostaglandins appear to alter not only the function of the uveoscleral pathway(s) but also the structure. They produce extracellular matrix remodeling, widening of intermuscular spaces along the longitudinal ciliary muscle bundles, and dissolution of collagen types I and III.[81,82]

The observed ultrastructural changes are most likely the anatomic counterpart to the functional improvement in uveoscleral outflow associated with the clinical use of the prostaglandins. While improvement in uveoscleral outflow may be the most obvious mechanism by which these agents work, studies at the cellular level suggest that some other intracellular metabolic changes may also contribute to the overall effect.[83,84]

Most scientists agree that the mechanism of action for increased uveoscleral outflow involves activation of the FP class of prostaglandin receptors found at the iris root and ciliary body. Stimulation of these receptors results in the up-regulation of matrix metalloproteinases (which are similar to collagenases that in turn result in a remodeling of extracellular matrix and widening of intermuscular spaces in the ciliar body. Aqueous may then more easily exit the eye around the cellular structures.[81,82,85] A study in

FP-receptor-deficient mice, with presumed functional uveoscleral outflow pathways, showed no affect of any of the four hypotensive lipids on reduction of intraocular pressure.

Controversy exists, however, as to the exact mechanism of action of bimatoprost. While clinically it seems to work in the same way, evidence suggests that there may be some differences in the way it acts.[86] Bimatoprost by itself seems to have little effect on prostaglandin receptors. The manufacturer of bimatoprost (Allergan, Irvine, California) has significant evidence that it is derived, at least in part, from and mimics the action of a seemingly parallel group of autocoids called prostamides. These hypotensive lipids are derived from the endocannabinoid family. Bimatoprost also seems to inhibit enzymes that metabolize prostaglandins.[87] On the other hand, research from a rival company's laboratories suggested that all of the currently available agents are direct prostaglandin FP agonists in tissue cultures of human trabecular meshwork cells.[88] Because of the lack of clarity as to the mechanism of action of bimatoprost and perhaps unoprostone, the terms 'prostanoids' and 'hypotensive lipids' have been used to designate the entire group.

Efficacy

Double masked clinical trials comparing latanoprost 0.005 percent once daily to timolol 0.5 percent twice daily in over 800 patients showed that latanoprost reduced IOP by 25 to 35 percent. This effect was sustained over the full 6-month study period.[89-91] In patients who continued latanoprost in an unmasked manner, this IOP reduction persisted for 1 to 2 years without tachyphylaxis,[92] whereas wash-out studies following chronic therapy showed that this effect could persist for several days to weeks after discontinuation.[93] The addition of 0.005 percent latanoprost, once daily, in a double-masked fashion to patients maintained on oral acetazolamide produced a further IOP decrease of 21 percent following 18 days.[94,95] Generally, The HLs have relatively flat IOP curves over 24 h, demonstrating both low circadian IOP fluctuation and, unlike the beta-blockers, effective diurnal and nocturnal IOP control.[77,78,96] They do not evidence short-term escape or long-term drift.[97,98]

Side Effects

Ocular Side Effects

Initial studies in human eyes showed that PGs caused burning, stinging, and marked conjunctival hyperemia. Because of this, subsequent development of PG analogs for ocular treatment concentrated on preserving the pressure lowering effect and minimizing external ocular side effects.

The well-established ocular side effects of PG administration include an increase in iris pigmentation changes. All evidence suggests that this change in color is due solely to an increase in melanin pigment within each melanocyte.[99] With perhaps rare exceptions, iris pigmentation does not change in patients with uniformly blue or brown irides.[100] Latanoprost can also increase the length and pigmentation of eyelashes.[101] These primarily cosmetic changes are most noticeable (and disturbing) with monocular use.

Several reports of iritis and CME with latanoprost,[102,103] and the other PG analogs[104] have surfaced. These include case reports and case series in which some eyes, mostly aphakic and pseudophakic, have developed CME or iritis. However, only one report demonstrated a consistent recurrence of moderate iritis upon rechallenge with latanoprost in five eyes of four patients.[103] Use of a topical nonsteroidal agent in conjunction with these drugs may be considered in these situations.[105]

Systemic Side Effects

Despite a single report of facial rash associated with its use,[106] it seems unlikely that these agents can cause systemic side effects. Latanoprost has a systemic half-life of 17 minutes, is rapidly converted to an inactive metabolite in the liver, and is excreted primarily in the urine.[107] The fact that no contralateral IOP-lowering effect was found in clinical trials further supports this lack of systemic action.

To conclude, prostanoids as a group are very well tolerated with side effects being relatively mild and local; serious side effects are infrequent and systemic ones rare.

Drugs in Clinical Use

The first usable prostaglandin was developed in Japan. Isopropyl unoprostone (Rescula) is a prodrug that is derived from a pulmonary metabolite of PGF2, lowers IOP in a dose-dependent fashion with twice daily dosing, and was reported to be well tolerated.[108] Major progress was made with the development of a 17-phenylsubstituted PGF2-isopropyl ester (PHXA34), which is considerably more potent than the PGF2 without the phenyl substitution.[109] PHXA41 (latanoprost) has the same chemical structure as PHXA34 but is a solution of only the R epimer. One would expect it to be more potent, and it is!

Latanoprost

Latanoprost is marketed under the trade name Xalatan as a 0.005 percent solution and includes 0.02 percent benzalkonium chloride preservative plus various inert ingredients. Each drop delivers approximately of latanoprost. It is a very potent IOP lowering medication and has become one of the most useful antiglaucoma agents. In initial trials, latanoprost 0.005 percent reduced IOP by 25–35 percent with a single daily dose.[110,111] The 0.005 percent dose seems to be the most efficient with the best balance of efficacy versus side effects.[112] Furthermore, unlike most drugs, more is not better; once-daily dosage appears to be superior to twice daily.[113,114]

Dosing one drop every 24 hours is recommended at bedtime, based on the phase III Scandinavian trial,[91] in which evening administration produced the maximal effect. Though the conventional thought is to minimize cosmetic consequences of hyperemia by evening closing, such as advantage is not proven. Latanoprost is superior in pressure lowering to once-daily timolol gel throughout the day from 8 am to 12 midnight.[115] Latanoprost produced a higher incidence of conjunctival hyperemia than timolol, but the hyperemia was mild in all cases. No patients developed miosis or signs of intraocular inflammation. Latanoprost had no effect on heart rate or blood pressure, whereas timolol did slow the pulse an average of 2–3 beats per minute. It has also been shown to be superior in diurnal IOP control to brimonidine.[116] In a study comparing latanoprost with timolol, betaxalol and brimonidine, latanoprost had the best IOP-lowering effect, the least systemic side effects, and very few significant local side effects.[117] Latanoprost has been shown to have no adverse effect on the respiratory system, even in patients with significant, steroid-dependent asthma.[118]

Because latanoprost (and the other PGF2 analogs) works by significantly increasing the outflow of aqueous through the uveoscleral pathways, its effects on IOP should be additive to any agent that decreases aqueous formation. PGF2-isopropyl ester is additive to beta-blocker therapy, causing a further decrease in IOP of 17 percent compared with timolol alone.[119,120] In a subsequent study of patients whose conditions were uncontrolled with timolol, the addition of PGF2-isopropyl ester reduced IOP an additional 6–9 mm Hg below the level produced by timolol alone.[121] Latanoprost is also additive with carbonic anhydrase inhibitors (CAIs), topical CAIs, topical adrenergic agonists.[94,95,122]

In summary, topical latanoprost was the first of the potent prostaglandin ocular hypotensive agents. It has been shown to be better than any of the other classes of drugs in terms of monotherapy, with additivity to most, if not all, of the other types of ocular hypotensive agents.

Bimatoprost

Numerous studies have shown bimatoprost effectiveness in lowering IOP and its superiority in maintaining 24-hour control compared to timolol and dorzolamide.[123,124,114–116] Like its chemical cousin, bimatoprost as monotherapy seems to be superior in flattening the diurnal curve to timolol alone and to timolol combined with dorzolamide.

Most published studies to date have shown that when compared to latanoprost, bimatoprost seems to offer slightly improved pressure control or works in a greater percentage of patients.[125,126] Similarly, bimatoprost seems to have a slight edge in IOP control over travoprost.[127]

In summary, bimatoprost, seems to be, by a slight margin, the most potent of these agents but with a concomitant increase in local side effects.

Travoprost

Travaprost is a highly selective FP receptor agonist.[128] Like latanoprost, it is a very effective agent when used once daily for lowering IOP in most species including human; unlike latanoprost, it is more effective when used twice daily compared to once daily but, of course, side effects, especially conjunctival hyperemia, increase proportionately when that happens.[129] The obligatory studies comparing travoprost to timolol showed that both the 0.0015 percent and 0.004 percent solutions were superior in pressure lowering activity by about 2 mm Hg over 9 months versus timolol.[130] Compared to latanoprost, travoprost shows similar IOP levels over a 24-hour period but may have a greater duration of action—over 40 hours from a single dose[77]

Like the other prostaglandin and prostaglandin-like agents, travoprost works well with timolol and other topical antiglaucoma medications.[131]

CARBONIC ANHYDRASE INHIBITORS

Carbonic anhydrase inhibitors (CAIs) continue to be the only systemic agents used for the long-term treatment of glaucoma, if only occasionally. A topical version introduced more than 40 years after the introduction of the systemic agent moved the oral agents quite far down on the list of practical options for the chronic treatment of glaucoma. These drugs are all derivatives of sulfonamides and were introduced into clinical practice as diuretics. Even with chronic use, their diuretic action is only effective for 1–2 weeks. CAIs reduce intraocular pressure (IOP) by decreasing aqueous humor formation. As such they are useful in essentially all forms of glaucoma, even when the anterior chamber angle is sealed or the outflow facility is very low.

Mechanism of Action

Carbonic anhydrase inhibitors decrease IOP by inhibiting aqueous humor formation (Chapter 3). Inhibition of this enzyme may diminish aqueous humor production by altering the local pH in the nonpigmented epithelium. This could cause a malfunction of enzymes that catalyze ion secretion into the intercellular clefts.[132] The systemic acidosis induced by these drugs may also depress aqueous humor formation.[133] The observed ocular hypotensive effect of CAIs is probably produced by both local action on the ciliary epithelium and the induced systemic acidosis.

Topical CAIs appear somewhat less effective and usually reduce flow less than 20 percent. In contrast to betablockers, which do not reduce flow during sleep, oral CAIs inhibit night time flow by 24 percent.[134]

Dorzolamide has been shown to improve fluorescein flow in the macula and optic nerve head of normal volunteers.[135] In 26 eyes of 26 glaucoma patients, dorzolamide increased peak-systolic central retinal artery velocity, and increased end-diastolic velocity in the ophthalmic and central retinal arteries, with a reduction in the resistance index.[136] In addition, both brinzolamide and dorzolamide significantly increased optic nerve head blood flow in rabbits, with minimal systemic acid–base disturbances.[137] The benefit of these effects for optic nerve protection in the treatment of chronic glaucoma remain to be evidence based.

Side Effects

Ocular

The side effects of the topical CAIs are largely ocular in nature. Stinging on administration is the most common especially with dorzolamide.[138] Some patients experience actual ocular pain.[139] Brinzolamide often produces a transient blurring of vision. Presumably because of their sulfonamide derivation, the topical agents are associated with a relatively high rate of allergic reactions (about 10 %), as are the oral agents. Contact dermatitis may be seen on the eyelids.[140,141]

As can happen with any sulfa-derived medication, choroidal detachments with induced myopia and hypotony have been reported.[142,143]

Systemic

Systemic side effects prevent the long-term usage of systemic CAIs in the majority of glaucoma patients, particularly the elderly. Up to 50 percent of patients cannot tolerate these agents.[144] All of the commonly used oral CAIs produce similar side effects and IOP reduction when used in equipotent doses. However, individual variations do exist, and one drug may be more tolerable than another, in certain patients.

Although paraesthesias occur in two-thirds of patients, they do diminish with time. Half of patients note anorexia and weight loss, and 25 percent report fatigue, malaise, and transient diarrhea. Patients should be warned of potential side effects and told that many side effects will diminish in severity after a few days to a few weeks of treatment. Patients prepared in this manner are more trusting of the physician and are more ready to accept problems when they occur. Older patients are generally less tolerant of oral CAIs.[145]

Drugs in Clinical Use

Acetazolamide (Diamox)

The first available CAI, acetazolamide remains the most frequently used oral glaucoma agent. It has been supplied as 125 and 250 mg tablets, and 500 mg sustained release (SR) capsules. Effective IOP reduction can be achieved with a dose as low as 62.5 mg twice daily, with maximal benefit seldom achieved by more than 1 gram daily. Once-daily SR capsules may be effective throughout the 24-hour cycle for a proportion of patients, and may be better tolerated than the tablets.

Methazolamide (Neptazane)

Supplied in some countries in 25 and 50 mg tablets, dosing of methazolamide ranges from 25 to 100 mg twice daily. More frequent administration is probably not beneficial because it has a plasma half-life of 14 hours. The dose is proportional to both the IOP efficacy and induced side effects, and can be titrated appropriately.[146] Because of its pharmacodynamics, methazolamide, 50 mg daily, is probably safer than acetazolamide in patients with renal disease, and it is less likely to produce fatigue, drowsiness, and depression.

Dorzolamide

The glaucoma community was pleased when, 41 years after Becker first used acetazolamide to treat glaucoma, effective topical CAIs were introduced. Dorzolamide first appeared in 1995.[147,148] and differs from the oral agents in that it has both a free sulfonamide group and a second amine group, which adds the right amount of lipid and aqueous solubility for good corneal penetration.[147] dorzolamide has been reported with twice-daily instillation to reduce IOP by 21 and 13 percent at peak and trough times, respectively.[149] Dosing t.i.d. improves the trough effect, and this regimen is recommended when this drug is used alone.

In pediatric practice, dorzolamide, although not quite as effective as oral therapy, clinically worked in most of the children tested, produced much less side effects, and was better tolerated than acetazolamide.[150] While probably not as effective as the prostaglandin analogs over the 24-hour period, dorzolamide appears comparable in pressure lowering activity to both timolol and brimonidine when used three times daily in monotherapy.[151]

Surprisingly, dorzolamide is additive to other aqueous suppressants such as timolol, both clinically and in measurements of aqueous formation,[152,153] and to drugs acting on the outflow system such as pilocarpine and prostaglandins.[154] Dorzolamide has been used successfully in a fixed combination with timolol.[155]

Brinzolamide

Brinzolamide was a known CAI that was irritating when used topically in solution because of its low pH and had a disappointing effect due to poor corneal penetration. Placing the compound in a suspension rather than in the traditional solution was found to improve its ability to get across the cornea, reduce the surface irritation, increase its pressure-reducing activity, and prolong the duration of action.[156]

As a 1 percent suspension, brinzolamide demonstrates good corneal penetration with enhanced ocular hypotensive efficacy, prolonged duration of action, and reduced surface irritation compared with its solution. It is at least as effective as thrice-daily dorzolamide when administered at b.i.d. or t.i.d. frequency, achieving an IOP reduction of between 15 and 22 percent.[138] When added to twice-daily timolol maleate 0.5 percent, brinzolamide lowered IOP a further 13 to 16 percent. This is statistically equivalent to the adjunctive effect of dorzolamide with timolol.[157]

Sympathomimetic Agonists

Along with pilocarpine, epinephrine was one of the first agents used to treat glaucoma and was used as ocular hypotensive agents since 1900 when Darier treated glaucoma patients with subconjunctival injections of epinephrine. The sympathomimetic agonists used to treat glaucoma can be divided into those that are nonselective and activate both alpha and beta receptors, and those that are selective for alpha receptors alone. The nonselective drugs are represented by epinephrine compounds and dipivefrin HCl, while the available selective sympathetic agonists consist of various preparations of apraclonidine and brimonidine.

Epinephrine

Alpha adrenergic stimulation reduces ultrafiltration because of vasoconstriction and decreased ciliary body blood flow. These early effects diminish in several hours. The predominant effect of epinephrine is an increase in both conventional (trabecular meshwork) and unconventional (uveoscleral) outflow facility for a net reduction in IOP. Some investigators ascribe the effect of epinephrine on trabecular outflow to β-adrenergic receptors,[158] and others to β-adrenergic receptors.[159] It is important to stress that the IOP lowering mechanism of epinephrine is controversial. In these as well as other aspects.[160-162]

Epinephrine frequently causes ocular irritation (toxic rather than allergic reactions) with follicular conjunctivitis. Rebound conjunctival hyperemia occurs several hours after administration; first, the musculature lining the conjunctival blood vessel contracts causing blanching, then, the muscles relax past their "neutral" tone and fill with blood causing the hyperemic appearance.

Oculosympathetic innervation in the orbit includes Mueller's muscle, which when stimulated by epinephrine may cause eyelid retraction. Similarly, stimulation of the iris dilator muscles by epinephrine causes mydriasis. Epinephrine (and dipivefrin) should not be used to treat open angle glaucoma in patients who also have narrow anterior chamber angles because of the potential for papillary block with drug-induced iris dilation. Epinephrine has been associated with a significant percentage (up to 30 percent) of cystoid macular edema (CME) when used in aphakes[163] or in pseudophakes with torn or opened posterior capsules (the Irvine–Gass Syndrome[164]). This CME is usually clinically apparent as reduced acuity and contrast sensitivity.

Dipivefrin

Dipivefrin is a prodrug, which means that it must undergo biotransformation before exhibiting its pharmacologic effect. It was produced to reduce the frequency and magnitude of some of the side effects of epinephrine eye drops. Two pivaloyl groups were added to the basic epinephrine molecule. This increases the lipid solubility of the compound by 600 times and the ocular penetration by 17 times when compared with epinephrine.[165] Dipivefrin is effective at a clinically available concentration of 0.1 percent, 10 to 20 times less concentrated than commercial epinephrine eye drops. While all of the ocular and systemic side effects of epinephrine eye drops can and do occur with Propine, they do so to a lesser extent.[166]

α2-ADRENERGIC AGONISTS

The α2-adrenergic agonists reduce IOP largely by decreasing aqueous formation.[167] Topical α2 agonists have been studied and used for their ability to lower IOP for over a quarter of a century. The selective alpha agonist agents used to treat glaucoma are modifications of the clonidine molecule. Clonidine, developed to control systemic blood pressure, easily crosses the blood–brain barrier. When used topically, the raw clonidine molecule does lower IOP, but it also gets absorbed systemically in sufficient concentration to cause systemic hypotension.[168,169] Two topical alpha-adrenergic agonists are available for glaucoma therapy, apraclonidine which is relatively nonselective for alpha1 and alpha2 receptors, and that is more selective for alpha2 than alpha1 receptors.

Apraclonidine

A derivative of clonidine, apraclonidine was found to act similarly to clonidine without the systemic side effects.[170] It is sometimes used to block postoperative rises in IOP after glaucoma laser surgery, including peripheral iridotomies (YAG and Argon),[171,172] trabeculoplasties (both ALT and SLT), and YAG posterior capsulotomies.[170]

Brimonidine

More recently, another α2-adrenergic agonist, brimonidine, has been identified as a potent ocular hypotensive agent.[173] Brimonidine is much more selective than clonidine and apraclonidine for α2-receptors. It has significantly fewer of the problems found with apraclonidine because of its increased selectivity for the α2 receptor.[174] It decreases IOP by reducing aqueous formation; in addition, it acts by increasing uveoscleral outflow.[64] IOP control with brimonidine was comparable to that of timolol at peak drug effect, although not quite as good at the trough (4.3 mm Hg vs 6.0 mm Hg).[175] In a 3-month clinical trial comparing brimonidine 0.2 percent with betaxolol 0.25 percent b.i.d., the IOP-lowering efficacy of brimonidine was significantly greater at both peak and trough effect.[176] It is also believed that it has some neuroprotective functions in addition to lowering IOP. These include neuroprotection to the inner retina following mechanical and ischemia/reperfusion injury, at concentrations may be achieved in the posterior segment with topical therapy.[177-179]

Brimonidine has been combined with timolol in a fixed combination with comparable results to the separate, concomitant medications.[180]

Side Effects

Although generally better tolerated than apraclonidine, the most common ocular side effect with brimonidine is ocular allergy, which is reported in 5 to 25 percent of patients.[176,181] This can range from mild conjunctival injection to occasionally severe follicular conjunctivitis and blepharoconjunctivitis. Brimonidine was first marketed in a 0.2 percent solution. However, more recently it has been produced in a 0.15 percent marketed as Alphagan P. This solution seems to be equally effective as the 0.2 percent solution with possibly reduced systemic and topical side effects. In addition, the use of preservatives other than benzalkonium chloride (e.g. polyquaternarium, purite™) seems to reduce some of the topical side effects of brimonidine.[182] Brimonidine can produce cardiovascular instability, sleepiness and in children and thus these agents should be avoided in those under 15 years of age.[183]

CHOLINERGIC DRUGS

The cholinergic drugs are the oldest effective medical treatment for glaucoma. More than 100 years ago, Laqueur used physostigmine (eserine), an extract from the Calabar or ordeal bean, for the treatment of glaucoma. They are applied topically for the treatment of glaucoma because of their effect on parasympathetic receptors in the iris and ciliary body. Cholinergic agents all lower intraocular pressure (IOP) by improving aqueous outflow. These medications differ, however, by the manner in which they stimulate ciliary muscle contraction. The most commonly used cholinergic agent is pilocarpine, which directly stimulates the cholinergic receptor.

Cholinesterase inhibitors, such as echothiophate and physostigmine, work indirectly by inhibiting the enzyme acetylcholinesterase and thus prolonging the duration of action of endogenous acetylcholine. Carbachol has both a direct and an indirect effect. The most notable side effects of miotics (myopia, brow ache, and miosis) limit the widespread use of these agents for treating chronic glaucoma. However, they remain effective pressure-lowering agents and still can play an important role in managing specific glaucoma situations.

Mechanisms of Action

Angle-closure Glaucoma

Cholinergic drugs are useful for the short-term management of angle-closure glaucoma associated with pupillary block. Miotic agents help prepare an eye for iridotomy and are not a substitute for it in pupillary block angle-closure glaucoma. Cholinergic drugs constrict the pupillary sphincter, tighten the iris, decrease the volume of iris tissue in the angle, and pull the peripheral iris away from the trabecular meshwork. These changes reduce intraocular pressure (IOP) by allowing aqueous humor to reach the outflow channels. These changes reduce intraocular pressure (IOP) by allowing aqueous humor to reach the outflow channels. If the IOP is quite elevated (i.e. above 45 or 50 mm Hg), the pupillary sphincter may be ischemic and may not respond to cholinergic stimulation.[184]

Occasionally, standard miotic agents in high concentrations can produce sufficient miosis, forward movement of the lens, and vascular congestion to precipitate or aggravate angle-closure glaucoma.[185]

Open-angle Glaucoma

In open-angle glaucoma, the cholinergic agents reduce IOP by increasing the facility of outflow. Parasympathomimetic drugs stimulate the ciliary muscle, putting traction on the scleral spur and the trabecular meshwork, which separates the trabecular sheets and prevents Schlemm's canal from collapsing. This mechanical change in the configuration of the meshwork increases fluid conductivity.[186]

Side Effects

Ocular

Ocular side effects related to contraction of the iris and ciliary body are common with cholinergic agents and frequently lead to discontinuation of the medication. Miosis can degrade vision, particularly in elderly patients with cataracts. In patients with a posterior subcapsular cataract, the miosis exaggerates the effect of a central media opacity, whereas patients with nuclear cataracts may become more symptomatic in conditions of low illumination. Ciliary muscle contraction, particularly in young patients, can produce a severe headache and accommodative myopia. The induced myopia, which can exceed 5 diopters, results from axial thickening and forward displacement of the lens. This effect begins 15 minutes after instillation of 2 percent pilocarpine, peaks at 45 minutes, and lasts for 1 to 2 hours, making it difficult to provide stable vision for a young patient using a single spectacle correction.[185] To date, efforts have failed to dissociate the accommodative and miotic response of cholinergic agents from their beneficial effect on outflow facility.

Considerable circumstantial evidence linking miotic therapy and retinal detachment has been accumulated.[187] Anticholinesterase drugs initiate and speed the development of cataracts, especially in patients over age 50.[188] Cholinergic drugs produce hyperemia and congestion of the conjunctival and iris blood vessels and breakdown of the blood–aqueous barrier.[189] There are reports of apparent drug-induced iritis in patients treated with anticholinesterase agents. Chronic inflammation from long-term miotic use encourages posterior synechiae and can produce an adherent and miotic pupil, both of which can complicate cataract surgery.

Systemic

Cholinergic drugs can produce a variety of systemic side effects, including nausea, vomiting, diarrhea, abdominal cramping, salivation, sweating, bradycardia, hypotension, bronchospasm, muscle weakness, and central nervous system stimulation. Direct-acting miotics are more likely to produce these symptoms when instilled every few minutes during the treatment of acute angle-closure glaucoma.[190]

Drugs in Clinical Use

Direct-acting Agents

Pilocarpine: Pilocarpine is our most commonly used miotic. Today, it is rarely used as first-line therapy because other medications have either fewer ocular side effects or a more convenient dosing schedule. Its efficacy, cost, and lack of systemic effects, however, make pilocarpine attractive as a second-line agent in many patients.

Chronic use studies demonstrate that the response correlates with dosages ranging from 0.5 to 4 percent concentration, with an IOP reduction of approximately 20 percent.[191] Higher concentrations may provide added effect in patients with dark irides.[192]

Topical pilocarpine administration produces a reduction in IOP that begins in an hour and lasts for 4 to 8 hours.[191] Pilocarpine is prescribed for use four times daily (i.e. as close to every 6 hours as possible) to ensure good IOP control. When used in conjunction with other antiglaucoma medications, control can sometimes be obtained with administration three times (or even twice) daily.

Hyperosmotic Agents

Hyperosmotic agents, administered orally or intravenously, are used to treat acute, substantial elevations of intraocular pressure (IOP) that do not respond to topical ocular hypotensive medications and systemic carbonic anhydrase inhibitors. Because hyperosmotic agents are best tolerated for a limited duration, hyperosmotic agents are never used for the chronic control of glaucoma. They are useful for the short-term management of acute glaucoma.

These agents increase the osmolality of the blood, creating a high osmotic gradient between the systemic circulation and the vitreous. Water is "sucked" from the vitreous cavity and enters the general circulation, thereby reducing intraocular pressure. Large, rapid doses of these agents cause a greater osmotic difference, a greater removal of water from the vitreous, and a greater reduction of intraocular pressure. Their effects wear off quickly as there is a rapid re-equalization of the osmotic gradient between the blood and the vitreous cavity. Thus, it is important that some more definitive means of lowering intraocular pressure be achieved within several hours of administering these medications, as if nothing else is done, the intraocular pressure will again rise once the compartments have equilibrated.[193]

The hyperosmotic agent mannitol (Osmitrol, 20 and 50% solutions) is given parenterally (intravenously). There are two oral hyperosmotic agents, glycerin 50 percent (Osmoglyn) and isosorbide 40 percent solution (Ismotic). Oral glycerin should not be used in diabetic patients as it is metabolized to glucose. For these patients, isosorbide solution is preferred.[194]

Side Effects

Although most of the associated side effects are relatively mild, some are serious and even potentially fatal. These drugs should be administered with caution in patients with cardiac, renal, and hepatic disease. Headache, nausea, vomiting, and diuresis are the most frequent side effects and are seen with all of the agents in clinical use.[195]

Drugs in Clinical Use

Oral Agents

Glycerol: Glycerol (Glyrol, Osmoglyn), the most commonly prescribed hyperosmotic agent, is usually administered as a 50 percent solution in a dose of 1.5–3 ml/kg.[196] It begins to lower IOP in 10–30 minutes, reaches a maximum effect in 45–120 minutes, and has a duration of effect of 4–5 hours.[196,197] Glycerol has an intense, sweet taste and is more palatable when given in an iced unsweetened fruit juice or cola base.

Intravenous Agents

Mannitol: Mannitol is an effective hyperosmotic drug that is currently the agent of choice for intravenous administration. The usual dose is 2.5–7.0 ml/kg of the 20 percent solution. The drug begins to lower IOP in 15–30 minutes, reaches a maximum effect in 30–60 minutes, and has a duration of action of approximately 6 hours.[198] It is not necessary to administer the full dose of the drug; when IOP falls to the desired level, the infusion can be terminated.

REFERENCES

1. Jay JL, Allan D. The benefit of early trabeculectomy versus conventional management in primary open angle glaucoma relative to severity of disease, Eye. 1989;3(Pt 5):528-35.
2. Sherwood MB, Migdal CS, Hitchings RA, Sharir M, Zimmerman TJ, Schultz JS. Initial treatment of glaucoma: surgery or medications. Survey of Ophthalmology. 1993;37:293-305.

3. Feiner L, Piltz-Seymour JR, Collaborative Initial Glaucoma Treatment S. Collaborative Initial Glaucoma Treatment Study: a summary of results to date, Current Opinion in Ophthalmology. 2003;14:106-11.
4. Schulzer M, Drance SM, Douglas GR. A comparison of treated and untreated glaucoma suspects. Ophthalmology. 1991;98:301-7.
5. Wilson MR, Gaasterland D. Translating research into practice: controlled clinical trials and their influence on glaucoma management. Journal of Glaucoma. 1996;5:139-46.
6. Weinreb RN. Lowering intraocular pressure to minimize glaucoma damage. Journal of Glaucoma. 2001;10:S76-7.
7. Palmberg P. Evidence-based target pressures: how to choose and achieve them. International Ophthalmology Clinics. 2004;44:1-14.
8. Palmberg P. How clinical trial results are changing our thinking about target pressures. Current Opinion in Ophthalmology. 2002; 13:85-8.
9. Evidence-based management of glaucoma: recommendations of an expert panel. Edited by Coleman AL, Baerveldt G, Bournias TE. Montvale, NJ, Thomson-PDR, 2003.
10. Mishima S, Gasset A, Klyce SD Jr., Baum JL. Determination of tear volume and tear flow. Investigative Ophthalmology. 1966;5:264-76.
11. Lederer CM Jr., Harold RE. Drop size of commercial glaucoma medications. American Journal of Ophthalmology. 1986;101:691-4.
12. Mishima S. Clinical pharmacokinetics of the eye. Proctor Lecture, Investigative Ophthalmology and Visual Science. 1981;21:504-41.
13. Doane MG, Jensen AD, Dohlman CH. Penetration routes of topically applied eye medications. American Journal of Ophthalmology. 1978;85:383-6.
14. Zimmerman TJ, Kooner KS, Kandarakis AS, Ziegler LP. Improving the therapeutic index of topically applied ocular drugs. Archives of Ophthalmology. 1984;102:551-3.
15. Shell JW. Pharmacokinetics of topically applied ophthalmic drugs. Survey of Ophthalmology. 1982;26:207-18.
16. Brechue WF, Maren TH. pH and drug ionization affects ocular pressure lowering of topical carbonic anhydrase inhibitors. Investigative Ophthalmology and Visual Science. 1993;34:2581-7.
17. Katz LJ. Twelve-month evaluation of brimonidine-purite versus brimonidine in patients with glaucoma or ocular hypertension. Journal of Glaucoma. 2002;11:119-26.
18. March WF, Stewart RM, Mandell AI, Bruce LA. Duration of effect of pilocarpine gel. Archives of Ophthalmology. 1982;100:1270-1.
19. Shedden A, Laurence J, Tipping R, Timoptic XESG. Efficacy and tolerability of timolol maleate ophthalmic gel-forming solution versus timolol ophthalmic solution in adults with open-angle glaucoma or ocular hypertension: a six-month, double-masked, multicenter study. Clinical Therapeutics. 2001;23:440-50.
20. Shedden AH, Laurence J, Barrish A, Olah TV. Plasma timolol concentrations of timolol maleate: timolol gel-forming solution (TIMOPTIC-XE) once daily versus timolol maleate ophthalmic solution twice daily. Documenta Ophthalmologica Advances in Ophthalmology. 2001;103:73-9.
21. Armaly MF, Rao KR. The effect of pilocarpine Ocusert with different release rates on ocular pressure. Investigative Ophthalmology. 1973;12:491-6.

22. Alani SD, Hammerstein W. The ophthalmic rod—a new drug-delivery system II, Graefe's archive for clinical and experimental ophthalmology = Albrecht von Graefes Archiv fur klinische und experimentelle Ophthalmologie. 1990;228:302-4.
23. Gwon A, Borrmann LR, Duzman E, Robins DS, Shen D. Ophthalmic rods. New ocular drug delivery devices. Ophthalmology. 1986;93:82-5.
24. Phillips CI, Howitt G, Rowlands DJ. Propranolol as ocular hypotensive agent. The British Journal of Ophthalmology. 1967;51:222-6.
25. Elliot MJ, Cullen PM, Phillips CI. Ocular hypotensive effect of atenolol (Tenormin, I.C.I.). A new beta-adrenergic blocker. The British Journal of Ophthalmology. 1975;59:296-300.
26. Krieglstein GK, Sold-Darseff J, Leydhecker W. The intraocular pressure response of glaucomatous eyes to topically applied bupranolol. A pilot study, Albrecht von Graefes Archiv fur klinische und experimentelle Ophthalmologie Albrecht von Graefe's archive for clinical and experimental ophthalmology. 1977;202:81-6.
27. Katz IM, Hubbard WA, Getson AJ, Gould AL. Intraocular pressure decrease in normal volunteers following timolol ophthalmic solution. Investigative Ophthalmology. 1976;15:489-92.
28. Coakes RL, Brubaker RF. The mechanism of timolol in lowering intraocular pressure. In the Normal Eye, Archives of Ophthalmology. 1978;96:2045-8.
29. Wayman L, Larsson LI, Maus T, Alm A, Brubaker R. Comparison of dorzolamide and timolol as suppressors of aqueous humor flow in humans. Archives of Ophthalmology. 1997;115:1368-71.
30. Sonntag JR, Brindley GO, Shields MB. Effect of timolol therapy on outflow facility. Investigative Ophthalmology and Visual Science. 1978;17:293-6.
31. Zimmerman TJ, Harbin R, Pett M, Kaufman HE. Timolol and facility of outflow. Investigative Ophthalmology and Visual Science. 1977;16:623-4.
32. Tieri O, Polzella A. Clinical use and action mechanism of propranolol, Ophthalmologica Journal International d'ophtalmologie International Journal of Ophthalmology Zeitschrift fur Augenheilkunde. 1975;170:36-42.
33. Reiss GR, Lee DA, Topper JE, Brubaker RF. Aqueous humor flow during sleep. Investigative Ophthalmology and Visual Science. 1984; 25:776-8.
34. Radius RL, Diamond GR, Pollack IP, Langham ME. Timolol. A new drug for management of chronic simple glaucoma. Archives of Ophthalmology. 1978;96:1003-8.
35. Zimmerman TJ, Kaufman HE. Timolol, dose response and duration of action. Archives of Ophthalmology. 1977;95:605-7.
36. Urtti A, Salminen L. A comparison between iris-ciliary body concentration and receptor affinity of timolol. Acta Ophthalmologica. 1985;63:16-8.
37. Teping C, Wiedemann B. [The COMOD system. A preservative-free multidose container for eyedrops], Klinische Monatsblatter fur Augenheilkunde. 1994;205:210-7.
38. Schoenwald RD, Stewart P. Effect of particle size on ophthalmic bioavailability of dexamethasone suspensions in rabbits. Journal of Pharmaceutical Sciences. 1980;69:391-4.

39. Miller-Meeks MJ, Farrell TA, Munden PM, Folk JC, Rao C, Schoenwald RD. Phenylephrine prodrug. Report of clinical trials, Ophthalmology. 1991;98:222-6.
40. Greaves JL, Wilson CG, Rozier A, Grove J, Plazonnet B. Scintigraphic assessment of an ophthalmic gelling vehicle in man and rabbit. Current Eye Research. 1990;9:415-20.
41. Laurence J, Holder D, Vogel R, Gross RL, Haik BG, Karp DW, Koby MM, Zimmerman TJ. A double-masked, placebo-controlled evaluation of timolol in a gel vehicle. Journal of Glaucoma. 1993; 2:177-82.
42. Soll DB. Evaluation of timolol in chronic open-angle glaucoma. Once a day vs twice a day. Archives of Ophthalmology. 1980; 98:2178-81.
43. Schlecht LP, Brubaker RF. The effects of withdrawal of timolol in chronically treated glaucoma patients. Ophthalmology. 1988; 95:1212-6.
44. Weinreb RN, Caldwell DR, Goode SM, Horwitz BL, Laibovitz R, Shrader CE, Stewart RH, Williams AT. A double-masked three-month comparison between 0.25 percent betaxolol suspension and 0.5 percent betaxolol ophthalmic solution. American Journal of Ophthalmology. 1990;110:189-92.
45. Mills KB, Wright G. A blind randomised cross-over trial comparing metipranolol 0.3 percent with timolol 0.25 percent in open-angle glaucoma: a pilot study. The British Journal of Ophthalmology. 1986;70:39-42.
46. Broadway DC, Grierson I, O'Brien C, Hitchings RA. Adverse effects of topical antiglaucoma medication. II. The outcome of filtration surgery. Archives of Ophthalmology. 1994;112:1446-54.
47. Harris LS, Greenstein SH, Bloom AF. Respiratory difficulties with betaxolol. American Journal of Ophthalmology. 1986;102:274-5.
48. Nies AS, Evans GH, Shand DG. Regional hemodynamic effects of beta-adrenergic blockade with propranolol in the unanesthetized primate. American Heart Journal. 1973;85:97-102.
49. Drance SM. [Primary chronic open angle glaucoma—are there vascular risk factors?], Klinische Monatsblatter fur Augenheilkunde. 1996;208:A9-13.
50. McMahon CD, Shaffer RN, Hoskins HD Jr., Hetherington J Jr. Adverse effects experienced by patients taking timolol. American Journal of Ophthalmology. 1979;88:736-8.
51. Duch S, Duch C, Pasto L, Ferrer P. Changes in depressive status associated with topical beta-blockers. International Ophthalmology. 1992;16:331-5.
52. Mastropasqua L, Carpineto P, Ciancaglini M, Gallenga PE. A 12-month, randomized, double-masked study comparing latanoprost with timolol in pigmentary glaucoma. Ophthalmology. 1999;106:550-5.
53. Hong YJ, Shin DH, Ahn BH, McCarty B. Intraocular pressure after a two-week washout following long-term timolol or levobunolol. Journal of Ocular Pharmacology and Therapeutics: The Official Journal of the Association for Ocular Pharmacology and Therapeutics. 1995;11:107-12.
54. Orzalesi N, Rossetti L, Invernizzi T, Bottoli A, Autelitano A. Effect of timolol, latanoprost, and dorzolamide on circadian IOP in glaucoma or ocular hypertension. Investigative Ophthalmology and Visual Science. 2000;41:2566-73.

55. Nordmann JP, Mertz B, Yannoulis NC, Schwenninger C, Kapik B, Shams N, Unoprostone Monotherapy Study Group EU. A double-masked randomized comparison of the efficacy and safety of unoprostone with timolol and betaxolol in patients with primary open-angle glaucoma including pseudoexfoliation glaucoma or ocular hypertension. 6 month data. American Journal of Ophthalmology. 2002;133:1-10.
56. Brandt JD, VanDenburgh AM, Chen K, Whitcup SM, Bimatoprost Study G. Comparison of once- or twice-daily bimatoprost with twice-daily timolol in patients with elevated IOP: a 3-month clinical trial. Ophthalmology. 2001;108:1023-31; discussion 1032
57. Fellman RL, Sullivan EK, Ratliff M, Silver LH, Whitson JT, Turner FD, Weiner AL, Davis AA, Travoprost Study G. Comparison of travoprost 0.0015 percent and 0.004 percent with timolol 0.5 percent in patients with elevated intraocular pressure: a 6-month, masked, multicenter trial. Ophthalmology. 2002;109:998-1008.
58. Hass I, Drance SM. Comparison between pilocarpine and timolol on diurnal pressures in open-angle glaucoma. Archives of Ophthalmology. 1980;98:480-1.
59. Merte HJ, Merkle W. [Experiences in a double-blind study with different concentrations of timolol and pilocarpine (author's transl)], Klinische Monatsblatter fur Augenheilkunde. 1980; 177:443-50.
60. Smith RJ, Nagasubramanian S, Watkins R, Poinoosawmy D. Addition of timolol maleate to routine medical therapy: a clinical trial. The British Journal of Ophthalmology. 1980;64:779-81.
61. Kass MA, Korey M, Gordon M, Becker B. Timolol and acetazolamide. A study of concurrent administration, Archives of ophthalmology. 1982;100:941-2.
62. Berson FG, Epstein DL. Separate and combined effects of timolol maleate and acetazolamide in open-angle glaucoma. American Journal of Ophthalmology. 1981;92:788-91.
63. Toris CB, Zhan GL, Yablonski ME, Camras CB. Effects on aqueous flow of dorzolamide combined with either timolol or acetazolamide. Journal of Glaucoma. 2004;13:210-5.
64. Larsson LI. Aqueous humor flow in normal human eyes treated with brimonidine and timolol, alone and in combination. Archives of Ophthalmology. 2001;119:492-5.
65. Schuman JS. Effects of systemic beta-blocker therapy on the efficacy and safety of topical brimonidine and timolol. Brimonidine Study Groups 1 and 2. Ophthalmology. 2000; 107:1171-7.
66. Berry DP Jr., Van Buskirk EM, Shields MB. Betaxolol and timolol. A comparison of efficacy and side effects. Archives of Ophthalmology. 1984;102:42-5.
67. Stewart RH, Kimbrough RL, Ward RL. Betaxolol vs timolol. A six-month double-blind comparison. Archives of Ophthalmology. 1986;104:46-8.
68. Berrospi AR, Leibowitz HM. Betaxolol. A new beta-adrenergic blocking agent for treatment of glaucoma. Archives of Ophthalmology. 1982;100:943-6.
69. Feghali JG, Kaufman PL. Decreased intraocular pressure in the hypertensive human eye with betaxolol, a beta 1-adrenergic antagonist. American Journal of Ophthalmology. 1985;100:777-82.

70. Messmer C, Flammer J, Stumpfig D. Influence of betaxolol and timolol on the visual fields of patients with glaucoma, American journal of ophthalmology. 1991;112:678-81.
71. Collignon-Brach J. Long-term effect of ophthalmic beta-adrenoceptor antagonists on intraocular pressure and retinal sensitivity in primary open-angle glaucoma, Current eye research. 1992;11:1-3.
72. Gupta A, Chen HC, Rassam SM, Kohner EM. Effect of betaxolol on the retinal circulation in eyes with ocular hypertension: a pilot study, Eye. 1994;8 (Pt 6):668-71.
73. Harris A, Spaeth GL, Sergott RC, Katz LJ, Cantor LB, Martin BJ. Retrobulbar arterial hemodynamic effects of betaxolol and timolol in normal-tension glaucoma, American journal of ophthalmology. 1995;120:168-75.
74. Brubaker RF. Mechanism of action of bimatoprost (Lumigan), Survey of ophthalmology. 2001;45 Suppl 4:S347-51.
75. Bahler CK, Howell KG, Hann CR, Fautsch MP, Johnson DH. Prostaglandins increase trabecular meshwork outflow facility in cultured human anterior segments, American journal of ophthalmology. 2008;145:114-9.
76. Lim KS, Nau CB, O'Byrne MM, Hodge DO, Toris CB, McLaren JW, Johnson DH. Mechanism of action of bimatoprost, latanoprost, and travoprost in healthy subjects. A crossover study. Ophthalmology. 2008;115:790-5 e794.
77. Dubiner HB, Sircy MD, Landry T, Bergamini MV, Silver LH, Darell Turner F, Robertson S, Andrew RM, Weiner A, Przydryga J. Comparison of the diurnal ocular hypotensive efficacy of travoprost and latanoprost over a 44-hour period in patients with elevated intraocular pressure. Clinical Therapeutics. 2004;26:84-91.
78. Walters TR, DuBiner HB, Carpenter SP, Khan B, VanDenburgh AM, Bimatoprost Circadian IOPSG: 24-Hour IOP control with once-daily bimatoprost, timolol gel-forming solution, or latanoprost: a 1-month, randomized, comparative clinical trial. Survey of Ophthalmology. 2004;49 Suppl 1:S26-35.
79. Diaz E, Goldberg GR, Taylor M, Savage JM, Sellen D, Coward WA, Prentice AM. Effects of dietary supplementation on work performance in Gambian laborers. The American Journal of Clinical Nutrition. 1991;53:803-11.
80. Ziai N, Dolan JW, Kacere RD, Brubaker RF. The effects on aqueous dynamics of PhXA41, a new prostaglandin F2 alpha analogue, after topical application in normal and ocular hypertensive human eyes. Archives of Ophthalmology. 1993,111:1351-8.
81. Lutjen-Drecoll E, Tamm E. Morphological study of the anterior segment of cynomolgus monkey eyes following treatment with prostaglandin F2 alpha. Experimental Eye Research. 1988;47:761-9.
82. Lindsey JD, Kashiwagi K, Kashiwagi F, Weinreb RN. Prostaglandin action on ciliary smooth muscle extracellular matrix metabolism: implications for uveoscleral outflow. Survey of Ophthalmology. 1997;41 Suppl 2:S53-9.
83. Zhan GL, Camras CB, Opere C, Tang L, Ohia SE. Effect of prostaglandins on cyclic AMP production in cultured human ciliary muscle cells. Journal of Ocular Pharmacology and Therapeutics : The Official Journal of the Association for Ocular Pharmacology and Therapeutics. 1998;14:45-55.

84. Zhao X, Pearson KE, Stephan DA, Russell P. Effects of prostaglandin analogues on human ciliary muscle and trabecular meshwork cells. Investigative Ophthalmology and Visual Science. 2003;44:1945-52.
85. Gaton DD, Sagara T, Lindsey JD, Weinreb RN. Matrix metalloproteinase-1 localization in the normal human uveoscleral outflow pathway. Investigative Ophthalmology and Visual Science. 1999; 40:363-9.
86. Krauss AH, Woodward DF. Update on the mechanism of action of bimatoprost: a review and discussion of new evidence. Survey of Ophthalmology. 2004;49 Suppl 1:S5-11.
87. Koda N, Tsutsui Y, Niwa H, Ito S, Woodward DF, Watanabe K. Synthesis of prostaglandin F ethanolamide by prostaglandin F synthase and identification of Bimatoprost as a potent inhibitor of the enzyme: new enzyme assay method using LC/ESI/MS. Archives of Biochemistry and Biophysics. 2004;424:128-36.
88. Sharif NA, Kelly CR, Crider JY. Human trabecular meshwork cell responses induced by bimatoprost, travoprost, unoprostone, and other FP prostaglandin receptor agonist analogues. Investigative Ophthalmology and Visual Science. 2003;44:715-21.
89. Camras CB. Comparison of latanoprost and timolol in patients with ocular hypertension and glaucoma: a six-month masked, multicenter trial in the United States. The United States Latanoprost Study Group. Ophthalmology. 1996;103:138-47.
90. Watson P, Stjernschantz J. A six-month, randomized, double-masked study comparing latanoprost with timolol in open-angle glaucoma and ocular hypertension. The Latanoprost Study Group. Ophthalmology. 1996;103:126-37.
91. Alm A, Stjernschantz J. Effects on intraocular pressure and side effects of 0.005 percent latanoprost applied once daily, evening or morning. A comparison with timolol. Scandinavian Latanoprost Study Group. Ophthalmology. 1995;102:1743-52.
92. Camras CB, Alm A, Watson P, Stjernschantz J. Latanoprost, a prostaglandin analog, for glaucoma therapy. Efficacy and safety after 1 year of treatment in 198 patients. Latanoprost Study Groups. Ophthalmology. 1996;103:1916-24.
93. Linden C, Nuija E, Alm A. Effects on IOP restoration and blood-aqueous barrier after long-term treatment with latanoprost in open angle glaucoma and ocular hypertension. The British Journal of Ophthalmology. 1997;81:370-2.
94. Rulo AH, Greve EL, Hoyng PF. Additive ocular hypotensive effect of latanoprost and acetazolamide. A short-term study in patients with elevated intraocular pressure. Ophthalmology. 1997, 104:1503-7.
95. Hoyng PF, Rulo A, Greve E, Watson P, Alm A. The additive intraocular pressure-lowering effect of latanoprost in combined therapy with other ocular hypotensive agents. Survey of Ophthalmology. 1997;41 Suppl 2:S93-8.
96. Gross RL, Peace JH, Smith SE, Walters TR, Dubiner HB, Weiss MJ, Ochsner KI. Duration of IOP reduction with travoprost BAK-free solution. Journal of Glaucoma. 2008;17:217-22.
97. Goldberg I. Comparison of tropical travoprost eye drops given once daily and timolol 0.5 percent given twice daily in patients with open-angle glaucoma or ocular hypertension. J. Glaucoma. 2001;10:414-22, Journal of Glaucoma 2002, 11:275

98. Bayer A, Weiler W, Oeverhaus U, Skrotzki FE, Stewart WC, Xplore Observation G. Two-year follow-up of latanoprost 0.005 percent monotherapy after changing from previous glaucoma therapies. Journal of Ocular Pharmacology and Therapeutics: The Official Journal of the Association for Ocular Pharmacology and Therapeutics. 2004;20:470-8.
99. Selen G, Stjernschantz J, Resul B. Prostaglandin-induced iridial pigmentation in primates. Survey of Ophthalmology. 1997;41 Suppl 2:S125-8.
100. Wistrand PJ, Stjernschantz J, Olsson K. The incidence and time-course of latanoprost-induced iridial pigmentation as a function of eye color. Survey of Ophthalmology. 1997;41 Suppl 2:S129-38.
101. Wand M. Latanoprost and hyperpigmentation of eyelashes. Archives of Ophthalmology. 1997;115:1206-8.
102. Ayyala RS, Cruz DA, Margo CE, Harman LE, Pautler SE, Misch DM, Mines JA, Richards DW. Cystoid macular edema associated with latanoprost in aphakic and pseudophakic eyes. American Journal of Ophthalmology. 1998;126:602-4.
103. Fechtner RD, Khouri AS, Zimmerman TJ, Bullock J, Feldman R, Kulkarni P, Michael AJ, Realini T, Warwar R. Anterior uveitis associated with latanoprost. American Journal of Ophthalmology. 1998;126:37-41.
104. Wand M, Shields BM. Cystoid macular edema in the era of ocular hypotensive lipids. American Journal of Ophthalmology. 2002; 133:393-7.
105. Miyake K, Ota I, Maekubo K, Ichihashi S, Miyake S. Latanoprost accelerates disruption of the blood-aqueous barrier and the incidence of angiographic cystoid macular edema in early postoperative pseudophakias. Archives of Ophthalmology. 1999; 117:34-40.
106. Rowe JA, Hattenhauer MG, Herman DC. Adverse side effects associated with latanoprost. American Journal of Ophthalmology. 1997;124:683-5.
107. Stjernschantz J. Studies on ocular inflammation and development of a prostaglandin analogue for glaucoma treatment. Experimental Eye Research. 2004;78:759-66.
108. Takase M, Murao M, Koyano S, Okita M, Ueno R. [Ocular effects of topical instillation of UF-021 ophthalmic solution in healthy volunteers]. Nihon Ganka Gakkai zasshi. 1992;96:1261-7.
109. Alm A, Villumsen J. PhXA34, a new potent ocular hypotensive drug. A study on dose-response relationship and on aqueous humor dynamics in healthy volunteers. Archives of Ophthalmology. 1991;109:1564-8.
110. Alm A, Villumsen J, Tornquist P, Mandahl A, Airaksinen J, Tuulonen A, Marsk A, Resul B, Stjernschantz J. Intraocular pressure-reducing effect of PhXA41 in patients with increased eye pressure. A one-month study. Ophthalmology. 1993;100:1312-6; discussion 1316-7
111. Nagasubramanian S, Sheth GP, Hitchings RA, Stjernschantz J. Intraocular pressure-reducing effect of PhXA41 in ocular hypertension. Comparison of dose regimens. Ophthalmology. 1993;100:1305-11.
112. Lusky M, Ticho U, Glovinsky J, Weinberger D, Nesher R, Yassur Y, Melamed S. A comparative study of two dose regimens of latanoprost in patients with elevated intraocular pressure, Ophthalmology. 1997;104:1720-4.

113. Linden C, Alm A. Effects on intraocular pressure and aqueous flow of various dose regimens of latanoprost in human eyes. Acta Ophthalmologica Scandinavica. 1997;75:412-5.
114. Diestelhorst M, Roters S, Krieglstein GK. The effect of latanoprost 0.005 percent once daily versus 0.0015 percent twice daily on intraocular pressure and aqueous humour protein concentration in glaucoma patients. A randomized, double-masked comparison with timolol 0.5 percent, Graefe's archive for clinical and experimental ophthalmology = Albrecht von Graefes Archiv fur klinische und experimentelle Ophthalmologie. 1997;235:20-6.
115. Harasymowycz P, Hutnik CM, Nicolela M, Stewart WC. Latanoprost versus timolol gel-forming solution once daily in primary open-angle glaucoma or ocular hypertension. Canadian Journal of Ophthalmology Journal Canadien d'ophtalmologie. 2007;42:75-81.
116. Einarson TR, Kulin NA, Tingey D, Iskedjian M. Meta-analysis of the effect of latanoprost and brimonidine on intraocular pressure in the treatment of glaucoma. Clinical Therapeutics. 2000; 22:1502-15.
117. Waldock A, Snape J, Graham CM. Effects of glaucoma medications on the cardiorespiratory and intraocular pressure status of newly diagnosed glaucoma patients. The British Journal of Ophthalmology. 2000;84:710-3.
118. Hedner J, Svedmyr N, Lunde H, Mandahl A. The lack of respiratory effects of the ocular hypotensive drug latanoprost in patients with moderate-steroid treated asthma. Survey of Ophthalmology. 1997;41 Suppl 2:S111-5.
119. Villumsen J, Alm A. The effect of adding prostaglandin F2 alpha-isopropylester to timolol in patients with open angle glaucoma, Archives of ophthalmology. 1990;108:1102-5.
120. Diestelhorst M. The additive intraocular pressure-lowering effect of latanoprost 0.005 percent daily once and pilocarpine 2 percent t.i.d. in patients with open-angle glaucoma or ocular hypertension. a 6-month, randomized, multicenter study. German Latanoprost Study Group, Graefe's archive for clinical and experimental ophthalmology = Albrecht von Graefes Archiv fur klinische und experimentelle Ophthalmologie. 2000;238:433-9.
121. Rulo AH, Greve EL, Hoyng PF. Additive effect of latanoprost, a prostaglandin F2 alpha analogue, and timolol in patients with elevated intraocular pressure. The British Journal of Ophthalmology. 1994;78:899-902.
122. Maruyama K, Shirato S. Additive effect of dorzolamide or carteolol to latanoprost in primary open-angle glaucoma: a prospective randomized crossover trial. Journal of Glaucoma. 2006;15:341-5.
123. DuBiner H, Cooke D, Dirks M, Stewart WC, VanDenburgh AM, Felix C. Efficacy and safety of bimatoprost in patients with elevated intraocular pressure: a 30-day comparison with latanoprost. Survey of Ophthalmology. 2001;45 Suppl 4:S353-60.
124. Coleman AL, Lerner F, Bernstein P, Whitcup SM. A 3-month randomized controlled trial of bimatoprost (LUMIGAN) versus combined timolol and dorzolamide (Cosopt) in patients with glaucoma or ocular hypertension. Ophthalmology. 2003; 110:2362-8.
125. Choplin N, Bernstein P, Batoosingh AL, Whitcup SM, Bimatoprost/Latanoprost Study G. A randomized, investigator-

masked comparison of diurnal responder rates with bimatoprost and latanoprost in the lowering of intraocular pressure. Survey of Ophthalmology. 2004;49 Suppl 1:S19-25.
126. Konstas AG, Katsimbris JM, Lallos N, Boukaras GP, Jenkins JN, Stewart WC. Latanoprost 0.005 percent versus bimatoprost 0.03 percent in primary open-angle glaucoma patients. Ophthalmology. 2005; 112:262-6.
127. Cantor LB, WuDunn D, Cortes A, Hoop J, Knotts S. Ocular hypotensive efficacy of bimatoprost 0.03 percent and travoprost 0.004 percent in patients with glaucoma or ocular hypertension. Survey of Ophthalmology. 2004;49 Suppl 1:S12-8.
128. Sharif NA, Kelly CR, Crider JY, Williams GW, Xu SX. Ocular hypotensive FP prostaglandin (PG) analogs: PG receptor subtype binding affinities and selectivities, and agonist potencies at FP and other PG receptors in cultured cells. Journal of Ocular Pharmacology and Therapeutics: The Official Journal of the Association for Ocular Pharmacology and Therapeutics. 2003; 19:501-15.
129. Hellberg MR, McLaughlin MA, Sharif NA, DeSantis L, Dean TR, Kyba EP, Bishop JE, Klimko PG, Zinke PW, Selliah RD, Barnes G, DeFaller J, Kothe A, Landry T, Sullivan EK, Andrew R, Davis AA, Silver L, Bergamini MV, Robertson S, Weiner AL, Sallee VL. Identification and characterization of the ocular hypotensive efficacy of travoprost, a potent and selective FP prostaglandin receptor agonist, and AL-6598, a DP prostaglandin receptor agonist. Survey of Ophthalmology. 2002;47 Suppl 1:S13-33
130. Goldberg I, Cunha-Vaz J, Jakobsen JE, Nordmann JP, Trost E, Sullivan EK, International Travoprost Study G. Comparison of topical travoprost eye drops given once daily and timolol 0.5 percent given twice daily in patients with open-angle glaucoma or ocular hypertension. Journal of Glaucoma. 2001;10:414-22.
131. Orengo-Nania S, Landry T, Von Tress M, Silver LH, Weiner A, Davis AA, Travoprost Study G. Evaluation of travoprost as adjunctive therapy in patients with uncontrolled intraocular pressure while using timolol 0.5 percent. American Journal of Ophthalmology. 2001; 132:860-8.
132. Berggren L. Direct Observation of Secretory Pumping *in Vitro* of the Rabbit Eye Ciliary Processes. Influence of Ion Milieu and Carbonic Anhydrase Inhibition. Investigative Ophthalmology. 1964;3:266-72.
133. Bietti G, Virno M, Pecori-Giraldi J. Acetazolamide, metabolic acidosis, and intraocular pressure. American Journal of Ophthalmology. 1975;80:360-9.
134. McCannel CA, Heinrich SR, Brubaker RF. Acetazolamide but not timolol lowers aqueous humor flow in sleeping humans, Graefe's archive for clinical and experimental ophthalmology = Albrecht von Graefes Archiv fur klinische und experimentelle Ophthalmologie. 1992;230:518-20.
135. Harris A, Arend O, Arend S, Martin B. Effects of topical dorzolamide on retinal and retrobulbar hemodynamics. Acta Ophthalmologica Scandinavica. 1996;74:569-72.
136. Martinez A, Gonzalez F, Capeans C, Perez R, Sanchez-Salorio M. Dorzolamide effect on ocular blood flow. Investigative Ophthalmology and Visual Science. 1999;40:1270-5.
137. Barnes GE, Li B, Dean T, Chandler ML. Increased optic nerve head blood flow after 1 week of twice daily topical brinzolamide

treatment in Dutch-belted rabbits. Survey of Ophthalmology. 2000;44 Suppl 2:S131-40.
138. Silver LH. Ocular comfort of brinzolamide 1.0 percent ophthalmic suspension compared with dorzolamide 2.0 percent ophthalmic solution: results from two multicenter comfort studies. Brinzolamide Comfort Study Group. Survey of Ophthalmology 2000, 44 Suppl 2:S141-5.
139. Stewart WC, Stewart JA, Leech JN. Acute and chronic ocular symptoms of dorzolamide 2 percent compared with placebo. Journal of Glaucoma 2003, 12:151-5.
140. Aalto-Korte K. Contact allergy to dorzolamide eyedrops. Contact Dermatitis 1998, 39:206
141. Kalavala M, Statham BN. Allergic contact dermatitis from timolol and dorzolamide eye drops. Contact Dermatitis 2006, 54:345
142. Fineman MS, Katz LJ, Wilson RP. Topical dorzolamide-induced hypotony and ciliochoroidal detachment in patients with previous filtration surgery. Archives of Ophthalmology 1996, 114:1031-2.
143. Callahan C, Ayyala RS. Hypotony and choroidal effusion induced by topical timolol and dorzolamide in patients with previous glaucoma drainage device implantation. Ophthalmic Surgery, Lasers and Imaging: The Official Journal of the International Society for Imaging in the Eye 2003, 34:467-9.
144. Berson FG, Epstein DL, Grant WM, Hutchinson BT, Dobbs PC. Acetazolamide dosage forms in the treatment of glaucoma. Archives of Ophthalmology 1980, 98:1051-4.
145. Shrader CE, Thomas JV, Simmons RJ. Relationship of patient age and tolerance to carbonic anhydrase inhibitors. American Journal of Ophthalmology 1983, 96:730-3.
146. Maren TH, Haywood JR, Chapman SK, Zimmerman TJ. The pharmacology of methazolamide in relation to the treatment of glaucoma. Investigative Ophthalmology and Visual Science 1977, 16:730-42.
147. Balfour JA, Wilde MI. Dorzolamide. A review of its pharmacology and therapeutic potential in the management of glaucoma and ocular hypertension. Drugs and Aging 1997, 10:384-403
148. Pfeiffer N. Dorzolamide: development and clinical application of a topical carbonic anhydrase inhibitor. Survey of Ophthalmology 1997, 42:137-51.
149. Lippa EA, Carlson LE, Ehinger B, Eriksson LO, Finnstrom K, Holmin C, Nilsson SE, Nyman K, Raitta C, Ringvold A, et al. Dose response and duration of action of dorzolamide, a topical carbonic anhydrase inhibitor. Archives of Ophthalmology 1992, 110:495-9.
150. Portellos M, Buckley EG, Freedman SF. Topical versus oral carbonic anhydrase inhibitor therapy for pediatric glaucoma. Journal of AAPOS: The Official Publication of the American Association for Pediatric Ophthalmology and Strabismus/American Association for Pediatric Ophthalmology and Strabismus 1998, 2:43-7.
151. Whitson JT, Henry C, Hughes B, Lee DA, Terry S, Fechtner RD. Comparison of the safety and efficacy of dorzolamide 2 percent and brimonidine 0.2 percent in patients with glaucoma or ocular hypertension. Journal of Glaucoma 2004, 13:168-73.
152. Wang RF, Serle JB, Gagliuso DJ, Podos SM. Comparison of the ocular hypotensive effect of brimonidine, dorzolamide,

latanoprost, or artificial tears added to timolol in glaucomatous monkey eyes. Journal of Glaucoma 2000, 9:458-62.
153. Wayman LL, Larsson LI, Maus TL, Brubaker RF. Additive effect of dorzolamide on aqueous humor flow in patients receiving long-term treatment with timolol. Archives of Ophthalmology. 1998; 116:1438-40.
154. Le HH, Chang MR, Cheng Q, Lee DA, Hartenbaum D. The effectiveness and safety of dorzolamide 2 percent in addition to multiple topical antiglaucoma medications. Journal of Ocular Pharmacology and Therapeutics: The Official Journal of the Association for Ocular Pharmacology and Therapeutics. 1999; 15:305-12.
155. Strohmaier K, Snyder E, DuBiner H, Adamsons I. The efficacy and safety of the dorzolamide-timolol combination versus the concomitant administration of its components. Dorzolamide-Timolol Study Group. Ophthalmology. 1998;105:1936-44.
156. Iester M. Brinzolamide ophthalmic suspension: a review of its pharmacology and use in the treatment of open angle glaucoma and ocular hypertension. Clinical Ophthalmology. 2008;2:517-23.
157. Shin D. Adjunctive therapy with brinzolamide 1 percent ophthalmic suspension (Azopt) in patients with open-angle glaucoma or ocular hypertension maintained on timolol therapy. Survey of Ophthalmology. 2000;44 Suppl 2:S163-8.
158. Schenker HI, Yablonski ME, Podos SM, Linder L. Fluoro-photometric study of epinephrine and timolol in human subjects. Archives of Ophthalmology. 1981;99:1212-6.
159. Erickson K, Liang L, Shum P, Nathanson JA. Adrenergic regulation of aqueous outflow. Journal of Ocular Pharmacology. 1994; 10:241-52.
160. Kupfer C, Gaasterland D, Ross K. Studies of aqueous humor dynamics in man. II. Measurements in young normal subjects using acetazolamide and L-epinephrine. Investigative Ophthalmology. 1971;10:523-33.
161. Mittag T, Tormay A. Desensitization of the beta-adrenergic receptor-adenylate cyclase complex in rabbit iris-ciliary body induced by topical epinephrine. Experimental Eye Research. 1981; 33:497-503.
162. Langham ME, Krieglstein GK. The biphasic intraocular pressure response of rabbits to epinephrine. Investigative Ophthalmology. 1976;15:119-27.
163. Mackool RJ, Muldoon T, Fortier A, Nelson D. Epinephrine-induced cystoid macular edema in aphakic eyes. Archives of Ophthalmology. 1977;95:791-3.
164. Gass JD, Norton EW. Cystoid macular edema and papilledema following cataract extraction. A fluorescein fundoscopic and angiographic study. Archives of Ophthalmology. 1966;76:646-61.
165. Mandell AI, Stentz F, Kitabchi AE. Dipivalyl epinephrine: a new pro-drug in the treatment of glaucoma. Ophthalmology. 1978; 85:268-75.
166. Mills KB, Jacobs NA. A single-blind randomised trial comparing adrenaline 1.0 percent with dipivalyl epinephrine (propine) 0.1 percent in the treatment of open-angle glaucoma and ocular hypertension. The British Journal of Ophthalmology. 1988;72: 465-8.

167. Gharagozloo NZ, Relf SJ, Brubaker RF. Aqueous flow is reduced by the alpha-adrenergic agonist, apraclonidine hydrochloride (ALO 2145), Ophthalmology. 1988;95:1217-20.
168. Harrison R, Kaufmann CS. Clonidine. Effects of a topically administered solution on intraocular pressure and blood pressure in open-angle glaucoma. Archives of Ophthalmology. 1977;95:1368-73.
169. Petursson G, Cole R, Hanna C. Treatment of glaucoma using minidrops of clonidine. Archives of Ophthalmology. 1984; 102:1180-1.
170. Brown RH, Stewart RH, Lynch MG, Crandall AS, Mandell AI, Wilensky JT, Schwartz AL, Gaasterland DE, DeFaller JM, Higginbotham EJ. ALO 2145 reduces the intraocular pressure elevation after anterior segment laser surgery. Ophthalmology. 1988;95:378-84.
171. Robin AL, Pollack IP, deFaller JM. Effects of topical ALO 2145 (p-aminoclonidine hydrochloride) on the acute intraocular pressure rise after argon laser iridotomy. Archives of Ophthalmology. 1987;105:1208-11.
172. Del Priore LV, Robin AL, Pollack IP. Neodymium: YAG and argon laser iridotomy. Long-term follow-up in a prospective, randomized clinical trial. Ophthalmology. 1988;95:1207-11.
173. Serle JB, Steidl S, Wang RF, Mittag TW, Podos SM. Selective alpha 2-adrenergic agonists B-HT 920 and UK14304-18. Effects on aqueous humor dynamics in monkeys. Archives of Ophthalmology. 1991;109:1158-62.
174. Gordon-Bennett PS, Ioannidis AS, Papageorgiou K, Andreou PS. A survey of investigations used for the management of glaucoma in hospital service in the United Kingdom. Eye. 2008;22:1410-18.
175. Katz LJ. Brimonidine tartrate 0.2 percent twice daily vs timolol 0.5 percent twice daily: 1-year results in glaucoma patients. Brimonidine Study Group. American Journal of Ophthalmology. 1999;127:20-6.
176. Serle JB. A comparison of the safety and efficacy of twice daily brimonidine 0.2 percent versus betaxolol 0.25 percent in subjects with elevated intraocular pressure. The Brimonidine Study Group III. Survey of Ophthalmology. 1996;41 Suppl 1:S39-47.
177. Evans DW, Hosking SL, Gherghel D, Bartlett JD. Contrast sensitivity improves after brimonidine therapy in primary open angle glaucoma: a case for neuroprotection. The British Journal of Ophthalmology. 2003;87:1463-5.
178. Sponsel WE, Paris G, Trigo Y, Pena M, Weber A, Sanford K, McKinnon S. Latanoprost and brimonidine: therapeutic and physiologic assessment before and after oral nonsteroidal anti-inflammatory therapy. American Journal of Ophthalmology. 2002; 133:11-8.
179. Burke J, Schwartz M. Preclinical evaluation of brimonidine, Survey of ophthalmology. 1996;41 Suppl 1:S9-18.
180. Craven ER, Walters TR, Williams R, Chou C, Cheetham JK, Schiffman R, Combigan Study G. Brimonidine and timolol fixed-combination therapy versus monotherapy: a 3-month randomized trial in patients with glaucoma or ocular hypertension. Journal of ocular pharmacology and therapeutics: the official journal of the Association for Ocular Pharmacology and Therapeutics. 2005; 21:337-48.

181. LeBlanc RP. Twelve-month results of an ongoing randomized trial comparing brimonidine tartrate 0.2 percent and timolol 0.5 percent given twice daily in patients with glaucoma or ocular hypertension. Brimonidine Study Group 2. Ophthalmology. 1998;105:1960-7.
182. Whitson JT, Ochsner KI, Moster MR, Sullivan EK, Andrew RM, Silver LH, Wells DT, James JE, Bosworth CF, Dickerson JE, Landry TA, Bergamini MV, Brimonidine 0.15 percent Study G. The safety and intraocular pressure-lowering efficacy of brimonidine tartrate 0.15 percent preserved with polyquaternium-1. Ophthalmology. 2006; 113:1333-9.
183. Al-Shahwan S, Al-Torbak AA, Turkmani S, Al-Omran M, Al-Jadaan I, Edward DP. Side-effect profile of brimonidine tartrate in children. Ophthalmology. 2005;112:2143.
184. Tyner GS, Scheie HG. Mechanism of the miotic-resistant pupil with increased intraocular pressure. AMA Archives of Ophthalmology. 195;50:572-9.
185. Abramson DH, Chang S, Coleman DJ, Smith ME. Pilocarpine-induced lens changes. An ultrasonic biometric evaluation of dose response. Archives of Ophthalmology. 1974;92:464-9.
186. Flocks M, Zweng HC. Studies on the mode of action of pilocarpine on aqueous outflow. American Journal of Ophthalmology. 1957; 44:380-6; discussion 387-8.
187. Beasley H, Fraunfelder FT. Retinal detachments and topical ocular miotics. Ophthalmology. 1979;86:95-8.
188. Axelsson U, Holmberg A. The frequency of cataract after miotic therapy. Acta Ophthalmologica. 1966;44:421-9.
189. Stocker FW. Experimental studies on the blood-aqueous barrier; electrophotometric measurements of fluorescein content of aqueous after intravenous injection of fluorescein, the eye being under the influence of physostigmine, pilocarpine, neostigmine or atropine. Arch Ophthal. 1947;37:583-90.
190. Greco JJ, Kelman CD. Systemic pilocarpine toxicity in the treatment of angle closure glaucoma. Ann Ophthalmol. 1973; 5:57-9.
191. Drance SM, Nash PA. The dose response of human intraocular pressure to pilocarpine. Canadian Journal of Ophthalmology Journal Canadien d'ophtalmologie. 1971;6:9-13.
192. Harris LS, Galin MA. Effect of ocular pigmentation on hypotensive response to pilocarpine. American Journal of Ophthalmology. 1971;72:923-5.
193. Mehra KS, Singh R, Char JN, Rajyashree K. Lowering of intraocular tension. Effects of isosorbide and glycerin. Archives of Ophthalmology. 1971;85:167-8.
194. Bruckner HL. Glycerol versus isosorbide. Ann Ophthalmol. 1972; 4:629-33.
195. Becker B, Kolker AE, Krupin T. Isosorbide. An Oral hyperosmotic agent. Archives of Ophthalmology. 1967;78:147-50.
196. Drance SM. Effect of oral glycerol of intraocular pressure in normal and glaucomatous eyes. Archives of Ophthalmology. 1964;72:491-3.
197. Thomas RP. Glycerin. An Orally Effective Osmotic Agent. Archives of Ophthalmology. 1963;70:625-8.
198. Barry KG, Khoury AH, Brooks MH. Mannitol and isosorbide. Sequential effects on intraocular pressure, serum osmolality, sodium, and solids in normal subjects. Archives of Ophthalmology. 1969;81:695-700.

Antiallergy Therapy

NR Biswas, GK Das, Harivenkatesh N, Ashok Garg (India)

INTRODUCTION

Allergic ocular disease is one of the most common problems seen by ophthalmologists worldwide. The allergic disease can involve several type of reactions which varies from mild intermittent tearing characteristics of seasonal and perennial allergic conjunctivitis (SAC) to more constant itching and mucoid discharge of vernal keratoconjunctivitis (VKC) and ultimately to the vision threatening corneal scarring of atopic keratoconjunctivitis (AKC). New and effective treatment of allergic conjunctivitis depends on clear understanding of the underlying pathophysiology. Ocular allergy represents a variety of problems that are primarily type-1 hypersensitivity reactions (IgE mediated) with the cell mediated or type IV hypersensitivity response playing a role in some of these disorders. Patients with atopic disease may also have deficient immunoregulation with depressed T cell function that results in systemic involvement. Appropriate treatment should be prescribed to the ocular and systemic involvement and should consider this underlying defect in T cell function.

Histamine release can cause a variety of uncomfortable symptoms and sometime life-threatening complications. Drug therapy is successful in satisfactorily relieving associated signs and symptoms when ocular tissues are affected. Pathophysiology of allergic ocular diseases is being mentioned here for better understanding of ocular allergy and antiallergy medication.

TYPE 1 HYPERSENSITIVITY REACTIONS

It is also known as anaphylactic, immediate or IgE mediated reactions which occur when an antigen such as a pollen, drug is reintroduced into the individual who has been previously exposed to the antigen. Upon initial exposure to antigen, IgE antibodies are produced which get attached to mast cells and make the cells susceptible to rupture when the patient is again exposed to same antigen. Disruption of mast cells cause a release of large quantities of inflammatory mediators including histamine and histamine activates H_1 receptors on blood vessels causing vasodilation. These dilated vessels leak fluid causing tissue to swell. Common clinical signs and symptoms of type-1 reaction include redness swelling and itching. Such reactions occur in allergic conjunctivitis.

The following ophthalmic diseases are characterized by type-1 hypersensitivity reactions.

Hay Fever Conjunctivitis

Seasonal perennial allergic conjunctivitis and atopic conjunctivitis constitute 50 percent of all allergic conjunctivitis and are often associated with hay fever. Allergic conjunctivitis can result from a variety of exogeneous antigens and is component of more widespread allergic states. Airborne pollens, dust and other environmental contaminants constitute the largest single group of agents responsible for the disorder. Ophthalmic drugs are not uncommon causes of allergic conjunctivitis. It includes neomycin, sulphonamides, atropine and thiomersal.

Vernal Conjunctivitis

Vernal conjunctivitis is usually a bilateral inflammation affecting mainly adolescent males. It involves upper tarsal conjunctiva and limbal conjunctiva. This disease is seasonal and has peak activity during the warm months of the year. This type of conjunctivitis is more common in tropical countries. It is specially characterized by the formation of large papillale having the appearance of cobble stone on the upper tarsal conjunctiva. Symptoms include intense itching during warm months and often a thick ropy discharge.

Atopic Keratoconjunctivitis

Atopic keratoconjunctivitis represents a hypersensitivity state caused by predispositional, constitutional or hereditary factors rather than by acquired hypersensitivity to specific antigens. Such patients usually have a family history of allergy specially asthma or hay fever. Ocular findings are conjunctival hyperemia and chemosis. Corneal involement is not uncommon.

Giant Papillary Conjunctivitis

Giant papillary conjunctivitis (GPC) is a specific conjunctival inflammatory reaction to soft contact lens materials but also has been reported in patients wearing methyl methacrylate ocular prosthesis. This condition is characterized by papillary hypertrophy primarily affecting the upper tarsal conjunctiva. It probably represents a chronic conjunctival inflammatory reaction to denatured proteins that are adherants to anterior lens surface. Lens thickness and diameter may also play a role.

ANTIALLERGY MEDICATION

Since much of the symptomatic picture of type-1 hypersensitivity reactions is caused by histamine release from mast cells, antihistaminics are usually effective in relieving annoying symptoms. These agents are usually given with decongestants and

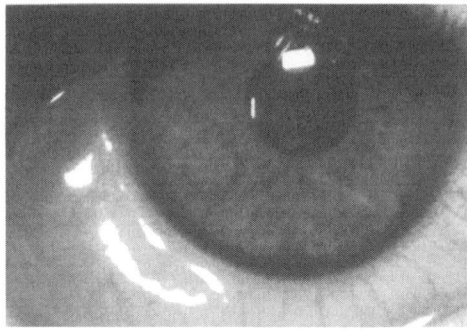

Fig. 12.1A: Seasonal allergic conjunctivitis
(*Courtesy*: Allergan India Limited)

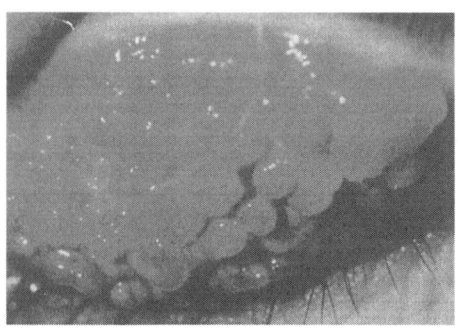

Fig. 12.1B: Vernal keratoconjunctivitis
(*Courtesy*: Allergan India Limited)

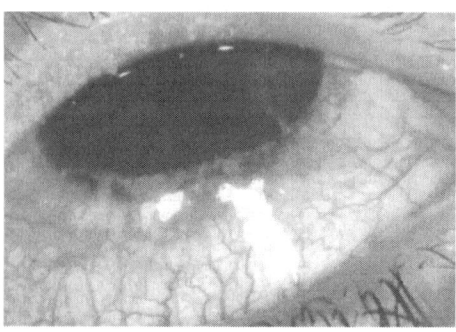

Fig. 12.1C: Atopic keratoconjunctivitis
(*Courtesy*: Allergan India Limited)

are given topically or systemically depending upon the degree of involvement. Mast cell stabilizers are also very effective and can be given prophylactically.

Current treatment options include nondrug therapy, pharmacotherapy and immunotherapy. Initially attention is directed at identifying the offending allergen and eliminating it whenever possible.

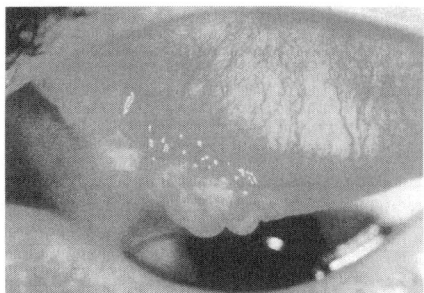

Fig. 12.1D: Giant papillary conjunctivitis
(*Courtesy*: Allergan India Limited)

Mild symptoms of itching and discomfort can be relieved with cool compresses and artificial tear/saline irrigation of the eyes (nondrug therapy). More intense signs and symptoms usually require pharmacotherapy, immunotherapy or both.

Current ocular therapy emphasises the use of topical medication to alter mediator production, release or end organ. Although more potent mediator antagonists are becoming available, simultaneous control of all mediators is difficult. The antiallergy medication is broadly classified into following categories:

1. Topical mast cell stabilizers.
2. Antihistamines combinations.
    i. Topical antihistamines—vasoconstrictor
    ii. Topical high potency antihistamines
    iii. Oral antihistamines
3. NSAIDs
    i. Topical NSAIDs
    ii. Systemic NSAIDs
4. Topical steroids
5. Topical immunosuppressors.

TOPICAL MAST CELL INHIBITORS

Topical mast cell inhibitors are one of the most commonly used antiallergy agent in the ophthalmology worldwide.

Mast cell stabilizers act by preventing calcium influx into the mast cells and basophills thus preventing the cascade that results in degranulation.

These are potent H_1 receptor antagonists. Once these mast cell inhibitors are bound to a membrane receptor, they prevent IgE cross linking and thus stabilises the entire excitation process. Their mechanism of action also involve increasing intracellular cyclic adenosine monophosphate levels thereby reducing calcium influx or by inhibiting the enzyme nucleosides disphosphate kinase in the cytoplasm.

Mast cell stabilizers can also act by inhibiting the release of neuropeptides from sensory nerve endings. The various agents of this group used in ophthalmology are as follows.

Cromolyn Sodium (Sodium Cromoglycate)

Indications in the treatment of allergic ocular disorders including vernal keratoconjunctivitis giant papillary conjunctivitis, vernal keratitis and allergic keratoconjunctivitis.

Cromolyn sodium inhibits the degranulation of sensitized mast cells and basophills which occur after exposure to specific antigens thus inhibiting the release of histamine and SRS-A (Slow reacting substance of anaphylaxis) from the mast cell. It has no intrinsic vasoconstrictors, antihistamines or anti-inflammatory activity.

Cromolyn sodium is poorly absorbed and approximately 0.03 percent of cromolyn is absorbed following topical administration to the eye. Systemically absorbed drug is excreted unchanged in the urine.

Contraindications: Hypersensitivity to cromolyn or to any component of its product. Patients are advised not to wear soft contact lenses during cromolyn sodium treatment.

Dosage: It is available as topical ophthalmic solution in strength of 2 percent and 4 percent (in 5 ml and 10 ml vials) usual dosage is to instill 1-2 drops in each eye 4-6 times a day at regular intervals till the desired effect is obtained. It is effective alone or in combination with other antiallergy drugs (Topical or systemic).

Symptomatic response to the therapy is usually evident within few days but treatment should be given up to six weeks or more. Effect of therapy depends upon administration at regular intervals. Continue therapy as long as needed to sustain clinical improvement. Topical corticosteroids can be used concomitantly with cromolyn sodium.

Adverse reactions: The most frequent adverse reaction reported is ocular stinging or burning sensation upon instillation which

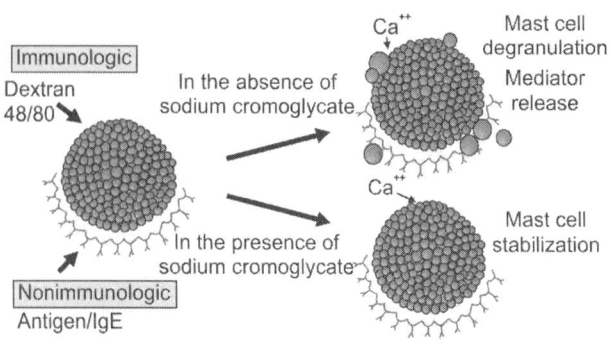

The protective effect of sodium cromoglycate on the mast cell from the immunologic and nonimmunologic triggers

Fig. 12.2: Mechanism of action of sodium cromoglycate
(*Courtesy*: Cipla Ltd)

usually regresses with continued use. So patient should be initially warned about this reaction before starting the treatment. Other adverse effects reported are conjunctival injection, watery, itchy and puffy eyes, dryness around eyes, irritation styes.

Disodium Cromoglycate

Disodium cromoglycate (DSCG) is the prototype mast cell stabilizer. It is used widely and is effective to varying extents in different ophthalmic allergic disorders. In vernal keratoconjunctivitis DSCG is more effective in treating signs and symptoms in children and adults. This agent is also effective in other forms of allergic conjunctivitis (GPC and AKC). It is safe and well-tolerated. It is given topically.

It has been shown that DSCG can prevent the reflex stimulation of primary afferent nerve fiber endings initiated by capsaicin a compound capable of causing the release and depletion of neuropeptides. DSCG is also known to inhibit activation of neutrophils, eosinophils and monocytes and to prevent neutrophil chemotaxis.

Lodoxamide

It is most potent topical mast cell inhibitor. Lodoxamide is 2500 times more potent than cromolyn sodium. It effectively prevents histamine release from mast cells during immediate hypersensitivity reactions.

Lodoxamide significantly reduces recruitment of neutrophils and eosinophils and prevents mast cell degranulation. Inhibition of leukocyte, monocyte and eosinophils activation by mast cell stabilizers is important in modifying the allergic inflammatory response. It stabilizes the mast cell response in vernal conjunctivitis and has dual mechanism of action.

Indications: It is highly effective in treatment of vernal keratoconjunctivitis (VKC), giant papillary conjunctivitis (GPC) and atopic keratoconjunctivitis (AKC). Lodoxamide is more efficacious than DSCG with earlier improvement of signs and symptoms. It is most effective in VKC and for sustained relief of signs and symptoms and treatment of corneal complications.

Dosage: It is available as 0.1 percent ophthalmic suspension (Lodoxamide tromethamine) usual dosage is to instill 1–2 drops in the affected eyes 4 times a day throughout the year.

Adverse reactions: No serious adverse effects have been reported with topical lodoxamide use except for transient burning and stinging sensation, ocular itching, dry eye, blurred vision tearing/discharge, hyperemia, crystalline deposits, foreign body sensation, rarely chemosis, corneal abrasion, keratitis, blepharitis, allergy, etc. which regresses with regular and continuous use of lodoxamide. Topical preparation should be instilled at regular intervals for better response.

Other new mast cell inhibitors that are on trials and shall be available commercially shortly.

Nedocromil

It is a disodium salt of pyranoquinoline dicarboxylic acid.

It has been reported more effective in vernal keratoconjunctivitis. Nedocromil prevents chemotactic and inflammatory mediator release from the effector cells such as granulocytes, monocytes, macrophages and mast cells. In comparison to DSCG, nedocromil is more effective in controlling symptoms of VKC and SAC. In GPC nedocromil is effective in reducing itching and mucous discharge.

It is tried in conc of 1 percent to be given 1–2 drops 4 times a day. No serious side effects have been reported with the use of this drug.

Ketotifen Fumarate

Ketotifen is a relatively selective, noncompetitive histamine antagonist (H_1 receptor and mast cell stabilizer). Ketotifen inhibits the release of mediators from cells involved in hypersensitivity reactions. Decreased chemotaxis and eosinophil activation have also been shown.

Indications: It is indicated for the treatment of allergic conjunctivitis of diverse etiology.

Dosage: It is available as 0.025 percent topical solution (0.25 mg/ml—0.345 mg/ml ketotifen fumarate) in 5 ml and 7 ml packs.

Recommended dose is to instill one drop in each affected eye every 8–12 hours. This solution is for topical ophthalmic use only. It is not recommended for injection or oral use.

It is contraindicated in patients, who are hypersensitive to any component of the product.

Adverse reactions: Generally topical ketotifen solution is safe for ophthalmic use. However, in less than 5 percent of patients following ocular adverse affects may appear.

Burning or stinging sensation, allergic reaction, conjunctivitis, discharge, dry eyes.

Keratitis, lacrimation disorder, photophobia and rash. General adverse effects may include flu syndrome, pharyngitis.

In pregnant, lactating mothers and children below 3 years of age, its use is not generally recommended.

Olopatadine Hydrochloride

Olopatadine is a new agent that exerts both mast cell stabilization effect and an antihistaminic effect. It is highly potent and a relatively selective H_1-receptor antagonist that inhibits *in vivo* and *in vitro* the type-I immediate hypersensitivity reaction. It has no effect on alpha-adrenergic dopamine muscarinic type 1 and 2 and serotonin receptors.

Olopatadine has been reported to have low systemic exposure following topical ocular administration. Clinical trials have shown that it has more than 90 percent inhibition of basophil and mast cell degranulation and histamine induced conjunctival vascular permeability.

Olopatadine is indicated for the treatment of allergic conjunctivitis of diverse etiology.

Dosage and administration: Olopatadine is available as 0.1 percent topical ophthalmic solution in 5 ml vial. The recommended dose is 1-2 drops in each affected eye 3-4 times per day (every 6-8 hours).

Olopatadine ophthalmic solution is available for topical use only. Not for injection. It is contraindicated in those patients, who are hypersensitive to any component of this product.

Patients are instructed not to wear contact lenses during treatment with olopatadine. In pregnant, lactating mothers and children below 3 years of age, its use is not generally recommended.

Adverse reactions: Ophthalmic adverse effects reported are burning or stinging sensation, dry eye, foreign body sensation, hyperemia, keratitis, lid edema and pruritus.

Systemic effects include headache, asthenia, cold syndrome, pharyngitis, sinusitis and taste perversion.

Azelastine Hydrochloride

Azelastine is a phthalazinone derivative of noval with histamine H_1 receptor antagonist activity, which also inhibits mast cell histamine release, has some leukotriene and platelet aggregating factor (PAF) antagonistic activity and inhibits IgE-mediated inflammation *in vivo*.

While the inhibition of itching of the eyes in allergic patients by azelastine eyedrops is certainly due to inhibition of the release and actions of histamine, the inhibition of conjunctival redness is likely to be the result of a combination of the various anti-inflammatory actions of azelastine. Due to its multiple activities azelastine is classified as an antiallergic and anti-inflammatory agent rather simply as an antihistamine.

Azelastine is a highly selective H_1 receptor blocker with a very low affinity for both β-receptors and muscarinic receptors. Topical azelastine reduces the neutrophil and eosinophil infiltrate following a single antigen challenge in patients with seasonal allergic diseases. Interleukocyte—adhesion molecule-1 (ICAM-1) expression is also reduced on epithelial cells.

Desmethyl azelastine, a metabolite of azelastine is pharmacologically active and probably contributes to the activity of the parent compound.

Indications: Azelastine is indicated for the treatment of seasonal allergic conjunctivitis.

Dosage and administration: It is available as 0.05 percent topical ophthalmic solution in 5 ml vial.

Recommended dosage is to instill one drop in each affected eye twice daily. Dose can be increased to four times a day depending upon the severity of the condition. Topical azelastine is generally not recommended for pregnant, lactating mothers and children.

Adverse reactions: Local adverse effects include burning and tingling sensation, local irritation, etc.

Systemic effects include metallic or bitter taste in mouth (Dysgeusia), hot flushes, epistaxis, etc. Bitter taste may disappear quickly.

The other mast cell inhibitors that are on ophthalmic clinical trials are:
- Nicotinamide
- Picumast
- Calmodulin antagonists.

Hopefully these compounds shall appear in commercial market shortly.

ANTIHISTAMINES

Antihistamines are histamine H_1-receptor antagonists and cause sympathomimetic vasoconstriction. First and second generation antihistamines are being used either topically or systemically in the treatment of various ocular allergic disorders.

H_2 receptors have also been indentified on the ocular surface.

H_1 receptors are involved primarily with neuronal tissue and H_2 receptor with vascular tissue, thus combination drops containing both H_1 and H_2 receptor antagonists have been found more useful in treatment of allergic eye diseases.

Various topical antihistamine available in combination for ophthalmic use are pheniramine maleate, pyrilamine maleate, antazoline and levocabastine.

1. Pheniramine maleate 0.3 percent ophthalmic solution in combination with 0.025 percent naphazoline HCl (in 10 ml and 15 ml packs).
2. Pheniramine maleate 0.5 percent ophthalmic solution with 0.125 percent phenylepherine HCl (in 10 ml and 15 ml packs).
3. Pyrilamine maleate 0.1 percent ophthalmic solution with 0.12 percent phenylephrine HCl and 0.1 percent antipyrine (in 10 ml and 15 ml packs).
4. Antazoline 0.5 percent ophthalmic solution with 0.05 percent naphazoline HCl (in 15 ml packs).
5. Topical levocabastine HCl 0.05 percent ophthalmic suspension available without decongestant.
6. Tetrahydozoline 0.05 percent ophthalmic solution with zinc sulphate (0.25%).
7. Emedastine difumarate topical ophthalmic solution (0.05%).

Usual dosage for various topical antihistamines combinations is to instill 1–2 drops in the affected eyes 3–4 times daily till the desired response is obtained.

Levocabastine Hydrochloride

Levocabastine is a potent, selective histamine H_1-receptor antagonist for topical ophthalmic use. It has rapid onset and long duration of action.

It has been shown to effectively control the symptoms of allergic conjunctivitis. It is 15000 times more potent than pheniramine and more effective than cromolyn sodium. It provides relief within minutes and block histamine the primary mediatory for type, response to allergy and is safe and comfortable.

It is indicated for use in the treatment of seasonal allergic conjunctivitis.

Dosage and administration: Levocabastine is available as 0.05 percent ophthalmic suspension in 2.5, 5 and 10 ml bottles. The recommended dosage is to instill one drop in the affected eye four times daily. Treatment may be continued up to two weeks. Levocabastine instilled four times daily is significantly more effective than its vehicle in reducing ocular itching associated with allergic conjunctivitis.

In pregnant, lactating mothers and in children below 12 years topical levocabastine is generally not recommended.

Adverse reactions: The most frequent ocular adverse reactions reported with it are mild transient stinging and burning sensation, visual disturbances, eye pain or eyelid edema.

Systemic effects include headache, dry mouth, fatigue, pharyngitis, cough, nausea and dyspnea.

Emedastine Difumarate

Emedastine is a relatively selective histamine H_1 antagonist. Clinical studies have shown concentration dependent inhibition of histamine induced increase in conjunctival vascular permeability in the conjunctiva following topical ocular administration.

Following topical administration emedastine has low systemic exposure.

Indications: Emedastine is indicated for topical use in the treatment of allergic conjunctivitis.

Dosage and administration: Emedastine is available as topical 0.05 percent ophthalmic solution in 5 ml opaque plastic dispenser.

Recommended dosage is to instill one drop in the affected eye four times a day.

It is generally not recommended for use in pregnant, lactating mothers and children below three years of age.

Adverse reactions: Headache, asthenia, blurred vision, burning or stinging sensation, corneal infiltrates, corneal staining, discomfort, dry eyes, keratitis, pruritus, sinusitis and hyperemia.

Topical impiramine which has H_1 and H_2 receptor blocking activity is on trials. It has been shown to be highly effective in reducing signs and symptoms in the conjunctival challenge test in patients with seasonal allergic conjunctivitis.

A variety of topical antihistamine and decongestant (vasoconstrictor) combinations are available. But with the emergence of high potency H_1 receptor antagonists, these agents are playing a lesser role in the treatment of allergic eye diseases. Before discussing systemic antihistamines, it is worthwhile to discuss decongestants used in treating allergic disorders in combination with topical antihistamines.

Decongestants

These are adrenergic agonists with direct vasoconstrictive activity. This vasoconstrictor effect (Phenylephrine and imidazole derivatives) makes them useful as topical ocular decongestants. Following instillation, the conjunctival vessels constrict within minutes causing the eye to normal white color.

Due to relatively low concentrations required for ocular decongestion, phenylephrine and imidazole derivatives generally do not cause systemic side effects.

Phenylephrine

It is a synthetic amine structurally similar to epinephrine and is present in several topical commercial preparations. Concentration of 0.12 percent or 0.125 percent cause vasoconstriction with little or no pupillary dilation in eyes with intact corneal epithelium.

Phenylephrine is contraindicated in eyes predisposed to angle closure glaucoma. Prolonged or excessive use may result in rebound conjunctival hyperemia. Phenylephrine solution can exhibit variable effectiveness since they are subject to oxidation on exposure to air, light or heat. Antioxidants like sodium bisulfite may be added to it prolong shelf life.

Imidazole Derivatives

The imidazoline derivatives used topically are naphazoline, tetrahydrozoline and oxymetazoline differ structurally from phenylephrine by replacement of benzine ring with an unsaturated ring. Concentrations used for ocular vasoconstriction do not alter pupil size or raise IOP in the normal eye.

These agents are generally more stable in solution than phenylephrine and have a longer shelf life and longer duration of action. Following instillation, the balancing effect, occurs within minutes and may last up to several hours. The solutions may sting upon initial instillation.

In addition to vasoconstrictor substances, ocular decongestants may also contain antihistamines, viscosity increasing agents, preservative, buffers and astringents. Various topical combination products with antihistamines as already mentioned are available commercially (Table 12.1).

TABLE 12.1: Ophthalmic decongestants		
Vasoconstrictor	Concentration (percent)	Duration (hr)
Epinephrine	0.1	1-3
Phenylephrine	0.12	0.5-1.5
Oxymetazoline	0.025	< 6 hours
Naphazoline	0.012-0.1	2-3
Tetrahydrozoline	0.05	2-3

Individual drug monograph of various decongestants is as follows:

Phenylephrine HCl: Used as a decongestant either alone or in combination with topical antihistamine to provide relief from symptoms of mild ocular allergy disorder (relief of eye irritation caused by hay fever, colds, dust, wind, sun, smog or hard contact lenses).

Contraindications: Hypersensitivity to any of its components, narrow angle glaucoma because the mydriatic action of phenylephrine may precipitate angle block.

Dosage: It is available as topical ophthalmic solution in strength of 0.125-0.12 percent usual dosage is to instil 1-2 drops of 0.12 percent solution in eyes 2-4 times daily.

Adverse reactions: On topical use it may cause transitory stinging on initial instillation, blurring of vision, rebound miosis and decreased mydriatic response to therapy.

Naphazoline HCl: It is used as topical vasoconstrictor to soothe, refresh, moisturize and removes redness due to mild ocular allergic disorder or minor eye irritation.

Dosage: It is available in various topical ophthalmic preparations in concentrations varying from 0.012 to 0.1 percent. It is also available as topical ophthalmic solution alone.

Usual dosage is to instill 1-2 drops into the conjunctival sac of the affected eyes every 2-4 hours.

Contraindications: Like phenylephrine it is also contraindicated in patients with narrow angle glaucoma, unstable systemic hypertension and individuals using MAO inhibitors. Over use can produce rebound hyperemia.

Adverse reactions are similar to those mentioned in phenylephrine section.

Tetrahydrozine HCl: It is also used as topical ocular decongestant. It is available as topical ophthalmic solution either alone or in combination with antihistamines in the strength of 0.05 percent. Usual dosage is to instill 1-2 drops into the affected eyes 2-4 times a day.

Adverse reactions and contraindications are similar to as described in phenylephrine section.

Oxymetazoline HCl: It is a imidazoline derivative and is sympathomimetic drug that acts to constrict blood vessels. Its effect is due to direct action of the drug upon the alpha (postsynaptic) receptors of vascular smooth muscles. Oxymetazoline is characterized by an early onset of action, a relatively long duration of action and a low tendency to rebound congestion.

Indications: It is indicated for use as a long-acting topical ocular vasoconstrictor for symptomatic relief of allergic conjunctivitis, non-infectious conjunctivitis and ocular congestion caused by conditions such as allergy, dry eyes, swimming, smog, contact lens wear and eye strain.

Contraindications: It is contraindicated in patients in whom pupillary dilation should be avoided, e.g. angle closure glaucoma or those with critically narrow angles and hypersensitivity to the drug.

It should be used with caution in patients using systemic MAO inhibitors as an increase in blood pressure may occur. In children it may cause sedation and hence use with caution.

Dosage: It is available as liquifilm sterile ophthalmic solution in conc of 0.025 percent usual dosage is 1-2 drops in the affected eyes every 8 hourly.

Adverse reactions: Pupillary dilation may occur in susceptible individuals and may be associated in IOP rise. Other ocular effects are transient burning and stinging sensation.

Oxymetazoline is best topical decongestant of this group which has been shown to be more potent and effective than naphazoline HCl, tetrahydrozoline HCl and xylometazoline HCl.

Oxymetazoline slow elimination rate ensures that more drug stays in contact with superficial blood vessels for longer time period.

It produces a marked and prolonged reduction of hyperemia with the onset of effect occurring with in 1-5 minutes of instillation.

Its liquifilm character protects the tear film and prevents development of an iatrogenic dry eye. Liquifilm soothes and comforts inflamed ocular tissue.

It has no systemic side effects.

Rose petal aqueous infusion: It is also used to provide relief from mild ocular allergic irritation of the eye. It is available as topical solution (aqueous infusion in 7.5 ml with 0.01 percent thiomersal) usual dosage is to instill one drop in the affected eye twice-thrice a day. If irritation persists or increases, discontinue the use of infusion immediately.

Oral pseudoephedrine: (30 and 60 mg oral tablets) and topical ephedrine solution (0.05%) are also used in relieving ocular irritation.

Emedastine: It is a benzimidazole derivative and is a new high potency, high affinity H_1 selective histamine receptor antagonist that effectively inhibited allergic conjunctivitis in trial patients.

It displays a rapid onset and good duration of action. Its action starts within 10 minutes of topical instillation and effect last for 4 hours. This agent appears to be a promising new drug for the treatment of ocular allergic diseases.

ORAL ANTIHISTAMINES

Oral antihistamines are prescribed in conjunction with topical antiallergy agents in severe cases of ocular allergic disorders where topical therapy alone is insufficient to achieve desired effects.

Although systemic antihistamines such as chlorpheniramine, clemastine, dexchlorpheniramine, diphenhydramine, promethazine and triprolidine relieve ocular allergic symptoms, but they have greater CNS penetration and increased anticholinergic side effects like dryness and drowsiness. While second generation H_1-receptor antagonists such as terfenadine, fexofenadine, astemizole, cetrizine and loratadine do not cross blood-brain barrier to any appreciable extent and thus are minimally sedating.

In addition to blocking H_1-receptors, terfenadine and loratadine have been found to inhibit histamine release.

Astemizole and cetrizine have been found to be effective in reducing symptoms of seasonal allergic conjunctivitis. Loratadine has been found to protect against the clinical and cellular early phase and late phase reactions.

The onset of action of these oral antihistamines is approximately one hour after administration, but maximal antagonism at their sites of action takes several hours longer.

These agents are useful in ocular allergic disorders specially when eyelid edema and chemosis are significant.

The various systemic antihistamines given orally are always prescribed in conjunction with standard topical antiallergy agents to be more effective in relieving the symptoms.

Levocetirizine

It is a new highly effective and well-tolerated antihistamine. Levocetirizine being the potent single isomer of cetrizine binds twice as strongly to histamine H_1 receptors and has a highly consistent and predictable antihistamine action.

It is available as 5 mg tablet.

Dosage: 5 mg orally once or twice daily. It is indicated for the treatment of allergic conjunctivitis.

Desloratadine

It is active metabolite of loratadine and is indicated for use in seasonal allergic conjunctivitis. Desloratadine possesses pharmacodynamic activity similar to that of loratadine but has a relative potency 10–20 times greater than loratadine.

It is available as 5 mg tablet. Dosage is 5 mg orally once daily.

The dosage of various systemic antihistamines is given in Table 12.2.

TABLE 12.2: Oral antihistamine dosages

Drug name	Dose (mg)	Dose interval (h)	Max daily dose (mg)	Antihistamine activity
Chlorpheniramine	4	4-6	24	Moderate
Dexchlorpheniramine	2	4-6	12	High
Clemastine	1	12	08	Moderate
Diphenhydramine	25-50	6-8	400	Moderate
Promethazine	12.5-25	6-24	100	High
Triprolidine	2.5	4-6	10	High
Astemizole	10	24	10	High
Brompheniramine	04	4-6	24	High
Cetrizine	10	24	10	High
Loratadine	10	24	10	High
Pyrilamine	25-50	6-8	200	Moderate
Terfenadine	60	12	120	High
Fexofenadine	60	12	120	High
Tripelennamine	25-50	4-6	300	Moderate
Hydroxazine	50 mg	6-8	400	High

Although second generation H_1 receptor antagonist antihistamines are relatively free of systemic adverse reactions yet rare adverse effect of ventricular tachycardia can occur with terfenadine and astemizole if their metabolism is inhibited by hepatic disease or drugs such as erythromycin and certain antifungal agents.

Fexofenadine

It is a newer second generation nonsedating specific antihistamine (H_1 blocker). It is a hydrochloride salt of terfenadine active metabolites.

It has been shown to have a good clinical efficacy and tolerability in the treatment of vernal keratoconjunctivitis and seasonal allergic conjunctivitis.

Fexofenadine is truly nonsedating and safe antihistamine.

Dosage: It is available as 60 mg and 120 mg tablets. Usual dosage is 60 mg twice a day or 120 mg OD for 14–21 days till the desired response is obtained.

It is usually given in combination with topical antiallergy drops.

Adverse reactions: Generally, the drug is well-tolerated. However, the common adverse effects seen are headache, throat irritation, viral infection, nausea, dysmenorrhea, drowsiness, dyspepsia and fatigue.

Drug interactions: Fexofenadine is least likely nonsedating antihistamines to interact with other medications.

Fexofenadine does not impair driving performance, a usual precaution advised with other antihistamines.

NSAIDs (ANTIPROSTAGLANDIN THERAPY)

One of the oral nonsteriodal anti-inflammatory drugs (NSAIDs), aspirin (a cyclooxygenase inhibitor) has been proved effective in controlling symptoms in patients of vernal keratoconjunctivitis (VKC) unresponsive to DSCG and corticosteroids. Clinical studies have shown dramatic improvement in conjunctival and episcleral redness limbal infiltration and epithelial keratitis with systemic aspirin therapy. Standard oral dosage of aspirin is 0.5–1.5 gm daily for 4–6 week period. With oral aspirin there is marked symptomatic improvement, e.g. reduced palpebral papillae size, decreased punctate keratopathy and decreased limbal inflammation.

Topical NSAIDs which are effective in ocular allergy are as follows:
1. Topical suprofen (1%) is effective in managing the signs and symptoms of giant papillary conjunctivitis and vernal keratoconjunctivitis. Usual dosage is to instill 1–2 drops in the affected eye three times a day for 4–6 weeks.
2. The most effective topical NSAIDs used commonly in treating ocular allergic disorder is: Topical ketorolac tromethamine solution (0.5%). Topical ketorolac is the itch buster in allergic conjunctivitis.

   The salient features of topical ketorolac solution is:
   - It stops allergic itch promptly—start immediately after instillation.
   - Provides relief from allergic symptoms—itching, tearing, redness and swelling.
   - Breaks the itch-rub cycle. It inhibits prostaglandin formation by blocking enzyme cyclooxygenase putting an end to further cycle of irritation and discomfort.
   - Provides relief from acute flare ups with no need for prophylactic use. The recommended dosage is to instill one drop in the conjunctival sac four times a day for relief of ocular itching due to seasonal allergic conjunctivitis.
   - In patients with allergic conjunctivitis the most frequent adverse effect reported with the use of topical ketorolac solution is transient burning and stinging sensation on instillation. Otherwise, it is a safe medication in ocular allergy disorder.

TOPICAL STEROIDS

Glucocorticoids exert a potent anti-inflammatory effect in allergic ocular disorders but are reserved for refractory cases unresponsive to other know antiallergy agents because of their potential side effects specially risk of cataract formation, steroid induced glaucoma and decreased resistance to infection.

Topical loteprednol (0.5%), rimexolone (1%), fluorometholone FML (0.3%) are new potent steroid with marked anti-inflammatory properties but with a reduced propensity to elevate intraocular pressure (an important side effect with previous generation topical steroids, e.g. dexamethasone, betamethasone, hydrocortisone and prednisolone).

- Topical loteprednol, rimexolone and FML effectively suppresses inflammation in allergic conjunctivitis.
- They inhibit leukocyte accumulation better than dexamethasone.
- Microfine suspension helps in uniform distribution and rapid absorption
- Proven safety in children also.

TOPICAL IMMUNOSUPPRESSORS

Topical immunosuppressor therapy in ocular allergic disorders is recently introduced anti-allergy agent with promising results.

Cyclosporine

It is a cyclic peptide that exerts a potent immunosuppressive effect by acting specifically on lymphocytes particularly CD4+ T cells. Cyclosporine inhibits transcription of interleukin-2 (IL-2) as well as other cytokines such as interferon, gamma and other interleukins. Decreased IL-2 production by CD4+ cell results in decreased activation and in decreased levels of cytokines which in turn results in inhibition of cell mediated immunity.

Topical cyclosporine 2 percent has been clinically tried with a dosage of (instill one drop in the affected eye four times a day) in patients of vernal keratoconjunctivitis and atopic keratoconjunctivitis (AKC). There was complete improvement in symptoms of ocular allergic disorders in 6 weeks of treatment in more than 80 percent of patients. Cyclosporine is also effective in reducing signs and symptoms of atopic keratoconjunctivitis. In a recent study topical cyclosporine therapy was correlated with a significant reduction in numbers of T-cells and plasma cells in the conjunctiva of patients with vernal keratoconjunctivitis.

Unlike systemic cyclosporine, topical preparation is relatively free of adverse effects and holds a promising future in the treatment of various ocular allergic disorders.

RECENT ADVANCES IN IMMUNOSUPPRESSIVE THERAPY

- Active research is going on competitive inhibition of IgE binding to effector cells using Fc fragments from human IgE. Isolation of the specific binding site and fragment production with recombinant DNA technology may allow selective inhibition of mast cells or eosinophils in ocular allergic disorders.

- Adhesion molecules are proteins that allow cells to interact with one another. In patients of SAC and VKC, there is a marked increase in conjunctival expression of ICAM-1, ICAM-3 and other adhesion molecules when compared to normal.

    Intensive efforts are going on in developing specific therapeutic agents that can modulate these adhesion molecule (proteins) and diminish the allergic response.
- Clinical trials are going on in development of suitable therapeutic agents that could modulate the actions of cytokines such as IL-3, IL-5 and GM-CSF suppressing aspects of the immune response that are not strongly affected by current available medications. A better clinical understanding of the role of specific cytokines in the different ocular allergic disorders shall stimulate the development of tailoring therapeutic agents to each of these entities.

Liposomes

New drug delivery systems may offer advantages in future therapy for ocular allergic disorders. Liposomes are vesicles consisting of lipid bilayers alternating with aqueous compartments. They may provide several advantages over current therapeutic modalities in ocular diseases.

- These allow prolonged contact between the medication and ocular tissue by preventing excessive rapid drug removal via tears.
- Changes in lipid composition and liposome structure can alter the amount of intraocular drug absorption.
- Incorporation of monoclonal antibodies into outer lipid bilayer of the liposome would transport the liposome to the target tissue or cell type where the drug is required.

A safe liposome system is now available for ocular use. Cationic lipids such as BDSA can be added to the outer surface of liposomes thereby increasing the contact time of medication with ocular tissues. This liposome system cause minimal eye irritation and may prove valuable in clinical treatment of ocular allergy.

BIBLIOGRAPHY

1. Agarwal A. Textbook of Ophthalmology, 1st edn. New Delhi: Jaypee Brothers Medical Publishers, 2002.
2. Bartlett JD. Clinical Ocular Pharmacology, 4th edn. Boston: Butterworth-Heinemann, 2001.
3. Bartlett JD. Ophthalmic Drug Facts, Lippincott – William and Wilkins, 2001.
4. Bartlett JD, Ross RN. Primary Care of Ocular Allergy. J Am Optom Assoc. 1990; 61: S3-46.
5. Ciprandi G, et al. Drug Treatment Allergic Conjunctivitis: Drugs, 1992;43:154.
6. Crick RP, Trimble RB. Textbook of Clinical Ophthalmology, Hodder and Stoughton, 1986.

7. Duane TD. Clinical Ophthalmology, 4th edn. Butterworth – Heinemann, 1999.
8. Duvall. Ophthalmic Medications and Pharmacology, Slack Inc, 1998.
9. Ellis PP. Ocular Therapeutics and Pharmacology, 7th edn. CV Mosby, 1985.
10. Fechner. Ocular Therapeutics, Slack Inc., 1998.
11. Fraunfelder. Current Ocular Therapy, 5th edn. WB Saunders, 2000.
12. Garg A. Current Trends in Ophthalmology, 1st edn. New Delhi: Jaypee Brothers Medical Publishers, 1997.
13. Garg A. Manual of Ocular Therapeutics, 1st edn. New Delhi: Jaypee Brothers Medical Publishers, 1996.
14. Garg A. Ready Reckoner of Ocular Therapeutics, 1st edn. New Delhi: 2002.
15. Goodman LS, Gilman A. Pharmacological Basis of Therapeutics, 7th edn, New York: Macmillan, 1985.
16. Havener's. Ocular Pharmacology, 6th edn. CV Mosby, 1994.
17. Kanski. Clinical Ophthalmology, 4th edn. Butterworth – Heineman, 1999.
18. Kershner. Ophthalmic Medications and Pharmacology, Slack. Inc., 1994.
19. Olin BR, et al. Drugs Facts and Comparisons: Facts and Comparisons, St. Louis, 1997.
20. Onofrey. The Ocular Therapeutics; Lippincott-William and Wilkins, 1997.
21. Rhee. The Wills Eye Drug Guide, Lippincott–William and Wilkins, 1998.
22. Steven Podos. Textbook of Ophthalmology, New Delhi: Jaypee Brothers Medical Publishers, 2001.
23. Zimmerman. Textbook of Ocular Pharmacology, Lippincott and William and Wilkins, 1997.

Local Anesthetic Agents

Ashok Garg (India)

INTRODUCTION

In modern ophthalmology with the preponderance of elderly patients (due to increased life expectancy) and the move towards the hightech outpatient surgical care, there is a growing emphasis and need of local anesthesia.

Local anesthesia is lifeline of modern ophthalmic surgery and is safer and should always be used unless there are specific indications for general anesthesia. Local anesthesia in the eye may be achieved by topical application of anesthetic drops or by infiltration of the sensory nerves with anesthetic solution (injectables).

LOCAL ANESTHETICS (INJECTABLES)

Local anesthetics prevent the generation and conduction of nerve impulses by reducing sodium permeability increasing the electrical excitation threshold slowing the nerve impulses propagation and reducing the rate of rise of the action potential.

Indications

Local injectable anesthetics are indicated for infiltration anesthesia in any kind of intraocular surgery.

Contraindications

Hypersensitivity to local anesthetics, para-aminobenzoic acid or parabens. Do not use large doses of local anesthetics in patients with heart block.

Precautions during Local Injectable Anesthesia

- Use local anesthetic with caution when there is inflammation or sepsis in the region of proposed injection.
- Monitor cardiovascular respiratory vital signs and state of consciousness after each injection.
- Local anesthetic should be injected with great care in debilitated or elderly patients, acutely ill patients, children and patients with increased intra-abdominal pressure or patients with severe shock or heart block.

- Many drugs used during local anesthesia are considered as potential triggering agents for familial malignant hyperthermia hence the arrangement for supplemental general anesthesia should be there.
- Use solutions containing a vasoconstrictor with great caution in patients with history of hypertension, peripheral vascular disease, arteriosclerotic heart disease, cerebral vascular insufficiency, heart block, thryotoxicosis diabetes. These patients may exhibit exaggerated vasoconstrictor response.
- Watch for hypersensitivity reactions including anaphylaxis to any component of local anesthetics.
- Administer ester type local anesthetics cautiously to patients with abnormal or reduced levels of plasma esterases.
- Some of these anesthetic products contain sulfites which may cause allergic type reactions in certain susceptible patients. Although prevalence of sulfite sensitivity is low.
- Use amide type local anesthetics with care in patients with impaired hepatic function.
- Use local anesthetics with caution in patients with renal disease.
- Exercise caution regarding toxic equivalence when mixtures of local anesthetics are employed.
- Do not use disinfecting agents containing heavy metals for skin (Periorbital area) disinfection.
- Do not use local anesthetics in any condition in which a sulphonamide drug is employed.
- Patients should be asked to avoid touching or rubbing the eye until the anesthesia is worn off.

Adverse Reactions of Local Injectable Anesthetics

The most common acute adverse reactions are related to the CNS and cardiovascular systems. These are generally dose related and may result from rapid absorption from the injection site, from diminished tolerance or from unintentional intravascular injections.

CNS Adverse Reactions

Restlessness, anxiety, dizziness, tinnitus, blurred vision, tremors, convulsions, nausea, vomiting, chills, pupil constriction excitement may be transient or absent.

Depressive effects: These may or may not be preceded by the excitatory symptoms. These are: drowsiness, sedation, generalized CNS depression, unconsciousness, coma, apnea and respiratory depression and even death from respiratory arrest.

Cardiovascular Symptoms of Toxicity

- Peripheral vasodilation
- Hypertension and tachycardia
- Decreased cardiac output

- Hypotension
- Bradycardia
- Methemoglobinemia
- Heart block, ventricular arrhythmias
- Circulatory collapse.

Allergic Adverse Reactions

- Cutaneous lesions of late onset
- Erythema, angioneurotic edema
- Sneezing, syncope
- Excessive sweating
- Elevated temperature and anaphylactoid symptoms.

Overdosage

Acute emergencies from local injectable anesthetics are generally related to high plasma levels encountered during therapeutic use or to unintended subarachnoid injection overdosage can lead to:
- Convulsions, apnea and under ventilation
- Circulatory depression.

If not treated promptly, convulsions and cardiovascular depression can result in hypoxia, acidosis, bradycardia, arrhythmias and cardiac arrest. Various local injectable anesthetics used in ophthalmology are classified as follows:

Esters
- Procaine
- Chloroprocaine
- Tetracaine.

Amides
- Lidocaine
- Prilocaine
- Mepevacaine
- Bupivacaine
- Etidocaine
- Centbucridine

Individual drug monographs are described as follows:

ESTERS

Procaine

Procaine is para-aminobenzoic acid ester of diethylaminoethanol. It was first prepared in 1905. Its chemical structure is shown in Figure 13.1.

Indication: Procaine is used for infiltration anesthesia prior to any intraocular surgery. It is not used topically.

Dosage: It is available as 1 percent (2 ml) ampoules. It has rapid onset of action (2-5 minutes) with an average duration of action one hour.

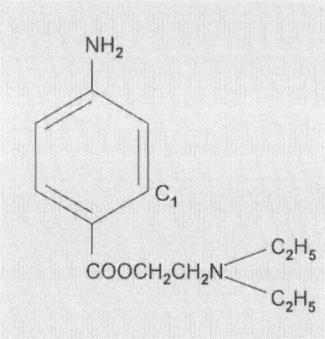

Fig. 13.1: Chemical structure of procaine

Concentration of 0.5–2 percent are used with a maximum dose of 14 mg/kg body weight.

Detoxification occurs by hydrolysis to para-amino-benzoic acid and dietheylaminoethanol through the enzyme pseudocholinesterase in the plasma.

Solution for infiltration anesthesia is freshly prepared. To prepare 60 ml of 0.5 percent solution (5 mg/ml) dilute 30 ml of 1 percent solution with 30 ml sterile distilled water.

Add 0.5–1 ml of epinephrine (1:1000 per 100 ml anesthetic solution for vasoconstrictive effect (1:200000 to 1:100000).

Precautions and adverse reactions have already been described in general monograph section of local injectable anesthetics.

Chloroprocaine

Chloroprocaine is a 2 chloro–4 aminobenzoate ester of b-diethyl aminoethanol. It was introduced in 1952 as an analog of procaine. Its chemical structure is shown in Figure 13.2.

Chloroprocaine is used for infiltration anesthesia in concentrations of 0.5–2 percent. Onset of anesthesia is very rapid (2–5 minutes) and the average duration of action lasts for 1½ hours. It is twice as potent as procaine and has similar pharmacological properties. Metabolism is largely through hydrolysis by pseudocholinesterase in the plasma.

Tetracaine (Amethocaine)

Tetracaine is a para-butylaminobenzoic acid ester of dimethylaminoethanol. It was first prepared in 1933. Its chemical structure is shown in Figure 13.3.

Tetracaine is used for infiltration as well as topical anesthesia.

Dosage: It is available in conc of 0.25–2 percent solutions. Tetracaine is a potent and toxic local anesthetic and dangerous over dosage may occur if it is given in doses higher than 1.5 mg/kg body weight.

It should be given with caution for infiltration anesthesia purpose.

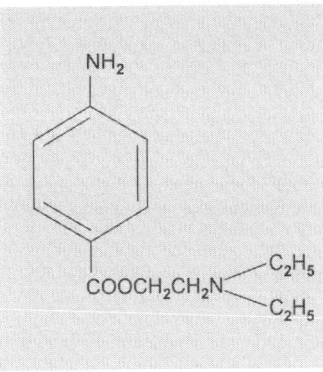

Fig. 13.2: Chemical structure of chloroprocaine

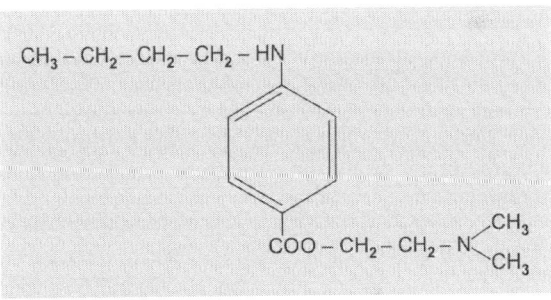

Fig. 13.3: Chemical structure of tetracaine

AMIDES

Lidocaine

It is one of the most common local injectable anesthetic agent used in ophthalmic surgery worldwide.

Lidocaine is 2-diethylamino-2'-6'-acetoxylidide. It was first prepared in 1948. Its chemical structure is shown in Figure 13.4.

Indication: Lidocaine 2 percent is used for infiltration anesthesia prior to any type of intraocular surgery.

Dosage: It is available in conc of 0.5–4 percent as lidocaine hydrochloride (2, 5 ml ampoules and 30 ml and 50 ml vials). For infiltration anesthesia generally 1 percent and 2 percent solutions are used (In 2 ml, 5 ml and 10 ml ampoules; 30 and 50 ml vials). It has rapid onset of action (0.5–2 minute) and average duration of action lasts for 1½ – 2 hours.

Lidocaine is metabolized in the liver to xylidine and diethyl amino acetic acid or is directly excreted into the urine and bile.

For infiltration anesthesia it is generally given with mixture of adrenaline and hyaluronidase to prolong the anesthetic effect and

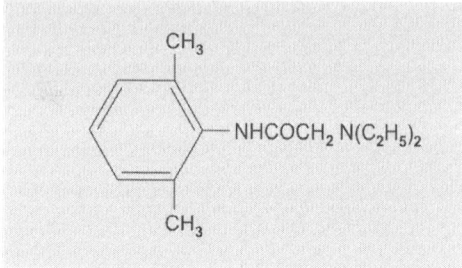

Fig. 13.4: Chemical structure of lidocaine

better diffusion to the ocular tissue. Hyaluronidase is an enzyme capable of depolymerizing hyaluronic acid found in interstitial spaces and when it gets depolymerized, fluid passes more easily between the tissues. Preferably 1:100000 solution of adrenaline conc is used and it causes sufficient vasospasm to reduce signficantly the rate of removal of local anesthetic agent. A correctly placed Retrobulbar or peribulbar injection of this solution causes complete akinesia and anesthesia of the globe. Hyaluronidase is also mixed with 2 percent lidocaine and adrenaline injection for better diffusion of solution into the tissues. It increases the effective area of anesthesia by 40 percent though inevitably of shorter duration.

Various lidocaine combinations available commercially are:
- Lidocaine HCl 0.5–2 percent with 1:100000 to 1:200000 epinephrine (in 5 ml and 10 ml ampoules, 20, 30 and 50 ml vials).
- Lidocaine HCl 1.5–5 percent with 7.5 percent dextrose (in 2 ml ampoules).

Safe dose for lidocaine HCl is — 7 mg/kg body weight with vasoconstrictors and 2.9 mg/kg body weight without vasoconstrictors. Recently preservative free 1 percent lidocaine hydrochloride (0.5 ml) ampoules have been available commercially for intracameral use during intraocular surgery.

Usual dosage is to inject 0.25 cc of 1 percent preservative free lidocaine into the anterior chamber through the cannula through 1 mm stab incision made in the peripheral cornea, 5 seconds later eye is anesthetized.

Advantages of intracameral injection of lidocaine:
- It relieves all discomfort and apprehension of the patient.
- It decreases the need of sedation.
- Surgery is quicker and less tense and patient respond faster with no complications or adverse effects.
- Has an excellent deeper depth of anesthesia.
- Eliminates blocks and their potential complications.
- Has good effect in conjunction with topical anesthesia.

Prilocaine

Prilocaine is a-propylamino – 2 methyl proprionanilide. It was first prepared in 1960. Its chemical structure is shown in Figure 13.5.

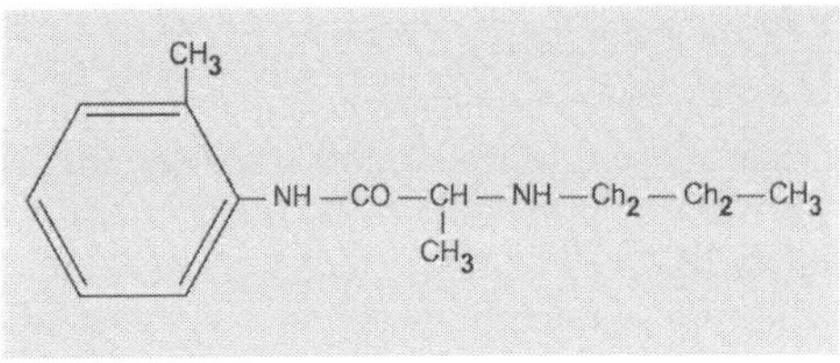

Fig. 13.5: Chemical structure of prilocaine

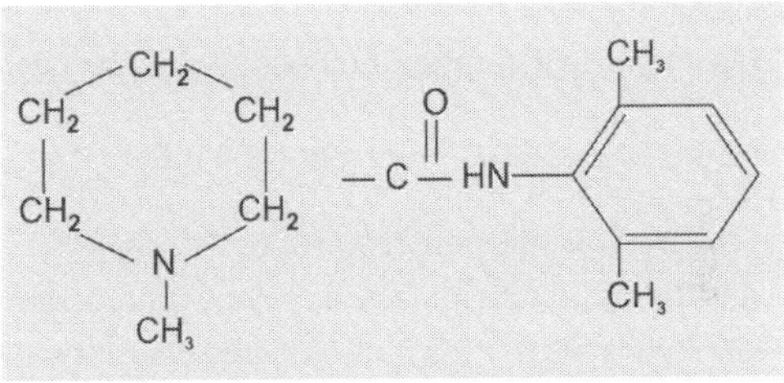

Fig. 13.6: Chemical structure of mepivacaine

Its pharmacological properties are similar to those of lidocaine and its onset of action takes 5–15 minutes and duration of action lasts for 1–3 hours.

It is used for infiltration and regional nerve block anesthesia. It is available in conc of 0.5–3 percent. The suggested maximum dose is 10 mg/kg body weight.

An unusual toxic effects are seen after administration of large doses (more than 800 mg) is cyanosis due to methemoglobinemia.

Mepivacaine

It is N-methyl pipecolic acid 2,6 dimethyl anilide. It was first prepared in 1956. Its chemical structure is shown in Figure 13.6. Mepivacaine has pharmacological properties similar to those of lidocaine. Notable exception is its effect on blood vessels. It is shown to have mild vasoconstrictor effect which reduces its absorption. The effect of mepivacaine on the peripheral circulation is a potentiation of the action of norepinephrine on nerve endings. The onset of action starts within 3–5 minutes and duration of action is from 2–2½ hours (with epinephrine). The suggested maximum dose is 7.0 mg/kg body weight.

It is used for infiltration and nerve block anesthesia.

Dosage: It is commercially available as mepivacaine HCl 1–2 percent injectable solutions (in 20, 30 and 50 ml vials). For infiltration anesthesia 1 percent conc is used.

Bupivacaine

It is structurally similar to mepivacaine and is one of the common anesthetic agent used in the ophthalmology for infiltration anesthesia. It was first prepared in 1963. Its chemical structure is shown in Figure 13.7.

Bupivacaine is 3-4 times more potent than lidocaine. Its onset of action starts within 5-10 minutes and duration of action lasts for 3-5 hours (with epinephrine).

Dosage: It is available as bupivacaine HCl injectable solution in conc of 0.25-0.75 percent (in 2 ml ampoules and 10, 30 and 50 ml vials). For retrobulbar or peribulbar injection 0.75 percent strength solution is used.

It is also available in combination with epinephrine commercially.

Bupivacaine HCl 0.25-0.75 percent (in 2 ml ampoules, 10 ml, 30 ml and 50 ml vials).

The maximum safe dose is 2.0 mg/kg body weight.

Practically for infiltration anesthesia prior to intraocular surgery, it is used in combination of 2 percent lidocaine to produce complete akinesia and anesthesia of globe for more than 2 hours. Usually 50:50 percent of both solutions (0.5% bupivacaine HCl and 2% lidocaine HCl in addition to adrenaline and hylase) are used to produce anesthesia for major ocular surgeries.

Etidocaine

It is used for infiltration anesthesia in ophthalmic surgery.

It is available as 0.5-1 percent injectable solutions (in 30 ml vials and 20 ml ampoules). Its onset of action starts in 5-15 minutes and duration of action lasts for 3-5 hours. It is also available commercially with epinephrine. Etidocaine HCl 1.0-1.5 percent with 1:20000 epinephrine (30 ml vials).

Centbucridine

It is 4-N-butylamino-1,2,3,4, tetrahydroacridine hydrochloride. It is recently introduced anesthetic agent. It has been shown 5-8 times more potent than lidocaine.

It is used for infiltration anesthesia and topical anesthesia.

Dosage: It is available as 0.5 percent centbucridine injectable solution (in 10 ml and 30 ml vials).

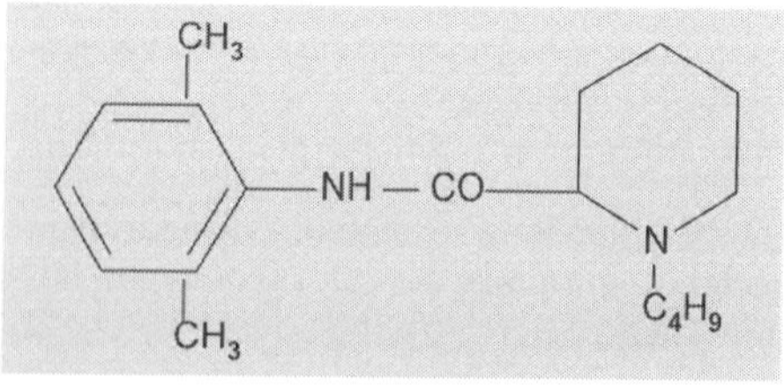

Fig. 13.7: Chemical structure of bupivacaine

Its onset of action starts in 2–5 minutes and duration of action lasts for 1–1½ hours.

LOCAL ANESTHETICS (TOPICAL)

Topical anesthesia is mainstay of modern ophthalmic surgery. Topical anesthesia is now widely used from superficial minor surgery of conjunctiva and cornea to hightech phacoemulsification, Excimer laser PRK and lasik surgery. Topical anesthetic agents produce their effect by blocking nerve conduction in the superficial cornea and conjunctiva. The physiological effect of all topical anesthetic agents occurs in a similar fashion. They work at the level of cell membrane by preventing the sodium flux by closing the pores through which the ions migrate in the lipid layer of nerve cell membrane. The anesthetics agents block conduction of afferent nerve impulses thereby abolishing sensation and producing local anesthetic action.

Indications

Corneal anesthesia of short duration for any diagnostic and surgical procedure on the eye.

Contraindications

Known hypersensitivity to the drug or to any other ingradient in these preparations. Prolonged used specially for self-medication is not recommended.

Precautions

These anesthetic agents are for topical ophthalmic use only. Prolonged use is not recommended as it may diminish duration of anesthesia, retard wound healing and cause epithelial erosions. It may produce permanent corneal opacification with accompanying visual loss, severe keratitis, scarring or corneal perforation, if signs of sensitivity develops discontinue the use.
- Tolerance varies with the status of the patient. Give debilitated, elderly or acutely ill patients reduced doses commensurate with their weight, age and physical status.
- Use with caution in patients with abnormal or reduced levels of plasma esterases.
- Use with caution in patients with known allergies, cardiac disease or hyperthyroidism.
- Protection of the eye from irritating chemicals, foreign bodies and rubbing during the period of anesthesia is important.

Adverse Reactions

On topical use these anesthetic agents may cause:
- Mild stinging and burning sensation, vasodilation
- Shortening of tear break-up time

- Decreased blinking
- Corneal edema
- Decreased epithelial mitosis and migration
- Slow epithelial healing
- Punctate epithelial keratitis
- Epithelial desquamation
- Allergic reactions of lid and conjunctiva
- Iritis.

Various anesthetic agents used in ophthalmology as topical agents are:
- Benoxinate
- Proparacaine
- Tetracaine
- Lidocaine
- Centbucridine
- Cocaine
- Phenacaine
- Dimethocaine
- Piperocaine
- Dibucaine
- Naepaine
- Butacaine.

In today ophthalmic surgery and in diagnostic procedures proparacaine, benoxinate and tetracaine are commonly used. Their action starts within 15–20 seconds and effects last for 15–20 minutes.

Other topically applied anesthetic agent is 4 percent xylocaine, its use is becoming lesser and lesser due to problems with irritation, allergy, etc.

Individual drug monograph of topical anesthetic agent is as follows:

Benoxinate HCl (Oxybuprocaine)

It is a para-aminobenzoic acid ester. Its chemical structure is shown in Figure 13.8.

It is available as 0.4 percent topical solution. Its action starts within 10 seconds of topical instillation and effect last for 15 minutes. 1 to 2 drops of 0.4 percent solution is sufficient to anesthetize the cornea. For deep anesthesia 3 instillations at 90 second interval is sufficient. Because of high degree of safety, it is most suitable for topical use.

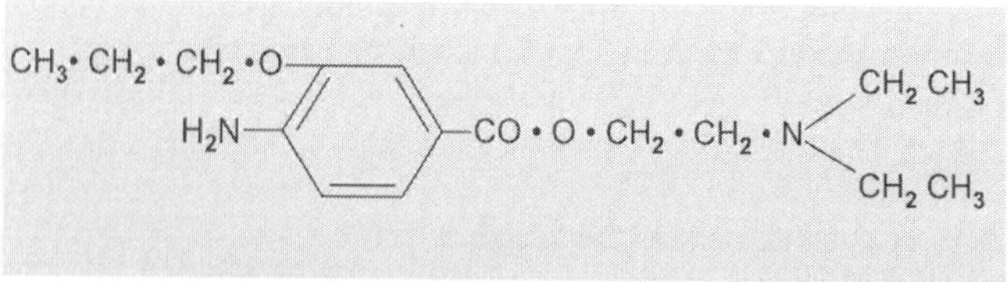

Fig. 13.8: Chemical structure of benoxinate

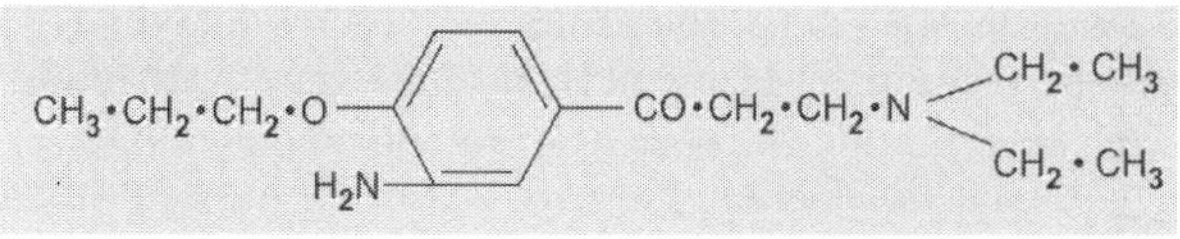

Fig. 13.9: Chemical structure of proparacaine

It is also available as 0.4 percent benoxinate HCl solution with 0.25 percent fluorescein sodium (in 5 ml pack). It is associated with less irritation on instillation.

Another topical anesthetic agent having properties and uses similar to benoxinate is proxymetacaine (0.5%).

Proparacaine

It is one of the most common topical anesthetic agent used for topical anesthesia in intraocular surgery (phacoemulsification, cataract surgery, excimer laser PRK and lasik surgery).

Proparacaine is a benzoic acid ester. Its chemical structure is shown in Figure 13.9.

Proparacaine is available as 0.5 percent and 0.75 percent topical solution. It is used 2-5 minutes prior to intraocular surgery.

Its effect starts within 15-20 seconds and lasts for 15 minutes. Potency is similar to that of tetracaine. Maximum Dose is 10 mg (About 20 drops of 0.5 percent solution on topical instillation).

Due to higher degree of potency and safety, it is most appropriate choice for topical ocular anesthesia. It is available as 0.5 percent proparacaine HCl solution and 0.25 percent fluorescein sodium.

Tetracaine

It is parabutylaminobenzoic acid ester of dimethy lamino ethanol.

It is one of the most popular topical anesthetic agent currently used in ophthalmology.

It is available as 0.25-1 percent topical solution usually 0.5 percent strength is used for topical anesthesia.

Tetracaine HCl penetrates tissue more deeply than proparacaine and benoxinate.

Its action starts in 20 seconds and last for 10-12 minutes after topical instillation. It is instilled 2-5 minutes prior to the surgery. 1-2 drops are instilled topically 2-3 times at 60 second duration. Maximum dose is 5 mg (10 drops to each eye of 0.5% solution).

On topical instillation however it produces stinging sensation for 30 seconds.

Lidocaine HCl

Lidocaine is 2-diethyl amino, 2,6 acetoxylidine.

Prior to introduction of topical benoxinate, proparacaine and tetracaine anesthetic agents 4 percent lidocaine HCl was commonly used for topical anesthesia.

One drop of 4 percent lidocaine solution renders the cornea anesthetized within 30–60 seconds and effect lasts for 10 minutes.

It is rapidly acting and does not cause dilation of pupil.

On topical instillation however it causes marked stinging sensation for 30 seconds.

Due to its stinging sensation problem, it is now less commonly used for topical anesthesia purpose.

Centbucridine

It is recently introduced topical anesthetic agent.

It is available as one percent topical solution and effect lasts for 15 minutes.

It causes very less stinging than four percent. Lidocaine and is safe on topical use. Usual dosage is one drop to be instilled topically and sufficient to produce topical anesthesia.

Cocaine

It is an alkaloid of erythoxylon coca. It was first introduced in 1884. Its chemical structure is shown in Figure 13.10.

Cocaine was quite extensively used in late fifties of last century. It is available as topical solution in concentration of 1–10 percent as cocaine HCl. One drop of 2 percent solution renders the cornea anesthetize within 30 seconds and effect lasts for 12 minutes.

Maximum dose is 20 mg (about 10 drops to each eye of 2% solution). It is however toxic directly to corneal epithelium. It may be used to aid penetration of the other drugs (like cycloplegics) into the cornea and anterior chamber. Cocaine causes mydriasis and when absorbed systemically it may be associated with dangerous drug interactions and hypertensive crisis and CNS stimulation. Toxic doses of coccaine cause fatal circulatory and respiratory collapse. It is now not commonly used for topical purpose as better topical agents are available.

Phenocaine

It is derivative of phenetiden. It is N, N, bis (p-ethoxy-phenyl) acetamidine. Its chemical structure is shown in Figure 13.11.

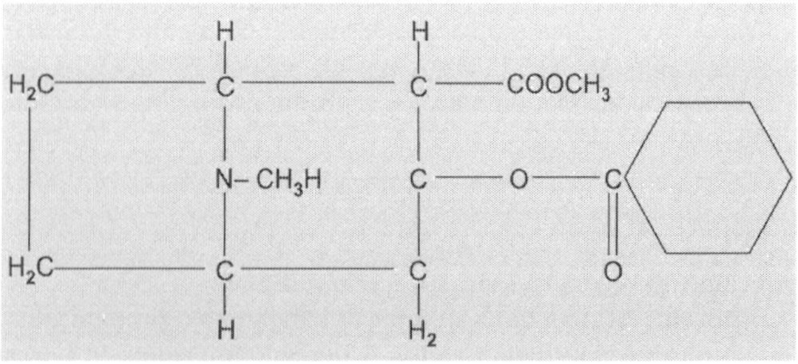

Fig. 13.10: Chemical structure of cocaine

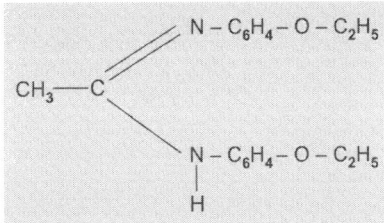

Fig. 13.11: Chemical structure of phenocaine

As it is not an ester, it can be considered as an alternative agent for use in patient sensitive to ester group.

It is used as 1 percent topical solution for instillation. Phenacaine is no longer used because it causes excessive irritation and highly toxic.

Dimethocaine

It was first prepared in 1932. It is 3-diethylamino, 2,2 dimethyl propyl p-aminobenzoate. Its chemical structure is shown in Figure 13.12. It has been used in ophthalmology as topical agent in conc of 2-5 percent. It is derivative of para-aminobenzoic acid.

Piperocaine

It is benzoic acid ester of methyl piperidinopropanol. Its chemical structure is shown in Figure 13.13. It is used as topical 2 percent solution for topical anesthesia. It has effect of regeneration of corneal epithelium.

Piperocaine alongwith lidocaine are the only agents associated with normal healing of the cornea.

Dibucaine

Dibucaine is 2 butoxy-N (2-diethyl aminoethyl) cinchoninamide. It is quinolone derivative and is not an ester. Its chemical structure is shown in Figure 13.14

Dibucaine is probably the most potent local anesthetic agent but its use has declined because of toxicity. It is used as 0.1 percent topical solution for instillation.

Naepaine

It is mono-n-amylaminoethyl-p-aminobenzoate. Its chemical structure is shown in Figure 13.15.

One topical use, it does not cause mydriasis or alteration in intraocular pressure not it is associated with local irritation. It is derivative of para-aminobenzoic acid and is used as 2-4 percent topical ophthalmic solution.

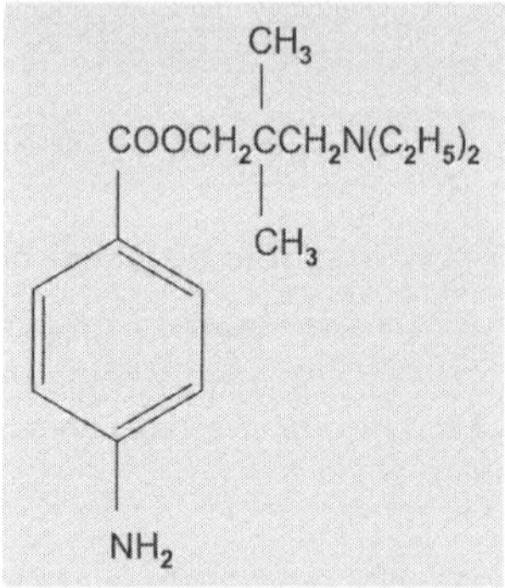

Fig. 13.12: Chemical structure of dimethocaine

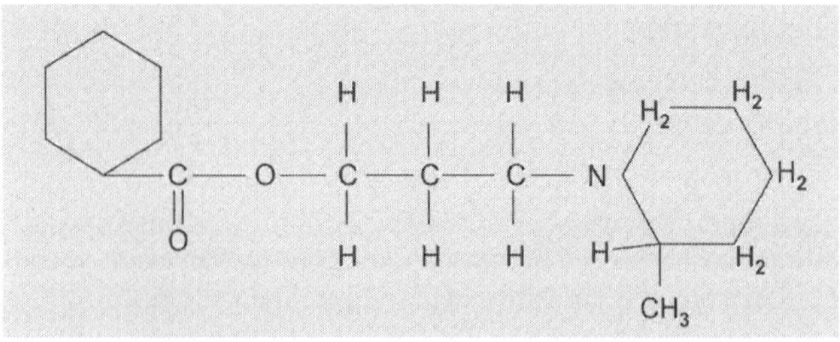

Fig. 13.13: Chemical structure of piperocaine

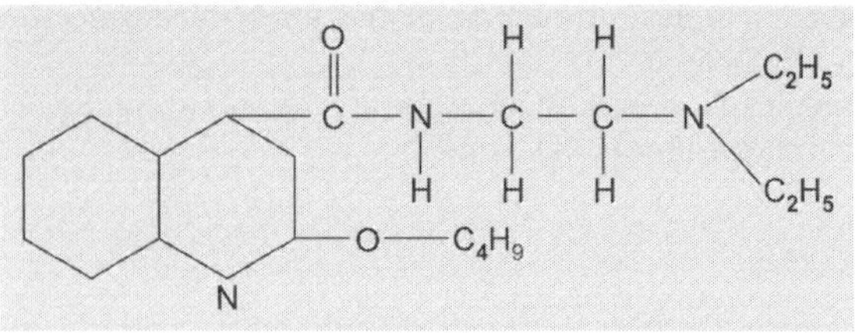

Fig. 13.14: Chemical structure of dibucaine

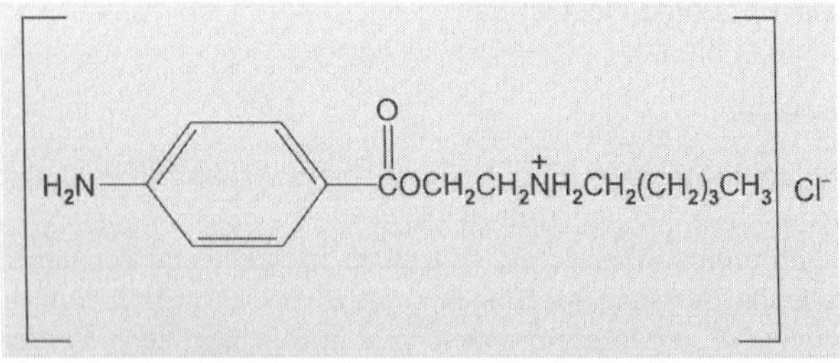

Fig. 13.15: Chemical structure of naepaine

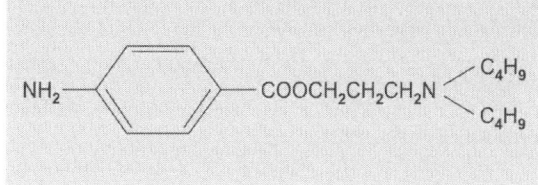

Fig. 13.16: Chemical structure of butacaine

Butacaine

It is para-aminobenzoic acid ester of dibutylamino- propanol. Its chemical structure is shown in Figure 13.16.

It is used topically as 2 percent solution.

SYNOPSIS OF OPHTHALMIC USES OF LOCAL ANESTHETICS

Local Injectable Anesthetics

- Facial nerve block
- Retrobulbar anesthesia
- Peribulbar anesthesia
- Eyelid infiltration.

Topical Anesthetics

For intraocular surgery like:
- Cataract surgery
- IOL implantation
- Phacoemulsification
- Excimer laser PRK and lasik surgery
- Gonioscopy
- Tonometry
- Fundus contact lens biomicroscopy
- Evaluation of corneal abrasions
- Forced duction testing
- Schirmer tear testing
- Electroretinography
- Lacrimal dilation and irrigation
- Contact lens fitting
- Superficial foreign body removal
- Minor surgery of conjunctiva
- Suture removal
- Corneal epithelial debridement.

BIBLIOGRAPHY

1. Agarwal A. Textbook of Ophthalmology, 1st edn. New Delhi: Jaypee Brothers Medical Publishers, 2002.

2. Bartlett JD. Clinical Ocular Pharmacology, 4th edn. Boston: Butterworth-Heinemann, 2001
3. Bartlett JD. Ophthalmic Drug Facts: Lippincott–William and Wilkins, 2001.
4. Bryant JA. Local and Topical Anesthetics in Ophthalmology, Surv. Ophthalmol, 1969;13:263.
5. Crick RP, Trimble RB. Textbook of Clinical Ophthalmology, Hodder and Stoughton, 1986.
6. Duane TD. Clinical Ophthalmology, 4th edn. Boston: Butterworth-Heinemann, 1999.
7. Duvall. Ophthalmic Medications and Pharmacology, Slack Inc, 1998.
8. Ellis. PP. Ocular Therapeutics and Pharmacology, 7th edn. CV Mosby, 1985.
9. Fechner. Ocular Therapeutics, Slack Inc., 1998.
10. Forrest. Anesthesia in Ophthalmic Surgery: Butterworth – Heinemann, 1997.
11. Fraunfelder. Current Ocular Therapy, 5th edn. WB Saunders, 2000.
12. Garg A. Current Trends in Ophthalmology, 1st edn. New Delhi: Jaypee Brothers Medical Publishers, 1997.
13. Garg A. Manual of Ocular Therapeutics, 1st edn. New Delhi: Jaypee Brothers Medical Publishers, 1996.
14. Garg A. Ready Reckoner of Ocular Therapeutics, 1st edn. New Delhi: 2002.
15. Gills. Ophthalmic Anaesthesia, Slack. Inc., 1993.
16. Goodman LS, Gilman A. Pharmacological Basis of Therapeutics, 7th edn. New York: Macmillan, 1985.
17. Greenbaum. Ocular Anaesthesia, WB Saunders, 1992.
18. Havener's. Ocular Pharmacology, 6th edn. CV Mosby, 1994.
19. Kanski. Clinical Ophthalmology, 4th edn. Butterworth – Heineman, 1999.
20. Kershner. Ophthalmic Medications and Pharmacology: Slack. Inc., 1994.
21. Mcgol drick. Ophthalmic Anaethesia, W.B. Saunders, 1992.
22. Olin BR, et al. Drugs Facts and Comparisons: Facts and Comparisons, St. Louis, 1997.
23. Onofrey. The Ocular Therapeutics; Lippincott-William and Wilkins, 1997.
24. Rhee. The Wills Eye Drug Guide, Lippincott–William and Wilkins, 1998.
25. Sobol WM, et al. Ocular Anaesthetic Properties and adverse reactions: Int. Ophthalmol. Clinic 1989; 29: 195.
26. Steven Podos. Textbook of Ophthalmology, New Delhi: Jaypee Brothers Medical Publishers, 2001.
27. Webster RB. Local Anaesthetics for Ophthalmic Use: Aust J Optom. 1974: 57: 399.
28. Zimmerman, Textbook of Ocular Pharmacology, Lippincott and William and Wilkins, 1997.

14

Ophthalmic Viscosurgical Devices and Other Ocular Surgical Adjuncts

Ashok Garg (India)

INTRODUCTION

Viscoelastic agents, irrigating solutions and enzymes are adjuncts to a variety of ophthalmological procedures and surgeries. These are vital components of any type of intraocular surgery.

First let me discuss various viscoelastic substances used in the ophthalmology.

VISCOELASTIC SUBSTANCES

The development of modern ophthalmic microsurgery has dramatically changed the facet of ocular surgery in many ways. But the increasing number of surgical steps also involves a greater risk of involuntary tissue damage. The field of microsurgery strategy is therefore not only the desired action on the tissue but also the prevention of undesired side effects on the surrounding tissue [Precision tissue specific action (PTSA)]. For this purpose space tactics are used.

Space tactics is a more active protection against touch by providing sufficient space for manipulation within the eye. It is accomplished by space maintaining or enlarging devices such as hydrodynamic flow systems or viscoelastic substances.

The term viscosurgery was coined by Prof Endre Balasz of USA to describe the use of solutions with viscous elastic, pseudoplastic properties during and after ocular surgery. Viscosity makes a material protective and lubricating while elasticity provides protection from vibrating instruments and other mechanical impacts. Pseudoplasticity allows the material to deform and may be used to safely manipulate tissue. While we perform intraocular viscosurgery. We actually use a viscoelastic agent as a fluid or soft surgical instrument because the molecules of a true viscoelastic can deform and reform.

CRITERIA FOR SELECTION OF VISCOELASTIC MATERIAL

Optical Properties

Materials suitable for intraocular use should not impair the visibility of the operation field. Transparency is primary prerequisite. A color slightly different from aqueous is useful for distinction.

Surface Tension

The specific weight of the injected material determines whether the bubble will raise or descend in the aqueous and whether it can be used to elevate or to depress the surrounding tissue.

Viscosity

Viscous fluids are ideal surface tools since layers deposited onto tissue implant surface will remain there. As space tactical tools viscous fluids are suitable in walled off cavities with small orifices (anterior chamber).

Elasticity

Elastic materials are resistant against deformation and therefore stable as to their shape. They are ideal space tactical tools since their action is independent of flow conditions.

Viscoelasticity

The viscoelastic solutions, the viscous and elastic responses to a mechanical force depends on the velocity of the impact. The optimal solution for surgical purposes is a substance with a transition from viscous to elastic behavior at relatively low velocities.

Miscellaneous

Viscoelastic agent should be easy to inject, (inert, non-inflammatory, nontoxic). No particles or clumps, causes less rise of IOP with low molecular weight viscoelastics. It must be hydrophilic enough and able to be diluted and should not prevent the movement of metabolites and waste products.

ROLES OF VISCOELASTIC SUBSTANCES

Roles of viscoelastic substances in intraocular surgery are:
- To maintain an anatomical situation created by surgeon and maintenance of anterior chamber
- To lubricate
- To protect and isolate newly created or restored tissue surfaces
- To prevent the formation of undesirable fibrin coagulum
- Protection of corneal endothelium from mechanical trauma
- To enable easy manipulation of tissues in the eye
- To provide coating ability to implants, instruments and corneal epithelial surface.

INDICATIONS FOR VISCOELASTIC SUBSTANCES

- Phacoemulsification
- IOL implantation
- Congenital cataract surgery
- Extracapsular cataract surgery

- For breaking synechiae as a soft instrument
- Posterior segment surgery
- Penetrating trauma surgery
- Strabismus surgery
- Corneal surgery
- Plastic surgery for congenital ptosis surgery.

COMMERCIALLY AVAILABLE VISCOELASTIC SUBSTANCES

Hyaluronic Acid

It is a natural compound of connective tissue. In the ocular cavities it is a major component of the vitreous and occurs as covering layer on the tissue surface of the anterior segment. Hyaluronic acid is not metabolized or degraded within the eye. It passes unaltered through the trabecular meshwork as a large molecule and is transported then with the blood flow to the liver. Hyaluronic acid is a linear polysaccharide composed of sodium glucuronate and N-acetyl glucosamine. The chain is unbranched and contains no intermolecular bridges.

Sodium Hyaluronate

Sodium hyaluronate (NaH), a large polysaccharide molecule is a viscoelastic substance. It is a natural biological product present nearly in all the connective tissues in living organisms from bacteria to human tissue. It stabilizes cells and tissues and hence protects cell from permanent deformation.

Various biological sources including the umbilical cord, bovine vitreous and rooster comb contain a large amount of sodium hyaluronate. Low molecular weight sodium hyaluronate may also be produced from streptococci by microbial fermentation. It is component of capsular material around streptococcal organisms. In the eye concentration of sodium hyaluronate is highest in cortical gel and trabecular angle and low in the aqueous humor and covering the endothelium.

Sodium hyaluronate has two fractions H3 inflammatory (if-Na-Ha) and noninflammatory (Nif-Na-Ha). For intraocular purpose noninflammatory fraction is used.

The molecular weight of sodium hyaluronate varies dramatically depending on the sources. The viscosity of sodium hyaluronate solution is influenced by the molecular weight, concentration and shear rate. At higher shear rate, the resistance of flow decreases and it remains constant at low shear rate. This typical pseudoplasticity is exhibited by sodium hyaluronate only. In 1980, Mitter and Stegmann introduced sodium hyaluronate for anterior segment surgery.

One percent sodium hyaluronate is true viscoelastic agent. It is highly viscous, elastic and pseudoplastic of very high molecular weight ($1.1 - 1.8 \times 10^6$). Its viscosity is 100,000–300,000 centi poise and molecular weight is about 4 million Daltons. It is non-allergic and clear. It is 1 percent solution of highly purified sodium hyaluronate from dermis of rooster combs. It consists of very large hyaluronic acid chains with high molecular weight. One of its greater advantage is that the transition from viscous to elastic behavior occurs even at low concentration and low velocities. Owing to its elasticity it can be injected through a 30 G cannula and still retains its original shape in aqueous. Besides space tactics tools, sodium hyaluronate also inhibits migration of lymphocytes, granulocytes and macrophages. It also inhibits phagocytic activity, synthesis and release of prostaglandins by macrophages during phagocytosis.

Sodium hyaluronate preparation is a specific fraction development for use in anterior segment and vitreous procedures as a viscoelastic agent. It is nonantigenic, does not cause inflammatory or foreign body reactions and has a high viscosity.

The 1 percent solution is transparent and remains in the anterior chamber for less than 6 days. It protects chamber for less than 6 days. It protects corneal endothelial cells and other ocular strucutres. It does not interfere with epithelization and normal wound healing.

Indications

It is used as ophthalmosurgical aid in various anterior segment procedures like:
- Phacoemulsification
- IOL implantation
- Facilitates capsulorrhexis
- Corneal transplant surgery
- Glaucoma surgery
- Reconstructive surgery following eye injury
- Various procedures of ocular microsurgery
- Vitreous replacement after retinal detachment surgery.

It is also used as surgical aid in posterior segment surgery to gently separate, maneuver and hold tissues.

It also creates a clear field of vision therapy facilitating photocoagulation and intra- and postoperative inspection of the retina.

It has also been used in the treatment of refractory dry eye syndrome.

Administration and Dosage

It is available as preloaded syringe with 27 G or 30 G cannula containing sodium hyaluronate 10 mg/ml or 14 mg/ml strength (in 0.25, 0.50, 0.80, 2 ml and 4 ml syringes). Store at 2–8°C and remains unaltered after 3–5 years at this temperature. Do not freeze. Use the drug at room temperature (Acclimatization at room temperature is necessary).

Dosage

For phacoemulsification/IOL implantation/ECCE during cataract surgery as soon as the anterior chamber is entered, the role of

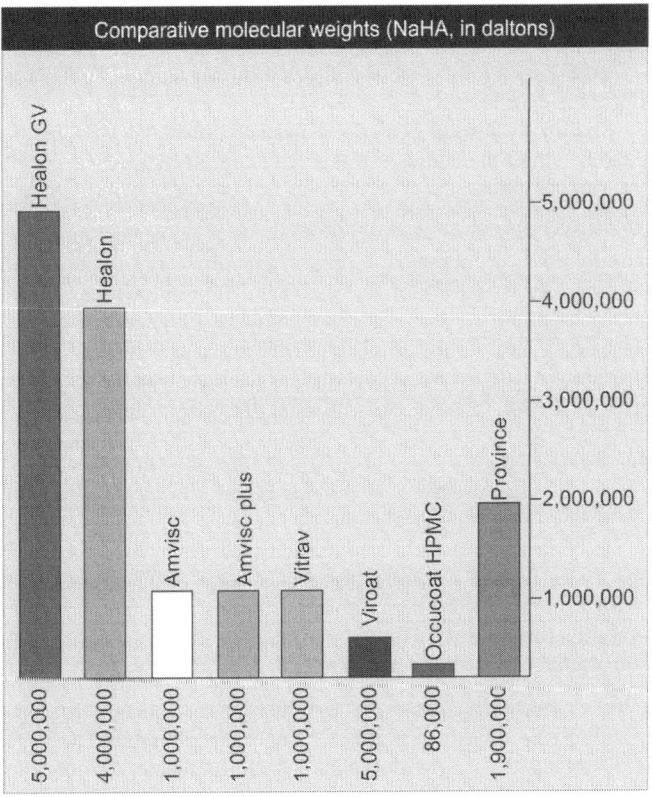

Fig. 14.1: Sodium hyaluronate and corneal endothelial protective mechanisms

viscoelastic begins. It fills, maintains and cushions the anterior chamber. During anterior capsulotomy it prevents scrolling up of margins.

Hydraulic separation of nucleus and cortex, synechiae (anterior or posterior) release can be easily done with sodium hyaluronate. When placed over the pupil, it gets dilated mechanically. It tamponades the bleeding vessels on iris or in wound. After capsulotomy it helps in viscoexpression of nucleus (after continuous curvilinear capsulorrhexis). It helps in plugging posterior capsule break and after dry aspiration. It makes phacoemulsification successful by coating corneal endothelial cells.

It protects anterior chamber angle during anterior chamber IOL insertion. It also acts as surgical instrument during anterior, posterior or iris clip lenses.

A sufficient amount is slowly introduced (using 27 G cannula or needle) into the anterior chamber.

Inject either before or after delivery of the lens. Injection before lens delivery protects the corneal endothelium from possible damage arising from removal of the cataractous lens. It may be used to coat surgical instruments and the IOL prior to the insertion.

Additional amount can be injected during surgery to replace any of the drug lost.

Sodium hyaluronate can be easily distinguished from vitreous. Vitreous sticks to cellulose sponge and cannot be washed out of anterior chamber.

Glaucoma filtration surgery: Intraoperative and postoperative maintenance of depth of anterior chamber and patency of filtering site is important for successful filtering surgery. Both are maintained by viscoelastic substances of high viscosity and elasticity. If left into the anterior chamber it also avoids hypotony and choroidal detachment postoperatively. It restores flat chamber after glaucoma. Injected early into the trabeculectomy it protects corneal endothelial cell loss. Sodium hyaluronate maintains full anterior chamber and normal IOP in eyes with ciliary block after glaucoma surgery. It also helps in anterior capsulotomy in presence of anterior capsule tear.

In conjunction with the performance of the trabeculectomy, inject slowly and carefully through a corneal paracentesis to reconstitute the anterior chamber. Further injection can be given to allow it to extrude into the subconjunctival filtration site through and around the sutured outer scleral flap.

Corneal transplant surgery: In penetrating keratoplasty, it helps in filling the anterior chamber prior to trephination. It coats and protects the new endothelial cells and delicate surrounding structures. Anterior and posterior synechiae can be released easily with its use.

After removal of corneal button, fill the anterior chamber with the drug, then suture the donor graft in place. An additional amount may be injected to replace the lost amount as a result of surgical manipulation. It has also been used in the anterior chamber of the donor eye prior to trephination to protect the corneal endothelial cells of the graft. Sodium hyaluronate facilitates the separation of deep stroma during dissection of stroma. It is known as viscodelamination of cornea.

Retinal reattachment surgery: Sodium hyaluronate is slowly introduced into the vitreous cavity. By directing the injection, it can be used to separate membranes away from the retina for safe excision and release of traction. It also serves to maneuver tissues into the desired position and aids in holding the retina against the sclera for reattachment.

A new viscoelastic gel, i.e. poly (1-vinyl-2-pyrrolidinone) hydrogel has been recommended as vitreous substitute.

VES like healon have been used as a surgical tool in maneuvering tissues, i.e. in dissection of epiretinal membranes in cases of proliferative diabetic retinopathy and macular pucker.

Healon yellow, its color facilitate injecting the viscoelastic substance under the membranes and simplified its removal at the end of surgery. Its use also helps in stopping the bleeding and reposition of a detached retina.

Strabismus surgery: There is role for sodium hyaluronate in adjustable strabismus surgery. The force needed to adjust suture postoperatively is less with viscoelastic substances specially with sodium hyaluronate. It lubricates the muscle and may decrease scarring in epimuscular tissue postoperatively.

Plastic surgery: During dacryocystorhinostomy (DCR) VES helps in identifying lacrimal sac and cut ends of a severed lacrimal canaliculus. It also lubricates fascia lata strips during congenital ptosis surgery.

Other uses: In postoperative suprachoroidal hemorrhage the intraocular use of sodium hyaluronate 10 percent facilitate hemorrhage drainage from sclerotomies site. It produces even distribution of hydraulic forces and hence pushes choroidals to its place.

The use of sodium hyaluronate has been shown in delineating the extent of cyclodialysis cleft. It reforms the chamber and provides maximum access for argon laser treatment.

Sodium hyaluronate is useful in dry eye, would healing and chemical burns. When placed on cornea it helps in preventing drying of cornea and surface.

Advantages of Hyaluronic Acid in Ophthalmic Viscomicrosurgery

- It ensures to maintain anterior chamber depth and visibility.
- It minimizes interaction between tissues and acts as temponade and vitreous substitute during retinal reattachment surgery.
- It also preserves tissue integrity and good visibility when use to fill the anterior and posterior segments of the eye following open sky procedures.
- It is a natural component of the tissues and is extremely well tolerated.
- It tends to counter-balance the vitreous thrust.
- It efficiently protects the intraocular structures.
- It is eliminated in relatively short time with no significant increase in postsurgical intraocular pressure.
- It does not have inflammatory reactions in the eye.
- It does not interfere with the physiological circulatory dynamics of the aqueous humor.
- It enhances the visibility of surgical field.
- It facilitates the insertion and the implantation of intraocular lenses and foldable lenses following phacoemulsification.
- Due to its lubricating and viscoelastic properties, transparency and ability to protect corneal endothelial cells is maintained.

At present there is no contraindications except for hypersensitivity reactions to the use of sodium hyaluronate solution when recommended for use in intraocular surgery.

Adverse Reactions

Although well-tolerated, a transient postoperative increase in IOP has been reported. Sometimes postoperative inflammatory reactions (iritis, hypopyon) corneal edema and corneal decompensation are also seen.

Precautions

Postoperative intraocular pressure may be elevated as a result of pre-existing glaucoma and by operative procedures and sequelae including enzymatic zonulysis, absence of an iridectomy, trauma to filtration structure and by blood and lenticular remnants in the anterior chamber.

- Do not overfill the anterior chamber, remove some of the preparation by irrigation or aspiration at the close of surgery (except in glaucoma surgery).
- Carefully monitor IOP specially during immediate postoperative period. Treat significant rise in IOP appropriately.
- In posterior segment surgery monitor rise in IOP after injection of large amounts of the drug (specially in aphakic diabetes).
- Hypersensitivity reactions as this preparation is extracted from avian tissues and contains minute amounts of protein, so potential risk of hypersensitivity may exist.
  Other preparations of sodium hyaluronate available commercially are as follows:

Hyalectin (IAL)

It is highly viscous 1 percent solution of sodium hyaluronate of lower molecular weight—1 million Daltons. It is less viscous and less elastic than Healon. It has special features like:
- It is eliminated in relatively short time with no increase in postsurgical intraocular pressure. Therefore there is no need to remove IAL after the operation.
- It does not give inflammatory reactions.
- It is a specialty whose active ingradient is a specific fraction of the hyaluronic acid sodium salt which is obtained by unique methodology based on sequential molecular ultrafiltration stages. This procedure allows the exclusion of low molecular weight fractions and gives a product characterized by a mean molecular weight in the range of 500000–730000 and with a very high degree of purity.
- The isotonic 1 percent aqueous solution of hyalectin (20 mg/2 ml) exhibits particular viscous characteristics which make it specially suitable for intraocular viscomicrosurgery.
- It provides an effective protection to ocular tissues vulnerable to surgical manipulations and it allows to preserve anatomical form and relationship among the various structures of the eye.
- IAL favorably differentiates from hyaluronic acid with very high molecular weight whenever such substances are left in the anterior chamber. IAL does not cause rise in postoperative IOP in comparison to hyaluronic acid with high molecular weight (which cause significant rise in postoperative IOP).
- It physically shields corneal endothelium, the lens and the angle structures during surgical procedures.

- IAL sets apart from each other traumatized tissues enhancing surgical repair and preventing formation of anterior and posterior synechiae.
- It helps in restoration and preservation of the ocular volume in reconstructive surgery following eye injury.

It is available as 1 percent solution in preloaded disposable syringes (2 ml).

Sodium Hyaluronate and Chondroitin Sulfate Solution

Viscoat

It is highly viscous but less elastic and pseudoplastic than 1 percent sodium hyaluronate. It is available as solution of (3:1 mixture of) 3 percent sodium hyaluronate and 4 percent chondroitin sulfate with 0.45 mg sodium dihydrogen phosphate hydrate, 2.65 mg disodium hydrogen phosphate and 4.3 mg NaCl (in 0.5 ml pack).

It is used as surgical aid in the anterior segment procedures including cataract extraction and IOL implantation. The molecular weight of sodium hyaluronate is 500000 and the chondroitin sulfate 50000. It is produced by genetic engineering. Because of its stickiness, it is claimed to be quite effective in protecting endothelium but does not maintain anterior chamber as healon.

The disadvantage is that it is difficult to aspirate, tends to trap small air bubbles, less cohesive and requires refrigeration.

Chondroitin Sulfate

It is a biological polymer and is a proteoglycan.

Chondroitin sulfate from shark cartilage was introduced in 1980 as a coating for intraocular lenses. It is a natural compound of hard connective tissue such as cartilage in humans and one of the major glycosaminoglycans of the corneal stroma.

The physical and chemical properties and molecular structure of chondroitin sulfate is quite similar to hyaluronic acid with the difference of presence of sulfur and double negative charges per molecular subunit.

The molecular size is $5 \times 100 \times 10^3$ centistokes, thus being much smaller than hyaluronic acid. The sugar moieties occur as repeating disaccharide subunits consisting of glucuronic acid in B-1, 3 linkage with N-acetyl galactosamine for chondroitin sulfate.

Double negative charge of chondroitin sulfate coats the positively charged tissue or implant surface and thus decreases the electrostatic interaction between the implant and the endothelium.

Chondroitin sulfate alone has a low viscosity because of which it cannot maintain space. If concentration of chondroitin sulfate is increased to 50 percent, it improves the viscosity but causes endothelial cell damage due to dehydration, sticks of lens surface and does not wash away easily.

Due to these problem chondroitin sulfate is generally combined with another biological polymer-sodium hyaluronate.

This formulation makes it a good viscous substance which increases its coating ability and cell protection.

When used alone, it is available as 20 percent solution which can be injected through 30 G cannula. Chondroitin sulfate is more a surface than a space tactical tool. Chondroitin sulfate is available in combination with HPMC which has a good coating property and does not require refrigeration.

Methylcellulose

It was introduced in 1976 for coating of intraocular lenses. It is an artificial compound in the eye. Its viscosity is 3000–4000 centipoise approximately and an average molecular weight of 86000, an osmolarity of 285 mOsm and a pH of 7.2.

It is somewhat viscous, low cost but not truly viscoelastic. It is water soluble, inert substance and nontoxic to the endothelium, transparent and nonpyrogenic. It is basically used as lubricant and maintain anterior chamber but not so well.

It is two percent solution of hydroxy propyl methyl cellulose suitable for intraocular use. It is highly purified brand of hydroxy propyl methyl cellulose. Hydroxy propyl and methyl groups increases the hydrophilicity of the compound. It is designed as such to serve as an acid in ophthalmic procedures of the anterior segment.

Injection of methyl cellulose serves to support a deep anterior chamber during intraocular surgery and allows through manipulation with less trauma to corneal endothelium and other surrounding tissues. It impedes vitreous leakage into the anterior chamber thereby decreasing the possibility of postoperative flat chamber.

Indications for Use of Methylcellulose

- Cataract surgery
- IOL implantation
- Keratoplasty
- Filtering surgery for glaucoma
- Vitrectomy
- Retinal detachment surgery
- Strabismus surgery
- Plastic surgery.

Precautions

- Do not overfill the anterior chamber with methyl cellulose.
- Remove as much possible of methyl cellulose by irrigation/aspiration at the close of surgery for preventing corneal endothelial cell loss as a result of performed procedure.
- Carefully monitor IOP specially during the immediate postoperative period.
- Instillation of methyl cellulose should be done so as to avoid trapping of air bubble behind methyl cellulose.

- Carefully examine the solution for rubber particles that may have been aspirated with repeated washing of sterile water for injection.
- Concurrent presence of medication in the chamber or associated ocular structures should be avoided as it may interact with methyl cellulose to cause clouding.

Presentation

It is available as 2 percent HPMC solution in 2 ml vials or prefilled sterilized disposable. Syringes with sterile 27 G cannula. Administration route and technique is same as discussed in sodium hyaluronate section.

Adverse Reactions

Methyl cellulose is tolerated extremely well after injection into human eyes. However, transient rise in intraocular pressure postoperatively has been reported.

Isolated incidence of postoperative inflammatory reactions (Iritis, hypopyon) as well as corneal edema and corneal decompensation have been reported.

The main advantage of methyl cellulose is its availability at a very low cost in comparison to sodium hyaluronate specially in, developing countries. HPMC main advantages are its availability, ease of preparation, storage at room temperature, ability to withstand autoclaving and potential for low cost.

The disadvantage of this viscoelastic substance is its low viscosity because of which it is not able to maintain anterior chamber and requires large bore cannula.

Polyacrylamide

It is a linear, long chain and high molecular weight synthetic polpymer. It has repeated acrylamide units without protein or other molecular contamination. Acrylamide monomer units are highly reactive and toxic substances but in polymer form, it is highly stable and nontoxic. Polyacrylamide has a low contact angle because of which it possesses good surface wetting and coating properties.

Orcolon (Low concentration poly acrylamide 4.5 mg/ml) is commercially available.

It has molecular weight of one million dalton and high and stable viscosity of approximately 40000 cps with good elastic and pseudoplastic properties. The osmolality is 340 mOsm and the pH is 7.2. It is injected through 27 G cannula and can be stored at room temperature.

Delayed sustained increase in intraocular pressure secondary to the use of polyacrylamide in the anterior chamber has been reported. The cause may be related to presence of small particles of viscoelastic which could lead to compromised trabecular meshwork.

Collagen

Collagen constitutes an important bulk of connective tissues. There are different types of collagen, i.e. I, II, III and IV, etc. Collagel (1.4% collagen type IV) was viscoelastic introduced in 1990. It is obtained from human placental tissue.

It has a molecular weight of approximately one million daltons and a viscosity of 500,00 centipoise (Zero shear rate), an osmolality of 300 mosm and a pH of 6.2.

It has been clinically compared with healon and no significant difference in IOP, corneal thickness, endothelial cells and postoperative visual acuity have been observed. It is commercially available for use.

FUTURE VISCOELASTICS

A new polymer, poly-TEGMA 40 percent (triethylenglycol monomethacrylate) and poly-GLYMA (glycerol monomethacrylate) have been evaluated in rabbits and preclinical studies as potential viscoelastic substances for intraoperative use in anterior segment surgery. These are highly swelling and hydrophilic polymers. Poly-GLYMA and poly-TEGMA 40 percent are characterized by high biological tolerance after its implantation into the anterior chamber. Poly-TEGMA 40 percent is potential viscoelastic substance and shall be commercially available in short future.

Provisc has been recommended as a safe and effective visoelastic substance in modern surgery of cataract.

IRRIGATING SOLUTIONS

Irrigating solutions are aqueous solutions used to cleanse and to maintain moisture of ocular tissues. Ideally, these solutions are isotonic. The optimum pH is 7.4. A pH less than 7 or greater than 8 has caused callular stress and death when the tissues have been exposed to prolonged period of time.

Two types of irrigating solutions are available for use in ophthalmolgoy.

Intraocular Irrigating Solutions

The commercially available intraocular irrigating solutions (e.g. BSS and BSS plus) are used during ocular surgery to protect the lens and cornea in patients. Unlike physiological saline and Ringer lactate solution, these balanced salt solutions provide magnesium and calcium ions as cellular nutrients.

These nutrients are required for intercellular and intracellular function during prolonged ocular, surgery. In addition to magnesium and calcium, bicarbonate, glucose and glutathione are present in these perfusion solutions (BSS plus). These components help to maintain a deturgesced or thin cornea by avoiding corneal clouding. Various commercially available intraocular irrigating solutions are:

BSS solution containing 0.64 percent NaCl, 0.075 percent KCl, 0.03 percent magnesium chloride, 0.043 percent calcium chloride, 0.39 percent sodium acetate, 0.17 percent sodium citrate and sodium hydroxide or hydrochloric acid in (15,30,300 and 500 ml sterile packs).

BSS plus (Mix aspastically just prior to use)

Part I—480 ml containing 7.44 mg NaCl, 0.395 mg KCl, 0.433 mg sodium phosphate, 2.19 mg sodium bicarbonate, hydrochloric acid or sodium hydroxide/ml.

Part II—20 ml containing 3.85 mg calcium chloridedihydrate, 5 mg magnesium chloride hexahydrate, 23 mg dextrose and 4.6 mg glutathione disulfide/ml.

It is preservative free (500 ml pack) and 30 ml pack. Its pH is at or near the optimal 7.4 level (pH of human aqueous humor).

Salient Features of BSS Plus Solution

- It is iso-osmotic with intraocular tissues.
- BSS plus solution provides uncompromised endothelial nourishment even during phacoemulsification.
- In addition to supplying fine essentials ions (Sodium, potassium, magnesium, calcium and chloride) this solution provides the endothelium with three additional constituents.
- Sodium bicarbonate for normal endothelial pump function to help reduce corneal swelling. It is vital for maintaining endothelial barrier integrity and is activating agent for endothelial cell metabolic pumps for maintaining corneal clarity.
- Dextrose is an energy source for endeothelial cell metabolism and is essential for acrobic metabolism of endothelial cells and helps to maintain transparency of cornea and lens.
- Oxidized glutathione to protect cell against oxidative stress and maintain integrity of the blood aqueous barrier to minimize inflammation. It maintains functional complexes of endothelial cells.
- BSS plus solution does not contain alien ingredients such as acetate or citrate which can chelate free calcium ions. Calcium ions help to maintain the corneal endothelium's vital barrier function.

Compound sodium lactate solution (in 500 ml pack): Compound sodium chloride solution (in 5 ml and 500 ml packs).

Extraocular Irrigating Solutions

Extraocular irrigating solutions are sterile isotonic solutions for general ophthalmic use.

Ocular uses include irrigating procedures following tonometry, gonioscopy, foreign body removal or use of Fluorescein. They are also used to soothe and clense the eye and in conjunction with hard contact lenses. As these solutions have short contact time with the eye, they do not need to provide nutrient to the cells. Unlike intraocular irrigants, irrigants for extraocular use contain preservatives which prevent bacteriostatic contamination. However, the preservatives are exceedingly toxic to the corneal endothelium and intraocular use of extraocular irrigating fluids is contraindicated.

Various commercial preparations of extraocular fluids available are:

Extraocular irrigating solution containing (EIS): 0.49 NaCl, 0.075 KCl, 0.048 percent calcium chloride, 0.03 percent magnesium chloride, 0.39 percent sodium acetate and 0.17 percent sodium citrate with 0.013 percent benzalkonium chloride (in 30 ml and 120 ml sterile packs).

EIS containing: Boric acid and sodium borate with 0.004 percent phenylmercuric nitrate or 0.002 percent thimerosal (in 15,30, 120 and 180 ml packs).

EIS containing: 0.49 percent NaCl, 0.075 percent KCl, 0.03 percent magnesium chloride, 0.048 percent calcium chloride, 0.39 percent sodium acetate, 0.17 percent sodium citrate, 0.013 percent benzalkonium chloride and sodium hydroxide or hydrochloric acid in (30 ml and 120 ml packs).

EIS containing: 1.2 percent boric acid, 0.38 percent KCl, 0.014 percent sodium carbonate anhydrous, 0.05 percent EDTA and 0.01 percent benzolkonium chloride (in 30 ml and 120 ml packs).

EIS containing: 0.05 percent tetrahydrozoline HCl with NaCl, sodium borate, boric acid, 0.01 percent benzalkonium chloride and 0.1 percent EDTA (in 15 ml pack).

EIS solution containing: NaCl, sodium proprionate, sodium borate, boric acid, glycerin, rose and camphor water, extract of witch hazel, berbrine bisulfate and benzalkonium chloride (in 120 ml pack).

EIS solution containing: 0.49 NaCl, 0.4 percent sodium biphosphate and 0.45 percent sodium phosphate with 0.005 percent banzolkonium chloride (in 180 ml pack).

SURGICAL ENZYMES

Various chemical enzymes used in ophthalmology are:

Alpha Chymotrypsin

It is a proteolytic enzyme. The principal proteolytic effect is exerted by the splitting of peptide bonds of amino acids in the zonular fibers and ocular tissues.

Indication: It is mainly used for enzymatic zonulysis for intracapsular lens extraction particularly in young patients.

Destruction of the equatorial pericapsular membrane of the lens occurs in 5 minutes. Zonular fibers are lysed with in 10-15 minutes of application and complete lysis of the entire zonular membrane occurs in 30 minutes.

However, it does not have any effect on the vitreolenticular adhesions found in such patients in whom ECCE is the treatment of choice.

Contraindications: Significant anterior displacement of lens-iris diaphragm with impending vitreous loss.

High vitreous pressure, gaping incisional wound, congenital cataracts, hypersensitivity to chymotrypsin or any component of the preparation.

Administration and dosage: Fresh solution of alpha chymotrypsin is prepared just before use.

Commercially it is available as powder for ophthalmic solution containing 150 units or 300 units with 2 ml sodium chloride diluent per dual chamber univial.

It is also available as 750 units per vial with 9 ml BSS diluent. Reconstitute solution before use. The 750 units vial may be reconstituted with 5 ml (150 units/ml) or 10 ml (75 units/ml) of the diluent provided. A solution of 150 units/ml is equivalent to a 1:5000 dilution. The 300 units vials reconstituted with 2 ml of diluent yield a 1:5000 solution.

When used for intracapsular cataract extraction, a fresh solution of alpha-chymotrypsin is injected into the anterior chamber immediately prior to the removal of lens (intracameral injection) and within 3–5 minutes will have sufficiently weakened the lens zonules. Usually 0.2–0.5 ml of freshly prepared 1:5000 solution injected slowly behind the lens into the posterior chamber. This enzyme is rapidly in activated in the presence of serum and blood however drugs used routinely in cataract surgery like adrenaline (1:100000) does not inhibit the enzyme activity.

Adverse reactions: The adverse effects include transient rise in IOP, moderate uveitis corneal edema, striation. Delayed healing of incisions has also been reported. Other adverse effects are wound disruption, vitreous loss.

Urokinase

It is useful for dissolving blood clot of coagulated hyphema. Usual dosage is 5,000 units of urokinase are dissolved in 2 ml of normal saline (pH 7.2–7.6) and injected into the anterior chamber through a small keratome incision. It causes liquefaction of the clot which can then be washed out with Ringer lactate solution.

Hyaluronidase

This enzyme is prepared from mammalian testes and acts by depolymerizing hyaluronic acid an essential component of the intercellular ground substance which determines the permeability of tissue.

The enzyme hyaluronidase is commonly used in conjunction with local anesthetics lignocaine (2%) with adrenaline for infiltration and regional local anesthesia. Hyaluronidase is also indicated for subconjunctival hemorrhage for hasten reabsorption

and for cortisone therapy when given subconjunctivally for early pterygium resolution. The advantages it brings to local injection are:
1. Quicker diffusion and a more effective action of lignocaine and adrenaline in promoting akinesia of orbicularis oculi and extraocular muscles.
2. The swelling at the site of injection is appreciably lessened by its presence. The duration of anesthesia is about the same as without the use of hyaluronidase provided that adrenaline is used.

   The effect of the injection is hastened by the massage of the infiltrated area.
3. Hyaluronidase increases the area of anesthesia by 40 percent.
4. It is nontoxic to the ocular tissues.

Dosage: It is available as an odorless, fluffy powder containing 300 units of activity per mg.

It is freshly prepared just before use. For local anesthesia, it is directly reconstituted in 2 percent lidocaine solution 1 ampoule of hyaluronidase containing 1500 IU (each ml) is directly mixed into 30 ml vial of 2 percent lidocaine and adrenaline. Hyaluronidase can also be obtained by dissolving the contents of one ampoule in 10 ml sterile distilled water and withdrawing 1 ml of it.

Adverse reactions: Generally, there are no signs of local or systemic tissue therapy.

Hyaluronidase is antigenic and may sometime produce allergic reactions. Because of danger of spreading the infection, the enzyme should not be injected into or around an infected area.

Ocular malignancy is also considered as a contraindication for hyaluronidase for similar action.

Solutions of hyaluronidase rapidly lose their viscosity reducing activity at room temperature. Fresh solution should be used certainly within 12 hours.

SURGICAL ADJUNCTS

Fractionated Purified Silicone Oil

Fractionated purified silicone oil is purified, sterile and apyrogenic silicone oil designed to be injected into the vitreous space for prolonged tamponade after surgical treatment for retinal pathologies.

Fractionated purified silicone oil has following salient features:
- It is free from low molecular weight components (MWC) and other impurities (confirmed by gas chromatography) which cause toxicity and inflammation when applied intraocularly.
- Absence of toxic residual polymerization catalysts.
- It has viscosity 1300 + 100 centistrokes.
- Specially developed by fractionation process free from residual polymerization catalysts which can cause adverse ocular reactions.

Indications: It is indicated for use as prolonged tamponade in retinal detachment surgery specially retinal detachment with giant tear, retinal detachment with proliferative vitreal retinopathy, proliferative diabetic retinopathy and traumatic retinal detachment.

Contraindications: Pseudophakic patients with silicone intraocular lens as silicone oil can chemicaly interact and opacify silicone elastomers.

Dosage and administration: It is available as 10 ml vial with special flip off seal in a sterile pouch. Store it at 8-24°C. This vial is available for single use only and should not be resterilized. Another preparation polydimethyl siloxane (Silicon oil) is also available as single use 10 and 15 ml vials.

Direction for use: Fractionated purified silicone oil can be used in conjunction with or following standard retinal surgical procedures including scleral buckle surgery, membrane peeling, vitrectomy, retinotomy or relaxing retinectomy.

In aseptic conditions decant the contents of the vial into a sterile syringe to avoid introduction of air bubble into the oil. Oil can be injected into the vitreous from the syringe by placing the syringe in a syringe driver or via a single use cannulated infusion line. Plug in the infusion terminal to the tip of the syringe. Inject it slowly subretinal fluid can be drained with a flute needle during silicone oil infusion. The vitreous cavity can be filled with oil between 80-100 percent while exchanging for fluid or air taking special care to avoid high intraocular pressure from developing during the exchange. As silicone oil is less dense than eye aqueous fluid, a basal iridectomy at 6 o' clock meridian is generally recommended (Andoiridectomy) to minimize oil induced pupillary block and early angle closure glaucoma.

Silicone oil should be removed at an appropriate interval with in one year following instillation provided retina is stable, attached and without significant remanant of proliferation.

Silicone oil can be removed from the posterior chamber by withdrawl with a normal 10 ml syringe and 1 mm cannula (wide bore). By repeated oil fluid exchange most of the remaining silicone oil droplets can be removed from the eye. Avoid leaving silicone bubbles in the vitreoretinal cavity. As there are chances of migration of silicone oil into the anterior chamber and appearance of corneal changes like edema, hazing or opacification and descemet folds. Patient corneal status should be regularly monitored and early corrective action including oil extraction from anterior chamber should be taken.

Visual Outcome and Clinical Results

Successful reattachment of the retina occur in 65-80 percent of the patients using fractionated silicone oil. This rate may vary depending on the specific etiology off the disease and severity of the condition.

Regarding visual acuity status 50-75 percent of patients show improvements in visual acuity at 6 months. In 15-25 percent of patients visual acuity do not change while in 10-20 percent of cases visual acuity deterioration occurs which is mainly related to redetachment of retina, further progression of retinal disease and cataract complications.

Precautions: As with any surgical procedure, posterior segment surgery using fractionated purified silicone oil, potential risk must be evaluated by ophthalmic surgeon.

Adverse reactions: Most common adverse reactions reported are cataract, keratopathy, glaucoma and anterior chamber oil migration.

Other adverse reactions include redetachment, optic nerve atrophy, rubeosis iridis, temporary IOP increase, macular pucker, vitreous hemorrhage, traction detachment, angle block, subretinal silicone oil, choroidal detachment, PVR reproliferation and cystoid macular edema.

Botulinum Toxin Type A

Pharmacokinetics

Botulinum toxin is a sterile lyophilized form of purified botulinum toxin type A produced from a culture of the Hall strain of Clostridium botulinum grown in special medium containing N-Z amine and yeast extract. Botulinum toxin type A blocks neuromuscular conduction by binding to receptor sites on motor nerve terminals, entering the nerve terminals and inhibiting the release of acetyl choline. When injected IM at therapeutic doses botulinum toxic type A produces a localized chemical denervations muscle paralysis. The paralytic effect on muscles injected is useful in reducing the excessive, abnormal contractions associated with blepharospasm. Botulinum toxin type A is also used in the treatment of strabismus. It affects muscle pairs by inducing an atrophic lengthening of the injected muscle and corresponding shortening of the muscles antagonist.

Indications: It is specially used for the treatment of strabismus and blepharospasm associated with dystonia including benign essential blepharospasm or VII nerve disorders in patients.

Contraindications: Hypersensitivity to any ingradient in the formulation.

Dosage and administration: Botulinum toxin type A (Botox) is available as powder for injection (lyophilized) containing 100 units of lyophilized Clostridium botulinum toxin type A along with 0.05 mg albumin (human) and 0.9 mg sodium chloride in vials (Preservative free).

Administration

Strabismus Botulinum toxin type A is intended for injection into extraocular muscles utilizing the electrical activity recorded from the tip of the injection needle as a guide to placement within target muscle.

The volume of botulinum toxin type A injected for the treatment of strabismus should be between 0.05–0.15 ml per muscle.

Preparation

An injection of botulinum toxin type A is prepared by drawing into a sterile 1 ml tuberculin syringe an amount of the properly diluted Toxin (See dilution table) slightly greater than the intended dose.

Air bubbles in the syringe are expelled and the syringe is attached to the electromyographic injection needle preferably at 1½ inch 27 gauge needle. Excess volume than intended dose is expelled through the needle into waste container use a new sterile needle and syringe to enter the vial on each occasion for dilution or removal of botulinum toxin.

Eye must be prepared before giving injection. Put several drops of topical anesthesia and an ocular decongestant several minutes prior to injection initial doses of diluted botulinum toxin type A create paralysis of injected muscles beginning 1–2 days after injection and increasing in intensity during the first week. The paralytic effect lasts for 2–6 weeks and gradually resolves over a similar time period.

The recommended doses for strabismus are:
  i. For vertical muscles and horizontal strabismus <20 prism diopters use 1.25–2.5 U in any one muscle.
  ii. For horizontal strabismus of 20–50 diopters use 2.5–5 U in any muscle.
  iii. For persistent VI nerve palsy of more than one month duration use 1.25–2.5 U in the medial rectus muscles.

Re-examine the patients 7–14 days after each injection to assess the effect of that dose subsequent injections should be given only when the effects of previous dose have dissipated.

Maximum recommended dose for a single injection for any one muscle is 25 U.

Blepharospasm: Diluted botulinum toxin type A is injected using a 27 gauge needle without electromyographic guidance. Initially 1.25–2.5 U (0.05–0.1 ml volume at each site) should be injected into the medial and lateral pretarsal orbicularis oculi of the upper lid and into the lateral pretarsal orbicularis oculi of the lower lid.

In general, effect of injection is seen in 3 days and reaches to peak at 1–2 weeks post-treatment. Each treatment lasts for three months following which the procedure may be repeated.

Dose can be increased to two-fold in repeat treatment sessions if initial dose is considered insufficient.

The cumulative dose of botulinum toxin type A should not exceed 200 U in a 30-day period.

Dilution Technique

For dilution use sterile normal saline without preservative 0.9 percent sodium chloride injection is generally recommended. Since botulinum toxin type A is denatured by bubbling or violent agitation, inject the diluent into the vial gently.

Administer preferably within 4 hours after reconstitution. Store reconstituted botulinum toxic type A in a refrigerator at 2–8°C and solution should be clear, colorless and free of particulate matters.

These dilutions are calculated for an injection volume of 0.1 ml.

Store the Lyophilized product in a freezer at –5°C Administer within 4 hours after the vial is removed from freezer and reconstituted.

Precautions

- Safe and effective use of botulinum toxin type A depends upon proper storage of the product, selection of the correct dose and proper reconstruction and administration technique.
- During administration, care should be taken about retrobulbar hemorrhage development which may compromise the entire process.
- Caution should be taken for reduced blinking from botulinum toxin type A injection of the orbicularis muscle which can lead to corneal exposure, persistent epithelial defect and corneal ulceration specially with patients of VII nerve disorders. This may require protective drops, ointments, therapeutic soft contact lenses or patching.
- Exercise caution when botulinum toxin type A is injected into those patients who are taking aminoglycosides as effect of botulinum toxin may be potentiated by aminoglycosides antibiotics.

Adverse Reactions

Ocular adverse reactions reported are as follows:

Strabismus: Strabismus induced paralysis of one or more extraocular muscles which may lead to spatial disorientation, diplopia or past pointing. Other adverse effects may be ptosis and vertical deviation in horizontal strabismus injection.

TABLE 14.1: Dilution	
Dilution of botulinum toxin type A diluent added 0.9% sodium chloride (Preservative free)	Resulting dose
1 ml	10 units
2 ml	5 units
4 ml	2.5 units
8 ml	1.25 units

Blepharospasm: Adverse reactions reported are ptosis irritation/tearing, lag ophthalmos, photophobia, ectropion, keratitis, diplopia and ecchymosis.

Absorbable gelatin film: It is a sterile absorbable gelatin film for use in ophthalmic surgery.

Pharmacokinetics

In dry state, it resembles in appearance and texture of cellophane of equivalent thickness, when moistened it acquires a rubbery consistency and can then be cut to desired size and shape fitted to rounded or irregular surfaces. The rate of absorption after implantation varies form 1-6 months depending upon the size and site of implant. Usually pleural and muscle implants are completely absorbed in 8-14 days while dural and ocular implants require 2-5 months for complete absorption. Dural and ocular implants have specific characteristics of absence of undue tissue reactions with the consequent decreased development of adhesions.

Indications: Absorbable gelatin film is indicated for use in ocular surgery specially in glaucoma filtration operations (like iridenclesis and trephination), extraocular muscle surgery, diathemy and scleral buckling operations for retinal detachment. There is an appreciable lack of cellular reaction to the film implanted subconjunctivally or used as a seton into the anterior chamber. Implants also help to prevent the formation of adhesions between contiguous ocular structures.

Contraindications: Do not implant in infective conditions of the eye.

Dosage and administration: Gelatin film is commercially available in 100 mm × 125 mm, and 25 mm × 50 mm sizes. Store it at room temperature (15-30°C). To ensure sterility use immediately after withdrawal from the envelope.

Before use immerse gelatin in sterile saline solution soak until quite pliable cut to the desired size and shape and apply according to the site.
- In iridencleisis, this film is used as seton. Put a small piece (4 mm × 10 mm) over the prolapsed iris pillar parallel to the limbus. Tenon capsule and the conjunctiva are then closed with continuous absorbable sutures closely spaced to ensure tight wound closure.
- For diathermy and scleral buckling operations place film over the sclera, then suture the muscle and conjunctiva over the underlying film.
- In extraocular muscle surgery place film over and beneath the muscle before Tenon's capsule and the conjunctiva are closed in layers.

CHELATING AGENTS, COLLAGENASE INHIBITORS AND MUCOLYTICS

Collagenase is an enzyme which has been shown to be secreted by damaged epithelial cells of the cornea. It is capable of destroying collagen and is responsible for destruction of stromal tissue in alkali burns of cornea and possibly in other chronic ulcerative conditions of the cornea. Chelating agent used in ophthalmology are:

Ethylenediaminetetra Acetate

Ethylenediaminetetra acetate (EDTA) is available either as sodium or calcium salts. It forms stable and highly water soluble complexes with many divalent and trivalent metallic ions and owe their therapeutic applications to this chelating property.

Sodium EDTA is converted to calcium EDTA in the presence of calcium. The most common use of sodium EDTA is in the removal of calcium deposits from the corneal stroma. Sodium EDTA will not penetrate the corneal epithelium and this should be mechanically removed before hand.

Sodium EDTA 0.01 percent solution can be used for 15-20 minutes of continuous corneal irrigation and as much 100 ml of solution may be used without causing apparent toxic corneal changes. EDTA is also an effective collagenase inhibitor and immediate irrigation of the eye with sodium EDTA following alkali burns may reduce the alkali damage. Calcium EDTA topical drops may be used at a conc of 0.2 percent and given every hour in day for up to 2-3 weeks.

Laevo-cysteine

It has powerful anticollagenase action. It exerts its action by binding to the zinc.

Laevo-cysteine may be used frequently and hourly dose is recommended. It is used in the conc of 0.1-0.2 molar L-cysteine has been shown to be of value in the prevention of stromal destruction by collagenase specially in cases of alkali burns. L. cysteine is less toxic than calcium EDTA.

Acetylcysteine

It is also used as collagenase inhibitor. It is less toxic and more stable than L-cysteine. Acetylcysteine is available as eyedrops in conc of 5 percent, 10 percent and 20 percent. The 20 percent solution is most effective.

It is mainly used for its mucolytic properties. Mucus filaments occurs in keratoconjunctivitis sicca and in superior limbal keratitis. Five percent solution of acetyle cysteine is relatively free of ocular discomfort and irritation.

CAUSTIC PREPARATIONS IN OPHTHALMOLOGY

Caustic preparations like carbolic acid and absolute alcohol are used in treating certain type of corneal ulcers (Dendritic type) and painful blind eye respectively.

Carbolic Acid

Pure carbolic acid is a phenol with potent bactericidal and fungicidal actions. It probably acts by denaturing the bacterial proteins. It rapidly penetrates ocular tissue and acts as local anesthetic. Pure carbolic acid is applied on pointed stick and touched on the corneal ulcer edges. Excess of drug is removed with filter paper and eye is washed with normal saline.

Alcohol

One hundred percent alcohol is used in relieving pain in blind eye. 1 ml of absolute alcohol is given by slow retrobulbar or peribulbar route.

Hydrogen Peroxide

It is colorless, odorless liquid used mainly as an antiseptic. It owes its action to its ready release of nascent oxygen when applied to the tissue. The application causes on effervescence which mechanically removes the tissue debris from other inacessible area. It has short duration of action and poor penetration. It is used in the conc of 2 percent for cleansing eyelid margins in the cases of squamous and ulcertive blepharitis. For this purpose, it is applied with a glass rod with wrapped cotton wool.

CYANOACRYLATE TISSUE ADHESIVES IN OPHTHALMOLOGY

Tissue adhesives represent a major advance in the treatment of corneal perforations of diverse etiology. The first human patient treated with tissue adhesive was reported in 1968 by Webster. Tissue adhesives allow convenient immediate closure of perforations avoiding and delaying surgical interventions. The glue spontaneously falls off when the lesion heals.

Indications

- It is the most efficient method of immediate wound closure in corneal perforations up to 3 mm in length
- In corneal thinning (Due to herpes simplex infectious ulcers)
- All types of corneal melts and various types of wound leaks
- Mooren's ulcer
- Marginal ulceration (S/p cataract surgery with perforation)
- Post-PK traumatic perforation
- Skin closure in upper lid blepharoplasty procedure.

N-butyl-2 cyanoacrylate can successfully seal a perforation without excess ocular toxicity. It is necessary that epithelium and necrotic stroma be debrided to allow firm adhesion of the cyanoacrylate glue to surrounding healthy basement membrane.

Dosage and Application

The application of cyanoacrylate tissue adhesive is done with topical proparacaine or benoxinate anesthesia either at slit-lamp or under the operating microscope. A lid speculum is placed. The epithelium is debrided from the site of the perforation or descemetocele and from the surrounding cornea and dries the ulcer and periulcer area of debris and loose cells with weckcell sponges (cellulose sponges). Liquid tissue adhesive in short stokes or concentric spots is placed using a 25-gauge needle on a tuberculin syringe. It polymerizes instantly to the tissue then perforation is checked to be sure that it is sealed. Sterile saline is dripped on the eye and a therapeutic soft contact lens is applied. Prophylactic topical antibiotic drops are given 2–3 times daily following application of tissue adhesive. If needed for inflammation steroids may be used with greater safety. The cornea normally heals and dislodge the glue in 1–3 months usually leaving the eye quiet but scarred and amenable to transplant if vision is significantly compromised.

If there is a persistent perforation or impending perforation, the patient can undergo either reapplication of the tissue adhesive or surgical procedure to close the perforation.

During tissue adhesive application, it is essential to observe the patient closely to be sure the anterior chamber has reformed and there is no associated superinfection. When therapeutic contact lens or adhesive therapy is inadequate, surgical patch grafting will usually be successful. For moderate size perforations a small lamellar button may be sutured into the debrided defect. In the event of large perforations, it may be preferable to perform penetrating keratoplasty.

Adverse Effects

It should not be applied too thickly as the heat generated by the adhesive polymerization process may cause injury to the adjacent tissue. Adhesive avoids connective tissue healing and is only slowly absorbed.

BIBLIOGRAPHY

1. Agarwal A. Textbook of Ophthalmology, 1st edn. New Delhi: Jaypee Brothers Medical Publishers, 2002.
2. Bartlett JD. Clinical Ocular Pharmacology, 4th edn. Boston: Butterworth-Heinemann, 2001
3. Bartlett JD. Ophthalmic Drug Facts, Lippincott-William and Wilkins, 2001.
4. Buratto. Viscoelastics in Ophthalmic Surgery: Slack. Inc., 2000.
5. Crick RP, Trimble RB. Textbook of Clinical Ophthalmology, Hodder and Stoughton, 1986.
6. Dich. Viscoelastics in Ophthalmic Surgery, Springer-Verlag, 2000.
7. Duane TD. Clinical Ophthalmology, 4th edn. Butterworth-Heinemann, 1999.
8. Duvall. Ophthalmic Medications and Pharmacology, Slack Inc., 1998.

9. Ellis PP. Ocular Therapeutics and Pharmacology, 7th edn. CV Mosby, 1985.
10. Fechner. Ocular Therapeutics, Slack Inc., 1998.
11. Fraunfelder. Current Ocular Therapy, 5th edn. WB Saunders, 2000.
12. Garg A. Current Trends in Ophthalmology, 1st edn. New Delhi: Jaypee Brothers Medical Publishers, 1997.
13. Garg A. Manual of Ocular Therapeutics, 1st edn. New Delhi: Jaypee Brothers Medical Publishers, 1996.
14. Garg A. Ready Reckoner of Ocular Therapeutics, 1st edn. New Delhi, 2002.
15. Goodman LS, Gilman A. Pharmacological Basis of Therapeutics, 7th edn. New York: Macmillan, 1985.
16. Havener's, Ocular Pharmacology, 6th edn. CV Mosby, 1994.
17. Kanski. Clinical Ophthalmology, 4th edn. Butterworth-Heineman, 1999.
18. Kershner. Ophthalmic Medications and Pharmacology, Slack. Inc., 1994.
19. Olin BR, et al. Drugs Facts and Comparisons: Facts and Comparisons, St Louis, 1997.
20. Onofrey. The Ocular Therapeutics; Lippincott-William and Wilkins, 1997.
21. Rhee. The Wills Eye drug Guide, Lippincott-William and Wilkins, 1998.
22. Steven Podos. Textbook of Ophthalmology, New Delhi: Jaypee Brothers Medical Publishers, 2001.
23. Zimmerman. Textbook of Ocular Pharmacology, Lippincott and William and Wilkins, 1997.

15

Mydriatics and Cycloplegics

Ashok Garg (India)

INTRODUCTION

Mydriatics are drugs which dilate the pupil while cycloplegics are agents which causes paralysis of ciliary muscle (paralysis of accommodation). Mydriatics usually produce paralysis of ciliary muscle in greater or lesser degree.

All these drugs when instilled into the conjunctival sac are rapidly absorbed through the cornea and become effective in the inner eye.

Currently two classes of drugs: (i) adrenergic agonist and (ii) cholinergic antagonist, are available for mydriatic purpose. For most dilation procedures the adrenergic or anticholinergic agents can be used either alone or in combination for maximum mydriasis. Anticholinergic agents used topically in the eye for the purpose of inhibiting accommodation are termed cycloplegics. Their primary use is for cycloplegic refraction and in the treatment of uveitis. Since these agents also inhibit action of the iris sphincter muscle they are effective mydriatics and are commonly used for routine pupillary dilation.

MYDRIATIC ADRENERGIC AGENTS (SYMPATHOMIMETIC AGENTS)

The effect of sympathomimetic agents on the eye include pupil dilation, increase in the outflow of aqueous humor and vasoconstriction (α-adrenergic effects), relaxation of ciliary muscle and decrease in the formation of aqueous humor. The various agents of this group used in ophthalmology are as follows:

Adrenaline (Epinephrine)

It acts on dilator fibers and directly produces dilation after the instillation of four drops of 1:1000 solution.

The instillation being repeated in 5 minutes. It is mainly used in the treatment of open angle glaucoma.

Adrenaline may be combined with procaine and atropine as a subconjunctival injection to achieve mydriasis in severe cases of iritis.

Coccaine Hydrochloride

It is an alkaloid and is used as coccaine hydrochloride 2 and 4 percent drops.

It acts as mydriatic by inhibiting the action of amine oxidase. It is toxic to the cells of corneal epithelium and this effect may be used to advantage in that the damage to the epithelium allows a greater penetration of drugs through the cornea.

It does not cause dilatation of pupil and pupil continue to react to light even after prolonged application. It is therefore ineffective when the sympathetic nerve is paralyzed.

Phenylephrine

It is one of the most common sympathomimetic agents (α-adrenergic stimulant) used in ophthalmology for dilation purposes. It is used in the form of hydrochloride. It acts directly on the alpha receptors of the dilators pupillae causing pupil dilatation. Following topical instillation it acts on iris dilator muscle and smooth muscles or conjunctival arterioles causing pupillary dilation and balancing of conjunctiva. Its action can be reversed by thymoxamine 0.1 percent.

Indications: For pupil dilatation in diagnostic purposes (for complete fundus exam) and in various pathological conditions of the eye [in uveitis (Posterior synchiae)], open angle glaucoma in conjunction with miotics, refraction, ophthalmoscopic examination and before intraocular surgery.

Contraindication: Hypersensitivity to any of these agents, narrow angle glaucoma, patients with long-standing insulin dependant diabetes, hypertensive patients receiving reserpine or guanthedine, aneurysm, cardiac diseases, debilitated and elderly patients and patients with IOL implantation.

Dosage: For pupillary dilation commercial concentrations of 2.5 percent and 10 percent (in 2.5 ml and 15 ml packs) ophthalmic solutions are available. Maximum dilation occurs in 45-60 minutes depending upon the concentration used and number of drops instilled. The pupil size usually returns to predrug levels within 4-6 hours. Since phenylephrine has little or no effect on the ciliary muscle mydriasis occurs without cycloplegia.

Phenylephrine 1 percent solution can be used in diagnosis of Horner's syndrome. Significantly mydriasis can occur in the eye with a postganglionic lesion as compared to normal innervation.

The mydriatic response may be affected in cases of injury to corneal epithelium (Corneal abrasions and trauma). Concentration as small as 0.125 percent present in decongestants solution have been reported to cause mydriasis if the corneal epithelium is damaged. In general, 2.5 percent topical concentration is used for routine dilation specially in children and elderly patients because 10 percent concentration has clinical ocular and systemic side effects.

For diagnostic purpose usual dosage is 1 drop of 2.5 percent solution in each eye followed by one drop more in 5-10 minutes. Sufficient mydriasis is produced in 15-30 minutes and effect lasts for 4-6 hours. For pathological condition, usual dosage is 1 drop of 2.5 percent or 10 percent solution (depending upon the condition) three times a day till the desired result is obtained.

Topical phenylephrine can be used alone or in combination of other mydriatic/cycloplegic agents in diagnostic procedures and pathological conditions of the eye.

Adverse reactions: On topical use, it may cause transient stinging on initial instillation, blurring of vision and rarely maculopathy with a central scotoma results from use in aphakic patients.

Prompt reversal generally follows discontinuation.

Phenylephrine may cause rebound miosis and decreased mydriatics response to therapy in older persons.

Systemic side effects include CVS effects like palpitation, tachycardia, extrasystole, cardiac arrhythmia, extrasystole, cardiac arrhythmia, hypertension, headache and browache but usually diminishes as the treatment is continued.

Other effects include reflex bradycardia, pulmonary embolism, myocardial infarction, stroke and death associated with cardiac reactions. Sometimes 10 percent phenylephrine on conjunctival instillation may cause significant elevation of blood pressure. Exercise caution with elderly patients and children and carefully monitor the blood pressure in such cases.

Hydroxyamphetamine

It is an indirect acting adrenergic agonist. Its pharmacological action is primarily due to release of nor-epinephrine from postganglionic adrenergic nerve terminals. It has very little effect on accommodation.

Indications: To dilate the pupil for diagnostic procedure and ophthalmoscopic examination of the eye.

Dosage: It is available as 1 percent topical solution (15 ml pack). It has mydriatic effect comparable to 2.5 percent phenylephrine. Maximum pupillary dilatation occurs in 25-40 minutes and effect last for 4-6 hours.

Since the drug stimulates the release of norepinephrine from adrenergic nerve terminals, its mydriatic effect depends on the integrity of the adrenergic innervation to the pupil. A pupil with postsympathetic ganglion lesion will fail to dilate.

Hydroxyamphetamine can be used to differentiate clinically postganglionic Horner's syndrome from one that is central or preganglionic. Hydroxyamphetamine is a slightly weaker mydriatic in young children and infants because the adrenergic innervation to the iris is not yet full developed in this age group. Adverse effects are similar to those reported with phenylephrine.

CHOLINERGIC ANTAGONIST AS MYDRIATIC AGENTS

Cholinergic antagonist especially tropicamide differs from phenylephrine and hydroxyamphetamine in its mechanism of action. Tropicamide blocks the effects of acetylcholine released from cholinergic nerve endings at the iris sphincter and ciliary muscle. The drug therefore causes mydriasis and cycloplegia. Compared to other cycloplegics, the accommodative effect of tropicamide is less pronounced and of shorter duration.

Dosage: Following topical instillation of 0.5 percent or 1 percent ophthalmic preparation. Mydriasis occurs within 20-30 minutes and effect lasts for 6-8 hours. The advantage of tropicamide over adrenergic mydriatics is that mydriasis with it is more pronounced and bright illumination has no signicant effect on pupil size. The mydriatic effect appears independently of iris pigmentation.

Adverse reactions to tropicamide are quite rare. Since it is devoid of vasopressor action, it is safe for use in patients with cardiac disease and hypertension. Due to its relatively faster onset, short duration and intensity of mydriatic action, tropicamide is presently the drug of choice for pupil dilation. For clinical situations where maximum pupillary dilation is desirable, tropicamide is combined with phenylephrine or hydroxyamphetamine. Various commercial combinations are available. The details are given at the end of this chapter.

CYCLOPLEGIC MYDRIATICS

Cycloplegic mydriatics are commonly used for both objective and subjective refractive procedures.

In different pathological conditions of the eye as treatment, specially strabismus in children (Esotropia), uveitis (Anterior and posterior uveitis) these agents are commonly used.

Parasympatholytic agents are commonly used as cycloplegic mydriatics.

Mechanism of Action

Anticholinergic agents block the responses of the sphincter muscle of the iris and the muscles of the ciliary body to cholinergic stimulation producing pupillary dilation (mydriasis) and paralysis of accommodation (cycloplegia).

Indications

For cycloplegic refraction and for dilation of pupil in the inflammatory conditions of the iris and uveal tract.

Contraindications

Narrow angle glaucoma, sensitivity to belladona alkaloids or any component. In elderly patients specially with atropine where undiagnosed glaucoma or extensive pressure in the eye may be present.

Precautions

- Avoid excessive systemic absorption by compressing the lacrimal sac by digital pressure for 1–2 minutes after instillation.
- Permanent mydriasis may occur in patients with keratoconus.
- Use with caution longer-acting agents (atropine and scopolamine) and they may cause posterior synechiae formation when treating anterior segment inflammation.
- Acute hypersensitivity reaction, discontinue use and have 1:1000 epinephrine solution available.
- Sulfite sensitivity.
- Avoid potentially hazardous tasks (observe caution while driving or performing other tasks requiring alertness).
- Do not exceed recommended dosages.
- Excessive use in children and susceptible cases should be avoided.

Adverse Reactions of Parasympatholytic Agents

On topical use adverse effects reported are increased IOP, transient stinging and burning sensation, allergic lid reactions, hyperemia, follicular conjunctivitis vascular congestion, edema, exudate, photophobia and eczematoid dermatitis.

Systemic adverse effects include systemic atropine toxicity manifested by flushing and dryness of the skin, blurred vision, photophobia with or without corneal staining, dryness of mouth and nose, anhidrosis, fever, rapid pulse, bladder distension, hallucinosis, loss of neuromuscular coordination. Severe reactions are manifested by hypotension with progressive respiratory depression, coma, medullary paralysis and death.

Other adverse effects reported are cardiac dysrhythmias specially in patients undergoing surgery for glaucoma, headache, parasympathetic stimulation, allergic reactions and toxic manifestations of anticholinergic drugs.

In addition use of cyclopentolate and tropicamide has been associated with psychotic reactions and behavioral disturbances in children. CNS disturbances like ataxia incoherent speech,

TABLE 15.1: Cycloplegic mydriatics

Drug	Mydriasis		Cycloplegia		Solution Available
	Onset (minutes)	Duration (hours/days)	Onset (minutes)	Duration (hours)	
Atropine	30–40	7–10 d	60–90	7–10	0.5–3%
Homatropine	40–60	1–3 d	30–60	1–3	2–5%
Scopolamine	20–30	3–7 d	30–60	5–7	0.25%
Cyclopentolate	30–60	1 d	20–45	1 d	0.5–2%
Tropicamide	20–40	4–8 hours	20–30	4–8 hours	0.5–1%

restlessness, seizures, disorientation to time and place and failure to recognize peoples.

Overdosage

When symptoms of atropine toxicity develops (see adverse reactions) administer parenteral physostigmine.

Various parasympatholytic agents used in ophthalmology as cycloplegic mydriatics are:
- Atropine
- Homatropine
- Scopolamine
- Cyclopentolate
- Tropicamide.

Individual drug monograph is as follows:

Atropine Sulfate

It is a potent parasympatholytic agent for use in producing cycloplegia and mydriasis.

It is the strongest mydriatic for common use in ophthalmology.

It completely paralysis the sphincter pupillae and ciliary muscle. It takes considerable time to cause complete paralysis.

It is an alkaloid used in water soluble form (Atropine sulphate).

Indication: Atropine sulphate is used both for its cycloplegic and mydriatic effects for cycloplegic refraction or for pupil dilation in acute inflammatory conditions of the iris and uveal tract. For cycloplegic refraction its use is on decline due to the availability of faster acting, short duration parasympatholytic agents.

Dosage: It is available as topical ophthalmic solution in concentration of 0.5 percent, 1 percent, 2 percent and 3 percent. Atropine ointment is available in 0.5 percent and 1 percent concentrations.

A single drop of 1 percent atropine solution results in maximal mydriasis in about three hours and effect of single dose last for 3–7 days.
- For uveitis treatment, usual dosage is to instill 1-2 drops of 1 percent solution into the eyes four times daily while in children recommended dosage is to instill 1-2 drops of 0.5 percent solution three times a day.
- For refraction, instill one drop of 1 percent solution into the eye twice a day 1-2 days prior to examination. While in children recommended dosage is 1-2 drops of 0.5 percent solution twice daily 1-3 days before the examination and one hour before examination.

Ophthalmologists consider atropine as first drug of choice for the first drug of choice for the first refraction in all children under the age of seven years or when there is risk of convergent strabismus. It may also be used as type of occlusion in amblyopia, latent nystagmus and in difficult cases of accommodative spasms.

Atropine is drug of choice in severe anterior segment inflammation reducing the risk of posterior synechiae.

Adverse reactions: Generalized adverse reactions of parasympatholytic agents are already discussed in this chapter. As atropine has potential local and systemic side effects. It is necessary to discuss these effects separately.

Ocular adverse effects: Atropine may cause local irritation, accommodative spasm, anterior movement of lens-iris diaphragm, breakdown of blood aqueous barrier, decreased anterior chamber depth, drug induced cicatrizing conjunctivitis, hyperemia, corneal toxicity, increased intraocular pressure, cataract formation, allergic blepharoconjunctivitis, twitching of orbicularis oculi, iris cyst, miosis, increased peripheral vitreal traction.

Systemic effects: Dose related side effects.

Homatropine

It is semisynthetic alkaloid prepared from atropine. It is used in its water soluble form homatropine hydrobromide.

Indications: It is moderately long-acting mydriatic and cycloplegic for refraction and in treatment of inflammatory conditions of the uveal tract, for preoperative and postoperative states when mydriasis is required and as an optical aid in certain cases of axial lens opacities.

Dosage: It is available as 2 percent and 5 percent ophthalmic solution.

For refraction, instill 1–2 drops of 2 percent solution into the eyes and repeat it 5–10 minutes, if necessary.

For uveitis, instill 1–2 drops of 2 percent solution into the eyes every 3–4 hours interval.

It acts more quickly than atropine, mydriasis being usually complete with in 40 minutes and cycloplegia after one hour of instillation. The duration of action is shorter than atropine and recovery occurs in about 24 hours.

Adverse effects have already been covered in general monograph of parasympatholytic agents.

	TABLE 15.2: Dose-related side effects of atropine	
	Dose	*Effects*
a.	0.5–2 mg (1–4 drops of 1% solution)	Tachycardia dry mouth Mydriasis/cycloplegia
b.	5 mg (10 drops, 1% solution)	In addition to above one speech disturbance. Restlessness confusion. Hot/dry skin Decreased GI motility urinary retention
c.	>10 mg (20 drops or more of 1% solution)	Above side effect and ataxia Hyperexcitability Hallucination Coma Convulsion Death

Scopolamine

It is used in its water soluble form of scopolamine hydrobromide.

Indications: It is an anticholinergic agent for use in producing cycloplegia and mydriasis, for preoperative and postoperative states in the treatment of iridocyclitis.

Dosage: It is available as 0.25 percent ophthalmic solution.

Usual dosage for refraction is instill 1-2 drops into the eye one hour before refraction.

For uveitis, instill 1-2 drops four times daily into the affected eyes.

Its mydriatic effect starts in 20-30 minutes and cycloplegic effect appears in 30-60 minutes and duration of effect last for 3-7 days.

Cyclopentolate HCl

It is a synthetic mydriatic and cycloplegic agent. It is very effective and short-acting.

Indications: It is used for mydriasis and cycloplegia in diagnostic procedures.

Dosage: It is available as 0.5, 1 percent and 2 percent ophthalmic solution.

Maximal mydriasis occurs in 30 minutes and cycloplegia is usually complete in 40 minutes.

To ensure complete cycloplegia two applications of cyclopentolate HCl are used at 10 minutes interval.

Recovery of accommodation usually occurs in 8-24 hours.

Recommended dosage in adults—instill one drop of 1 percent solution, repeat in 5-10 minutes. Although complete recovery occurs in 24 hours time, yet 1-2 drops of 1 percent or 2 percent pilocarpine reduces recovery time to 3-6 hours in most eyes.

In children usual dosage is to instill 1 drop of 0.5 percent, 1 percent or 2 percent solution in each eye followed 5 minutes later by second application. Observe patient closely for at least 30 minutes following instillation.

Tropicamide

It is another rapidly acting mydriatic and cyclopegic agent and act faster than cyclopentolate (short-acting anticholinergic agent).

It blocks the parasympathetic fibers and causes relaxation of sphincter pupillae muscle of the iris producing mydriasis.

Indications: For mydriasis and cycloplegia for diagnostic purposes, when short-acting mydriatic is needed for some preoperative and postoperative states.

It prevents constriction of pupil caused by intense light stimulation during indirect ophthalmoscopy or retinal photography.

TABLE 15.3: Relative efficiency of cycloplegics

Drug	% Efficiency
1% Atropine	100%
1% Cyclopentolate	92%
1% Tropicamide	80%
5% Homatropine	54%
0.25% Scopolamine	48%

Dosage: It is available as 0.5 percent and 1 percent ophthalmic solutions.

Recommended dosage for refraction is to instill 1–2 drops of 1 percent solution into the eyes, repeat after 5 minutes an additional drop to prolong mydriatic effect.

For fundus examination, instill 1–2 drops of 0.5% solution 15–20 minutes prior to examination.

On account of its short latency, brief duration and effective mydriasis, it is perhaps the best mydriatic for the usual fundus examination.

Due to shorter duration of action, it is used as provocative test for acute glaucoma though under strictly controlled conditions.

It is used alone or in combination of sympathomimetic agent (Phenylephrine) to produce much better response and mydriatic effect persists to facilitate ocular examination.

Some other drugs of this group were previously used for mydriatic and cycloplegic effect but now not is use.
1. Duboisine (0.1 – 1.0% drops)
2. Lachesine or E3 (0.5 drops)

MYDRIATIC COMBINATIONS

Phenylephrine is commonly used with tropicamide, cyclopentolate or scopolamine to induce mydriasis which is greater than of either drug alone.

Phenylephrine 5% and cyclopentolate HCl 1%: Instill 1 drop into each eye every 5–10 minutes not to exceed three times.

Phenylephrine 10% and scopolamine 0.3%: For mydriasis, cycloplegia and to break posterior synechiae in iritis.

Dosage: For mydriasis 1–2 drops into the eye and repeat in 5 minutes, if necessary. Postoperatively, 1–2 drops into the eyes 3–4 times daily.

Phenylephrine 5% with tropicamide 0.8%
- For short-acting mydriasis in refraction and in pre- and postoperative states.
- For refraction instill 1–2 drops and repeat at 5 minutes interval, if necessary.
- For postoperative stage instill 1–2 drops three times a day.

Cyclopentolate HCl 1% with dexamethasone sodium phosphate 0.1%: For postoperative inflammation where mydriatic and inflammatory therapy is simultaneously required.

Dosage: Instill 1-2 drops into the affected eyes three times a day.

Atropine sulphate 1% solution with dexamethasone sodium phosphate 0.1%: For postoperative inflammation and anterior and posterior uveitis where mydriatic and inflammatory therapies are required in conjunction.

Dosage: Instill 1-2 drops into the affected eyes three times a day.

Phenylephrine (5%) and tropicamide (0.8%) combination is commonly used in ophthalmology today. The major advantage of this combination is that it produces quick mydriasis and mydriatic effect persists to facilitate ocular examination.

Indications: This preparation is mainly indicated for:
- Ophthalmoscopic examination
- Slit lamp examination
- Retinal photography
- Prior to ocular surgery and other diagnostic procedures.

It is also used:
- As an adjunct in the treatment of anterior uveitis
- In the management of anterior segment burns (to dilate the pupil and prevent iris adhesions to the lens)
- In cycloplegic refraction
- For the management of iridocyclitis associated with stromal keratitis
- For the management of uveal inflammation associated with fungal keratitis.

Dosage: This combination is available as topical ophthalmic solution (in 5 ml pack). For ophthalmological examinations 1-2 drops in the eye 15-30 minutes prior to the procedure are advised. For other indications frequency should be as per direction of ophthalmologists.

This preparation is contraindicated in patients suffering from closed angle glaucoma and hypersensitivity to any ingradient of this formulation.

Adverse reactions: On topical application there may be transient burning or stinging sensation and lacrimation. Blurred vision, photophobia and allergic reactions may occur.

BIBLIOGRAPHY

1. Agarwal A. Textbook of Ophthalmology, 1st edn. New Delhi: Jaypee Brothers Medical Publishers, 2002.
2. Bartlett JD. Administration of Cycloplegic Agents. Am J Optom. Physical Optics 1978;55:227.
3. Bartlett JD. Clinical Ocular Pharmacology, 4th edn. Boston: Butterworth-Heinemann, 2001
4. Bartlett JD. Ophthalmic Drug Facts. Lippincott: William and Wilkins, 2001.

5. Crick RP, Trimble RB. Textbook of Clinical Ophthalmology. Hodder and Stoughton, 1986.
6. Duane TD. Clinical Ophthalmology, 4th edn. Butterworth Heinemann, 1999.
7. Duvall. Ophthalmic Medications and Pharmacology. Slack Inc, 1998.
8. Ellis PP. Ocular Therapeutics and Pharmacology, 7th edn. CV Mosby, 1985.
9. Fechner. Ocular Therapeutics. Slack Inc., 1998.
10. Fraunfelder. Current Ocular Therapy, 5th edn. WB Saunders, 2000.
11. Garg A. Current Trends in Ophthalmology, 1st edn. New Delhi: Jaypee Brothers Medical Publishers, 1997.
12. Garg A. Manual of Ocular Therapeutics, 1st edn. New Delhi: Jaypee Brothers Medical Publishers, 1996.
13. Garg A. Ready-Reckoner of Ocular Therapeutics, 1st edn. New Delhi: Jaypee Brothers Medical Publishers 2002.
14. Goodman LS, Gilman A. Pharmacological Basis of Therapeutics, 7th edn. New York: Macmillan, 1985.
15. Havener's. Ocular Pharmacology, 6th edn. CV Mosby, 1994.
16. Kanski. Clinical Ophthalmology, 4th edn. Butterworth-Heineman, 1999.
17. Kershner. Ophthalmic Medications and Pharmacology. Slack. Inc., 1994.
18. Olin BR, et al. Drugs Facts and Comparisons: Facts and Comparisons. St Louis, 1997.
19. Onofrey. The Ocular Therapeutics. Lippincott: William and Wilkins, 1997.
20. Rhee. The Wills Eye Drug Guide. Lippincott: William and Wilkins, 1998.
21. Steven Podos. Textbook of Ophthalmology. New Delhi: Jaypee Brothers Medical Publishers, 2001.
22. Zimmerman. Textbook of Ocular Pharmacology. Lippincott: William and Wilkins, 1997.

16

Ophthalmic Dyes

Ashok Garg (India)

INTRODUCTION

Ophthalmic dyes are one of the most useful diagnostic agents used in the detection and management of disorders of the visual system.

Various dyes used in ophthalmology are:
- Fluorescein sodium
- Fluorexon
- Rose bengal
- Lissamine green
- Indocyanine green.

Individual drug monograph is as follows:

FLUORESCEIN SODIUM

Fluorescein sodium is a yellow water soluble dibasic acid dye of the xanthine series that produce intense green fluorescent color in alkaline solution. Chemically it is $C_2H_{12}O_5Na$ (Molecular weight 376.27). It is orange red in powder and yellow in solution.

It fluoresces yellow green in blue light and is most common staining agent used in the ophthalmology.
- Its peak absorption: 465–490 nm
- Peak emission: 520–530 nm

Fluorescence increases with greater concentration up to 0.001 percent and with greater pH up to pH 8. But at very high concentrations quenching occurs. It dimerises, polymerizes and emission shifts to longer wavelengths. Fluorescein is used to demonstrate defects of corneal epithelium. It does not actually stain the tissues but is used as an indicator dye.

The normal precorneal tear film appears yellow or orange with fluorescein. The intact corneal epithelium prevents penetration of water soluble fluorescein and is not colored by it. Any break in the epithelium barrier permits rapid fluorescein penetration occurring due to any trauma, infection and other causes. Epithelial defects or cornea appear bright green and is easily visualized. If epithelial loss is severe, topical fluorescein penetrates into the aqueous and is readily visible biomicroscopically as a green flare.

Fluorescein sodium exhibits a high degree of ionization at physiological pH. Therefore, it does not penetrate the intact corneal epithelium. Break down of epithelium allows for stromal penetration. When exposed to light, fluorescein absorbs certain wavelengths and emits fluorescent light of longer wavelength. At pH 8 fluorescein reaches its maximum intensity.

Clinical Characteristics

- Stains epithelial defects bright green
- Diffuses into intercellular spaces
- Will not stain devitalized cells or mucus
- Tear film appears yellow orange
- Can exhibit pseudoflare, Fischer-Schweitzer mosaic
- Promotes growth of *Pseudomonas* in solution
- Will stain soft contact lenses.

Indications: Fluorescein sodium is used for (Figs 16.1 to 16.6):

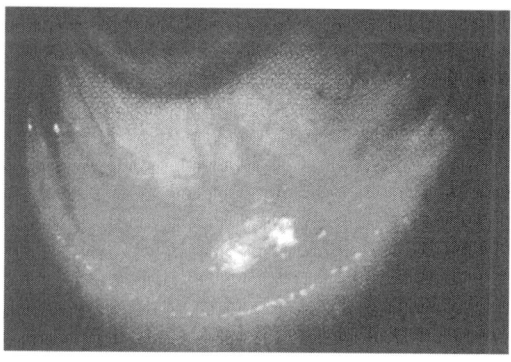

Fig. 16.1: Fluorescein strips for evaluation of conjunctival injuries and infections

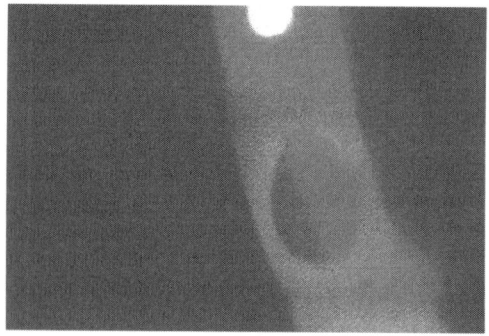

Fig. 16.2: Fluorescein strips for dry eye disorder (break-up time, BUT)

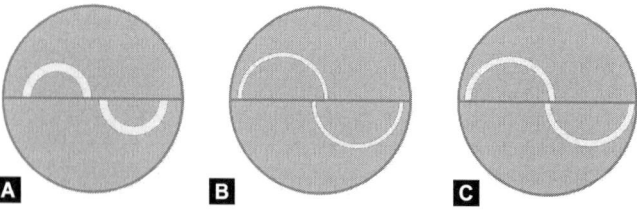

Figs 16.3A to C: Fluorescein strips for applanation tonometry
(*Courtesy:* FDS Limited)

Ophthalmic Dyes

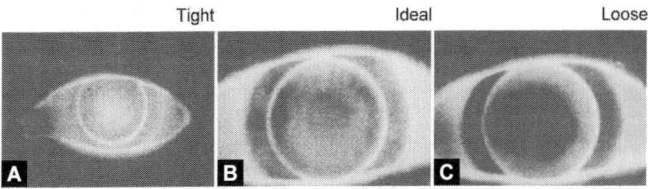

Figs 16.4A to C: Fluorescein strips for evaluation of contact lens fitting

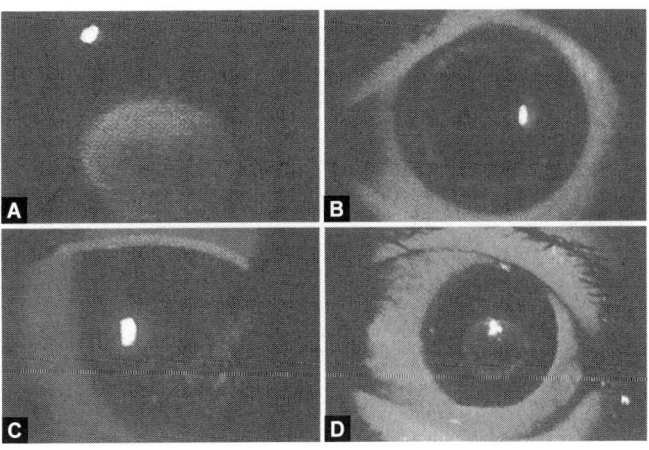

Figs 16.5A to D: Fluorescein strips for evaluation of corneal injuries and infections

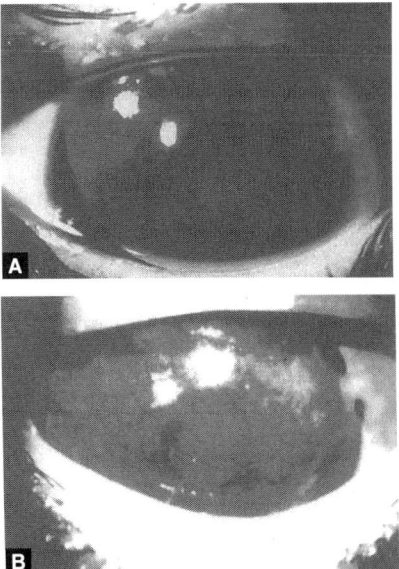

Figs 16.6A and B: Fluorescein dye test
(*Courtesy*: FDS Limited)

Topical

- Lacrimal testing (TBUT, Jones test)
- Detection of corneal epithelial defects
- Detection of penetration of globe (Seidel's sign)
- Applanation tonometry
- Contact lens/corneal fitting relationship
- Fitting of rigid contact lenses
- Retinal angiography.

Injection

- Vitreous fluorophotometry.
- Diagnostic aid in ophthalmic angiography including examination of fundus, evaluation of iris vasculature, distinction between viable and nonviable tissue, observation of aqueous flow, differential diagnosis of malignant and non-malignant tumors, determination of circulation time and adequacy.

Unlabeled Use

It can be administered orally as a diagnostic aid in the detection of certain retinal vascular diseases.

Contraindications

- Hypersensitivity to active ingradient or any other components
- Do not use topically with soft contact lenses as lenses may get discolored.

Administration and dosage: For topical use fluorescein may be administered as a topical solution or by fluorescein impregnated paper strips. Since fluorescein in solution is susceptible to bacterial contamination, multidose formulations are dispensed with a preservative such as chlorobutanol or thimerosal. For diagnostic purposes such as applanation tonometry, a local anesthetic is included in the formulation.

Topical Formulations

a. In topical solution it is available as 2 percent solution in (1, 2 and 15 ml packs).
   To detect foreign bodies, corneal abrasions instill 1–2 drops of 2 percent solution. Allow a few seconds for staining. Washout excess with sterile irrigating solution.
b. Topical solution containing
   0.25 percent fluorescein sodium
   0.1 percent proparacaine hydrochloride
   0.01 percent thimerosal preservative
   } in 5 ml pack
c. 0.25 fluorescein sodium
   0.50 percent proparacaine hydrochloride
   0.01 percent thimerosal with povidone,
   } in 5 ml pack

boric acid and polysorbate 80
0.25 percent fluorescein sodium   ⎤ 0.4
percent benoxinate hydrochloride   ⎥ in 5 ml
1 percent chlorobutanol, povidone buffers pack ⎦

Fluorescein strips: Fluorescein impregnated strips are useful for routine procedures such as contact lens fitting, lacrimal system evaluation. Bacterial contamination is minimized since the strips are stored in dry state. When wetted with water or an irrigating solution, the dye is released from the strips and can be applied to the eye by gently touching the conjunctiva with sterile filter paper impregnated with fluorescein of 1 or 2 percent solution.

Various fluorescein strips preparations are:
1. 1 mg strips (boric acid, polysorbate 80 and 0.5 percent Chlorobutanol).
2. 9 mg strips (boric acid, polysorbate 80 and 0.5 percent Chlorobutanol).
3. 0.6 mg and 1 mg strips.
4. High molecular fluorescein (Higlo) strips for soft. Contact lenses and it does not stain soft lenses.

Intravenous fluorescein (Fluorescein angiography): It is used for the detection of vascular abnormalities of fundus. Following injection into antecubetal vein, the dye appears in central retinal artery. Integrity of retina and choroid as well as arm to retinal circulation time may be determined. For IV use fluorescein is available as 10 and 25 percent injections (in 2 ml, 5 ml ampoules and in 10 ml disp. syringe).

Oral fluorescein: It can be administered by mixing fluorescein powder or several vials of 10 percent injectables fluorescein in a citrus drink. Time of onset of maximal fluorescence is 45-60 minutes as compared to seconds *via* the injectable route. Oral fluorescence can be used to study disorders characterized by late leakage of dye such as cystoid macular edema, to study retinal vascular abnormalities in young diabetic patients and to document retinal pigment epithelial detachment, central serous choroidopathy and optic disk edema.

Adverse reactions: Topical application of fluorescein has minimum adverse effects. Injection administration may cause nausea, headache, GI distress, vomiting, syncope, hypotension, signs of hypersensitivity, thrombophlebitis at the injection site, severe shock, convulsions, temporary yellowish skin discoloration, itching, anaphylaxis, pyrexia, urticaria, puritis, angioneurotic edema. Discoloration of skin disappear in 6-12 hours and urine. Fluorescence fades in 24-36 hours. Extravasation at the injection site causes intense pain, at the site and dull aching pain in the injection arm.

Precautions

- Exercise great caution in administering to patients with a history of hypersensitivity, allergy or asthma.

- Avoid extravasation during injection. The high pH of the solution can result in severe local tissue damage, sloughing of skin, superficial phlebitis, subcutaneous granuloma and toxic neuritis along with median curve in the antecubital area.
- Avoid parenteral administration, in pregnant patients specially in the first trimester.

FLUOREXON

It is N, N-bis (Carboxymethyl)–aminoethyl, fluorescein tetra-sodium salt. Its molecular weight is 710.

With a molecular size nearly twice that of fluorescein, it penetrates hydrophilic contact lens at a much slower rate.

Upon ocular instillation, it yeilds a pale yellow brown color.

Fluorexon is less brilliant than fluorescein and does not increase linearly with increasing concentration.

It stains epithelial defects, devitalized cells and mucin (less than fluorescein or rose bengal). It does not stain most soft contact lenses and may stain high water (more than 60%) contact lenses.

It promotes the growth of *Pseudomonas*. Fluorexon is not recommended for use with high water soft contact lenses since the chances of discoloration are greater and more difficult to reverse than with lower water content contact lenses.

For optimal fluorescence, a special yellow filter is recommended. It generally causes little or no discomfort when instilled into the eye. Due to its large molecular size it is less effective stain for epithelial defects, erosions and contact lens induced effects than fluorescein.

Indications: Diagnostic and fitting aid for patients with hydrogel (soft) contact lenses. Use in eye with or without lens in place when fluorescein is contraindicated to avoid staining lenses.
- Evaluation of corneal integrity of patients wearing hydrogel contact lenses.
- Can be used in the place of sodium fluorescein when conducting the tear break-up time (BUT) test.
- For performing the applanation tonometry without removing the lens.
- For detecting the lathe-cut index markings (Toric lenses).

Dosage: It is available as 0.35 percent topical solution (in 0.5 ml pipettes). Instill one drop of fluorexon on the concave surface of the lens and place the lens immediately on the eye.

Alternatively instill 1–2 drops in the lower cul-de-sac and ask the patient to blink several times. Additional drop may be necessary during a prolonged examination. Rinse both the eyes and lens with sterile irrigating solution or saline following examination.

As the dye passes under the lens, observe a central dark zone of 6-9 mm in diameter which forms after each blink. The lens may be reinserted immediately as compare to the long waiting period required after the use of fluorescein.

Examination should be started immediately after instillation of fluorexon drops because this material tends to dissipate

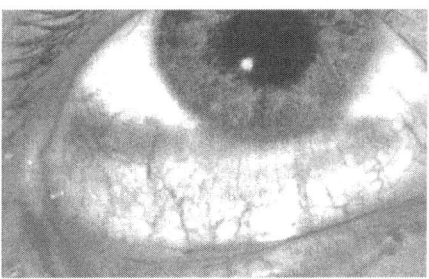

Fig. 16.7: Rose bengal staining test
(*Courtesy*: FDS Limited)

readily with the tear flow leading to a progressive reduction in fluorescence.

Precaution: Do not use solutions containing hydrogen peroxide to clean or sterilize lenses until all traces of fluorexon are removed. Hydrogen peroxide can bind fluorescein molecules to the lens.

ROSE BENGAL

It is Iodine derivative of fluorescein chemically it is 4,5,6,7, tetrachloro – 2,4,5,7 tetraiodo fluorescein sodium.

It stains devitalized cells and mucin a brilliant red. It also stains the mucus of precorneal tear film (Fig. 16.7).

Rose bengal stains the nucleus more than the cytoplasm and higher concentration stain more distinctly and highlight more subtle defects. When applied as solution or from a moistened filter paper strip, this dye is an effective aid in the evaluation of keratoconjunctivitis sicca, herpes simplex keratitis, corneal abrasions and detection of foreign bodies. A correlation may exist between intensity of staining and severity of cellular defect.

There is no need of actual break in the epithelium for positive staining with rose bengal. It has also antiviral properties.

Indications: As diagnostic agent for routine ocular examination on when superficial corneal or conjunctival tissue change is suspected. Effective aid for diagnosis of keratitis, corrosions or abrasions and in detection of foreign body. Contraindication is known hypersensitivity to rose bengal.

Dosage: It is available as topical 1 percent solution containing 1 percent rose bengal with povidone, sodium borate, PEG p-isooctylphenyl 10 and 0.01 percent thimerosal in 5 ml pack. It is also available as 1.3 mg strip. Topically instill 1–2 drops into the conjunctival sac before examination.

Strips: Thoroughly saturate tip of strip with sterile irrigating solution, remove excess before application. Touch conjunctiva or lower fornix with moistened strip. The patient should blink several times after application.

Adverse reaction: Rose bengal can cause marked ocular irritation and discomfort following instillation specially in more severly diseased eyes and with the use of higher concentrations of dye. A topical anesthetic shall be used to alleviate the discomfort specially topical solution formulation is applied. Application of dye using commercially available filter paper strip usually results in less discomfort. Rose bengal stains a line along the ciliary margin on conjunctival tarsus in normal eyes.

Rose bengal can stain eyelids, cheeks, fingers and clothing in a concentration dependent manner. Keep the amount of dye at the minimum and irrigating the eye help circumvent this problem.

LISSAMINE GREEN

Lissamine green stains degenerated cells, dead cells and mucus fibrils in the same manner as rose bengal. The cell nucleus is stained more intensely than the cytoplasm. Vacuoles in the mucus thread remains unstained.

Indications: As diagnostic agent for routine ocular examination on when supercial corneal or conjunctival tissue change is suspected. Helpful in the diagnosis of keratitis, corrosions or abrasions and in detection of foreign body.

Contraindication is known hypersensitivity to Lissamine green.

Dosage: It is available as sterile ophthalmic strips. Each strip contain approx 15 mg of Lissamine green (pack of 100 strips).

Direction for use: Moisten impregnated tip with sterile water or normal saline. While the patient looks-up, stroke the tip across the bulbar conjunctiva. The patient should than blink several times to obtain best results.

Adverse reactions: It can cause ocular discomfort and irritation following instillation.

INDOCYANINE GREEN

It is a unique ophthalmic dye due to its high protein binding capacity and near infrared fluorescence. It is a sterile, water soluble tricarbocyanine dye with a peak spectral absorption at 800-810 nm in blood or blood plasma. Chemically indocyanine green, contains < 5 percent sodium iodide.

Indocyanine green has unique characteristic for recording of indicator-dilution curves for both diagnosis and research purposes independent of oxygen saturation fluctuations. In dye dilution curves dye is injected as a single bolus as rapidly as possible.

Pharmacokinetics: The peak absorption and emission of indocyanine green lie in 800–850 nm where transmission of energy by the pigment epithelium is more efficient than in the visible light energy region. Indocyanine green is about 98 percent bound to plasma protein so excessive dye extravasation does not take place in the highly fenestrated choroidal vasculature. It is highly useful in both absorption and fluorescence infrared angiography of the choroidal vasculature when using proper filters and film in a fundus camera.

Following IV injection indocyanine green is rapidly bound to plasma protein of which albumin is the principle carrier (95%). Indocyanine green undergoes no significant extrahepatic or enterohepatic circulation. Indocyanine green is taken-up from the plasma almost exclusively by the hepatic parenchymal cells and is secreted entirely into the bile.

Indications

- Indocyanine green is used for ophthalmic angiography.
- It is indicated for digital indocyanine green video-angiography (ICG-V) and ICG-angiography guided laser photocoagulation.
- ICG-V is a new technique using indocyanine green as fluorescein dye that enhances imaging of choroid, its associated pathology and has been shown to be useful in better delineating occult choroidal neovascularization into well demarcated ones. This enhanced imaging of choroid and well demarcation of choroidal neovascularization is specifically due to indocyanine green special properties of high protein binding capacity and near infrared fluorescence.
- Indocyanine green videoangiography is a predictive indicator of future exudative changes in eyes with drusen
- ICG-V can detect subgroups of patients with drusen who are at higher risk of having exudative changes developed.
- Indocyanine green angiography guided laser photocoagulation increases the proportion of patients with well defined or treatable neovascularization in cases of ARMD. ICG angiography may allow identification and treatment of feeder vessel in a small percentage of eyes with subfoveal neovascularization which may allow treatment and resolution of neovascularization of previously untreatable eyes. ICG provides additional information regarding the presence, location, filling patterns and leakage from choroidal neovascularization.

Administration and dosage: It is available as powder for injection in 25 mg and 50 mg strengths alongwith aqueous solvents (pH 5.5-6.5) in 10 ml ampoules aqueous solvent is specially prepared sterile water for injection to dissolve indocyanine green.

Dosage: Generally 40 mg dye in 2 ml of aqueous solvent is given. Immediately follow the injected dye bolus with a 5 ml bolus of normal saline. This injection regimen provides the optimal concentration of spatially limited dye bolus to the choroidal vasculature following IV injection. This dye is nontoxic on IV administration. In certain patients half the volume of ICG has been found to produce angiograms of comparable resolution.

Compatibility must be ensured before injecting indocyanine green. Use only the aqueous solvent (pH 5.5-6.5) provided with the dye which is specially prepared sterile water of injection to dissolve indocyanine green because there are certain reports of incompatibility with certain commercially available water for injections.

Indocyanine green is unstable in aqueous solution and should be used within 10 hours. However, dye is stable in plasma and whole blood. Use sterile techniques in handling the dye solution and in the performance of the dilution curves.

Indocyanine green powder may cling to the vial or lump together because it is freeze dried in vials. This is certainly not due to the presence of water.

Precautions

- As indocyanine green contains sodium iodide so use it with caution in individuals who have history of allergy to iodides.
- Excessive caution should be taken when indocyanine green is administered in pregnant woman or to a nursing woman. Give ICG only if clearly indicated.
- Do not perform radioactive iodine uptake studies for atleast a week following the use of indocyanine green.
- Heparin preparations containing sodium bisulfite reduce the absorption peak of indocyanine green in blood and hence contraindicated.

Adverse reactions: Anaphylactic or urticarial reactions have been reported in patients without history of allergy to iodides. If such reactions occur treat with suitable agents (e.g. Epinephrine, antihistamines or corticosteroids).

TRYPAN BLUE

Trypan blue is a dye which safely stains the anterior lens capsule and is mainly used in cataract surgery (ECCE, IOL surgery and phacosurgery).

Trypan blue is a capsule stainer which reduces the risk of complication due to unrecognized radial capsule by facilitating the performance of the capsulorehexis in the absence of red fundus reflex specially in the cases of matured cataract. Special feature of trypan blue is that it stains the anterior capsule without affecting the corneal endothelium. So blue stained capsule can be easily identified from the underlying unstained lenticular tissue. It helps the eye surgeon to see capsule clearly thus eliminates the chances of hitting the outline with the phacotip during phacoemulsification.

Mechanism of action: Trypan blue is used to enhance the visualization of the anterior lens capsule of the eye during removal of cataractous lens replacement procedures. Trypan blue provides a clear, visible staining at low amounts without diffusing into or through concerned tissues. So it facilitates the controlled opening of anterior capsule and reduces the risk of inadvertent damage to the capsule specially radial tear towards or beyond the equator of the lens. Besides, it has low toxicity profile.

Pharmacokinetics: Trypan blue solution concentration is more preferred in the range of 0.01–0.1 percent. In this range an optimal staining effect is achieved, while at the same time the risk of possible damage to the eye or any part thereof due to the toxicity of the dye is minimized. After few drops instillation of trypan blue dye on to anterior lens capsule, it selectively stains the anterior lens capsule whereas the lenticular material beneath the anterior lens capsule is not stained. No traces of the dye are present in ocular tissues shortly after the cataract extraction procedure has been completed.

Indications: Trypan blue is indicated for facilitating surgical procedures for cataract extraction (IOL surgery and phacosurgery) and as a staining agent.

Administration and dosage: It is available as 1 ml single use ampoule commercially. Each ml contains 0.6 mg trypan blue, 1.9 mg of sodium mono-hydrogen orthophosphate, 0.3 mg of sodium dihydrogen orthophosphate, 8.2 mg of sodium chloride and sodium hydroxide for adjusting the pH and water for injection.

For trypan blue administration, first step of procedure is to inject air into the anterior chamber using a 26 gauge needle in the area where the second site is made. This prevents the water like dilution of the trypan blue. Then trypan blue is withdrawn from the ampoule into the tuberculin syringe and is injected by needle into the anterior chamber between the airbubble and the lens capsule. Use the bevel down of the needle and see to it that the injection is made in a drop format so that the whole capsule gets stained. If some portion is left unstained, inject a drop in that area till it gets stained. It is kept lie in this position for a minute for complete staining of the anterior capsule to occur. Thereafter viscoelastic is injected into the anterior chamber. This will distend the eye so that during clear corneal incision eye shall be tense and one can create a good valve. Now one can use a straight rod to stabilize the eye with the left hand and with the right hand clear corneal or scleral incision can be made. Inject viscoelastic inside the eye to remove the air bubble and trypan blue. Now rhexis can be started with a needle or Forceps (Surgeon choice). One can see the contrast between the capsule which has been stained and the cortex which is unstained. The rhexis is continued and finally completed. After rhexis completion we can see the stained anterior capsule lying in the anterior chamber.

Contraindication: Trypan blue is contraindicated in patients with a hypersensitivity to the dye or any of its components.

Adverse reactions:
- Clinical literature reports are not certain if extended contact of trypan blue with the corneal endothelium produces corneal damage or not. At present no case has been reported as the trypan blue is washed off with the viscoeleastic and the BSS fluid.
- Mild postsurgical inflammatory reactions and some bullous keratopathy have been reported to occur after using trypan blue in certain cases.
- Trypan blue solution should be given to a pregnant woman only if the benefits clearly outweigh any possible risks.

- On the whole trypan blue is well tolerated following injection into the anterior chamber of the eye during cataract surgery.

VERTEPORFIN (VISUDYNE)

Visudyne (Verteporfin) is a photosensitive second generation porphyrin (benzoporphyrin), mono acid derivative which has been recently approved by FDA (Food and Drug Administration) USA for the photodynamic therapy (PDT) the drug/light combination for the treatment of wet age related macular degeneration (ARMD).

Pharmacokinetics: Veteporfin is a chlorin type molecule and exists as an equal mixture of two regio isomers each of which consists of an enantiomeric pair that demonstrate similar pharmacological activity *in vitro* and *in vivo*. It has a molecular formula of $C_{41}H_{42}N_4O_8$ and a molecular weight of 718.81 (Fig. 16.8). Verteporfin is formulated in a lipid-based preparation that augments solubility in the blood.

It is a lipophilic molecule that selectively accumulates in vascular endothelial cells such as the neovascular tissues of AMD possibly due to increased concentration of low density lipoprotein (LDL) receptors in the membrane of these cells.

Verteporfin has a long absorption wavelength with several peaks including a strong absorption peak in the 680–695 mm region. It absorbs light efficiently at a wavelength of 689 nm (red light) which can penetrate a thin layer of blood, melanin or fibrotic tissue. This absorption peak does not interfere with any of the absorption peaks of naturally presents substances. Due to its peak absorption at a long wavelength enables the laser light to penetrate deep into the target tissue.

Association of verteporfin with lipoprotein provides selectivity for neovascular tissues and enhances the photodynamic effect. It is cleared rapidly from the plasma with an elimination half-life of 5-6 hours. Verteporfin is excreted almost exclusively in the feces primarily within 24 hours of administration.

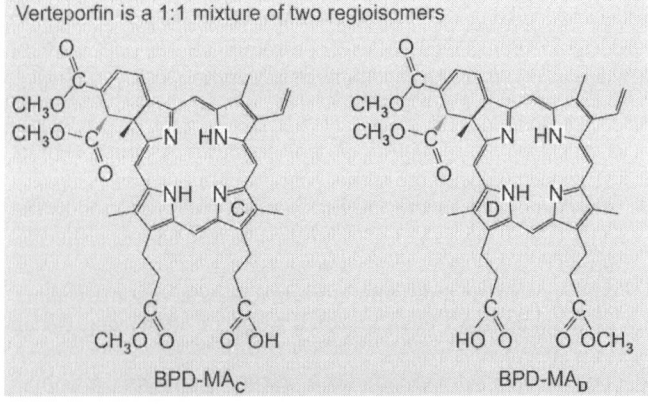

Fig. 16.8: Chemical structure of verteporfin
(*Courtesy*: Novartis ophthalmics)

Ophthalmic Dyes

The selective uptake and retention of verteporfin in CNV (Chroidal neovascularization) is important because it limits the extent of damage to surrounding normal healthy tissues uptake of verteporfin is rapid reaching maximum levels within 30 minutes.

Indications: Verteporfin is indicated for the treatment of age-related macular degeneration in patients with predominantly classic subfoveal choroidal neovascularization (Wet type).

Administration and dosage: Verteporfin (Visudyne) is commercially available in single use 15 mg vials as a sterile, lipid-based, freeze dried powder that requires reconstitution with sterile water and dilution with 5 percent dextrose solution before administration. It is available for intravenous infusion only. Verteporfin should be stored at room temperature between 20–25°C and shall be protected from light.

Reconstitution: For a total volume of 7.5 ml of reconstituted drug 7.0 ml of sterile water for injection has to be injected into the verteporfin vial which should then be gently agitated until the powder is completely dissolved. The reconstituted solution must be protected from light and used within 4 hours. Saline solution should not be used because verteporfin precipitates in saline.

Dilution: Further dilution with 5 percent dextrose for injection is required to achieve a drug dose of 6 mg/m_2 BSA and a total infusion volume of 30 ml. BSA can be determined using a nomogram or a graphic algorithm.

Dosage and mechanism of action: Verteporfin therapy is a two-step process involving administration of a nontoxic light activated drug and its subsequent activation by a specific wavelength of light using a nonthermal diode laser device.

Verteporfin is activated at a long wavelength that optimizes energy absorption of the drug (Figs 16.9 to 16.11). The most suitable light source for verteporfin therapy is diode laser operating at a wavelength of 689 + 3 nm. At the power used to activate verteporfin the laser causes no thermal damage to retinal tissues. The laser beam is delivered through a slit lamp to the affected area in the retina and the light is targeted to the desired area by means of a low intensity helium-neon (HeNe) beam through a standard ophthalmological contact lens.

The optimal regimen of verteporfin therapy recommended internationally is as follows:

Verteporfin

Dose	:	6 mg/m_2 body surface area (BSA)
Infusion rate	:	3 ml/min
Duration of infusion	:	10 minutes
Formula for m^2 BSA	:	$\dfrac{\text{Height (m)} \times \text{weight (kg)}}{6}$
Light application	:	Interval after start of verteporfin infusion: 5 min.

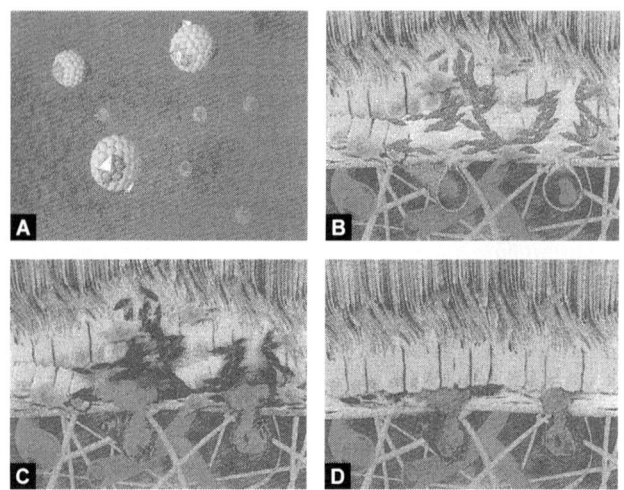

Figs 16.9A to D: Schematic illustration of 4 stages of mechanism of action of verteporfin: (A) Circulating visudyne complexes with LDL; (B) Visudyne selectively accumulates in neovascular tissue which is rich in LDL receptors; (C) Light-activated visudyne produces reactive forms of oxygen which cause structural and functional cell damage; (D) Visudyne selectively occludes neovascular tissue, while sparing overlying retinal cells and Bruch's membrane (*Courtesy*: Novartis ophthalmics)

Wavelength	:	689 nm
Dose	:	50 J/cm^2
Intensity	:	600 mw/cm^2
Resulting duration of light application	:	835

Strict adherence to this regimen is necessary for safe and effective treatment.

Mechanism of action of verteporfin: Verteporfin is a potent photosensitizer which is administered intravenously as a liposomal preparation. Immediately after intravenous administration, verteporfin partitions into the lipoproteins in the blood, particularly the LDL fraction. It selectively accumulates within neovasculature including neovascular endothelial tissue probably due to increased uptake of LDL and increased expression of LDL receptors on rapidly proliferating cells. Once verteporfin has bound to surface receptors on endothelial cell membranes, it is taken-up into the cell and binds to intracellular or cytoplasmic components. This is thought to be a major mechanism of selective accumulation and retention of verteporfin in these tissues.

Application of the nonthermal diode laser to the target tissues (689 nm) causes verteporfin to transform from a ground singlet state to an excited triplet state. Verteporfin initiates photochemical reactions either directly *via* the formation of reactive free radicals (type-I mechanism) or indirectly *via* the transfer of its energy into

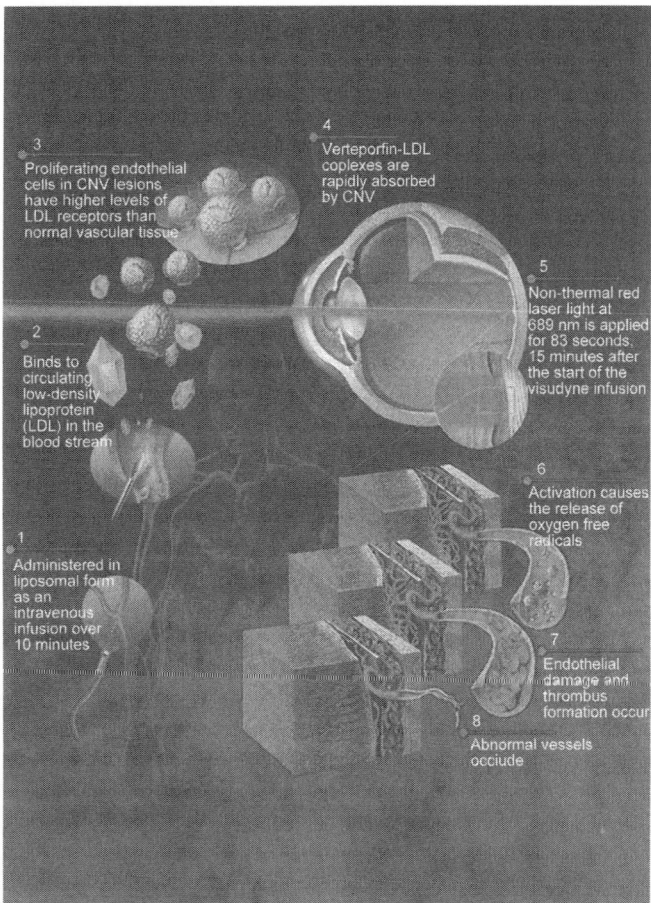

Fig. 16.10: Verteporfin mechanism of action
(*Courtesy*: Novartis ophthalmics)

ground state oxygen ($3O_2$) and highly reactive singlet oxygen ($1O_2$) type-II mechanism.

Both photochemical reactions can occur simultaneously and both causes direct cytotoxicity. Both reactions cause damage or death to cells in which verteporfin has accumulated. Damage to endothelial cells leads to platelet adhesion, platelet aggregation and thrombus formation and this process results in occlusion of the leaking CNV. Occlusion of CNV can be safely reproduced without any negative effect on the overlying retinal tissue.

So the primary mechanism of visudyne therapy may be damage to the fibrovascular tissue through the induction of neovascular occlusion. Histologically the endothelial cells lining the vessels are damaged, they are swollen and the nuclear membrane breaks. Other nearby vessels remain intact and there is minimal damage to adjacent retinal structures such as overlying photoreceptors and RPE, therapy maintaining function of the retina and helps to increase the chances of stable vision.

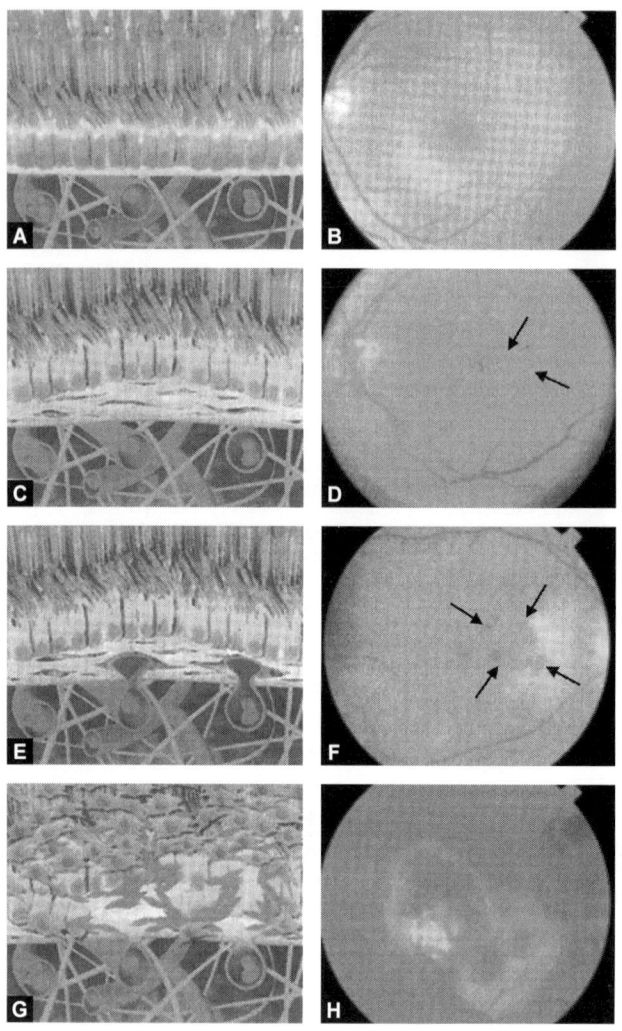

Figs 16.11A to H: Pathophysiology of AMD
(*Courtesy*: Novartis ophthalmics)

The abnormal blood vessels may return after several months. However, verteporfin therapy can be reapplied at up to 3 months intervals if necessary.

Adverse reactions: Usually verteporfin therapy is well tolerated. Most adverse events are mild to moderate and transient in nature.

a. Ocular adverse events
   - Transient vision disturbances (Decreased vision and visual field defects)
   - Cataract
   - Conjunctivitis
   - Eye pain
   - Lacrimation disorder

- Photophobia
- Subretinal hemorrhage
- Vitreous hemorrhage.

  Patients in whom such symptoms appear should therefore not drive or operate machinery for as long as these symptoms persists.

  To provide safe and effective treatment the recommended light dose of 50 J/cm^2 should not be exceeded.

b. Systemic adverse reactions
   - Back pain
   - Abdominal pain
   - Asthenia
   - Flu syndrome
   - Headache
   - Injection site adverse reactions like edema, extravasation, fibrosis, hemorrhage, hypersensitivity, inflammation and pain
   - Photosensitivity reactions
   - Digestive adverse reactions like diarrhea, dyspepsia, nausea and vomiting
   - Metabolic and nutritional adverse reactions like glycosuria, hypokalemia, ketosis and hypercholesterolemia
   - Dizziness
   - Rhinitis and pruritus.

     Injection site adverse events can be limited by compliance with IV procedures. Photosensitivity reactions can be limited by compliance with precautionary, guidelines immediately after verteporfin therapy patients should take the following precautions:
   - Avoid exposure to direct sunlight or bright indoor lighting
   - Wear dark sunglasses while outdoors during the first 48 hours
   - Reschedule dental or elective hospital surgery to avoid exposure to powerful operating lights
   - Exposure to low levels of indoor light should be encouraged to promote photobleaching and rapid drug elimination.

Contraindications: Verteporfin therapy is contraindicated in patients with porphyria or patients with known hypersensitivity to verteporfin or any other component of the lipid-based formulation.

Precautions: Caution should be taken in treating patients with uncontrolled hypertension, unstable cardiovascular disease, active hepatitis or moderately severe or severe liver disease. Advanced cataracts and retinal tears should be treated before initiation of verteporfin therapy.

Overdose: Overdose of drug and/or light in the treated eye may result in nonperfusion of normal retinal vessels with the possibility of a severe decrease in vision that could be permanent. An overdose of visudyne may also result in the prolongation of the period during which the patient remains photosensitive to bright light. In such cases photosensitivity precautions are extended for a time proportional to the overdose.

BIBLIOGRAPHY

1. AAO. Ophthalmology Monograph on Fluorescein and Indocyanine Green, 2001.
2. Agarwal A. Textbook of Ophthalmology, 1st edn. New Delhi: Jaypee Brothers Medical Publishers, 2002.
3. Bartlett JD. Clinical Ocular Pharmacology, 4th edn. Boston: Butterworth-Heinemann, 2001
4. Bartlett JD. Ophthalmic Drug Facts, Lippincott–William and Wilkins, 2001.
5. Berkow JW, et al. Fluorescein and Indocyanine Green Angiography Techniques, 2nd edn. American Academy of Ophthalmology, 1997.
6. Crick RP, Trimble RB. Textbook of Clinical Ophthalmology, Hodder and Stoughton, 1986.
7. Duane TD. Clinical Ophthalmology, 4th edn. Butterworth–Heinemann, 1999.
8. Duvall. Ophthalmic Medications and Pharmacology, Slack Inc, 1998.
9. Ellis PP. Ocular Therapeutics and Pharmacology, 7th edn. CV Mosby, 1985.
10. Fechner. Ocular Therapeutics, Slack Inc., 1998.
11. Feenstra, et al. Comparison of Fluorescein and Rose Bengal Staining, Arch. Ophthalmol., 1992;99:605.
12. Fraunfelder. Current Ocular Therapy, 5th edn. WB Saunders, 2000.
13. Garg A. Current Trends in Ophthalmology, 1st edn. New Delhi: Jaypee Brothers Medical Publishers, 1997.
14. Garg A. Manual of Ocular Therapeutics, 1st edn. New Delhi: Jaypee Brothers Medical Publishers, 1996.
15. Garg A. Ready Reckoner of Ocular Therapeutics, 1st edn. New Delhi: 2002.
16. Goodman LS, Gilman A. Pharmacological Basis of Therapeutics, 7th edn. New York: Macmillan, 1985.
17. Havener's. Ocular Pharmacology, 6th edn. CV Mosby, 1994.
18. Kanski. Clinical Ophthalmology, 4th edn. Butterworth–Heineman, 1999.
19. Kershner. Ophthalmic Medications and Pharmacology, Slack. Inc., 1994.
20. Olin BR, et al. Drugs Facts and Comparisons: Facts and Comparisons, St. Louis, 1997.
21. Onofrey. The Ocular Therapeutics; Lippincott-William and Wilkins, 1997.
22. Reichel. Atlas of Indocyanine Green Angiography, Lippincott–William and Wilkins, 1995.
23. Rhee. The Wills Eye Drug Guide: Lippincott–William and Wilkins, 1998.
24. Steven Podos. Textbook of Ophthalmology, New Delhi: Jaypee Brothers Medical Publishers, 2001.
25. Yannuzzi LA, et al. Digital Indocyanine Green Video Angiography and Choroidal Neovascularization, Retina, 1992;12:191.
26. Zimmerman. Textbook of Ocular Pharmacology, Lippincott–William and Wilkins, 1997.

17

Ocular Lubricants and Artificial Tear Solutions

Ashok Garg (India)

INTRODUCTION

Dry eyes (Keratoconjunctivitis Sicca) is one of the most common causes of chronic low grade burning, irritation and discomfort of the eyes specially in elderly population. It is lacrimal insufficiency although reflex tearing can decrease with advancing age, a variety of diseases can also diminish basal tear secretion. Diseases which cause hyposecretion include: Drug induced hyposecretion, Sjögren's syndrome, erythema multiforme, pemphigoid lupus erythematosis, scleroderma, polyarteritis nodosa, sarcoidosis, Mikulicz's syndrome, polymyositis, etc.

A number of artificial tears and ophthalmic lubricants are available to treat this condition. Ophthalmic lubricants represents the cornerstone of the management of ocular surface disease. A number of new formulations have arrived commercially which have recognized the importance of limiting preservative toxicity while enhancing epithelial cell growth.

Availability of synthetic polymers suitable for ocular use has helped in development of artificial tear solutions, ointments and other formulations to help in alleviating ocular discomfort and maintain integrity of surface epithelium. Practically, formulations for dry eyes should be compatible with and substitute for components of tear film layer including lipid, aqueous and mucin.

Individual monograph of various ophthalmic preparations available commercially is as follows:

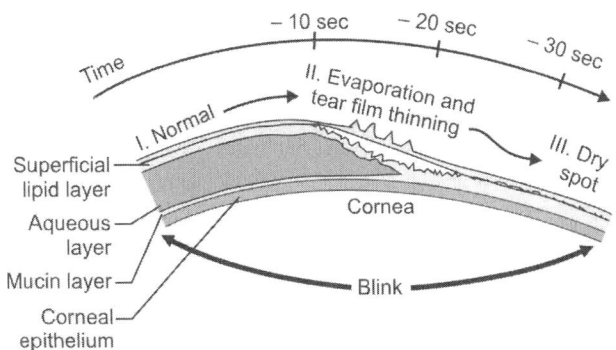

Fig. 17.1: Mechanism of tear film break-up [In dry eye upper yellow line (tear film) thins out and dry spots forms] (*Courtesy*: Allergan India Ltd)

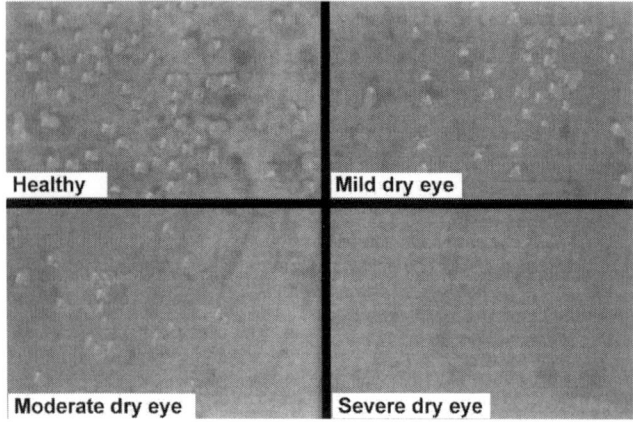

Fig. 17.2: Impression cytology mapping (in dry eye conditions cells appear fewer, irregular in size and shape and take up staining less uniformly) (*Courtesy:* Allergan India Ltd)

ARTIFICIAL TEAR SOLUTIONS

Lubricants preparations formulated as artificial tear solutions usually contain inorganic electrolytes, preservatives and water soluble polymeric system. Sodium chloride, potassium chloride, calcium and magnesium chloride, various other ions and boric acid help to maintain tonicity and pH of the formulations. Preservatives include: Benzalkonium chloride, Chlorobutanol, thimerosal, EDTA, methylparaben and ethyl paraben are used in multidose preparations to prevent bacterial contamination. Methylcellulose and its derivatives like Hydroxypropyl methylcellulose, Hydroxy ethylcellulose, carboxy methylcellulose, polyvinyl alcohol (PVA), povidone, dextran, propylene glycol and other mucoadhesive increased viscosity agents can enhance viscosity and promote tear film stability.

In addition to polymers, lipids and vitamin A have also been added into new ocular lubricants. Several commercial topical preparations are available containing phospholipid derivative and retinol (vitamin A). Vitamin A topical preparations have been shown to be effective in superior limbic keratoconjunctivitis and severe forms of dry eye syndrome.

Artificial tear solutions available commercially contain:
- Balanced amount of salts to maintain ocular tonicity (0.9% NaCl equivalent)
- Buffers like Boric acid to adjust pH of the formulation
- Viscosity agents to prolong eye contact time
- Preservatives to maintain solution sterility.

Indications: Hypotonic topical tear solutions are indicated for the relief of dry eyes and ocular irritation associated with deficient tear production. These solutions are also used as ocular lubricants for artificial eyes.

Contraindications: Hypersensitivity to any of the component of artificial tear solution.

Dosage and preparations: Usual dosage is to instill 1–2 drops into the eyes at the frequency of four to six hours. However, depending upon severity of the symptoms, they may be used as often as hourly interval.

Artificial tear solutions are broady classified on following pattern:

Methylcellulose or Ethylcellulose Base

Solutions Containing

- Hydroxypropyl methylcellulose 0.5 percent or 1 percent with 0.01 percent benzalkonium chloride (in 10, 15 ml vials).
- Hydroxypropyl methylcellulose 0.5 percent, gelatin A, Chlorobutanol 0.5 percent, NaCl and polysorbate 80 (in 10, 15 ml and 30 ml vials)
- Methylcellulose 1 percent, propylene glycol, NaCl, boric acid and parabens (in 10, 15 ml vials).
- Hydroxypropyl methylcellulose 0.5 percent, Dextran 40 (0.1%) with benzalkonium chloride 0.01 percent, EDTA, NaCl and Boric acid (in 10, 15 ml vials).
- Hydroxypropyl methylcellulose 0.5 percent, Dextran 70 (0.1%), benzalkonium chloride (0.01%) and EDTA (0.05%) (in 15 ml vials).
- Hydroxy ethylcellulose (0.5%) 1.67 percent povidone with water soluble polymers, Thimerosal 0.004 percent and EDTA (1%) (in 10,15 ml vials).
- Hydroxy ethylcellulose 0.5 percent, Polyvinyl alcohol 1 percent and 0.01 percent benzalkonium chloride, EDTA and NaCl (in 15 ml vials).
- Hydroxy ethylcellulose in a hypertonic base with 0.25 percent sorbic acid and 0.1 percent EDTA (in 10 ml and 15 ml packs).
- Hydroxy ethylcellulose with sodium chloride in conc. of 0.44 percent and 0.35 percent.
- A new topical artificial tear solution of methylcellulose group is available commercially.

It contains—Carboxy methylcellulose sodium in conc. of 0.5 percent or with Purite preservative.

The added advantages of this tear solution over already available solutions containing Hydroxypropyl methylcellulose and Hydroxy ethylcellulose are:

- Carboxymethylcellulose (CMC) possesses strong mucoadhesive bonding—closely adheres to the epithelial surface.
- Being negatively charged it mimics the mucin layer in natural tears.
- The strong mucoadhesive force provides prolonged retention and comfort.
- CMC solution closely resembles the composition of natural tears—contains electrolytes present in normal tears.
- It maintains the ocular health of the patient as it has little or no effect on corneal tissue and goblet cell density.

- Purite in this solution is a unique preservative which breaks down into the natural tear component sodium and water when instilled into the eye minimizing preservative induced irritation and maximum comfort and maintains the integrity of corneal tissue.
- CMC solution does not affect cellular membrane integrity and least effect on conjunctival goblet cell density.
- Definitely safer than already available methyl—cellulose based tear solutions.
- Another topical artificial tear solution containing Carboxy-methylcellulose sodium 0.5 percent with unique preservative sodium perborate which breaks down to water and oxygen upon contact is commercially available.
- Carboxymethylcellulose (Carmellose) is also available commercially in 1.0 percent topical ophthalmic solution (preservative free). Its unpreserved formulation is closer to natural tears. Carmellose (Celluvisc) has full electrolyte complement and sodium lactate which flush debris, relieves lacrimal gland stress and does not effect cellular integrity. Its viscosity is more optimal for contact lens use. Carmellose (1%) is ideal for the treatment of post-LASIK dry eye conditions and leads to more rapid recovery of the ocular surface. Greater viscosity of Carmellose is ideal for postsurgical/LASIK recovery.

POLYVINYL ALCOHOL BASE SOLUTIONS

- Polyvinyl alcohol 1.4 percent and Povidine 0.6 percent (10 ml and 15 ml packs) and Chlorbutanol 0.5 percent and NaCl.
- Polyvinyl alcohol 1.0 percent, NaCl, 0.01 percent benzalkonium chloride and EDTA (15 ml pack).
- Polyvinyl alcohol 1 percent, PEG 8000, Dextrose, benzalkonium chloride and EDTA (15 ml pack).
- Polyvinyl alcohol 3 percent with 0.002 percent thimerosal, NaCl and EDTA (15 ml pack).
- Polyvinyl alcohol 1 percent, Hydroxy ethylcellulose, NaCl, PEG-300, Thimerosal (0.004 percent) and EDTA (0.02%) (15 ml pack).
- Polyvinyl alcohol (1%) with povidone, Benzalkonium chloride, Dextrose, EDTA, KCl, Sodium bicarbonate, NaCl, Sodium citrate and Sodium phosphate (15 ml and 30 ml packs).

Out of these PVA combinations (polyvinyl alcohol and Povidone tops in mucoadhesive strength making them a better choice. The other features of this combination are:

1. Two polymers (polyvinyl alcohol and povidone) enhance comfort and maintain corneal health.
2. Specific properties of polyvinyl alcohol are: It smoothes and cool dry, irritated scratchy eyes, provide needed moisture to dry ocular surface, does not cause blurring of vision, lubricates to prevent further irritation and enhances patient comfort.
   - Povidone has specific effects like mucomimetic action and enhances and spreadability of tear film.

- PVA and povidone solution supplements natural human tears and provides a substitute coating to protect and nourish the surface of the eye.
- Relatively safe on prolonged use.
- PVA and povidone topical ophthalmic solution can be used as tear substitute in cases of lacrimal secretion deficiency, Dry eye syndrome, etc.
- PVA and povidone together adhere to the corneal epithelium and prolong tear break up time and prevents further dry spots.
- Their synergistic action promotes tear stability.
- It prevent corneal dehydration and abrasive mechanical damage.
- PVA and povidone solution contains preservative Chlorbutanol which has been clinically proved to be safer than thimerosal and Benzalkonium chloride (BAK) on long term use.
- Chlorobutanol does not cause conjunctival or corneal damage.

LONGER LASTING MUCOADHESIVE OR INCREASED VISCOSITY AGENTS

- Polycarbophil and Dextran
- Methylcellulose

Both these ophthalmic solutions are preservative free (thus preservative associated adverse effects are removed).

On topical instillation these solutions have better duration of action than previously mentioned tear solutions.

POLYVINYL PYRROLIDONE POLYMER BASE TEAR SOLUTION

- Adsorbonac sodium chloride 2 percent or 5 percent ophthalmic solutions (Hyperosmotic).

    Other topical artificial tear solutions available are:
    a. Salt solution with Zinc and Glycerin
    b. Electrolyte based solution.

Adverse Reactions of Artificial Tear Solutions

On topical instillation these solutions are relatively safe, yet the ocular side effects reported are:
- Redness
- Mild stinging or temporary blurring of vision
- Ocular Discomfort
- Hypersensitivity reactions.

Intensive research is going on possible use of immunomodulators in severe dry eye disorders. Initial clinical results are found encouraging.

OINTMENTS

The second most common method for ocular lubrication is petrolatum, lanolin and mineral oil topical ointments. When instilled into the eye, they dissolve at the temperature of the ocular tissue and disperse with tear fluids. A major advantage is that ointment is retained in the cul-de-sac longer than artificial tear solutions.

Ointments are generally applied directly to the inferior conjunctival sac a 0.25 to 0.50 inch ribbon. Ointment can also be given by placing on a cotton tipped applicator and apply it to the upper lid margin and lashes. Both ocular irritation and blurring of vision are minimized with this method of instillation.

Dosage: Lubricant ointments are generally preferred for bed time use. However, depending upon the severity of the condition, it can also be used more frequently during the day. Since ointments block the access of solutions should be instilled prior to ointment application. These ointments serve as lubricants and emollients.

Indications: For protection and lubrication of the eye in exposure keratitis, decreased corneal sensitivity, recurrent corneal erosions, Keratitis Sicca specially for bed time use, after removal of Foreign body, during and following surgery.

Contraindications: Hypersensitivity to any component use of contact lens is contraindicated during the course of treatment.

Preparations

- Ointment containing white petrolatum, mineral oil and Lanolin, preservative free (in 3.5 gm packs).
- White petrolatum preservative free (in 0.5 gm pack)
- White petrolatum, anhydrous liquid lanolin and mineral oil, preservative free (in 3.5 gm pack).
- White petrolatum 55.5 percent, 42.5 percent mineral oil and 2 percent petrolatum/lanolin alcohol, preservative free (in 0.7 gm pack).
- Fifty-five percent white petrolatum, 42.5 percent mineral oil, 2 percent non-ionic lanolin derivative and 0.5 percent chlorobutanol (in 3.5 gm and 7 gm packs).
- Five thousand IU vitamin A, polysorbate 80, NaCl and 0.05 percent EDTA (in 15 ml packs).
- White petrolatum and Mineral oil, preservative free (in 1 ml pack).
- White petrolatum and light mineral oil, preservative free (in 3.5 gm pack).
- White petrolatum, mineral oil, Lanolin and methyl paraben/ Ethyl paraben (in 3.5 gm pack).
- Ocular Lubricant Ointment containing Hydroxy propylmethyl-cellulose (2%) with sodium chloride, potassium chloride, calcium chloride, magnesium chloride, sodium acetate and Sodium citrate, preservative free (5 gm pack). It presents prolonged corneal mucoadhesive and clear film. It is versatile

gel which provides protective coat to all topical surface of the eye.

For treatment of moderate to severe dry eye a new Lubricant eye gel is commercially available. It is not an ointment or a drop but it is clear gel that liquefies and spreads rapidly upon contact with the eye.

It contains Carbopal 980 (polyacryclic acid) a gelling agent with high water binding power that transforms from gel to liquid upon contact with the ocular tissue.

It minimises blurring and streaking common with thick tears and ointments. It is available in a 10 ml tube.

Adverse reactions: Topical ointments are safe on prolonged use yet ocular side effects reported are ocular irritation, redness or hypersensitivity reaction.

If ocular pain, change in vision, continued redness or irritation occurs or conditions persists/worsen more than 72 hours, discontinue the use and consult the ophthalmologist.

OCULAR INSERTS (SOLID DEVICES)

For the relief of dry eye symptoms, another route is the use of preservative free water soluble polymeric insert (Lacriset). The cylindrical rod which contains 5 mg hydroxy propylmethylcellulose is placed in lower cul-de-sac (slow dissolving polymers). It then imbibes fluid and swells. It starts dissolving within 6-8 hours releasing the polymer to the ocular surface for 12-24 hours.

Indications: This device can be beneficial in dry eye syndromes such as keratitis sicca, exposure keratitis, decreased corneal sensitivity and recurrent corneal erosions. It is comfortable and well accepted. Disadvantage is that manual dexterity is required for placement in the cul-de-sac and cost to the patient is considerably greater than solutions and ointments.

A common problem reported by the patients is blurred vision as the rod dissolves causing the tear film to thicken. Adding fluid drops (isotonic saline) can reduce viscosity and minimise visual complaints.

Contraindications: Hypersensitivity to hydroxy propyl-methyl-cellulose.

Adverse reactions: Ocular adverse reactions are mild and transient and includes transient blurring of vision, ocular irritation and discomfort, matting or stickiness of eyelashes, photophobia, hypersensitivity, edema of eyelids and hyperemia.

If improperly placed in the inferior cul-de-sac corneal abrasion may result. So patient should practice insertion and removal of insert.

Patient should exercise caution while operating hazardous machinery or driving a vehicle. If symptoms worsen, remove insert and consult the ophthalmologist. Commercially it is available as 5 mg hydroxy propylcellulose ophthalmic insert (Lacriset). It is preservative free.

SOFT CONTACT LENS THERAPY

Hydrophilic bandage lenses often provide a tear reservoir but it should be used in conjunction with replacement tears. Caution should be taken because such patients are prone to contact lens intolerance and super infections. Forniceal scarring may dislodge the lenses.

PUNCTAL PLUGS

Mechanical occlusion of the lacrimal puncta has become an accepted method to block tear drainage and thereby prolong action of natural tears along with artificial tear preparations. Two types of punctal plug are currently used.
- Silicon based plug
- Temporary absorbable collagen implant.
a. Punctal plug is usually inserted directly into the inferior puncta. This procedure requires topical anesthesia and punctal dilation prior to the placement.
b. The temporary intracanalicular collagen implant consists of 0.2, 0.3 and 0.4 mm diameter inserts packaged at the edge of a foam strip. The implants are placed halfway into the punctal opening and advanced into the horizontal canaliculus with the aid of forceps and magnification. The procedure can be done with or without Local anesthesia. Following placement, the implant swells impeding tear flow up to 2 weeks before the implant are totally absorbed. Punctal occlusion can benefit patients whose symptoms are not relieved by topical therapy alone.
c. Punctum silicone plugs are available in 1.6, 2 and 2.8 mm sizes (Packs of 2 or 10 plugs with inserter tool). These silicone plugs are flexible and blocks the puncta and eliminate tear loss by this route.

Contraindications: Hypersensitivity to silicone—Precautions should be taken that do not press the finger on or near the eyelid and do not attempt to replace a plug which has fallen out. Relief may not occur immediately after insertion. Some discomfort and tearing may occur for few days.

COLLAGEN IMPLANTS

Indications: For the relief of dry eyes and secondary abnormalities such as corneal ulcer, pterygium, blepharitis, conjunctivitis, keratitis, red lid margins, recurrent chalazion, recurrent corneal erosion, filamentary keratitis and other external eye diseases.

Contraindications: Tearing secondary to chronic dacryocystitis with mucopurulent discharge.

It is commercially available as absorbable intracanalicular collagen implant in 2, 3 and 4 mm sizes.

Implant should be inserted by the ophthalmologist. Placement of implant in all four canaliculi is recommended to prevent a false negative response.

Patient should be informed that relief may not occur immediately after insertion and no removal is necessary if implant dissolve within 5–7 days.

Successful treatment may indicate a need for permanent treatment (e.g. nondissolvable silicone plugs).

MISCELLANEOUS PREPARATIONS

- Topical solution containing 2.5 percent hydroxy propylmethylcellulose with boric acid, EDTA and 0.01 percent benzalkonium chloride (in 15 ml pack) for professional use in gonioscopic examinations.
- Topical solution containing hydroxy ethylcellulose with 0.004 percent thimerosal and 0.1 percent EDTA for bonding gonioscopic prisms to the eye (in 15 ml pack).
- Topical solution containing 0.25 percent tyloxapol and 0.02 percent benzalkonium chloride (in 15 ml pack) for use as a cleaning, wetting and lubricating agent for artificial eye wearers.

    Usual dosage is to instill 1–2 drops on to artificial eye 3–4 times daily.

RECENT ADVANCES IN NEW POLYMERS FOR DRY EYE SYNDROME

Stimulation of Tears

Several drugs such as Bromhexine has been clinically tried to stimulate tear production. Such compounds require the presence of normal Lacrimal gland that responds to stimulation. However, in many patients with Dry eye Syndrome, the lacrimal gland is destroyed by the disease process or the ducts are occluded by the cicatrization due to conjunctival involvement. In such cases stimulation of tear production is not possible because of the pathology of lacrimal glands on their draining channels.

New Artificial Tear Preparations

Several new artificial tear preparations are in various stages of development. All are preservative free and contains viscoelastic materials which has significant role in realization of the mucin layer in maintaining tear film integrity. The following preparations shall be available commercially in near future.

Hyaluronic acid: It is commonly used in cataract surgery and penetrating keratoplasty for the prevention of endothelial damage. 0.1 percent hyaluronic acid is being clinically evaluated for the treatment of dry eye with initial encouraging results.

RGD peptide: RGD consists of three amino acids—Arginine, Glycine and Aspartate that forms the binding site for fibronectin.

A new artificial tear compound containing 18 peptides with the RGD sequence combined with chondroitin sulfate has shown initial positive response in treating dry eye.

High viscosity methylcellulose: Recently topical ophthalmic solution containing very high concentration of Methylcellulose have been clinically tried in the treatment of dry eye with certainly positive results.

Besides these preparations, immunotherapy in the form of Cyclosporine A and α-interferon are also in investigational stage. Preliminary favorable subjective and objective patient response. Immunotherapy appears to have a place in the treatment of dry eye and offers the possibility of directly treating the underlying pathology.

New Polymers

An ideal topical artificial tear replacement should be well tolerated, have low surface tension, be nonirritating, contains no toxic preservatives and have a long residance time on the cornea and conjunctiva. Some new polymers for use in dry eye syndrome are good prospects in such direction.

Recently carbomer gel has been clinically evaluated. Carbomer gel has markedly longer residance time and has significant increase in the tear film break up time at 10 minutes.

So these strong advocation for the concept of replacement of tears with a substance that prolongs the residance time, improves the tear film break up time and is superior to tear replacement fluids that are of low viscosity and quickly are washed away from the ocular surface after blinking.

BIBLIOGRAPHY

1. Agarwal A. Textbook of Ophthalmology, 1st edn. New Delhi: Jaypee Brothers Medical Publishers, 2002.
2. Bartlett JD. Clinical Ocular Pharmacology, 4th edn. Boston: Butterworth-Heinemann, 2001
3. Bartlett JD. Ophthalmic Drug Facts: Lippincott-William and Wilkins, 2001.
4. Crick RP, Trimble RB. Textbook of Clinical Ophthalmology: Hodder and Stoughton, 1986.
5. Duane TD. Clinical Ophthalmology, 4th edn. Butterworth-Heinemann, 1999.
6. Duvall. Ophthalmic Medications and Pharmacology: Slack Inc, 1998.
7. Ellis PP. Ocular Therapeutics and Pharmacology, 7th edn. CV Mosby, 1985.
8. Fechner. Ocular Therapeutics: Slack Inc., 1998.
9. Fraunfelder. Current Ocular Therapy, 5th edn. WB Saunders, 2000.
10. Garg A. Current Trends in Ophthalmology, 1st edn. New Delhi: Jaypee Brothers Medical Publishers, 1997.
11. Garg A. Manual of Ocular Therapeutics, 1st edn. New Delhi: Jaypee Brothers Medical Publishers, 1996.
12. Garg A. Ready Reckoner of Ocular Therapeutics, 1st edn. New Delhi: 2002.
13. Goodman LS, Gilman A. Pharmacological Basis of Therapeutics, 7th edn. New York: Macmillan, 1985.

14. Havener's. Ocular Pharmacology, 6th edn. CV Mosby, 1994.
15. Holly FJ. Tear Film Physiology: Int. Ophthalmol Clin 1987; 27: 2.
16. Kanski. Clinical Ophthalmology, 4th edn. Butterworth-Heineman, 1999.
17. Kershner. Ophthalmic Medications and Pharmacology: Slack. Inc., 1994.
18. Korb. The Tear Film: Butterworth-Heinemann, 2001.
19. Lemp MA. Recent Developments in Dry Eye Management: Surv. Ophthalmol 1987;94:1299.
20. Olin BR, et al. Drugs Facts and Comparisons: Facts and Comparisons, St. Louis, 1997.
21. Onofrey. The Ocular Therapeutics; Lippincott-William and Wilkins, 1997.
22. Rhee. The Wills Eye Drug Guide: Lippincott-William and Wilkins, 1998.
23. Steven Podos. Textbook of Ophthalmology, New Delhi: Jaypee Brothers Medical Publishers, 2001.
24. Tuberville AW, et al. Punctal Occlusion in Tear Deficiency Syndrome. Ophthalmology 1982;89:1170.
25. Zimmerman. Textbook of Ocular Pharmacology: Lippincott and William and Wilkins, 1997.

18

Topical Immune Therapy

Ashok Garg (India)

INTRODUCTION

Topical immune therapy is relatively a latest addition in ocular therapeutic armamentarium to treat iatrogenic inflammation following any type of intraocular surgery and to make up the decreased levels of ocular immunoglobulins vital for the ocular defence system against external infections during postoperative phase following intraocular surgery.

Before discussing the topical immune therapy monograph let me discuss in nutshell about the ocular defence system and immunity.

OCULAR DEFENSE SYSTEM AND IMMUNITY

As we know that protection from disease results from the detection and subsequent elimination of substances recognized as foreign by the body. This active protection system is called immunity. Immunology is the study of those systems responsible for protection of the individual against external and internal assault.

The eye can manifest virtually any type of immune response as it possesses a number of unique anatomical, physiological and biochemical features, these responses often have a distinct character.

The optical integrity and normal protection function of the eye depends on an adequate supply of fluid covering its surface. The exposed part of the ocular globe—the cornea and the bulbar conjunctiva is covered by a thin fluid film known as preocular tear film. Tears refer to fluid present as precorneal tear film and in conjunctival sac.

Tear film is complex trilaminar structure consisting of aqueous layer delimited on both sides by layer of surface active substances. Tear film is directly in contact with the environment and is critically important for protecting the eye from external influences.

The chemical composition of human tears is quite complex as it contains proteins, lipids, metabolites, enzymes, electrolytes and other elements dissolved in fluid secretions of lacrimal gland which play an important role in the defence of the outer eye.

The tear protein fraction forms the first line of ocular defence against external infections.

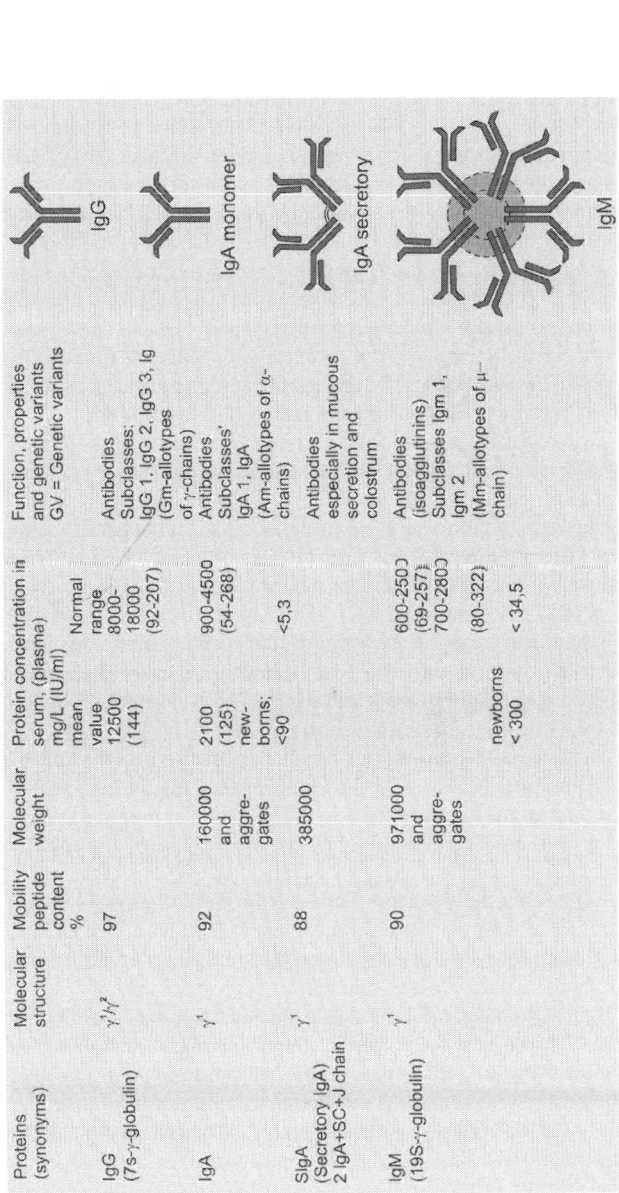

Fig. 18.1: Structural formulas of various immunoglobulins present in tears

The antibacterial properties of immunoglobulins, lysozyme, lactoferrin and b-lysin have been well-documented by research scientists.

Immunoglobulins (IgA and IgG) are the major immunoglobulins present in the tears. A small fraction of IgM is also present in the normal tears. Normal tears contains an average of 14 mg percent of IgA, 17 mg percent of IgG and 5–7 mg percent of IgM.

IgA and IgG may act to modulate the normal flora of the ocular adnexa allowing saprophytic growth which prevents less favorable flora from colonizing the ocular surface. They also prevent adherance of bacteria to the mucosal surface, agglutinate bacteria and neutralize viruses and toxins. In the original state any immunoglobulins found in ocular tissues are likely to the mainly derived from the circulating plasma but on the initial exposure to antigen the urea and limbal conjunctiva acquire antibody producing cells, some of which tend to persist.

The conjunctiva has the property of mucous membrane elsewhere in being rich with IgA. IgA present in tears is likely to be derived from both the conjunctiva and the lacrimal gland.

Early diffusion of IgG in the cornea due to its small molecular size in comparison to IgA and IgM is probably responsible for the preponderance of IgG in the cornea. Small quantity of IgM is probably due to blood aqueous and blood retinal barriers. During acute inflammation of the eye, IgG is the most predominant immunoglobulin present in concentration five times more than that of IgA. This significant increase is associated with increased local synthesis and increased vascular permeability resulting serum IgG spitting into the tears. Similarly there is increased concentration of IgM in tears following acute inflammation due to transudation of serum proteins into the tears.

Extensive research studies conducted in the last decade by the author and his team had shown the interesting findings which are of paramount importance in relation to ocular defence system during immediate postoperative period following intraocular surgery. These are:

- In the immediate postoperative period (up to 7 days following intraocular surgery of any type, there is significant decrease in globulin levels of tears predisposing the eye an added risk of infections due to low tissue immunological defense.
- There is tremendous increase in tear secretion rate (confirmed by Schiremer's test) during the immediate postoperative period resulting in a more dilution of immunoglobulins. This increased tear secretion rate is due to mild trauma caused by surgical interference. At this juncture local tissue response to microbial invasion is severely compromised.
- During the critical period of immediate postoperative phase (1–7 days) the host ocular tissue remains immunocompromised.
- Meticulous aseptic care and suitable topical anti-inflammatory therapy is needed to protect the eye from external influences and to beef up immunocompromised ocular defence system due to iatrogenic inflammation of the eye.

Generally during this critical period topical steroid preparations are advised which have their own ocular and systemic side effects.

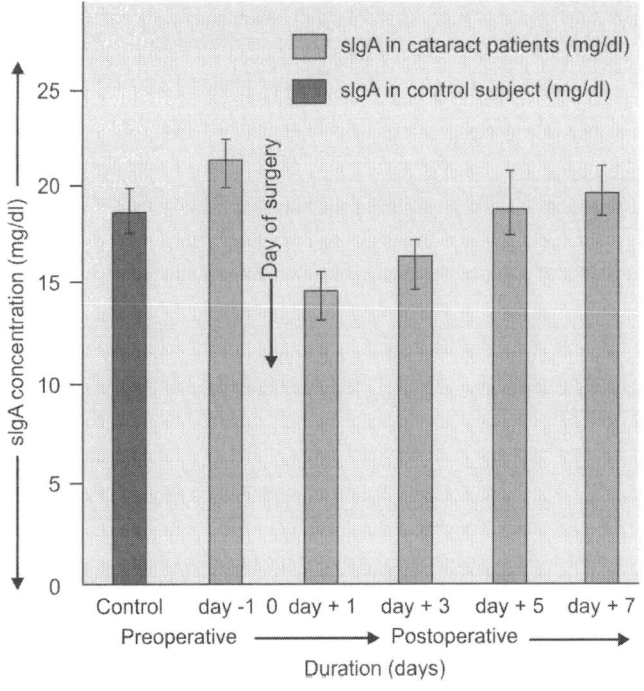

Fig. 18.2: Tear IgA concentration before and after iatrogenic inflammation of the eye

Based on above crucial findings. Author prepared a topical nonsteroidal immune therapy to be supplemented locally to beef up compromised immune defence system of the eye. Extensive biochemical and clinical trials were conducted of this topical immune therapy before it became commercially available. Trials were conducted in two phases:
1. In phase I trials were conducted in rabbit's eye to ascertain the efficacy of topical globulin eyedrops and their possible use in human beings.
2. On getting encouraging response from animal studies (Phase II), extensive biochemical and clinical trials were conducted in human beings.

INDICATIONS FOR TOPICAL IMMUNE THERAPY

- Cataract surgery (ICCE or ECCE)
- Filtering surgery for glaucoma
- IOL implantation and phacoemulsification
- Keratoplasty
- Vitrectomy and posterior segment surgery
- Ocular surgery following trauma
- Lasik surgery
- Squint surgery.

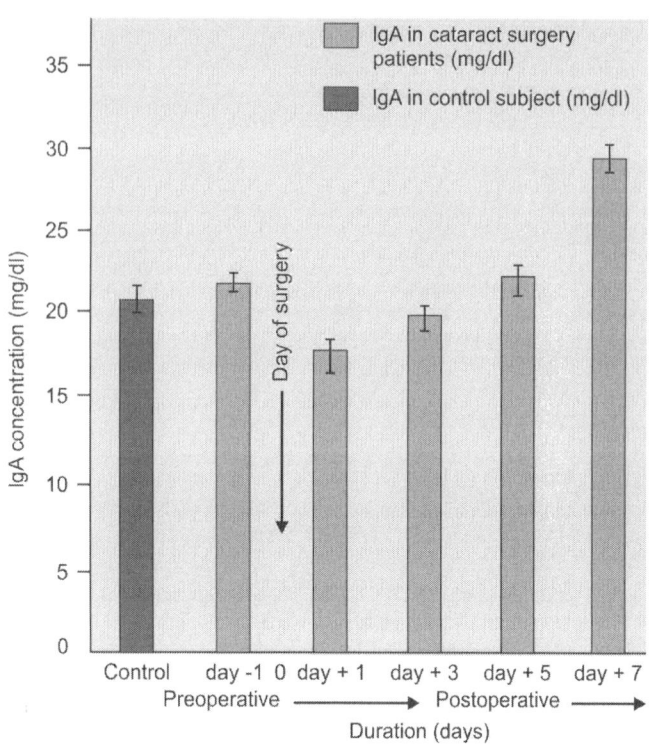

Fig. 18.3: Tear IgG concentration before and after iatrogenic inflammation of the eye

Mechanism of Action

Topical globulin eyedrops (immune therapy) acts by augmenting the severely depleted immunoglobulin levels of tear during immediate postoperative period of 1–7 days following intraocular surgery. It supplements the immunoglobulins present in the tears to fight against external influences.

<u>DOSAGE</u>

It is available as topical ophthalmic solution (Aspac). It contains 0.1 percent each of IgG and IgA and 0.05 percent of IgM in fixed concentrations (available in 5 ml pack). Needs to be refrigerated (2–8°C) when vial is not opened. Once opened for topical use, the vial can be stored at room temperature.

Usual dosage is to instil 1–2 drops in the affected eye three to four times a day for a week and then gradual tapering over next 7 days.

Topical immune therapy in optimum dose is advocated for a postoperative (1–7 days) because after a week natural globulin levels come back to preoperative levels. This rise in level of natural globulins may be partially due to fall in tear secretion rate and

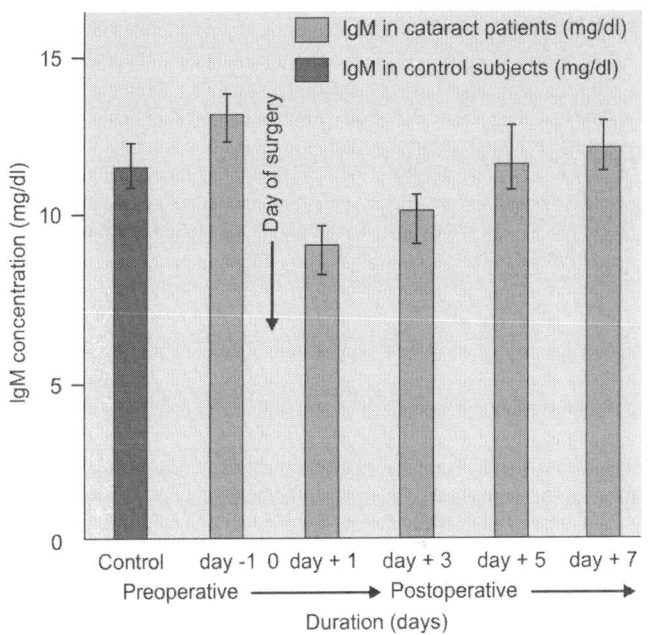

Fig. 18.4: Tear IgM concentration before and after iatrogenic inflammation of the eye

due to enhanced local globulin production from tear glands. This increase in globulin level is also due to exudation of serum globulins through the blood tear barrier.

A raised clinical score of inflammation during this period is indication of supporting the same view. Topical immune therapy is well-tolerated and its intraocular penetration is high.

CONTRAINDICATION

Known hypersensitivity to any of its components.

ADVERSE REACTIONS

On topical use it will be tolerated and has least side effects.

However, ocular side effects reported are transient burning sensation, irritation, stinging and foreign body sensation, conjunctival injection and hypersensitivity reactions.

SUMMARY

Keeping in view of enormous clinical value of topical immune therapy, it will be wonder drug of ophthalmology in near future specially for treating iatrogenic inflammation of the eye.

BIBLIOGRAPHY

1. Agarwal A. Textbook of Ophthalmology, 1st edn. New Delhi: Jaypee Brothers Medical Publishers, 2002.
2. Bartlett JD. Clinical Ocular Pharmacology, 4th edn. Boston: Butterworth-Heinemann, 2001.
3. Bartlett JD. Ophthalmic Drug Facts. Lippincott-William and Wilkins, 2001.
4. Crick RP, Trimble RB. Textbook of Clinical Ophthalmology. Hodder and Stoughton, 1986.
5. Duane TD. Clinical Ophthalmology, 4th edn. Butterworth – Heinemann, 1999.
6. Duvall. Ophthalmic Medications and Pharmacology. Slack Inc, 1998.
7. Ellis PP. Ocular Therapeutics and Pharmacology, 7th edn. CV Mosby, 1985.
8. Fechner. Ocular Therapeutics, Slack Inc., 1998.
9. Fraunfelder. Current Ocular Therapy, 5th ed. WB Saunders, 2000.
10. Garg A. Current Trends in Ophthalmology, 1st edn. New Delhi: Jaypee Brothers Medical Publishers, 1997.
11. Garg A. Manual of Ocular Therapeutics, 1st edn. New Delhi: Jaypee Brothers Medical Publishers, 1996.
12. Garg A. Ready Reckoner of Ocular Therapeutics, 1st edn. New Delhi: 2002.
13. Garg A. Tear Immunoglobulins Status in Iatrogenic Inflammation of the Eye. Internationale Ophthalmologica, 1989;14:1-28.
14. Goodman LS, Gilman A. Pharmacological Basis of Therapeutics, 7th edn. New York: Macmillan, 1985.
15. Havener's. Ocular Pharmacology, 6th edn. CV Mosby, 1994.
16. Kanski. Clinical Ophthalmology, 4th edn. Butterworth – Heinemann, 1999.
17. Kershner. Ophthalmic Medications and Pharmacology. Slack. Inc., 1994.
18. Koevary. Ocular Immunology in Diseases. Butterworth–Heinemann, 1999.
19. Olin BR, et al. Drugs Facts and Comparisons, Facts and Comparisons. St Louis, 1997.
20. Onofrey. The Ocular Therapeutics. Lippincott-William and Wilkins, 1997.
21. Rhee. The Wills Eye Drug Guide. Lippincott – William and Wilkins, 1998.
22. Steven Podos. Textbook of Ophthalmology. New Delhi: Jaypee Brothers Medical Publishers, 2001.
23. Zimmerman. Textbook of Ocular Pharmacology. Lippincott–William and Wilkins, 1997.

19

Topical Hyperosmotic Agents

Ashok Garg (India)

INTRODUCTION

Corneal edema is relatively common condition seen in various anterior segment disorder. It initially manifests itself in epithelium which becomes steamy due to accumulation of fluid between the cells. At the same time fluid accumulates between the Lamellae and produces haziness throughout the cornea due to alterations in the refractive condition.

Corneal deturgescence is achieved when pump function of the corneal endothelium balance the fluid accumulating effect of intraocular hydrostatic pressure and corneal swelling pressure. Disturbance of this balance or disruption of the limiting membranes of the cornea (epithelium and endothelium) results in corneal edema. Epithelial edema, results in significant visual impairment and painful surface break down.

MAJOR CAUSES OF CORNEAL EDEMA

A. Elevated intraocular pressure in:
   - Acute angle closure glaucoma
   - Congenital glaucoma
B. Trauma in:
   - Birth trauma (forceps injury)
   - Nonsurgical contusion injury
   - Penetration of a foreign body
   - Surgical trauma (intraocular surgery).
C. Dystrophy:
   - Endothelial dystrophies
   - Anterior membrane dystrophies
   - Acute hydrops.
D. Endothelial dysfunction secondary to inflammation:
   - Intraocular inflammation
   - Uveitis
   - Focal keratitis (bacterial, fungal or viral)
   - Corneal graft rejection.
E. Epithelial damage due to:
   - Mechanical injury
   - Chemical injury
   - Radiation injury.

The treatment for persistent corneal edema is penetrating Keratoplasty. Topical hyperosmotic agents are helpful in treating short-term corneal edema of diverse etiology. These agents are used clinically to consider corneal edema as stromal, epithelial or both. Stromal edema is usually caused by endothelial dysfunction and is not well correlated with increased intraocular pressure. Epithelial edema is influenced by both these factors. Clinically epithelial edema is more responsive to topical hyperosmotic therapy. Stromal edema is reduced by such agents but it does not seem to be as responsive as epithelial edema. However epithelial edema is much greater deterrant to good vision.

Mechanism of Action

All hyperosmotic agents work according to the same basic principle. An osmotic gradient is induced between the epithelium and the tear film by introducing a medication that is hyperosmolal to the tissue fluid (about 300 mOsm/kg). Water is then drawn towards the more highly osmotic compartment (i.e. the tear film) and is thus eliminated from the epithelium and stroma. This osmotic effect assumes that the epithelium is a true semipermeable membrane that allows water but not electrolytes to pass. This assumption cannot always be made specially in patients whose epithelium has been damaged or traumatized.

VARIOUS TOPICAL HYPEROSMOTIC AGENTS USED IN OPHTHALMOLOGY

a. Hypertonic salt agents:
   - Topical NaCl solution (2% and 5%)
   - Topical NaCl ointment (6% gel)
   - Topical NaCl solution with methyl cellulose.
b. Topical glycerine solution (50%).
c. Glucose 40 ophthalmic ointment with petrolatum and lanolin.
d. Polyoxythylene (0.4%) emulsion with silicone oil.
e. Hypertonic salt agents like 2 and 5 percent topical sodium chloride solutions are commonly used to treat corneal edema of various etiology (acute and chronic) including bullous Keratitis. Usual dosage is to instill 1–2 drops in the affected eyes 3–4 times a day till the desired response is achieved.
   Topical preparations available commercially are:
   1. Two and 5 percent NaCl solution is povidone with two water soluble polymers, 0.004 percent thimerosal and 0.1 percent EDTA.
   2. Two or 5 percent solution with hydroxy propyl methyl cellulose and parabens. Five percent solution also contains propylene glycol, sodium borate and boric acid.

Recently 6 percent sodium chloride ophthalmic gel has been commercially available (containing petrolatum and lanolin). Topical gel is considered superior to topical 5 percent Nacl solution in term of efficacy and tolerability. Recommended dosage of ophthalmic gel is to apply 1–2 times a day. Usually bed time dosage is preferred for better results and compliance. An average reduction in corneal thickness of 28 percent is noted at the peak of effect with gel. Adverse side effect reported with topical sodium chloride solution or gel is ocular discomfort and tingling sensation.

Glycerine Solution

Anhydrous glycerol a topical 50 percent solution of glycerol or propylene glycol with 0.55 percent chlorobutanol is most effective in clearing corneal edema. This solution is very effective in reducing corneal stromal edema and is helpful for short-term use. It is generally used to clear a cornea clouded because of angle closure glaucoma. To be most effective it is not applied as single drop but as a slow drip in which many drops are instilled several seconds apart until the cornea clears usually within 2–3 minutes. If a single drop is used the osmolality of the medication immediately begins to decrease as a consequence of dilution from imbibed water. Glycerol is quite irritating in the eye and should be given only after a topical anesthetic.

- Glucose 40 percent ophthalmic ointment is (40%) ointment in petrolatum and lanolin (3.5 g pack). It is also used for treatment of acute corneal edema. Usual dosage is to apply once at bed time till the desired response is obtained.
- Recently an emulsion of polyoxyethylene (0.4%) and silicone oil has been clinically tried in corneal edema cases.

    The polyoxyethylene molecule is a long chain consisting of alternating hydrophillic and hydrophobic segments. This drug when applied in the eye turns its hydrophilic part toward the cornea and its hydrophobic part towards the silicone. The dehydration that occurs is an osmotic effect while the silicone oil acts like a chemical contact lens and smooths out minor surface irregularities.

- For corneas with damaged or traumatized epithelium such as can result from ruptured edema blebs, these hyperosmotic agents having low molecular weight (Sodium chloride glucose) are not very useful. Because in such a case, the cornea imbibes isotonic or even hypertonic saline because the semi permeable barrier is absent. Hyperosmotic agents are of little value when managing corneal edema existing concurrently with traumatized epithelium. Solutions of macromolecule polymers of sufficiently large size to prevent diffusion into the stroma are effective at controlling edema despite absent or traumatized epithelium.
- In the past Research scientists have also tried 30 percent sulfacetamide in polyvinyl alcohol, 5 percent gum cellulose solution and corn syrup. These agents were found not very effective.

    Commercially today only 5 percent sodium chloride solution and 6 percent Nacl ointment containing petrolatum and lanolin are the most effective, hyperosmotic agents for reducing corneal edema and are commonly prescribed worldwide with good results.

BIBLIOGRAPHY

1. Agarwal A. Textbook of Ophthalmology, 1st edn. New Delhi: Jaypee Brothers Medical Publishers, 2002.
2. Bartlett JD. Clinical Ocular Pharmacology, 4th edn. Boston: Butterworth-Heinemann, 2001.
3. Bartlett JD. Ophthalmic Drug Facts, Lippincott-William and Wilkins, 2001.
4. Becker B, et al. Oral Hyperosmotic Agents. Arch Ophthalmol, 1967; 78: 147.
5. Crick RP, Trimble RB. Textbook of Clinical Ophthalmology, Hodder and Stoughton, 1986.
6. Duane TD. Clinical Ophthalmology, 4th edn. Butterworth-Heinemann, 1999.
7. Duvall. Ophthalmic Medications and Pharmacology, Slack Inc, 1998.
8. Ellis PP. Ocular Therapeutics and Pharmacology, 7th edn. CV Mosby, 1985.
9. Fechner. Ocular Therapeutics: Slack Inc., 1998.
10. Fraunfelder. Current Ocular Therapy, 5th edn. WB Saunders, 2000.
11. Garg A. Current Trends in Ophthalmology, 1st edn. New Delhi, Jaypee Brothers Medical Publishers, 1997.
12. Garg A. Manual of Ocular Therapeutics, 1st edn. New Delhi: Jaypee Brothers Medical Publishers, 1996.
13. Garg A. Ready Reckoner of Ocular Therapeutics, 1st edn. New Delhi, 2002.
14. Goodman LS, Gilman A. Pharmacological Basis of Therapeutics, 7th edn. New York, Macmillan, 1985.
15. Havener's. Ocular Pharmacology, 6th edn. CV Mosby, 1994.
16. Kanski. Clinical Ophthalmology, 4th edn. Butterworth-Heineman, 1999.
17. Kershner. Ophthalmic Medications and Pharmacology, Slack. Inc., 1994.
18. Kolker AE. Hyperosmotic Agents in Glaucoma. Invest Ophthalmol 1970; 9: 418.
19. Lambert DW. Topical Hyperosmotic Agents. Am J Ophthalmol 1980, 20: 163.
20. Olin BR, et al. Drugs Facts and Comparisons, Facts and Comparisons, St. Louis, 1997.
21. Onofrey. The Ocular Therapeutics. Lippincott-William and Wilkins, 1997.
22. Rhee. The Wills Eye Drug Guide, Lippincott-William and Wilkins, 1998.
23. Steven Podos. Textbook of Ophthalmology, New Delhi: Jaypee Brothers Medical Publishers, 2001.
24. Zimmerman. Textbook of Ocular Pharmacology, Lippincott and William and Wilkins, 1997.

Antiretroviral Drug Therapy of Ocular Infections in AIDS

Ashok Garg (India)

INTRODUCTION

Since its first recognition and detection in 1981 in USA, AIDS (Acquired immunodeficiency syndrome) has assumed a threatening role of a single largest disease worldwide. It has emerged as a global health problem of extraordinary proportion and unprecedented emergency. According to a World Health Organization report it is estimated that currently around 30 million people including 2.5 million children have been infected with human immunodeficiency virus (HIV) worldwide and projected prevalence of 40 million infected by 2000 AD. HIV is undoubtedly is a major pandemic of this century. Out of these 90 percent infected people live in developing countries. In India more than 2 million people are estimated to be infected with HIV and it is projected that India will harbor the highest number of cases by 2000 AD.

The problem related to this pandemic are not only 100 percent fatality but also a worldwide distribution, social stigma that is enormous and genetic variations in replication of virus which has made development of an effective treatment still elusive.

Acquired immunodeficiency syndrome rapid spread is a cause of great concern. Till such time when effective cure becomes available and early diagnosis can help prevent it further transmission, AIDS will continue to plague mankind.

Ocular involvement is seen in more than 50 percent of AIDS patients and includes various clinical presentations. These ocular manifestations can be the presently signs of a systemic infection in an otherwise asymptomatic HIV positive cases. As a result, the role of the ophthalmologist in the prevention, detection and management of AIDS afflicted eyes assume great significance. Hence a correct diagnosis by the ophthalmologist may be vital for prolonging the life of the patient by early initiation of treatment.

The severity of ophthalmic sequelae of HIV infection increases as immunocompetency decreases while the presumed HIV related asymptomatic ocular lesions occur in the earlier stage, the relentless, destructive and blinding infections specially opportunistic ones occur in the late stage of AIDS. The ocular manifestations of HIV infection can be broadly divided into following categories.

a. HIV-related retinopathy
b. Opportunistic infections of the eye.
c. Nonopportunistic infections

d. Tumor involvement
e. Cutaneous hypersensitivity reactions
f. Presence of HIV in ocular structures
g. Specific features in infants and children.

The details of various ocular manifestations has been discussed in a separate chapter of this book. However, here I am mentioning by specific signs and symptoms of each group of ocular manifestations necessary to understand the pharmacokinetics of antiretroviral drugs being prescribed in these conditions in a better way.

HIV-RELATED RETINOPATHY

Cotton wool spots are most common sign of HIV infection and these are seen in 50-70 percent of AIDS patients. Non-infectious retinopathy also includes hemorrhage and other microvascular abnormalities. These are indistinguishable from those observed in diabetes, hypertension, anemia and collagen diseases. They are usually located at the posterior pole and may disappear spontaneously in the course of few weeks. Dot hemorrhages which may come and go are seen in 20-40 percent of AIDS patients. Microaneurysms, telangiectasia and focal areas of nonperfusion

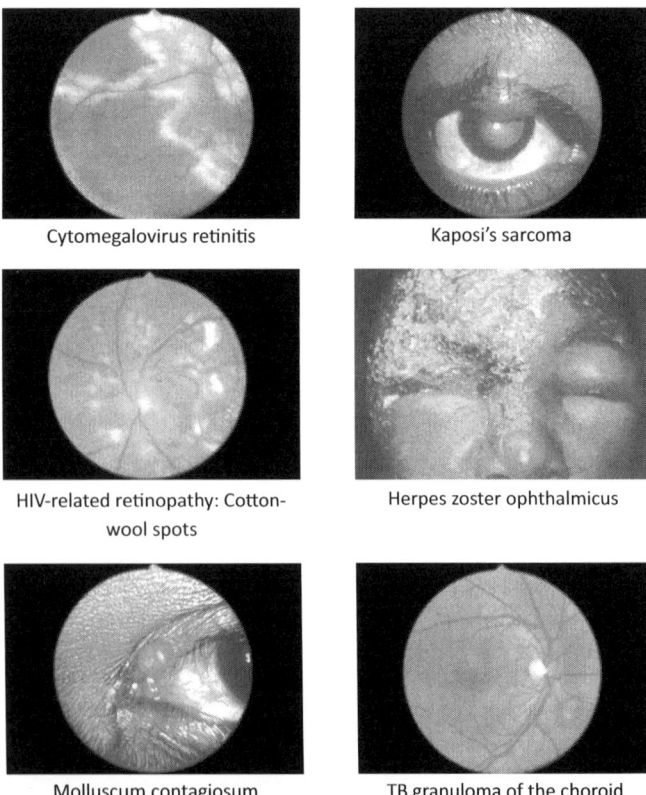

Fig. 20.1: Various ocular manifestations of AIDS

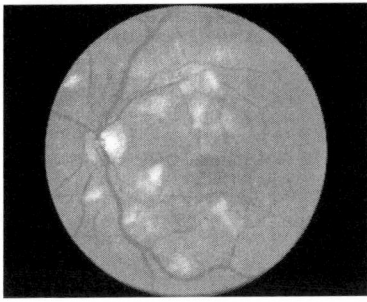

Fig. 20.2: Ocular manifestations of AIDS (cotton-wool spots)

are detected in most AIDS patients undergoing fluorescein angiography and are final common expression of vaso-occlusion. Usually this non-infectious retinopathy does not interfere with vision and does not necessitate treatment.

OPPORTUNISTIC INFECTIONS OF THE EYE

Infectious agents capable of producing intraocular infection in AIDS patients include cytomegalovirus, *Cryptococcus neoformans, Pneumocystis carinii, Mycobacterium avium intracellulare, Toxoplasma gondii, Histoplasma capsulatum* and *Candida albicans*. The various ocular infections caused by these agents are:

Cytomegalovirus Retinitis

It is by for the most common opportunistic infection of the eye and the major cause of visual loss in AIDS patients. It is most common end organ disease in patients with cytomegalovirus (CMV) infections accounting for 70-85 percent of all CMV diseases. It is commonly seen in patients with very low CD4 + lymphocyte counts (below $50 \times 10^6/l$). It is bilateral in 50 percent of cases and often starts at the posterior pole. As it causes irreversible retinal destruction early detection and institution of appropriate therapy is a desirable goal.

The earliest findings are white lesions simulating cotton-wool spots followed by appearance of geographic yellow white granular areas representing full thickness retinal necrosis later these lesions coalesce and are associated with retinal hemorrhage and vasculitis eventually involving entire retina causing total retinal atrophy.

It is associated with mild inflammatory reaction in the anterior segment and the vitreous cavity. This mild reaction is attributed to the inability to mount sufficient immunological responses. CMV retinitis is relentlessly progressive and destroys the whole retina within 6 months.

Cryptococcal Infection

Cryptococcus neoformans is the most common life-threatening fungal pathogen. The combination of low grade papilledema and headaches in an HIV positive patient even in the absence of

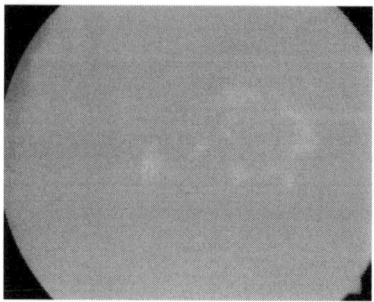

Fig. 20.3: Ocular manifestations of AIDS cytomegalovirus retinitis

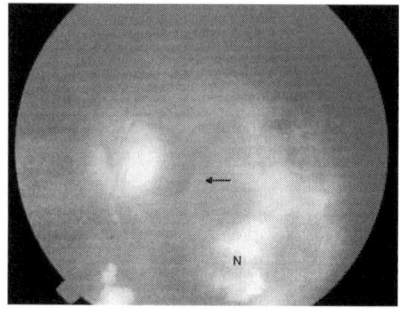

Fig. 20.4: Fundus photograph of AIDS patient with CMV retinitis (notable features are multiple large area of yellow white intraretinal necrosis (N) and flame-shaped hemorrhages (arrow)

fever and neck stiffness should alert the ophthalmologist to the possibility of cryptococcal meningitis.

Toxoplasma Infection

Toxoplasma gondii retinochoroiditis in AIDS is characterized by lesions that are larger, less frequently associated with healed scars more commonly bilateral and may be difficult to distinguish from other opportunistic infectious retinitis. Antitoxoplasma regime has to be continued life long even if retinitis resolves.

Pneumocystis carinii Choroiditis

Unlike *Pneumocystis carinii* infection of the lung which occurs in 80 percent of AIDS patients infection of choroid is uncommon. Lesions appear like yellowish white elevated plaques.

NONOPPORTUNISTIC INFECTIONS

Certain infectious diseases whose natural history is well known in immunocompetent patients will take on different characteristics or will occur with greater frequency in the HIV seropositive host.

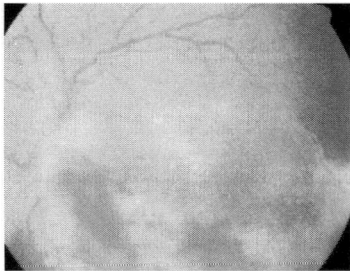

Fig. 20.5: Ocular manifestation of AIDS (CMV retinitis—hemorrhagic) necrosis of retina with exudates and periphlebitis)

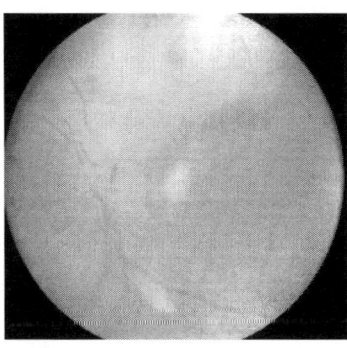

Fig. 20.6: Fundus photograph of the left eye showing cotton-wool spot and necrotizing retinitis with areas of hemorrhage along the superior temporal vascular arcades

Herpes Zoster Ophthalmicus

PORN or progressive outer retinal necrosis is caused by the herpes virus. Cutaneous zoster may or may not be feature. In early stages they are difficult to distinguish from CMV retinitis. A rapid progression in a circumferential pattern with sparing of the retinal vasculature distinguishes it from ARN and CMV retinitis.

This disease tends to run a severe course in HIV positive patients in terms of corneal involvement and postherpetic pain. Severe scarring of the eyelids and the conjunctiva may lead to trichiasis, conjunctival surface disorders or cicatricial ectropion with corneal exposure.

Herpes Simplex

Recurrent herpes simplex keratitis has been seen in AIDS patients. These dendritic corneal ulcers tended to be peripheral, resistant to therapy and have a high recurrence rate.

Viral Disease of Eyelids

Both molluscum contagiosum and verrucae of the eyelids are common cutaneous manifestations of HIV infections. Multiple verrucae around the eyelids are suggestive of HIV infection.

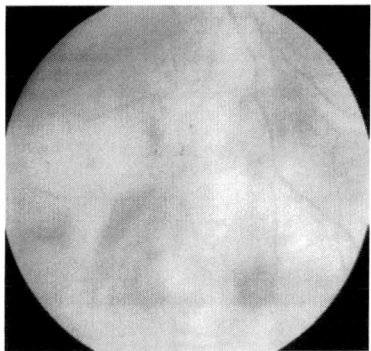

Fig. 20.7A: Fundus photograph of the left eye showing necrotizing retinitis with secondary retinal detachment

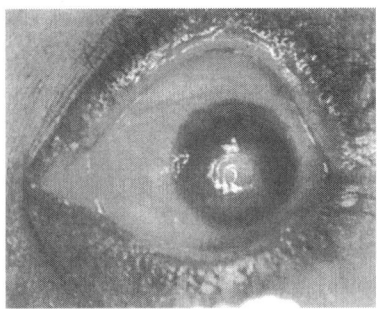

Fig. 20.7B: Ocular manifestations of AIDS (herpes zoster ophthalmicus)

Syphilitic Uveitis

Syphilitic disease may progress more rapidly in HIV infected patients. Serological testing for syphilis should be performed on all HIV seropositive patients with ocular inflammation. Ocular manifestations of syphilis in HIV patients include uveitis, retinitis and neuroretinitis, papillitis, optic neuritis and retrobulbar neuritis.

Choroidal Tuberculosis

There is an alarming rise in the prevalence of tuberculosis since the advent of the HIV/AIDS epidemic. Ocular lesions in AIDS patients due to TB include disseminated choroiditis, phylectenulosis and solitary choroidal granulomas.

TUMOR INVOLVEMENT

Kaposi's sarcoma, B-cell lymphoma and squamaous cell carcinoma are the most common malignancies reported in association with AIDS patients.

Kaposi's Sarcoma

Kaposi's sarcoma has become a major cause of morbidity and mortality in HIV infected patients. About 20 percent of patients with systemic Kaposi's sarcoma have ocular involvement. It may develop on eyelids, conjunctiva and rarely within the orbit. On the eyelids it appears as deep purple red nodules while conjunctival lesions are bright red and resemble subconjunctival hemorrhage. The lower fornix is more often affected than the upper fornix.

Lymphoma of Orbit

Certain cases of lymphoma of orbit have been reported specially in western patients.

Squamous Cell Carcinoma of Conjunctiva

There has been marked increase in the cases of conjunctival neoplasms. HIV infection is a risk factor for the development of squamous cell dysplasia and neoplasia of the conjunctiva. About 75-80 percent of patients with these lesions are HIV positive.

NEURO-OPHTHALMOLOGICAL MANIFESTATIONS

Human immunodeficiency virus infection may be associated with a large variety of neurophthalmological manifestations including optic nerve disease (edema, inflammation or atrophy), retrobulbar neuritis, visual field defects, cortical blindness, pupillary defects and ocular motor nerve palsies. Most of these disorders are due to infectious lesions of central nervous system. Neurosyphilis, cryptococcal meningitis and central nervous system toxoplasmosis are the first pathogens to be suspected in such cases.

CUTANEOUS HYPERSENSITIVITY REACTIONS

It has been shown that TB patients infected with HIV have an increased risk of developing hypersensitivity reactions when treated with thiacetazone. About 75 percent of the patients admitted with Steven's Johnson syndrome in African countries are HIV positive.

HIV IN OCULAR STRUCTURES

HIV has been isolated from tears, conjunctiva, cornea, aqueous humor, retinal vascular endothelium and other ocular tissues. In areas where corneal transplantation is performed, it is imperative to rule out HIV infection in the donor.

OCULAR MANIFESTATIONS OF HIV INFECTIONS IN CHILDREN

Cotton wool spots and CMV retinitis seem to be less common than in adults. Decreased lacrimation is a frequent finding and is probably due to the same pathological process as the salivary gland enlargement which occurs in children with AIDS. Retinal perivasculities in the peripheral vessels has been reported in 40 percent of children with AIDS in African countries.

ANTIRETROVIRAL THERAPY OF OCULAR INFECTIONS IN AIDS PATIENTS

The currently approved antiretroviral drugs fall into three categories.

Nucleoside Reverse Transcriptase Inhibitors (NRTIs)

The primary mechanisms of action of this class drugs is by inhibition of viral reverse transcriptase and termination of the growing DNA chain.

Drugs of NRTI group are:
- Zidovudine
- Didanosine
- Lamivudine
- Stavudine
- Zalcitabine.

Non-nucleoside Reverse Transcriptase Inhibitors (NNRTIs)

These drugs inhibit reverse transcriptase but are not incorporated into the viral DNA.

Drugs of NNRTs group are:
- Nevirapine
- Delavirdine.

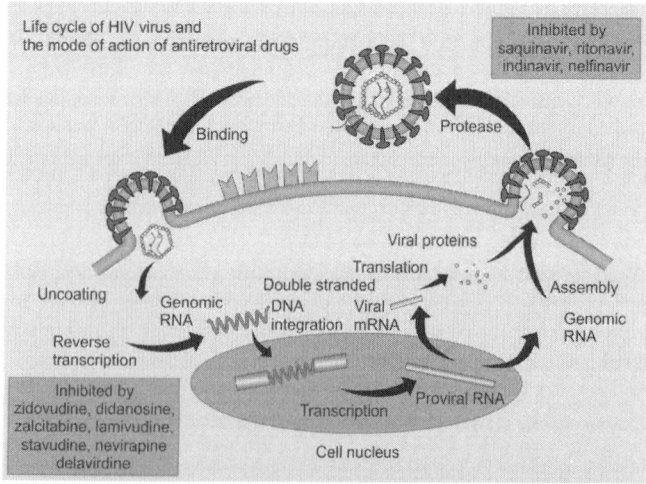

Fig. 20.8: Mechanism of action of antiretroviral drugs and life cycle of HIV

Protease Inhibitors

The activity of the protease enzyme is critical for the maturation of newly formed virions. Protease inhibitors (PIs) specific for HIV-1 inhibit this enzyme thereby preventing the maturation of virions capable of infecting other cells.

Drugs of this group are:
- Saquinavir
- Indinavir
- Ritonavir.

Antiviral Metabolites

- Ganciclovir
- Foscarnet
- Cidofovir/zidovovir (HPMPC).

HIV infection is associated with an incredibly high rate of replication, even during the asymptomatic phase of infection. Secondly replication is highly error prone. Every base pair of the genome mutates on a daily basis. Mutations coding for resistance to antiretroviral drugs can potentially arise during this process.

So the drug regimen has to be highly active-potent enough to completely suppress viral replication in order to prevent selection of resistant mutants. The overall potency of the regimen is more important than the absolute number of agent. With currently available drugs this usually translates into a regimen containing at least 3 agents—generally two nucleoside analog reverse transcriptase inhibitors and a protease inhibitor with high potency. Even a highly active regimen must be initiated early in the course of the disease.

Drug selection, administration and dosage in individual ocular infection in AIDS patients is being described here.

CYTOMEGALOVIRUS INFECTION

Drugs of choice for treatment of CMV retinitis are ganciclovir, foscarnet and cidofovir.

Ganciclovir

It is a nucleoside analog of 2′-deoxyguanosine and acts by preventing DNA elongation. The active form is the triphosphate form. It can be given by intravenous injection form, oral, intervitreal and ganciclovir implant forms.

Intravenous Dosage

An intravenous loading dose of 5 mg/kg every 12 hourly IV for 14–21 days and then reduced to maintenance dose of 6 mg/kg OD 5 days a week IV or 5 mg/kg OD on all seven days of the week. Maintenance therapy however does not prevent relapse from occurring but it will serve to prolong the interval until relapse by several weeks or months. Recurrence is reported in 30–40 percent of patients during maintenance therapy. If relapse occurs, patients usually respond to reinduction with ganciclovir. It is given slow IV (over one hour in 100 ml of 0.9% normal saline). During the treatment period, it is necessary to check:

- Complete hemogram (twice a week during treatment phase) and every two weeks during maintenance phase.
- Liver function tests LFT/renal function (including twice a week during treatment phase and every two weeks during maintenance phase.
- *Dilated fundoscopy:* After two weeks during treatment phase and once a month during maintenance phase.

Stop ganciclovir and introduce foscarnet if:
- Neutrophil count $< 0.5 \times 10^9/l$
- Platelet count $< 50 \times 10^9/l$.

Oral Ganciclovir

Recent studies indicate a role of oral ganciclovir as a prophylactic agent against CMV retinitis.

The bioavailability of oral ganciclovir administered in a dosage of 3000 mg/day with food is 9 percent. However, serum levels of 0.5 µg/ml are obtained at this dosage which are virostatic for most CMV isolates. This level of systemic drug is adequate to suppress both visceral and ocular CMV infections. It has been shown that difference between oral and intravenous ganciclovir in prophylaxis treatment is not statistically significant.

Mean time to progression is 68 days vs 96 days with IV route. Oral ganciclovir is recommended for:
- Maintenance therapy
- Primary prophylaxis of CMV end organ disease
- Peripheral disease (not Juxtapapillary or macular).

Intravitreal Injection of Ganciclovir

Intravitreal injections of ganciclovir are used to treat patients who are intolerant of systemic therapy. Dosage of intravitreal ganciclovir is 200–400 µg/dose given 1–2 times per week providing higher intravitreal concentrations than systemic therapy. Much higher doses of intravitreal ganciclovir (2000 µg) result in excellent control of retinitis and require only weekly injection.

Though intravitreal injections provide intraocular therapy for CMV retinitis yet these injections can be complicated by endophthalmitis, vitreous hemorrhage, retinal detachment and cataract. When CMV retinitis is unilateral, local intravitreal therapy provides no prophylaxis against the development of retinitis in the fellow eye, the probability of which may be 50 percent during the first 6 months of treatment if systemic therapy is not undertaken concurrently. Intravitreal administration do not provide systemic protection against CMV dissemination.

Recently liposome encapsulated ganciclovir intravitreal injection is commercially available for use. It reduces the number of intravitreal injections, stabilizing CMV retinitis and maintain higher intravitreal dose of ganciclovir for a longer duration.

Ganciclovir Implant (Intravitreal Devices)

The ganciclovir implant was developed to derive the advantage of local therapy, i.e. delivery of concentrated drug directly to the infected retina without the risk of systemic drug toxicity or an indwelling catheter. Moreover implant offers the advantage of sustained intraocular release of ganciclovir obviating the need for repeated intravitreal injections.

It consists of central pellet of ganciclovir 4.5 mg encased in a polyvinyl alcohol (PVA) polymer that is water permeable. PVA is surrounded partially by an impermeable polymer, ethylene vinyl acetate which restricts the surface area available for drug diffusion. Finally the implant is coated with an additional layer of PVA. It is then heat treated which changes the crystalline structure of the PVA, modifying the overall drug release rate. Depending upon ganciclovir release implant can provide therapeutic levels of ganciclovir up to eight months but release rates vary among individuals.

It is surgically implanted in the vitreous cavity by making 5 mm incision in pars plana positioned 4 mm posterior to limbus. A small strut on the implant is sutured to side of the scleral incision after

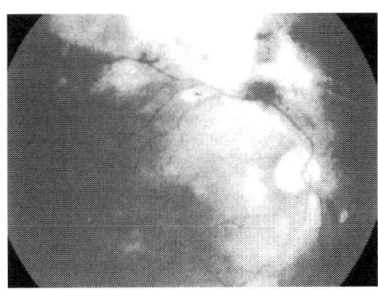

Fig. 20.9: Ocular manifestation of AIDS in right eye (Initial visit before intravitreal ganciclovir injection)

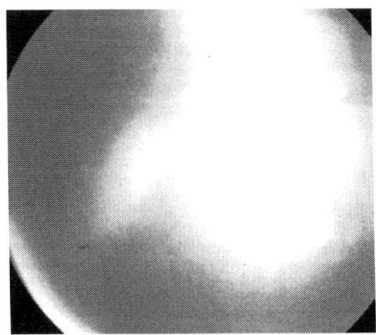

Fig. 20.10: Right eye one day after treatment with intravitreal liposome encapsulated ganciclovir injection

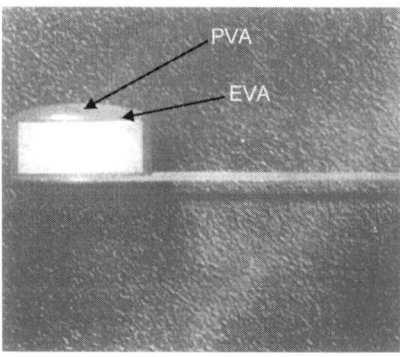

Fig. 20.11: Ganciclovir implant design

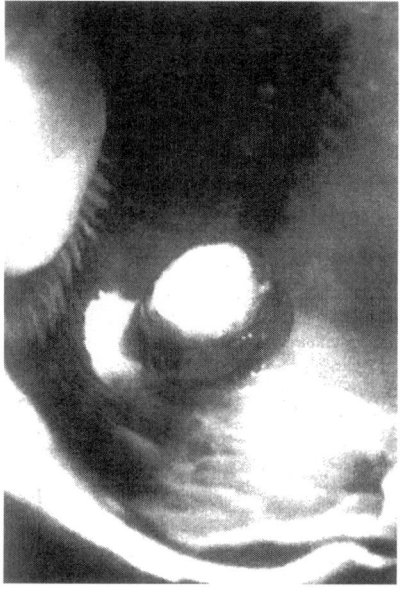

Fig. 20.12: Gross appearance of ganciclovir implant

a vitrectomy performed at the incision site. The incision is closed and eye reformed with BSS. The implant slowly release the drug at a rate of approximately 1.4–1.9 µg per hour over an 8 months period. Clinical studies have shown the regression of CMV retinitis up to a period of three years with repeated implantation every eight months. Use of implant has been advocated for treatment of both newly diagnosed and recurrent CMV retinitis. Median time for progression of peripheral disease is 226 days. No device related complications except alteration in electrophysiological tests have been reported.

Ganciclovir resistance: Drug resistance is an emerging problem of great concern because of limited number of available agents effective against cytomegalovirus. Cytomegalovirus UL 97 mutations have been detected in polymorphonuclear leukocytes of 31 percent of patients treated with ganciclovir for three months or more and in none of those treated less than three months. The mutation is associated with an increase CMV DNA viral load in the blood as well as with progression of CMVR.

If there is no response despite three weeks of treatment:
- Consider combined ganciclovir and foscarnet treatment if macula is threatened.
- Stop zidovudine if being used during induction phase with ganciclovir.

Other drug interactions are:
- Ganciclovir + Zidovudine – increased nephrotoxicity
- Ganciclovir + Imipenam – Cilastin – increased generalized seizures.

Toxicities of ganciclovir include bone marrow suppression with neutropenia, thrombocytopenia, neurological dysfunction, abnormal liver, function tests, etc. The most serious side effect is neutropenia which can occur in up to 35 percent of the patients.

Foscarnet

It exerts its antiviral action by a selective inhibition at the pyrophosphate binding site on virus specific DNA polymerase and reverse transcriptase at a concentration that does not affect cellular DNA polymerase. CMV strain resistant to ganciclovir may be sensitive to foscarnet.

Dosage: The treatment of CMV retinitis is started with an induction dosage regimen of 90 mg/kg IV BD for 14–21 days (depending on fundus review) followed by daily maintenance regimen at dose ranging from 90 mg/kg IV OD. Foscarnet can also be given by intravitreal injection in the dose of 2.4 mg every week.

How to administer: Foscarnet solution 24 mg/kg is to be given over 2 hours with 1000 ml of normal saline as hydration fluid (use 5% Dextrose if NA^+ levels are high) concurrently. This also prevents risk of thrombophlebitis.

Monitor schedule is same as for ganciclovir. The major adverse effect reported with Foscarnet is nephrotoxicity. Other side effects include hypocalcemia and seizures.

Treatment Efficacy

Ganciclovir
- Response rate   80–100 percent
- Remission rate   60–80 percent
- Median time to remission   21–38 days

Foscarnet
- Response rate   80–100 percent
- Remission rate   40–80 percent
- Median time to remission   58–90 days

BREAKTHROUGH RETINITIS

It is relapse while on maintenance therapy.
Treatment of breakthrough retinitis can be:
a. Foscarnet alone or high dose ganciclovir
b. Combination of ganciclovir and foscarnet

Clinical studies have shown that median time to progression in patients treated with foscarnet is 1.3 months, with high dose ganciclovir is two months and with combination therapy of ganciclovir and foscarnet is 4.3 months. While morbidity and mortality is same in three groups.

Newer Modalities

Cidofovir/Zidofovir (HPMPC)

It is 1, 3-Hydroxy–2-Phosphonyl Methoxy propyl (HPMPC) is latest nucleotide analogue active against cytomegalovirus. It can be administered by intravenous or intravitreal injection.

Cidofovir operates by being incorporated in retinal cells where it blocks the enzymes the virus need to reproduce. Ganciclovir and foscarnet also prevent the virus from replicating but cidofovir action lasts far longer and it is about 100 times more potent than ganciclovir.

Intravenous treatment dosage of 5 mg/kg per week for first two weeks followed by injection. 5 mg/kg/alternate week as maintenance therapy along with probenecid.

Main advantage of this therapy is of long duration of effect. Concurrent probenecid administration is necessary to decrease nephrotoxicity.

Standard intravitreal dosage is 20 mg dose injected every six weeks. With this regimen retinitis does not reactivate. The incidence of iritis after intravitreal injection is sharply decreased with concomitant oral probenecid.

Uveitis and hypotony are reported side effects with both routes of delivery.

Protease Inhibitors in CMVR

It is commonly seen that CMV retinitis patients have a very low CD4+ Lymphocyte count (below $50 \times 10^6/l$).

Protease inhibitors can change the classical picture of CMV retinitis. Recent studies have shown that triple drug combination lead to decreased plasma HIV-RNA levels below the detection limit of currently available assay in over 90 percent of individuals overall incidence of CMVR is dramatically decreased. Recurrence free intervals are prolonged.

There are reports of sustained increase in CD4 counts and reach the value of $100 \times 10^6/l$ or more after 12–16 weeks of treatment. The elevated levels are maintained during the whole follow-up period.

New investigational compound on trial for CMV retinitis are:
- Lobucavir an antisense oligonucleotide 1515-2922.
- Anti CMV monoclonal antibody MSL-109.

- Halogenated benzamidozole—20 times more potent than ganciclovir.

TOXOPLASMA INFECTION

Toxoplasma gondii, retinochoroiditis in AIDS is characterized by lesions that are Larger, less frequently associated with healed scars, more commonly bilateral and may be difficult to distinguish from other opportunistic infectious retinitis.

Anti-*Toxoplasma* regimen has to be continued life long even if retinitis resolves. Evaluation for cerebral or disseminated toxoplasmosis is necessary.

Most of the these patients respond to standard anti-*Toxoplasma* treatment within 6 weeks first choice of treatment is:
- Sulphadiazine + Pyrimethamine + Folinic acid
- Second choice is Clindamycine + Pyrimethamine + Folinic acid
- Third choice is Atovaquone + Pyrimethamine + Folinic acid.
- Primary prophylaxis is not recommended.

For secondary prophylaxis and chronic suppressive therapy above mentioned drugs are used.

Dosage: Sulphadiazine – For treatment 2 gm tds PO/IV and for maintenancc 1g tds PO.

Pyrimethamine: For treatment 200 mg PO on day 1 in divided doses and then 50 mg OD.

Clindamycin: For treatment 600 mg PO/IV eight hourly and for maintenance 450 mg PO/IV eight hourly. Folinic acid (Given to decrease risk of myelosuppression)

Dosage: 15 mg PO daily (treatment and maintenance)
- Atovaquone—for treatment 750 mg four times daily (has to be given with food).
- Sulphadiazine when given IV has to be diluted in 100 ml normal saline and given over one hour.

Pyrimethamine is given orally in tablet form. Clindamycin when given IV has to be diluted in normal saline five percent Dextrose and given over 20 minutes (in 100 ml).

During treatment period close monitoring is required for hemogram, urinary and serum electrolytes and LFT.

Complications

- Sulphadiazine   Crystalluria
- Pyrimethamine   Myelosuppression
- Clindamycin   *Corynebacterium difficile enterocolitis*
- Atovaquone   Rash and neutropenia.

HERPES ZOSTER OPHTHALMICUS

Start with IV acyclovir 10 mg/kg or 500 mg/sqm eight hourly for 7–10 days.

How to administer: Dilute with normal saline and give over one hour. Diluted solutions should not have more than 5 mg/ml of acyclovir.

After that switch to oral therapy. Oral dosage is 800 mg five times daily.

During treatment period monitor hemogram once weekly and electrolytes twice a week. Main adverse effect with acyclovir therapy is nephrotoxicity. Tailor dose according to creatinine clearance.

Topical one percent Foscarnet sodium solution five times/day or topical one percent Trifluoridine solution five times/day can also be given. Extensive epithelium debridement alongwith prolonged antiviral therapy may be helpful.

MYCOBACTERIUM TUBERCULOSIS

First choice of treatment is:

Rifampicin + INH + pyrazinamide. Add ethambutol if resistance suspected.

Dosage

Rifampicin	600 mg PO (>50 kg body wt.) daily
	450 mg PO (<50 kg body wt.) daily
INH	300 mg PO daily
Pyridoxine	10 mg PO daily
Pyrazinamide	2 g PO daily (750 kg body wt)
1.5 g PO daily	(<50 kg body wt)
Ethambutol	15 mg/kg PO daily.

Take as single dose before breakfast. During treatment period monitor LFT twice weekly at first, then monthly, renal (creatinine clearance) weekly at start, then monthly, hemogram (monthly) and eye examination if ethambutol indicated.

MYCOBACTERIUM AVIUM INTRACELLULARE

First choice of treatment:
- Rifampicin: 600 mg PO daily (> 50 kg body wt)
  450 mg PO daily (< 50 kg)
- Rifabutin: 450 mg PO daily (> 50 kg wt)
  300 mg PO daily (< 50 kg)
- Ethambutol: 15 mg/kg PO daily
- Clarithromycin: 500–1000 ug PO × 12 weeks
- Amikacin (Given when there is no resolution of symptoms) or above regimen
  – 7.5 mg/kg/day IV/IM as single dose × 14 days.

Second choice of treatment:
Substitute any one of the above with either
  – Ciprofloxacillin – 500 mg PO daily bd
  – Clofazimine - 100 mg PO daily.

OCULAR SYPHILIS

Treat it as neurosyphilis usually higher doses are recommended. Recommended dosage is 10-24 million IU of aqueous pencillin IV daily × 10-14 days + probencicid 50 mg PO daily.

If allergy than skin test and desensitize. Ceftriaxone has been found to very effective. Retreat if CSF cell count does not decline by 6 months or normalize by 2 years.

ACUTE RETINAL NECROSIS

Varicella-zoster virus (VZV) is the causative organism of both acute retinal necrosis (ARN) and progressive outer retinal necrosis. ARN is devastating, rapidly progressive necrotizing retinitis.

Start with acyclovir 7.5-10 mg/kg IV daily for 10-14 days. Long-term suppression therapy with oral acyclovir is 500 mg PO five times daily for several months. However, the emergence of acyclovir resistant strains of herpes virus is problematic specially in AIDS patients.

Other recommended drug is intravenous foscarnet 40-60 mg/kg three times daily.

In severe cases intravitreal ganciclovir and foscarnet can be given.

PNEUMOCYSTIS CARINII CHOROIDITIS

Treatment: Trimethoprim/Sulphamethoxazole or Pentamidine. Most lesions disappear in 3-12 weeks following treatment.

Fungal Infections

Fungal infections like those of *Candida, Cryptococcus, Aspergillus, Coccidioidomycosis* and *Histoplasmosis* are more often seen in AIDS patients as compare to normal population and has to be treated by systemic antifungal agents.

AIDS though not curable yet certainly manageable. Apart from intensive antiretroviral medication, prophylactic treatment and close monitoring, once the diagnosis is confirmed patient should be encouraged to carry on the routine of daily life.

RECENT ADVANCES IN ANTIRETROVIRAL DRUG THERAPY

Fomivirsen Sodium (Vitravene)

Fomivirsen sodium is recently introduced antiretroviral drug. It is a phosphorothioate oligonucleotide that inhibits human cytomegalovirus (CMV) replication through an antisense mechanism. The nucleotide sequence of Fomivirsen is complementary to a sequence in mRNA transcripts of CMV. Binding of Fomivirsen to the target mRNA results in the inhibition of IE2 protein synthesis subsequently inhibiting replication.

The antisense mechanism of action and molecular target of fomivirsen are different from that of other inhibitors of CMV replication which function by inhibiting the viral DNA polymerase. Fomivirsen is very potent against clinical CMV isolates which are resistant to ganciclovir, foscarnet or cidofovir.

Fomivirsen is cleared from the vitreous over the course of 7–10 days by a combination of tissue distribution and metabolism. Metabolism is the primary route of elimination from the eye. Fomivirsen ocular concentrations are maximum in the retina and iris. It is detected in the retina within hours after injection and concentration increases over 3–5 days.

Indications: Fomivirsen is indicated in cytomegalovirus retinitis. Fomivirsen is given as local treatment of CMV retinitis in patients with AIDS who are intolerant or have a contraindication to other treatments for CMV retinitis.

Route of administration and dosage: Fomivirsen is given intravitreally for ophthalmic use. It is not recommended for use in patients who have recently (2–4 weeks) been treated with either IV or intravitreal cidofovir because of risk of exaggerated ocular inflammation.

The recommended induction dose is 0.05 ml (330 mcg) as a single intravitreal injection on alternate week for two doses followed by maintenance doses of 330 mcg (0.05 ml) once every four weeks. Fomivirsen is administered by intravitreal injection (0.05 ml/eye) into the affected eye following application of standard topical or local anesthetics and antimicrobials using 30 gauge needle or a low volume syringe.

Postinjection monitoring includes light perception and optic nerve head perfusion. If not completely perfused by 7–10 minutes perform anterior chamber paracentesis with a 30 gauge needle at the slit lamp. Store the fomivirsen between 2 and 25°C.

Adverse reactions: The most observed ophthalmic adverse reactions include ocular inflammation (uveitis) including iritis and vitritis (in 25% of patients). Other local adverse reaction reported are transient rise in IOP, blurred vision, cataract, conjunctival hemorrhage, photophobia, desaturation of color vision, floaters, retinal edema and hemorrhage, vitreous opacities and retinal detachment.

Systemic adverse reactions include abdominal pain, asthenia, diarrhea, fever, infection, nausea, rashes, vomiting, abnormal liver function, neuropathy, neutropenia, sweating, thrombocytopenia, anorexia, decreased weight and dehydration.

Precautions: Patients receiving fomivirsen should have regular eye follow-up examinations. CMV may exist as a systemic disease in addition to CMV retinitis. Therefore, careful monitoring of patients for extraocular CMV infections (e.g. colitis, pneumonitis and retinitis in the opposite eye if single eye is being treated).

BIBLIOGRAPHY

1. Agarwal A. Textbook of Ophthalmology, 1st edn. New Delhi: Jaypee Brothers Medical Publishers, 2002.
2. Bartlett JD. Clinical Ocular Pharmacology, 4th edn. Boston: Butterworth-Heinemann, 2001
3. Bartlett JD. Ophthalmic Drug Facts, Lippincott-William and Wilkins, 2001.
4. Crick RP, Trimble RB. Textbook of Clinical Ophthalmology, Hodder and Stoughton, 1986.
5. Duane TD. Clinical Ophthalmology, 4th edn. Butterworth-Heinemann, 1999.
6. Duvall. Ophthalmic Medications and Pharmacology, Slack Inc, 1998.
7. Ellis PP. Ocular Therapeutics and Pharmacology, 7th edn. CV Mosby, 1985.
8. Fechner. Ocular Therapeutics, Slack Inc., 1998.
9. Fraunfelder. Current Ocular Therapy, 5th edn. WB Saunders, 2000.
10. Garg A. Current Trends in Ophthalmology, 1st edn. New Delhi: Jaypee Brothers Medical Publishers, 1997.
11. Garg A. Manual of Ocular Therapeutics, 1st edn. New Delhi: Jaypee Brothers Medical Publishers, 1996.
12. Garg A. Ready Reckoner of Ocular Therapeutics, 1st edn. New Delhi: 2002.
13. Garg A. Synopsis of AIDS, 2nd edn. New Delhi; Jaypee Brothers Medical Publishers, 1992.
14. Goodman LS, Gilman A. Pharmacological Basis of Therapeutics, 7th edn. New York: Macmillan, 1985.
15. Havener's. Ocular Pharmacology, 6th edn. CV Mosby, 1994.
16. Kanski. Clinical Ophthalmology, 4th edn. Butterworth-Heineman, 1999.
17. Kershner. Ophthalmic Medications and Pharmacology, Slack. Inc., 1994.
18. Olin BR, et al. Drugs Facts and Comparisons, Facts and Comparisons, St. Louis, 1997.
19. Onofrey. The Ocular Therapeutics; Lippincott-William and Wilkins, 1997.
20. Rhee. The Wills Eye Drug Guide, Lippincott-William and Wilkins, 1998.
21. Steven Podos. Textbook of Ophthalmology, New Delhi: Jaypee Brothers Medical Publishers, 2001.
22. Zimmerman. Text book of Ocular Pharmacology, Lippincott-William and Wilkins, 1997.

21

Sterilization, Disinfection and Antiseptics in Ophthalmology

Ashok Garg (India)

Sterilization is defined as the process by which an article, surface or medium is freed of all microorganisms either in vegetative or spore state.

Disinfection is defined as destruction of all pathogenic organisms or organisms capable of giving rise to infection.

Chemical disinfectants which can safely be applied to skin or mucous membrane surfaces and are used to prevent infection by inhibiting the growth of bacteria are called antiseptics. Bactericidal agents are those which are able to kill bacteria.

Bacteriostatic agents are those which only prevent the multiplication of bacteria which may remain alive. A particular chemical may be bactericidal or bacteriostatic at different concentrations.

Sterilization methods depend on the purpose for which sterilization is carried out, the material which has to be sterilized and the nature of microorganisms that are to be removed or destroyed. The most important factor in decision-making is to recognize that the methods of sterilization and disinfection chosen must be appropriate to the individual situation, in terms of cost and availability as well in terms of clinical needs. Re-evaluation is necessary from time to time because, inspite of most stringent following of rules and safest of practice, complications still occur, sometimes to the deteriment of patient care and staff safety. Various methods of sterilization and disinfection used in ophthalmology are as follows:

PHYSICAL METHODS

1. Dry heat
2. Moist heat
3. Filtration
4. Ionizing radiation.

Dry Heat

Flaming

Inoculating wires, loops, points of forceps and searing spatulas may be held in bunsen flame till they become red hot for sterilizing them.

TABLE 21.1: Sterilization and disinfection methods

Methods	Achieves	Time	Kills	Advantages	Disadvantages/Cautions	Power source	Suitable for	Min. Temp.
General autoclave	Sterilization	Approx 45 minutes Follow manufacturer's instructions	• Bacteria • Spores • Viruses • Fungi	• Low running cost • Minimal maintenance • Suitable for busy unit • Drying cycle	• Difficult to obtain spare parts in developing countries	• Electric (single or three phase) • Kerosene • Paraffin	• All metal instruments • Drapes • Gowns • Dressings • Toughened plastic • Glass	121°C
'Little Sister' autoclave	Sterilization	20 minutes cycle	• Bacteria • Spores • Viruses • Fungi	• Quick and efficient • Small-bench top size • Suitable for busy unit	• High running cost • Difficult to obtain spare parts in developing countries • No drying cycle • Sensitive to voltage fluctuations	• Electric (single phase)	• All metal instruments • Toughened plastic • Glass	134°C
Portable autoclave/ Domestic cooker	Sterilization	Minimum of 15 minutes Follow manufactures instructions	• Bacteria • Spores • Viruses • Fungi	• Low running cost • Quick and efficient • Suitable for mobile units • Minimal maintenance	• Drying cycle unreliable • Sensitive to voltage fluctuations • Relatively small • Various manufacturers whose instructions must be followed	• Electric (single phase) • Gas • Kerosene • Paraffin • Charcoal • Wood	• All metal instruments • Drapes • Gowns • Dressing • Toughened plastic • Glass	121°C
Hot air ovens	Sterilization	2 hour cycle	• Bacteria • Spores • Viruses • Fungi	• Drying cycle • Minimal maintenance	• Expensive • Slow • Instruments get extremely hot and can not be used immediately • Must not be used in confined space	• Electric (single phase)	• All metal instruments • Toughened plastic • Glass	180°C

Contd...

Contd...

Methods	Achieves	Time	Kills	Advantages	Disadvantages/Cautions	Power source	Suitable for	Min. Temp.
Ionizing irradiation	Sterilization	According to manufacturers	• Bacteria • Spores • Viruses • Fungi	• Bulk quantities • Suitable for delicate items and items which must be kept dry and not soaked	• Usually only available commercially and used by large manufacturing companies	• Gamma rays	• Needles • Syringes • Sutures • Toughened plastic	
Boiling	High level disinfection	Minimum of 10 minutes	• Bacteria • Viruses • Fungi	• Low running cost • Quick and efficient • Easy to teach • Suitable for all situations • Minimal maintenance • Readily available	• Does not kill spores • Blunts scissors and knives • Causes rusting of instruments	• Electric (single phase) • Gas • Kerosene • Paraffin • Charcoal • Wood	• 'Heavy' metal instruments • Plastic • Glass • Sutures • Needles	100°C
Ethylene oxide C_2H_4O	Sterilization	According to manufacturers	• Bacteria • Spores • Viruses • Fungi	• Bulk quantities • Suitable for delicate items and items which must be kept dry and not soaked	• Very expensive • Dangerous-explosive • Carcinogenic • Only suitable for large tertiary centers with appropriate facilities	• Electric with C_2H_4O gas cartridges	• Plastic eye shields • Ophthalmic instruments and probes • Delicate tubing	Varies with type of equipment used
Formalin	Sterilization	12 hours	• Bacteria • Spores • Viruses • Fungi	• Low running costs • Suitable for delicate items susceptible to rust • A cabinet can hold a large quantity of instruments • Formalin tablets usually readily available	• Airtight containers required • Irritant to skin, eyes and if inhaled • Gloves and eye protection advisable • Items must be rinsed in sterile water before use • Slow	• Electric (single phase) if an old refrigerator is adapted as a cabinet	• All metal instruments • Toughened plastic • Glass • Delicate • Tubing	*Room temperature 20°C Well ventilated

Contd...

Contd...

Methods	Achieves	Time	Kills	Advantages	Disadvantages/Cautions	Power source	Suitable for	Min. Temp.
Glutaraldehyde 2%	Sterilization in 10 hours Disinfection in 10 minutes	Follow manufacturers instructions several trade names now available	• Bacteria • Spores • Viruses • Fungi	• Becoming more readily available	• Relatively expensive • Irritant to skin, eyes and if inhaled • Gloves and eye protection advisable • May leave greasy residue • Items must be rinsed and lumen irrigated thoroughly before use	• All metal instruments • Airways and endo-tracheal tubes • Plastic • Glass		
Isopropyl Alcohol 70%	Disinfection	10 minutes Note: The quantity used for soaking must be changed daily	• Bacteria • Spores • Viruses (see exceptions*)	• Low cost • Readily available	• Good for use on indirect ophthalmoscope lenses as evaporation avoids smearing	• Highly inflammable • Corrosive—do not leave metal instruments soaking longer than 10 minutes • Tonometry items must be rinsed and wiped dry before use • Evaporates • Does not kill entero and adeno viruses*	• All metal instruments • Wiping Schiotz tonometer plate and applanation prism tip • Indirect ophthalmoscope lenses	

Contd...

Contd...

Methods	Achieves	Time	Kills	Advantages	Disadvantages/Cautions	Power source	Suitable for	Min. Temp.
Sodium hypochlorite	Disinfection	10 minutes Note: The quantity used for soaking must be changed daily	• Bacteria • Spores • Viruses	• Becoming more readily available • Reasonable cost	• Highly volatile and corrosive—do not use metal container to soak items • Bleach • Applanation prisms must be rinsed and wiped dry before use	• Indirect ophthalmoscope lenses • Applanation prism tip only may 'sit' in solution		
Chlorhexidine	Disinfection	10 minutes Note: The quantity used for soaking must be changed daily	• Bacteria • Spores • Fungi	• Low cost • Readily available	• Evaporates • Does not kill viruses • Blunts scissors and knives	• Plastic • Rubber • Metal instruments • Wiping Schiotz tonometer plate and applanation prism tip		
Povidone iodine	Disinfection	10 minutes Note: The quantity used for soaking must be changed daily	• Bacteria • Spores • Fungi • Viruses (see exceptions*)	• Low cost • Readily available • Versatile	• Stains fabric and surfaces • Discolors instruments • Solution is dark—difficult to see items in soak • Irritant to skin • Does not kill entero or adeno virus*	• All metal instruments • Sutures • Blades		

Authors: Sue Stevens and Ingrid Cox, First published in Journal of Community Eye Health, Volume 9, issue no. 19, 36–41, 1996. [*Courtesy:* DANPCB (Danish Assistance to the National Programme for control of Blindness)] Indian Supplement, New Delhi.

TABLE 21.2: Sterilization methods in ocular surgery

Sterilization methods		OT sterilization	
Linen (gowns, caps, masks, drapes)	Autoclaving	Method 1	
Glassware (e.g. syringes)	Hot air oven (Dry heat), ETO	Wash theater with copious amount of water	
Metal instrument: Moisture labile (sharp instruments) (Vannas scissors/ keratome)	Dry heat/ETO	Fumigate with formalin vapour (30 ml of 40% formalin dissolved in 90 ml of clean water for 1000 cu. ft)	
Moisture resistant	Autoclaving/ETO		
Plastic instruments (Components)	ETO	Keep room closed for 6 hours	
Intraocular implants	ETO	Carbolize with 2 percent carbolic acid (takes about 24 hours for the pungent smell of formalin and carbolic acid to dissipate)	
Sutures (including monofilament nylon)	Can be autoclaved	Method 2	
Diathermy/Cautery electrodes	Autoclaving	Dissolve 325 ml of aldekol (6% formaldehyde + 6% glutaraldehyde + 5% benzalconium chloride) in 150 ml of water. Spray as aerosol for 30 min.	
Endoilluminators/Probes	ETO	Close room for 2 hours	
Lenses (Indirect/Optical)	Chemical disinfection	Allow fumes to clear (turn on exhaust/air conditioning)	
Silicone buckles/sponges	Autoclaving	(Takes only about 3 hours to sterilize the OT).	
Silicone oil	Hot air oven		
Perfluorocarbon liquids	ETO/Millipore filter (0.2 µl)		
Recommended temperature, pressure and duration			
Autoclave 121°C	15–30 lb psi	45 min	
Flash autoclave 134°C		20 min	
Hot air oven 150°C		2 hours	
ETO	55 lb psi		
Cidex	Bactericidal 10–30 min Sporicidal 3–10 hours		
Sterile technique: Principles			
Keep microorganism load to an irreducible minimum if they cannot be fully eradicated		Gowns are considered sterile only from waist to shoulder in front and up to the sleeves	
If there is any doubt regarding sterility of any article, consider it to be unsterile		Keep nonsterile personnel or visitors to a minimum	
Only sterile personnel should touch sterile articles.		Don't	
Sterile persons should avoid leaning over an unsterile area, while nonsterile persons should avoid reaching over a sterile field		—	Rush through while scrubbing.
		—	Wear same footwear from an unrestricted area to a restricted area
Tables are sterile only at table level		—	Let a mask hang loose around the neck and reuse the same
The edge of anything that encloses sterile contents is not considered sterile		—	Wear a cap that does not fully cover the scalp hair and a mask that does not snugly cover the nose
Sterile persons should keep well within the sterile area; nonsterile persons should keep away from the sterile area		—	Move about with hands folded or within gown pockets
Moisture is a potential source of contamination; so avoid using moisture soaked linen packages		—	Throw around soiled linen and unsterile covers

Incineration

This method is used for rapidly destroying materials such as soiled dressing, waste and animal caracases.

Hot Air Oven

This is one of the most widely used method for sterilization by dry heat in ophthalmology. These fan-assisted ovens sterilize by dry heat and are often used in larger and central medical centers. The sterilizing time is 2 hours but complete cycle is 4 hours. Hot air ovens are useful for drying washed instruments. For sterilization static temperature of 160°C for 1 hour is used.

It can be used to sterilize:
- Glassware
- Sharp instruments
- Forceps, scissors, scalpels and all glass syringes
- Swabs, fats, grease, etc.

Rubber materials should not be sterilized as they will not stand this high temperature. For sharp instruments sterilization time is 2 hours at static 150°C (Control by thermostat) is recommended to prevent blunting. The oven must be allowed to cool slowly for about 2 hours the door is opened.

Moist Heat

Temperature below 100°C

The temperature employed is either 60°C for 30 minutes or 72°C for 15–20 minutes (Flash method) followed by rapid cooling. By this process all nonsporing pathogens such as *Mycobacterium brucella* and *Salmonella* are destroyed.

Temperature at 100°C

Boiling high level disinfection is achieved by boiling. Vegetative bacteria are killed almost immediately at 90–100°C but sporing bacteria require considerable period of boiling. Boiling is not recommended for sterilization of instruments used for surgical procedure. Nothing short of autoclaving at high pressure can destroy spores and ensure sterilization.

Instruments must be completely immersed in already boiling water in a container preferably with a lid. Boil at 100°C for at least 10–20 minutes.

Although boiling is the most readily available method it has the distinct disadvantage of blunting instruments. Instruments must not be placed on top of each other. A silicon mat on the bottom of container will help to protect the instruments. Silicone tubing will also protect the tips of fine instruments.

Boiling kills bacteria, fungi, viruses including the AIDS virus but not spores. Chelate forceps are used to remove articles from boiler.

TABLE 21.3: Autoclave sterilization

Steam pressure Lb/in²	Temperature in 0°C	Holding time for sterilization (min.)
0	100	—
10	115	45
15	121	15
30	134	3

Steaming at 100°C: An atmosphere of steam is used to sterilize culture media which may decompose if subjected to higher temperature.

Temperature above 100°C (Autoclaving): The principal of autoclave is that when pressure inside a closed vessel increases, the temperature at which water boils and that of steam it forms also increases. Saturated steam has great penetrative power. The temperature setting and sterilizing time is dependant on the type of autoclave and articles being treated. The condensed water insures moist condition for killing the microbe present. Sterilization by steam under pressure is carried out at temperature between 108–147°C.

By using the appropriate time and temperature, a variety of materials such as dressings, instruments, laboratory ware, media, pharmacological products and OT clothes can be sterilized. Heat is conducted through the walls of sealed containers until the temperature of the material inside is in equilibrium with the steam outside.

The complete cycle can take up to 45 minutes which includes drying time. Articles can be placed in metal sterilizing drums with holes to allow for steam penetration.

If dampness of drapes and gowns, etc. is noted when they are removed from the autoclaves they must not be used as this indicates a faulty cycle and sterility has not been achieved.

'Little sister' autoclaves are also available for sterilization using steam under pressure. These autoclaves are small enough to place on a work surface, bench top, shelf or trolly and are specially useful for resterilizing instruments during operating sessions, e.g. if contamination occurs or for subsequent cases.

Portable autoclaves are also useful in theaters for sterilizing sets of instruments. They are very quick, efficient and popular in rural and camp areas.

Precautions during Autoclaving

- Because of varying sterilization times for different items it is recommended that similar items are placed together.
- Instruments must not be left in an autoclave for longer than necessary as it will cause corrosion.
- The steam must penetrate the contents so autoclave must not be packed tightly.
- Instruments tips should be protected with silicone tubing.

- Sterilizing drums must open during the cycle and closed on completion.
- Porous load items must be double wrapped.
- Spare parts shall always be available.

Filtration

This method is used to sterilize heat labile liquids. This is useful for antibiotic solutions, sera, carbohydrate solutions, etc.
Various types of filter used are:
- Berkefeld earthenware candles
- Asbestos disk filters
- Sintered glass filters
- Colloiden or membrane filters.

Ionizing Radiation

This method of sterilization is used commercially by large companies specially for syringes, needles and suture material. Nonionizing and ionizing radiations are being widely used for mass sterilization. Infrared and ultraviolet rays are of nonionizing type while gamma ray and high energy electrons are of high energy ionizing type.

Gamma radiation is used for sterilization of most plastics, syringes, swabs, culture plates, various types of rubber products, card board, fabric metal, foils, etc.

CHEMICAL METHODS

It includes:
- Gas
- Vapour
- Soaking in liquid chemicals.

There are a large number of chemical agents available for use as antiseptics and disinfectants. Their main mode of action is:
- Proteins coagulation
- Disruption of cell membrane
- Removal of free sulphydryl groups which are essential for functioning of the cell
- Substrate competition

The factors which determine the potency of disinfectants are:
- Concentration of substance
- Time of action
- pH of medium
- Temperature
- Nature of the organisms
- Presence of extraneous material.

Ethylene Oxide (C_2H_4O)

It is a colorless liquid with a boiling point of 10.7°C and at normal temperature and pressure it is very penetrating gas with a sweet smell. It is highly inflammable and in concentration greater than 3 percent in air, it is highly explosive. Its explosive tendency is eliminated by mixing it with inert gases such as CO_2 or nitrogen in 10 percent concentration.

It is lethal to microorganisms due to its power of alkylating the amino, carboxyl, hydroxyl and sulphadryl group in the protein molecule. In addition it reacts with DNA and RNA.

It diffuses through many types of porous materials and readily penetrates the plastics. It is specially used for sterilizing:
- Sutures
- Intraocular lenses
- Clothing
- Glassware
- Plastic products.

This gas is effective for almost all instruments and materials and specially for those which do not tolerate heat sterilization or soaking in chemicals. It is used for eye shields, ophthalmic probes, tubing and vitrectomy equipment. The sterilizing cycle is lengthy (12 hours) and it is enormously expensive to setup and run.

All microorganisms are destroyed including the AIDS virus.

Formalin

Formaldehyde (Formalin) in aqueous solution is markedly bactericidal and sporicidal and also has an effect on viruses. Formalin is mainly used for sterilizing (Fumigating) operation theater rooms. Ten percent formalin is used to sterilize clean metal instruments. Formalin gas is used for sterilizing heat sensitive catheters, sick room wards and laboratories. Under properly controlled conditions, clothing, bedding, furniture, cryoprobe, various parts of operating microscopes are satisfactorily disinfected. This gas is irritant to the eyes and skin and precautions must be taken in handling. It is known carcinogenic. Eye protection if available should be worn.

Precautions When using Formalin

- Instruments must be dismantled where possible
- Requires 7 gram of formalin per cubic meter
- Room temperature must be kept at 20°C
- Instruments must be rinsed in sterile water before use
- Good practice achieves destruction of all microorganisms including the AIDS virus.

SOAKING IN LIQUID CHEMICALS

This method is used when alternative methods are unavailable or known to damage instruments and other materials. On long-term use it can cause staining, corrosion and blunting of instruments. Soaked instruments should be rinsed under a stream of sterile water before being used. It is not advisable to use chemical soaking for syringes, needles and other skin cutting instruments.

Here, I am discussing commonly used liquids in ophthalmic practice.

Glutaraldehyde

Two percent glutaraldehyde is used when heat sterilization is impractical and other methods are unavailable. It has an action similar to formaldehyde. It is less toxic and irritant to the eyes and skin. It has no deleterious effect on lenses of instruments, rubber anesthetic tubes, plastic wares, polythene tubine, etc.

Items must be totally immersed with no air bubbles present in a covered container for a minimum of 10 minutes which achieves disinfection. Sterilization take 10 hours. Thorough rinsing under stream of sterile water is important. Because glutaraldehyde is a corrosive chemical and severe irritant if its vapour is inhaled or it comes into contact with skin. The area should be well ventilated. Corneal edema has been reported in patients following the use of glutaraldehyde to sterile cannulae used during cataract surgery. These cannulae and all lumens should be thoroughly irrigated and rinsed.

Shelf life (once activated) is 14–28 days. It disinfects in just 10 minutes killing both gram-positive and gram-negative microorganisms and viruses including HIV and hepatitis B. It sterilizes in 4 hours killing all forms of microbial life including resistant bacterial spoks. It is highly resistant to inactivation by organic soil and is compatible with common surgical materials including carbon, steel, copper, brass, nickel, chrome plate and aluminum.

Isopropyl Alcohol

Isopropyl alcohol 70 percent and ethyl alcohol (ethanol) are commonly used as skin antiseptics. These act by denaturing bacterial protein. Methyl alcohol is also effective against fungal spores.

Isopropyl alcohol 70 percent is available at low cost and ready to use for disinfecting indirect ophthalmoscope lenses and metal instruments including sharps. It can also be used to disinfect the plunger and plate of a Schiotz tonometer and the tip of applanation prisms.

Isopropyl alcohol swabs are commercially available for use as skin disinfectant when soaking, it is a rapid method taking only 2 minutes in a covered container. The quantity used for soaking must be changed daily. Extreme caution should be taken as this agent is highly inflammable. It kills bacteria, spores some viruses including AIDS virus but not entero or adenoviruses or fungi.

Sodium Hypochlorite

It is readily available commercially. It is prepared by adding 500 ml of sodium hypochlorite 1 percent to 1 liter of boiled water. This makes a total quantity of 1.5 liters. Shelf life is 7–14 days. The quantity used for soaking must be changed daily. Use plastic or glass containers only metal containers for shelf or soaking storage are not suitable as sodium hypochlorite is a bleach, highly volatile and corrosive. It should not be used for disinfecting Schiotz tonometer.

Items must be completely immersed in a covered container for a minimum of 10 minutes and rinsed under a stream of sterile water before use.

Sodium hypochlorite kills bacterias, spores and viruses including the AIDS virus but not fungi.

Biguanides (Polyhexanide and Chlorhexidine) (Fig. 21.1)

The biguanides were first synthesized in 1940. Chlorhexidine was first developed in 1950 and polyhexa methylene biguanide (polyhexanide), PHMB was developed in 1960s.

Commercial preparations of PHMB may be composed of a mixture of various lengths of polymer chains. The degree of polymerization may relate to microbicidal activity.

The optimal antiamebic concentration for ocular use has not been determined yet 0.02 percent concentration is commonly used. A 0.00005 percent concentration of PHMB in contact lens disinfectant (ReNu) is present and that is too low concentration.

Chlorhexidine is commercially available as a skin disinfectant in a detergent or alcohol and for use as a mucosal rinse. A concentration of 0.02 percent in isotonic saline or artificial tears has been used successfully in treating *Acanthamoeba* keratitis.

Biguanide disinfectants interrupt microbial DNA function by complexing with intracellular phosphated molecules such as adenosine triphosphate and nucleic acids.

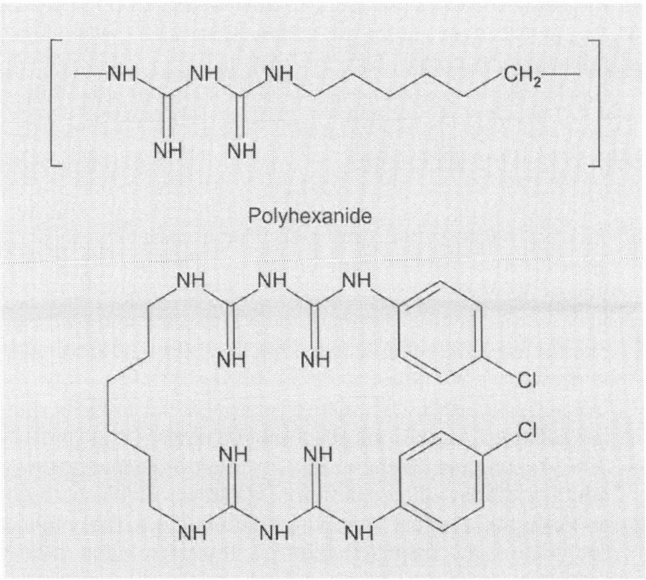

Fig. 21.1: Chemical structures of chlorhexidine and polyhexanide

It is suitable for disinfecting plastic, rubber and metal instruments but can cause blunting of scissors and knives. Items shall be completely immersed in a covered container for a minimum of 10 minutes and they must be rinsed under a stream of sterile water before use.

Four percent chlorhexidine has broad spectrum kill. It is effective in presence of organic matter. It has reduced surfactant content so no damage to skin. No-animal fat emollients keeps the skin soft and protects it from detergents. It is effective against bacteria, spores and fungi but does not kill viruses.

Povidone Iodine (Halogens)

Iodine is aqueous and alcoholic solutions has been used as skin disinfectant. It is an active bactericidal agent with a moderate activity against spores. Chlorine and its compounds have been used as disinfectants. Commercially it is available as 5 percent sterile ophthalmic prep solution. It contains 5 percent povidone iodine (0.5% available iodine) stabilized by glycerin.

It is indicated in the eye for prepping of the periocular region (lids, brow and cheek) and irrigation of the ocular surfaces (cornea, conjunctiva and palpebral fornices) prior to any ocular surgery.

This topical solution is an isotonically balanced preoperative microbicidal solution that can safely be used directly on the cornea and conjunctival cul-de-sac as well as on periocular region. This solution is strictly used for external use only. It is not used for intraocular injection or irrigation.

Salient features of this topical solution are:
- Assure asepsis in less than 60 seconds and stained skin is virtually impossible to reinfect for at least 1 hour.
- It is nontoxic, has excellent skin tolerance and does not burn the skin.
- It has broad spectrum of action sporicidal, bactericidal, antimycotic, viricidal and protozocidal.
- It decreases the incidence of postoperative endophthalmitis.

How to Use this Solution

- First squeeze the entire content of bottle into a sterile prep cup.
- Saturate sterile cotton tipped applicator or sponge to prep lashes and lid margins using one or more applicators per lid. Repeat once.
- Saturate sterile prep sponge to prep lids, brow and cheek in circular ever expanding fashion until the entire field is covered. Repeat prep three times.
- Irrigate the cornea, conjunctiva and palpebral fornices with this solution using a sterile disposable syringe.
- After the prepping solution has been left in contact for two minutes. Sterile saline solution in a syringe should be used to flush the residual prepping solution from the cornea, conjunctiva and palpebral fornices. Topical solution is safe and effective for use and occasional local sensitivity reaction has been reported.

Povidone-iodine is effective against bacteria, spores, fungi, some viruses including AIDS virus but not entero or adenovirus.

It is also available commercially as following:
i. Betadine antiseptic solution 10 percent for prepping skin sites.
ii. Betadine surgical scrub 7.5 percent—a soap used for hand scrubbing.

Phenols

Phenols cause cell membrane damage causing lysis and are powerful microbial substances lysol and cresols are good general disinfectants.

Acetone

Acetone is one of the most commonly used potent bactericidal agent. It is used for sterilization of sharp cutting instruments. It has wide action against gram-positive and gram-negative microorganisms.

Cetrimide

It is used as 10 percent cetrimide solution (in 1:10 dilution) for disinfection of hands in routine OPD procedure in ophthalmology.

Betapropiolactone

It is condensed product of Ketane and formaldehyde with a boiling point of 163°C. It has rapid biocidal action. 0.2 percent betapropiolactone (BPL) solution is used for sterilization of biological products. It is capable of killing all microorganisms and is very active against viruses.

Alcoholic Rub-in Hand Disinfectant

It is a liquid disinfectant containing:
(Each 100 ml contains)

2 - propanol	45.0 g
1 - propanol	30.0 g
Ethyl – hexadecyl – dimethyl Ammonium – ethylsulfate	0.2 g

(Skin protection substance).

It is broad spectrum bactericidal, fungicidal and viricidal. It is also effective against AIDS virus and hepatitis B virus.

It is entirely new concept in hand disinfection, completely eliminating the need for frequent washing. The liquid is rubbed on hands which penetrates deep into the skin forming an inner protective film that does not affect sweating functions while destroying transient pathogens and resident skin flora. It is gentle on skin, acts instantaneously and provides optimally sustained activity without requiring a soap scrub before hand. It penetrates the crypts of the skin into the lower lying horny layers and there forms a defensive barrier against microbes with the result germ count on the hands remains low for several hours.

Alcoholic rubs contain specific quaternary ammonium compounds which are related to its broad spectrum of action for disinfection of hands in ocular surgery.

Alcoholic rubs assure asepsis, protection of natural skin film and skin lipids and prevents spread of nosocomial infections. Ideally rub 3 ml of alcoholic rub disinfectant in one push well over hands and nail grooves for 30 seconds. It is used with a specially designed elbow dispenser to prevent contamination. This pump is calibrated to dispense the exact dosage required. Such 3 consecutive pushes are taken and rub into hands, grooves and up to elbows for 5 minutes. It is nonsticky and give comfortable feel and total protection in perforated gloves also.

Commercially it is available as 100 ml and 500 ml bottle packs.

Cutasept

It is an ideal two component antiseptic for skin.
Each 10 g contains:
2- Propanol   63 g
Benzalkonium cl   0.025 g

It is an ideal surgical antiseptic which serves to clean the skin as disinfect it. Its two components have a synergistic effect on each other. 2-Propanol is a potent broad spectrum microbicidal serves as the glide path for Benzalkonium chloride which has residual effect, inhibiting intraoperative bacterial growth. It has potent action against microbes, viruses including HIV and hepatitis B, fungi bacteria.

It has rapid onset and good residual effect and deep penetration inhibits intraoperative bacterial growth in the incision folds of the skin.

It is mainly used in ophthalmology for periocular prep preparation. Cutasept is painted in operative and perioperative area for 2 minutes with a sterile swab dipped in the solution. Allow the area to dry or about 30 seconds, repaint the entire area as before and allow to dry. Cover the disinfected area with sterile eyesheet leaving the incision site open.

Commercially it is available as 100 ml and 500 ml bottle packs.

Concentrated Cold Sterilizer

It is an ideal solution for sterilization of thermolabile and thermostable instruments like metals, glass, stainless steel, porcelain, plastic, ceramics and rubber. Due to high degree of compatibility of this solution with material surfaces, it can be used for disinfection/sterilization of all kinds of precleaned instruments.

Each 100 g contains:
- Glutaraldehyde   7 g
- 1,6 Dihydroxy 2-5   8.2 g
  Dioxahexane

- Polymethyl urea derivatives   17.6 g
- Rust inhibitors

Usually 5 and 10 percent dilution solutions are used. Five percent solution gives disinfection within one hour while 10 percent solution provides disinfection in 15 minutes. For total sterilization immerse the items in 10 percent solution for 5 hours.

This solution has potent bactericidal, fungicidal, sporicidal and viricidal activity. It is effective again AIDS virus and hepatitis B virus. This solution has long shelf life and rapid action suitable for emergency disinfection.

Commercially it is available as 250 and 500 ml bottle packs.

Bacillocid

It is specially used as concentrated surface and environmental disinfectant with cleansers. It is recommended in 2 and 0.5 percent dilution specially for disinfection/fumigation of operation theaters. It has broad spectrum of activity and is a bactericidal MRSA, sporicidal, fungicidal, tuberculocidal, viricidal including hepatitis B and HIV virus. As it contains corrosion inhibitors so it is safe for all surfaces. It is effective within 30-60 minutes. Commercially it is available as 100 ml and 500 ml packs.

Bacillol 25

It is aldehyde free, quick acting alcoholic spray surface disinfectant. Chemically each 100 gms of the spray contains:

    Ethanol   10 gm
    2-Propanol   9 gm
    1-Propanol   6 gm and corrosion inhibitors.

It is recommended for disinfection of tonometers, operating microscopes, scan probes and operation theaters in between surgeries. Bacillol is effective against all types of bacteria, fungi, viruses including HIV and rota virus.

Contact time for the spray on the surface is 25 seconds to 5 minutes. Commercially it is available as 250 ml bottle with spray.

Baktolin 5.5

It is complete and effective hygenic nonsoap wash lotion which does not disturb the natural pH of the skin. It is specially designed for frequent hand washes.

Chemically it contains—sodium laureth sulfate, sodium chloride, PEG-7/glyceryl cocoate, cocamidopropyl betaine, glycerin, Disodium laureth, Sulfosuccinate, PEG-120/Methyl glucose dioleate, Sodium benzoate, Sodium Salicyclate, Propylene glycol, Parfum and Sodium citrate.

These combinations of ingradients produce a germ inhibiting effect (RF.3 log).

Baktolin has same pH as that of skin (no change in natural balance of skin pH) so the skin remains smooth and well nourished even after prolonged use (unlike use of soaps which may strip the skin of its protective lipid layer and deplete the acid mantle and skin may become dry and cracked and more susceptible to infections).

Commercially, it is available as 500 ml bottle with dispenser. Recommended dosage for each hand wash is 0.5 ml.

AIDS AND DISINFECTION IN RELATION TO OPHTHALMOLOGY

Recently, the media worldwide has devoted considerable space to the problem of AIDS leading to insecurity and panic in persons outside the group of those at risk. Fear of AIDS spread has risen specially among peoples employed in health care profession — Doctors, dentists, nurses and laboratory personnel. Every health professional is prospectively subjected to contact with AIDS patients and thus with carriers of HIV virus. Classified as a lipophilic retrovirus, the HIV virus may be considered labile. Outside the host organism, it quickly loses its activity. Due to its sensitivity the virus is very quickly destroyed by virucidal disinfectants outside the body. Twenty-five percent ethyl alcohol, 1 percent glutaraldehyde and 0.2 percent sodium hypochlorite are adequate disinfectants for instruments and contaminated surfaces. These findings have led to development of preparations containing alcohol or aldehyde and aldehyde derivatives are well suited for disinfection in AIDS prophylaxis.

The presence of HIV particles in tear fluid, on the conjunctival surface or in the contact lenses of patients has made it necessary to establish better guidelines for decontamination of instruments during ophthalmological procedures. Following decontamination procedures should be followed during ophthalmological procedure:

a. The applanation tonometer prisms are cleaned by wiping them gently with cotton, moistened with isopropanol. After cleaning tonometer is wiped dry.

   After each working day the prisms are kept dry in the holder after rinsing them in 0.15 percent glutaraldehyde solution for 5 minutes.

b. The Schiotz tonometer is disinfected in the autoclaves using ethylene oxide. Alternative method is to immerse in isopropyl alcohol for 5 minutes or in 1:10 dilution of sodium hypochlorite for 5–10 minutes or 1:1000 merthiolate wiped dry and then emerged in pure water, carefully rinsed and again wiped dry. All present disinfection solutions known to be effective against HIV are toxic to the cornea. They are easily retained by Schiotz tonometer after immersion, autoclave disinfection is the measure of choice.

c. Goldman's and other contact lenses and gonioscopes are washed in running water and then gently wiped with cotton moistened with 70 percent isopropyl alcohol or 3 percent hydrogen peroxide. Following this the lens is again rinsed with water and wiped dry.

   Neither tonometers nor contact lenses can be emerged in isopropanol without serious damage to the instruments.

d. Gloves are not used in routine examinations but if the patient is known to be an HIV carrier and whenever the skin of the investigator is not intact the use of gloves is recommended. When an HIV positive patients is examined, use of a face mask during the examination is also advised. Disinfection of the hands is the most important step for prevention of infection. Hands should be disinfected following every cutaneous contact with AIDS patients and contaminated instruments. The safest, simplest method for skin is alcoholic rubs. This enables hands to be disinfected hygienically at any time independent from wash basin and water faucet.

Suitable disinfectant for HIV prophylaxis contains 45 g 2-propanol, 30 g 1-propanol and 0.2 g mecetronium ethylsulfate (INN), application 3 ml for 1 minute.

e. Instruments that come into direct contact with external surfaces of the eye should be wiped clean and disinfected by 5-10 minutes exposure to a fresh solution of 3 percent hydrogen peroxide or a fresh solution containing 5000 parts per

TABLE 21.4: Disinfection process vs items

	Item group classification	Process classification
1.	Critical (Enters sterile tissue)	Sterilization by sporicidal chemical
2.	Semicritical (Touches mucous membrane)	High level disinfection by sporicidal chemical
3.	Noncritical (Touches intact skin)	Intermediate or low level disinfection

TABLE 21.5: Disinfectant classification and recommended concentration

		Recommended concentration
a.	*High level*	
	Glutaraldehyde	2 percent
	Formaldehyde	6 percent
	Hydrogen peroxide	6 percent
	Demand release chlorine dioxide	MR
b.	*Intermediate level*	
	Chlorine 1000 ppm	MR
	Phenol	MR
	Iodophor	MR
c.	*Lower level*	
	Alcohol	70–90 percent
	Sodium hypochlorite 100 ppm	MR
	Phenoli and Iodophoric germicidal detergent	MR
	Quaternary ammonium compounds	MR

*MR - Manufacturers recommendations.

million (mg/l) free available chlorine—1:10 dilution of sodium hypochlorite or 70 percent ethanol or 70 percent isopropanol. The device should be thoroughly rinsed in tap water and dried before use.
f. Contact lenses used in trial fittings should be disinfected between each fitting by following regimens:
   i. Disinfection of soft lenses with a commercially hydrogen peroxide contact lens disinfecting system. Alternatively soft lenses can be disinfected with the standard heat disinfection (78–80°C for 10 minutes).
   ii. Rigid gas permeable (RGP) trial fitting lenses can be disinfected using hydrogen peroxide disinfection system. RGP lenses may warp if they are heat disinfected.
g. Whenever possible, perform tonometry with Schiotz tonometer and then sterilize (autoclave or ethylene oxide) prior to the subsequent use.
h. If it is necessary to perform applanation tonometry, remove the applanation tonometer prism and wash it with warm water and a surface cleaner 0.004 percent thimerosal. Protein cleaning is beneficial before glutaraldehyde treatment which would denature proteins at the tonometer surface.

The clean tonometer prism is then soaked for 10 minutes in 2 percent glutaraldehyde. The tonometer prism is removed after 10 minutes. Thoroughly rinse the prism with water and thimerosal until the surface is no longer slippery. This rinse is extremely important and should continue till all the disinfectant is removed to prevent potential ocular damage. When the prism is clean it can be dried with cotton and replaced in the tonometer holder.

The decontamination procedures selected for ophthalmological examinations should be estimated to be effective enough. Spread of infections bacterial and viral is known through the use of diagnostic ophthalmic equipment like tonometers and Gonioscopes. Spread of adenovirus, HSV, AIDS virus and hepatitis virus is possible.

BIBLIOGRAPHY

1. Agarwal A. Textbook of Ophthalmology, 1st edn. New Delhi: Jaypee Brothers Medical Publishers, 2002.
2. Bartlett JD. Clinical Ocular Pharmacology, 4th edn. Boston: Butterworth-Heinemann, 2001.
3. Bartlett JD. Ophthalmic Drug Facts, Lippincott-William and Wilkins, 2001.
4. Crick RP, Trimble RB. Textbook of Clinical Ophthalmology, Hodder and Stoughton, 1986.
5. Duane TD. Clinical Ophthalmology, 4th edn. Butterworth–Heinemann, 1999.
6. Duvall. Ophthalmic Medications and Pharmacology, Slack Inc, 1998.
7. Ellis PP. Ocular Therapeutics and Pharmacology, 7th edn. CV Mosby, 1985.
8. Fechner. Ocular Therapeutics, Slack Inc., 1998.
9. Fraunfelder. Current Ocular Therapy, 5th edn. WB Saunders, 2000.

10. Garg A. Current Trends in Ophthalmology, 1st edn. New Delhi: Jaypee Brothers Medical Publishers, 1997.
11. Garg A. Manual of Ocular Therapeutics, 1st edn. New Delhi: Jaypee Brothers Medical Publishers, 1996.
12. Garg A. Ready Reckoner of Ocular Therapeutics, 1st edn. New Delhi: Jaypee Brothers Medical Publishers, 2002.
13. Goodman LS, Gilman A. Pharmacological Basis of Therapeutics, 7th edn. New York: Macmillan, 1985.
14. Havener's. Ocular Pharmacology, 6th edn. CV Mosby, 1994.
15. Kanski. Clinical Ophthalmology, 4th edn. Butterworth-Heinemann, 1999.
16. Kershner. Ophthalmic Medications and Pharmacology, Slack. Inc, 1994.
17. Olin BR, et al. Drugs Facts and Comparisons: Facts and Comparisons, St Louis, 1997.
18. Onofrey. The Ocular Therapeutics; Lippincott-William and Wilkins, 1997.
19. Rhee. The Wills Eye Drug Guide, Lippincott-William and Wilkins, 1998.
20. Steven Podos. Textbook of Ophthalmology, New Delhi: Jaypee Brothers Medical Publishers, 2001.
21. Zimmerman. Text book of Ocular Pharmacology, Lippincott-William and Wilkins, 1997.

Miscellaneous Drugs in Ophthalmology

Ashok Garg (India)

INTRODUCTION

In this chapter, I shall discuss those drugs/preparations which are commonly used in various ophthalmic conditions yet they do not fall in any specific category of drug classification.

LID SCRUBS

Blepharitis is mainly treated by careful eyelid hygiene. It can be easily done by the patient at home. Several eyelid cleansers are now commercially available to treat this condition. These eyelid cleansers are reported to be effective with potentially less ocular stinging, burning sensation and toxicity.

Commercial lid scrubs are prepared to aid in the removal of oils, debris or desquamated skin associated with the eyelid inflammation.

Indications

- For eyelid cleansing and hygiene to help in the removal of oils, debris, white plaques at eyelashes and desquamated skin.
- For hygienic eyelid cleansing in contact lens wearers.

Dosage and Administration

Lid (eye) scrubs are available as solution containing:
- PEG–200 glyceryl tallowate, disodium laureth sulfosuccinate, cocamidopropylamine oxide, PEG-78, glyceryl cocoate, benzyl alcohol and EDTA.
  It is commercially available in LID 30s (pads) and kit form (120 ml and 60 pads).
- Another preparation containing PEG-80 sorbitan Laurate, sodium trideceth, PGE-150 distearate, cocoamindopropyl hydroxysultaine, Lauroam phocarboxy glycinate, sodium laureth–13 carboxylate, PGE-15 tallow polyamine, quaternium-15 which is alcohol and dye free and is available in LID 30s (pads), 30, 120 and 240 ml and compliance kit (120 ml and 100 pads).

For scrub solution administration patient is asked to close the eyes and gently scrub on eyelids and lashes using lateral side-to-side strokes rinse thoroughly. These scrub solutions are designed to be used in full strength on eyelid tissue but shall not be instilled directly into the eyes. These commercial eye scrub solutions are packaged with gauze or cotton pads which provide an abrasive action to augment the cleansing properties of the detergent solution.

ASTRINGENT OPHTHALMIC SOLUTION

Astringent ophthalmic solutions are available for the relief of eye irritation and eye strain of diverse etiology. Such solutions provide immediate soothing effect to the eye.

Indications

Astringent ophthalmic solutions are indicated for minor non-specific irritation due to pollution, eye glare and asthenopia (eyestrain) due to TV viewing, excessive close work and people working on computers. In today's fast and modern life, excessive and large scale use of computers in office and home has led to development of computer vision syndrome (CVS). Such people usually complain of foreign body sensation, redness of eye, irritation and dry eye (due to reduced blinking).

In such situations astringent ophthalmic solutions provide immediate relief from the symptoms.

Administration and Dosage

Various topical ophthalmic solutions are available as astringent. These include solutions containing:
- Zinc sulphate 0.12 percent, boric acid 1.25 percent, naphazoline HCl 0.056 percent and chlorpheniramine maleate 0.01 percent in 10 ml and 5 ml packs.
- Zinc sulphate 0.25 percent, tetrahydrozoline 0.05 percent, EDTA and benzalkonium chloride (0.004%) in 15ml and 10 ml packs.
- Zinc sulphate 0.1 percent, borax 0.05 percent, boric acid 1.9 percent.

  Sodium chloride 0.45 percent, potassium chloride 0.45 percent and hydroxypropyl methylcellulose 0.7 percent in 10 ml packs and 120 ml pack (eye lotion).

  Recommended dosage is to instill 1-2 drops into the affected eyes 4 times daily. If solutions become cloudy, discard it and do not use. Astringent solution is also available as an eye lotion with cup to wash the tiring eyes. Put the solution in eye shaped cup and wash/immerse the affected eye in the cup for few minutes. After that clean the eyes with fresh water.

OPHTHALMIC DIAGNOSTIC TEAR TEST STRIPS

Various types of ophthalmic diagnostic test strips are available for use in ophthalmic diseases specially related to dry eye, corneal ulceration and tear assay in iatrogenic inflammations of the eye.

Indications

Schirmer Tear Test Sterile Strips

Graduated sterile Schirmer test strips are available to check tear levels and measurement of the total secretion (Reflex and Basal). Tear secretion Schirmer test strips are made of Whatman's filter paper no 41 and cut into specific dimensions of 5×30 mm.

Test I: Schirmer tear test I is performed to diagnose dry eye syndrome to evaluate lacrimal gland function specially in contact lens wearers, to check tear production prior to eyelid surgery and prior to corneal transplantation and cataract and IOL surgery.

Test II: Schirmer's tear test II is usually performed to assess the adequacy of reflex lacrimation specially in iatrogenic inflammation of eye following cataract surgery, IOL surgery and phaco surgery.

Sno Test Strips

Tear test is performed on eye before any topical medication specially (anesthetic or antibiotics) is administered or other extraocular procedures are carried out (manipulation of eyelids).

Zone-quick Thread Test

This is usually done to assess tear volume. In this test no topical anesthesia is required. If any topical ophthalmic drops have been instilled into the eye then perform the test after 5–10 minutes. This test can be done even during contact lens wear.

Administration and Dosage

- Schirmer sterile tear test strips are available in a pack of 100 and 250 pouches of 1 sterile strip each.

    Schirmer test is usually performed in dim light room. Patient is seated on chair and strips are placed at the junction of the middle and temporal one-third of lower eyelid margin. Avoid to touch the cornea as it may stimulate reflex lacrimation and pain. Patient is asked either to keep the eyes open and look up or to close eyes gently. After 5 minutes the strip is removed and amount of wetting measured. Test is considered at normal level when wetting is 15 mm over the graduated sterile strips between 5 and 10 mm it is graded borderline while cutoff point is 6 mm between normal and abnormal tear secretions.
- Sno-strips are commercially available as sterile tear flow test strips in pack of 100 pouches of one sterile strip each. Sno-strips are usually applied to temporal lid margin of the eye. The distance between notch (ridge) and shoulder of strip is 10 mm which should be wetted in about 3 minutes. Repeat the test for 5–10 minutes indicating the reduced tear secretion.
- Zone-quick are available as phenol red threads (PRT) in 50 aluminium packing sets (100 threads).

    For zone-quick test, one eye should be evaluated at a time. Thread is generally placed on the palpebral conjunctiva.

Patient is asked to look straight ahead and blink normally for 15 seconds. After 15 seconds gently pull the lower eyelid down and remove the thread with upward motion. Measure entire length of red portion of thread in millimeters.

Precautions

- In zone-quick thread test tear volume may vary. Repeat test on different days shall give a more accurate volume measurement.
- Zone-quick test may induce a slight mechanical irritation leading to excessive lacrimation in some cases. In such patients perform another tear test in addition to zone-quick test.

HAMAMELI'S OPHTHALMIC SOLUTION

This topical solution has been reported to be useful for the treatment of optic opacity caused by cataract.

Commercially it is available as aqueous and glycerin solution of senecio compositae, Hamameli's water and boric acid in 7 ml packing.

Recommended dosage is to instill 2 drops morning and night into the affected eyes.

BORIC ACID

It is available as ophthalmic powder for treating squamous blepharitis. Boric acid is generally prescribed to remove white plaques and crusts deposited on eye-lashes in blepharitis cases.

Boric acid is also used as buffer to maintain ophthalmic products in the range of pH 6–8 which is comfortable range for ocular instillation.

It is also used in contact lens solutions. For blepharitis put few quicks of boric acid in a small bowl of light warm water. Ask the patient to clean the eyelids margins for plaques and crusts with cotton swabs dipped in boric acid water with side-to-side (lateral movement).

INACTIVE INGREDIENTS IN OPHTHALMIC PRODUCTS

A number of following inactive yet useful agents may be present in various ophthalmic preparations (solutions and ointments).

Preservatives

Preservatives are added to ophthalmic products to destroy or inhibit multiplication of microorganisms which are introduced to product by chance. Each preservative may induce epithelial toxicity specially when more than 12 drops are instilled into the eye per day.

Various preservatives used in ophthalmic solutions and ointments are:

- Benzalkonium chloride
- Benzethonium chloride
- Cetylpyridinium chloride
- Cetylthonium chloride
- Chlorobutanol
- EDTA (Ethylenediamine tetra acetate).
- Phenylmercuric nitrate
- Phenylmercuric acetate
- Phenyl ethyl alcohol
- Polyaminopropyl biguanide
- Polyquad
- Thimerosal
- Methyl/propyl parabens
- Sodium benzoate
- Sodium propionate
- Sorbic acid.

Viscosity-stimulating Agents

Viscosity increasing agents help to slow drainage of the product from the eye thus increasing retention time of the active drug and increased bio-availability may result.

Various viscosity stimulating agents used in ophthalmic products are:
- Carboxymethyl cellulose sodium
- Dextran 70
- Gelatin
- Glycerin
- Hydroxyethyl cellulose
- Hydroxypropyl methylcellulose
- Methylcellulose
- PEG
- Poloxamer 407
- Polysorbate 80
- Propylene glycol
- Polyvinyl alcohol
- Polyvinyl pyrrolidone (povidone).

Antioxidants

Antioxidants play an useful role in preventing or delaying deterioration of ophthalmic products by oxygen in the air various antioxidants used are:
- EDTA
- Sodium bisulfite
- Sodium metabisulfite
- Sodium thiosulfate
- Thiourea.

Wetting Agents

The main function of wetting agents is to reduce surface tension allowing drug solution to easily spread into the eye.

Various wetting agents used are:
- Polysorbate 20 and 80
- Poloxamer 282
- Tyloxapol.

Buffers

Buffers play a crucial role in maintaining ophthalmic products in the range of pH 6–8 which is an ideal range for ophthalmic instillation.

Various buffer agents used are:
- Acetic acid
- Boric acid
- Hydrochloric acid
- Phosphoric acid
- Potassium bicarbonate
- Potassium borate, carbonate, citrate, phosphate and tetraborate
- Sodium acetate
- Sodium bicarbonate, biphosphate, borate, carbonate, citrate, hydroxide and phosphate.

Tonicity Agents

These agents help the ophthalmic product solution to be isotonic with preocular tear film. Products containing sodium chloride equivalence range of 0.9 percent + 0.2 percent are graded isotonic and shall help to prevent ocular irritation and tissue damage. Generally a range of 0.6 to 1.8 percent is considered ideal for ophthalmic use.

Various tonicity agents used are:
- Buffers
- Dextran 40 and 70
- Dextrose
- Glycerin
- Potassium chloride
- Propylene glycol
- Sodium chloride.

Aminocaproic Acid

Aminocaproic acid is an antifibrinolytic drug recommended for the treatment of excessive bleeding from systemic hyperfibrinolysis. This drug may be useful for the treatment of traumatic hyphema. Recommended dosage is 100 mg/kg body weight every 4 hours to a maximum dose of 30 g daily. It can also be administered in one half of this dosage to reduce side effects while maintaining efficacy.

Liquid Perfluorocarbons

Dr Stanley Chang (USA) introduced a heavier than water liquid for tamponading the retina and it was N-perfluorocarbon amine. The basic principle of these liquids is that they are heavier than water, so they would flatten the retina or unfold a giant tear.

There are 4 types of perfluorocarbon liquids being used in posterior segment surgery.
a. Perfluoro-N-Octane
b. Perfluoro–Decaline
c. Perfluoro–Tributylamine
d. Perfluoro–Phenanthrene

Liquid perfluorocarbons are heavier than water. These are generally used to push the retina against the back of the eye with the patient lying in the supine position. These liquids are clear, with low viscosity and surface tension and are immiscible with water liquid perfluorocarbons have refractive indices very close to aqueous so it is difficult to see the interface between perfluorocarbon and the aqueous. However, a clear miniscus is visible between the perfluorocarbon and the intraocular fluids or BSS. Some perfluorocarbons are intended for intraoperative use only while others are left in eyes for a prolonged period of time.

Indications and Administration

Liquid perfluorocarbons are ideally suited for unrolling the flap of a giant retinal tear. After vitrectomy the perfluorocarbons can be injected through the cannula whose tip is positioned posterior or under the flap of giant tear. As the perfluorocarbon flows into the eye, it gets settled on the back of retina pushing it against the posterior choroid. Subretinal fluid shall be displaced anteriorly and flow into central vitreous cavity through the giant retinal tear as the perfluorocarbon is injected. Usually a partial fill is used to partially unroll the tear, further vitrectomy is done to relieve traction on the anterior edge of the tear and then more perfluorocarbon is added to further flatten the retina. Endolaser can be given through the perfluorocarbon. Gas is then infused into the eye through the pars plana infusion port as the perfluorocarbon is aspirated.

Perfluorocarbons are also heavier than intraocular lenses. Hence, these liquids can be used to float a displaced intraocular lens off the posterior retina making it safer and easier to reposition or remove. The injection of perfluorocarbon may be useful when there is a concomitant retinal detachment as it will simultaneously push the retina against the back of the eye holding it away from IOL instruments and lift the intraocular lens anteriorly.

Perfluorocarbons can be used to push the retina posteriorly in detachments complicated by fibrovascular tissue proliferation as in proliferative diabetic retinopathy or by pre-retinal fibrous membranes as in eyes with massive periretinal proliferation. This can make the membranes easier to visualize and dissect.

Some perfluorocarbons are left in the eyes to provide prolong tamponade of the inferior retina. Finally, the perfluorocarbon liquid must be removed in a second operation.

<u>VISCOSURGICAL DEVICES</u>

Sodium hyaluronate and chondroitin sulfate are approved as vitreous replacement substances and for use during intraocular surgery to protect the corneal endothelium. Recently sodium hyaluronate is prepared as 0.1 percent topical ophthalmic solution in saline for treating severe dry eye syndrome. The beneficial effects of sodium hyaluronate are due to its viscoelastic properties which lubricate and protect the ocular surface. Most patients achieve control of symptoms with topical instillation up to 4-6 times daily.

BIBLIOGRAPHY

1. Agarwal A. Textbook of Ophthalmology, 1st edn. New Delhi: Jaypee Brothers Medical Publishers, 2002.
2. Bartlett JD. Clinical Ocular Pharmacology, 4th edn. Boston: Butterworth-Heinemann, 2001.
3. Bartlett JD. Ophthalmic Drug Facts, Lippincott-William and Wilkins, 2001.
4. Crick RP, Trimble RB. Textbook of Clinical Ophthalmology. Hodder and Stoughton, 1986.
5. Duane TD. Clinical Ophthalmology, 4th edn. Butterworth - Heinemann, 1999.
6. Duvall. Ophthalmic Medications and Pharmacology. Slack Inc, 1998.
7. Ellis PP. Ocular Therapeutics and Pharmacology, 7th edn. CV Mosby, 1985.
8. Fechner. Ocular Therapeutics. Slack Inc, 1998.
9. Fraunfelder. Current Ocular Therapy, 5th edn. WB Saunders, 2000.
10. Garg A. Current Trends in Ophthalmology, 1st edn. New Delhi: Jaypee Brothers Medical Publishers, 1997.
11. Garg A. Manual of Ocular Therapeutics, 1st edn. New Delhi: Jaypee Brothers Medical Publishers, 1996.
12. Garg A. Ready Reckoner of Ocular Therapeutics, 1st edn. New Delhi: 2002.
13. Goodman LS, Gilman A. Pharmacological Basis of Therapeutics, 7th edn. New York: Macmillan, 1985.
14. Havener's. Ocular Pharmacology, 6th edn. CV Mosby, 1994.
15. Kanski. Clinical Ophthalmology, 4th edn. Butterworth - Heinemann, 1999.
16. Kershner. Ophthalmic Medications and Pharmacology, Slack. Inc, 1994.
17. Olin BR, et al. Drugs Facts and Comparisons: Facts and Comparisons. St Louis, 1997.
18. Onofrey. The Ocular Therapeutics. Lippincott-William and Wilkins, 1997.
19. Rhee. The Wills Eye Drug Guide. Lippincott – William and Wilkins, 1998.
20. Steven Podos. Textbook of Ophthalmology. New Delhi: Jaypee Brothers Medical Publishers, 2001.
21. Zimmerman. Textbook of Ocular Pharmacology. Lippincott and William and Wilkins, 1997.

23

Ocular Drug Toxicity: Complications

Ashok Garg (India)

INTRODUCTION

Ocular tissue undesired side effects have been seen by every ophthalmologists in their practice involving various drugs used topically and systemically for the treatment of various ocular problems. An adverse drug reaction (ADR) is an undesirable response to a drug occurring during or following a course of therapy. The types of adverse effects of drugs on the eye may be mild and transient like temporary decrease in vision, abnormal pupillary responses, Accommodation impairment, color vision disturbance, abnormal eye movements to serious side effects like cataract, glaucoma and retinal damage which may seriously disrupt in ocular functions.

It is essential for every ophthalmologist to have complete insight to recognize and prevent vision threatening complications from adverse effects of drug reactions. It is essential for the ophthalmologist to obtain a careful history with special attention to particular medication used. The clinicians shall be fully aware of certain oculotoxic drugs and their side effects to detect the drug related ocular disorder.

Before going into details of complications of various topical ocular formulations, let me remind you that for certain drugs with potential ocular toxicity a careful pre-treatment examination should be performed before the drug is administered especially, if:
- The drug shall be used for a long period of time.
- It is known to have established severe toxic effects.

Patients taking such drugs should undergo frequent monitoring examinations so that if the symptoms do arise, the drugs can be withdrawn immediately.

Often reversible effects are observed while the patient is off the drug and later after resolution of the effects, the drug regimen may be restarted at a lower dose. The pre-treatment examination should include following parameters:

Visual acuity: Check visual acuity for near and distance vision with and without pin hole testing and spectacles (if required).

Pupillary responses: Check pupil size, briskness of reactions (direct and consensual) to light and convergence reflex.

Ocular motility examination: Check complete motility in all field directions of gaze with ductions, versions and convergence.

Intraocular pressure monitoring: Periodic tonometry should be done as intraocular pressure rise is sensitive adverse effect of certain topical formulations.

Slit-lamp examination is essential as certain drugs affect the conjunctiva, cornea and lens.

Ophthalmoscopy: Perform ophthalmoscopy (direct and indirect) with dilation as certain drugs may produce changes in the retina, macula and the optic nerve.

Specific retinal function examinations: These examinations include
- Electroretinography (ERG)
- Fundus photography
- Visual field analysis
- Color vision tests
- Visual evoked potential (VEP)
- Fluorescein angiography

Generalized Ocular Manifestations of Drug Toxicity

- Reduced visual acuity due to transient changes in refractive errors, anterior and posterior segment toxicity.
- Blurring of vision may be caused by mydriasis and cycloplegia as well as anterior and posterior segment toxic changes.
- Color vision disturbances that may include hallucination, altered perception and diminished sensitivity.
- Ocular movement abnormalities include neuromuscular myesthenic block, paralytic strabismus, diplopia and oculogyric crisis.
- Severe conjunctival inflammation and corneal opacification.
- Glaucoma
- Cataract development
- Optic nerve pathology (optic neuritis)
- Exophthalmos, retinal hemorrhage, vasculopathy, retinal pigment epitheliopathy and macular edema.

Ocular adverse drug reactions (OADR) may be predictable and unpredictable. In 80–90 percent of cases OADR caused by drugs can lead to complete loss of vision also. The causes of adverse drug reactions are summarized as follows:
- Exaggeration of intended pharmacological effects
- Concomitant administration of drugs with synergistic effects
- Immunological mechanism
- Idiosyncratic reactions
- Cytotoxic reactions
- Genetically determined enzymatic defects
- Error in self-administration of the drugs

Here in this chapter, I shall discuss the main systemic and local complications due to the use of various topical ocular formulations and ocular surgery adjuncts prescribed by ophthalmologists in their day-to-day practice. In modern hightech scenario it is important to have complete insight into the complications of prescribing ophthalmic formulations.

COMPLICATIONS OF TOPICAL ANTIMICROBIAL AGENTS

Topical anti-microbial drugs-antibiotics, anti-fungals, anti-virals and anti-parasitics are the most common drugs prescribed by ophthalmologists. These drugs used to treat a wide variety of infectious diseases ranging from mild conditions to vision threatening infections such as corneal ulceration and endophthalmitis. Topical antimicrobial agents are often used in postocular surgical phase for the prophylasis of infections. Although these drugs are effective, however, in some cases complications may arise from their use. In this chapter the common and serious complications of the use of topical antimicrobial drugs are reviewed.

Systemic Complications

A major advantage of the topical use of drugs is that, high local drug level can be achieved with minimal systemic absorption, However, idlosyncratic and immunological reactions can occur with exposure to minute quantities of drugs. Two such reactions that may occur related to the use of topical antimicrobial drugs are aplastic anemia and Stevens-Johnson syndrome.

Aplastic Anemia

It is a well-known, potentially fatal complication of the ingestion of drugs. Chloramphenicol a commonly used topical ophthalmic antibiotic is the most common cause of drug related aplastic anemia. Bacterial break down product of chloramphenicol may be responsible for this complication in susceptible individuals.

Chloramphenicol has two known effects on the bone marrow.
1. Dose-related reversible suppression of the bone marrow affecting mainly the red blood cell line.
2. Progressive marrow aplasia.

Stevens-Johnson Syndrome

It is an acute dermatitis with severe mucous membrane involvement that most commonly occurs in association with *Mycoplasma pneumoniae* infection or as a reaction to variety of drugs. In the milder form of disease there is symmetrical involvement with skin lesions affecting mainly the extremities. Mucous membrane involvement is mild and generally limited to one surface. The disease generally resolves in 1 to 4 weeks without any sequelae.

In major form cutaneous eruptions are more variable in morphological features, area of extent of involvement.

Lesions may become confluent, bullar may form and there may be toxic epidermal necrolysis.

Drug induced cases of STS generally occur after 7-14 days of drug therapy but may occur within hours if patients had previous exposure to the drug. Sulfonamides are the drugs most commonly complicated as causes of SJS followed by penicillin.

Phenylbutazone and barbiturates. Patients should be questioned about previous exposure to sulfonamides and specially about any reaction to these drugs before ophthalmic sulphonamide preparations are prescribed.

Local Complications

Most of the complications of topical antimicrobial drugs affect only local structure. They may be immunological or allergic in origin, related to toxicity of the drug or reflect a lack of specificity of effect against the organism being treated. Local side effects may be caused by preservatives which are combined in commercially available antimicrobials.

Nonspecific Local Complications

Contact Dermatoconjunctivitis

It is a cell-mediated reaction and most commonly related to the use of topical ophthalmic medications. Patients are usually sensitized to previous exposure to the drug. Because of popularity of topical neomycin-polymixin B-bacitracin combination, many individuals are sensitized to neomycin, a common cause of this condition. This disease begins 24–72 hours following repeated instillation of the drug.

The patient complains of itching. Chronic changes include thickening of skin and hyperpigmentation and sometimes mild ectropion may occur.

Initially findings will be more apparent in the lower conjunctiva and eyelid but eventually the entire eye and upper lid are involved in the process.

Conjunctival involvement takes the form of papillary conjunctivitis.

The diagnosis of contact dermatoconjunctivitis is generally made on the basis of clinical appearance of the patient. In patients taking several topical ophthalmic drugs, the specific offender can be identified by cutaneous patch testing.

In addition to neomycin other drugs that may cause CDC are topical gentamicin, tobramycin, idoxiuridine trifluridine, natamycin, atropine and commonly used preservatives like thiomersal and EDTA. The treatment of CDC requires identification and discontinuation of the offending agent.

Chronic Follicular Conjunctivitis

CFC may occur as a complication of the long-term topical use of the drug. Affected patients complain of chronic redness and mild discharge. In general, follicular reaction involves both the upper and lower palpebral conjunctiva but it is most apparent in the lower fornix.

Drug-related CFC is a diagnosis of exclusion.

Idoxiuridine is the most common cause of CFC among the antimicrobial drugs. Sulfonamides are also another cause for

CFC. The conjunctivitis resolve in 6 weeks after discontinuation of offending drug.

Punctate Marginal Keratitis

It occurs either during the acute stages of infectious conjunctivitis or as a hypersensitivity reaction to topical drugs. The most common topical antimicrobial drug implicated is gentamicin but several other drugs like atropine, mydriatics and epinephrine may also cause.

PKM treatment involves the discontinuation of the offending agent. In addition topical steroids may be useful.

Keratitis Medicamentosa

It refers to corneal epitheliopathy related to the use of certain topical medications. In milder form KM may affect only the lower cornea. In more severe forms, the entire corneal epithelium may become involved. The epithelium may slough and superficial stromal edema and necrosis may lead to corneal scarring and vascularization. KM must be suspected in any patient with epithelial keratitis of any degree. The antivirals appear to be most common cause of medication induced epithelial Keratitis. A 2-week course of idoxuridine or trifluridine will nearly always cause KM. Among the antibiotics the aminoglycoside, neomycin, gentamicin and Tobramycin appears to be drugs that may cause KM. Preservative benzalkonium commonly used in preparation of topical antibiotics may also cause desquamation of the outer two layers of the corneal epithelium.

The treatment of KM is discontinuation of all topical medications. Early recognition of the problem is essential since advanced disease may take 2–3 months to clear. The use of non-preserved artificial tears may ameliorate symptoms. In extreme causes, use of bandage soft contact lenses may relieve pain until the epithelium begin to heal. Patient should understand the nature of disease as prolonged time may be required for disease resolution.

Inhibition of Epithelial Wound Healing

Antimicrobial drugs exert their effects by one of two broadly defined mechanisms of action: (i) Disruption of cell wall (ii) Inhibition of intracellular metabolic process.

To heal an epithelial defect, the bordering epithelium must replicate and slide to fill the defect. In addition epithelial defects may persist following any type of corneal infection and antibiotics, antifungals or antivirals may be used beyond the period that is needed to eradicate the infecting organisms. Antimicrobial drugs that inhibit intracellular metabolic processes may have a deleterious effect on healing of corneal epithelium.

Although topical antimicrobials may not have an appreciable effect on the healing of healthy epithelium following a mechanical injury but these agents may have a markedly deleterious effect on the healing of persistent epithelial defects that occur in neurotrophic, postsurgical and postinfections corneas and in corneas that have suffered chemical injuries.

The first step in treating such cases is to assess the patients topical medications and to eliminate or reduce to lowest possible level of all those might interfere with epithelial healing.

Specific Local Complications

Sulfonamides

Calcific band-shaped keratopathy has been reported with use of topical sulfonamides. This was most likely complication caused by the preservative since band keratopathy is known to be caused by chronic exposure to organic mercurials.

Amphotericin B

Salmon colored subconjunctival nodules have been seen following S/C injection of amphotericin B in doses greater than 5 mg. Histological examination of nodules revealed numerous histiocytes in an area of fibrosis in addition to lymphocytes and plasma cells. The lesions eventually resolved but permanent yellowing of conjunctiva remains.

Idoxuridine

IDU has been reported to cause punctal or canalicular stenosis. It has been attributed to cicatricial changes occurring in patients who have had a CFC related to the drug.

Propamidine

Propamidine isoethionate is a nonspecific conjunctivitis remedy. It can cause intraepithelial microcystic lesions related to the use of topical preparation. The lesions are asymptomatic and resolved without sequelae following discontinuation of the drug.

COMPLICATIONS OF STEROIDS

Corticosteroids are important therapeutic agents that are used to treat ocular inflammation commonly.

Complications of steroids are related to dose and duration of therapy. The clinician must consider all the possible complications when counseling and treating patients with vision threatening disease.

Corticosteroids

Few adverse effects of steroids occur with short-term therapy. Most problems occur with long-term therapy. However, long-term and short-term adverse effects are grouped together. In general, the lower the maintenance dose, lesser the side effects. These adverse effects are produced both by topical and systemic steroid therapy.

Topical Steroids

Dermatitis

Periocular dermatitis resulting from long-term use of fluorinated steroid drops or ointment have been reported. This dermatitis is similar to perioral dermatitis and should not be confused with allergic contact dermatitis.

Infection and Ulceration

Inappropriate use of topical steroids by patient and registered medical practitioners lead to infectious keratitis specially herpetic keratitis. Reactivation of herpes simplex virus in patients who have undergone penetrating keratoplasty is specially common in patients who were previously treated with steroid antibiotic combination.

Delayed Wound Healing

Corneal wound healing may be inhibited by proliferation of fibroblasts and new vessels. Ocular surgery may be carried out but the surgeon may use interrupted suture techniques and delay suture removal for few weeks.

Cataracts

Cataract development specially posterior subcapsular type has shown to occur after prolonged treatment with steroid drops and ointments. With the stoppage of the steroids, some of these changes are either partially or totally reversible. Visual impairment is variable. Once visual impairment has taken place, complete resolution of lenticular opacification cannot be expected. The pathophysiology of steroid induced cataract formation is by mechanism affecting water transport by increasing cation influx. This leads to excess water in cells. Causing intumescence of the cell and a disparity of refractive index from the surrounding medium.

The steroids also bind to specific amino acids groups within the lens cell fibers. These combined factors are responsible for the lost in transparency.

Elevated IOP (Steroid-induced Glaucoma)

Prolonged use of corticosteroids may cause an elevation of intraocular pressure, leading to optic nerves damage and visual field. Changes synonymous with chronic open angle glaucoma.

As ophthalmologists we are familiar with abuse of long-term steroids use for minor inflammation by patient himself. So, ophthalmologists should monitor all patients on steroids, no matter what preparation or initial IOP to watch for any increase in IOP. The elevation of IOP can occur within days of starting therapy or it can occur months later on. Patients with myopia greater than 5 diopters or a history of glaucoma are more susceptible to this

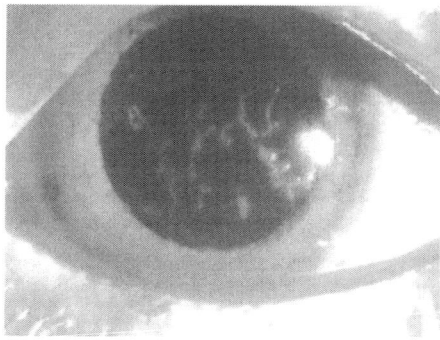

Fig. 23.1: Fluorescein stain of dendritic ulcer with numerous branches made worse by the use of topical steroid eyedrops

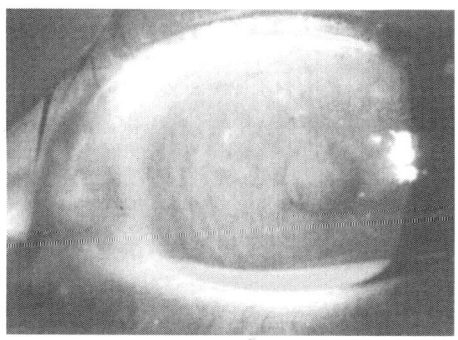

Fig. 23.2: Steroid-induced dendritic keratitis. Fluorescein stain of dendritic ulcer

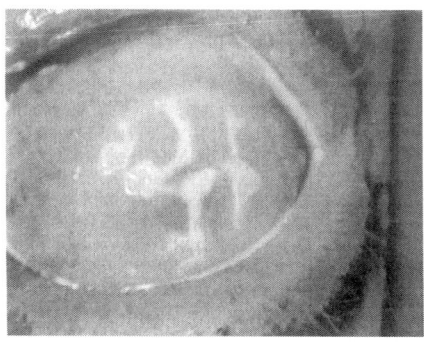

Fig. 23.3: Steroid-induced dendritic keratitis, dendritic ulcer under magnification with fluorescein stain (*Courtesy:* Kanski Clinical Ophthalmology, Butterworth International Edition)

complication. Raised IOP by steroids is related to cytoplasmic and nuclear receptors for steroids that have been shown in trabecular meshwork.

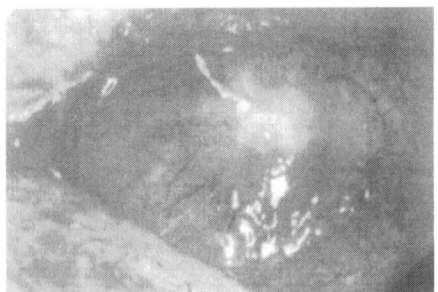

Fig. 23.4: Steroid-induced fungal keratitis (*Courtesy:* Kanski Clinical Ophthalmology, Butterworth International Edition)

Steroid-induced elevations in IOP appear to be secondary to decreased facility of aqueous outflow. The mechanisms include accumulation of glycosaminoglycans or an increase in debris in the trabecular meshwork due to inhibition of phagocytosis.

The frequency and severity of IOP rise is greater with topical application than with systemic administration.

The patient is usually asymptomatic unless the intraocular pressure increases enough to cause corneal edema (Decreased vision, halos, photophobia or pain). Clinical signs of prolonged elevation of IOP include optic nerve cupping and visual field defects.

Steroid induced IOP elevations almost always respond within days to weeks of stopping the steroids. It is not always possible to abruptly stop steroids because of underlying ocular condition being treated.

It is important to note that although most patients will respond to hypotensive agents, the hypertensive effect can occur in susceptible individuals who are already on hypotensive agents when steroids are added for either ocular or systemic diseases.

In those patients in whom hypotensive agents are unable to control IOP in steroid induced glaucoma Argon laser trabeculoplasty and glaucoma filtering surgery are necessary treatment modalities.

Periocular Steroids

One of the rare but most dangerous complications of injections behind Tenon's capsule is penetration of globe and accidental intraocular injection, substantial retinal damage has also been reported when the vehicles in which steroids are commonly packed react. The preservatives and the osmolality of the vehicle can cause retinal degeneration, pre-retinal membrane formation, cataract formation. Other complications of injection itself includes retrobulbar hemorrhage, proptosis of globe and fibrosis of extraocular muscles.

Increased IOP may also occur with depot injections of long acting steroids. Injections of long acting steroids are not indicated in patients with episcleritis and scleritis.

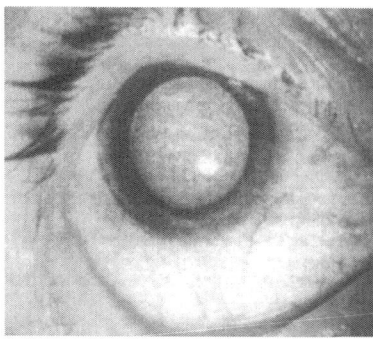

Fig. 23.5: Steroid-induced cataract (mature type)

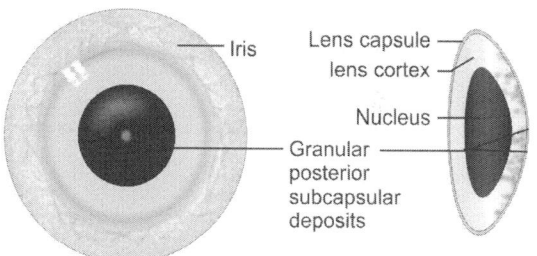

Fig. 23.6: Steroid-induced cataract (posterior subcapsular type)

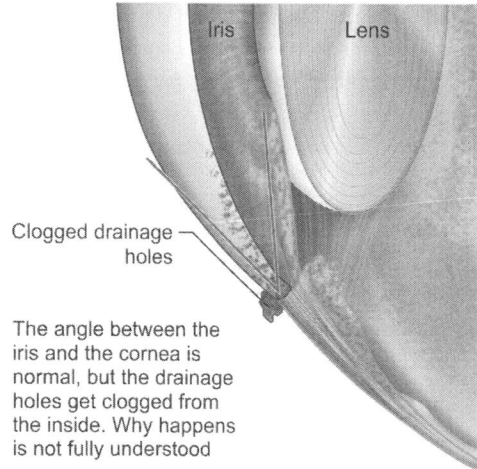

Fig. 23.7: Steroid-induced glaucoma (chronic open angle type)
(*Courtesy:* Allergan India Limited)

Systemic Steroids

Systemic steroids affect patients in many ways. A number of side effects seem to occur early on, in the treatment. The classical clinical triad that contributes to the moon-face appearance of some patients using systemic steroids comprises ptosis, chemosis and swelling of the periorbital tissues.

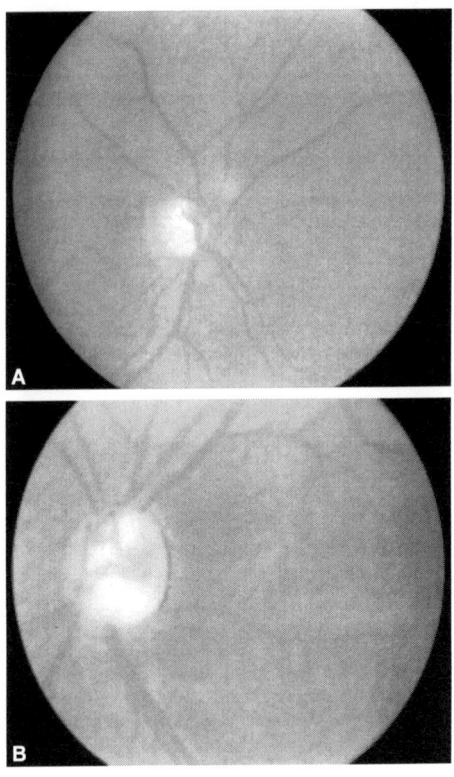

Figs 23.8A and B: Steroid-induced glaucoma (large terminal glaucomatous cup with C/D ratio 1.0 and optic atrophy)

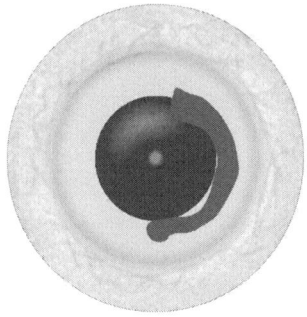

Fig. 23.9: Steroid-induced glaucoma visual field loss (arcuate scotoma in early glaucoma)

Various Adverse Effects

Abnormalities of the hypothalmic-pituitary adrenal axis: Soon after start of steroid therapy abnormalities of hypothalmic-pituitary gland adrenal axis including decreased cortisol, adrenal axis response to ACTH and blunted response to insulin induced hypoglycemia can occur. Long-term therapy may blunt this effect.

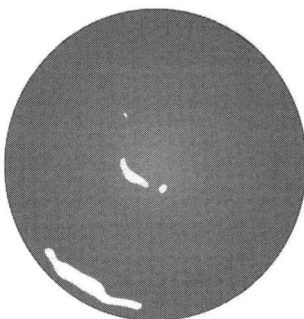

Fig. 23.10: Steroid-induced glaucoma, severe visual field loss in advanced glaucoma

However, low dose maintenance and alternate day therapy will minimize this effect.

Steroids should be withdrawn slowly as quick tapering often result in flare up of ophthalmic disease and can leave the patients with adrenal suppression. Too rapid a decrease in steroids can also result in pseudorheumatism. Systemic steroids can also cause retardation of growth in children and secondary amenorrhea in females.

Mood changes: Steroids induce euphoria depression, headache, halucination and psychosis. Suicidal tendencies may also increase. Previous history of psychiatric problems is not believed to increase the tendency for patients to manifest such behavioral disturbances during therapy.

Increased intracranial pressure: Steroids may cause benign increase in intracranial pressure. Pseudotumor cerebri is most commonly indicated by headache while the patient is taking steroids.

Ophthalmic changes: Studies have shown the presence of exophthalmos induced by exogenous steroids. Other ocular effects are:
- Ocular palsy due to extraocular muscles myopathy
- Thining and thickening of sclera
- Refractive changes due to electrolyte and water shifts
- Posterior subcapsular cataracts
- Elevation of IOP
- Papilledema, visual fields changes like scotoma, constriction and glaucoma field defects
- Ptosis, subconjunctival hemorrhage
- Visual hallucinations, mydriasis, ciliary body epithelial microcysts
- Color vision defects, myopia, diplopia
- Myesthenic block and toxic amblyopia
- Central serous retinopathy
- Herpes keratitis activation
- Retinal hemorrhages, edema, abnormal ERG and VEP
- Pseudotumor cerebri.

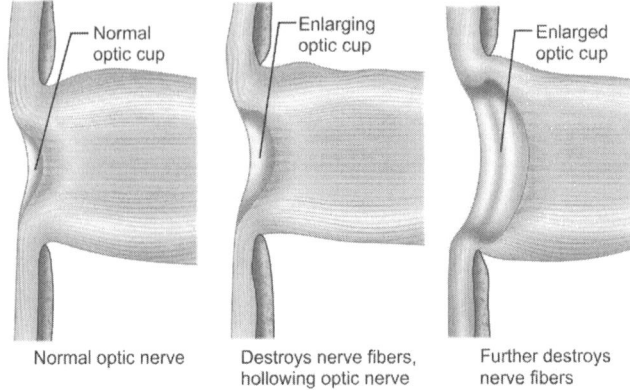

Fig. 23.11: Progression of glaucoma (steroid-induced)

Diabetes: Systemic steroids induce glucose intolerance owing to increased hepatic gluconeogenesis and decreased peripheral utilization.

Previously, healthy non-diabetic patients can develop hyperosmolar, hyperglycemic nonketotic coma.

Such patients may be treated with diet restriction, weightloss, oral hypoglycemic agents and if necessary by insulin. By halting the steroids-induced diabetes will resolve however it may take several months.

Infections: Steroids make patients more susceptible to infections. These include bacterial, viral, fungal and parasitic infections.

Alternations in Lipid Metabolism

Steroids have two effects on lipid metabolism:
1. Marked redistribution of body fat resulting in classic cushingoid appearance of a patient with moon face, buffalo hump and wasting of the extremities.
2. Facilitation of lipolysis of the triglycerides of adipose tissue.

Coronary Risk Factors

Hypertension is commonly found in patients treated with systemic streoids with an increased incidence in patients with underlying impaired renal function. The exact mechanism that causes hypertension is not clear. Researchers believe that an increased in plasma serum volume, glomerular filtration and decrease in plasma renin concentration and increase in renal vascular resistance may cause hypertension.

Dermatological Effects

Hirsutism and acne occur in about 10 percent of patients on long-term systemic steroid therapy.

GIT Disorders

Superficial punctate gastric erosions with hemorrhage may occur and are reversible with cessation of steroid therapy. So patients are advised to use antacid cover when taking oral steroids. Steroids used for more than 30 days or short-term use of large doses may cause peptic ulcers. The incidence of peptic ulcers is 1.8 percent. This risk is also dependent on the patients underlying disease state, age, nutritional status and concomitant drug use and past history of ulcers.

Other GIT effects are:
- Visceral perforation
- Pancreatitis
- Nausea
- Increased appetite.

Osteoporosis

Patients on prolonged therapeutic regimes of steroids often develop osteoporosis. Postmenopausal women, elderly people and immobilized patients are more susceptible to this complication. Osteoblastic activity is inhibited and bone resorption increases leading to the loss of trabecular bone specially in spine, rib and distal radii. Steroids may cause increased urinary calcium loss and decreased enteric absorption which may lead to secondary hyperparathyroidism and bone resorption. Aseptic necrosis of femoral head can be devastating.

Myopathy

Muscle weakness with wasting of proximal limb and girdle occurs more readily with fluorinated steroids than with other steroids. Most patients improve with the cessation of the medication but recovery may be slow and incomplete.

Leukocytic and Platelet Aberrations

Use of steroids tends to be accompanied by an increase in the no of circulating WBC which is due to increased rate of entrance of polymorphonuclear leukocytes into the blood from the bone marrow.

Thrombocytosis and thrombocytopenia have also been reported to increase.

Hematological Changes

- Ecchymosis
- Purpura
- Easy bruising.

These are common in elderly patients and are believed to be caused by diminished phagocytosis and alterations of connective tissue.

Subconjunctival and retinal hemorrhage may also be seen in patients who develop purpura and ecchymosis.

Anaphylaxis

A rare but serious complication of IV steroids is an anaphylactoid reaction in asthmatics. CNS manifestations associated with IV steroids include headache, lethargy, confusion, seizures, hemiplegia and loss of vision.

Renal Effects

These are:
- Sodium retention, potassium loss
- Hypokalemic alkalosis
- Fluid retention.

General Effects

- Increased sweating
- Subcutaneous tissue atrophy.

SYSTEMIC ADVERSE REACTIONS OF GLAUCOMA MEDICATIONS

Following major classes of drugs are currently used to treat various types of glaucomas:
- Miotics
- Beta-adrenergic blockers
- Alpha-adrenergic agonists
- Carbonic anhydrase inhibitors
- Sympathomimetics
- Parasympathomimetics
- Prostaglandins
- Hyperosmotic agents
- Calcium channel blockers
- Antimetabolites
- Neuroprotective agents.

Both local and systemic side effects may occur secondary to glaucoma medications and these adverse reactions may be severe or fatal. Ophthalmologists are becoming increasingly aware of these systemic side effects, although some of the adverse reactions are idiosyncratic and non-dose related. Ophthalmologists play a major role in the monitoring of glaucoma patients for potential adverse reactions.

In this chapter, systemic adverse reactions related to these anti-glaucoma drugs are discussed to offer some guidelines for the use of these medications. The local adverse effects have been given in antiglaucoma therapy chapter already.

Beta-adrenergic Blockers

There are currently five beta-adrenergic blocking agents which are main ocular hypotensive agents commonly used worldwide. These are timolol, betaxolol, carteolol, metipranalol and levobunolol. These agents are generally well-tolerated following topical application to the eye, however adverse systemic reactions may occasionally be severe enough to require discontinuation of the drug.

Of the possible adverse reactions, due to beta-blockers, about 50-70 percent are systemic side effects. The important adverse systemic side effects reported secondary to the use of topical ocular beta-adrenergic blocking agent. The systemic side effects reported so far as follows:

Cardiovascular System Effects

- Arrhythmia
- Bradycardia
- Cardiac arrest
- Cerebral ischemia
- CVS accident
- CHF
- Heart Block
- Hypotension
- Palpitation
- Syncope.

Central Nervous System Effects

- Asthenia
- Ataxia
- Depression
- Dizziness and fatigue
- Hallucinations
- Headache, insomnia
- Lethargy
- Myasthenia
- Paresthesia.

Dermatological Effects

- Alopecia
- Pruritis
- Urticaria
- Nail pigmentary changes.

Gastrointestinal Effects

Diarrhea and nausea.

Endocrine and Metabolic Effects

- Glucose imbalance
- Potassium imbalance.

Respiratory Effects

- Asthma
- Bronchospasm
- Dyspnea
- Respiratory failure.

Urogenital Effects

Sexual dysfunction.

To reduce beta-blocker toxicity, nasolacrimal occlusion and eyelid closure in addition to the use of least amount of medication (1 drop per application) with lowest concentration of medication are indicated.

Carbonic Anhydrase Inhibitors

The incidence and severity of many adverse reactions to carbonic anhydrase inhibitors (CAI) are dose-related and usually respond to lowering of dosage or withdrawal of drug. Many patients unable to tolerate one CAI may be able to tolerate another serious effects are infrequent specially during short-term therapy.

Various systemic side effects of CAI are:

Central Nervous System Effects

- Asthenia, ataxia
- Confusion, depression
- Convulsion
- Dizziness, fatigue
- Fever
- Headache
- Tinnitus
- Paresthesia of extremities
- Tremor
- Numbness
- Vertigo.

Dermatological Effects

- Alopecia
- Erythema multiforme
- Photosensitivity
- Pruritis
- Urticaria.

Gastrointestinal Tract Effects

- Metallic taste
- Anorexia
- Constipation
- Melena
- Nausea, vomiting
- Weight loss.

Hematological Effects

- Blood dyscrasia
- Agranulocytosis
- Bone marrow depression
- Hemolytic anemia
- Leukopenia
- Thrombocytopenia.

Urogenital Effects

- Crystalluria
- Glycosuria
- Hematuria
- Polyuria
- Renal calculi
- Renal colic
- Urinary frequency
- Sexual dysfunction.

Sympathomimetic Agents

Adverse effects generally occur less frequently with sympathomimetic agents and are milder following topical ocular application of dipivefrin than epinephrine. The decreased incidence of adverse systemic effects seen may be due to its prodrug nature.
Systemic effects are:
- Arrhythmia
- Hypertension
- Palpitation
- Syncope
- Tachycardia
- Ventricular extrasystole
- Headache
- Sweating
- Asthma.

Parasympathomimetic Agents

The adverse effects of topically applied miotics are generally more severe and prolonged with the long acting anti-cholinesterasis. Topical pilocarpine is generally better tolerated than the other miotics. Adverse effects of miotics are reduced, if therapy is started with a low concentration of the drug, the concentration is increased gradually and daily dose is instilled in the eye at the bed time. Adverse side effects subside after the first few days of therapy or treatment of with miotics is discontinued temporarily.
Systemic toxicity usually occurs only after very frequent administration of drug.
The most common effects are:
- Abdominal pain
- Diarrhea
- Nausea, vomiting

- Asthma
- Bronchospasm
- Dyspnea
- Pulmonary edema
- Urinary incontinence
- Arrhythmia
- Asthenia
- Headache
- Tremor
- Sweating and vasodilation.

Alpha-adrenergic Agonists

Drugs of this group used in glaucoma therapy are clonidine, apraclonidine, brimonidine and dapirazole usually these drugs are well-tolerated on topical use. However, following systemic adverse effects have been reported with long use of these medications.

Systemic adverse effect reports are:
- Bradycardia
- Vasovagal attack
- Palpitation, anxiety, syncope
- Orthostatic hypotension
- Gastrointestinal reactions
- Insomnia, irritability
- Decreased libido
- Abnormal taste
- Depression
- Hypertension.

Prostaglandins

Latanoprost and unoprostone are recently launched antiglaucoma therapy of prostaglandin group. These are quite effective and well-tolerated. The systemic side effects reported are:
- Upper respiratory tract infection
- Cold, flu, pain in chest muscles
- Joint back pain
- Rashes and allergic reactions, angina pectoris.

Hyperosmotic Agents

Systemic hyperosmotic agents like glycerin, mannitol, isosorbide are used for immediate control of intraocular pressure in acute glaucoma cases. Systemic adverse effects reported with systemic hyperosmotic agents are:
- Hypertension aggravation
- Nausea, vomiting
- Marked diuresis
- Urinary retention
- Confusion
- Congestive heart failure
- Fluid and electrolyte imbalance
- Dry mouth acidosis

- Chills, urticaria
- Fever, pulmonary edema
- Diabetic hyperglycemia.

Antimetabolites

Antifibroproliferative agents used in glaucoma therapy are 5-fluorouracil (5Fu), mitomycin C and daunorubicin.

Adverse side effects of these antimetabolites are frequent at full doses and lesser at lower doses.

COMPLICATIONS OF TOPICAL OCULAR ANESTHETIC AGENTS

Topical ocular anesthetics play an important role in the diagnosis and treatment of ocular diseases. Although these anesthetics are generally safe, complications do arise from their use. In addition the potential for their abuse exists, causing significant ocular morbidity. The complications of topical anesthetics must be recognized because such complications often can be treated or reversed proper recognition of these complications may reduce the incidence of ocular morbidity. The ophthalmologist must be aware of the possibilities for complications both ocular and systemic and how to deal with those that arise.

Adverse Effects

Direct Corneal Effects

Topical anesthetic agents can affect the eye in many ways, including the alteration of lacrimation and tear film stability and direct epithelial toxicity. Endothelial toxicity may occur in cases of perforating injury. Moreover, agent and its vehicle may serve as reservoir of microbial contamination with the potential for causing an infection.

Alteration of lacrimation: Topical anesthetics can cause decreased stability of tear film and decreased aqueous reflex tear production by virtue of their own properties or properties of preservatives. Anesthetics by disrupting the surface microvilli of the epithelial cells cause a decrease in mucous adherence, poor wettability of cornea and shortening of tear break up time. Ocular surface anesthesia block conduction in the different loop of reflex tearing pathway causing decreased aqueous tear production in response to noxious stimuli. Further these agents cause the blink rate to decrease. All these factors cause an increased rate of tear evaporation facilitating deterioration of the ocular surface.

Epithelial toxicity: Direct epithelial toxicity can occur when an epithelial defect is present, topical ocular anesthetics slow down the healing process. Chronic use of topical ocular anesthetics causes delayed healing of epithelial defects by mechanism of disruption of the vinculin-based epithelial cell motility complexes.

In the intact epithelium topical proparacaine 0.5 percent has been shown to increase the sloughing rate of epithelial cells.

Endothelial toxicity: Endothelial toxicity may be caused by exposure to topically applied anesthetic agents when a transcorneal portal of entry (perforating injury) is present. Intracameral BAC the primary preservatives used in topical anesthetics (0.025 to 0.05%) causes irreversible corneal edema data on individual toxicities of topical agents to the endothelium are not available yet.

Microbial contamination: The possibility of multidose vial contamination has been reported in some cases. The squeeze bottles of topical anesthetic agents had recoverable bacterial contamination in the cap areas.

Systemic and Noncorneal Effects

Lethal toxicity: Although the topical ocular anesthetic are in general a fairly safe group of drug, but they have been reported to cause important systemic reactions.

Coccaine is the most potent in terms of the systemic reactions, in that topical application can be lethal. Coccaine poisoning may occur with doses as small as 20 mg.

Allergy and idiosyncratic reactions: Idiosyncratic and allergic reactions occur as well. The most common is contact dermatitis. Proparacaine is one of the most common topical agent causing contact dermatitis. Manifestations include periocular swelling, erythema and the typical rashes of contact dermatitis.

Stevens-Johnson syndrome may also be either caused or precipitated by the application of topical agents.

The most common systemic adverse reactions of local injectable anesthetics are related to the CNS and CVS systems. These are generally dose related and may result from rapid absorption from the injection site, from diminished tolerance or from unintentional intravascular injections.

Central Nervous System—Adverse Reactions

- Restlessness, dizziness anxiety, tinnitus, blurred vision, tremors, convulsions, nausea, vomiting, chills, pupil constriction and excitement which may be transient.
- *Depressive effects:* These may or may not be preceded by the excitatory symptoms. These are drowsiness, sedation, generalized CNS depression, coma, unconsciousness, apnea, respiratory depression and even death from respiratory arrest.

Cardiovascular symptoms: These are:
- Peripheral vasodilation
- Hypertension and tachycardia
- Decreased cardiac output
- Hypotension
- Bradycardia
- Methemoglobinemia
- Heart block, ventricular arrhythmias
- Circulatory collapse.

Allergic adverse reactions
- Cutaneous lesions of late onset
- Erythema, angioneurotic edema
- Sneezing, syncope
- Excessive sweating
- Elevated temperature and anaphylactoid symptoms.

Secondary Adverse Effects

Interference with Diagnostic Tests

Hypofluoroscence of fluorescein: All ocular surface anesthetics can cause interference with and distoration of diagnostic test results. It can cause decrease in the fluoroscence of sodium fluorescein. Use of artificial tears solutions, or sterile sodium chloride as a vehicle for the fluorescein will avoid this decrease in fluorescence.

Variability in Schirmer's Testing

The use of topical anesthetic agents diminishes the reliability of Schirmer's testing. This effect is due to fact that variability in the density of anesthesia may cause a variability of reflex tearing. One can avoid this condition by increasing the density of anesthesia.

Reduction of Microbial Recovery

Topical anesthetic drugs have been reported to decrease the recoverability of organisms in ocular surface culturing.

Preclusion of Sequential Testing

Topical agents may preclude necessary diagnostic testing. In case of disorders such as Horner's syndrome, the use of topical anesthetic agents can distort the results of subsequent cocaine and hydroxyamphetamine testing. In diseases caused by herpes zoster or simplex, with strong neurotrophic components, topical anesthetic may mask significant diagnostic clues. The order of instillation of drops in diagnostic testing must be carefully planned.

Surface Keratopathy

Punctate keratitis is a hypersensitivity reaction caused by topical anesthetic agents themselves.

Topical agents precipitate intraepithelial proteins or globulins. This punctate keratitis is frequently absent immediately after the instillation of topical anesthetic agent, but it may appear about 5–20 minutes later.

Alterations of Ocular Response to Other Topical Agents

Changes in Epithelial Permeability

Topical anesthetics may cause the eye to respond differently to other topically applied agents by changing the permeability of the ocular surface to such agents altering their bioavailability. The alteration in permeability of the ocular surface to various agents may involve a direct effect on the epithelium. These agents cause a loosening of the desmosomal area of cell-cell adhesion. When this condition occurs other pharmaceutical agents are more able to penetrate this normally poorly permeable layer.

Prolonged Surface Contact

The bioavailability of topically applied agents may be altered by an additional mechanism. Anesthetics decrease the reflex secretion of tears causing an increase in length of time required for tear wash out. This allows topically applied agents to be in contact with the epithelial surface for a prolonged period of time.

Abuse of topical ocular anesthetics: Topical ocular anesthetic abuse is a serious disorder causing keratitis and persistent epithelial defect. It is generally accepted that frequent use of topically applied agents cause poor healing of epithelial defects, leading to corneal stromal infiltration. This infiltrate appears ring-shaped. The presence of a prolonged epithelial defect may also give rise to an increased susceptibility to secondary infections.

Various ocular adverse effects reported with topical anesthetic agents are summarized as below:
- Mild stinging and burning sensation
- Vasodilation
- Shortening of tear break-up time
- Decreased blinking
- Corneal edema
- Decreased epithelial mitosis and migration
- Slow epithelial healing
- Punctate epithelial keratitis
- Epithelial desquamation
- Allergic reactions of lid and conjunctiva
- Iritis.

TOXICITY OF SURGICAL SOLUTIONS

Surgical solutions play an important role in many aspects of anterior and posterior segment ocular surgery. They include preoperative antiseptics, irrigating solutions viscoelastic substances, mydriatics and miotics and a number of other agents designed to enhance intraocular operations. All surgical solutions and additives have the potential for injuring the tissues they contact like cornea, lens, trabecular meshwork, uvea, vitreous and retina. This potential for injury is more, when solution is used inside the eye rather than applied externally because the concentration to which the sensitive intraocular tissues are exposed are much higher. Because of potential for toxicity there should always be specific indication for the use of an intraocular solution or medication.

Antiseptic Solutions

Cleaning of periocular skin area with an antiseptic scrubbing solution is a routine step in the preparation of the eye for operation and is designed to reduce the risk of bacterial contamination. Toxicity of these solutions is related to inherent toxicity of the antiseptic itself, concentration, presence of a detergent and contact time.

Recent reports of keratitis resulting from accidental exposure to chlorhexidine highlight the potential for toxicity of the scrubbing solution is allowed to enter the cojunctival sac.

Pain and decreased vision following chlorhexidine exposure, this was associated with
- A large corneal epithelial defect
- Punctate keratitis
- Stromal edema and vascularization
- Intrastromal hemorrhages
- Irreversible bullous keratopathy

In chlorhexidine exposure limited to epithelial involvement, the patients recovered without sequelae within 5 days.

The adverse effects have also been seen following use of following antiseptics:
- Tincture of iodine
- Hexachlorophene 3 percent with detergent
- 70 percent ethanol
- 7.5 percent povidone iodine with detergent (Betadine)

Toxicity of these antiseptics can lead to:
- Marked corneal de-epithelization
- Conjunctival chemosis
- Anterior stromal edema

Corneal toxicity is a potential for corneal exposure to scrubbing solution cannot be completely eliminated. It is advised to use 10 percent povidone–iodine solution without detergent (Betadine solution). This solution is germicidal against a broad range of gram-positive and gram-negative bacteria, yeast, fungi and protozoa.

In addition conjunctival sac can be irrigated with BSS after the skin has been prepared.

Irrigating Solutions Toxicity

An essential component in most intraocular surgical procedures is a safe irrigating solution. The irrigants keep the globe inflated and maintains normal pressure volume relationships intraoperatively. The increase in the number of intraocular surgical procedures being performed over the last decade has been paralleled by an increase in the number of commercially available irrigating solutions.

The potential for damage to the corneal endothelium and other tissues is related to the chemical composition, pH and osmolality of the solution that bathes those tissues.

The most physiological solution is the one that most closely matches the chemical composition of human aqueous humour. BSS plus is an ideal solution. Endothelial barrier and pump functions both may be adversely affected by nonphysiological solutions. The key advantage of BSS plus lie in its physiological bicarbonate buffer and the presence of glucose and glutathione.

Patients at Increased Risk

Patients with low cell densities or morphological abnormalities of the endothelium (diabetes, endothelial dystrophies) are known to be more susceptible to surgical trauma and other stresses such as contact lens wear that might result in corneal decompensation. Diabetics are also more likely than others to require cataract extraction or vitrectomy.

A physiological irrigating solution becomes even more important as intraocular manipulations become more complex and the duration and volume of irrigation increases.

Formulation Problems and Toxicity

There have been reports of irrigating solution toxicity most of which are related to microbial contamination, inadequate packaging or improper formulation. Filamentous fungi yeasts and anerobic bacteria have been isolated from various irrigating solutions and corneal stroage media in recent years.

Container failures and manufacturing errors have been implicated as source of contamination.

A single lot of contaminated irrigating solutions can result in widely dispressed cases of postoperative endophthalmitis many of which may be delayed in onset or difficult to diagnose.

Poor packaging of irrigating solutions can result in widely dispressed cases of postoperative endophthalmitis many of which may be delayed in onset or difficult to diagnose.

Poor packaging of irrigating solutions may lead to corneal decompensation.

Improper formulation and variations in quality control result in intraoperative endothelial cell edema and temporary corneal clouding.

Reuse

I strongly advise against reuse of irrigating solution because of the increased risk of contamination. Irrigating solutions contain no preservatives, and designed to be used once after opening. Reuse contradicts all standard infection control principles and increase the chances of error in the operation theater.

Viscoelastic Solutions

Viscoelastic solutions are used increasingly for protection of corneal endothelium and manipulation of tissues during anterior segment surgery. Generally these solutions are effective and well-tolerated in most instances. Clinical problems associated with these solutions have been related to increased intraocular pressure formulation problems and intraocular inflammation as well as corneal edema and corneal decompensation.

Intraocular Pressure

All viscoelastic solutions have the potential of raise the IOP to dangerous levels. The pressure usually peaks in less than 12 hours after administration. The mechanism responsible for the increased pressure is probably related to decrease outflow facility. Anterior chamber washout does not eliminate the decrease in outflow facility but it does decrease the level and duration of the postoperative pressure rise.

I, therefore, recommend washout or aspiration of viscous solutions at the end of surgery in all cases. I also recommend using intracameral carbachol, topical apracolonide (Iopidine) or a systemic carbonic anhydrase inhibitor for pressure control during the first 24 hours postoperatively.

Formulation Problems and Toxicity

Currently available viscoelastics solution are formulated in phosphate buffered saline and non-buffered saline (Amvisc). All appear nontoxic to the endothelium. However, calcium precipitation due to excessive phosphate concentration in the viscoat vehicle have been seen.

Intraocular Inflammation

Commercially available, highly purified viscoelastic solutions are non-antigenic in human beings. However in some cases postoperative intraocular inflammation has been seen (Iritis and Hypopyon). It is probably due to the presence of endotoxins or other protein impurities in the viscoelastic material.

New Viscoelastic Solutions

A host of new viscous solution based on sodium hyaluronate, chondroitin sulphate, hydroxy propyl methyl cellulose, polyacrylamide and collagen and being developed. An ideal viscoelastic solution should effectively protect and manipulate tissues. It should be uniform, inexpensive and easy to manufacture and purify. It also should not contain antigenic proteins. Finally it should be formulated in a BSS that resembles as closely as possible the composition of aqueous humour.

Mydriatics and Miotics

Control of pupil during intraocular surgery can be accomplished using a variety of mydriatics and miotics. Almost all drugs formulated for topical, intravenous use contains preservatives and other chemicals that are toxic to the endothelium or that may adversely affect the physiological balance of the ocular irrigant.

Mydriatics

A well-dilated pupil facilitates many surgical maneuvers. Intraocular epinephrine has been the mydriatic of choice for most ophthalmologists. Studies have shown the corneal edema after intraocular administration of epinephrine. Toxicity of 1:1000 and 1:10000 solutions is due to sodium bisulfite (preservative), an acidic pH and non-physiological citrate buffer.

Miotics

A miotic pupil facilitates corneal trephine centration, peripheral iridectomy, anterior chamber lens insertion and a variety of other intraocular manipulations. Most surgeons prefer a miotic pupil at the end of cataract surgery to ensure lens centration and to protect the endothelium from the lens implant. Pilocarpine is toxic to the endothelium, so its intraocular use should be avoided. Currently available intraocular miotics include acetyl choline chloride (miochol) and carbachol.

Some reports have shown the corneal swelling and endothelial changes during perfusions of human cornea with miochol. When carbachol use may lead to reversible corneal swelling.

Other Agents

Preservatives

Preservatives like sulfites, parabens, benzalkonium, benzyl alcohol, chlorhexidine and thiomersal have been shown to affect endothelial structure and function adversely and their use should be avoided benzalkonium chloride is particularly toxic.

Another potential source of preservative toxicity is reuse of instruments and irrigating tubings. Ethyline oxide gas sterilization of plastics may cause release of complex compounds that can combine with sterilant residues, resulting in toxicity or inflammation. Iritis and corneal decompensation have been reported as a result of toxicity from thiomersal residues in reused viscoelastic cannulas.

Thrombin

Commercial preparations of bovine thrombin designed for topical application have been added to irrigating solutions and used during vitrectomy for diabetic retinopathy and trabeculectomy for neovascular glaucoma. These thrombins have been shown with 20 percent incidence or severe postoperative inflammation with sterile hypopyon formation and fibrin deposition.

Alpha-Chymotrypsin

It is a proteolytic enzyme mainly used for enzymatic zonulysis for intracapsular lens extraction specially in young patients.

The adverse effects reported with alpha chymotrypsin include transient rise in IOP, corneal edema, striation, moderate uveitis, delayed healing of incisions, wound disruption and vitreous loss.

Hyaluronidase

The enzyme hyaluronidase is commonly used in conjunction with local anesthetic (Lignocaine 2% with adrenaline) for infiltration and regional local anesthesia.

Hyaluronidase is antigenic and may sometimes produce allergic reactions. Because of danger of spreading infection the enzyme should not be injected into or around an infected area.

COMPLICATIONS OF CONTACT LENS SOLUTIONS

Todays, contact lens professionals have not only many different lenses at their disposal but also a great no of sophisticated contact lens solutions. Recent datas for possible sources of eye irritation, increased incidence of allergic sensitivity, chemical and physical changes in lens integrity and discoloration or lens spoilage have been traced to problems related to contact lens solutions. The most prominent complications are related to:
- Solution stability
- Patient sensitivity
- Chemical and lens binding
- Product compatibility.

Solution Stability

The composition of contact lens solutions are from simple salt solutions to complex disinfecting formulas. The possibility of complications with their use is always present in the hands of typical contact lens wearer.

Many of the ingredients of the contact lens solutions change with time and precipitate undesirable reactions. An example of an undesired reaction in contact lens solutions is changed in sorbic acid, a popular preservative for such solutions which when in fresh state performs satisfactorily but when allowed to degrade produces mixed aldehyde that can discolor protein deposits on the lenses. Consequently, the useful life is shortened. Many contact lens solution can develop physical stability problems, i.e. precipitates, unnatural odour or color, evaporation under a variety of conditions. Both hot and cold weather are responsible in this process.

Patient Sensitivity

Sensitivity reactions can be grouped as allergic responses to either specific chemicals or contact lens deposits. The typical sensitivity to thiomersal has been well-documented.

Once a contact lens wearer recognizes his or her sensitivity to thiomersal, the wearer should avoid products containing this preservative.

Most wearers can tolerate sorbic acid preserved products much better than thiomersal preserved products From the first day, they are worn, contact lenses collect deposits consisting of complex mixtures of protein, lipid and mucin. Workers have shown that giant papillary conjunctivitis is an autoimmune response of the conjunctiva to contact lens deposits. This condition is a significant contributor to the contact lens drop out rate.

Chemical and Lens Binding

Some of the ingredients of contact lens solutions are attracted to external and internal surfaces of the lenses. This phenomenon severely limits the types of chemicals for contact lens formulations.

Benzalkonium chloride (BAC) is the most widely used preservative of ophthalmic and hard contact lens solutions. In soft lens reaction BAC was found to bind very strongly to HEMA material. This binding leads to concentration of BAC in the lenses which then renders the lenses potentially damaging to the eye.

This complications lead to search for low binding/non-binding chemicals. Chlorhexidine, an antibacterial disinfecting and preservative agent was found to have a much lower binding to HEMA than BAC. As a result chlorhexidine is widely used as both preservative and a disinfecting agent for soft contact lenses but the accumulative binding of chlorhexidine to protein deposits is undesirable. Thus regular cleaning of HEMA lenses become specially important.

This leads to the use of hydrogen peroxide (H_2O_2). The chemical degradation route of H_2O_2 is very well defined.

The advantage of H_2O_2 for soft contact lenses is that there is no undesirable action.

Product Compatibility

Contact lens wearers have too many care products from which to choose many wearers mixing and matching these products indiscriminately. For example, a wearer might use a cleaner of one company and disinfecting solution from other company. Although many contact lens solutions are reasonably compatible with other company products. The use of combinations of contact lens solutions may lead to variety of problems ranging in severity from minor to major. Further failure of the user to read directions for use, Carefully and to comply with these directions can lead to unfortunate circumstances.

Recently Bausch and Lomb and Allergan have come up with an excellent multipurpose solution for soft and RGP lenses which contains no chlorhexidine and thiomersal. It can be used safely for cleaning, rinsing disinfecting and storing soft lenses without any side effects. Compatibility and stability of solution is very good. There is no binding and sensitivity reactions reported with multipurpose solution.

COMPLICATIONS OF INTRAVENOUS FLUORESCEIN

Fluorescein angiography is performed using an intravenous injection of a dye, sodium Fluorescein followed by serial fundus photography. Sodium fluorescein is a relatively low molecular weight, highly water soluble compound that exhibits the physical property of fluorescence. When exposed to a light of wavelength between 165-490 nm (green yellow), using properly matched exciting and barrier filters, the retinal and choroidal vasculature as well as fundus abnormalities can be assessed. Although IV injection of fluorescein are fairly safe yet several side effects have been reported.

CLASSIFICATION OF ADVERSE REACTIONS

Adverse reactions are categorized as mild, moderate and severe depending on their duration, the need for medical intervention and the final outcome. A mild effect is defined as a transient effect requiring no treatment and eventuating in a rapid and complete resolution. The vast majority of side effects to fluorescein are of the mild variety.

A reaction is considered moderate if despite its transient nature, resolutions is more gradual and occasionally requires medical intervention.

Severe adverse reactions are complication that are associated with prolonged effects requiring intensive treatment.

Mild Adverse Reactions

Nausea and Vomiting

The single most common side effects of intravenous fluorescein is nausea which is reported to occur in 3-18 percent of patients. The origin of nausea remains uncertain. An inverse relationship has been shown between the rapidity with which injection is given and the incidence of nausea. Therefore it is recommended that injection should be given as briskly as it is safe and practical.

Psychogenic factors play an important role in the development of nausea. Nausea appears to be more common in the young, highly anxious patients.

Pretreatment of patients with antiemetics has been tried with variable results.

Extravasation

FA requires the injection of sodium fluorescein into an accessible vein usually in the anticubital region. Intravenous injections carry with them the risk of inadvertent extravasation of the medication into the perivascular tissues. Since patients most likely to undergo this procedure are elderly and diabetic, vessel fragility and accessibility are of definite concerns. Certainly the incidence will depend on the skill and expertise of person giving the injection, the technique used and individual patient factors. If extravasation of dye is detected or suspected, the injection should be stopped immediately. If sufficient dye has reached the blood stream before extravasation the angiogram may be continued. If extravasation is detected early, symptoms may vary from none to mild discomfort that can be easily controlled. In severe extravasation, symptoms will be more pronounced. The injection site may become very painful requiring a specific treatment.

Inadvertent Intra-arterial Injections

Fluorescein dye may inadvertently be injected intra-arterially following attempted venipuncture. Additionally the use of tourniquet may dampen arterial pulsations making the distinction between vein and artery more difficult. However, several other useful signs may be employed to recognize an arterial puncture with the use of butterfly needle the bright red glow of refluxed arterial blood can be seen within clear tubing. Immediate treatment consists of pressure over the puncture site to prevent hematoma formation. Fortunately no adverse long-term sequelae have been reported.

Other Minor Reactions

It includes sneezing, pruritis, paresthesias of tongue and lips and abdominal cramps. An immediate and temporary yellowish discoloration of skin and conjunctiva occurs to a varying degree in every patient and it may as for several hours. This is actually not a side effect.

Moderate Adverse Reactions

Of greater concern to the patient and eye surgeon are moderate reactions those requiring some form of medical therapy. These reactions are:

Skin Eruption

The development of a skin eruption represents the most common of the moderate reactions.

Most frequent skin reaction to fluorescein is urticaria. It occurs in about 1 percent of patients undergoing angiography.

The onset of signs and symptoms occur in 10–15 minutes after the administration of the dye. The reaction is typically self-limiting usually resolving within few hours. Oral or IV low dose of antihistaminic provides relief.

Syncope

Intravenous injection alone can cause a vasovagal response which can lead to light headedness, dizziness and syncope.

In such situation monitoring of the patients vital sign is essential. Generally the syncope episode is short lived and requires only minimal supportive care.

Skin Necrosis

The extravasation of the dye can lead to a marked localized reaction with the development of necrosis and sloughing of the overlying skin. The pathophysiological features are believed to be related to local inflammation and vasospasm causing ischemia and tissue damage. The relative risk of skin necrosis is proportional to the volume of dye extravasated. The earliest sign of necrosis is the development of a white avascular patch of skin.

Severe Adverse Reactions

Cardiovascular Complications

Cardiovascular system complications are rare with fluorescein angiography. An incidence of one in 5000 patients have been reported.

Cardiovascular system effects include myocardial infarction and cardiac arrest. In addition to these CVS shock, chest pain have also been shown.

Respiratory Complications

Respiratory complications due to fluorescein angiography are also not common incidence is 14,000 patients.

A severe anaphylactic response to the dye, leading to laryngeal edema and bronchospasm can seriously compromise oxygen exchange. It can also lead to respiratory arrest. These life-threatening reactions require prompt intervention by experienced medical personal for successful treatment.

Death

Though rarely reported, IV fluorescein angiography can cause a fatal cardiopulmonary reaction. This has been noted to occur as rapidly as 30 seconds following the injection but most commonly occurs within several hours.

DRUG-INDUCED OCULAR CICATRIZATION

Drug-induced ocular pemphigoid or drug induced cicatrization of the conjunctiva is clinically identical to this disease and occurs secondary to long-term use of topical ocular medications. Topical ocular therapy can produce many side effects, i.e. scarring with shrinkage of conjunctiva although less common, but is a deleterious complication of long-term use of certain topical ocular medications. Drugs that have been shown to produce such effect include epinephrine, pilocarpine, idoxuridine, timolol, echothiophate iodide, demecarium bromide and various preservatives in topical eyedrops. Kristensen and Norn were first to suggest an association between long-term topical drug use and ocular cicatrization.

Clinical Manifestations

Differential Diagnosis

The early diagnosis of drug-induced ocular cicatrization is difficult. The early manifestations—Chronic conjunctivitis with irritation, burning and tearing are similar to those of ocular cicatrical pemphigoid. Later on dry eye symptoms develop. Corneal dessication leads to foreign body sensation, photophobia and reduced visual acuity from scarring. Terminal stage disease is characterized by ocular surface Keratinization and ankyleoblepharon. The Diagnosis is missed unless the fornices of patients using long-term topical medications are examined for shortening or shrinking. The diagnosis of drug induced ocular pemphigoid is made both by excluding other causes of conjunctival shrinkage and by obtaining a thorough history of topical medication use. The differential diagnosis of ocular scarring and shrinkage must be kept in the mind. These can be:

- Chemical, thermal or radiation burns
- Severe membranous conjunctivitis
- Stevens-Johnson syndrome
- Sjögren's syndrome
- Sarcoidosis
- Trachoma
- Bullous pemphigoid
- Pemphigus.

Ocular cicatrical pemphigoid is a chronically progressive disease and if untreated can have a variable and asymmetrical course that may or may not be progressive. It can occur as non-progressive toxic reaction that is self-limiting once the offending topical medication is stopped or it can be relentlessly progressive. In progressive cases an immunological factors has been suggested.

Disease Stages

Although there is no uniformly accepted classification for ocular cicatrical pemphigoid, yet, Foster has described following four stages:

Stage I: It consists of conjunctival inflammation, mucoid discharge, rose bengal staining of the conjunctival epithelium and subepithelial fibrosis with fine white subepithelial striae.

Stage II: It continues with conjunctival shrinkage and foreshortening of the inferior fornix.

Stage III: It includes frank symblepharon and a wide variety of other ocular changes including keratopathy, corneal neovascularization, trichiasis and tear insufficiency.

Stage IV: It is end stage disease marked by severe sicca syndrome, ocular surface keratinization and ankyloblepharon.

Drug induced ocular pemphigoid appears pathologically identical to idiopathic, ocular cicatrical pemphigoid. There is chronic conjunctival subepithelial inflammation with an invasion of the submucosal tissue by newly formed connective tissue which subsequently contracts. Ocular cicatricial pemphigoid is associated with a diminished and unstable tear film caused by destruction of conjunctival goblet cells. The chronic dry eye condition and exposure results in Keratinization of the ocular surface.

Treatment

The treatment criteria to patients with ocular irritation and conjunctival shortening of recent onset should be careful and methoidical with primary stoppage of all topical medications. Every effort should be made to eliminate other causes of conjunctival cicatrization. Patients with ocular irritation may need only artificial tear lubricants and mild topical steroids for comfort. If preservatives are potential cause of cicatrization then preservative free artificial tear should be prescribed.

In addition to it, a soft bandage contact lens can be given to keep patients comfortable by protecting the cornea from excessive drying. Topical all transretinoic ointment can be given to reverse the surface disorder especially keratinization.

All patients must be followed regularly for disease progression. Reduction in tear flow with an accumulation of thick stingy discharge leads to blepharitis in many patients. Such patients are managed with frequent warm eyelid scrubs with mild soap followed by application of antibiotic ointment.

Secondary bacterial conjunctivitis is known to occur in this condition. If suspected then following culture test, treat specific pathogens with suitable antibiotic drops.

If the conjunctival scarring and shrinkage progress ectropion and trichiasis may occur. Trichiasis can be controlled by electrolysis or cryotherapy. Surgical eyelid procedures should be avoided because of poor results and the risk of exacerbating the condition. Systemic steroids have been found helpful in the treatment of acute exacerbations of ocular cicatrical pemphigoid.

Systemic immunosuppressive therapy consisting of cyclophosphamide or azathioprine both with or without prednisone has been used with success. Cytotoxic therapy is indicated for those patients with documented progressive conjunctival shortening which can lead to symblepharon and total blindness.

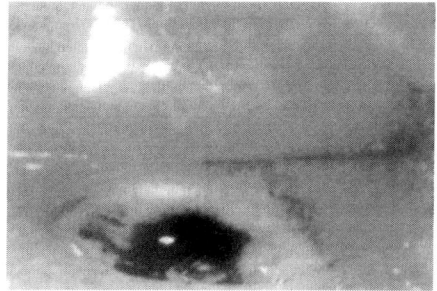

Fig. 23.12: Drug-induced ocular cicatricial pemphigus

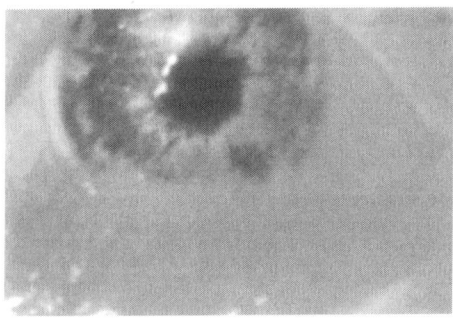

Fig. 23.13: Drug-induced Stevens-Johnson syndrome

SYSTEMIC DRUGS CAUSING OCULAR TOXICITY

The eye due to relatively small size, multiple tissue characteristics and rich blood supply are highly vulnerable to toxic substances. Systemically administered medications have potential to produce adverse ocular effects and almost all the structures of the eye are susceptible. Although list of systemically administered drug is very big here in this section, I shall describe the most common used systemic drugs that have been reported to cause ocular toxicity, giving in nutshell the salient features of ocular adverse effects.

Antimalarial Drugs

Chloroquine, Quinacrine and Hydroxychloroquine on prolong use can cause following changes in the cornea.
- In early phase diffuse punctate deposits develop in the corneal epithelium and later these deposits aggregate to form curved lines which converge and coalesce below the central cornea.
- Corneal changes lead to visual symptoms like halos around light, glare and photophobia.
- On discontinuation of drug therapy these objective and subjective corneal signs disappear.
- Other adverse effects include night blindness, visual hallucinations, cataract (Posterior subcapsular, optic neuritis/atrophy and toxic amblyopia).

Chlorpromazine

Out of phenothiazine derivatives chlorpromazine is the only drug that produce changes in cornea and lens.
These changes include:
- Lenticular pigmentation which may vary from fine dot like optics on anterior lens surface to central pearl like light pigmented aggregation surrounded by small pigment clump.
- Corneal pigment changes may also develop in those patients who have concomitant lens opacities. Corneal pigmentation is noticed at the level of endothelium and Descemet's membrane in inter palpebral fissure area.

- Such patient may complain of glare, halos around bulb and hazy vision.
- On discontinuation of drug therapy these pigment deposits remain static and irreversible.
- Other effects include discoloration of conjunctiva and sclera.

Analgesics

Analgesics are most commonly used in diverse conditions of systemic disorders.

Non-narcotic analgesics may produce following adverse ocular effects:
- Decrease in visual acuity and color vision
- Visual hallucinations
- Lid/conjunctival irritation, edema.
- Mydriasis.

Narcotic analgesics may produce:
- Decrease in vision.
- Visual hallucinations
- Diplopia, myopia
  Photophobia and color vision defects
- Lid edema
- Dry eyes
- Mydriasis or anisocoria
- Accommodative paralysis
- Optic atrophy
- Nystagmus and visual field scotomas.

Antiarthritic Drugs

Gold salts: Following prolonged administration gold salts can be deposited in various tissues of body including eye, known as chrysiasis.

Ocular chrysiasis can involve the conjunctiva, cornea and lens. Various ocular adverse effects are:
- Gold deposits (red, brown or violet) in lid, conjunctiva, pancorneal and lens.
- Diplopia
- Extraocular muscles paresis
- Ptosis
- Myasthenic block
- Iritis
- Papilledema and retinal hemorrhages.

Antigout
- Decreased visual acuity
- Scleritis
- Corneal: Keratitis, ulcers, scarring, dellen
- Macular edema and retinal hemorrhages
- Diplopia
- Extraocular muscle paresis.

Corticosteroids

Systemic steroids can produce posterior subcapsular cataracts (PSC) that are clinically difficult to distinguish from complicated cataracts and age-related PSC cataracts.

These cataracts remain unchanged even on discontinuation or decrease in the dose of the drug. Other adverse effects include:
- Decreased vision
- Myopia, diplopia
- Color vision defects
- Delayed wound healing
- Mydriasis
- Retinal hemorrhages and edema
- Papilledema
- Exophthalmos
- Extraocular muscle paralysis
- Toxic amblyopia
- Visual fields scotomas
- Glaucoma.

Nonsteroidal Anti-inflammatory Drugs (NSAIDs)

- Decrease in vision
- Red green color vision defect
- Visual hallucinations
- Myopia, Photophobia
- Diplopia and extraocular muscle paralysis
- Dry eye
- Keratitis
- Mydriasis
- Accommodative paralysis
- Serous retinopathy
- Retinal hemorrhages
- Corneal deposits
- Macular edema, papilledema
- Optic neuritis/atrophy
- Toxic amblyopia and nystagmus.

General Anesthetic Agents

General anesthesia is given in a wide variety of surgeries. It is important to know the ocular adverse effects of general anesthetic agents (commonly used drugs include chloroform, ether, ketamine, methoxy flurane, nitrous oxide, trichloroethylene, halothane).

The ocular adverse effects reported are:
- Visual hallucinations
- Decrease in vision
- Diplopia and color vision defects
- Mydriasis (on light anesthesia)
- Miosis (on deep anesthesia)
- Eso or exotropia

- Nystagmus
- Scotomas.

Antihistamines

H1 antihistamines have varying degree of atropine like actions including the ability to alter tear film integrity. Both aqueous and mucin production may decrease with use of systemic antihistamines. Other adverse effects include:
- Decreased visual acuity
- Diplopia
- Dry eyes
- Punctate keratitis
- Visual hallucinations
- Anisocoria
- Mydriasis
- Accommodative paralysis
- Nystagmus
- Retinal hemorrhages.

Anti-infective Agents

Systemic Antibiotics

Systemic antibiotics are widely prescribed both in medical and surgical conditions of diverse etiology.

Aminoglycosides
- Diplopia
- Color vision defects
- Decrease in vision
- Ptosis
- Brow loss
- Visual hallucinations
- Papilledema and retinal hemorrhages
- Optic neuritis
- Toxic amblyopia
- Pseudotumor cerebri
- Scotomas.

Cephalosporins
- Diplopia
- Visual hallucinations
- Corneal peripheral edema
- Subconjunctival hemorrhage
- Retinal hemorrhages
- Papilledema
- Retinal pigment epithelium disturbances
- Nystagmus.

Chloramphenicol
- Decrease vision and color vision defects
- Lid or conjunctival allergy
- Mydriasis

- Retinal edema, hemorrhages
- Optic atrophy
- Toxic amblyopia
- Retrobulbar or optic neuritis.

Erythromycin and Related Drugs
- Photosensitivity
- Subconjunctival hemorrhage
- Retinal hemorrhage
- Color vision defects
- Extraocular muscle paralysis.

Colistin
- Diplopia
- Mydriasis
- Extraocular muscle paralysis

Nitrofurantoins (Nalidixic acid)
- Glare
- Scintillating scotomas
- Mydriasis
- Accommodative paralysis
- Retinal hemorrhages
- Papilledema
- Lid or conjunctival photosensitivity
- Extraocular muscle paralysis
- Nystagmus.

Penicillins
- Diplopia, blepharoconjunctivitis
- Photosensitivity
- Subconjunctival hemorrhage
- Ptosis
- Edema
- Extraocular muscle paralysis
- Allergy.

Antifungals

Penicillin derivatives (Griseofulvin)
- Subconjunctival hemorrhage
- Keratitis, ulcers, scarring
- Macular edema
- Scleritis
- Photosensitivity
- Ulceration.

Polyenes Derivatives
- Retinal exudates/hemorrhages
- Optic neuritis
- Extraocular muscle paralysis
- Diplopia.

Imidazoles
- Photophobia
- Shimmering lights

- Visual hallucinations
- Diplopia
- Corneal vortex whorls
- Superficial punctate Keratitis
- Iritis
- Optic neuritis or atrophy
- Oculogyric crisis.

Antileprosy Drugs

Phenazines
- Corneal polychromatic crystals
- Macular retinal pigment epithelium mattle
- Hyperpigmentation
- Decrease in vision.

Sulfones
- Visual hallucinations
- Lid edema
- Hyperpigmentation
- Optic atrophy
- Retinal hemorrhages
- Decrease in vision.

Antiparasitics

Amebicides
- Corneal opacities
- Diplopia
- Optic atrophy/neuritis
- Macular degeneration
- Macular edema
- Decrease in vision
- Toxic amblyopia.

Antihelminthics
- Variable color vision
- Color vision defects
- Flashing lights
- Dry eyes and punctate keratitis
- Corneal multicolor deposits
- Nonreactive pupils
- Punctate keratitis
- Iritis
- Chorioretinitis
- Scotomas
- Mydriasis
- Yellow sclera
- Yellow or black pigmentation of conjunctiva
- Decreased visual acuity
- Toxic amblyopia.

Antituberculosis Drugs

Ethambutol
- Visual field constriction
- Hemianopia
- Extraocular muscle paralysis
- Retinal or macular edema
- Vascular dilation
- Photophobia
- Scotomas: Annular, central, cecocentral
- Color vision defects.

Para-aminosalicylates
- Red green color defect
- Accommodative paralysis
- Retinal hemorrhage
- Scotomas
- Lid inflammation, edema.

Cycloserine
- Flickering vision
- Visual hallucinations
- Photosensitivity
- Retinal hemorrhage.

Isoniazid, Ethionamide
- Keratitis
- Mydriasis
- Retrobulbar neuritis
- Red green color defects
- Diplopia, photophobia
- Visual hallucinations
- Extraocular muscle paresis
- Visual field hemianopia
- Diplopia, photophobia
- Nystagmus.

Rifampicin, Capreomycin
- White vision
- Angioneurotic edema
- Flashing lights
- Conjunctival hyperemia
- Iritis
- Decrease in vision
- Visual hallucinations
- Blepharoconjunctivitis.

Antivirals (Systemic)
- Lid spasm
- Erythema
- Subconjunctival hemorrhage
- Retinal hemorrhage
- Decreased visual acuity.

Antineoplastic Drugs

Alkaloids
- Nonspecific pain, burning
- Pseudotumor cerebri
- Optic neuritis/atrophy
- Lid edema
- Dry eyes
- Photophobia
- Hyperpigmentation
- Eyelash or brow loss
- Papilledema.

Antibiotics—Antineoplastics
- Decrease in vision
- Photophobia
- Retinal hemorrhages
- Subconjunctival hemorrhage
- Toxic amblyopia.

Antimetabolites
- Diplopia, Photophobia
- Lid edema, pain, cicatricial ectropion
- Hyperpigmentation
- Photosensitivity
- Subconjunctival hemorrhage
- Color vision defects
- Nystagmus
- Eyelash or brow loss
- Ulcer.

Thiotepa
- Lid edema
- Eyelash or brow loss
- Iritis
- Retinal hemorrhage.

Folic Acid Antagonists
- Keratitis
- Periorbital edema
- Extraocular muscle paralysis.

Heavy Metals
- Oculogyric crisis
- Orbital pain
- Cortical blindness
- Hemianopia
- Extraocular muscle paralysis.

Interferon
- Abnormal oculography
- Visual hallucinations
- Eyelash or brow growth
- Papilledema
- Retinal hemorrhage.

Nonsteroidal Antiestrogens (e.g. Tamoxifen, Temorifen)
- White or yellow refractile opacities in the macular and paramacular area
- Reduced visual acuity.
- Abnormal visual fields.
- Subepithelial corneal whorl opacities
- Paracentral scotomas
- Retinal pigment epithelium disturbances.

Vinca Alkaloids (e.g. vinblastine, vincristine)
- Corneal ulcers or deposits
- Decreased dark adaptation
- Iritis, scleritis
- Hemianopia
- Cortical blindness
- Visual field constriction
- Central or paracentral scotomas.
- Nystagmus.

Antianginal Drugs

- Photophobia, halos
- Myopia, Diplopia, reduced visual acuity
    - Yellow or blue vision due to nitrates
    - Color vision defect
    - Dry eyes
    - Corneal ulcers
    - Periorbital edema
    - Papilledema and optic neuritis
    - Nystagmus
    - Lid edema, eyelashes loss
    - Pseudotumor cerebri.

Antiarrhythmics

Anticholinergics
- Dryness of mucous membrane
- Marked mydriasis
- Pupillary dilatation and cycloplegia
- Dry eyes
- Accommodative paralysis
- Photophobia, diplopia
- Reduced vision
- Visual hallucinations

Beta-adrenergic Blockers
- Reduced tear secretion
- Photophobia
- Ptosis
- Conjunctival edema
- Decreased corneal sensation
- Severe dry eye

- Yellow or white corneal stromal opacities
- Ocular pain
- Ocular Pseudotumor
- Accommodative paralysis

Quinidine
- Diplopia, photophobia
- Night blindness
- Dry eyes
- Corneal deposits
- Iritis
- Mydriasis
- Retinal hemorrhage
- Optic neuritis
- Toxic amblyopia
- Reduced vision.

Antihypertensives

Alpha-adrenergic Agonists
- Visual hallucinations
- Lid edema
- Decreased vision
- Toxic miosis
- Retinal or macular degeneration
- Visual hallucinations.

Beta-adrenergic Blockers
- Dry eyes
- Hemianopia
- Extraocular muscles paralysis
- Retinal hemorrhages
- Diplopia, photophobia
- Reduced vision
- Ocular pain and subconjunctival hemorrhage

Angiotension-converting Enzymes Inhibitors
- Visual hallucinations
- Lid edema, brown discoloration
- Photosensitivity
- Accommodative paralysis
- Reduced vision.

Ganglionic Blockers
- Red green color vision defect
- Ptosis
- Dry eyes
- Conjunctival edema
- Mydriasis
- Macular edema
- Optic atrophy
- Retinal vasodilation.

Monoamine Oxidase Inhibitors
- Reduced vision, photophobia
- Diplopia, nystagmus

- Blepharospasm, dry eyes
- Accommodative paralysis
- Toxic amblyopia, oculogyric crisis.

Rauwolfia Alkaloids
- Yellow vision and reduced vision
- Tearing
- Mydriasis, iritis
- Retinal hemorrhages
- Oculogyric crisis
- Abnormal conjugate gaze
- Jerky pursuit.

Antimigraine Agents

- Red green color vision defect
- Visual hallucinations and reduced vision
- Miosis
- Accommodative paralysis
- Retinal vascular spasm
- Optic neuritis
- Lid edema
- Scotomas, hemianopia

Cardiac Glycosides

- Change in color vision
- Impairment of vision
- Snowy vision
- Photophobia and visual hallucinations
- Mydriasis
- Accommodative spasm
- Retrobulbar or optic neuritis
- Scotomas central or paracentral
- Toxic amblyopia.

Peripheral Vasodilators

- Ptosis
- Miosis
- Retinal hemorrhages
- Lid edema.

Bronchodilators

- Color vision defect
- Reduced vision
- Photophobia and diplopia
- Mydriasis
- Rebound redness
- Hemianopia
- Horizontal nystagmus.

Alcohols

- Miosis/Mydriasis
- Tearing
- Ptosis, diplopia
- Accommodative paralysis
- Nystagmus
- Blue vision
- Toxic amblyopia
- Strabismus oscillopsia
- Central scotomas

Alcohol Antagonists

- Visual hallucinations
- Color vision defects
- Mydriasis, anisocoria
- Retrobulbar or optic neuritis
- Toxic amblyopia
- Extraocular muscles paralysis
- Nystagmus
- Scotomas.

Anorexiants (Amphetamines)

- Reduced vision
- Blue vision
- Eyelash loss
- Blepharospasm
- Mydriasis
- Decreased pupil reflex and convergence
- Retinal vein occlusion
- Nystagmus.

Muscles Relaxants (Benzodiazepines)

- Decreased depth perception
- Reduced vision
- Diplopia, visual hallucinations
- Color vision defects
- Oculogyric crisis
- Nystagmus
- Retinal hemorrhage.

Anticonvulsants

- White snow vision
- Night blindness
- Diplopia, photosensitivity
- Scotomas, nystagmus
- Retinal hemorrhages.

Antidepressants

- Impaired vision
- Color vision defects
- Diplopia
- Jerky pursuit, tearing
- Blepharospasm
- Dry eyes
- Accommodative paralysis
- Toxic amblyopia.

Antipsychotics and Tranquilizers

- Night blindness
- Visual hallucinations
- Color halos
- Yellow or brown vision
- Corneal hyperpigmentation
- Miosis/mydriasis
- Cataract, diplopia
- Nystagmus, oculogyric crisis
- Papilledema
- Optic atrophy
- Scotomas
- Exophthalmos.

Psychedelic Drugs

- Visual hallucinations
- Color vision defect
- Yellow or violet vision
- Flashing colored lights
- Prolonged after images
- Ptosis
- Miosis, anisocoria.

Sedatives and Hypnotics

- Reduced vision and color vision defects
- Visual hallucinations
- Yellow or green vision
- Diplopia, photophobia
- Blepharoclonus
- Oscillopsia
- Vertical gaze palsy
- Dry eyes
- Accommodative paralysis
- Anisocoria, miosis
- Optic neuritis, papilledema
- Toxic amblyopia
- Optic atrophy.

Dermatological Preparations

Hexachlorophene
- Reduced vision, diplopia
- Mydriasis/Miosis
- Absent pupil light reflex
- Retinal hemorrhages
- Papilledema, optic atrophy
- Pseudotumor cerebri.

Chrysarobin
- Ocular irritation (nonspecific)
- Brown violet lid discoloration
- Keratoconjunctivitis
- Punctate keratitis
- Gray corneal opacities.

Retinoids
- Impaired vision
- Myopia
- Dry eyes
- Decreased dark adaptation
- Lid inflammation, edema
- Corneal opacities
- Hyperpigmentation
- Papilledema and optic neuritis.

Psoralen Therapy
- Photophobia
- Dry eyes
- Keratitis
- Pigmentary glaucoma
- Central scotomas
- Photosensitivity.

Diuretics

Spironolactone
- Reduced vision
- Myopia
- Lid redness

Ethacrynic Acid
- Impaired vision
- Subconjunctival hemorrhage
- Retinal hemorrhage
- Nystagmus.

Sulfonamides
- Yellow vision
- Visual hallucinations
- Photophobia
- Accommodative paralysis
- Retinal hemorrhage
- Contact lens intolerance.

Thiazides
- Myopia, yellow vision
- Dry eyes
- Visual hallucinations
- Photosensitivity
- Retinal Hemorrhage
- Cortical blindness.

Hyperosmotics

- Visual hallucinations
- Impaired vision
- Nystagmus
- Retinal hemorrhage
- Lid edema
- Decreased IOP.

Gastrointestinal Drugs

Antacids
Bismuth salts may produce:
- Toxic impaired vision
- Visual hallucinations
- Corneal deposits
- Lid blue discoloration.

Histamine H_2 blockers may produce:
- Visual hallucinations
- Mydriasis
- Decreased pupil light reflex
- Retinal hemorrhages.

Antiemetics
- Impaired vision
- Color vision defect
- Tearing
- Lid edema
- Mydriasis
- Decreased pupil light reflex
- Photophobia, diplopia
- Strabismus

Antispasmodics
- Photophobia, diplopia
- Micropsia
- Visual hallucinations
- Flashing lights
- Dry eyes
- Mydriasis
- Accommodative paralysis
- Red vision
- Eyelash loss.

Hormonal Drugs

Androgens
- Cataract
- Papilledema
- Pseudotumor cerebri
- Visual field defects
- Impaired vision, diplopia

Corticosteroids
- Cataract (Posterior subcapsular)
- Glaucoma
- Myopia, Diplopia
- Visual Hallucinations
- Delayed wound healing
- Ciliary body microcysts
- Retinal edema and hemorrhage
- Papilledema
- Exophthalmos
- Toxic amblyopia
- Visual field defects (scotomas)
- Myasthenic block

Antihyperglycemics

Insulin
- Mydriasis
- Absent pupil light reflex
- Extraocular muscle paralysis
- Strabismus
- Nystagmus
- Decreased vision, diplopia.

Sulfonylureas
- Photophobia, diplopia
- Color vision defect
- Central or cecocentral scotomas
- Retinal hemorrhage
- Retrobulbar or optic neuritis.

Antithyroid Drugs

Iodines
- Impaired vision
- Green vision, visual hallucination
- Mydriasis
- Punctate keratitis
- Hypopyon, iritis
- Vitreous floaters
- Retinal or macular degeneration
- Exophthalmos
- Visual field defects
- Toxic amblyopia
- Retrobulbar neuritis.

Thiouracils
- Conjunctival depigmentation
- Dry eyes, keratitis
- Exophthalmos
- Nystagmus
- Retinal hemorrhages

Thyroid Replacement Therapy
- Visual hallucinations
- Cataract
- Papilledema
- Optic neuritis/atrophy
- Impaired vision
- Myasthenic block
- Visual field constriction
- Central scotomas
- Hemianopias.

Oral Contraceptives

Estrogen-Progesterone Combination
- Impaired vision, diplopia, myopia, color vision defects blue vision, colored halos
- Dry eyes, iritis
- Mydriasis, anisocoria
- Cataract
- Retinal vascular occlusion
- Macular edema
- Optic or retrobulbar neuritis
- Papilledema
- Visual field constriction
- Scotomas
- Nystagmus
- Pseudotumor cerebri.

Nonsteroidal Antiestrogens
- Flashing or colored lights
- Glare image distortion
- Phosgene stimulation
- Prolonged after images
- Photophobia, diplopia
- Posterior subcapsular cataracts
- Retinal vasospasm
- Optic neuritis
- Visual field constriction.

Immunosuppressant Drugs
- Visual hallucinations
- Retinal hemorrhage
- Retinal pigment epithelium disturbances
- Cortical blindness
- Hypertrichosis.

Neuromuscular Drugs

Polyalcohols
- Impaired vision
- Diplopia
- Ptosis, ciliary flush
- Nystagmus
- Extraocular paralysis

Anticholinergics
- Impaired vision
- Visual hallucinations
- Mydriasis
- Accommodative paralysis
- Retrobulbar neuritis.

Baclofen
- Impaired vision, diplopia
- Lid photosensitivity
- Corneal edema, punctate keratitis
- Mydriasis, miosis
- Strabismus
- Oculogyric crisis.

Myasthenia Gravis Drugs

- Impaired vision, Diplopia
- Miosis
- Ptosis
- Blepharoclonus
- Tearing.

Vaccines (DPT, Polio, Measles, Mumps-rubella, Smallpox, Rabies, Tetanus)

- Decreased vision
- Photophobia, Diplopia
- Visual hallucinations
- Iritis, mydriasis
- Accommodative paralysis
- Papilledema
- Optic neuritis
- Myasthenic block
- Nystagmus
- Visual field defects
- Scotomas
- Pseudotumor cerebri.

Vitamins

Vitamin A
- Diplopia, yellow vision
- Red dyschromatopsia
- Calcium deposits in conjunctiva, cornea and sclera

- Miosis
- Retinal hemorrhages, optic atrophy
- Papilledema, exophthalmos
- Strabismus, nystagmus
- Scotomas
- Pseudotumor cerebri

Vitamin D
- Diplopia
- Visual hallucinations
- Calcium deposits in cornea, sclera
- Decreased pupil light reflex
- Cataract
- Retinal hemorrhages
- Papilledema
- Optic atrophy/Neuritis
- Small optic disc
- Strabismus
- Narrowed optic foramina
- Nystagmus
- Hemianopia
- Extraocular muscle paresis.

Sildenafil (Viagra)

It can cause:
- Retinal dysfunction
- Affect visual function for about 5 hours
- Visual disturbances include bluish color tinge, light sensitivity and blurred vision.

Vigabatrin

- Symptomatic or asymptomatic field loss
- Bilateral peripheral concentric constriction
- Visual field defects
- Tunnel vision.

Isotretinoin

- Impaired dark adaptations
- Glare sensitivity
- Blepharoconjunctivitis
- Dry eye
- Contact lens intolerance
- Subepithelial corneal opacities.

Thioridazine

- Reduced visual acuity
- Color vision changes
- Disturbances in dark adaptation
- Pigmentary retinopathy.

Amiodarone

- Optic neuropathy or optic neuritis
- Visual impairment
- Keratopathy
- Bilateral corneal deposits
- Whorl like corneal opacity
- Lenticular opacity
- Glare and halos around light.

BIBLIOGRAPHY

1. Agarwal A. Textbook of Ophthalmology, 1st edn. New Delhi: Jaypee Brothers Medical Publishers, 2002.
2. Bartlett JD. Clinical Ocular Pharmacology, 4th edn. Boston: Butterworth-Heinemann, 2001
3. Bartlett JD. Ophthalmic Drug Facts. Lippincott: William and Wilkins, 2001.
4. Crick RP, Trimble RB. Textbook of Clinical Ophthalmology. Hodder and Stoughton, 1986.
5. Duane TD. Clinical Ophthalmology, 4th edn. Boston: Butterworth-Heinemann, 1999.
6. Duvall. Ophthalmic Medications and Pharmacology, Slack Inc, 1998.
7. Ellis PP. Ocular Therapeutics and Pharmacology, 7th edn. CV Mosby, 1985.
8. Fechner. Ocular Therapeutics, Slack Inc., 1998.
9. Fraunfelder. Current Ocular Therapy, 5th edn. WB Saunders, 2000.
10. Garg A. Current Trends in Ophthalmology, 1st edn. New Delhi: Jaypee Brothers Medical Publishers, 1997.
11. Garg A. Manual of Ocular Therapeutics, 1st edn. New Delhi: Jaypee Brothers Medical Publishers, 1996.
12. Garg A. Ready Reckoner of Ocular Therapeutics, 1st edn. New Delhi: Jaypee Brothers Medical Publishers 2002.
13. Goodman LS, Gilman A. Pharmacological Basis of Therapeutics, 7th edn. New York: Macmillan, 1985.
14. Havener's. Ocular Pharmacology, 6th edn. CV Mosby, 1994.
15. Kanski. Clinical Ophthalmology, 4th edn. Butterworth-Heinemann, 1999.
16. Kershner. Ophthalmic Medications and Pharmacology, Slack. Inc., 1994.
17. Olin BR, et al. Drugs Facts and Comparisons: Facts and Comparisons. St. Louis, 1997.
18. Onofrey. The Ocular Therapeutics. Lippincott: William and Wilkins, 1997.
19. Rhee. The Wills Eye Drug Guide, Lippincott-William and Wilkins, 1998.
20. Steven Podos. Textbook of Ophthalmology, New Delhi: Jaypee Brothers Medical Publishers, 2001.
21. Zimmerman. Textbook of Ocular Pharmacology, Lippincott: William and Wilkins, 1997.

24

Topical and Systemic Ophthalmic Drugs with Common Dosages

Ashok Garg (India)

ANTIBIOTIC THERAPY

Topical Antibiotic Solutions and Ointments

Usual Dosage

Topical drops: Three to four times a day depending upon severity of the infection.

Ointment: One time preferably at bedtime, dosage can be increased depending upon severity of the infective condition.

- Gentamicin solution or ointment 0.3 percent
- Tobramycin solution or ointment 0.3 percent
- Amikacin solution 0.3 percent
- Sisomycin solution or ointment 0.3 percent
- Neomycin solution 0.17 percent and ointment 5 mg/g
- Framycetin solution or ointment 0.5 percent and 1.0 percent
- Chloramphenicol solution 0.4-1 percent and ointment 0.5 percent
- Erythromycin ointment 0.5 percent
- Polymyxin B solution 0.5-1.0 percent in combination with neomycin 0.35 percent ointment 1-1.5 mg/g with neomycin
- Polymyxin B 10000 units and bacitracin 500 units/g in ointment
- Sulfacetamide solution 10 percent, 20 percent, 30 percent and ointment 10 percent
- Sulfisoxazole solution or ointment 4 percent
- Tetracycline ointment or suspension 1 percent
- Chlortetracycline ointment 1 percent
- Trimethoprim 0.1 percent and polymyxin B 10000 units/ml
- Norfloxacin solution or ointment 0.3 percent
- Ciprofloxacin solution or ointment 0.3 percent
- Ofloxacin solution or ointment 0.3 percent
- Pefloxacin solution or ointment 0.3 percent
- Lomefloxacin solution or ointment 0.3 percent
- Sparfloxacin solution or ointment 0.3 percent
- Levofloxacin solution 0.5 percent
- Gemifloxacin solution 0.3 percent (under trials)
- Moxifloxacin solution 0.3 percent (under trials)
- Gatifloxacin solution 0.3 percent (under trials).

Systemic Antibiotics in Ophthalmology

Dosage

Standard dosage of systemic antibiotics is mentioned alongwith individual drug. However, dosage may vary depending upon type and severity of ocular infection being treated.

- Benzyl penicillin (penicillin G)—parenteral IM/IV 4–30 million units/24 hours in divided dosage 4–6 hourly.
- Phenoxymethyl penicillin—orally 200–500 mg 6 hourly
- Methicillin—parenteral IM/IV 1–2 g 4 hourly
- Cloxacillin—orally 250–500 mg 6 hourly
- Carboxypenicillin—parenteral 400–500 mg/kg/day 4 hourly
- Ampicillin—orally 250–500 mg 4–6 hourly or by parenteral route
- Amoxicillin—orally 250–500 mg 4–6 hourly
- Cefazolin—parenteral dose 1–6 g/day 6–8 hourly
- Cephalothin—parenteral dose 2–12 g/day 6–8 hourly
- Cephapirin—parenteral 1–2 g every 4 hours
- Cephaloridine—parenteral 2–4 g/day 6 hourly
- Cephradine—oral, IM/IV: 0.5–1 g 6 hourly
- Cephalexin—oral 0.5–1 g 6 hourly
- Cefadroxil—oral 1 g 12 hourly
- Cefaclor—oral 0.5–1 g 8 hourly
- Cefamandole—parenteral 1 g 4 hourly
- Cefoxitin—parenteral 1–2 g 4 hourly
- Cefuroxime—parenteral 750 mg–1.5 g 8 hourly
- Cefonicid—parenteral 1–2 g 24 hourly
- Ceforanide—parenteral 1 g 12 hourly
- Cefotiam—parenteral 1 g 12 hourly
- Cefotetan—parenteral 1 g every 12 hourly
- Cefotaxime—parenteral 1–2 g 4–6 hourly
- Cefoperazone—parenteral 1–4 g 4–8 hourly
- Cefixime—200–400 mg/day
- Cefsulodin—parenteral 0.5–1 g 6–12 hourly
- Ceftazidime—parenteral 1–2 g 8–12 hourly
- Ceftizoxime—parenteral 1–2 g 8–12 hourly
- Netilmicin—parenteral 3–6.5 mg/kg/day 8 hourly
- Kanamycin—parenteral 15 mg/kg/day 8 hourly
- Doxycycline—oral 100–200 mg/dose 2–24 hourly
- Chlortetracycline—oral 250–500 mg/dose 6 hourly
- Methacycline—oral 150–300 mg/dose 6–12 hourly
- Minocycline—parenteral 200 mg/dose
- Oxytetracycline—oral 500 mg 6 hourly
- Sulfonamides—parenteral 100 mg/kg/day 6–8 hourly, oral dose 2–4 g/day 6 hourly
- Erythromycin—oral 1–2 g/day 6 hourly, parenteral 1–4 g/day continuous drip
- Roxithromycin—oral 150 mg BD before food intake
- Clindamycin—parenteral 1–3 g/day 6 hourly, oral 600 mg–1.8 g/day 6 hourly
- Vancomycin—parenteral 2 g/day 6–12 hourly
- Spiramycin—oral 6–9 million IU/day in 2–3 divided doses

- Azithromycin—oral 500 mg–1 g once daily
- Clarithromycin—oral 200–500 mg BD
- Norfloxacin—oral 400 mg BD, parenteral 200–400 µg/day 12 hourly
- Ciprofloxacin—oral 500–1500 mg/day 6 hourly, parenteral 5–10 mg/kg/day 12 hourly
- Ofloxacin—oral 200–400 mg 6 hourly, parenteral 100–200 mg/day/12 hourly, IV infusion—200 mg infusion over 30 minutes BD
- Pefloxacin—oral 400 mg BD, IV infusion 400 mg in 100 ml of 5 percent dextrose solution infusion over one hour
- Lomefloxacin—oral 400 mg once daily
- Sparfloxacin—oral 400 mg in divided doses
- Gemifloxacin—oral 400 mg in divided doses
- Moxifloxacin—oral 400 mg in divided doses
- Levofloxacin—oral 500 mg in divided doses
- Gatifloxacin—oral 400 mg in divided doses
- Metronidazole oral 400–800 mg every 8 hourly, infusion 15 mg/kg infusion over 30–60 minutes BD
- Cotrimoxazole oral 1 tablet (double strength BD (trimethoprim 160 mg and sulfamethoxazole 800 mg), parenteral 20 mg TMP/kg/day 8 hourly.

TOPICAL ANTI-INFLAMMATORY THERAPY

Corticosteroids

Dosage: Disease specific

- Hydrocortisone
Acetate suspension	0.5–2.5 percent
Acetate solution	0.2 percent
Acetate ointment	1.5 percent
- Prednisolone
Acetate suspension	0.12 percent, 0.25 percent and 1.0 percent
Sodium phosphate solution	0.12 percent, 0.5 percent and 1.0 percent
Phosphate solution	0.5 percent
Phosphate ointment	0.25 percent
- Dexamethasone
Sodium phosphate solution	0.1 percent, 0.05 percent and 0.01 percent
Suspension	0.1 percent
Sodium phosphate ointment	0.05 percent
- Betamethasone
Sodium phosphate solution	0.1 percent
Sodium phosphate ointment	0.1 percent
- Triamcinolone acetonide
Suspension	0.1 percent
Ointment	0.1 percent
- Progesterone-like agents
Medrysone suspension	0.1 percent

- Fluorometholone
  Suspension   0.1 and 0.25 percent (FML forte)
  Ointment   0.1 percent
- Fluorometholone acetate
  suspension   0.1 percent
- Rimexolone suspension   0.1 percent
- Loteprednol etabonate
  solution   1 percent and 0.5 percent

Corticosteroid Antibiotic Combinations

Dosage: Based on desired corticosteroid dose and disease specific

- Dexamethasone (0.1%) with neomycin (0.5%) in the form of ophthalmic solution.
- Dexamethasone (0.1%) with neomycin (0.35%) and polymyxin B (10000 units/ml) suspension or ointment.
- Dexamethasone (0.1%) with chloramphenicol (0.5-1%) solution.
- Dexamethasone (0.1%) with ciprofloxacin (0.3%) solution.
- Dexamethasone (0.1%) with lomefloxacin (0.3%) suspension.
- Dexamethasone (0.1%) with sparfloxacin (0.3%) suspension.
- Dexamethasone (0.1%) with framycetin (0.3%) suspension.
- Dexamethasone (0.1%) with tobramycin (0.3%) suspension.
- Dexamethasone (0.1%) with chloramphenicol (1%) and polymyxin B 5000 IU solution and ointment.
- Dexamethasone (0.1%) with gentamicin (0.3%) solution.
- Betamethasone (0.1%) with neomycin (0.5%) solution.
- Betamethasone (0.1%) with chloramphenicol (0.5%) in solution and ointment.
- Betamethasone (0.1%) with gentamicin (0.3%) solution.
- Hydrocortisone (0.5%) with neomycin (0.5%) ointment and solution.
- Hydrocortisone (1.5%) and neomycin (0.5%) ointment.
- Hydrocortisone (10 mg/g), polymyxin B 0.5 mg/g, bacitracin 400 units/g and neomycin 5 mg/g ointment.
- Hydrocortisone (1%) with gentamicin (0.3%) suspension.
- Hydrocortisone (0.5%) with chloramphenicol (1.0%) ointment.
- Hydrocortisone (0.5%) with chloramphenicol (0.5%) solution.
- Prednisolone (1%) with gentamicin (0.3%) suspension.
- Prednisolone (0.2%) with sulfacetamide (10%) and phenylephrine (0.12%) solution.
- Fluorometholone (0.1%) with neomycin (0.35%) in solution.
- Fluorometholone (0.1%) with gentamicin (0.9%) in solution.
- Fluorometholone (0.1%) with tobramycin (0.3%) in solution.
- Prednisolone (0.5%) neomycin (0.35%) and polymyxin B 10,000 units/ml suspension.

Topical Nonsteroidal Anti-inflammatory Drugs (NSAIDs)

- Flurbiprofen—0.03 percent solution
  Dosage 1 drop every 30 minutes, 2 hours preoperatively (total dose—4 drops) to prevent intraoperative miosis.

- Diclofenac—0.1-1 percent solution
  Dosage 3-4 times a day for 2 weeks for postoperative inflammation and also useful qid for several weeks in cystoid macular edema (CME).
- Suprofen—1.0 percent solution
  Dosage 2 drops at 1, 2 and 3 hours preoperatively or every 4 hours while awake on the day of surgery.
- Ketorolac—0.5 percent solution
  Dosage 3-4 times a day till the desired effect is obtained.
- Indomethacin
  Suspension—0.5-1.0 percent
  Solution—0.1 percent
  Dosage Four times a day.
- Aspirin—1 percent solution, four times a day
- Acetyl salicyclic acid—0.03 percent solution, four times a day.
- Diflunisol—0.03 percent solution, four times a day.
- Oxyphenbutazone—10 percent ointment, 1-2 times.
- Phenylbutazone—10 percent ointment, 1-2 times.

Immunosuppressive Agents in Ophthalmology

Alkylating Agents

- *Cyclophosphamide:* Usual dose is 150-200 mg/day (1-2 mg/kg/day) to be taken orally empty stomach. After 7 days (WBC count) dosage may be reduced by 25-50 mg to stabilize the WBC at about 3000 cells/μl.
- *Chlorambucil:* Start at 0.1-0.2 mg/kg/day orally and increase every 3-4 day to a total dosage of 10-12 mg/day.

Antimetabolites

- *Azathioprine:* Orally start at 1-2 mg/kg/day and gradually increase to 2.5 mg/kg/day.
- *Methotrexate:* Dose is variable due to high drug toxicity for first 1-4 weeks orally then IM/IV dose of 2.5-15 mg is given over 36-48 hours.

Cyclosporin A

Oral 2.5-5 mg/kg/day in an olive oil with milk or juice. Maximum dose 10 mg/kg/day.

ANTIVIRAL THERAPY

Idoxuridine
Solution—0.1 percent and ointment—0.5 percent

Usual dose: Solution one drop every hour during day and every 2-3 hours at night.
Ointment can be applied 4-6 times a day.

Vidarabine (Ara-A)
Ointment—0.3 percent

Intravenous infusion—200 mg/ml
Topical ointment to be applied 5 times a day for 14–21 days.

Trifluridine (TFT)
Solution 1 percent
Dose: 6–9 times a day for 14 days.

Cytarabine
Ointment—1 percent
Injection form 100 mg/500 mg/1000 mg/ml
Ointment to be put in 6–9 times a day for 14 days
Systemic form dose is 100 mg/ml/24 hours.

Acyclovir
- Ointment 3 percent
  Dose: 5 times a day for 4 days
- Oral tablet—200 mg, 400 mg and 800 mg.
  Dose: 200–800 mg is given 5 times a day for 10 days.
- For IV preparation 250 mg powder is available.
  Dose: 5 mg/kg body weight 8 hourly for 5–10 days.

BVDU (Bromovinyldeoxyuridine)
- Solution—0.1 percent
  Dose: 1–2 drops 8–9 times a day.
- Injection 7.5–15 mg/kg/day in 3 divided doses for 5 days.

Interferons
Parenteral—30–400 million/ml once or twice a day for 14 days.

Zidovudine (AZT) Oral capsule 100 mg
Dose: 100–200 mg 8 hourly.

Famciclovir
Dose: 500–700 mg three times a day for 7 days.

Ganciclovir
Parenteral (IV)—5 mg/kg body weight for 14–21 days followed by a maintenance dose of 5 mg/kg/day for 5 days a week.
Orally—500 mg 6 hourly or 1 g three times a day.

Foscarnet
Dose: IV 60 mg/kg over 1 hour, 8 hourly for 14–21 days. Maintenance dose is 90–120 mg/kg IV over 2 hours once daily.

Cidofovir (HPMPC)
Parenteral IM/IV 20–100 µg

Lobucavir
Oral 400 mg twice daily.

Indinavir
Oral 800 mg 8 hourly empty stomach.

Ritonavir
Oral 600 mg/12 hours immediately after food.

Saquinavir
Oral 600 mg every 8 hours to be taken within 2 hours following meals.

Nelfinavir
Oral 750 mg three times a day.

Valaciclovir
Oral 1000 mg thrice a day for 7 days.

ANTIFUNGAL THERAPY

Nystatin
Topical ointment containing 100000 IU of nystatin.
Dose: 4–5 times a day till the ulcer heals.

Amphotericin B
Topical solution—0.075–0.3 percent in distilled water or dextrose 5 percent in water solution.
Dose: To be instilled at hourly interval.

Natamycin
Ophthalmic suspension—5 percent
Dose: 1–2 drops 4–6 times a day for 14 days.

Clotrimazole
Topical solution 1 percent
Dose: One drop on hourly basis over the days.

Miconazole
Ophthalmic solution and applicaps—1 percent
Dose: One drop every hour.

Econazole
Ointment—1 percent
Fresh ophthalmic solution—1 percent
Dose: 4–6 times a day.

Ketoconazole
- Oral in tablet form
  Dose: 200–800 mg/24 hours as a single daily dose
- Fresh topical preparation (1–5%).

Fluconazole
- Ophthalmic solution—0.3 percent
  Dose: One drop at every 4 hour interval
- Oral tablet—200–600 mg/day for 21 days.

Itraconazole
Oral—200 mg twice daily for a week.

Flucytosine
- Oral as 250 mg and 500 mg capsules
  Dose: 50–150 mg/kg/day divided in 4 doses for a week.
- Topical solution 1 percent
  Dose: One drop every hour.

Silver Sulfadiazine
Ophthalmic solution and applicaps—1 percent
Dose: One drop at hourly interval initially then tapering to 4 times a day over 14–21 days.

Terbinafine
Oral as 125 mg and 250 mg tablets
Dose: 250 mg once a day for 2-4 weeks.

ANTIGLAUCOMA THERAPY

Miotics

Acetylcholine: Available as powder and fresh ophthalmic solution (1:100) is prepared before use.
Dose: 0.5-2 ml of this solution is given through intracameral route to produce good miosis.

Pilocarpine
- Pilocarpine hydrochloride as topical solution in strengths of 0.25 percent, 0.50 percent, 1 percent, 2 percent, 3 percent, 4 percent, 6 percent, 8 percent and 10 percent.
- Pilocarpine nitrate in strength of 1 percent, 2 percent and 4 percent eyedrops.
  Dose: Normally 0.5-4 percent concentrations are used and dosage is one drop three times a day.
- Pilocarpine ocusert P20 and P40
- Pilocarpine 4 percent gel (at bedtime)
- Piloplex (twice a day has more effect than plain pilocarpine)
- Pilocarpine and epinephrine combination.
  Solution (pilocarpine strength varies from 1-6 percent and epinephrine 1% solution)
  Dose: To instill 1-2 drops in the affected eyes 1-4 times a day.
- Pilocarpine—physostigmine combination. Topical solution containing pilocarpine 2 percent and physostigmine 0.25 percent.
  Dose: Instill 1-2 drops 4 times a day.
- Pilocarpine nitrate 1 percent with clonidine 0.125 percent.

Carbachol: Topical solution in strengths of 0.75 percent, 1.5 percent, 2.25 percent and 3 percent.
Dose: 1-2 drops in the eyes up to 3 times a day. Intracameral dose is 0.5 ml into the anterior chamber during ocular surgery. For intracameral use it is available in the concentration of 0.01 percent in 1.5 ml ampoules.

Physostigmine: Topical solution 0.25 percent and 0.5 percent
Dose: Instill 2 drops 4 times a day.

Demecarium: Solution—0.125 and 0.25 percent
Dose: 1-2 drops twice a day.

Echothiophate: Solution—0.03 percent, 0.06 percent, 0.125 percent and 0.25 percent.
Dose: 1-2 drops twice day.

Isofluorophate: Ointment 0.025 percent in polyethylene mineral oil gel.
Dose: Instill 0.25 inch strip oint once every night.

Alpha-adrenergic Agonists

Apraclonidine: Solution—0.5 and 1 percent
Dose: One drop 1 hour before laser surgery and one drop immediately after the procedure or three times a day as adjunct to other glaucoma therapy.

Clonidine: Solution: 0.125 percent, 0.25 percent and 0.50 percent
Dose: One drop three times a day.

(a) Brimonidine (Alphagan): Topical solution 0.2 percent
Dose One drop two times daily.

(b) Alphagan P: Topical brimonidine purite solution 0.2 percent
Dose: One drop two times daily.

(c) Topical Brimonidine (0.2%) solution with Timolol Maleate: (0.5%)
Dose: One drop two times daily.

Dapirazole
Dose: Two drops followed 5 minutes later by 2 drops to reverse mydriasis by phenylephrine and tropicamide.

Sympathomimetics

Epinephrine: Available as the hydrochloride, borate and bitartrate salts as topical solution in strengths of 0.5–2 percent.
Dose: 1 drop three times a day.

Dipivefrine: Topical solution 0.1 percent
Dose: One drop two times a day.

Adrenergic Blocking Agents (Beta-blockers)

Usual dose: Two times a day

Betaxolol: Solution—0.25 percent and 0.5 percent

Carteolol: Solution—0.1 percent

Levobunolol: Solution—0.25 percent and 0.5 percent
Dose: 1–2 drops once a day.

Metipranol: Solution—0.1 percent, 0.3 percent and 0.6 percent

Timolol: Solution—0.25 percent and 0.5 percent, and ophthalmic gel—0.25 percent and 0.5 percent.

Carbonic Anhydrase Inhibitors

Acetazolamide
- Oral tablets 125 mg, 250 mg, and 500 mg sustained release capsules.
  Dose: 250 mg 6 hourly or 500 mg capsule twice a day.
- Parenteral dose—250–500 mg powder/5–10 ml distilled water.
- Topical ophthalmic solution—5 percent
  Dose: One drop 2–3 times a day.

Dichlorphenamide: Oral tablet of 50 mg
Dose: 100 mg every 12 hourly.

Methazolamide: Oral as 25 mg and 50 mg tablets.
Dose: 50–100 mg 2–3 times a day.

Dorzolamide
- Topical ophthalmic solution—2 percent
- Combination of topical dorzolamide (2%) with timolol maleate (0.5%).
  Dose: One drop three times a day for solo dorzolamide 2 percent solution.
- One drop two times a day for combination drop.

Brinzolamide: Ophthalmic suspension—1 percent
Dose: One drop three times a day.

Ethoxazolamide: Oral as 125 mg tablets
Dose: 125 mg tablet four times a day.

Prostaglandins

Latanoprost (Xalantan): Topical ophthalmic solution—0.005 percent.
Dose: One drop once daily preferably in the evening.

Xalcom: Topical latanoprost 0.005 percent and timolol maleate 0.5 percent solution.
Dose: 1 drop once daily preferably in the evening.

Unoprostone (Rescula): Topical ophthalmic solution—0.12 percent.
Dose: One drop twice daily.

Bimatoprost (Lumigan): Topical ophthalmic solution 0.03 percent
Dose: 1 drop once daily preferable at bedtime.

Travoprost (Travatan): Topical ophthalmic solution 0.004 percent
Dose: 1 drop once daily preferable at bedtime.

Ocular Hypotensive Lipids

Topical ophthalmic solution—0.01 percent.
Dose: One drop twice daily.

Hyperosmotic Agents

Glycerin: Oral solution as 50 percent and 75 percent lime flavored.
Dose: 1.0–1.5 gm/kg body weight given 1–1.5 hours before surgery.

Isosorbide: Oral solution as 45 percent mint flavored.
Dose: 1–2 g/kg given 2–4 times a day.

Mannitol: As solution in 5–25 percent.
Dose: 0.5–2.0 g IV body weight given as usual 15–20 percent solution over a period of as short as 30 minutes.
Urea powder: As 30 percent solution.
Dose: 0.5–2 g/kg IV.

Antimetabolites/Antifibroproliferative Agents

5-Fluorouracil (5 FU)
Dose: For subconjunctival route freshly prepared during filtering surgery, 0.5 cc of solution containing 5 mg of 5 FU (prepared from commercially available 50–10 mg/ml in physiological saline).

Postoperatively 5 mg of 5 FU injection is given subconjunctivally over a 2-week period.

Mitomycin C
Dose: Applied once at the time of glaucoma surgery. 3 × 2 mm cellular sponge moistened with a 0.02–0.04 mg/ml (0.02–0.04%) mitomycin C applied to the bed of trabeculectomy flap for 4–5 minutes.

Daunorubicin
Dose: Intraoperatively it is given on 4 × 4 mm cellulose sponge soaked in daunorubicin (0.2 mg/ml) 0.25 ml is applied below the conjunctival flap over the proposed site of trabeculectomy for 4 minutes.

Neuroprotective and Neuroregenerative Agents

Alpha-2 Agonists

Brimonidine (Alphagan)
Dosage: Already mentioned.

N-methyl-O-aspartate antagonists (on trials)
- Memantine
- Eliprodil
- Riluzole
- L-Deprenyl.

ANTIALLERGY THERAPY

Topical Mast Cell Inhibitors

Cromolyn sodium: Topical ophthalmic solution as 2 percent and 4 percent.
Dose: 1–2 drops 4–6 times a day.

Disodium cromoglycate (DSCG): Solution—2 percent.
Dose: 1–2 drops 3–4 times a day.

Lodoxamide: Ophthalmic suspension—0.1 percent.
Dose: 1–2 drops 4 times a day.

Nedocromil: Ophthalmic solution—1 percent.
Dose: 1–2 drops 4 times a day.

Olopatadine: Solution in 0.05 percent. and 1 percent.
Dose: 1–2 drops 3 times a day.

Azelastine hydrochloride: Ophthalmic solution 0.05 percent
Dose: 1–2 drops 2–4 times a day.

Ketotifen (Topical): Solution in 0.025 percent
Dose: 1–2 drops 2 times a day.

Drugs on trials:
- Nicotinamide
- Picumast
- Calmodulin.

Antihistamines

Usual Dose

1–2 drops 3–4 times a day.

Pheniramine maleate: 0.3 percent ophthalmic solution with 0.025 percent naphazoline HCl.

Pheniramine maleate: 0.5 percent ophthalmic solution with 0.125 percent phenylephrine HCl.

Pyrilamine maleate: 0.1 percent solution with 0.12 percent phenylephrine HCl and 0.1 percent antipyrine.

Antazoline: 0.5 percent solution with 0.05 percent naphazoline HCl.

Topical levocabastine: HCl 0.05 percent suspension available without decongestant.

Tetrahydrozoline: 0.05 percent solution with zinc sulfate (0.25%).

Levocetrizine: It is a new highly effective and well-tolerated antihistamine. Levocetrizine being the potent single isomer of cetrizine binds twice as strongly to histamine H1 receptors and has a highly consistent and predictable antihistamine action.
It is available as 5 mg tablet.
Dosage: 5 mg orally once or twice daily. It is indicated for the treatment of allergic conjunctivitis.

Desloratadine: It is active metabolite of loratadine and is indicated for use in seasonal allergic conjunctivitis. Desloratadine possesses pharmacodynamic activity similar to that of loratadine but has a relative potency 10–20 times greater than loratadine. It is available as 5 mg tablet.
Dosage: Is 5 mg orally once daily.

Decongestants

Phenylephrine HCl: Topical solution of 0.125 percent.
Dose: 1–2 drops 2–4 times daily (0.12 solution).

Naphazoline HCl: Topical solution as 0.012–0.1 percent.
Dose: 1–2 drops every 2–4 hours.

Tetrahydrazoline: Topical solution alone or in combination with antihistamines in concentration of 0.05 percent.
Dose: 1–2 drops 2–4 times a day.

Oxymetazoline HCl: Topical solution as 0.025 percent.
Dose: 1–2 drops every 8 hourly.

Rose petal aqueous infusion: Topical solution (aqueous infusion in 7.5 ml with 0.1% thiomersal).
Dose: 1–2 drops thrice a day.

Ephedrine: Topical solution 0.05 percent.
Dose: 1–2 drops 3 times a day.

Emedastine: Topical solution 1–2 drop 3 times a day.

Topical NSAIDs

Suprofen: Topical solution—0.1 percent.
Dose: 1–2 drops three times a day.

Ketorolac: Topical solution—0.5 percent.
Dose: 1–2 drops 3–4 times a day.

Topical Steroids

Usual dose: 1–2 drops 3–4 times a day
- Loteprednol (0.5%) solution
- Rimexolone (1%) solution
- Fluorometholone (0.3%) solution.

Topical Immunosuppressors

- *Cyclosporine:* Topical ophthalmic solution 2 percent.
  Dose: One drop 4 times a day.
- Competitive inhibitors of IgE binding to effector cells (on trials).
- Adhesion protein molecules (on trials)
- Cytokine modulators (on trials).

LOCAL ANESTHETIC AGENTS

Injectable Agents

Esters

Procaine: Available as 1 percent (2 ml) ampoules.
Dose: 14 mg/kg body weight (in concentration of 0.5–2%).

Chloroprocaine: Solution in concentration of 0.5–2 percent.

Tetracaine: Solution as 0.25–2 percent.
Dose: 1.5 mg/kg body weight.

Amides

Lidocaine: Solution in concentration of 0.5–4 percent.
  For infiltration anesthesia generally 1–2 percent concentration are used.

Various lidocaine combinations available are:
- Lidocaine HCl 1.5–5 percent with 7.5 percent dextrose
- Preservative free 1 percent lidocaine HCl ampoules (0.5 ml) for intracameral use during intraocular surgery.

Prilocaine: Solution as 0.5–3 percent.
Dose: 10 mg/kg body weight.

Mepivacaine: Injectable solution as 1–2 percent.
Dose: 7.0 mg/kg body weight.

Bupivacaine: As bupivacaine injectable solution in concentration of 0.25–0.75 percent.
Dose: 2.0 mg/kg body weight.

Etidocaine: Solution as 0.5–1 percent.
 Combination (etidocaine 1.0–1.5% with 1:20000 epinephrine).

Centbucridine: Solution as 0.5 percent.

Topical Anesthetic Agents

Usual dose: 1–2 drops for temporary (15–20 minutes) anesthesia to allow ocular examination and manipulation
- Benoxinate HCl (0.4%) topical solution
- Proparacaine (0.5 and 0.75%) solution
- Tetracaine (0.25–1%) solution
- Lidocaine HCl (4%) solution
- Centbucridine (1%) solution
- Cocaine (2%) solution
- Phenocaine (1%) solution
- Dimethocaine (2.5%) solution
- Piperocaine (2%) solution
- Dibucaine (0.1%) solution
- Naepaine (2–4%) solution
- Butacaine (2%) solution.

Out of these practically topical benoxinate, proparacaine, tetracaine, lidocaine and centbucridine ophthalmic solutions are used in day-to-day practice.

MYDRIATICS AND CYCLOPLEGICS

Mydriatic Adrenergic Agents

Adrenaline (epinephrine)
Dose: It produces dilation after the instillation of 4 drops of 1:1000 solution.

Cocaine HCl: Solution as 2 percent and 4 percent drops.

Phenylephrine: Topical solution in concentration of 2.5–10 percent.
Dose: One drop 2–3 times.

Hydroxyamphetamine: Topical solution 1 percent.
Dose: One drop 2–3 times.

Cholinergic Antagonist as Cycloplegic Mydriatics

Atropine sulfate: Topical solution in concentration of 0.5 percent, 1 percent, 2 percent and 3 percent.
 Ointment—5 percent and 1 percent concentration
 Dose: 1 drop 2-4 times as needed
 Ointment 1-2 times as required

Homatropine: Topical solution 2 percent and 5 percent
Dose: One to 2 drops 3-4 times as required

Scopolamine: Solution—0.25 percent
Dose: One drop 2-4 times for 7 days

Cyclopentolate HCl: Topical solution : 0.05 percent, 1 percent and 2 percent
Dose: One drop 3-4 times as required

Tropicamide: Topical solution—0.5 percent, 1 percent
Dose: One drop 3-4 times as needed.

Mydriatic Combinations

Usual dose: One drop 3-4 times as required
- Phenylephrine 5 percent and cyclopentolate HCl 1 percent
- Phenylephrine 10 percent and scopolamine 0.3 percent
- Phenylephrine 5 percent and tropicamide 0.8 percent
- Cyclopentolate HCl 1 percent with dexamethasone sodium phosphate 0.1 percent
- Atropine sulfate 1 percent solution with dexamethasone sodiumphosphate 0.1 percent.

ARTIFICIAL TEARS AND LUBRICANTS

Methylcellulose or Ethylcellulose Base

- *Hydroxypropylmethylcellulose* 0.5 percent or 1 percent with 0.01 percent *benzalkonium chloride*
- *Hydroxyethylcellulose* 0.5 percent with *povidone* and water soluble polymers, thiomerosal 0.004 percent and EDTA 1 percent
- *Carboxymethylcellulose (CMC)* in concentration of 0.5 percent preservative free

 Usual dosage: 1-2 drops 4-6 times a day

Polyvinyl Alcohol-base Solutions

- *Polyvinyl alcohol:* 1.4 percent and povidone 0.6 percent with chlorbutanol 0.5 percent and NaCl
 Dose: 1-2 drops 4-6 times a day

Longer Lasting Mucoadhesive or Increased Viscosity Agents

- Polycarbophil and dextran
- Methylcellulose
  These solutions are preservative free
  Dose: 1–2 drops 4–6 times a day.

Polyvinylpyrrolidone Polymer-base Tear Solution

1. Adsorbonac sodium chloride 2 percent or 5 percent solutions
2. Salt solution with zinc and glycerin
   - Electrolyte-based solution
   Dose: 1–2 drops 4 times a day.

Ointments

- Containing petrolatum (55.5%), lanolin (2%) and mineral oil (42.5%) (preservative free)
  Dose: Apply 0.25–0.50 inch ribbon of ointment preferably at bedtime
- Ocular lubricant ointment (gee) containing hydroxypropyl-methylcellulose (2%) with, NaCl, KCl, CaCl, $MgCl_2$, sodium acetate and sodium citrate (preservative-free).
- Lubricant gel carbopal 980 (polyacryclic acid) which transforms from gel to liquid upon contact with the ocular tissue.

Ocular Inserts (Solid Devices)

- Preservative-free water-soluble polymeric insert (Lacrisert) containing 5 mg of hydroxypropylmethylcellulose.

Punctal Plugs

- Silicone plug in 0.3, 0.5, 0.6, 0.7 and 0.8 mm sizes alongwith inserter tool
- Collagen implants—in 0.2, 0.3, 0.5 and 0.6 mm sizes.

Miscellaneous Preparations

- Topical solution containing 2.5 percent hydroxypropylmethyl-cellulose with boric acid, ethylene diaminetetra-acetic acid (EDTA) and 0.01 percent benzalkonium chloride for gonio-scopic examinations.
- Topical solution containing 0.25 percent tyloxapol and 0.02 percent benzalkonium chloride for use as cleaning, wetting and lubricating agent.

Dose: Instill 1–2 drops on to artificial eye 3–4 times a day.

OPHTHALMIC VISCOSURGICAL DEVICES

- *Sodium hyaluronate:* Available as preloaded syringe with 27G, 30G cannula containing sodium hyaluronate 10 mg/ml or 14 mg/ml, store at 2–8°C. Do not freeze. Use the drug at room temperature only.
- *Hyalectin:* Highly viscous 1 percent solution of sodium hyaluronate of lower molecular weight
- Solution containing combination (3:1 mixture) of 3 percent sodium hyaluronate and 4 percent chondroitin sulfate with 0.45 mg sodium dihydrogen phosphate and NaCl.
- Chondroitin sulfate as 20 percent solution with 30G cannula
- Hydroxypropyl methylcellulose 2 percent solution in 2 ml vials or prefilled sterilized disposable syringes with 27G cannula
- Polyacrylamide: Orcolon (low concentration polyacrylamide 4.5 mg/ml) solution with 27G cannula
- Collagen (1.4% collagen type IV) viscoelastic agent.

New Agents on Trial

- *Poly-TEGA* 40 percent (triethyleneglycol monomethacrylate)
- *Poly-GLYMA* (glycerol monomethacrylate).

IRRIGATING SOLUTIONS

Intraocular Irrigating Solutions

BSS Containing

- 0.64 percent NaCl, 0.75 percent KCl, 0.03 percent magnesium chloride.
- 0.043 percent calcium chloride, 0.39 percent sodium acetate.
- 0.17 percent sodium citrate and sodium hydroxide.

BSS Plus (Mix aseptically before use)

Part I—480 ml containing 7.44 mg NaCl, 0.395 mg KCl, 0.433 mg sodium phosphate, 2.19 mg sodium bicarbonate, sodium hydroxide/ml.

Part II—20 ml containing 3.85 mg calcium chloride dihydrate, 5 mg magnesium chloride hexahydrate, 23 mg dextrose and 4.6 mg glutathione disulfide/ml.

These solutions are used during any type of intraocular surgery including phacoemulsification.

Extraocular Irrigating Solutions

These solutions are used for general ophthalmic use including short procedure (excluding intraocular surgery). EIS containing 0.49 NaCl, 0.075 KCl, 0.048 percent CaCl, 0.03 percent magnesium chloride, 0.39 percent sodium acetate, 0.17 percent sodium citrate with 0.013 percent benzalkonium chloride.

SURGICAL ENZYMES

Alpha-chymotrypsin: Available as powder for ophthalmic solution containing 150 units or 300 units with 2 ml sodium chloride diluant per dual chamber univial. Available as 750 units per vial with 9 ml BSS diluant.

Urokinase
Dose: 5000 units of urokinase are dissolved in 2 ml of normal saline. Useful for dissolving blood clot of coagulated hyphema.

Hyaluronidase: Available as odorless fluffy powder containing 300 units of activity per mg. Freshly prepared before use for local ocular anesthesia.

Chelating Agents and Mucolytics

- Sodium EDTA (0.01% solution)
- Laevocysteine (0.1–0.2 molar concentration)
- Acetylcysteine (as eyedrops in concentration of 5%, 10% and 20%).

Caustic Preparations

- Pure carbolic acid
- 100% alcohol
- Hydrogen peroxide (2%).

Cyanoacrylate Tissue Adhesive

N-butyl-2 cyanoacrylate tissue adhesive is used for immediate wound closure in corneal perforations up to 3 mm in length.

SURGICAL ADJUNCTS

Fractionated Purified Silicone Oil

Fractionated purified sterile, apyrogenic silicone oil is commercially available for prolonged temponande after surgical treatment for severe retinal detachment specially retinal detachment with giant tears, proliferative vitreal retinopathy and traumatic retinal detachment.

It is available as 10 ml vial with special flip off seal in a sterile pouch. (Store it as 8–24°C). This vial is for single use only. Do not resterilize it. This purified silicone oil is free from toxic residual polymerization catalysts.

Polydimethyl Siloxane (Silicone Oil)

It is available as single use 10 and 15 ml vials (injections). It is used for retinal detachment surgery.

Povidone Iodine

It is used prior to eye surgery to prep the periocular region and irrigate the ocular surface.

It is available as 5 percent solution in 50 ml and 15 ml packs. Povidone iodine is indicated for external use only. It is not recommended for intraocular injection or irrigation.

Absorbable Gelatin Film

It is sterile film available in 100 mm × 125 mm and 25 mm × 50 mm sizes.

It is used in many surgical procedures including glaucoma filtration operations, extraocular muscle surgery, diathermy and scleral buckling operations.

Botulinum Toxin Type A

It is available as powder for injection (Lyophilized).

100 units of lyophilized *Clostridium botulinum* toxin type A.

It is supplied in vials (Preservative free) containing 0.05 mg albumin (human), 0.9 mg sodium chloride.

It is mainly used in the treatment of blepharospasm (to reduce excessive abnormal contractions).

TOPICAL IMMUNE THERAPY

Ophthalmic solution (Aspac) containing 0.1 percent each of IgG, IgA and 0.05 percent of IgM in fixed concentrations.

Store in refrigerator at 2–8°C when the vial is not opened. Once opened it can be stored at room temperature.

Dose: Instill 1–2 drops three to four times a day for a week postoperatively and then gradual tapering over next 7 days.

TOPICAL HYPEROSMOTIC AGENT

Hypertonic Salt Agent

- Topical NaCl solution as 2 percent and 5 percent with two water soluble polymers, 0.004 percent thimerosal and 0.1 percent EDTA.
- Topical NaCl solution 2 percent or 5 percent with hydroxypropylmethylcellulose and parabens.
- Five percent solution also contains propylkeneglycol sodium borate and boric acid.
  Usual dosage: 1–2 drops 4–6 times a day as required.
- Topical 6 percent NaCl ophthalmic gel with petrolatum and lanolin.
  Dose: 0.25 inch ribbon of ointment 1–2 times a day.

Glycerine Solution

Available as 50 percent solution of glycerol or propylene glycol with 0.55 percent chlorobutanol.

Dose: It is applied as slow drip in which many drops are instilled several seconds apart.

Glucoser 40 percent ophthalmic ointment in petrolatum and lanolin.

Emulsion of polyoxyethylene (0.4%) and silicone oil.

ANTICATARACT THERAPY

Topical Agents

- Aspirin 1 percent topical solution
- Sulindac 1 percent solution
- Glutathione 1 percent solution
- Benzyl alcohol—0.07 percent solution
- Catalin
  Topical ophthalmic solution in concentration of 0.75 mg/15 ml of solvent
- Cineraria maritima ophthalmic solution (15 ml)
- Topical solution containing—potassium iodide (3.3%), sodium chloride (0.83%) and calcium chloride (1.0%).

Usual dosage: 1-2 drops 3-4 times till required.

Systemic Therapy

Vitamin E Therapy

Dose: 200 mg capsules.

Antioxidant Therapy

- Mixcarotin soft gel capsules containing 15.44 mg of mixed carotenoids in oily suspension (alpha-carotene, beta-carotene, lutein, cryptoxanthin and zeaxanthin) equivalent to 25,000 IU of vitamin A.
  Dose: One capsule daily preferably at bedtime.
- Antioxidant capsule containing—zinc 30 mg, copper 1.5 mg, selenium 60 µg, manganese 5 mg, vitamin A 6000 IU, vitamin B_{12} 20 mg, vitamin C 200 mg and vitamin E 60 IU.
  Dose: One capsule daily preferably at bedtime.

Other Systemic Agents on Trials

- Sodium salicylate
- Clinoril
- GSH
- Cyclopenthiazide
- Tetramethylglutaric acid
- Spirohydantoin
- NSAIDs like naproxen, ansam, indomethacin, ibuprofen, oxyphenbutazone and paracetamol.

MEDICAL THERAPY FOR ARMD (AGE-RELATED MACULAR DEGENERATION)

Antioxidants

Mixcarotin soft gel capsules containing 15.44 of mixed carotenoids (alpha-carotene, beta-carotene, lutein, cryptoxanthin and zeaxanthin).
Dose: One capsule daily at bedtime.

Antiangiogenic Agents

- Interferon
- Thalidomide
- Retinoids
- Amitoride
- Beta-cyclodextrin
- AGM 1470.

Growth Factors

- *Isotretinoin*
- *VEGF.*

MEDICAL THERAPY FOR DIABETIC RETINOPATHY

- *D400*—available as tablet
  Dose: One tablet three times a day till required
- *Antioxidants*—containing beta-carotene, vitamin E, zinc
- *Aldose reductase inhibitors*
  - Sulindac (250 mg twice daily)
  - Ponalrestat (600 mg daily)
  - Indomethacin and sorbin (on trials).
- *Cyclooxygenase* inhibitors
  - Aspirin (325 mg twice daily)
  - Dipyridamole (225 mg daily)
  - Ticlopidine (500 mg daily).
- Cyclandelate 400 mg 4 times daily.
- Miscellaneous drugs (on trials)
  - Calcium dobesilate (Doxium)
  - Sulfonyl ureas
  - Pentoxyphylline
  - Antiangiogenic agents like interferon, retinoids, amiloride, thalidomide, VEGF inhibitor antibodies, isotretinoin and growth factors
  - Metabolic inhibitors
  - Vitamin E.

OPHTHALMIC DYES

Fluorescein Sodium

- Topical solution available as 2 percent solution
  Dose: Instill 1–2 drops of 2 percent solution for detection of foreign bodies and corneal abrasions

Topical solution contains:
- 0.25 percent fluorescein sodium
- 0.1 percent proparacaine HCl
- 0.01 percent thimerosal preservative.

Fluorescein strips—available as
- 1 mg strips (boric acid, polysorbate 80 and 0.5 percent chlorobutanol)
- 9 mg strips
- 0.6 mg and 1 mg strips
- High molecular fluorescein (Higlo) strips for soft lenses.

Intravenous fluorescein—for IV use it is available as 10 percent and 25 percent injections.

Oral fluorescein—can be given by mixing fluorescein powder or vial of 10 percent injectable fluorescein in a citrus drink.

Fluorexon

Available as 0.35 percent topical solution (in 0.5 ml pipettes)
Dose: Instill 1–2 drops.

Rose Bengal

Available as topical 1 percent solution containing 1 percent rose bengal with povidone, sodium borate
- PEG and 0.01 percent thimerosal
- Also available as 1.3 mg strip
  Dose: Topically instill 1–2 drops.
- *Lissamine green:* Available as sterile ophthalmic strips. Each strip contains approximately 15 mg of lissamine green.
- *Indocyanine green:* Indicated for digital indocyanine green videoangiography (ICG-V) and ICG-angiography-guided laser photocoagulation.
   It is available as powder for injection in 25 mg and 50 mg strengths alongwith aqueous solvent (pH 5.5–6.5).
   Aqueous solvent is specially prepared sterile water for injection to dissolve indocynanine green.
   Dosage: Use 40 mg dye in 2 ml of aqueous solvent. Immediately after injected dye bolus (IV) with a 5 ml bolus of normal saline. This injection regimen provides the optimal concentration of dye to the choroidal vasculature following IV injection. This dye is nontoxic on IV administration.
- Trypan blue is a dye which safely stains the anterior lens capsule during cataract surgery (ECCE, IOL surgery and phaco surgery). Trypan blue is a capsule stainer which reduces the risk of complication due to unrecognized radial capsule by facilitating the performance of the capsulorhexis in the absence of red fundus reflex specially in cases of matured cataract. Special feature of trypan blue is that it stains the anterior capsule without affecting the corneal endothelium. So blue stained capsule can be easily identified from the underlying unstained lenticular tissue.

It is available as 1 ml ampoule commercially. Each ml contains 0.6 mg trypan blue, 1.9 mg of sodium monohydrogen orthophosphate, 0.3 mg of sodium dihydrogen orthophosphate, 8.2 mg of sodium chloride and sodium hydroxide for adjusting the pH and water for injection.
- Visudyne (verteporfin) is a photosensitive second generation porphyrin (benzoporphyrin). Monoacid derivatives which has been recently approved by FDA (Food and Drug Administration) USA for the photodynamic therapy (PDT)—the drug/light combination for the treatment of wet age-related macular degeneration (ARMD). It requires a special diode laser for activation.
  - It has been launched commercially recently.
  - Dosage range is 6 mg/m^2
  - Fluence range—50 J/cm^2 and irradiation time is 15 min.

CONTACT LENS CARE PRODUCTS

Storage/soaking solutions: Solution containing polyvinyl alcohol with 0.01 percent benzalkonium chloride and 0.2 percent EDTA.

Wetting solution: Solution containing hydroxypropylmethylcellulose, polyvinyl alcohol, 0.004 percent benzalkonium chloride and 0.01 percent, EDTA.

Cleaning/soaking/wetting solution: Solution containing hydroxypropylmethylcellulose, boric acid, nonoxynol 15, 0.01 percent benzalkonium chloride and 0.01 percent EDTA.

Rewetting solutions: Solution containing povidone, water soluble polymers with 0.004 percent thimerosal and 0.1 percent EDTA.

Cleaning solutions and gel: Isotonic solutions polymeric cleaning agent, hydroxyethylcellulose, polysorbate 21, 0.1 percent EDTA and 0.01 percent polyquaternium-1.

Rigid Gas Permeable (RGP) Contact Lens Products

Disinfecting/wetting/soaking solution: Isotonic solution with polyvinyl alcohol, 0.003 percent chlorhexidine gluconate and 0.002 percent EDTA.

Cleaning/soaking solutions
- Solution containing hydrophilic polyelectrolyte, polyvinyl alcohol, hydroxyethylcellulose with chlorhexidine gluconate and EDTA.
- Tablet containing papain, NaCl, sodium carbonate, sodium borate and EDTA.

Soft (Hydrogel) Contact Lens Products

Rinsing/storage solutions: Isotonic buffered solution of NaCl, sodium hexametaphosphate, sodium borate, boric acid with 0.1 percent sorbic acid.

Surfactant cleaning solutions
- Isotonic polymeric cleaning agent, hydroxyethylcellulose, polysorbate 21. 0.1 percent EDTA and 0.01 percent polyquaternium 1.
- Solution with 20 percent isopropyl alcohol, poloxamer 407 and amphoteric 10.

Enzymatic cleaners: Tablet containing papain, NaCl, sodium carbonate, sodium borate and EDTA.

Rewetting solutions
- Isotonic solution with polyhexamethylene biguanide 0.001 percent, tromethamine 12 mg/ml, tyloxapol and disodium edetate.
- Isotonic solution with polyvinyl alcohol and 0.002 percent thimerosal and 0.01 percent EDTA.

Chemical disinfection systems: Solution containing 0.013 percent tris tallow ammonium chloride, 0.002 percent thimerosal, bis tallow ammonium chloride, sodium bicarbonate, sodium phosphate, propylene glycol, polysorbate 80 and special soluble poly-HEMA.

Multiaction disinfecting solution containing isotonic solution with NaCl, sodium borate, boric acid, poloxamine, 0.0005 percent polyaminopropyl biguanide and EDTA.

Topical comfort/complete eyedrops: It is isotonic polymeric aqueous solution consisting of EDTA, sodium chloride, potassium chloride with sorbic acid and boric acid. These topical eyedrops are used to relieve minor irritation, discomfort and blurring during soft, semisoft or hard contact lenses wear.

RECENT MULTIPURPOSE SOFT LENS CARE SYSTEMS

- *Multipurpose solution (Renu)* containing sterile isotonic solution with boric acid, disodium edetate, sodium borate and sodium chloride. Active ingredients are dymed 0.001 percent and hydranate 0.03 percent, poloxamine 1 percent.

This MP solution is used for cleaning, rinsing, disinfecting, lubricating and storing the soft contact lens. It cleans, disinfects and removes protein every day due to hydranate a unique agent.

Multipurpose solution containing (complete)
- Polyhexamethylene biguanide (PHMB) 0.001 percent
- Tyloxapol 0.025 percent
- Tromethamine 1.2 percent
- Edetate sodium 0.05 percent

This MP solution does not contain chlorhexidine, thimerosal or other mercury containing ingredients. In this MP solution PHMB acts as disinfectant. Tyloxapol acts as surfactant and lubricant. While tromethamine is biological buffer. This MP solution can be used for cleaning, rinsing, disinfecting, lubricating, storing and rewetting the soft contact lenses.

ANTIRETROVIRAL DRUGS IN OPHTHALMIC INFECTIONS

The currently approved antiretroviral drugs fall into following categories:

Nucleoside Reverse Transcriptase Inhibitors

Drugs of Nucleoside reverse transcriptase inhibitors (NRTIs) group are:
- Zidovudine
- Didanosine
- Lamivudine
- Stavudine
- Zalcitabine.

Non-nucleoside Reverse Transcriptase Inhibitors

Drugs of Non-nucleoside reverse transcriptase inhibitors (NNRTIs) group are:
- Nevirapine
- Delavirdine.

Protease Inhibitors

Drugs of this group are:
- Saquinavir
- Indinavir
- Ritonavir.

Antiviral Metabolities

- Ganciclovir
- Foscarnet
- Cidofovir/zidofovir (HPMPC).

Drug selection, administration and dosage in individual ocular infection in AIDS patients is described as follows:

Cytomegalovirus Infection

Retinitis is the most common manifestation of CMV infection in AIDS patients. Drugs of choice are:

Ganciclovir: It can be given by intravenous injection form, oral, intravitreal and ganciclovir implant forms.

Intravenous dosage: Loading dose of 5 mg/kg every 12 hourly IV for 14-21 days then reduce to maintenance dose of 6 mg/kg OD 5 days a week. Dose is given slow IV (over an hour in 100 mg of 0.9 percent normal saline).

Oral dosage: Ideal for maintenance therapy and primary prophylaxis of CMV end organ disease at a dose of 1g (three times a day).

Intravitreal injection: It is given to those patients who are intolerant of systemic therapy.

Dosage: 200–400 mg/dose given 1–2 times per week.
- Liposome encapsulated ganciclovir Intravitreal high dose injection (once a week, 2000 µg/dose) are commercially available.
- Ganciclovir implant (Intravitreal devices). It has advantage of sustained intraocular release of ganciclovir obviating the need for repeated intravitreal injections.
- It consists of central pellet of ganciclovir 4.5 mg encased in the polyvinyl alcohol (PVAs) polymer (water permeable). PVA is surrounded by impermeable ethylene vinyl acetate polymer. Finally the implant has a coating of PVA. It is surgically implanted in the vitreous cavity by making 5 mm incision in pars plana positioned 4 mm posterior to the limbus. The implant slowly release the drug at a rate of about 1.4–1.9 mg per hour over an 8 months period.
- During ganciclovir therapy, following investigations are mandatory
- Complete hemogram (twice a week)
- Liver function tests/renal function tests (twice a week)
- Dilated fundoscopy (at 2 weeks interval).

Foscarnet: Dosage Induction dose is 90 mg/kg IV 12 hourly for 14–21 days followed by daily maintenance dose of 90 mg/kg IVOD. Intravitreal dosage is 2.4 mg every week. Foscarnet is given over 2 hours with 100 ml of normal saline as hydration fluid (use 5% dextrose if Na^+ levels are high).

Cidofovir (HPMPC): It can be administered by IV or Intravitreal injection.

Dosage: IV treatment dose is 5 mg/kg per week for first two weeks followed by injection of 5 mg/kg/alternate weeks as maintenance therapy along with probenecid (to decrease nephrotoxicity). Standard intravitreal dosage is 20 mg injected every 6 weeks.

New investigational compounds on trial for CMV retinitis are:
- Protease inhibitor
- Lobucavir
- Anti-CMV monoclonal antibody MSL-109
- Halogenated benzimidazole 20 times more potent than ganciclovir.

Toxoplasma Infection

- *Toxoplasma gondii*, retinochoroiditis in AIDS is common in this group of infection.
- First choice of treatment is sulfadiazine + pyrimethamine and folinic acid.
- Second choice of treatment is clindamycin + pyrimethamine + folinic acid.

- Third choice of treatment is atovaquone + pyrimethamine + folinic acid.

Dosage
- *Sulphadiazine:* For treatment – 2 g tds PO/IV.
  For maintenance – 1 g tds PO.
- *Pyrimethamine:* For treatment 200 mg PO on day-1, in divided doses and then 50 mg OD.
- *Clindamycin:* For treatment 600 mg PO/IV 8 hourly and for maintenance 450 mg PO/IV 8 hourly.
- Folinic acid is given to decrease risk of myelosuppression. *Dosage* is 15 mg PO daily.
- *Atovaquone:* For treatment 750 mg 4 times a day (has to be given with food). Sulphadiazine and clindamycin when given IV have to be diluted in normal saline, 5 percent dextrose and to be given in 30 minutes – 1 hr duration.
  Close monitoring for hemogram, urinary and serum electrolytes and LFT are required during treatment period.

Herpes Zoster Ophthalmicus

- Treatment of choice is acyclovir.

Dosage: Start with IV 10 mg/kg or 500 mg/sqm 8 hourly for 7–10 days.
It is given slowly over a duration of 1 hour with normal saline.
After that switch to oral therapy 800 mg 5 times daily.
During treatment period monitor hemogram once weekly and electrolytes (twice a week).
Topical 1 percent foscarnet sodium solution 5 times/day or topical 1 percent trifluridine solution 5 times/day can also be given.

Mycobacterium Tuberculosis

First choice of treatment is Rifampicin + INH + pyrazinamide.

Dosage:
- Rifampicin : 600 mg PO (>50 kg body weight) daily
  450 mg PO (<50 kg body wt)
- INH : 300 mg PO daily
- Pyridoxine : 10 mg PO daily
- Pyrazinamide : 2 g PO daily (>50 kg body wt)
  1.5 g PO daily (< 50 kg body wt)
- Ethambutol : 15 mg/kg PO daily

During treatment period monitor hemogram, LFT, renal tests and ocular fundus examination (specially with Ethambutol).

Ocular Syphilis

Treat it as neurosyphilis and usually higher doses are recommended.

Dosage: 10-24 million IU of aqueous penicillin IV daily for 10-14 days + probenecid 50 mg PO daily.

Acute Retinal Necrosis

Varicella zoster virus (VZV) is causative organism of acute and progressive retinal necrosis.

Drug and dosage (1): Start with acyclovir 7.5-10 mg/kg IV daily for 10-14 days.
- Maintenance therapy with oral acyclovir 500 mg PO 5 times daily for several months.
- Intravenous foscarnet 40-60 mg/kg three times a day. In severe cases intravitreal ganciclovir and foscarnet can be given.

Fungal Infections

Candidiasis: It is extremly common in AIDS patients.

Treatment: Clotrimazole or nystatin 500,000 units for 7-14 days in divided doses. Usual therapy is fluconazole 200 mg on first day followed by 100 mg once daily for 7-14 days. Alternatively itraconazole 100 mg/day for 7-14 day can be given.

Cryptococcosis: It is second most common fungal infection in AIDS patients.

Treatment: Induction treatment is with amphotericin B 0.7 mg/kg/day IV and flucytosine 25 mg/kg four times a day for 8 weeks. Fluconazole is preferred choice for oral therapy with a dosage of 200 mg/day.

Pneumocystis carinii choroiditis: Trimethoprim-sulphamethoxazole (DS) orally is best treatment of choice.

Dosage: Two tablets given 8 hourly and to be continued for atleast 2-3 weeks.

Recent Advances in Antiretroviral Drug Therapy

Fomivirsen Sodium (Vitravene)

It is indicated for cytomegalovirus retinitis and is given intravitreally for ophthalmic use.

Dosage: Induction dose is 0.05 ml (330 mcg) as a single intravitreal injection on alternate week for 2 doses followed by maintenance dose of 330 mcg (0.05 ml) once every 4 weeks. It is given using 30 gauge needle or a low volume syringe.

Post-injection monitoring include light perception and optic nerve head perfusion. Store fomivirsen between 2°C-25°C.

OCULAR THERAPEUTICS IN REFRACTIVE SURGERY

Photorefractive Keratectomy

Preoperative Ocular Therapeutics

Patients undergoing excimer photorefractive keratectomy (PRK) are given preoperatively a combination of topical antibiotics (Lomefloxacin or sparfloxacin 0.3%) and NSAID diclofenac sodium (1%) drops, 24 hours prior to procedure. This combination is given at 4 hourly interval. A mild oral sedation (diazepam 5-15 mg) is also given to the patient to overcome anxiety due to the procedure.

PRK surgery is performed under topical anesthesia. Following topical anesthetic agents can be used:

- Proparacaine HCl   0.5 percent
- Benoxinate HCl   0.4 percent
- Tetracaine HCl   0.5 percent

However, proparacaine (0.5%) is most commonly used topical anesthetic agent. It is given 2-5 minutes before operation.

Dosage: Two drops in each eye 2-3 times repeated at the interval of 1 minute. Onset of anesthetic action starts with in 15-20 seconds and effect lasts for 15-20 minutes enough for completion of PRK surgery.

Postprocedure Ocular Therapeutic Module

Following PRK corneal sensation returns to basline with in 12 weeks. The various modalities for the management of pain are:
- Oral analgesic (Preferably NSAID oral diclofenac or nimesulide for 5 days. Tab diclofenac sustained released 75 mg BD or nimesulide tablet 100 mg BD for 5 days continuously relieves the PRK pain to great extent.
- Topical nonsteroidal anti-inflammatory drugs are also given locally. These drugs can be:
    - Topical diclofenac 1 percent drops 4 times a day or
    - Topical ketorolac 0.5 percent 4 times a day, or
    - Topical piroxicam 1 percent 4 times a day help in reducing the pain.
    - Topical lubricant eyedrops 4-5 times a day gives the patient a soothing sensation. Polyvinyl alcohol liquifilm tear drops and sustained release special gel ointment help in post PRK pain.

In excessive pain condition, topical anesthetics like proparacaine 0.5 percent drops 3-4 times a day helps the patient to overcome the pain.

Lasik Surgery

Preprocedure Therapeutic Medications

Preoperatively patient undergoing elective lasik surgery is given broad range topical antibiotic eyedrops (preferably quinolones like topical sparfloxacin (0.3%) or lomefloxacin (0.3%) at 4 hourly interval starting 24 hours prior to surgery.

A mild oral sedation (Diazepam 2–10 mg) is generally given to relieve the anxiety of the patient.

Lasik surgery is performed under topical anesthesia because of rapid onset of action and lesser irritation to the patient. Topical anesthetic agents used are:
- Proparacaine HCl   :   0.5 percent
- Benoxinate HCl   :   0.4 percent
- Tetracaine HCl   :   0.5 percent

Proparacaine (0.5%) is the most commonly used topical anesthetic agent. Its action starts within 15–20 seconds and effect last for 15–20 minutes sufficient for completion of lasik surgery.

Postprocedure Therapeutic Modulation

During the initial active postoperative phase, refractive surgeons prefer to give:
- Oral antibiotics (Preferably ciprofloxacin 500 mg BD for 5 days.
- Topical fluorometholone (0.1%) drops 4 times a day for two weeks.
- Topical lubricant like polyvinyl alcohol liquifilm tear drops 4 times a day for 2 weeks.
- Topical antibiotic (Sparfloxacin 0.3%) 4 times a day for a week.
- Oral analgesic (preferably NSAID like Tab diclofenac 75 mg SR BD for three days.

Recent Update in Post PRK/Lasik Surgery Therapeutic Module

Several new topical agents have been advised in an attempt to modify the stromal wound healing following PRK/lasik surgery:
- Topical ADL-2 or rofecoxib (0.3%) reduces the accumulation of prostaglandin E and inflammatory cells in the corneal stroma.
- The combination of mitomycin C with topical steroids like fluorometholone (0.1%) or rimexolone (0.1%) decreases the subepithelial fibrosis.
- Application of cytokines has been shown to reduce corneal haze and scarring recently.
- Topical Interferon eyedrops 4 times a day for 4–5 weeks reduces the corneal haze remarkably.
- Topical dexamethasone (0.1%) in combination with Interferon α_2 produce less haze.
- Topical β-FGF treatment given 4 times a day until complete epithelial wound healing occurs sharply reduces corneal haze.
- Application of topical anti-TGF-B_1 antibody reduces corneal fibrosis remarkably.
- Application of topical synthetic MMP inhibitor has been shown to reduce intrastromal epithelial migration after laser ablations.

BIBLIOGRAPHY

1. Agarwal A. Textbook of Ophthalmology, 1st edn. New Delhi: Jaypee Brothers Medical Publishers, 2002.
2. Bartlett JD. Clinical Ocular Pharmacology, 4th edn. Boston: Butterworth-Heinemann, 2001
3. Bartlett JD. Ophthalmic Drug Facts, Lippincott–William and Wilkins, 2001.
4. Crick RP, Trimble RB. Textbook of Clinical Ophthalmology, Hodder and Stoughton, 1986.
5. Duane TD. Clinical Ophthalmology, 4th edn. Butterworth–Heinemann, 1999.
6. Duvall. Ophthalmic Medications and Pharmacology, Slack Inc, 1998.
7. Ellis PP. Ocular Therapeutics and Pharmacology, 7th edn. CV Mosby, 1985.
8. Fechner. Ocular Therapeutics, Slack Inc., 1998.
9. Fraunfelder. Current Ocular Therapy, 5th edn. WB Saunders, 2000.
10. Garg A. Current Trends in Ophthalmology, 1st edn. New Delhi: Jaypee Brothers Medical Publishers, 1997.
11. Garg A. Manual of Ocular Therapeutics, 1st edn. New Delhi: Jaypee Brothers Medical Publishers, 1996.
12. Garg A. Ready Reckoner of Ocular Therapeutics, 1st edn. New Delhi, 2002.
13. Goodman LS, Gilman A. Pharmacological Basis of Therapeutics, 7th edn. New York: Macmillan, 1985.
14. Havener's. Ocular Pharmacology, 6th edn. CV Mosby, 1994.
15. Kanski. Clinical Ophthalmology, 4th edn. Butterworth – Heinemann, 1999.
16. Kershner. Ophthalmic Medications and Pharmacology, Slack. Inc., 1994.
17. Olin BR, et al. Drugs Facts and Comparisons: Facts and Comparisons, St Louis, 1997.
18. Onofrey. The Ocular Therapeutics, Lippincott-William and Wilkins, 1997.
19. Rhee. The Wills Eye Drug Guide, Lippincott-William and Wilkins, 1998.
20. Steven Podos. Textbook of Ophthalmology, New Delhi: Jaypee Brothers Medical Publishers, 2001.
21. Zimmerman. Textbook of Ocular Pharmacology, Lippincott and William and Wilkins, 1997.

Ocular Manifestations of Systemic Diseases

Ashok Garg (India)

INTRODUCTION

Systemic diseases are usually related to ocular manifestations. The eyes are frequently involved in diseases affecting the rest of the body.

Ocular manifestations in certain multisystem disorders may offer diagnostic clues to aid in identifying the systemic disease. This chapter provides quick reference for signs and symptoms of ocular disorders association with common systemic diseases when dealing with cases in which patients have eye symptoms without a known systemic disease, physician should refer those cases to ophthalmologists for a specific ocular diagnosis.

VARIOUS SYSTEMIC DISEASES

The specific disease entities are given below with their ocular manifestations:

Thermal, Chemical and Acid Burns

Ocular symptoms are:
- Lid scarring and burn
- Symblepharon
- Trichiasis
- Iritis and corneal epithelium erosion
- Cataract.

Alkali Burns

- Severe skin burns
- Conjunctival vessel blanching
- Glaucoma retinopathy
- Corneal perforation
- Corneal blindness
- Cataract
- Retinitis.

Ultraviolet Radiation

- Keratitis
- Pain and photophobia

- Corneal epithelial damage
- Moderate iritis
- Cataract.

Infrared Radiation

Eclipse blindness, snow blindness and laser burns lead to:
- Potential retinal and macular damage
- Corneal erosions and iritis
- Posterior subcapsular cataracts.

Atomic Radiation

- Iritis
- Posterior subcapsular cataract.

Atopic Dermatitis

- Conjunctivitis
- Erythema of lids
- Posterior subcapsular cataracts
- Keratoconus
- Redness and itching of skin of lids.

Atopic Eczema

- Conjunctivitis
- Keratoconus and dry eyes
- Cataract.

Hay Fever

- Conjunctivitis
- Seasonal iritis
- Hyperemia.

Asthma

- Conjunctivitis
- Steroid-induced cataract and glaucoma.

Urticaria

- Periorbital edema
- Conjunctivitis and erythema.

Acne Rosacea

- Keratitis
- Corneal ulcers and pannus
- Iritis and blepharitis.

Epidermolysis Bullosa

- Lid bullae
- Lacrimal duct stenosis
- Blepharitis
- Hypertrichosis
- Corneal erosion, perforation.

Cicatricial Pemphigoid

- Conjunctivitis
- Dry eyes and photophobia
- Symblepharon and trichiasis.

Erythema Multiforme (Stevens-Johnson Syndrome)

- Conjunctivitis
- Symblepharon and trichiasis
- Corneal perforation/ulcer
- Uveitis and optic neuritis.

Ichthyosis

- Cataract (posterior polar)
- Ectropion
- Corneal opacities/scarring
- Pigmentary retinitis.

Incontinentia Pigmentii

- Nystagmus
- Blue sclera
- Chorioretinitis.

Pemphigus

- Conjunctivitis
- Cataract
- Acantholysis.

Psoriasis

- Deposition of scales in conjunctival sac
- Corneal infiltrates/erosion
- Vascularization
- Silvery skin scales.

Vogt-Koyanagi-Harada Syndrome

- Poliosis
- Uveitis
- Chorioretinitis
- Retinal detachment.

Xeroderma Pigmentosum

- Lid malignancies
- Keratitis
- Lid lesions.

von Hippel's Disease

- Retinal angioma
- Retinal detachment.

Ataxia Telangiectasia

- Nystagmus
- Strabismus
- Partial ophthalmoplegia
- Conjunctival telangiectasia.

Encephalotrigeminal Angiomatosis

- Choroidal hemangioma
- Homolateral congenital glaucoma.

Neurofibromatosis

- Exophthalmos
- Congenital glaucoma
- Optic nerve glioma
- Thickened corneal nerves.

Wyburn Syndrome

- Proptosis (pulsatile)
- Nystagmus
- AVA of retina.

Ankylosing Spondylitis

- Iridocyclitis (bilateral)
- Acute and recurrent.

Dermatomyositis

- Lid edema and redness
- Diplopia
- Extraocular muscle palsy
- Retinal hemorrhage and exudates.

Reiter's Syndrome

- Episcleritis
- Marginal corneal ulcer
- Keratitis and uveitis

- Retinitis
- Optic neuritis.

Rheumatoid Arthritis

- Conjunctivitis
- Scleritis
- Keratitis sicca and band keratopathy
- Corneal melting and iritis
- Cataract or glaucoma.

Sarcoidosis

- Lacrimal gland swelling
- Sarcoid lid nodule
- Mutton fat KPs
- Corneal edema, uveitis and iritis
- Chorioretinitis.

Systemic Lupus Erythematosus

- Episcleritis
- Conjunctival hyperemia
- Keratitis and iridocyclitis
- Retinal edema and papilledema
- Retinal hemorrhage and exudates.

Varicella

- Lid vesicles
- Conjunctivitis
- Keratitis and iritis
- Optic neuritis.

Rubella (German Measles)

- Congenital microphthalmos
- Strabismus and nystagmus
- Corneal edema
- Iridocyclitis and aniridia
- Cataract
- Congenital glaucoma
- Chorioretinitis and optic atrophy.

Vaccinia

- Symblepharon or ankyloblepharon
- Lid infections
- Keratitis and corneal perforation
- Vitreous opacity
- Pseudoretinitis
- Choroiditis, optic neuritis.

Herpes Simplex

- Follicular conjunctivitis
- Limbal dendritis
- Dendritic keratitis and corneal edema
- Congenital cataract
- Herpetic chorioretinitis.

Herpes Zoster

- Vesicular rashes
- Scleritis and lid edema, ptosis
- Keratitis, corneal edema and iritis
- Optic neuritis
- Retinal vasculitis.

Mumps

- Scleritis, conjunctivitis
- Keratitis and iritis
- Optic neuritis
- Dacryoadenitis
- Optic neuritis and extraocular muscle palsy.

Infectious Mononucleosis

- Conjunctivitis
- Dacryocystitis
- Lid edema
- Uveitis and vitritis
- Papillitis
- Retinal periphlebitis
- Keratitis.

Influenza

- Extraocular muscle myalgia and palsy
- Microphthalmos
- Iritis, cataract
- Chorioretinitis
- Retinal hemorrhage and edema, optic neuritis.

Cytomegalic Inclusion Disease

- Iritis, cataract
- Chorioretinitis
- Optic atrophy.

Epidemic Keratoconjunctivitis

- Follicular conjunctivitis
- Pseudomembranes

- Punctate keratitis
- Uveitis.

Gonorrhea

- Purulent conjunctivitis
- Keratitis, iritis
- Orbital edema
- Lid edema and pseudomembranes.

Diphtheria

- Lid edema
- Corneal ulcer
- Membranous conjunctivitis
- Pseudomembranes.

Septicemia

- Conjunctival hemorrhage
- Iritis and iridocyclitis
- Endophthalmitis
- Retinal hemorrhage
- Chorloretinitis
- Roth's spots
- Endophthalmitis.

Leprosy

- Lid paralysis
- Corneal pannus
- Corneal perforation
- Iritis, nodules on iris
- Cataract
- Secondary glaucoma.

Tuberculosis

- Phlyctenular conjunctivitis
- Scleritis
- Uveitis
- Vitreous haziness
- Optic neuritis and diffuse choroiditis.

Lymphogranuloma Venereum

- Elephantiasis of lids
- Conjunctivitis
- Keratitis
- Retinal vessels dilatation.

Toxoplasmosis

- Conjunctivitis
- Strabismus
- Keratitis, uveitis
- Vitritis and chorioretinitis.

Candida albicans

- Dacryocystitis
- Lid thrush
- Keratitis, conjunctivitis
- Septic retinitis.

Histoplasmosis

- Lacrimal gland lesions
- Palpebral conjunctivitis
- Chorioretinitis.

Cryptococcus Infections

- Brow lesions
- Retinitis
- Papilledema
- Retinal detachment.

Cysticercosis

- Iritis
- Vitreous hemorrhage
- Retinal detachment
- Cataract.

Echinococcus (Hydatid Cyst)

- Proptosis
- Iritis
- Vitreous cyst
- Retinal cyst.

Toxocariasis

- Vitritis
- Choroiditis
- Leukokoria
- Macular scarring and optic neuritis.

Trichinosis

- Periorbital edema
- Painful eye movements
- Conjunctival chemosis.

Onchocerciasis

- Microfilarial invasion of ocular tissues
- Keratitis
- Cataract
- Conjunctivitis
- Secondary glaucoma
- Iritis and chorioretinitis
- Optic atrophy.

Turner's Syndrome

- Hypertelorism
- Strabismus
- Ptosis
- Oval-shaped cornea and corneal opacity
- Cataract
- Abnormal retinal pigmentation.

Anemias

- Subconjunctival hemorrhage
- Dilated retinal veins
- Retinal edema and exudates.

Leukemias

- Orbital infiltration
- Proptosis
- Exophthalmos
- Retinal edema and hemorrhage
- Papillitis
- Dilated retinal vessels.

Lymphomas

- Exophthalmos
- Ocular palsy
- Painless lid swelling
- Uveitis and vitritis
- Iritis.

Multiple Myelomas

- Crystals in conjunctiva and cornea
- Pars plana cysts
- Iris and ciliary body cysts
- Dilated retinal vessels
- Retinal hemorrhage
- Papilledema.

Sickle Cell Disease

- Comma-shaped conjunctival vessels
- Vitreous hemorrhage
- Papilledema
- Chorioretinal scars (black sunburst).

Thalassemia

- Epicanthal folds
- Sickle type retinopathy.

Thrombocytopenia

- Orbital hemorrhage
- Ocular palsy
- Retinal edema and exudates.

Arteriosclerosis

- Arcus senilis
- Lipid keratopathy
- Copper and silver wire appearance of retinal vessels
- Star maculopathy
- Retinal edema, hemorrhage and hard exudates
- Papilledema.

Hypertension

- Arcus senilis
- Lipid keratopathy
- Tortuous vessels
- Retinal hemorrhage and edema
- Papilledema
- Hard exudates.

Toxemia of Pregnancy

- Retinal hemorrhage and edema
- Papilledema.

Occlusive Vascular Diseases (Sudden)

- Amaurosis fugax
- Homonymous hemianopia
- Anisocoria
- Cherry red spot of macula.

Occlusive Vascular Diseases (Slow)

- Conjunctival vessel dilation
- Iritis
- Retinal vessel dilation

- Cotton-wool exudates
- Stasis retinopathy.

Venous Occlusive Diseases

- Rubeosis iridis
- Retinal venous congestion
- Branch vein occlusion.

Endocarditis

- Roth's spots
- Retinal hemorrhage and exudates
- Papillitis, iritis.

Aortic Arch Syndrome

- Dilated retinal vessels
- Retinal hemorrhage and exudates
- Cataract
- Papilledema
- Vitreous hemorrhage
- Glaucoma
- Corneal folds
- Ischemic iritis.

Adrenals Cushing's Disease

- Exophthalmos
- Hypertensive retinopathy
- Papilledema
- Retinal vessel tortuosity, hemorrhages and exudates.

Addison's Disease

- Hyperpigmentation of skin of lids and conjunctiva
- Papilledema
- Optic atrophy.

Diabetes Mellitus

- Fluctuations in refractive error
- Diplopia
- Optic neuritis and atrophy
- Third nerve palsy sparing pupil
- Cataract snowflake
- Vitreous hemorrhage
- Hard exudates and microaneurysm
- Corneal recurrent erosion
- Neovascularization of nerve head
- Rubeosis iridis
- Lipemia retinalis.

Hypoparathyroidism

- Photophobia
- Cataract
- Lid twitching
- Keratitis
- Cortical cataract
- Papilledema.

Hyperthyroidism

- Exophthalmos
- Orbital puffiness
- Lid retraction and lag
- Exposure keratitis
- Optic atrophy, papilledema
- Band keratopathy.

Alcoholism

- Optic neuritis
- Nystagmus
- Impaired conjugate gaze
- Ptosis and iridoplegia.

Liver Disease (Nutritional)

- Scleral icterus
- Night blindness
- Color vision impairment
- Dry eye
- Cataract
- Optic atrophy.

Malnutrition

- Xerophthalmia
- Night blindness
- Lid edema
- Keratopathy (necrotic)
- Chemosis.

Peptic Ulcer Diseases

- Iritis
- Glaucomatocyclic crisis.

Pancreatic Diseases

- Secondary glaucoma
- Cotton-wool exudates
- Retinal hemorrhages

Ulcerative Colitis

- Episcleritis
- Conjunctivitis, iritis
- Optic neuritis.

Vitamin A Deficiency

- Xerophthalmia
- Keratomalacia
- Bitot's spot on conjunctiva
- Dry cornea, perforation
- Retinal perivasculitis
- Degeneration of rod outer segment.

Vitamin B Deficiency

- Xerosis of cornea and conjunctiva
- Optic neuritis
- Central scotoma
- Retrobulbar neuritis.

Vitamin C Deficiency

- Subconjunctival hemorrhage.
- Retinal hemorrhage in severe cases.

Hypervitaminosis A, B and D

- Increased intracranial pressure
- Decreased vision
- Exophthalmos and diplopia
- Band keratopathy
- Zonular cataract
- Cystoid macular edema (CME) and papilledema
- Calcium deposits in conjunctiva and cornea.

Albinism

- Blond fundus
- Nystagmus and strabismus
- Prominent choroidal vessels
- Poor macular development.

Amyloidosis

- Extraocular muscle palsies
- Amyloid deposits in various tissues of eye
- Glaucoma, iritis
- Ptosis
- Vitreous opacity
- Retinal hemorrhage
- Optic nerve amyloid.

Galactosemia

Cataract—nuclear or zonular.

Gout

- Corneal, uric acid crystals
- Iridocyclitis
- Scleritis and episcleritis.

Marfan's Syndrome

- Lens dislocation (bilateral)
- Myopia
- Retinal detachment
- Multiple pupils
- Blue sclera.

Niemann-Pick Disease

- Cherry red spots
- Blindness.

Wilson's Disease

- Copper corneal ring
- Cataract (sunflower).

Craniofacial Syndromes

- Coloboma
- Exophthalmos
- Exposure keratitis
- Papilledema, optic atrophy.

Facial Deformity Syndromes

- Coloboma of lower lids
- Microphthalmos
- Nystagmus, strabismus
- Cataract.

Myasthenia Gravis

- Lid twitch sign
- Ptosis
- Diplopia
- Pupillary abnormalities
- Paradoxical lid retraction
- Pseudogaze palsy.

Muscular Dystrophy Disorders

- Cataract
- Ptosis
- External ophthalmoplegia
- Dry eyes
- Pigmentary retinopathy.

Bronchiectasis

Retinal vessels dilated, tortuous, edema, hemorrhages.

Bronchogenic Carcinoma

- Metastasis to choroid and retina
- Metastasis to iris.

Emphysema

- Retinal vascular dilatation
- Hemorrhage
- Papilledema
- Optic neuritis
- Cataract, secondary glaucoma.

Lowe's Syndrome

- Congenital cataract
- Congenital glaucoma.

Nephrotic Syndrome

- Mild retinopathy
- Retinal edema
- Mild papilledema.

Renal Transplantation

- Cataract (postsubcapsular)
- Glaucoma.

Wilms' Tumor

- Aniridia
- Orbital mass.

Breast Carcinoma

- Orbital metastasis frequent
- Iris or angle metastasis
- Choroidal and retinal metastasis.

Periarteritis Nodosa

- Nystagmus
- Extraocular muscle palsy
- Ptosis
- Nodular scleritis
- Peripheral ulcerative keratitis
- Uveitis
- Retinal hemorrhage
- Papilledema.

Scleroderma

- Lid margins scars and loss
- Keratitis
- Peripheral ulcerative keratitis
- Retinopathy.

Influenza

- Extraocular muscle myalgia and palsy
- Mild keratitis and iritis
- Retinal hemorrhage and edema
- Optic neuritis.

Malaria

- Conjunctivitis
- Keratitis
- Iritis
- Optic neuritis secondary to antimalarials.

Lymphomas

- Exophthalmos
- Proptosis
- Ocular palsy
- Lid edema
- Iritis
- Vitritis.

Thalassemia

Sickle type retinopathy.

Endocarditis

- Diplopia
- Ocular palsies
- Nystagmus
- Anisocoria
- Roth's spots
- Iritis

- Metastatic endophthalmitis
- Retinal hemorrhages, exudates
- Papillitis.

Malnutrition

- Xerophthalmia
- Night blindness
- Lid edema
- Chemosis
- Necrotic keratopathy.

Muscular Dystrophy Disorders

- Ptosis
- External ophthalmoplegia
- Dry eye
- Polychromatic cataract
- Pigmentary retinopathy.

Pneumonia

- Roth's spots
- Septic retinitis.

Renal Transplantation

Steroid induced cataract and glaucoma.

Breast Neoplasm

- Orbital metastasis
- Iris or angle metastasis
- Choroidal metastasis.

Lung Neoplasm

- Orbital metastasis frequent
- Choroidal and retinal metastasis.

Alkaptonuria

Dark pigmentation of sclera, conjunctiva and cornea.

BIBLIOGRAPHY

1. Agarwal A. Textbook of Ophthalmology, 1st edn. New Delhi: Jaypee Brothers Medical Publishers, 2002.
2. Bartlett JD. Clinical Ocular Pharmacology, 4th edn. Boston: Butterworth-Heinemann, 2001.
3. Bartlett JD. Ophthalmic Drug Facts, Lippincott-William and Wilkins, 2001.

4. Crick RP, Trimble RB. Textbook of Clinical Ophthalmology, Hodder and Stoughton, 1986.
5. Duane TD. Clinical Ophthalmology, 4th edn. Butterworth-Heinemann, 1999.
6. Duvall. Ophthalmic Medications and Pharmacology, Slack Inc, 1998.
7. Ellis PP. Ocular Therapeutics and Pharmacology, 7th edn. CV Mosby, 1985.
8. Fechner. Ocular Therapeutics, Slack Inc, 1998.
9. Fraunfelder. Current Ocular Therapy, 5th edn. WB Saunders, 2000.
10. Garg A. Current Trends in Ophthalmology, 1st edn. New Delhi: Jaypee Brothers Medical Publishers, 1997.
11. Garg A. Manual of Ocular Therapeutics, 1st edn. New Delhi: Jaypee Brothers Medical Publishers, 1996.
12. Garg A. Ready Reckoner of Ocular Therapeutics, 1st edn. New Delhi: Jaypee Brothers Medical Publishers, 2002.
13. Goodman LS, Gilman A. Pharmacological Basis of Therapeutics, 7th edn. New York: Macmillan, 1985.
14. Havener's. Ocular Pharmacology, 6th edn. CV Mosby, 1994.
15. Kanski. Clinical Ophthalmology, 4th edn. Butterworth-Heinemann, 1999.
16. Kershner. Ophthalmic Medications and Pharmacology, Slack Inc, 1994.
17. Olin BR, et al. Drugs Facts and Comparisons: Facts and Comparisons, St Louis, 1997.
18. Onofrey. The Ocular Therapeutics, Lippincott-William and Wilkins, 1997.
19. Rhee. The Wills Eye Drug Guide, Lippincott-William and Wilkins, 1998.
20. Steven Podos. Textbook of Ophthalmology, New Delhi: Jaypee Brothers Medical Publishers, 2001.
21. Zimmerman. Textbook of Ocular Pharmacology, Lippincott and William and Wilkins, 1997.

26

Quick Look Tabulated Ocular Therapeutics Information

Ashok Garg (India)

ANTIBACTERIALS

Drug name (Generic)	Dosage form/strength	Commercial packing
a. Aminoglycosides		
Gentamicin sulfate	Solution 0.3% (3 mg/ml)	In 5 and 10 ml dropper vials
	Ointment 3 mg/g	3.5 g and 5 g tubes
Tobramycin	Solution 0.3% (3 mg/ml)	In 3 and 5 ml dropper vials
	Ointment 3 mg/g	3 g and 5 g tubes
Sisomicin	Solution 0.3%	In 3 and 5 ml dropper vials
	Ointment 3 mg/g	3 g and 5 g tubes
Neomycin	Solution 0.17%	In 5 and 10 ml dropper vials
	Ointment 5 mg/g	3 g and 5 g tubes
Framycetin	Solution 0.5%	In 5 and 10 ml dropper vials
	Ointment 0.5 and 1%	3 and 5 g tubes
b. Tetracyclines	Solution 1%	In 5 ml dropper vial
	Ointment 1%	3 and 5 g tubes
Oxytetracycline	Ointment 1%	3 and 5 g tubes
c. Sulphacetamide	Solution 10,20, 30%	In 5 and 10 ml dropper vials
	Ointment 10 and 30%	3 and 5 g tubes
Sulfasoxazole diolamine	Solution 4%	In 10 and 15 ml dropper vials
d. Chloramphenicol	Solution 0.4–1%	3,5 and 10 ml dropper vials
	Ointment 5 mg/g and 10 mg/g	3 and 5 g tubes
	Powder for solution/ Injection 25 mg/vial	Preservative free 15 ml pack with diluent
e. Microlides		
Erythromycin	Ointment 0.5% (5 mg/g)	In 3 and 5 g tubes
Roxithromycin	Ointment 0.5%	In 3 and 5 g tubes
f. Polypeptides		
Polymixin B	Solution 0.5–1%	5 and 10 ml dropper vial
	Ointment 1–1.5 mg/g	3 and 5 g tubes
	Powder for solution 500,000 units	In 20 ml vial
Bacitracin	Ointment 500 units/g and 10000 units/g	Preservative free in 3 and 5 g tubes

Contd...

Contd...

Drug name (Generic)	Dosage form/strength	Commercial packing
g. Fluoroquinolones		
Norfloxacin	Solution 0.3%	In 5 and 10 ml dropper vials
	Ointment 3 mg/g (0.3%)	3 and 5 g tubes
Ciprofloxacin	Solution 0.3%	In 5 and 10 ml dropper vials
	Ointment 3 mg/g	3 and 5 g tubes
Ofloxacin	Solution 0.3%	In 5 and 10 ml dropper vials
	Ointment 3 mg/g	3 and 5 g tubes
Pefloxacin	Solution 0.3%	In 5 ml dropper vials
Lomefloxacin	Solution 0.3%	In 5 ml dropper vials
	Ointment 3 mg/g	3 and 5 g tubes
Sparfloxacin	Solution 0.3%	In 5 ml dropper vials
	Ointment 3 mg/g	3 g tubes
Levofloxacin	Solution 0.5%	In 5 ml dropper vials
Moxifloxacin	Solution 0.3%	Ophthalmic ointment 5 mg
Gemifloxacin	Solution 0.3%	
Gatifloxacin	Solution 0.3%	
Clinafloxacin	Solution 0.3%	
Besifloxacin	Suspension 0.6%	
Azithromycin	1% ophthalmic ointment	

COMBINATION ANTIBIOTICS

Bacitracin, Neomycin and Polymixin B	Combination solution/ Ointment containing	
	Polymixin B Sulfate 10000 units/g	In 5 and 10 ml dropper vials
	Neomycin sulfate 3.5 mg/g	In 5 mg tube
	Bacitracin 400 units/g	
Neomycin Sulfate,	Combination solution/ Ointment	In 5 and 10 ml
Polymixin B Sulfate	containing Polymixin B Sulfate 10000 units/g,	dropper vials
Gramicidin	Neomycin Sulfate 1.75 mg/g Gramicidin 0.025 mg/ml	In 3 and 5 g tubes
Bacitracin Zinc and	Combination solution/ Ointment	In 5 and 10 ml
Polymixin B Sulfate	Polymixin B Sulfate 10000 units/g	dropper vials
	Bacitracin Zinc 500 units/g	In 5 g tube
Polymixin B Sulfate and Oxytetracycline	Ointment containing Polymixin B Sulfate 10000 units/g and Oxytetracycline HCl 5 mg/g	In 3 and 5 g tubes
Trimethoprim Sulfate	Combination solution containing	
and Polymixin B	Polymixing B sulfate	In 5 and 10 ml dropper vials
	10000 units/g Trimethoprim: 1 mg/ml	
Sodium Sulphacetamide and Phenylephirine	Combination solution containing Sulphacetamide 15%	In 5 and 15 ml dropper vials
	Phenylephrine HCl 0.125%	

Contd...

Contd...

Drug name (Generic)	Dosage form/strength	Commercial packing
Gentamicin and Vancomycin	Combination solution containing Gentamicin 8 g/ml Vancomycin 20 m/ml	In 5 ml dropper vial

ANTI-INFLAMMATORY DRUGS

Topical Steroidal Agents

Drug name (Generic)	Dosage form/strength	Commercial packing
Hydrocortisone	as	
	Acetate solution 2%	3 and 5 ml dropper vials
	Acetate suspension 0.5–2.5%	3 and 5 ml dropper vials
	Acetate ointment 1.5%	3 and 5 g tubes
Prednisolone	as	
	Acetate suspension 0.12, 0.25 and 1%	5 ml dropper vial
	Sodium Phosphate solution 0.12, 0.5 and 1.0%	5 ml dropper vial
	Phosphate ointment-0.25%	3 and 5 g tubes
Dexamethasone	as	
	Sodium phosphate Solution-0.1%, 0.05 and 0.01%	5 ml dropper vial
	Suspension 0.1%, Sodium phosphate	5 ml dropper vial
	Ointment 0.05%	3 and 5 g tubes
Betamethasone	Sodium phosphate Solution 0.1%	In 5 and 10 ml dropper vials
	Sodium Phosphate Ointment 0.1%	3 and 5 g tubes
Triamcinolone acetonide	Suspension 0.1%	5 ml dropper vial
	Ointment 0.1%	3 and 5 g tubes
Medrysone	Suspension 1%	In 5 and 10 ml dropper vials
Fluorometholone	Suspension 0.1, 0.25%	In 5, 10 and 15 ml dropper vials
	Ointment 0.1%	3 and 5 g tubes
Rimexolone	Suspension 0.1%	5 ml and 10 ml dropper vials
Loteprednol etabonate	Solution 0.2 and 0.5%	In 2.5, 5 and 10 ml dropper vials

Nonsteroidal Anti-inflammatory Agents

Drug name (Generic)	Dosage form/strength	Commercial packing
Flurbiprofen	Solution 0.03%	in 2.5, 5 and 10 ml dropper vials
Ketorolac tromethamine	Solution 0.5%	In 5 ml dropper vial and single Use 0.4 ml unims
Suprofen	Solution 1%	In 2.5 and 5 ml dropper vials
Diclofenac sodium	Solution 0.1%	In 2.5 and 5 ml dropper vials
Indomethacin	Suspension 1% Solution 0.1%	In 3 and 5 ml dropper vials

Contd...

Contd...

Drug name (Generic)	Dosage form/strength	Commercial packing
Aspirin	Solution 1%	In 5 ml dropper vial
Fenoprofen	Solution 0.3%	In 5 ml dropper vial
Ibuprofen	Solution 0.5%	In 5 ml dropper vial
Ketoprofen	Solution 1.0%	In 5 ml dropper vial
Naproxen	Solution 0.5%	In 5 ml dropper vial
Piroxicam	Solution 1%	In 5 ml dropper vial
Diflunisol	Solution 0.03%	In 5 ml dropper vial
Phenylbutazone	Ointment 10%	3 and 5 g tubes
Oxyphenbutazone	Ointment 10%	3 and 5 g tubes
Bromfenac	Solution 0.09%	5 ml solution

TOPICAL STEROID-ANTIBIOTIC COMBINATIONS

Drug name (Generic)	Steroid per g/ml	Antibiotic per g/ml	Commercial packing
Dexamethasone Sodium Phosphate and Neomycin Sulfate	Solution 0.1%	0.5%	In 5 ml dropper vial
	Oint. 0.1%	0.5%	3 and 5 g tubes
Dexamethasone Sodium Phosphate Neomycin Sulfate and Polymixin B	Susp. 0.1%	0.35 (Neomycin) 10000 units/ml Polymixin B	In 5 ml dropper vial
	Ointment 0.1%	0.35 (Neomycin) 10000 units/ml Polymixin B	3 and 5 g tubes
Dexamethasone Sodium Phosphate and Chloramphenicol	Solution 0.1%	0.5–1%	In 5 ml dropper vial
Dexamethasone Sodium Phosphate and Framycetin	Susp. 0.1%	0.3%	In 5 ml dropper vial
Dexamethasone Sodium Phosphate and Tobramycin	Susp. 0.1%	0.3%	In 5 ml dropper vial
	Ointment 0.1%	0.3%	3 and 5 g tubes
Dexamethasone Sodium Phosphate, Chloramphenicol and Polymixin B Sulfate	Soln 0.1%	Chloramphenicol 1% Polymixin B 5000 IU	In 5 ml dropper vial
	Ointment 0.1%	Chloramphenicol 1% Polymixin B 5000 IU	In 3 and 5 g tubes
Dexamethasone Sodium Phosphate and Gentamicin	Solution 0.1%	0.3%	In 5 ml dropper vial
Dexamethasone Sodium Phosphate and Ciprofloxacin	Solution .0.1%	0.3%	In 5 ml dropper vial
	Ointment 0.1%	0.3%	In 3 and 5 g tubes
Dexamethasone Sodium Phosphate and Ofloxacin	Solution .0.1%	0.3%	In 5 ml dropper vial
Dexamethasone Sodium Phosphate and Lomefloxacin	Solution .0.1%	0.3%	In 5 ml dropper vial
Dexamethasone Sodium Phosphate and Sparfloxacin	Solution 0.1%	0.3%	In 5 ml dropper vial
Betamethasone with Neomycin	Solution 0.1%	0.5%	In 5 ml dropper vial
Betamethasone with Chloramphenicol	Solution 0.1%	0.5%	In 5 ml dropper vial
	Ointment 0.1%	0.5%	In 3 and 5 g tubes

Contd...

Contd...

Drug name (Generic)	Dosage form/strength		Commercial packing
Betamethasone and Gentamicin	Solution 0.1%	0.3%	In 5 ml dropper vial
Hydrocortisone and Neomycin	Solution 0.5%	0.5%	In 5 ml dropper vial
	Ointment 1.5%	0.5%	
	Ointment 0.5-1.5%	0.5%	3 and 5 g tubes
Hydrocortisone, Polymixin B, Bacitracin and Neomycin	Solution 10 mg/g 400 units/g 5 mg/g	0.5 mg/g Polymixin Bacitracin Neomycin	In 5 ml dropper vial
	Ointment 10 mg/g 400 units/g 5 mg/g	0.5 mg/g Polymixin Bacitracin Neomycin	In 5 g tube
Hydrocortisone and Gentamicin	Suspension 1%	0.3%	In 5 ml dropper vial
Hydrocortisone and Chloramphenicol	Solution 0.5%	1%	In 5 ml dropper vial
	Ointment 0.5%	1%	In 5 g tube
Hydrocortisone and Oxytetracycline	Suspension 1.5%	0.5%	In 5 ml dropper vial
	Ointment 1.5%	0.5%	In 3 and 5 g tube
Prednisolone and Gentamicin	Susp.1%	0.3%	In 5 ml dropper vial
Prednisolone and Sulphacetamide	Solution 0.2% to 0.5%	10% (Sulpha)	In 5 ml dropper vial
	Ointment 0.5%	10% (Sulpha)	In 3 and 5 g tubes
Prednisolone, Neomycin and Polymixin B	Suspension 0.5%	0.35% (Neomycin) 10000 units (Polymixin)	In 5 and 10 ml dropper vials
Fluorometholone and Neomycin	Solution 0.1%	0.35%	In 5 ml dropper vial
Fluorometholone and Gentamicin	Solution 0.1%	0.9%	In 5 ml dropper vial
Flurometholone and Tobramycin	Solution 0.1%	0.3%	In 5 ml dropper vial
Fluorometholone and Sodium Sulfacetamide	Suspension 0.1%	1%	In 5 and 10 ml dropper vials
Moxifloxacin and loteprednate	Suspension 0.5%	0.5%	Dropper vials
Moxifloxacin and Difluprednate	Solution 0.5% and 0.5 mg		5 ml solution

ANTIVIRAL THERAPY

First Generation Drugs

Indoxuridine (IDU)	Solution 0.1%	In 5 ml dropper vial
	Ointment 0.5%	3 and 5 g tubes
Vidarabine (Are-A)	Ointment 0.3%	In 5 g tubes
	Intravenous infusion 200 mg/ml	In 250 ml bottle
Trifluridine (TFT)	Solution 1%	In 5 and 10 ml dropper vials
Cytarabine	Ointment 1%	In 5 g tube
	Injection form -100 mg, 500 mg and 1000 mg/ml	1 and 2 ml ampoules and vials

Contd...

Contd...

Drug name (Generic)	Dosage form/strength	Commercial packing

Second Generation Drugs

Acyclovir	Ointment 3%	In 5 g tube
	Oral tablet 200 mg, 400 mg and 800 mg	Tablets in a pack of 50/100
	Powder 250 mg	In pack of 100 g/ 200 g/500 g
Bromo-vinyl deoxyuridine (BVDU)	Solution 0.1%	In 5 ml dropper vial
Interferons	Parenteral 30–400 Million/ml	In 2 and 5 ml vials
Zidovudine (AZT)	100 mg capsule	Pack of 50/100 cap.
Famiciclovir	100 and 200 mg tab.	In a pack of 50/100 tab.
Ganciclovir (DHPG)	Oral 250 mg capsule	in 100 cap pack
	Powder for injection Lyophilized 500 mg/vial	in 10 ml vial
	Ganciclovir sodium Intravitreal implant Minimum 4.5 mg	In individual unit boxes in a Sterile types package
Foscarnet sodium	Injection 24 mg/ml	In 250 and 500 ml bottles
Fomivirsen	Injection 6.6 mg/ml	In 0.25 ml single use vial
Cidofovir (HPMPC)	Injection 75 mg/ml	5 ml ampoule
Lobucavir	Oral 100 and 200 mg tab.	Box of 100 tablets
Indinavir	Oral 100 and 200 mg tab.	Box of 100 tablets
Ritonavir	Oral 100 and 200 mg tab.	Box of 100 tablets
Saquinavir	Oral 100 and 200 mg tab.	Box of 100 tablets
Nelfinavir	Oral 100 and 200 mg tab.	Box of 100 tablets
Valaciclovir	Oral 100 and 200 mg tab.	Box of 100 tablets
Ganciclovir	Ophthalmic gel	0.15%

ANTIFUNGAL THERAPY

Polyenes

Nystatin	Ointment containing 100000 IU of Nystatin	3 and 5 g tubes
Amphotericin B	Solution 0.75–3%	in 5 and 10 ml vials
Natamycin	Suspension 5%	in 5, 10 and 15 ml dropper vials

Imidazole Derivatives

Clotrimazole	Solution 1%	in 5 ml dropper vial
Miconazole	Solution 1%	in 5 ml dropper vial
	Applicaps 1%	In a pack of 30 applicaps
Econazole	Solution 1%	In 5 ml
	Ointment 1%	in 3 and 5 g tubes
Ketoconazole	Oral tab. 200 and 400 mg	In a pack of 100 tablet
	Fresh solution 1–5%	In 5 ml dropper vial
Fluconazole	Solution 0.3%	5 ml dropper vial
	Oral tab. 100 and 200 mg	Pack of 100 tablets
Itraconazole	Oral tablet 200 mg	Pack of 100 tablets

Contd...

Quick Look Tabulated Ocular Therapeutics Information

Contd...

Drug name (Generic)	Dosage form/strength	Commercial packing

Fluorinated Pyrimidines

Flucytosine	Oral as 250 and 500 mg capsules	Pack of 100 cap.
	Solution 1%	5 ml dropper vial

Silver Sulphadiazine

	Solution 1%	5 ml dropper vial
	Applicaps 1%	A pack of 30 applicaps

Terbinafine

	Oral tablet of 125 mg and 250 mg	A pack of 100 tablets

ANTI-ALLERGY THERAPY

Mast Cell Inhibitors

Cromolyn Sodium	Solution 2 and 4%	2, 5 and 10 ml dropper vials
Disodium Cromoglycate (DSCG)	Solution 2%	5 and 10 ml dropper vials
Lodoxamide Tromethamine	Solution 0.1% Suspension	5 and 10 ml dropper vials
Nedocromil	Solution 1%	5 ml dropper vial
Olopatadine HCl	Solution 0.05 and 1%	5 ml dropper vial
Azelastine HCl	Solution 0.05%	5 ml dropper vial
Ketotifen fumarate	Solution 0.025% (0.25 mg/ml)	5 and 7 ml dropper vials

Antihistamines

Levocarbastine HCl	Suspension 0.05%	In 2.5, 5 and 10 ml dropper vials
Emedastine Difumarate	Suspension 0.05%	5 ml opaque plastic Vial
Pheniramine maleate	Solution 0.3%	5 and 10 ml dropper vials
Levocetrizine	As 5 mg tablet (Dosage 5 mg orally once or twice daily)	In a strip of 10 tablets
Desloratidine	As 5 mg tablet (Dosage 5 mg orally once daily)	In a strip of 10 tablets
Ebastine	10 mg orally once daily	-do-

Decongestants

Phenyleprine HCl	Solution 0.125–0.12%	In 5, 10 and 15 ml dropper vials
Imidazole derivatives		
Naphazoline HCl	Solution 0.012–0.1%	In 5, 10 and 15 ml dropper vials
Tetrahydrozoline	Solution 0.05%	In 5, 10, 15 and 20 ml dropper vials
Oxymetazoline HCl	Solution 0.025%	In 10, 15 and 30 ml dropper vials
Ephedrine	Solution 0.05%	5 and 10 ml dropper vials

Contd...

Contd...

Drug name (Generic)	Dosage form/strength	Commercial packing
Rose petal aqueous Infusion	Solution (Aqueous infusion in 7.5 ml with 0.1% thimerosal)	In 5 and 10 ml dropper vials

Decongestants and Antihistamines Combination

	Antihistamine	Decongestant	
Pheniramine maleate and Naphazoline HCl	0.3% (Pheni)	0.025% (Napha)	In 5,10 and 15 ml dropper vials
Pheniramine maleate and Phenylephrine	0.5%	0.125%	In 5,10 and 15 ml dropper vials
Pyrilamine maleate, Phenylephrine HCl and Antipyrine	Pyrilamine 0.1% and Antipyrine (0.1%)	Phenylephrine 0.12%	In 5,10 and 15 ml dropper vials
Antazoline Phosphate and Naphazoline HCl	0.5% (Anta)	0.05% (Napha)	In 10 and 15 ml dropper vials
Tetrahydrozoline and Zinc Sulfate	0.25% (Zinc)	0.05% (Tetrahydrozoline)	In 10 and 15 ml dropper vials

Topical NSAIDs and Topical Steroids— See Anti-inflammatory Tables

Topical Immunosuppressors

Cyclosporine	Solution 2%	In 5 ml dropper vial

ANTIGLAUCOMA THERAPY

Miotics

Cholinergic Agents

Acetylcholine chloride	Fresh solution (1:100) acetycholrine when reconstitued	In 2 ml dual chamber univial alongwith diluent and sterile water
Pilocarpine HCl	Solution 0.25, 0.50%, 1, 2, 3, 4, 6, 8 and 10%	In 2,5, 10 and 15 ml dropper vials
Pilocarpine Nitrate	Solution 1, 2 and 4%	In 5,10 and 15 ml dropper vials
Pilocarpine HCl	Gel 4%	In 3 and 5 g tubes
Pilocarpine Ocular Therapeutic system (Ocusert)	Ocusert Pilo-20 releases 20 mcg pilocarpine per hour for one week	In a pack of 8 individual sterile system
	Ocusert Pilo-40 releases 40 mcg pilocarpine per hour for one week	In a pack of 8 individual sterile system
Pilocarpine Combinations		
Pilocarpine HCl and Epinephrine	Solution containing Pilocarpine 1–6% and and Epinephrine (1%) (Epilo1 – Epilo6)	In 5 and 10 ml dropper vials
Pilocarpine HCl and Physostigmine	Solution having Pilocarpine (2%) and Physostigmine 0.25%	In 5 ml dropper vial

Contd...

Contd...

Drug name (Generic)	Dosage form/strength	Commercial packing
Pilocarpine nitrate and clonidine	Solution having Pilocarpine nitrate (1%) and clonidine (0.125%)	In 5 ml dropper vial
Carbachol	Solution 0.75, 1.5, 2.25 and 3%	In 5,10 and 15 ml droptainers
	Intraocular solution 0.01%	In 1.5 ml ampoules/vials

Anticholinesterase Agents

Physostigmine sulfate	Solution 0.25 and 0.5%	5 ml dropper vial
	Ointment 0.25%	3.5 g tube
Demecarium bromide	Solution 0.125 and 0.25%	5 ml dropper vial
Echothiophate	as Powder for Reconstitution 1.5 mg to make Solution 0.03% other Strengths are 0.06%, 0.125 and 0.25%	Powder pack with 5 ml diluent
Isofluorophate	Ointment 0.025% in poly Ethylene mineral oil gel	3 and 5 g tubes
Citicoline	IM injection 1000 mg	Single packing

Alpha Adrenergic Agonists

Apraclonidine	Solution 0.5 and 1%	In 5 and 10 ml dropper vials
Clonidine	Solution 0.125, 0.25 and 0.5%	In 5 ml dropper vial
Brimonidine tartrate (Alphagan)	Solution 0.2%	In 5 and 10 ml dropper vials
Brimonidine purite (Alphagan P)	Solution 0.15%	In 5 and 10 ml dropper vials
Brimonidine tartrate and Timolol maleate	Solution having 0.2% Brimonidine and 0.5% Timolol maleate	In 5 ml dropper vial
Dapiprazole HCl	Powder Lyophilized 25 mg (0.5%) solution when reconstituted	In vial with 5 ml diluent and dropper

Sympathomimetics

Epinephrine	Solution 0.5%—2% Available as Epinephrine hydrochloride, Borate and bitartate	In 2, 7.5 and 10 ml dropper vials
Dipivefrin HCl	Solution 0.1%	In 2, 5, 10 and 15 ml dropper vials

Beta Blockers

Betaxolol HCl	Solution 0.25 and 0.50%	In 2.5, 5, 10 and 15 ml dropper vials
Carteolol HCl	Solution 1%	In 5 and 10 ml dropper vials
Levobunolol	Solution 0.25 and 0.50%	In 5, 10 and 15 ml dropper vials
Metipranolol HCl	Solution 0.1, 0.3 and 0.6%	In 5 ml and 10 ml dropper vials
Timolol maleate	Solution 0.25 and 0.5%	In 5,10 and 15 ml dropper vials
	Gel 0.25 and 0.5% (GFS)	5 g tube

Contd...

Contd...

Drug name (Generic)	Dosage form/strength	Commercial packing

Carbonic Anhydrase Inhibitors

Acetazolamide	Solution 5%	In 5 ml dropper vial
	Tablet 125 mg, 250 mg and sustained release (500 mg) capsule	In a pack of 100 tablets In 30 and 100 capsules packing in vials
	Powder for injection Lyophilized 500 mg	
Dichlorphenamide	Tablet 50 mg	Pack of 100 tablets
Methazolamide	Tablet as 25 mg and 50 mg	Pack of 100 tablets
Dorzolamide	Solution 2%	In 5 and 10 ml dropper vials
Dorzolamide and Timolol	Solution having 2% Dorzolamide and 0.5% Timolol	In 5 and 10 ml dropper vials
Brinzolamide	Suspension 1%	In 2.5, 5 and 10 and 15 ml dropper vials
Ethoxazolamide	Oral 125 mg tab.	In a pack of 100 tablets

Prostaglandins

Latanoprost (Xalantan)	Solution 0.005%	In 2.5 ml plastic Bottle with dropper tip
Latanoprost and Timolol (Xalcom)	Solution having 0.005% Latanoprost and 0.5% Timolol	In 3 ml plastic bottle with dropper vials
Unoprostone (Rescula)	Solution 0.15%	In 3 ml polypack with dropper tip
Bimatoprost (Lumigan)	Solution 0.03%	In 3 ml polypack with dropper tip
Travoprost (Travatan)	Solution 0.004%	In 3 ml polypack with dropper tip

Hyperosmotic Agents

Glycerine	Oral solution as 50 and 70%	In 7.5 and 15 ml pack
	Ointment 40%	In 3.5 g tube
Isosorbide	Oral solution as 45% (10 g per 220 ml)	In 220 ml pack
Mannitol	As injection solution 5–25%	In 50, 250, 500 and 1000 ml bottles
Urea powder	As 30% solution	In 100 ml bottle

Ocular Hypotensive Lipid (OHL)

	Solution 0.01%	In 5 and 10 ml dropper vials

Antimetabolites

5-Fluorouracil (5FU)	As powder and reconstituted solution (0.5 c.c. of solution contain 5 mgm of 5 FU)	Available as 50 mg/ml to 10 mg/ml in physiological saline
Mitomycin C	3 x 2 mm cellular Sponge moistened with 0.02–0.04 mg/ml of Mitomycin C	as powder with diluent

Contd...

Contd...

Drug name (Generic)	Dosage form/strength	Commercial packing
Daunorubicin	4 x 4 mm cellulose Sponge soaked in Daunorubicin (0.2 mg/ml)	Powder with diluent

LOCAL ANESTHETIC AGENTS

Injectable Agents

Esters

Procaine	Solution 1%	In 2 ml ampoule
Chloroprocaine	Solution 0.5–2%	2 ml ampoule
Tetracaine	Solution 0.25–2%	30 ml vial

Amides

Lidocaine HCl	Injection 0.5–4%	In 5 ml prefilled Syringe and 30 ml pack
	Ointment 5%	In 35 g tube
	Ampoule 1% (Preservative free) for intracameral use	2 ml ampoule
Lidocaine with Epinephrine	Combination Solution having 0.5–2% Lidocaine and 1:100000/vials 200000 epinephrine	In 10 ml ampoule and 20, 30 and 50 ml vials
Lidocaine with Dextrose	Combination solution containing 1.5–5% Lidocaine and 7.5% Dextrose	In 2 ml ampoule
Prilocaine	Solution 0.5–3%	In 2 ml ampoule and 30 ml vial
Mepivacaine	Injectable solution 1–2%	In 30 and 50 ml vials
Bupivacaine	Injectable solution 0.25–0.75%	In 30 ml vial
Bupivacaine and Epinephrine	Solution having 0.75% (Bupi) and 1:200000 Epinephrine solution	In 2 ml ampoule and In 30 ml vial
Etidocaine	as 0.5–1%	In 30 ml vial
Etidocaine and Epinephrine	Solution having 1.0–1.5% Etidocaine and 1:200000 Epinephrine	In 30 ml vial
Centbucridine	Injectable solution 0.5%	In 30 ml vial

Topical Anesthetic Agents

Benoxinate HCl	Topical solution 0.4%	In 5 and 15 ml dropper vials
Proparacaine HCl	Solution 0.5 and 0.75%	In 10 and 15 ml dropper vials
Tetracaine HCl	Solution 0.5 and 1%	In 10 and 15 ml dropper vials
Lidocaine HCl	Solution 4%	In 10 and 30 ml dropper vials
Centbucridine HCl	Solution 1%	In 10 and 15 ml dropper vials
Coccaine	Solution 2%	In 10 and 15 ml dropper vials
Phenocaine	Solution 1%	In 10 and 15 ml dropper vials
Dimethocaine	Solution 2.5%	In 10 ml dropper vial
Piperocaine	Solution 2%	In 10 ml dropper vial
Dibucaine	Solution 0.1%	In 5 and 10 ml dropper vials
Naepaine	Solution 2–4%	In 10 ml dropper vial
Butacaine	Solution 2%	In 10 ml dropper vial

Contd...

Contd...

Drug name (Generic)	Dosage form/strength	Commercial packing

LOCAL ANESTHETIC COMBINATIONS

Proparacaine and Fluorescein sodium	Combination solution having 0.5% Proparacaine and 0.25% Fluorescein sodium	In 5 ml dropper vial
Benoxinate and Fluorescein sodium	Combination solution having 0.4% benoxinate and 0.25% Fluorescein sodium	In 5 ml dropper vial

MYDRIATICS AND CYCLOPLEGICS

Mydriatic Adrenergic Agents

Adrenaline (Epinephrine)	Solution 1:1000	2 ml ampoule and 5 ml vials
Coccaine HCl	Solution 2 and 4%	5 and 10 ml dropper vials
Phenylephrine	Solution 2.5 and 10%	2, 5 and 15 ml dropper vials
Hydroxy amphetamine	Solution 1%	5 ml vial

Cholinergic Antagonist as Cycloplegic Mydriatics

Atropine sulphate	Solution 0.5, 1, 2 and 3% Ointment 0.5 and 1%	In 2,5 and 10 ml vials 3.5 and 5 g tubes
Homatropine	Solution 2 and 5%	2,5,10 and 15 ml dropper vials
Scopolamine	Solution 0.25%	In 5 and 15 ml dropper vials
Cyclopentolate HCl	Solution 0.05, 1 and 2%	2,5,10 and 15 ml dropper vials
Tropicamide	Solution 0.5, 1%	3, 5 and 10 ml dropper vials

Mydriatic Combinations

Phenylephrine HCl and Cyclopentolate HCl	Combination solution having 0.2–1% Cyclopentolate 1-5% phenylephrine	In 2 and 5 ml dropper vials In 2 and 5 ml dropper vials
Scopolamine HBr and Phenylephrine HCl	Combination solution having 0.3% scopolamine and 10% Phenylephrine	5 ml dropper vial
Tropicamide and Hydroxyamphetamine HBr	Combi Solution containing 1% hydroxyamphetamine and 0.25% tropicamide	In 5 and 15 ml dropper vial
Phenylephrine HCl and Tropicamide	Combination solution having Phenylephrine 5% and Tropicamide 0.8%	In 5 and 10 ml dropper vial
Cyclopentolate HCl and Dexamethasone Sodium phosphate	Combination solution having 1% cyclopentolate and 0.1% Dexamethasone	In 5 and 10 ml dropper vials

OPHTHALMIC VISCOSURGICAL DEVICES (OVD) AND SURGICAL ADJUNCTS

Viscoelastic Substances

Sodium Hyaluronate	Injection 10 mg/ml, 12 mg/ml, 14 mg/ml, 16 mg/ml and 30 mg/ml	In 0.4, 0.55, 0.85 and 2 ml preloaded disposable syringes with 27G or 30 G cannula

Contd...

Contd...

Drug name (Generic)	Dosage form/strength	Commercial packing
	Highly viscous 1% Solution of sodium Hyaluronate of lower Molecular weight	2 ml preloaded disposable syringe
Sodium Hyaluronate and Chondroitin sulfate	Injection Solution Containing (3.1 mixture) Of 3% sodium hyaluronate, 4% chondrotin sulfate with 0.45 mg sodium dihydrogen phosphate hydrate and 4.3 mg NaCl per ml	0.5 ml in preloaded disposable syringe
Sodium Hyaluronate and Fluorescein Sodium	Solution containing 10 mg Sodium Hyaluronate, 0.005 mg Fluorescein Sodium per ml	In 0.55 or 0.85 ml preloaded disposable syringe cannula
Chondrotin Sulfate	Injection solution 20%	In 2 ml vial with 30 G cannula
Polyacrylamide (oscolon)	Injection solution 4.5 mg/ml	2 ml vial with 27 G cannula
Hydroxy propyl methyl Cellulose (HPMC)	Injection solution 2 and 2.5%	In 2 or 15 ml vial or 2 ml prefilled sterile disposable syringe with 27G cannula
Poly TEGMA (Triethylenglycol monomethacrylate)	Injection solution as 40%	In 2 ml prefilled disposable syringe with cannula
Collagen	Injection solution 1.4% collagen type IV	In 2 ml disposable syringe with cannula

Irrigating Solutions

Intraocular Irrigating Solutions

BSS (Balanced Salt solution)	Solution containing 0.64 NaCl, 0.75% KCl, 0.3% magnesium chloride, 0.43% calcium chloride, 0.39% Sodium acetate 0.17% Sodium citrate and Sodium hydroxide	In 15,30, 300 and 500 ml sterile packs
BSS plus (Mix aseptically just before use)	Solution having Part-I (480 ml) containing 7.44 mg NaCl, 0.395 mg KCl, 0.433 mg Sodium Phosphate, 2.19 mg Sodium bicarbonate Hydrochloric acid or Sodium bicarbonate Hydrochloric acid or Sodium hydroxide/ml Part II (20 ml) containing 3.85 mg Calcium Chloride dehydrate, 5 mg magnesium chloride hexahydrate, 23 mg dextrose and 4.6 mg glutathione disulfide/ml	Preservative free in 10 ml, 30,50 and 500 ml packs

Extraocular Irrigating Solutions (EIS)

EIS Type I	Solution containing 0.49% NaCl, 0.075% KCl 0.048% Cacl, 0.03% mgcl	In 15, 30 and 120 ml

Contd...

Contd...

Drug name (Generic)	Dosage form/strength	Commercial packing
	0.39% Sodium acetate, 0.17% Sodium citrate and 0.013% Benzalkonium chloride	packs
EIS Type II	Solution containing Boric acid, Sodium borate With 0.004% phenyl Mercuric nitrate or 0.002% Thimerosal	In 15,30,120 and 180 ml packs
EIS Type III	Solution containing 1.2% Boric acid, 0.38% KCl, 0.014% Sodium carbonate anhydrous, 0.05% EDTA and 0.01% Benzalkonium Chloride	In 30 and 120 ml packs
EIS Type IV	Solution containing 0.05% tetrahydrozoline HCl with NaCl, Sodium Borate, Boric acid, 0.01% Benzalkonium Chloride and 0.1% EDTA	In 15 ml pack
EIS Type V	Solution containing NaCl, Sodium proprionate, Sodium borate, Boric acid, glycerin, Rose water, camphor, Extract of witch hazel, Berbrine bisulfate and Benzalkonium chloride	In 60 and 180 ml packs
EIS Type VI	Solution having 0.49 NaCl, 0.4% sodium biphosphate, 0.45% sodium phosphate with 0.005% Benzalkonium chloride	In 180 ml pack
Eye wash	Solution containing NaCl, mono or dibasic Sodium phosphate, Benzalkonium chloride and EDTA	In 120 ml pack with eye cup

Surgical Enzymes

Alpha Chymotrypsin	Available as powder Containing 150 units or 300 units of alpha Chymotrypsin with 2 ml sodium chloride diluent per dual chamber univial	As Powder pack of 750 units per vial with 9 ml BSS diluent
Urokinase	As powder 5000 units of Urokinase are dissolved in 2 ml normal saline	Powder pack with 9 ml BSS diluent
Hyaluronidase	Fluffy powder containing 300 units of activity/mg	Ampoule containing 1500 IU

Chelating Agents and Mycolytics

Sodium EDTA	Solution containing 0.01% sodium EDTA	In 5 and 10 ml dropper vials
Calcium EDTA	Solution containing 0.2% calcium EDTA	In 5 and 10 ml dropper vials

Contd...

Contd...

Drug name (Generic)	Dosage form/strength	Commercial packing
Acetyl cysteine	As solution in conc. of 5, 10 and 20% can be diluted in artificial tears or Physiological saline	In 10 and 15 ml dropper vials
Laevo cysteine	Solution in conc. of 0.1–0.2 molar of Laevocysteine	In 10 and 15 ml vials

Caustic Preparations

Pure alcohol	Solution as 100% alcohol	In 60 and 120 ml packs
Hydrogen peroxide	Solution as 2%	In 30 and 60 ml packs

Cyanoacrylate Tissue Adhesive

	As liquid tissue adhesive	In 15 and 30 g tubes

Surgical Adjuncts

Fractionated purified Silicone oil	Injection Silicone oil	10 ml vial with Special flip off seal In a sterile pouch (single use)
Polydimethyl siloxane (Silicone oil)	Injection (Polydimethyl Siloxane oil)	In sterile single use 10 and 15 ml vials
Botulinum toxin Type A	Powder for injection (Lyphilized) 100 units of Lyophilized *Clostridium* Botulinum Toxin Type A	Preservative free Powder in vial along with 0.05 mg albumin and 0.9 mg Sodium chloride in vials
Povidone Iodine	Solution containing 5% povidone iodine	In 15 and 50 ml packs
Absorbable gelatin film sterile	Sterile film in sizes of 100 x 125 mm and 25 x 50 mm	Single sterile pack and pack of 6 sterile films

<u>OPHTHALMIC DYES</u>

Fluorescein sodium	Topical solution 2% contains 0.25% Fluorescein sodium 0.1% Proparacaine HCl or 0.4% Benoxinate HCl 0.01% Thimerosal preservative	In 5 ml pack
	Topical solution 2% Fluorescein sodium plain	In 1, 2 and 15 ml packs
	Topical solution containing 0.25% Fluorescein sodium 0.05% Proparacaine HCl 0.01% Thimerosal with povidone, boric acid and polysorbate 80	In 5 ml pack
	Injection 10 and 25% Fluorescein sodium	In 1,2, 5, 10 and 15 ml packs
	Fluorescein strips as 0.6 mg, 1 mg and 9 mg strips (with Boric acid, polysorbate 80 and 0.5% Chlorbutanol) and High Molecular Fluorescein (Higlo) Strips for soft contact lenses	In a pack containing 100 or 300 strips Pack of 100 strips

Contd...

Contd...

Drug name (Generic)	Dosage form/strength	Commercial packing
Fluorexon	Solution as 0.35% (12N)	In 0.5 ml pipette
Rose Bengal	Topical solution 1% Containing 1% Rose Bengal with povidone, Sodium borate PEG10 and 0.01% thimerosal	5 ml dropper vial
	As 1.3 mg strip	Pack of 100 strips
Lissamine Green	Solution 0.1, 0.5 and 1%	5 ml dropper vial
	Sterile strips containing 15 mg of Lissamine green	Pack of 100 strips
Indocyanine Green	Powder for injection As 25 mg and 50 mg	Powder pack with 10 ml ampoule of aqueous solvent
Trypan Blue	Solution containing 0.6 mg Trypan Blue, 1.9 mg of Sodium mono hydrogen orthophosphate, 0.3 mg of sodium dihydrogen orthophosphate, 8.2 mg sodium chloride and sodium hydroxide	1 ml ampoule (Pack of 10 ampoules)
Verteporfin (Visudyne)	As Sterile lipid based Freeze dried powder Requires reconstitution With sterile water and Dilution with 5% Dextrose Before infusion	As single use 15 mg vial with sterile water and ampoules

LUBRICANTS AND ARTIFICIAL TEAR SOLUTIONS

Methylcellulose and Ethylcellulose Base

Hydroxypropyl methylcellulose (HPMC)	Solution containing 0.5 or 1% HPMC and 0.01% Benzalkonium chloride	In 10,15 ml dropper vials
	Solution containing 0.5% HPMC, Gelatin A, Chlorbutanol 0.5%, NaCl and polysorbate 80	In 10,15 and 30 ml vials.
	Solution containing 0.5% HPMC, boric acid, NaCl, KCl, Phosphoric acid and Sodium perborate	In 15 ml vial
	Solution containing 0.5% HPMC, Dextran 40 (0.1%). 0.01% Benzalkonium Cl EDTA, NaCl and Boric acid solution	In 10 and 15 ml vials
	0.5% HPMC, Dextran 70 (0.1%) Benzalkonium Chloride (0.01%) and EDTA	In 15 ml vial
	Solution: HPMC 1%, Propyleneglycol, NaCl, Boric acid and paraben	In 10 and 15 ml vials
	Solution 0.8% HPMC, 0.1%	Preservative free in 0.5 ml single dose containers (28s)

Contd...

Quick Look Tabulated Ocular Therapeutics Information

Contd...

Drug name (Generic)	Dosage form/strength	Commercial packing
	Dextran 70, Sodium phosphate, KCl, NaCl, Dextrose	
	Solution: 0.3 HPMC 2910, 0.1% Dextran 70, NaCl, KCl Sodium bicarbonate	Preservative free in single use 0.45 ml packs (28s)
	Solution: 0.4% HPMC 2910, Diabasic phosphate, potassium chloride, NaCl and 0.01% Benzalkonium Cl.	In 15 ml dropper vial
	Solution: 0.3% HPMC 2910, 0.1% Dextran, 0.01% polyquarterrnium-1 NaCl, KCl, Sodium borate	In 15 and 30 ml dropper vials
Hydroxyethyl cellulose (HEC)	Solution containing 0.5% hydroxy-ethylcellulose (HEC), 1.67% povidone with water soluble polymers, Thimerosal 0.004% and EDTA (1%)	In 10 and 15 ml vials
	Solution: 0.5% HEC, polyvinyl alcohol 1% and 0.01% Benzalkonium chloride, EDTA and NaCl	In 15 ml vial
	Solution: 0.5% HEC in a hypertonic base, 0.25% sorbic acid 0.01% EDTA	In 10 and 15 ml vials
	Solution: 0.5% HEC, 0.44% NaCl	In 10 and 15 ml vials
Carboxymethyl cellulose (CMC)	Solution containing 1% CMC, NaCl, KCl and sodium lactate	Preservative free in 0.3 ml unims (30 single dose pack)
	Solution: 0.25% sodium carboxymethyl cellulose, NaCl, KCl and sodium phosphate	Preservative free in 0.6 ml single dose containers
	Solution: 0.5% CMC, KCl, NaCl.	Preservative free containers in 0.3 ml single use
	Solution: 0.5% CMC, boric acid, Cacl, KCl, NaCl and magnesium chloride	In 15 ml vial

Polyvinyl Alcohol-base Solutions

	Solution containing 1.4% Polyvinylalcohol (PVA) and 0.6% Povidine, 0.5% Chlorbutanol and NaCl.	In 15 ml vial
	Solution: 1.4, 0.6% Povidone, retinyl palmitate, boric acid, 0.09% EDTA, 0.001% WSCP, NaCl, KCl.	In 15 ml dropper vial
	Solution: 1% PVA, PEG-400, 1% Dextrose, 0.01% Benzalkonium, EDTA	In 15 and 30 ml vials
	Solution: 1.4% PVA, 0.5% Chlorbutanol, NaCl	In 15 x 30 ml vials
	Solution: 0.5% PVA, 0.6% Povidone, Benzalkonium Cl, Dextrose, EDTA, NaCl, Sodium bicarbonate and Sodium phosphate.	In 15 and 30 ml vials

Contd...

Contd...

Drug name (Generic)	Dosage form/strength	Commercial packing
	Solution: 1.4% PVA, 0.6% povidone and NaCl	Preservative free in 0.3 ml single dose containers (30 and 50 UD)
	Solution: 3% PVA, 0.002% Thimerosal, NaCl and EDTA.	In 15 ml vial
Carmellose sodium	Opthalmic solution 10 mg	10 ml vial

Miscellaneous Artificial Tear Solutions

	Solution: Polysorbate 80, Sodium chloride, EDTA, Retinyl Palmitate, Mannitol, Sodium citrate and pyruvate	Preservative free in 10 and 15 ml packs
	Solution: 0.3% Glycerin, NaCl, KCl, Sodium citrate and Sodium phosphate	Preservative free in 0.3 ml (UD 32s)
	Solution: 0.25% Glycerin, EDTA, Sodium chloride and Benzalkonium Cl.	In 15 ml vial
	Adsorbonac NaCl 2 or 5% solution	In 5 and 10 ml vials
Ointments		
	Ointment containing petrolatum (55.5%) Lanolin (2%) and mineral oil (42.5%)	Preservative free in 3.5 and 5 g tubes
	Ointment: 2% HPMC, NaCl, KCl, CaCl, MgCl, Sodium acetate and Sodium citrate	Preservative free in 3.5 and 5 g tubes
	Lubricant gel Carbopal 980 (Polyacrylic acid) which Transforms from gel to liquid in contact with ocular tissue	In 5 g tube
	Gel: 0.3% HPMC	In 10 ml pack
	Ointment: 56.8% white petrolatum, 42.5% mineral oil, Chlorobutanol, Lanolin alcohols	In 3.5 and 7 g tubes
	Ointment: White petrolatum	Preservative free in 0.5 g pack
	Ointment: 55% white petrolatum, 32% mineral oil, boric acid, stearic acid and wheat germ oil	In 3.5 g tube
Ocular inserts		
lacriset	Polymeric insert having 5 mg of HPMC	Preservative free in 60s with applicator
Punctal plugs		
Collagen implant	Intracanalicular collagen implant consists of 0.2, 0.3, 0.4, 0.5 and 0.6 mm diameter inserts packed at the edge of a foam strip	In a pack of 10 or 72 plugs with inserter tool
Silicone plugs	Punctum silicone plug in 1.6, 2 and 2.8 mm sizes	In a pack of 2 or 10 plugs with inserter tool

Contd...

Contd...

Drug name (Generic)	Dosage form/strength	Commercial packing
Lubricant for artificial eyes	Solution containing 0.25% Tyloxapol and 0.02% Benzalkonium chloride	In 15 ml dropper vial
	Solution containing 2.5% HPMC with 0.004 Thimerosal and 0.1% EDTA	In 15 ml dropper vial for gonioscopic exam

TOPICAL IMMUNE THERAPY

Aspac (Topical)	Ophthalmic solution Containing 0.1% each of IgA, IgG and IgM in fixed concentrations	Preservative free In 5 and 10 ml dropper vial with controlled tip

TOPICAL HYPEROSMOTIC AGENTS

Sodium chloride (Hypertonic)	Solution as 2% or 5% NaCl with 0.004% water soluble polymer Thimerosal and 0.1% EDTA	In 10 and 15 ml dropper vials
	Topical NaCl solution 2% or 5% with HPMC and parabens	In 10 and 15 ml dropper vials
	Topical 5% NaCl solution with propylene glycol, sodium borate and boric acid	In 10 ml dropper vial
	Ointment containing 6% NaCl gel with petrolatum and Lanolin.	In 3.5 and 5 g tubes
Glycerine	Topical solution as 50% (0.6 g glycerine/ml) with 0.55% chlorobutanol	In 7.5 ml vial
	Ointment as 40% with petrolatum and lanolin parabens	
Sodium chloride	5% Ophthalmic solution 6% Ointment	

CONTACT LENS CARE PRODUCTS

Hard Lenses

Cleaning/Soaking/Wetting Solutions for Hard Lenses (Complete)

Total solution	Containing buffered Isotonic Polyvinyl alcohol, Benzalkonium chloride, EDTA	In 60 and 120 ml packs

Wetting Solutions (Hard Lenses)

	Solution containing 0.004% Benzalkonium Cl, EDTA, HPMC, NaCl, KCl and Polyvinyl alcohol	In 60 ml pack
	Solution: Buffered 0.1% EDTA, 0.01% Benzalkonium Cl	In 60 and 120 ml pack

Contd...

Contd...

Drug name (Generic)	Dosage form/strength	Commercial packing

Wetting/Soaking Solutions (Hard Lenses)

| | Solution containing buffered isotonic 0.1% EDTA and 0.05% Benzalkonium Cl | In 120 ml pack |
| | Solution: Buffered isotonic 0.003% Benzalkonium chloride, Polyvinyl alcohol and EDTA | In 120 and 180 ml pack |

Rewetting Solutions (Hard Lenses)

	Solution containing Povidone, water soluble polymers, sorbic acid and EDTA (Isotonic)	In 15 ml pack
	Solution (Isotonic) Hydroxyethyl cellulose sorbic acid, poloxamer 407, 0.1% EDTA, NaCl, KCl, Sodium borate, boric acid	In 5, 15 and 30 ml packs
	Solution: Isotonic 0.04%, thimerosal, 0.1%, EDTA, povidone and polyoxyethylene	In 15 ml pack
	Solution: Isotonic 0.1% EDTA, 0.001% polyquaternium-1, Dextran, NaCl, KCl and HPMC	Thimerosal free in 15 ml pack
	Solution: Buffered, isotonic Nacl, Carbamide, poloxamer 407, 0.2% EDTA, 0.15% Sorbic acid	In 15 ml pack
	Buffered solution with polyoxyl 40 stearate PEG 300 and 0.5% Chlorobutanol	In 15 ml pack

Cleaning Solutions (Hard Lenses)

	Solution with anionic sulfate surfactant, friction enhancing agents and NaCl	In 15 and 60 ml pack
	Solution: 15.7% isopropyl alcohol, poloxamer 407 and amphoteric 10	Preservative free in 12 ml
	Solution: Buffered isotonic Tween 21, polymeric cleaners, 0.1% EDTA and 0.001% polyquaternium-1.	Thimerosal free in 12 and 20 ml packs
	Buffered solution Cocoampho carboxy glycinate, sodium lauryl sulfate, hexylene glycol, Alkyl ether sulfate, fatty acid amide surfactants	Preservative free in 30 ml pack

Contd...

Contd...

Drug name (Generic)	Dosage form/strength	Commercial packing
	Solution: Cocoampho diacetate, glycol, 0.1% EDTA and 0.01% benzalkonium Cl.	In 60 ml pack
	Solution with poloxamer 188, 0.01% Benzalkonium Chloride and 0.2% EDTA	In 15 and 30 ml
	Solution with hydrophilic polyelectrolyte, polyvinyl alcohol, hydroxy ethyl cellulose, chlorhexidine gluconate and EDTA.	In 15 and 30 ml packs

Cleaning and Soaking Solution (Hard Lenses)

	Solution buffered surfactant cleaning agent with 0.004% Phenylmercuric nitrate	In 120 ml pack

Rigid Gas Permeable (RGP) Lenses

Wetting/Soaking Solutions (RGP Lenses)

	Buffered solution containing 0.0015% polyaminopropyl biguanide 0.05% EDTA, cationic cellular derivative polymer	In 120 ml pack
	Buffered solution low viscosity, 0.5% EDTA, 0.006% chlorhexidine gluconate, cationic cellulose derivative polymer as wetting agent	In 120 ml pack
	Solution having EDTA and Chlorhexidine	In 120 ml pack
	Solution: Isotonic hydroxyethyl cellulose, 0.006% polixetonium chloride	Thimerosal free in 120 ml pack
	Buffered solution: 0.005% chlorhexidine gluconate, 0.02% EDTA Octylphenoxy, ethanol, povidone, polyvinyl alcohol, propylene glycol and HEC, NaCl	In 120 and 240 ml packs
	Buffered solution: Sodium and potassium chloride, PVA, PVP, HEC, sodium bisulfite, 0.02%, Benzyl alcohol 0.1%, sorbic acid 0.05% and disodium edetate 0.1%	In 120 ml pack
	Buffered isotonic, 0.003% benzalkonium chloride, polyvinyl alcohol, EDTA	In 120 and 180 ml packs

Contd...

Contd...

Drug name (Generic)	Dosage form/strength	Commercial packing

Disinfecting/Cleaning Solutions (RGP Lenses)

	Buffered isotonic sterile saline solution having sodium edetate with biguanide copolymer 0.0031%	In 350 ml pack
	Solution: Lauryl sulfate salt of imidazoline octylphenoxy, 0.3% benzyl alcohol and 0.5% trisodium EDTA	Thimerosal free in 120 ml pack
	Solution: Lauryl sulfate salt, benzyl alcohol 0.1% and disodium edetate 0.5%	In 120 ml pack
	Buffered solution; sorbitan monolaurate, betaine surfactant, silicone glycol, polythylene glycol, 0.003% chlorhexidine gluconate, 0.005% polyamino propyl biguanide and 0.05% edetate disodium	In 120 ml pack

Surfactant Cleaning Solutions (RGP Lenses)

	Solution: Concentrated homogenous surfactant, alkyl ether sulfate, ethoxylated alkylphenol, cocoa-based phospholipid silica gel	In 30 ml pack
	Surfactant solution with alkyl ether sulfate silica gel	In 30 ml pack
	Buffered isotonic solution 0.004% thimerosal 0.1% EDTA, Tween 21, Hydroxyethyl cellulose and polymeric cleaners	In 12 and 20 ml packs
	Solution: Edetate disodium 0.1%, polyquad 0.001%, Tween 21, Polymeric cleaning agents	In 12 and 118 ml packs
	Buffered isotonic solution 0.1%, EDTA, 0.001% polyquaternium-1, Polymeric cleaners, Tween 21	Thimerosal free in 12 and 20 ml packs

Enzymatic Cleaners (RGP Lenses)

	Liquid containing subtilism and glycerol	Preservative free in 1 ml pack
	Tablets: Highly purified postpancreatin	Pack of 24 and 36 tablets

Contd...

Contd...

Drug name (Generic)	Dosage form/strength	Commercial packing
	Tablet: Papain, NaCl, sodium carbonate, sodium borate and EDTA	Pack of 16 and 24 tablets
	Liquid: Preservative free containing propylene glycol sodium borate and pancreatin	

Rewetting Solutions (RGP Lenses)

	Solution containing polyquad 0.1%, edetate disodium, citrate buffer dextran NaCl, KCl.	In 15 ml pack
	Solution: Sorbic acid 0.1%, edetate disodium 0.2%, HEC, sodium borate, boric acid and NaCl	In 15 ml pack
	Solution: Buffered, hypertonic 0.006%, Chlorhexidine gluconate, 0.05% EDTA, cationic cellulose derivative polymer as wetting agent	In 10 ml pack

Soft Lenses (Hydrogel)

Disinfection Nonhydrogen Peroxide Soft Lenses

	Buffered solution containing NaCl, 0.0001% polyhexamethylene biguanide, tromethamine, tyloxapol and EDTA	Thimerosal free 120 and 360 ml packs
	Buffered isotonic solution 0.005% chlorhexidine 0.1% EDTA, 0.001% Thimerosal, NaCl, sodium borate and boric acid	In 360 ml pack
	Buffered isotonic solution 0.05% EDTA, 0.001% polyquaternium-1 sodium citrate and NaCl	In 120 ml pack
	Solution: isotonic 0.00005% polyamino propyl biguanide, 0.01% EDTA, NaCl sodium borate, boric acid and poloxamine	In 120 and 355 ml pack

Disinfection Hydrogen Peroxide Soft Lenses

	Disinfectant/Soaking Solution 3% hydrogen peroxide, 0.85% stabilized	In 120, 240 and 360 ml packs

Contd...

Contd...

Drug name (Generic)	Dosage form/strength	Commercial packing
	with phosphonic acid, phosphate buffer and Cleaner/Rinser isotonic boric acid, sodium borate sodium perborate, 0.006% hydrogen peroxide	In 12 ml pack

Saline Solutions (Preserved) Soft Lenses

	Solution, buffered isotonic, 0.01% EDTA, 0.001% thimerosal, NaCl, sodium hexametaphosphate, boric acid and sodium borate	In 240 and 360 ml packs
	Solution: Isotonic 0.1% EDTA, 0.001% polyquaternium-1, NaCl, sodium borate	Thimerosal free in 360 ml pack
	Solution, Buffered isotonic 0.1% sorbic acid, 0.025% EDTA, NaCl, boric acid, sodium borate	Thimerosal free in 120, 240 and 360 ml packs
	Buffer solution 0.1% sorbic acid, boric buffer, EDTA, NaCl	In 60 and 360 ml packs
	Isotonic solution: NaCl, boric acid, sodium borate, sodium perborate, hydrogen peroxide, phosphoric acid	In 120, 240 and 360 ml packs

Preservative Free Saline Solutions (Soft Lenses)

	Buffer solution containing NaCl, boric acid and sodium borate	In 120, 240 and 360 ml packs
	Buffered isotonic solution: NaCl, catalytic neutralizing agent, EDTA, mono and dibasic sodium phosphates	In 15 ml single use containers

Rinsing/Storage Solutions (Soft Lenses)

	Solution containing NaCl, sodium hexametaphosphate, sodium hydroxide, boric acid, sodium borate 0.001% EDTA and 0.001% thimerosal	120 and 240 ml packs
	Isotonic buffered solution of NaCl, boric acid, 0.0003% polyaminopropyl biguanide and EDTA	In 120 and 340 ml packs
	Isotonic solution with 0.9% NaCl	Preservative free 120 and 240 ml packs
	Buffered isotonic with NaCl and EDTA or NaCl with boric acid and sodium borate	Preservative free 120 and 240 ml packs

Contd...

Quick Look Tabulated Ocular Therapeutics Information

Contd...

Drug name (Generic)	Dosage form/strength	Commercial packing

Surfactant Cleaning Solutions (Soft Lenses)

	Solution containing 0.001% thimerosal, EDTA	In 15 and 60 ml packs
	Buffered isotonic solution NaCl, sodium phosphate, tyloxapol, hydroxyl ethyl cellulose, polyvinyl alcohol, EDTA, sorbic acid	In 30 ml pack
	Solution with cocoamphor-carboxyglycinate, sodium lauryl sulfate, hexylene glycol, 0.1% sorbic acid, 0.2% EDTA	In 15 ml pack
	Solution: 15.7% isopropyl alcohol, poloxamer 407, amphoteric 10	Thimerosal free in 15 and 30 ml packs
	Solution: Buffered isotonic: 0.15% sorbic acid, 0.1% EDTA, boric acid, poloxamine, sodium borate, NaCl	In 240 ml pack
	Solution: Propylene glycol, sodium borate, highly purified porcine pancreatin enzymes	Preservative free in 5 and 10 ml packs
	Solution: 0.25% sorbic acid, 0.5% EDTA, NaCl, KCl, poloxamer 407	In 25 ml pack

Enzymatic Cleaners (Soft Lenses)

	Tablet containing papain, NaCl, sodium carbonate, sodium borate, EDTA	In pack of 12, 24, 36 and 48 tablets
	Tablet containing subtilisin A, polyethylene glycol, sodium carbonate, NaCl and tartaric acid	In pack of 8 tablets
	Tablets: Effervescing buffering and tableting agents subtilisin A. To make solution for soaking dilute in 3% hydrogen peroxide solution	In pack of 5,10,15 and 20 tablets

Disinfecting/Wetting/Soaking Solution (Soft Lenses)

ReNu multiplus	Solution containing Hydranate, boric acid, edetate sodium, sodium borate, NaCl, dymed (polyamino-propyl biguanide) 0.001% and 1% poloxamine	In 120, 240 and 360 ml packs
	Solution: 0.001% Polyhexamethylene	In 120, 240 and 360 ml packs

Contd...

Contd...

Drug name (Generic)	Dosage form/strength	Commercial packing
	Biguanide (PHMB), 0.025% tyloxapol, 1.2% tromethamine and 0.05% edetate disodium	

REWETTING SOLUTIONS (SOFT LENSES)

	Isotonic solution containing 0.25% sorbic acid, 0.1% EDTA, borate buffer, NaCl, HPMC and glycerin	Thimerosal free in 15 ml pack
	Isotonic solution NaCl, KCl, hydroxyethyl cellulose, poloxamer 407, sodium borate, boric acid, sorbic acid and EDTA	Thimerosal free in 5,15 and 30 ml packs
	Buffered isotonic solution NaCl, 0.0001% polyhexamethylene biguanide, tromethamine, tyloxapol, EDTA	In 15 ml pack
	Solution: Sorbic acid, 0.15% and edetate disodium 0.2%	In 15 ml pack
	Buffered isotonic NaCl, boric acid	Preservative free in 0.035 ml pack
	Isotonic solution: Citrate buffer, NaCl, 0.05% EDTA, 0.001% polyquaternium-1	In 10 and 20 ml packs
	Solution: Sorbic acid 0.1% and edetate disodium	In 15 ml pack
	Isotonic solution with NaCl, 0.13% potassium sorbate and 0.025% EDTA	Thimerosal free in 15 ml pack

NONSURGICAL ADJUNCTS

Lid Scrubs

	Solution containing PET-200 glyceryl tallowate, disodium laureth sulfosuccinate cocoamidopropylamine oxide, PEG-78 glyceryl cocoate, benzyl alcohol and EDTA	In a pack of 30/60 pads and solution (120 ml)
	Solution: PEG 80 sorbitan laurate, sodium trideceth sulfate, PEG-150 distearate, cocoamido propylhydroxy sutlaine, Lauroamphacarboxy-Glycinate, sodium laureth 13 carboxylate PEG-15 tallow polyamine, quaternium-15	Alcohol free. In 30,120 and 240 ml packs (120 ml and 100 pads)

Contd...

Contd...

Drug name (Generic)	Dosage form/strength	Commercial packing

Tear Test Strips

Schirmer test strip	Sterile test strips	Pack of 250 strips
Snostrips	Sterile tear flow test strips	In a pack of 100 strips
Zone quick	Phenol red threads (PRT)	In 50 aluminum packing sets (100 threads)

Hamameli's Water

	Solution containing aqueous and glycerin solution of senecio compositae, hamameli's water and boric acid	In 7 ml vial

Boric Acid

	As powder	In a pack of 15 g powder

Astringent Ophthalmic Solution

	Zinc sulphate 0.12% Boric acid 1.25% Naphazoline HCl 0.056% and Chlorpheniramine maleate 0.01%	In 5 and 10 ml dropper vials
	Zinc sulphate 0.25% Tetrahydrozoline 0.05% EDTA and benzalkonium Cl (0.004%)	In 10 and 15 ml dropper vials
	Zinc Sulphate 0.1% Bolax 0.05%, Boric acid 1.9%, Sodium chloride 0.45%, KCl 0.45, HPMC 0.7%	In 10 ml dropper vial and 120 ml bottle

Vitamin and Antioxidants

Vitamin A palmitate	Tablets/Cap. containing 5000 IU/10000 IU/ 15000 IU/ 25000 IU Vitamin A	In pack of 100/ 250 Tab./Cap.
Antioxidants	Capsule containing vitamin A 6000 IU, Zinc 30 mg, Copper 1.5 mg, Selenium 60 mcg, Manganese 5 mg, Vitamin B_{12} 20 mg Vitamin C 200 mg and Vitamin E 60 IU	In a pack of 100 capsules
	Mixcarotin cap. containing 15.44 mg Of mixed carotenoids in oily suspension (Alpha carotene,	Soft gel capsules (in a pack of 100 capsules)

Contd...

Contd...

Drug name (Generic)	Dosage form/strength	Commercial packing
	beta carotene, lutein, cryptoxanthin and Zeaxanthine) equivalent to 25000 IU of Vitamin A	
	Tablets containing 5000 IU betacarotene, 150 IU E, 20 mg B_1, B_2, B_6 each, 10 mcg B_{12}, 15 mg elemental Zn, 50 mcg, Selenium, 20 mg calcium pantothenate, 40 mg glutathion 40 mg B_3 100 mg C, 75 mg L-cysteine	In a pack of 100/250 tablets
	Capsule: 5000 IU Vitamin A, 400 mg C, 200 IU E, 40 mg Zn, 5 mg L-glutathione, 3 mg sodium pyruvate, 2 mg copper and 40 mcg selenium	In a pack of 60 capsules
	Capsules softgel: Vitamin A 5000 IU, 200 IU, Vitamin E, 200 mg Vitamin C, 7.5 mg Zinc, 1 mg copper, 15 mcg selenium and 1.5 mg Mn	In a pack of 50 capsules
	Tablets: 5000 vitamin A 30 IU Vitamin E, 60 mg Vitamin C, 40 mg Zinc, 2 mg copper and 40 mcg selenium	Film coated tablets in a pack of 60

Topical Anticataract Therapy

Catalin	Solution containing pyridophenoxazine (catalin) in concentration of 0.75 mg/15 ml solvent	Pack of Tablet alongwith 15 ml solvent
Cineraria	Solution containing large quantity of organic potassium	In 15 ml dropper vial
Anticataract solution	Solution containing 3.3% potassium iodide, 0.83% NaCl and 1.0% calcium chloride	In 10 ml dropper vial
Aspirin	Topical solution as 1%	In 15 ml dropper vial
Vitamin E therapy	Capsule containing 100/200 mg of vitamin E (alpha tocopherol)	In a pack of 100 capsules

Medical Therapy for Diabetic Retinopathy

D400	Tablet: Herbomineral preparation	In a pack of 100 tablets
Calcium debesilate	Capsule (500 mg)	In a pack of 50 capsules
Aspirin	Tablet (325 mg)	In a pack of 100 tablets
Dipyridamol	Tablet (225 mg)	In a pack of 60 tablets

Contd...

Contd...

Drug name (Generic)	Dosage form/strength	Commercial packing
Ticlopidine	Tablet (500 mg)	In a pack of 100 tablets
Cyclandelate	Capsule (400 mg)	In a pack of 100 capsules
Ponalrestat	Tablet (600 mg)	In a pack of 50 tablets
Sulindac	Tablet (250 mg)	In a pack of 100 tablets

Disinfective and Antiseptic Agents in Ophthalmology

Formaldehyde (Formalin)	As 10% aqueous solution	In 60 ml, 400 ml 1 liter and 5 liter packings
	As 10% tablets	In a pack of 60/100 tablets
Ethylene oxide	As 3% colorless liquid	In 400 ml and 1 liter packings
Glutaraldehyde	2% solution	As 60 ml, 400 ml and 1 liter packings
Sodium hypochlorite	As 1% solution	In 60 ml and 400 ml and 1 liter packings
Isopropyl alcohol	As 70% isopropyl alcohol	Presterilized individual swabs (A pack of 100 swabs)
Biguanides		
Polyhexanide (PHMB)	As stock 20% solution For ocular conditions diluted solution (1:1000) As 0.02% is prepared	In 60 ml, 100 ml and 400 ml packings
Chlorhexidine	As 5% stock solution 0.2% diluted solution is prepared in isotonic saline for ophthalmic use	In 100 ml, 400 ml and 1 liter packings
Povidone iodine (Halogens)	5% sterile prepared solution	In 5 ml, 15 ml dropper vials
Acetone	As 58.8% solution and 1 liter packings	In 60 ml, 100 ml and 400 ml
Cetrimide	10% solution	In 400 ml and 1 liter packings
Beta propiolactone (BPL)	0.2% solution/condensed product of ketone and formaldehyde	On 100 ml, 400 ml and 1 liter packings
Alcoholic rub-in-hand Disinfectant (Sterillium)	As solution containing 2-propanol 45.0 g 1- propanol 30.0 g Ethyl hexadecyl -2 g Dimethyl ammonium Ethyl sulfate	In 100 ml pack 100 ml
Cutasept (Antiseptic)	As solution containing 2-propanaol -63 g Benzalkonium Cl-0.025 g	100 and 500 ml packs 10 g
Korsolex disinfectant	As solution containing (Each 100 g contains) Glutaraldehyde 7.0 g Formaldehyde 8.2 g Polymethylol urea derivative 17.6 g	as 500 ml pack

Contd...

Contd...

Drug name (Generic)	Dosage form/strength	Commercial packing
Bacillol disinfectant	As solution (Each 100 g contains) Ethanol – 10 g 2-Propanol-9 g 1-Propanol- 6 g	As 200 ml pack with spray
Baktolin (Antiseptic)	As solution (Each 100 g contains) Propylene glycol 0.52% Sodium salicylate 0.46% Sodium lauryl Sulphate 4.08% Sodium benzoate 5.9% with cocoglucoside, PEG 120, glycerine, glycol stearate and sodium citrate	As 500 ml pack with dispenser
HIV disinfectant	Solution containing 45 g 2-propanol, 30 g 1-propanol, 0.2 g mecetronium ethyl sulfate (INN)	In 500 ml and 1 liter packs
Hydrogen peroxide	as stock solution (6%) For ophthalmic use can be diluted to 3%.	In 100 and 500 ml packs

Section 2

Applied Ocular Therapeutics in Ophthalmic Surgery

Comprehensive Review of Topical Ophthalmic Antibacterial Agents: Their Mechanisms of Action and Adverse Effects Including Long-Standing Drugs and the Most Recent Preparations

Renée Solomon, Eric Donnenfeld (USA)

BACTERIAL CONJUNCTIVITIS

Bacterial conjunctivitis is common, generally mild to moderate in severity, and usually self-limiting.[1] Treatment with topical ophthalmic antibiotics speeds resolution of the disease, decreases morbidity, prevents recurrence and spread of the disease to social contacts, decreases the incidence of permanent conjunctival changes, decreases the risk of corneal or intraocular infection when surgery is anticipated, and prevents the development of chronic conjunctivitis with its greater treatment challenges and risk of progression to corneal damage or disease.[2-4] The most frequently isolated pathogens in acute bacterial conjunctivitis are *Streptococcus pneumoniae* and *Haemophilus influenzae* in pediatric patients and *Staphylococcus epidermidis* in adult patients.[5,6]

Chronic conjunctivitis is defined as any case of conjunctivitis that lasts longer than 2 weeks. The most common pathogens associated with this condition are *Staphylococcus aureus* and *S. epidermidis*, the most common organisms found in normal lid and conjunctival flora. These pathogens produce toxins that can damage the conjunctiva and cornea, producing the superficial punctate keratopathy that is commonly seen. The punctate keratopathy characteristically involves the inferior cornea and conjunctiva. These organisms also commonly spread to other ocular structures, such as the meibomian orifices, lash follicles, and the lacrimal canaliculi, and may even breach the corneal epithelium.[2,3]

Other, more serious types of infectious conjunctivitis include hyperacute bacterial conjunctivitis, usually caused by *Neisseria gonorrhoeae* and *S. pneumoniae*. *Neisseria gonorrhoeae* is often associated with oropharyngeal infections and requires systemic and topical therapy.[2,3]

In the treatment of acute bacterial conjunctivitis, most physicians do not perform cultures, and therefore, prescribe broad-spectrum antibiotic agents. Because bacterial conjunctivitis is usually self-limiting, agents associated with a higher incidence of ocular toxicity or hypersensitivity reactions are best avoided. Combination products with gram-positive and gram-negative coverage are popular for their broad-spectrum of activity, but some contain agents that can be irritating or cause allergic reactions. Patient compliance is a common treatment challenge, particularly in pediatric patients, because they are reluctant to let anyone instill anything into their eyes and are sensitive to irritating agents.

BACTERIAL KERATITIS

Bacterial keratitis is an ophthalmic emergency that has the potential to cause significant vision loss secondary to corneal scarring and perforation. Rapid diagnosis and immediate treatment with appropriate antimicrobial therapy are necessary to limit the extent of tissue damage and to improve the visual prognosis.[3-7] Approximately 30,000 cases of microbial keratitis are diagnosed each year in the United States.[8] The most likely causative organisms depend on geographic location, pre-existing corneal disease, urban or rural environment, history of contact lens wear, and climate.[9-13]

Approximately 87 percent of all cases of bacterial keratitis in the United States result from infection by one of the following organisms: gram-positive infections are most commonly secondary to streptococci or staphylococci, whereas the gram-negative organisms include *Pseudomonas* species or *Enterobacteriaceae* (especially *Serratia marcescens* but also *Citrobacter, Klebsiella, Enterobacter*, and *Proteus* species).[14-16] Currently, the most common causes of microbial keratitis are *S. aureus* in the northern United States and *Pseudomonas* and *Streptococcus* species in the southern United States.[3,11,17] *Streptococcus pneumoniae* is the most common pathogen in many developing countries. *Staphylococcus* species are the most common organism associated with photorefractive keratectomy or LASIK.[18] *Pseudomonas* species are frequently associated with overnight contact lens wear, but may also be seen with daily-wear contact lenses.[19-27] In fact, *Pseudomonas* species have become a more common cause of bacterial keratitis in the southern United States than *S. aureus*.[28,29] In children younger than 3 years of age, *Pseudomonas* species have been identified as the most common bacterial cause of keratitis.[30,31]

Many ophthalmologists diagnose and treat bacterial keratitis based on their empirical observations and only perform a microbial analysis on particularly severe ulcers (e.g. those encroaching on or involving the visual axis). Most physicians choose what they think to be a broad-spectrum antibiotic and begin treatment immediately,[3,32,33] but the choice of agent may also be influenced by which pathogen is suggested by the disease presentation and the physicians' knowledge of pathogen prevalence in the local environment and patient population.[28,34-36] Care must be taken in the choice of a broad-spectrum antibiotic because certain commercially available agents may have significant gaps in the spectra of their antimicrobial efficacy, may poorly penetrate the cornea, or may be bacteriostatic rather than bactericidal. Any of these characteristics would make them unsuitable for the treatment of bacterial keratitis.

For approximately 25 years, the mainstay for the treatment of these infections has been dual therapy using topically administered fortified antibiotics.[37] These antibiotics are not commercially available and are specially formulated by hospital pharmacies or physicians when needed. Traditionally, one antibiotic provided coverage against gram-negative pathogens (an aminoglycoside such as tobramycin or gentamicin [13.6 mg/ml]), and the second antibiotic covered the spectrum of gram-positive bacteria (vancomycin [25 mg/ml], cefazolin [50 mg/ml], or bacitracin [10,000 U/ml]). Together, they provided an initial empirical regimen for the treatment of bacterial keratitis. During the past several years, the fluoroquinolone family of antibiotics has offered an alternative to fortified antibiotics as the mainstay of treatment for bacterial ulcerations. Two double-masked, controlled, clinical trials have supported the clinical efficacy of using the commercially available fluoroquinolones (ofloxacin 0.3% or ciprofloxacin 0.3%) as compared with fortified tobramycin and cefazolin.[38,39]

There are various routes for administering antibiotics in the treatment of ocular infections and include topical, subconjunctival, oral, intravenous, and intramuscular. Topical application of antibiotics is the preferred route of administration for bacterial conjunctivitis and keratitis because the drops provide therapeutically effective concentrations; the drops wash away bacteria and bacterial antigens; adverse systemic effects of the drugs are decreased or eliminated; and in reliable patients, they can be administered on an outpatient basis.[40-43] The factors that contribute to achieving effective therapeutic concentrations of the drug in the cornea include the frequency of administration, the concentration of the drug, the lipophilic nature of the drug where the epithelium is intact, the length of contact time of the drug with the cornea, and the lack of an intact corneal epithelium.[44,45] The next section deals with the individual characteristics of the various topical ophthalmic antibiotics used to treat bacterial conjunctivitis and keratitis.

PROPERTIES OF TOPICAL OPHTHALMIC ANTIBACTERIAL AGENTS

Fluoroquinolones

Chemistry, Ophthalmic Preparation, and Pharmacologic Action

The fluoroquinolones, the newest class of agents to be developed, are based on the prototype, nalidixic acid (1,8-naphthyridine), which was synthesized in 1962.[46] In the 1980s, the fluoroquinolones were created from nalidixic acid by adding a fluorine atom to position six of the molecule (Figs 27.1A to C). This addition widened the antibacterial spectrum of activity and resulted in decreased development of resistant organisms. The newer fluoroquinolones available for ophthalmic use include gatifloxacin

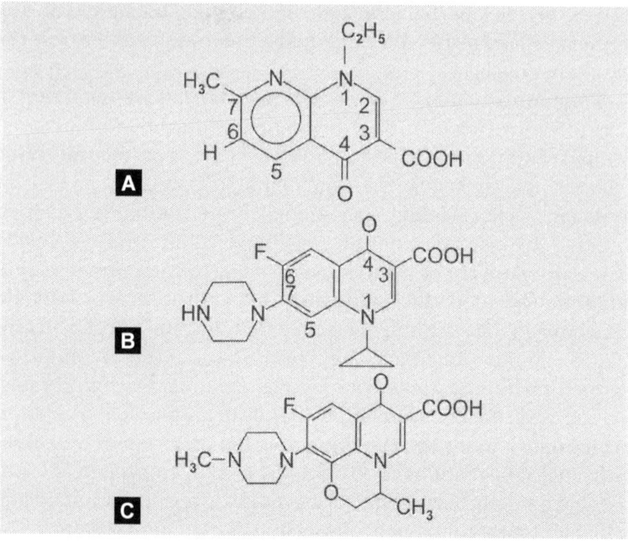

Figs 27.1A to C: Chemical structure of the nalidixic acid (A) from which the fluoroquinolones, including ciprofloxacin (B) and ofloxacin (C), were derived

ophthalmic solution 0.5 percent (Zymaxid®, Allergan, Inc., Irvine, CA), gatifloxacin 0.3 percent (Zymar®, Allergan, Inc.), moxifloxacin HCl ophthalmic solution 0.5 percent (Moxeza® Alcon Laboratories, Inc., Fort Worth, TX), moxifloxacin 0.5 percent (Vigamox®, Alcon Laboratories, Inc.), besifloxacin ophthalmic suspension 0.6 percent (Besivance™, Bausch and Lomb, Rochester, New York), levofloxacin ophthalmic solution 1.5 percent (Iquix®, Vistakon® Pharmaceuticals, LLC, Jacksonville, Florida), and levofloxacin ophthalmic solution 0.5 percent (Quixin, Vistakon® Pharmaceuticals, LLC). In addition to the fluoroquinolone eye drops, there is a fluoroquinolone ophthalmic ointment, ciprofloxacin (Ciloxan, Alcon Laboratories, Inc.) and generic formulations available of the prior generation fluoroquinolones, ofloxacin and ciprofloxacin. The previous generation fluoroquinolones predominantly either inhibit topoisomerase II (DNA Gyrase) or topoisomerase IV and therefore, only require one genetic mutation for bacteria to develop resistance.[47] Fourth-generation fluoroquinolones are equally effective against bacterial topoisomerase II and IV, which significantly expands their spectrum of action against gram-positive agents and atypical mycobacteria and Nocardia.[48,49] This duality of action of the fourth generation fluoroquinolones requires that for bacteria to become resistant to these agents, the bacteria must undergo two genetic mutations resulting in a significantly decreased chance of an organism developing resistance.[50] The fluoroquinolones are bactericidal by interfering with bacterial DNA replication, transcription, repair, and recombination.

Gatifloxacin differs from the prior generation ciprofloxacin in two positions, but the enhanced activity of the molecule compared to ciprofloxacin is due to a methoxy group at the 8-position of the fluoroquinolone structure. Moxifloxacin has the same group at the 8-position, but differs from gatifloxacin at the 7-position of the molecule. The 8-methoxy substitution yields the better coverage against gram-positive organisms, including resistant strains, while preserving the similar coverage against gram-negative organism seen in prior generations of fluoroquinolones.

Clinical Experience and Ophthalmic Uses for the Individual Ophthalmic Preparations of the Fluoroquinolones

The ophthalmic fluoroquinolones are indicated for the treatment of conjunctivitis. However, because of their broad spectrum antibacterial activity, they are also used to minimize the risk of postoperative endophthalmitis after cataract surgery, postoperative keratitis after keratorefractive procedures, and to treat bacterial keratitis. Minimum inhibitory concentrations determined *in vitro* suggest that fourth-generation fluoroquinolones are more effective than second-and third-generation fluoroquinolones against gram-positive bacteria, including Staphylococcal species found in endophthalmitis and bacterial keratitis cultures.[50,51] When selecting a fourth-generation fluoroquinolone, it is important to consider potency, ocular penetration, efficacy and safety. In addition, the acute management of bacterial corneal ulcers requires rapid access to therapy. The cost and toxicity of antibiotic therapy must also be considered. Fortified antibiotics are not commercially available and must be prepared on request. The fluoroquinolones are superior with respect to accessibility, cost, and low toxicity. The fluoroquinolones perform at least as well as, and often better than, the aminoglycosides in the treatment of gram-negative corneal ulcers. Prompt, appropriate treatment decreases the length of time to eradication of the infection, minimizes the risk of sequelae, helps prevent the spread of infection, and reduces the time away from daily activities.

Since there are two ophthalmic formulations of gatifloxacin and moxifloxacin, and no current generic formulations, brand names will be used in this section. The commercial ophthalmic formulations of gatifloxacin, Zymar® and Zymaxid®, and the commercial formulation of besifloxacin contain the preservative benzalkonium chloride (BAK) 0.005 percent, whereas the commercial ophthalmic formulations of moxifloxacin 0.5 percent, Vigamox® and Moxeza®, contain no BAK. As noted, Zymaxid® contains a higher concentration (0.5%) of the antibacterial agent, gatifloxacin, found in Zymar® (0.3%). In addition, Iquix is also a preservative-free formulation.

Gatifloxacin Ophthalmic Solution

The addition of the methoxy group at the 8-position of the ring structure increased the potency against gram-positive bacteria by four-fold from ciprofloxacin to gatifloxacin, resulting in a lower minimal inhibitory concentration (MIC). In comparing gatifloxacin to moxifloxacin, gatifloxacin was shown to be significantly more active against ocular isolates of *Pseudomonas aeurginosa* with a MIC_{90} of 1.28 versus 2.60 mg/ml for moxifloxacin. In addition, gatifloxacin was demonstrated to have slightly better activity than moxifloxacin against some gram-negative pathogens. As noted, Zymar® and Zymaxid® are formulated with the preservative BAK. The preservative is frequently included to prevent contamination of the bottle that could be picked up by skin flora if the bottle comes in contact with the skin during instillation. In addition, the antibiotic formulation is not anti-fungal, but the Zymar® and Zymaxid® formulation are resistant to contamination by fungi. It has been reported that BAK in the Zymar® and Zymaxid® formulations may enhance their antibacterial activity as shown by more rapid killing and lower MICs.

Moxifloxacin Ophthalmic Solution

Moxeza®[52] is a reformulation Vigamox® with a new vehicle, xanthan gum, which supports BID labeling because the new formulation allows the antibiotic to remain on the eye longer and increases penetration into the ocular tissues. Moxeza® is dosed two times per day for seven days and is indicated for patients four months of age and older.

A multicenter, vehicle controlled, randomized, double-masked, parallel group study was conducted on Moxeza to evaluate *in vivo* safety and efficacy.[52] The study group included clinically-diagnosed bacterial conjunctivitis in 1,180 patients aged >28 days (range 30 days to 92 years). Moxeza® or its vehicle was dosed one drop twice-daily for 3 days. Microbiological specimens were obtained from affected eyes on day 1, prior to the initial dose, and on day 4 after 3 days of dosing. All recovered bacteria were identified to the species level. The microbiological success rate for patients treated with Moxeza twice-daily for 3 days was 74.5 percent, compared with 56.0 percent of patients treated with its vehicle control ($P<0.0001$). Moxeza was also statistically more effective than vehicle in eradicating the three principle conjunctivitis pathogens, *Haemophilus influenzae* (98.5% vs 59.6%, respectively), *Streptococcus pneumoniae* (86.4% vs 50.0%, respectively), and *Staphylococcus aureus* (94.1% vs 80.0%, respectively) ($P<0.001$). This clinical study demonstrated that the use of Moxeza resulted in effective eradication of the three principle causative pathogens of bacterial conjunctivitis across all age groups when dosed twice-daily for 3 days.[52]

As indicated by Tauber, et al the majority of topical ophthalmic antibiotic products approved in the United States for the treatment of bacterial conjunctivitis have a 7- to 10-day treatment regimen, totaling a minimum of 21–42 or more drops over a course of therapy. A full course of therapy with Moxeza® is 14 drops over 7 days. Results from this Tauber's demonstrate that Moxeza®, when dosed topically twice daily for 3 days (total six drops per eye), was statistically superior to its vehicle in the percentage of patients classified as microbiological successes after 3 days of treatment (75% vs 56%, P<0.0001). Moxeza® was also significantly more effective than its vehicle in eradicating the three principle conjunctivitis pathogens. The eradication rate of *H. influenzae* was 98.5 percent for Moxeza® versus 59.6 percent for its vehicle; *S. pneumoniae* was 86.4 percent for Moxeza® compared with 50.0 percent for vehicle, and *S. aureus* was 94.1 percent for Moxeza® compared with 80.0 percent for vehicle.[52] BAK alone has significant *in-vitro* cytotoxicity to cultured ocular epithelial cells. As Moxeza® is preservative-free, there is no risk of corneal toxicity that may occur secondary to the BAK preservative. With respect to the issue of the potential of enhanced potency of Zymar due to BAK, some have argued that the BAK does not enhance potency because it is rapidly diluted in the tear film, weakening its ability to enhance potency when it reaches the ocular surface. In addition, it has been pointed out that the less concentrated ophthalmic formulation of moxifloxacin, Vigamox, does not need a preservative because of the intrinsic antibacterial and antifungal activities of its formulation.

Vigamox®: Studies have demonstrated that moxifloxacin has enhanced ocular penetration. *In vivo* studies have demonstrated that the conjunctival concentration of one drop of moxifloxacin twenty minutes prior to a conjunctival biopsy was greater than one drop of gatifloxacin, levofloxacin, ciprofloxacin and ofloxacin. In addition, the corneal concentration of moxifloxacin in the epithelium, stroma and endothelium in a patient undergoing penetrating keratoplasty was demonstrated to be higher than the concentration of gatifloxacin. A prospective, randomized, parallel, double-masked study of 50 patients undergoing cataract extraction were dosed preoperatively with Zymar or Vigamox every 10 minutes for 4 doses, beginning 1 hour prior to surgery. Mean concentrations measured in aqueous demonstrated that Vigamox achieved concentrations in aqueous humor 3.8 times greater than Zymar. The concentrations were 1.80 (+/- 1.21) micrograms/ml for Vigamox and 0.48 (+/- 0.34) micrograms/ml for Zymar. Furthermore, microbiologic dilution analyses of aqueous humor samples demonstrated that moxifloxacin was 4.9 times more microbiologically active against *S. epidermidis* (2.1 mg/ml) compared with gatifloxacin (0.4 mg/ml). The structure of moxifloxacin ophthalmic solution 0.5 percent may account for its enhanced penetration. Moxifloxacin is highly lipophilic and has high aqueous solubility at physiologic pH. 9 or the enhanced penetration may be as a result of the higher concentration of moxifloxacin than the concentration of other agents with which it was compared.

Besifloxacin: Besifloxacin ophthalmic suspension 0.6 percent is a chlorofluoroquinolone formulation which also indicated for the treatment of bacterial conjunctivitis.[53-55] Besifloxacin was developed solely for ophthalmic use, eliminating the contribution to resistance development from the selective pressure of systemic use. It has potent broad-spectrum bactericidal activity, especially against multidrug-resistant isolates.[56-58] The ophthalmic formulations for besifloxacin and azithromycin contain DuraSite® (polycarbophil, edetate disodium dihydrate and sodium chloride) (InSite Vision, Alameda, CA) a mucoadhesive polymer designed to prolong the drug's residence time on the ocular surface.[59] Besivance also contains 0.01 percent benzalkonium chloride (BAK) as a preservative, a compound that has been shown to have bacteriostatic and bactericidal activities of its own.[60,61]

Besifloxacin has been found to have good ocular penetration in monkeys, with rapid absorption and sustained concentrations in anterior ocular tissues through 24 hours after a single administration.[62] In a study to determine the concentrations of besifloxacin, moxifloxacin, and gatifloxacin in human aqueous humor after topical instillation of commercially available besifloxacin ophthalmic suspension 0.6 percent, moxifloxacin ophthalmic solution 0.5 percent, and gatifloxacin ophthalmic solution 0.3 percent, it was determined none of fluoroquinolones tested would likely be therapeutically effective in the aqueous humor against the most frequently identified drug-resistant staphylococcal isolates from recent cases of postoperative endophthalmitis.[63]

Levofloxacin: Levofloxacin is the L-enantiomer of its racemate ofloxacin. It was developed to address the increasing bacterial resistance to ofloxacin. Iquix is indicated for the treatment of corneal ulcers by susceptible strains. Iquix has the highest concentration available for any ophthalmic antibiotic. Therefore, it would not be surprising that studies have shown in the cornea, concentrations of levofloxacin were greater than those of gatifloxacin and moxifloxacin. Iquix has the highest aqueous solubility of the topically administered fluoroquinolones.

Adverse Effects

The fluoroquinolones have low rates of adverse effects.[64] The most frequently reported adverse events of Zymaxid® were worsening of the conjunctivitis, eye irritation, dysgeusia, and eye pain. For Zymar® the most frequently reported adverse reactions occurring in 5–10 percent of patients were conjunctival irritation, increased lacrimation, keratitis, and papillary conjunctivitis. Less frequently reported reactions found in 1–4 percent of patients were chemosis, conjunctival hemorrhage, dry eye, eye discharge, eye irritation, eye pain, eyelid edema, headache, red eye, reduced visual acuity and taste disturbance.

The most common side effects of Moxeza® are eye irritation, fever, and conjunctivitis. The most frequently reported ocular adverse events secondary to the use of Vigamox® found in 1–6 percent of patients were conjunctivitis, decreased visual acuity, keratitis, ocular discomfort, ocular hyperemia, ocular pain, ocular pruritis, subconjunctival hemorrhage and tearing.

The ocular adverse events occurring from use of Iquix® in 1–2 percent of patients included decreased/blurred vision, instillation site irritation/discomfort, ocular infection, and ocular pain/discomfort. The nonocular adverse events occurring in approximately 8–10 percent of patients were headache and taste disturbance. The most frequently reported adverse events, which occurred in 1-3 percent of patients, were transient decreased vision, fever, foreign body sensation, headache, transient ocular burning, ocular pain or discomfort, pharyngitis and photophobia. Other reactions that were reported in less than 1 percent of patients included allergic reactions, lid edema, ocular dryness and ocular itching. With respect to Besivance®, the most common adverse events in clinical trials were conjunctival redness, blurred vision, eye pain, eye irritation, eye pruritus and headache, reported in approximately 1-2 percent of patients one year and older.

In a randomized, masked, placebo-controlled animal study evaluating the anterior chamber toxicity of the two topical ophthalmic formulations containing DuraSite® (Besivance and Azithromycin), it has been determined that these two formulations are toxic to the anterior chamber. When injected into the anterior chamber the following side effects were noticed: conjunctival injection, moderate limbal vascularity, and severe, diffuse corneal edema, corneal ectasia and bullous keratopathy.[65] Because of the corneal edema, the anterior chamber could not be viewed, but vital staining and histopathologic evaluation revealed glaucomatous and toxic damage in eyes given DuraSite®-based medications, whereas the groups without the DuraSite® polymer showed minimal changes. Two mechanisms of damage were identified in the eyes injected with Besivance or AzaSite: acute glaucoma and direct toxic reaction. The authors noted besifloxacin and azithromycin are completely different classes of drugs, and that the concentrations of BAK are radically different in these two drugs, so they believe that it is reasonable to conclude that DuraSite is most likely responsible for the toxicity results. While further studies are warranted to determine if these problems are of clinical importance, the authors concluded that DuraSite® blocks the trabecular meshwork and may be additionally toxic when introduced as a large bolus. The authors recommended that until the safety of these medications is established with further studies using smaller injected volumes, that there should be placement of a suture over a clear corneal wound if DuraSite®-based medications are used.[65]

The most commonly reported adverse effect from topical ciprofloxacin treatment is the formation of a white crystalline precipitate in approximately 17 percent of treated eyes.[66-68] This results from precipitation of the drug (formulated at pH 4.5), which is poorly soluble at the near-neutral pH of the tear film. The relationship between this precipitate and antibacterial efficacy is unknown. The precipitate resolves spontaneously without sequelae after cessation of the medication. Like the 0.3 percent solution, the ciprofloxacin ointment has also been shown to cause a white precipitate that resolves spontaneously without sequelae after discontinuing it. Other adverse effects from the ointment include burning, punctate epitheliopathy, blurred vision, and tearing.[69]

EXTEMPORANEOUSLY COMPOUNDED FORTIFIED ANTIBIOTICS

Extemporaneously compounded fortified antibiotic eyedrop preparations contain high concentrations that are usually prepared from products formulated for intravenous use. A typical treatment regimen might consist of a combination of a cephalosporin (e.g. 50 mg/ml cefazolin) for gram-positive bacteria coverage and an aminoglycoside (e.g. 13 mg/ml tobramycin or gentamicin) for gram-negative bacteria coverage. However, these agents are not compatible when combined in the same solution and must be formulated separately and administered from different bottles. Another common extemporaneously fortified antibiotic is vancomycin 50 mg/ml.[70] Most need to be refrigerated after dispensing to the patient, because, being derived from intravenous products, they do not contain a preservative. Instillation of the two agents must be separated by intervals of several minutes or more (e.g. 15 minutes might be ideal) to prevent washout of the first agent by the second. The high concentrations used in these preparations exacerbate their epithelial toxic potential. This is a special concern for the aminoglycosides.

In the treatment of bacterial keratitis, fortified cefazolin-aminoglycoside preparations are as effective as the fluoroquinolones ofloxacin and ciprofloxacin, but are more difficult to obtain and use. Not all pharmacies are equipped to formulate extemporaneously-compounded agents and not all pharmacists are familiar with the procedures.

There has been some debate in the literature as to the efficacy of using a collagen shield as a vehicle to absorb and deliver drugs. Advocates argue that collagen shields soak up antibiotics and continuously deliver them to the cornea for several hours, enabling higher concentrations to be delivered for longer periods of time. However, some studies have found that collagen shields are not more efficacious than using fortified antibiotics alone.[71,72] According to several other studies, collagen shields are labor intensive yet as effective in treating bacterial keratitis, as frequent dosages of drops.[73-77]

AMINOGLYCOSIDES

Chemistry, Ophthalmic Preparation, and Pharmacologic Action

The two most commonly used aminoglycosides are tobramycin sulfate available as a 0.3 percent solution or ointment (AKTOB [Acorn, Inc, Buffalo Grove, IL], Defy, Tobrex [Alcon Laboratories, Fort Worth, TX]) and gentamicin sulfate (Figs 27.2A and B) available as a 0.3 percent solution (Garamycin, Genoptic [Allergan, Inc, Irvine, CA], Gentacidin, Gentak [Akorn, Inc, Buffalo Grove, IL], Ocumycin) and ointment (Garamycin, Genoptic). Neomycin [Bausch and Lomb Pharmaceutical, Inc, Tampa, FL] is also used, but is only available as a component of combination products, not as a single agent. The basic structure of aminoglycosides

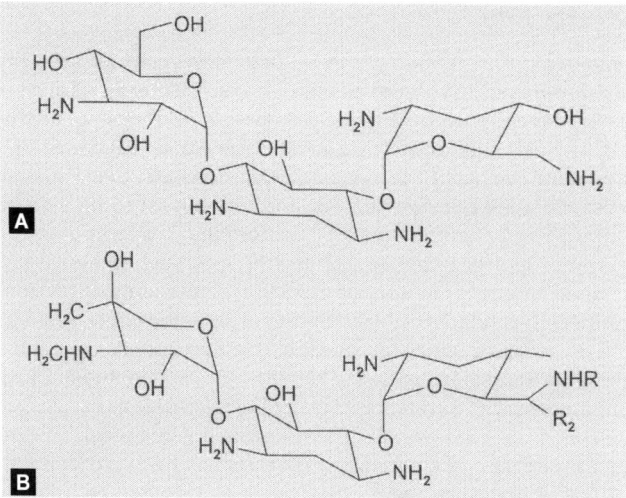

Figs 27.2A and B: The aminoglycosides, with some of the more commonly used ophthalmic formulations pictured, tobramycin (A), and gentamicin (B), which contain the characteristic two or more amino sugars connected by glycosidic bonds to a hexose nucleus

consists of two or more amino sugars connected by glycosidic bonds to a hexose nucleus. The individual characteristics of an aminoglycoside are determined by differences in the amino sugars attached to the nucleus.

The aminoglycosides cause bacterial cell death by irreversibly binding to 30S ribosomes and causing misreading of the genetic code and decreased or abnormal protein synthesis.[78] Aminoglycosides are valued in the treatment of external ocular infections because they are active against aerobic gram-negative organisms, including *Pseudomonas* species, *Proteus* species, *Klebsiella* species, *Escherichia coli*, *Salmonella* species, *Shigella* species, *S. marcescens*, *Haemophilus* species, and many gram-positive staphylococci.[79] *In vitro*, tobramycin is three times as effective as gentamicin against *Pseudomonas*[80] The aminoglycosides have limited use as broad-spectrum agents because of resistance caused by aminoglycoside-modifying enzymes. This occurs at an unacceptably high frequency (29%–41%).[81] Of particular concern is their lack of relative efficacy against *S. epidermidis* and *S. pneumoniae*.

Clinical Experience and Ophthalmic Uses

Gentamicin and tobramycin have been shown to be effective in the treatment of conjunctivitis, blepharoconjunctivitis, and bacterial keratitis.[78,82-84] The commercially-available concentrations are acceptable for the treatment of bacterial conjunctivitis, but the highly concentrated, fortified preparations are preferred for bacterial keratitis and are best used in conjunction with an antibiotic more active against gram-positive bacteria.

Adverse Effects

Gentamicin and tobramycin have been shown to be safe, but tobramycin may have fewer adverse effects.[85] The most significant safety concern with aminoglycosides is corneal epithelial toxicity.[81,86,87] This is especially so for neomycin and gentamicin.[86] Lass et al evaluated the concentration-dependent toxicities of neomycin, amikacin, gentamicin, and tobramycin using a rabbit epithelial cell culture model.[86] Subfortified concentrations of neomycin and gentamicin significantly inhibited epithelial cell metabolism after 5 minutes of exposure; all the aminoglycosides significantly inhibited cell metabolism at all tested concentrations after 30 and 60 minutes of exposure. Fortified doses may cause a reversible punctate epithelial keratitis or pseudomembranous conjunctivitis.[88,89] Several cases of conjunctival defects or necrosis have been reported with the use of fortified gentamicin,[87,90] and at least one case of conjunctival necrosis has been attributed to fortified tobramycin use.[87] Two cases of pseudomembranous conjunctivitis secondary to topical gentamicin have been reported: one case after use of commercial-strength gentamicin and one in response to fortified 1.36 percent gentamicin.[91] Neomycin has a high rate of associated allergic reactions; in one study, 18.5 percent of 27 patients with chronic conjunctivitis had patch test sensitivity to neomycin.[92] Other neomycin toxic manifestations are conjunctivitis, eyelid edema, punctate corneal erosions, and in high concentrations, reduced corneal sensation.[93]

BACITRACIN

Chemistry, Ophthalmic Preparation, and Pharmacologic Action

Bacitracin is a polypeptide antibiotic that contains a thiazolidine ring structure (Fig. 27.3). Bacitracin is bactericidal by binding to cell membranes[94] and is commercially produced as a topical ophthalmic ointment (AK-Tracin, Akorn, Inc, Buffalo Grove, IL) or in combination with polymyxin B (AK-poly-bac [Akorn, Inc, Buffalo Grove, IL], Polysporin, Polytracin [Medical Ophthalmics, Tarpon

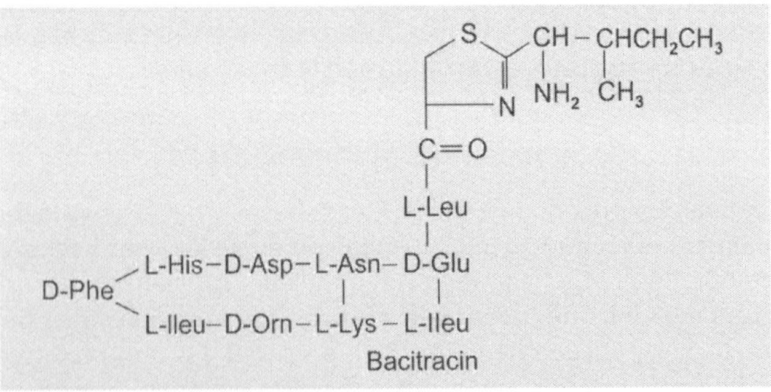

Fig. 27.3: Structural formula of bacitracin, the polypeptide antibiotic that contains a thiazolidine ring

Springs, FL]) or with polymyxin B and neomycin (AK-Spore [Akorn, Inc, Buffalo Grove, IL], Neosporin [Monarch Pharmaceuticals, Bristol, TN], Ocu-spor B). All these preparations contain bacitracin in a concentration of 500 U per gram of ointment. Unlike most of the other antibacterial agents discussed in this chapter, bacitracin is only available for topical use because of its systemic toxicity and poor solubility.

Clinical Experience and Ophthalmic Uses

Bacitracin is efficacious against most gram-positive organisms and select gram-negative organisms, including penicillinase-producing staphylococci, *Neisseria* species, *Haemophilus* species, and *Actinomyces* species. Bacitracin penetrates an intact cornea poorly, but its penetration may be increased by a corneal epithelial defect.[95]

Adverse Effects

Commercially-available preparations and fortified dosages of bacitracin generally do not irritate the ocular surfaces. Hypersensitivity reactions, namely skin eruptions, have been reported. There is one report of an acute anaphylactic reaction associated with topical application of bacitracin.[96]

BETA-LACTAM ANTIBIOTICS

Chemistry, Ophthalmic Preparation, and Pharmacologic Action

This class of antibiotics includes the penicillins and cephalosporins. Penicillins (Figs 27.4A and B) are composed of a thiazolidine ring connected to a beta-lactam ring to which a side chain is connected. The side chain is responsible for the individual characteristics of the penicillins. Like the penicillins, the cephalosporins (Figs 27.5A to C) contain a beta-lactam ring, are bactericidal, and inhibit cell

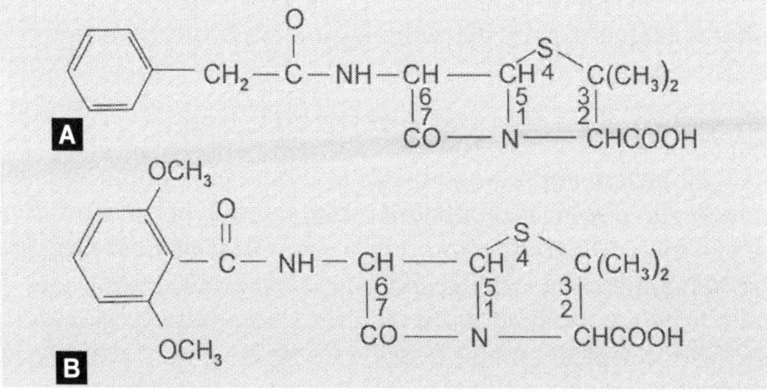

Figs 27.4A and B: Chemical formulas of the penicillin agents, which contain beta-lactam rings attached to thiazolidine rings (e.g. penicillin [A] and methicillin [B])

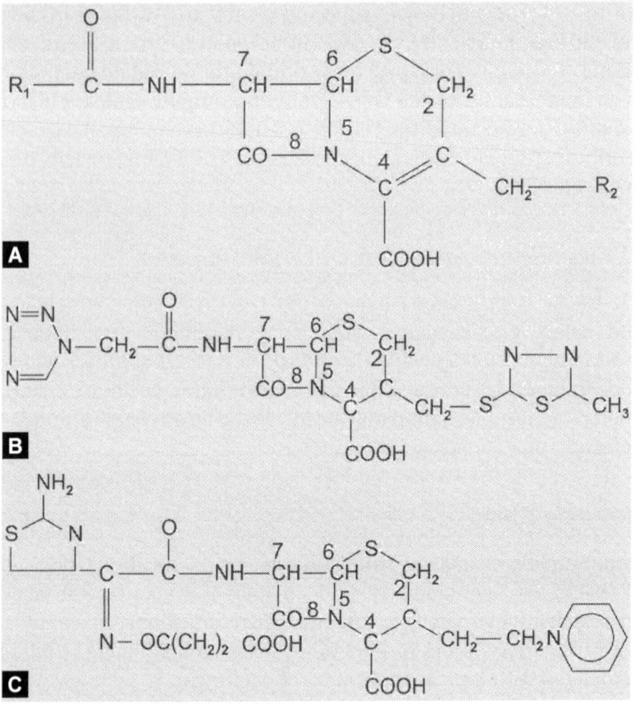

Figs 27.5A to C: Illustrations of the cephalosporins, which contain modifications to positions of the beta-lactam ring of cephalosporin (A), to create cefazolin (B), and ceftazidime (C)

wall synthesis. By preventing the synthesis of polysaccharides needed for bacterial cell wall structure, they cause bacterial death. They tend to be more active against gram-positive organisms, with increased gram-negative activity in the extended-spectrum penicillins and the second- and third-generation cephalosporins. Bacteria become resistant to penicillins by producing beta-lactamase; cephalosporins tend to be resistant to degradation by beta-lactamase. All methicillin-resistant *S. aureus* and enterococci are also resistant to cephalosporins. Approximately 10 percent of patients allergic to penicillin will also be allergic to cephalosporins.

Clinical Experience and Ophthalmic Uses

The beta-lactam antibiotics are not available in pharmaceutically manufactured topical ophthalmic preparations because of their poor stability. The most commonly used topical agent in this class is a first-generation cephalosporin, cefazolin 50 mg/ml, and is made from a parenteral preparation. As mentioned, cefazolin is used with a topical aminoglycoside in the treatment of bacterial keratitis. However, ceftazidime alone or in combination with an aminoglycoside or vancomycin has also been explored as an initial agent for topical therapy of bacterial keratitis.[97] A third-generation cephalosporin, ceftazidime, was found to be as effective as cefazolin in treating rabbit corneal ulcers caused by *S. aureus* and *S. pneumoniae* and as effective as tobramycin against *P. aeruginosa*.[98,99]

The cefazolin-aminoglycoside combination has been proven to be equivalent to monotherapy with ofloxacin and ciprofloxacin in bacterial keratitis. Topical cefazolin may also have an important role in combination with fluoroquinolones. Bower and coworkers[100] have predicted that 98.7 percent of their laboratory's ocular bacterial isolates would be susceptible to a fluoroquinolone-cefazolin combination versus 88.2 percent, 82.3 percent, and 80.4 percent, respectively, with ofloxacin, ciprofloxacin, and norfloxacin. Thus, in severe cases of bacterial keratitis, cefazolin may be a desirable addition to fluoroquinolone therapy, while culture results are pending and may supplant the need for fortified aminoglycosides.[101]

Adverse Effects

The most common adverse effects are allergic reactions to the penicillins with some cross-allergenicity with the cephalosporins. Topical penicillin can result in anaphylaxis, and less significantly, there is a high incidence of contact allergic blepharitis.[102] The cephalosporins have relatively few side effects,[102] and approximately only 5 percent of patients manifest allergic reactions.

CHLORAMPHENICOL

Chemistry, Ophthalmic Preparation, and Pharmacologic Action

Chloramphenicol, a nitrobenzene derivative (Fig. 27.6), available as a 1 percent ointment or a 0.5 percent solution (AK-Chlor, Chlormycetin [Monarch Pharmaceuticals, Bristol, TN], Chloroptic [Allergan, Inc, Irvine, CA], Ocu-Chlor), was the first broad-spectrum antibiotic with gram-positive and gram-negative coverage. It has been widely used in ointment form for the treatment of external ocular infection.[103]

Chloramphenicol inhibits bacterial protein synthesis by binding to the 50S ribosomal subunit. It is primarily bacteriostatic but may be bactericidal to some organisms (e.g. *H. influenzae*).

Clinical Experience and Ophthalmic Uses

Chloramphenicol has good antimicrobial activity against most gram-positive ocular isolates and limited gram-negative coverage.

$$O_2N-\underset{}{\bigcirc}-\underset{CHCH}{\overset{OH}{\underset{|}{C}}}-\underset{}{\overset{CH_2OH}{\underset{|}{C}}}-NH-\overset{O}{\underset{||}{C}}-CHCl_2$$

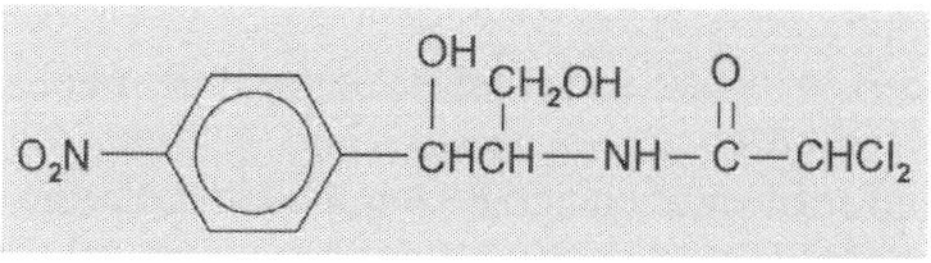

Fig. 27.6: Structure of chloramphenicol, a derivative of nitrobenzene

Chloramphenicol should not be used to treat infections in which gram-negative bacteria, especially *Pseudomonas* or *Serratia* species,[104] are suspected. Because it is usually bacteriostatic, not bacteriocidal, and because of its limited spectrum, chloramphenicol should not be used in vision-threatening circumstances.

In some studies, chloramphenicol has been shown to be as effective as ciprofloxacin, norfloxacin, and trimethoprim-polymyxin B in the treatment of bacterial conjunctivitis.[105-107]

Adverse Effects

Much has been written about a possible link between topical ophthalmic use of chloramphenicol and aplastic anemia. Oral chloramphenicol can affect the bone marrow in two ways; one is a dose-related, reversible bone marrow suppression and the other is an idiopathic, usually lethal effect. Topical chloramphenicol has been associated with dose-related and idiopathic bone marrow suppressions.[108-114] Chloramphenicol should best not be used in patients who have a family history of drug-related bone-marrow failure.[115,116] Concern about the risk of aplastic anemia and the development of more effective antibiotics have been sufficient to drastically reduce the use of chloramphenicol in the United States, although it is still widely used in other countries.

Burning may occur with topical instillation of chloramphenicol, but it is relatively nonirritating to ocular structures and allergic reactions are uncommon.

MACROLIDES

The macrolides include erythromycin, clarithromycin and azithromycin, the latter two which are semisynthetic. These antibiotics inhibit bacterial protein synthesis by irreversibly binding to the 50S ribosomal subunit.[117]

ERYTHROMYCIN

Chemistry, Ophthalmic Preparation, and Pharmacologic Action

Erythromycin 0.5 percent, is a macrolide antibiotic (Fig. 27.7) which is bacteriostatic in low concentrations, but can be bactericidal in high concentrations. Other determinants of its bactericidal activity include organism susceptibility, growth rate of the bacteria, and pH.[118] Erythromycin is only available in ointment form (0.5%) for topical ophthalmic use (Ak-mycin, Ilotycin, Romycin).

Clinical Experience and Ophthalmic Uses

Erythromycin is used as prophylaxis against neonatal conjunctivitis caused by *C. trachomatis* and *N. gonorrhoeae*. It is also used to treat mild bacterial conjunctivitis. Erythromycin is frequently employed in an ointment base as topical therapy for infections caused by gram-positive organisms or in combination

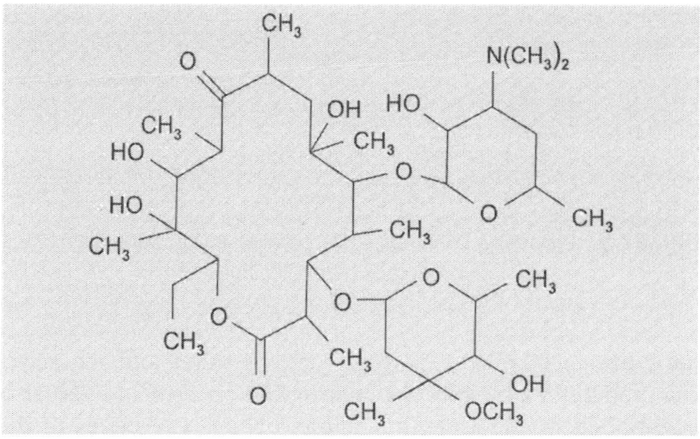

Fig. 27.7: Chemical structure of the macrolide antibiotic, erythromycin

with systemic tetracycline to treat *Chlamydia*. It has a broad-spectrum of antibacterial activity,[119] and is well tolerated by the ocular surface, but many resistant strains have developed. For example, several strains of *H. influenzae*, one of the most common pathogens in pediatric conjunctivitis, are resistant to erythromycin. In addition, the resistance of *Streptococcus* isolates is as high as 40 percent. Therefore, its usefulness in the treatment of external ocular infections is limited. Erythromycin is also used for infectious blepharitis and for nocturnal supplementation to topical eyedrops in the treatment of bacterial corneal ulcers.

Adverse Effects

Topical application of erythromycin is not usually irritating to ocular tissues.

AZITHROMYCIN

Chemistry, Ophthalmic Preparation, and Pharmacologic Action

Azithromycin ophthalmic solution 1 percent (AzaSite; Inspire Pharmaceuticals, Inc. a subsidiary of Merck and Company, Inc., Whitehouse Station, NJ) is another macrolide antibiotic which attacks bacterial protein synthesis. Azithromycin, a semi-synthetic molecule derived from the macrolide erythromycin (Fig. 27.8). Azithromycin differs from erythromycin by having a 15 member ring with an aza-methyl-substituted nitrogen in the aglycone ring The development of azithromycin expanded the indications for which macrolides could be used. The potential use in topical ocular anti-infective therapy has been quite limited until now, largely because of its chemical instability in an aqueous medium. Topical ophthalmic azithromycin is formulated in polycarbophil (the aqueous mucoadhesive polymer contained in DuraSite®) that delivers high and prolonged azithromycin concentrations in a variety of ocular tissues, including the cornea, conjunctiva

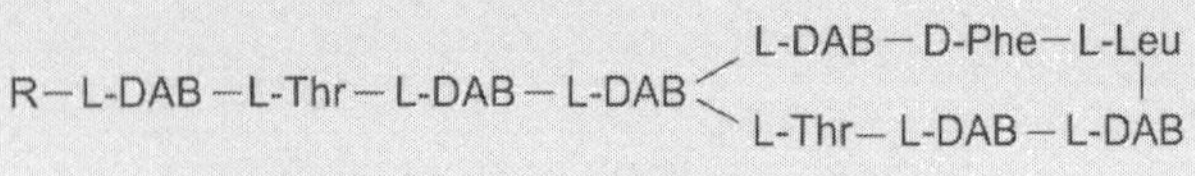

```
                                         L-DAB — D-Phe — L-Leu
R — L-DAB — L-Thr — L-DAB — L-DAB <                    |
                                         L-Thr — L-DAB — L-DAB

Polymyxin B₁: R= (+)-6-Methyloctanoyl
Polymyxin B₂: R= 6-Methylheptanoyl
DAB - α,γ-Diaminobutyric acid
```

Fig. 27.8: Polymyxin B sulfate, a polypeptide antibiotic, which is the most common polymyxin in clinical use

and p the eyelid.[120] The polymer entraps water and the active drug product in a bioadhesive matrix. The viscosity of the matrix is controlled by pH DuraSite® allows longer persistence of the active compound on the eye surface, by forming hydrogen bonds with glycosaminoglycans in mucus.[121] When a drop of AzaSite® is applied to the ocular surface, the polymer returns to a gel state. Thus, the azithromycin formulation in DuraSite stays in contact with the ocular surface, delivering the drug over a period of hours, increasing the overall bioavailability of azithromycin.[122] This property facilitates topical delivery of azithromycin and offers the benefit of a less-frequent dosing regimen.

Additionally, *in vitro* studies have shown that the killing spectrum of 1 percent azithromycin in DuraSite appeared to be enhanced compared to the solution without DuraSite. DuraSite was found to play a greater role in the inhibition of staphylococcal biofilm formation by AzaSite, compared to azithromycin which only had a moderate inhibitory effect. In a clinical trial, 1 percent azithromycin in DuraSite eliminated 82 percent of *Staphylococcus aureus*, including some species that were considered resistant to azithromycin.[123-124]

Clinical Experience and Ophthalmic Uses

Azithromycin ophthalmic solution 1 percent has been FDA approved for the treatment of bacterial conjunctivits caused by susceptible isolates of the CDC corneyform group G, *Haemophilus influenzae, Staphylococcus aureus, Streptococcus mitis group* and *Streptococcus pneumoniae*. Because of its spectrum of activity, it is particularly useful in treating pediatric bacterial eye infections. Azithromycin has potency up to four times higher than erythromycin against *Haemophilus influenzae* and *Neisseria gonorrhea*.[125] It is prescribed twice daily for the first two days and once daily for days 3 through 7.

Adverse Effects

The most frequently reported ocular adverse event reported in clinical trials was eye irritation, which occurred in 1 to 2 percent of patients. As noted above, in the "Adverse Effects" section for Besivance which is also formulated with DuraSite®, DuraSite® may be toxic to the anterior chamber causing an acute glaucoma and direct toxic reaction. The authors recommended that until the safety of medications with DuraSite® is established with further studies using smaller injected volumes, there should be placement of a suture over a clear corneal wound if DuraSite®-based medications are used.[65]

POLYMYXIN AND COMBINATION PRODUCTS

Chemistry, Ophthalmic Preparation, and Pharmacologic Action

Many of the combination products currently available in the United States contain polymyxin B sulfate (Figs 27.9A and B). It provides efficacy against commonly encountered gram-negative pathogens such as *H. influenzae*. Polymyxin is a bactericidal polypeptide antibiotic that interferes with cell wall synthesis and forms false pores in bacterial cell membranes. It is less effective against *Proteus, Providencia, Serratia,* and *Brucella* species. It came into use in

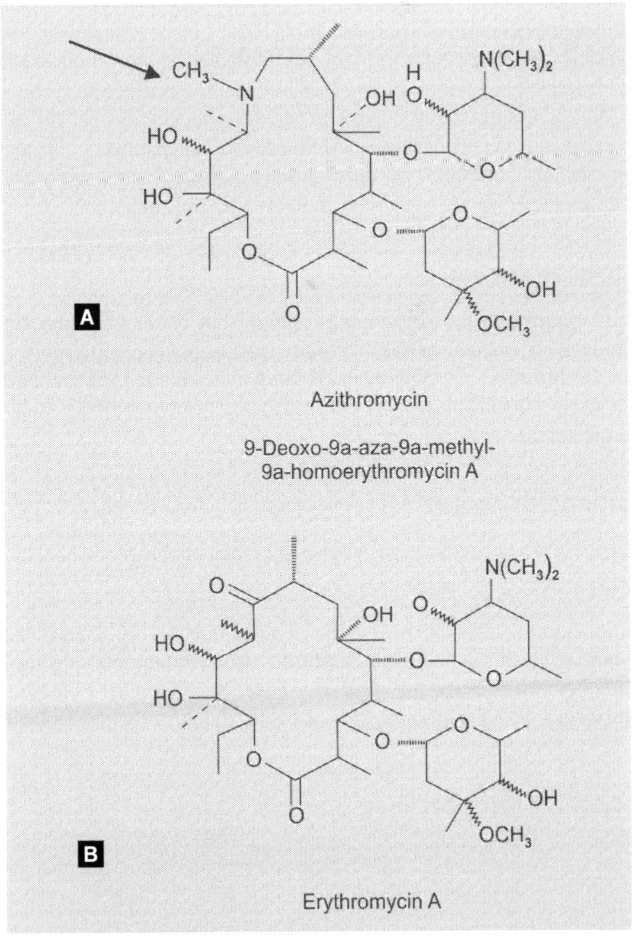

A

Azithromycin

9-Deoxo-9a-aza-9a-methyl-9a-homoerythromycin A

B

Erythromycin A

Figs 27.9A and B: Chemical structure of azithromycin

ophthalmology in the 1950s, when it was shown that polymyxin was effective in treating *Pseudomonas* corneal ulcers in rabbits.[126] The effectiveness of this agent was then shown in treating human corneal ulcers infected with *Pseudomonas* species.[127,128]

Combinations of polymyxin B with neomycin and gramicidin or trimethoprim are available as solutions, and combinations with bacitracin, neomycin, and bacitracin, or oxytetracycline are available as ointments only. The ointments contain 10,000 U per gram of polymyxin B.

Two antibiotics commonly combined with polymyxin are gramicidin and trimethoprim. Gramicidin alters bacterial cell wall permeability. Like bacitracin, it is only used topically because of systemic toxicity. Trimethoprim is a competitive inhibitor of bacterial dihydrofolate reductase, an enzyme that is necessary for purine synthesis.[129] The other compounds that polymyxin B are combined with are addressed elsewhere in this chapter.

Clinical Experience and Ophthalmic Uses

All polymyxin combination products have shown efficacy against bacterial conjunctivitis,[130,131] but no clinical studies of their use in the treatment of bacterial keratitis have been conducted. Clinical studies have shown that polymyxin B-trimethoprim and polymyxin B-neomycin-gramicidin are as effective as each other[132,133] and gentamicin sulfate,[134] sodium sulfacetamide,[134] and chloramphenicol[112,130] in the treatment of bacterial conjunctivitis.

Adverse Effects

Those combination antibiotic products that do not contain the highly allergenic agent neomycin are commonly recommended in the literature.[4,129,130] Polymyxin B rarely causes a hypersensitivity reaction. Chronic use of polymyxin B may result in toxic conjunctivitis.

SULFACETAMIDE

Chemistry, Ophthalmic Preparation, and Pharmacologic Action

Sulfacetamide (Fig. 27.10) 10 percent ointment (AK-Sulf, Cetamide, Sulamyd Sodium) and sulfacetamide 10 to 30 percent solutions (10% AK Sulf [Akorn, Inc, Buffalo Grove, IL], Bleph-10 [Allergan, Inc, Irvine, CA], Ophthacet, Ocusulf, Sulf-10 [CIBA Vision, Duluth,

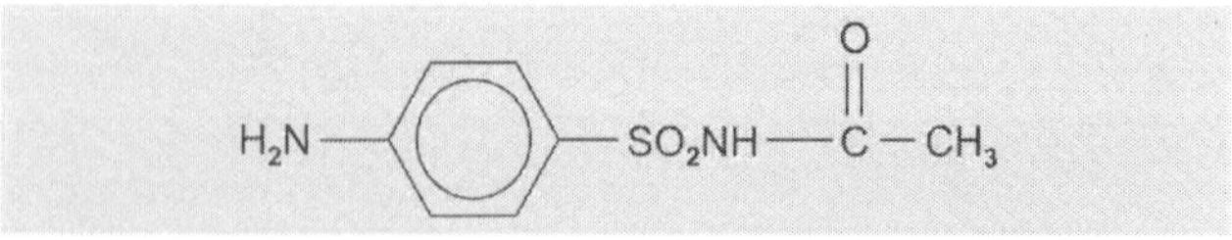

Fig. 27.10: Chemical structure of sulfacetamide one of the more commonly used sulfonamides in ophthalmic preparations

GA], Sulamyd Sodium, and Isopto Cetamide) act by preventing the incorporation of para-aminobenzoic acid into folic acid, thus inhibiting bacterial purine biosynthesis. Sulfonamides are bacteriostatic.

Clinical Experience and Ophthalmic Uses

Sulfonamides were used in the treatment of external ocular infections before the need to perform efficacy studies. It is difficult to find documentation of their value in the medical literature. In a study of 158 cases of culture-positive pediatric conjunctivitis, topical sulfacetamide was found to be equivalent in efficacy to trimethoprim-polymyxin B and gentamicin sulfate solutions.[134] Like erythromycin, sulfacetamides have a broad spectrum of antibacterial activity, but many strains of resistant bacteria have developed. Sulfacetamide is still effective against *H. influenzae*, but is ineffective against many staphylococcal isolates, *S. marcescens*, and *P. aeruginosa*, which makes it a poor choice as a first-line treatment for bacterial keratitis.[135] It remains a drug of choice for the treatment of *Nocardia* species.[136]

Adverse Effects

Topical sulfacetamide is generally well tolerated. However, there is a small but significant risk of Stevens-Johnson syndrome associated with the use of topical sulfacetamide.[137-139]

TETRACYCLINES

Chemistry, Ophthalmic Preparation, and Pharmacologic Action

Tetracycline (Fig. 27.11) inhibits bacterial protein synthesis by binding to the 30S ribosome, and it is among the broadest spectrum agents available. For most organisms, tetracycline is bacteriostatic.

Clinical Experience and Ophthalmic Uses

Systemic and topical (ointment) tetracycline are used concurrently to treat *C. trachomatis* conjunctivitis. Tetracycline can also be used for prophylaxis against ophthalmia neonatorum from

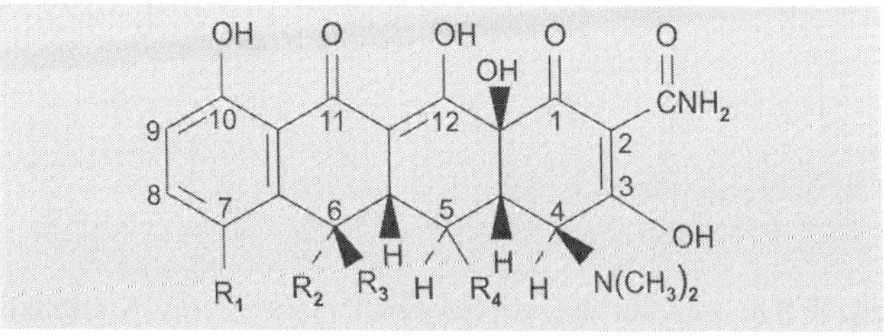

Fig. 27.11: The basis of the tetracyclines, shown above, is a four-ring naphthalene carboxamide

N. gonorrhoeae or chlamydial infections.[140,141] In newborns developing ophthalmia neonatorum, coexisting oropharyngeal involvement usually requires more than topical drug use.

Adverse Effects

Adverse reactions from tetracyclines, including deposition in the teeth and bones, may be seen with both systemic use and topical application.

VANCOMYCIN

Chemistry, Ophthalmic Preparation, and Pharmacologic Action

Vancomycin is a complex bactericidal tricyclic glycopeptide (Fig. 27.12) that inhibits bacterial cell wall synthesis.[142,143] It is active primarily against gram-positive bacteria, including methicillin-resistant *S. aureus, S. epidermidis*, and *Enterococcus* species.

Clinical Experience and Ophthalmic Uses

Topical vancomycin has been used successfully to treat chronic methicillin-resistant *S. aureus* in institutionalized patients.[144] Vancomycin has not been tested against other antibiotics in the treatment of bacterial keratitis, but there are numerous reported cases of keratitis caused by resistant organisms that resolved with topical vancomycin therapy.[145,146] Vancomycin 50 mg/ml has been tested against ciprofloxacin 0.3 percent in a rabbit model of methicillin-resistant *S. aureus* keratitis; ciprofloxacin was found to be more effective in that study.[147] These results have not been verified in clinical studies. Vancomycin should be considered as a first-line therapy in severe cases of keratitis in patients at high risk for infection by methicillin-resistant organisms, such as healthcare workers or institutionalized patients.

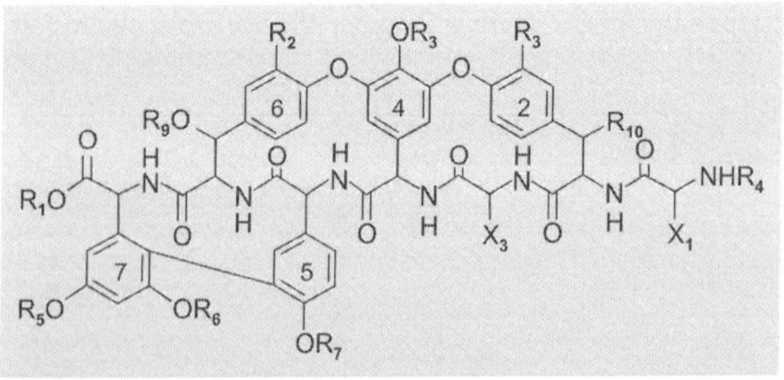

Fig. 27.12: Vancomycin is a complex bactericidal tricyclic glycopeptide

Adverse Effects

Vancomycin is rarely used in routine ocular infections because it is not commercially available in a topical ophthalmic form. Its use should be limited because of the risk of the development of bacterial resistance. Topical application of vancomycin produces discomfort because of its low pH in solution. Adverse effects include conjunctival injection, chemosis, papillary conjunctivitis, and superficial punctate keratopathy. In rabbits, topical application was noted to retard corneal epithelial wound healing.[148]

SELECTING THE OPTIMAL OPHTHALMIC ANTIBIOTIC

Goals of Treatment

In all bacterial infections, the goal of treatment is to rapidly eradicate the specific pathogen while minimizing adverse side effects and treatment costs. An ideal agent does not exist, and the choice of the most appropriate agent must be based on a rational compromise. The nature of this compromise must be patient- and disease-specific.

CLINICAL JUDGMENT IN CHOOSING AN OPHTHALMIC ANTIBIOTIC

In uncomplicated acute bacterial conjunctivitis, the need for treatment efficacy, though still important to limit the rate of recurrence and spread to personal contacts, must be balanced by a strong assurance of treatment safety and comfort, particularly in children, and a reasonable concern for treatment cost. A further consideration is to limit the use of antibiotics needed for systemic infections so that widespread resistance does not occur. The preparation chosen is usually commercially available in a topical ophthalmic form and has a broad-spectrum of efficacy against the most commonly implicated pathogens. The ophthalmologist and the patient can usually rest assured that they are dealing with a self-limited and usually benign process. In the treatment of acute bacterial conjunctivitis, no safety risks can be justified, and agents with known toxicity or a high incidence of hypersensitivity reactions should not be considered. However, in chronic or recurrent bacterial conjunctivitis, the ideal agent is the most effective broad-spectrum antibiotic available that the patient will tolerate, unless antibiotic susceptibility testing suggests that a specific narrow-spectrum agent may be more effective.

The sight-threatening nature of bacterial keratitis means that treatment speed and efficacy must take on more importance. Guidance in the choice of an antibiotic by knowing the specific organism and its sensitivity can be crucial to the outcome. The cost of treatment should only be taken into account if two or more treatment options are equal in efficacy and safety.[133]

BACTERIAL CONJUNCTIVITIS

Common Prescribing Practices

Physicians vary widely in their prescribing practices. Most cases of acute bacterial conjunctivitis are treated by nonophthalmologist physicians. Identification of the causative organism (e.g. by gram stain or culture) is rare. The use of a mild, broad-spectrum antibiotic preparation, such as one of the polymyxin B combination products (e.g. polymyxin B-trimethoprim or polymyxin B-zinc bacitracin) can be recommended. Sodium sulfacetamide is also commonly used, despite its bacteriostatic nature and limited spectrum because of its low cost and long clinical history. The use of chloramphenicol, because of the fear of aplastic anemia, and the use of neomycin, because of its relatively high rate of allergic reactions, are on the decline. Erythromycin cannot be recommended because of its lack of broad-spectrum and the emergence of resistant *H. influenzae*. In more serious cases, a fluoroquinolone may be indicated because of its broad-spectrum and efficacy against *H. influenzae*, as mentioned earlier, a common pathogen in pediatric conjunctivitis.

When bacterial conjunctivitis becomes chronic or recurrent culturing and sensitivity of the causative agent is recommended. In such cases, more aggressive treatment with a topical fluoroquinolone is recommended. Of the fluoroquinolones, ofloxacin followed by ciprofloxacin has the best coverage, and the lowest incidence of resistance. Their excellent tissue penetration capabilities will allow them to eradicate any bacteria that have breached the corneal epithelium and may also help reduce self-reinfection from pathogens sequestered in the meibomian orifices or lacrimal canaliculi.

BACTERIAL KERATITIS

Common Prescribing Practices

The medical literature documents the value of fortified antibiotics and the commercially available topical fluoroquinolone preparations in the treatment of bacterial keratitis. In a 1996 survey of 124 ophthalmologists from Florida, New York, and Illinois,[149] 82 percent reported that they would use a fluoroquinolone for initial treatment of less severe corneal ulcers, and 6 percent said that they would use fortified antibiotics. For more severe ulcers, prescribing practices shifted slightly toward fortified antibiotics, with 62 percent reporting that they would use fluoroquinolones for these cases and 23 percent stating that they would use fortified antibiotics. One common combination of extemporaneously-compounded fortified antibiotics is cefazolin 10 percent and tobramycin 1.5 percent administered as separate solutions. Vancomycin 50 mg/ml should be substituted for cefazolin for those cases in which antibiotic susceptibility testing suggests that it will be the most effective agent or there is a significant risk of methicillin-resistant *S. aureus*. *In vitro* susceptibility testing has shown that the use of a fluoroquinolone in combination with fortified cefazolin is effective against more ocular isolates than ofloxacin, ciprofloxacin, or norfloxacin used alone. Therefore, fortified tobramycin may be replaced with commercially-available ofloxacin or ciprofloxacin.[100] It is not known whether the precipitation of ciprofloxacin has any detrimental effect on efficacy. Norfloxacin is the least effective of the available fluoroquinolones and has not been shown effective in the treatment of bacterial keratitis.

NORFLOXACIN 0.3 PERCENT SOLUTION

Norfloxacin is the least potent of the topical fluoroquinolones.[150-152] It has been shown to be effective in the treatment of bacterial conjunctivitis[105] but not, with the exception of one small study, bacterial keratitis.[153] In conjunctivitis, it is comparable in efficacy to tobramycin 0.3 percent[155] and ciprofloxacin 0.3 percent.[67] Norfloxacin has also been shown to be as effective as gentamicin 0.3 percent in the treatment of blepharitis and conjunctivitis.[105,155-158] In the study by Miller and coworkers, norfloxacin suppressed or eliminated 89 percent of all organisms, based on pretreatment and post-treatment cultures. Norfloxacin has the highest rate of resistant bacteria among the fluoroquinolones based on *in vitro* testing with ocular isolates.[105,155-158]

REFERENCES

1. Mannis MJ, Plotnik RD. Bacterial conjunctivitis. In: Tasman W, Jaeger EA (Eds). Duane's Foundations of Clinical Ophthalmology, vol 4. Philadelphia, Lippincott Williams and Wilkins, 1998.
2. Foulks G. Bacterial infections of the conjunctiva and cornea. In: Albert DM, Jakobiec FA (Eds). Principles and Practice of Ophthalmology. Philadelphia, WB Saunders 1994. pp. 162–71.
3. Limberg MB. Review of bacterial keratitis and bacterial conjunctivitis. Am J Ophthalmol 1991;112:2S.
4. Lohr JA. Treatment of conjunctivitis in infants and children. Pediatric Annals 1993;22:11.
5. Gigliotti F, Williams WT, Hayden FG, et al. Etiology of acute conjunctivitis in children. J Pediatr 1981;98:531.
6. Seal DDV, Barratt SP, McGill JI. Aetiology and treatment of acute bacterial infection of the external eye. Br J Ophthalmol 1982;66:357.
7. Liesegang TJ. Bacterial keratitis. Inf Disease Clin N Am 1992;6:815.
8. Pepose JS, Wilhelmus KR. Divergent approaches to the management of corneal ulcers. Am J Ophthalmol 1992;114:630.
9. Erie JC, Nevitt MP, Hodge DO, Ballard DJ. Incidence of ulcerative keratitis in a defined population from 1950 through 1988. Arch Ophthalmol 1993;111:1665.
10. Upadhyay NP, Karmacharya PCD, Koirala AS, et al. Epidemiologic characteristics, predisposing factors, and etiologic diagnosis of corneal ulceration in Nepal. Am J Ophthalmol 1991;111:92.
11. Ormerod LD. Causation and management of microbial keratitis in subtropical Africa. Ophthalmology 1987;94:1662.
12. Mahajan VM. Ulcerative keratitis: an analysis of laboratory data in 674 cases. J Ocul Ther Surg. 1985;4:138.

13. Musch DC, Sugar A, Meyer RF. Demographic and predisposing factors in corneal ulceration. Arch Ophthalmol 1983;101:1545.
14. Jones DB. Strategy for the initial management of suspected microbial keratitis. New Orleans Academy of Ophthalmology Symposium on Medical and Surgical Diseases of the Cornea. St. Louis, CV Mosby 1980. p. 86.
15. Lass JF, Haaf J, Foster CS, Belcher C. Visual outcome in eight cases of *Serratia marcescens* keratitis. Am J Ophthalmol 1981;92:384.
16. Okumoto M. Enterobacteriaceae. In: Tasman W, Jaeger EA, (Eds). Duane's Foundations of Clinical Ophthalmology, Vol 2. Philadelphia: JB Lippincott, 1990.
17. Gudmundsson OG, Ormerod LD, Kenyon KR, et al. Factors influencing predilection and outcome of bacterial keratitis. Cornea 1989;8:115.
18. Donnenfeld ED, O'Brien TP, Perry HD, et al. Bacterial keratitis following photorefractive keratectomy (PRK). American Academy of Ophthalmology Final Program 1999;103:195.
19. Koidou-Tsiligianni A, Alfonso E, Foster RK. Ulcerative keratitis associated with contact lens wear. Am J Ophthalmol 1989;108:64.
20. Adams CP, Cohen EJ, Laibson PR, et al. Corneal ulcers in patients with cosmetic extended-wear contact lenses. Am J Ophthalmol 1983;96:705.
21. Weissman BA, Mondino BJ, Pettit TH, Hofbauer JD. Corneal ulcers associated with extended-wear soft contact lenses. Am J Ophthalmol 1984;97:476.
22. Hassman G, Sugar J. Pseudomonas corneal ulcer with extended-wear soft contact lenses for myopia. Arch Ophthalmol 1983;101:1549.
23. Lemp MA, Blackman HJ, Wilson LA, Leveille AS. gram-negative corneal ulcers in elderly aphakic eyes with extended-wear lenses. Ophthalmology 1984;90:60.
24. Galantine PG, Cohen EJ, Laibson PR, et al. Corneal ulcers associated with contact lens wear. Arch Ophthalmol 1984;102:891.
25. Schein OD, Ormerod LD, Barraquer E, et al. Microbiology of contact lens-related keratitis. Cornea 1989;8:281.
26. Cohen EJ, Laibson PR, Arentsen JJ, et al. Corneal ulcers associated with cosmetic extended wear soft contact lenses. Ophthalmology 1987;19:109.
27. Stein RM, Clinch TE, Cohen EJ, et al. Infected versus sterile corneal infiltrates in contact lens wear. Am J Ophthalmol 1988;105:632.
28. Liesegang TJ, Foster RF. Bacterial microbial keratitis in South Florida. Am J Ophthalmol 1980;90:38.
29. Ostler HB, Okumoto M, Wilkey C. The changing pattern of the etiology of central bacterial corneal (hypopyon) ulcer. Trans Pac Coast Otoophthalmol Soc 1976;57:235.
30. Cruz DA, Sabir SM, Capo H, Alfonso EG. Microbial keratitis in childhood. Ophthalmology 1993;100:192.
31. Ormerod LD, Gomez DS, Murphee AL, et al. Microbial keratitis in children. Ophthalmology 1986;93:449.
32. Baum JL, Jones DB. Initial therapy of suspected microbial corneal ulcers. I: Broad antibiotic therapy based on prevalence of organisms, II: Specific antibiotic therapy based on corneal smears. Surv Ophthalmol 1979;24:97.
33. Baum J. Therapy for ocular bacterial infection. Trans Ophthalmol Soc UK 1986;105:69.

34. Jones DB. Decision-making in management of microbial keratitis. Ophthalmology 1981;88:814.
35. McDonnell PJ, Nobe J, Gauderman WJ, et al. Community care of corneal ulcers. Am J Ophthalmol 1992;114:531.
36. Wilhelmus KR. Bacterial corneal ulcers. Int Ophthalmol Clin 1984;24:1.
37. Baum JL, Barza M, Weinstein L. Preferred routes of antibiotic administration in treatment of bacterial ulcers of the cornea. Int Ophthalmol Clin 1973;13:31.
38. O'Brien TP, Maguire MG, Fink NE, et al. Efficacy of ofloxacin vs cefazolin and tobramycin in the therapy for bacterial keratitis. Arch Ophthalmol 1995;113:1257.
39. Hyndiuk RA, Eiferman RA, Caldwell DR, et al. Comparison of ciprofloxacin ophthalmic solution 0.3 percent to fortified tobramycin-cefazolin in treating bacterial corneal ulcers. Ciprofloxacin Bacterial Keratitis Study Group. Ophthalmology 1996;103:1854.
40. Shell JW. Pharmacokinetics of topically applied ophthalmic drugs. Surv Ophthalmol 1982;26:207.
41. Lesar TS, Fiscella RG. Antimicrobial drug delivery to the eye. Drug Intell Clin Pharm 1985;19:642.
42. Barza M. Antibacterial agents in the treatment of ocular infections. Infect Dis Clin North Am 1989;3:53.
43. Groden LR, Brinser JH. Outpatient treatment of microbial corneal ulcers. Arch Ophthalmol 1986;104:84.
44. Kupferman A, Leibowitz HM. Topical antibiotic therapy of *Pseudomonas aeruginosa* keratitis. Arch Ophthalmol 1979;97:1699.
45. Davis SD, Sarff LD, Hyndiuk RA. Topical tobramycin therapy of experimental *Pseudomonas* keratitis: an evaluation of some factors that potentially enhance efficacy. Arch Ophthalmol 1978;96:123.
46. Lesher GY, Froelich ED, Gruet MD, et al. 1,8 Naphthyridine derivatives. A new class of chemotherapeutic agents. J Med Pharm Chem 1962;5:1063.
47. Jacoby GA. Mechanisms of resistance to quinolones. Clin Infect Dis 15;41 Suppl 2005;2:S120-6.
48. Smith A, Pennefather PM, Kaye SB, Hart CA. Fluoroquinolones: Place in ocular therapy. Drugs 2001;61(6):747-61.
49. Hooper DC. Mechanisms of fluoroquinolone resistance. Drug Rest Updat 1999;2(1):38-55.
50. Mather R, Karenchak LM, Romanowski EG, Kowalski RP. Fourth generation fluoroquinolones: New weapons in the arsenal of ophthalmic antibiotics. Am J Ophthalmol 2002;133(4):463-6.
51. Kowalski RP, Dhaliwal DK, Karenchak LM, et al. Gatifloxacin and moxifloxacin: An *in vitro* susceptibility comparison to levofloxacin, ciprofloxacin, and ofloxacin using bacterial keratitis isolates. Am J Ophthalmol 2003;136(3):500-5.
52. Tauber S, Cupp G, Garber R, Bartell J, Vohra F, Stroman D. Microbiological efficacy of a new ophthalmic formulation of moxifloxacin dosed twice-daily for bacterial conjunctivitis. Adv Ther 2001;28:566-74.
53. Karpecki P, Depaolis M, Hunter JA, White EM, Rigel L, Brunner LS, Usner DW, Paterno MR, Comstock TL. Besifloxacin ophthalmic suspension 0.6 percent in patients with bacterial conjunctivitis: a multicenter, prospective, randomized, double-masked, vehicle-

controlled, 5-day efficacy and safety study. Clin Ther 2009;31: 514-26.
54. Tepedino ME, Heller WH, Usner DW, Brunner LS, Morris TW, Haas W, Paterno MR, Comstock TL. Phase III efficacy and safety study of besifloxacin ophthalmic suspension 0.6 percent in the treatment of bacterial conjunctivitis. Curr Med Res Opin 2009;25:1159-69.
55. McDonald MB, Protzko EE, Brunner LS, Morris TW, Haas W, Paterno MR, Comstock TL, Usner DW. Efficacy and safety of besifloxacin ophthalmic suspension 0.6 percent compared with moxifloxcin ophthalmic solution 0.5 percent for treating bacterial conjunctivitis. Ophthalmology 2009;116:1615-23.
56. Haas W, Pillar CM, Zurenko GE, Lee JC, Brunner LS, Morris TW. Besifloxacin: A novel fluoroquinolone, has broad-spectrum *in vitro* activity against aerobic and anaerobic bacteria. Antimicrob Agents Chemother 2009;53:3552-60.
57. Carter NJ, Scott LJ. Besifloxacin ophthalmic suspension 0.6 percent. Drugs 2010;70:83-97.
58. Haas W, Pillar CM, Hesje CK, Sanfilippo CM, Morris TW. Bactericidal activity of besifloxacin against staphylococci, *Streptococcus pneumoniae* and *Haemophilus influenzae*. J Antimicrob Chemother 2010;65:1441-7.
59. Bowman LM, Si E, Pang J, Archibald R, Friedlaender M. Development of a topical polymeric mucoadhesive ocular delivery system for Azithromycin. J Ocul Pharmacol Ther 2009;25:133-9.
60. Blondeau JM, Borsos S, Hesje CK. Antimicrobial efficacy of gatifloxacin and moxifloxacin with and without benzalkonium chloride compared with ciprofloxacin and levofloxacin against methicillin-resistant *Staphylococcus aureus*. J Chemother 2007;19:146-51.
61. McDonnell G, Russell AD. Antiseptics and disinfectants: Activity, action, and resistance. Clin Microbiol Rev 1999;12:147-9.
62. Proksch JW, Granvil CP, Siou-Mermet R, Comstock TL, Paterno MR, Ward KW. Ocular pharmacokinetics of besifloxacin following topical administration to rabbits, monkeys, and humans. J Ocul Pharmcol Ther 2009;25:335-43.
63. Donnenfeld ED, Comstock TL, Proksch JW. Human aqueous humor concentrations of besifloxacin, moxifloxacin, and gatifloxacin after topical ocular application. Cataract Refract Surg 2011;37:1076-83.
64. Ball AP. Overview of clinical experience with ciprofloxacin. Eur J Clin Microbiol 1986;5:214.
65. Ness PJ, Mamalis N, Werner L, Maddula S, Davis DK, Donnenfeld ED, Olson RJ. An anterior chamber toxicity study evaluating Besivance, AzaSite, and Ciprofloxacin. Am J Ophthalmol 2010;150:498-504.
66. Gross RD, Hoffman RO, Lindsay RN. A comparison of ciprofloxacin and tobramycin in bacterial conjunctivitis in children. Clin Pediatr 1997;36:435.
67. Adenis JP, Brasseur G, Demailly P, et al. Comparative evaluation of efficacy and safety of ciprofloxacin and norfloxacin ophthalmic solutions. Eur J Ophthalmol 1996;6:287.
68. Adenis JP, Colin J, Verin P, Riss I, Saint-Blancat P. Ciprofloxacin ophthalmic solution in the treatment of conjunctivitis and

blepharitis: a comparison with fusidic acid. Eur J Ophthalmol 1996;6:368.
69. Wilhelmus KR, Hyndiuk RA, Caldwell DR, et al. 0.3 percent ciprofloxacin ophthalmic ointment in the treatment of bacterial keratitis. The Ciprofloxacin Ointment/Bacterial Keratitis Study Group. Arch Ophthalmol 1993;111:1210.
70. Fiscella RG. Extemporaneously compounded ophthalmic antibiotic solutions: survey of usage and costs, and pharmacoeconomic considerations. Hospital Pharmacy 1997;32:1240.
71. Finkelstein I, Trope GE, Menon IA, et al. Potential value of collagen shields as subconjunctival depot release system. Curr Eye Res 1990;9:653.
72. Assil KK, Zarnegar SR, Fouraker BD, Schanzlin DJ. Efficacy of tobramycin-soaked collagen shields vs tobramycin eyedrop loading dose for sustained treatment of experimental *Pseudomonas aeruginosa*-induced keratitis in rabbits. Am J Ophthalmol 1992;113:418.
73. Sawusch MR, O'Brien TP, Dick JD, Gottsch JD. Use of collagen corneal shields in the treatment of bacterial keratitis. Am J Ophthalmol 1988;106:27.
74. Phinney RB, Schwartz SD, Lee DA, Mondino BJ. Collagen-shield delivery of gentamicin and vancomycin. Arch Ophthalmol 1988; 106:1599.
75. Friedberg ML, Pleyer U, Mondino BJ. Drug delivery to the eye. Collagen shields, iontophoresis, and pumps. Ophthalmology 1991;98:725.
76. Hobden JA, Reidy JJ, O'Callaghan RJ, et al. Treatment of experimental *Pseudomonas* keratitis using collagen shields containing tobramycin. Arch Ophthalmol 1988;106:1605.
77. Hobden JA, Reidy JJ, O'Callaghan, et al. Quinolones in collagen shields to treat aminoglycoside-resistant pseudomonal keratitis. Invest Ophthalmol Vis Sci 1990;3:2241.
78. Edson RS, Terrell CL. The aminoglycosides. Mayo Clin Proc 1991; 66:1158.
79. Leibowitz HM, Hyndiuk RA, Smolin GR, et al. Tobramycin in external eye disease: a double-masked study vs gentamicin. Curr Eye Res 1981;5:259.
80. Gardner S. Treatment of bacterial keratitis. Ocular Ther Management 1990;3:1.
81. Wilhelmus KR, Gilbert Ml, Osato MS. Tobramycin in ophthalmology. Surv Ophthalmol 1987;32:111.
82. Laibson P, Michaud R, Smolin G, et al. A clinical comparison of tobramycin and gentamicin sulfate in the treatment of ocular infections. Am J Ophthalmol 1981;92:836.
83. Stewart RH, Smith RE, Cagle GD, et al. Tobramycin in the treatment of external ocular infections. A clinical study. Ocular Ther Surg 1982;1:72.
84. Timewell RM, Rosenthal AL, Smith JP, Cagle GD. Safety and efficacy of tobramycin and gentamicin sulfate in the treatment of external ocular infections of children. J Pediatr Ophthalmol Strabismus 1983;20:22.
85. Cagle G, Davis S, Rosenthal A, et al. Topical tobramycin and gentamicin sulfate in the treatment of ocular infections: multicenter study. Current Eye Res 1982;1:523.

86. Lass JH, Mack RJ, Imperia PS, et al. An *in vitro* analysis of aminoglycoside corneal epithelial toxicity. Curr Eye Res 1989; 8:299.
87. Davison CR, Tuft SJ, Dart JK. Conjunctival necrosis after administration of topical fortified aminoglycosides. Am J Ophthalmol 1991;111:690.
88. Petroutsos G, Guimaraes R, Giraud J, Pouliquen Y. Antibiotics and corneal epithelial wound healing. Arch Ophthalmol 1983; 101:1775.
89. Peoutsos G, Guimaraes R, Pouliquen Y. The effect of concentrated antibiotics on the rabbit's corneal epithelium. Int Ophthalmol 1984;7:65.
90. Nauheim R, Nauheim J. Bulbar conjunctival defects associated with gentamicin. Arch Ophthalmol 1987;105:1321.
91. Bullard SR, O'Day DM. Pseudomembranous conjunctivitis following topical gentamicin therapy. Arch Ophthalmol 1997; 115:1591.
92. Hatnen A, Terasvirta M, Fraki JE. Contact allergy to components in topical ophthalmologic preparations. Acta Ophthalmol (Copenh) 1985;63:424.
93. Wilhelmus KR. Antiparasitic drugs in ophthalmology. In: Tasman W, Jaeger EA (Eds). Duane's Foundations of Clinical Ophthalmology, Vol 2. Philadelphia: Lippincott-Williams and Wilkins, 1999.
94. Meleny FL, Johnson BA. Bacitracin. Am J Med 1949;7:794.
95. Bellows JG, Farmer CJ. Use of bacitracin in ocular infections; tolerance and permeability in rabbit eye. Am J Ophthalmol 1948; 31:1070.
96. Schechter JF, Wilkinson RD, Del Carpio J. Anaphylaxis following the use of bacitracin ointment. Report of a case and review of the literature. Arch Dermatol 1984;120:909.
97. Jones DB. New horizons in antibacterial antibiotics. Int Ophthalmol Clin 1993;33:179.
98. Mills RA, Osato MS, Pyron M, Jones DB. Efficacy of topical ceftazidime in experimental bacterial keratitis [abstract]. Invest Ophthalmol Vis Sci 1992;33:S935.
99. Kremer I, Robinson A, Braffman M, et al. The effect of topical ceftazidime on pseudomonas keratitis in rabbits. Cornea 1994; 13:360.
100. Bower KS, Kowalski RP, Gordon YJ. Fluoroquinolones in the treatment of bacterial keratitis. Am J Ophthalmol 1996;121:712.
101. Noe CA. Penicillin treatment of eyelid infections. Am J Ophthalmol 1947;30:477.
102. Gustaferro CA, Steckelberg JM. Cephalosporin antimicrobial agents and related compounds. Mayo Clin Proc 1991;66:1064.
103. Raynr SA, Buckley RJ. Ocular chloramphenicol and aplastic anemia. Is there a link? Drug Saf 1996;14:273.
104. Jensen HG, Felix C. *In vitro* antibiotic susceptibilities of ocular isolates in North and South America. *In vitro* Antibiotic Testing Group. Cornea 1998;17:79.
105. Miller IM, Wittreich JM, Cook T, Vogel R. The safety and efficacy of topical norfloxacin compared with chloramphenicol for the treatment of external ocular bacterial infections. The Norfloxacin-Chloramphenicol Ophthalmic Study Group. Eye 1992;6:111.

106. Power WJ, Collum LM, Easty DL, et al. Evaluation of efficacy and safety of ciprofloxacin ophthalmic solution versus chloramphenicol. Eur J Ophthalmol 1993;3:77.
107. Behrens-Baumann W, Quentin CD, Gibson JR, et al. Trimethoprim-polymyxin B sulfate ophthalmic ointment in the treatment of bacterial keratitis: a double-blind study versus chloramphenicol ophthalmic ointment. Curr Med Res Opin 1988;11:227.
108. Abrams SM, Degnan TJ, Vinviguerra V. Marrow aplasia following topical application of chloramphenicol eye ointment. Arch Intern Med 1980;140:576.
109. Carpenter G. Chloramphenicol eyedrops and marrow aplasia. Lancet 1975;2:326.
110. Fraunfelder FT, Bagby GC, Kelly DJ. Fatal aplastic anemia following topical application of ophthalmic chloramphenicol. Am J Ophthalmol 1982;93:356.
111. Brodsky E, Biger Y, Zeidan Z, Schneider M. Topical application of chloramphenicol eye ointment followed by fatal bone marrow aplasia. Isr J Med Sci 1989;25:5.
112. Fraunfelder FT, Morgan RL, Yunis AA. Blood dyscrasias and topical ophthalmic chloramphenicol. Am J Ophthalmol 1993; 115:812.
113. Scott JL, Finegold SM, Belkin GA, et al. A controlled double-blind study of the hematologic toxicity of chloramphenicol. N Engl J Med 1965;272:1137.
114. Rosenthal RL, Blackman A. Bone-marrow hypoplasia following use of chloramphenicol eye drops JAMA 1965;191:136.
115. Trobe GE, Lawrence JR, Hind VM, Bunney J. Systemic absorption of topically applied chloramphenicol eyedrops. Br J Ophthalmol 1970;163:690.
116. Apt L, Gaffney WL. Toxic effects of topical eye medication in infants and children. In: Tasman W, Jaeger EA, (Eds). Duane's Foundations of Clinical Ophthalmology, Vol 3. Philadelphia: JB Lippincott, 1990.
117. Mao JC, Putterman M, Wiegand RG. Biochemical basis for the selective toxicity of erythromycin. Biochem Pharmacol 1970; 19:391.
118. Sabath LD, Lorian V, Gerstein D, et al. Enhancing effect on alkalinization of the medium on the activity of erythromycin against gram-negative bacteria. Appl Microbiol 1968;16:1228.
119. Washington JA, Wilson WR. Erythromycin: a microbial and clinical perspective after 30 years of clinical use. Mayo Clin Proc 1985;60:271.
120. Utine CA. Update and critical appraisal of the use of topical azithromycin ophthalmic 1 percent (AzaSite) solution in the treatment of ocular infections. Clin Ophthalmol 2011;5:801-9.
121. Bowman L, Si E, Pang J, Archibad R, Friedlaender M. Development of a topical polymeric mucoadhesive ocular delivery system for azithromycin. J Ocul Pharmacol Ther 2009;25:133-9.
122. Akpek EK, Vittitow J, Verhoeven RS, et al. Ocular surface distribution and pharmacokinetics of a novel ophthalmic 1 percent azithromycin formulation. J Ocul Pharmacol Ther 2009; 25:433-9.
123. Wu EC, Kowalski RP, Romanowski EG, et al. AzaSite® inhibits *Staphylococcus aureus* and coagulase-negative Staphylococcus biofilm formation *in vitro* J Ocul Pharmacol Ther 2010;26:557-62.

124. Mitchell H Friedlaender1, Eugene Protzko. Clinical development of 1 percent azithromycin in DuraSite®, a topical azalide anti-infective for ocular surface therapy Clin Ophthalmol 2007; 1(1): 3-10.
125. Retsema J, Girard A, Schelkly W, et al. Spectrum and mode of action of azithromycin (CP-62, 993), a new 15-membered-ring-macrolide with improved potency against gram-negative organisms. Antimicrob Agents Chemother 1987;31;1939-47.
126. Wiggins RL. Experimental studies on eyes with polymyxin B. Am J Ophthalmol 1952;35:83.
127. Moorman LT. Treatment of *Pseudomonas* corneal ulcers. Arch Ophthalmol 1955;53:345.
128. McNeel JW, Wood RM, Senterfit LB. Effect of polymyxin B sulfate on *Pseudomonas* corneal ulcers. Arch Ophthalmol 1961;66:646.
129. Van Rensburg SF, Gibson JR, Harvey SG, Burke CA. Trimethoprim-polymyxin ophthalmic solution versus chloramphenicol ophthalmic solution in the treatment of bacterial conjunctivitis. Pharmatherapeutica 1982;3:274.
130. Abramowicz M. Trimethoprim-polymixin B for bacterial conjunctivitis. Med Lett Drugs Ther 1990;32:71.
131. The Trimethoprim-Polymyxin B Sulphate Ophthalmic Ointment Study Group: Trimethoprim-polymyxin B sulphate ophthalmic ointment versus chloramphenicol ophthalmic ointment in the treatment of bacterial conjunctivitis—a review of four clinical studies. J Antimicrob Chemother 1989;23:261.
132. Gibson JR. Trimethoprim-polymyxin B ophthalmic solution in the treatment of presumptive bacterial conjunctivitis—a multicenter trial of its efficacy versus neomycin-polymyxin B-gramicidin and chloramphenicol ophthalmic solutions. J Antimicrob Chemother 1983;11:217.
133. Genee E, Schlectweg C, Bauerreiss P, Gibson JR. Trimethoprim-polymyxin eye drops versus neomycin-polymyxin-gramicidin eye drops in the treatment of presumptive bacterial conjunctivitis—a double-blind study. Ophthalmologica 1982;184:92.
134. Lohr JA, Austin RD, Grossman M, et al. Comparison of three topical antimicrobials for acute bacterial conjunctivitis. Pediatr Infect Dis J 1988;7:626.
135. Syed NA, Hyndiuk RA. Infectious conjunctivitis. Infect Dis Clin N Am 1992;6:789.
136. Sridhar MS, Sharma S, Reddy MC, et al. Clinicomicrobiological review of *Nocardia* keratitis. Cornea 1998;17:17.
137. Genvet GI, Cohen EJ, Donnenfeld ED, Blecher MH. Erythema multiforme after use of topical sulfacetamide. Am J Ophthalmol 1985;99:465.
138. Rubin Z. Ophthalmic sulfonamide-induced Stevens-Johnson syndrome. Arch Dermatol 1977;113:235.
139. Gottschalk HR, Stone OJ. Stevens-Johnson syndrome from ophthalmic sulfonamide. Arch Dermatol 1976;112:513.
140. American Academy of Pediatrics Committee. Prophylaxis and treatment of neonatal gonococcal infections. Pediatrics 1980; 65:1047.
141. Periodic health examination, 1992 update. 4. Prophylaxis for gonococcal and chlamydial ophthalmia neonatorum. Canadian Task Force on the Periodic Health Examination. Am Med Assoc J 1992;147:1449.

142. Wilhelm MP. Vancomycin. Mayo Clin Proc 1991;66:1165.
143. Strominger JL, Tipper DJ. Bacterial cell wall synthesis and structure in relation to the mechanism of action of penicillins and other antibacterial agents. Am J Med 1965;39:707.
144. Brennan C, Mulder RR. Conjunctivitis associated with methicillin-resistant *Staphylococcus aureus* in a long-term-care facility. Am J Med 1990;88:14N.
145. Eiferman RA, O'Neill KP, Morrison NA. Methicillin resistant *Staphylococcus aureus* corneal ulcers. Ann Ophthalmol 1991;23:414.
146. Goodman DF, Gottsch JD. Methicillin-resistant *Staphylococcus epidermidis* keratitis treated with vancomycin. Arch Ophthalmol 1988;106:1570.
147. Callegan MC, Hill JM, Insler MS, et al. Methicillin-resistant *Staphylococcus aureus* keratitis in the rabbit: therapy with ciprofloxacin, vancomycin and cefazolin. Curr Eye Res 1992;11:1111.
148. Gigantelli JW, Torres Gomez J, Osato MS. *In vitro* susceptibilities of ocular Bacillus cereus isolates to clindamycin, gentamicin, and vancomycin alone or in combination. Antimicrob Agents Chemother 1991;35:201.
149. McLeod SD, DeBacker CM, Viana MA. Differential care of corneal ulcers in the community based on apparent severity. Ophthalmol 1996;103:479.
150. Wolfson JS, Hooper DC. The fluoroquinolones: structures, mechanisms of action and resistance, and spectra of activity *in vitro*. Antimicrob Agents Chemother 1985;28:581.
151. King A, Phillips I. The comparative *in vitro* activity of eight newer quinolones and nalidixic acid. J Antimicrob Chemother 1986;18(suppl):1.
152. Heesen FW, Mutyjens HL. *In vitro* activities of ciprofloxacin, norfloxacin, pipemidic acid, cinoxacin, and nalidixic acid against *Chlamyia trachomatis*. Antimicrob Agents Chemother 1984;25:123.
153. Vajapayee RB, Gupta SK, Angra SK, Munjal A. Topical norfloxacin therapy in *Pseudomonas* corneal ulceration. Cornea 1991;10:268.
154. Jacobson JA, Call NB, Kasworm EM, et al. Safety and efficacy of topical norfloxacin versus tobramycin in the treatment of external ocular infections. Antimicrob Agents Chemother 1988;32:1820.
155. Miller IM, Vogel R, Cook TJ, Wittreich J. Topically administered norfloxacin compared with topically administered gentamicin for the treatment of external ocular bacterial infections. The Worldwide Norfloxacin Ophthalmic Study Group. Am J Ophthalmol 1992;113:638.
156. Ross DL, Riley CM. Aqueous solubilities of some variously substituted quinolone antimicrobials. Int J Pharm 1990;63:237.
157. Jensen HG, Felix C. *In vitro* antibiotic susceptibilities of ocular isolates in North and South America. *In vitro* Antibiotic Testing Group. Cornea 1998;17:79.
158. Bower KS, Kowalski RP, Gordon YJ. Possible consequences of shaking hands with your patients with epidemic keratoconjunctivitis. Am J Ophthalmol 1996;121:711.

Preoperative and Postoperative Antibiotic Prophylaxis in Cataract Surgery

NR Biswas, Srujana Mohanty, GK Das, Madhurjya Gogoi (India)

Cataract extraction is one of the most commonly performed ophthalmic surgeries in the world. An infrequent but devastating complication is postoperative endophthalmitis, the reported prevalence in recent times being 0.04–0.26 percent.[1-3] Possible origins of infection include the ocular tear film, lids and adnexa; irrigating solutions and medications; surgical instruments including intraocular lenses; the respiratory and skin flora of the surgeon; and operating room air. Because sterile surgical techniques addresses many of these sources, it is now well-established that the source of most infecting agents is the endogenous ocular flora.[4,5] The most commonly recovered organisms have been gram-positive bacteria (coagulase-negative staphylococci, *Staphylococcus aureus*, and streptococci) with gram-negative organisms making up a small proportion of the total.[6] Surface flora routinely gain entry to the anterior chamber during cataract surgery. In one study, 13 of 59 eyes (22%) grew gram-positive organisms from aqueous cultures taken at the time of wound closure after intraocular surgery, and 8 of these eyes (62%) had organisms isolated from the eyelids and conjunctiva before or after disinfection.[7] In the endophthalmitis vitrectomy study,[6] a randomized multicentered prospective clinical study, confirmed microbiologic growth was demonstrated in 69.3 percent of patients with clinically suspected endophthalmitis. Gram-positive organisms were isolated from 94.2 percent patients. Two hundred twenty-six of the 323 isolates obtained (70%) gram-positive coagulase-negative micrococci, 32 (9.9%) *Staphylococcus aureus*, 29 (9.0%) *Streptococcus species*, 7 (2.2%) *Enterococcus species*, 10 (3.1%) miscellaneous gram-positives) and 19 (5.9%) gram-negative species.[4]

Given the ability of surface flora to enter the eye during surgery, many of the prophylactic techniques to decrease the risk of endophthalmitis aim to suppress their number and to limit the growth of those organisms that do enter the eye before the development of frank endophthalmitis. Administration of an effective antimicrobial forms a part of such prophylactic measures. Although there are no sufficient data to support a definitive role of antibiotics in preventing endophthalmitis, studies do report a reduction in ophthalmic flora with antibiotic use.[8,9] Further, before perioperative prophylactic antibiotics (and before the modern methods of cataract surgery), the risk of endophthalmitis after a cataract operation was 0.21–1.0 percent.[10] Thus, although the consequences of bacterial endophthalmitis support the use of perioperative prophylactic antimicrobials, a particular choice of antimicrobial agents has not been agreed upon.[8] Since systemically administered antibiotics have not demonstrated good intraocular penetration, various routes of administration have been tried, including preoperative topical, intraoperative infusion, and subconjunctival routes.

ANTIBIOTIC PROPHYLAXIS

A variety of options are available for preoperative, intraoperative, and postoperative antibiotic prophylaxis in cataract surgery, but a direct comparative evaluation is often not available, with a review even suggesting that only preoperative antisepsis with 5 percent povidone iodine may provide some benefit, abit limited.[4]

The ideal prophylactic antibiotic for cataract surgery should be broad spectrum, effective prophylactically, preservative (benzalkonium chloride) free, nontoxic and convenient to use. Presently, fluoroquinolones are the dominant family of ophthalmic antibiotics. The recently introduced fourth generation topical ophthalmic fluoroquinolones, levofloxacin, gatifloxacin, and moxifloxacinhave shown enhanced spectrum and potency for gram-positive cocci and possibly atypical mycobacterium, improved penetration into the anterior segment, and reduced drug resistance as compared to the older fluoroquinolones (norfloxacin 0.3%, ciprofloxacin 0.3%, and ofloxacin 0.3%).

Antibiotic sensitivity varies, but in one series, more than 90 percent of bacterial isolates were susceptible to cephalothin, vancomycin, chloramphenicol, ofloxacin and gatifloxacin; 70–90 percent were susceptible to gentamicin, cefotaxime, oxacillin and ciprofloxacin; and less than 70 percent were susceptible to neomycin. There was increased resistance among coagulase-negative staphylococci to both ciprofloxacin (20-38%) and cefazolin (19-40%).[11] Resistance to bacitracin, trimethoprim-sulfamethoxazole, and vancomycin remained unchanged. Vancomycin retained *in vitro* efficacy against more than 99 percent of gram-positive bacteria, and ceftazidime was effective against 100 percent of gram-negative bacteria tested, thus enabling their use in combination as reserve drugs (intravitreal injection) in the treatment of endophthalmitis.[12]

Preoperative prophylaxis for 3 days is effective in eliminating conjunctival microorganisms, and a number of antibiotics viz. fusidic acid, ofloxacin, gentamicin and cefmenoxime are useful.[13] Prophylactic preoperative antibiotics are most commonly used as eye drops. They are also used intraoperative intraocular (antibiotic infusion during surgery, intracamerally), intraoperative periocular [subconjunctivally (gentamicin, cefuroxime)], and postoperatively [aminoglycosides (neomycin, tobramycin, gentamicin) and fluoroquinolones].[14-16]

Intracameral bolus injection of cefazolin (1 mg in 0.1 ml solution), intracameral vancomycin (20 mg/ml), intracameral cefuroxime, and intracameral gentamicin (8 mg/ml) have been

Applied Ocular Therapeutics in Ophthalmic Surgery

TABLE 28.1: Antibiotics used commonly for prophylaxis in cataract surgery

Antibiotic	Topical	Subconjunctival	Intracameral
Ciprofloxacin	0.3%	—	—
Ofloxacin	0.3%	—	—
Gatifloxacin	0.3%	—	—
Moxifloxacin	0.5%	—	—
Cephazoline	5%	—	1 mg in 0.1 ml
Cefuroxime	—	—	1 mg
Vancomycin	2.5-5%	25 mg	Infusion = 10-50 mg/ml Capsular bag = upto 1 mg/ml
Gentamicin	0.3-1.4%	20-40 mg	8 µg/ml
Amikacin		20-50 mg	—
Tobramycin	0.3-1.4%	20-40 mg	
Chloramphenicol	0.5%	—	—

used at the time of cataract surgery with demonstrable efficacy and without apparent side effects.[17,18] Occasionally, the protective effect against postoperative endophthalmitis of intracameral prophylaxis is seen to be better with certain antibiotics (cefuroxime) as compared with topical antibiotics alone. Moxifloxacin 0.5 percent eye drop represents a first line antibiotic of choice for treating and preventing ophthalmic infections, but some have argued that it should be held in reserve (Table 28.1).

The ESCRS[19] endophthalmitis prophylaxis clinical trial is the latest and arguably the largest prospective European clinical study of antibiotic prophylaxis and the largest in ophthalmology on 35,000 cataract patients in 16 centers from 10 European countries. It showed a significant beneficial effect of cefuroxime injected intracamerally as compared to levofloxacin eye drops. Cefuroxime is a second generation bactericidal cephalosporin (β-lactam) antibiotic with activity against both gram-positive and gram-negative organisms, and is used only intracamerally.

Postoperatively, antibiotic may be used in combination with topical steroids as single preparation, without loss of efficacy, and it suffices in uneventful cataract surgeries. It reduces the number of eyedrops to be used, possibly increasing compliance, but does not allow each constituent to be tapered separately. The use of systemic antibiotics preoperatively, or postoperatively in uneventful surgeries, is no longer recommended. A preoperative conjunctival swab is no longer routine practice, with the possible exception of one eyed patients, and those with immunosuppression. Cost evaluation for the prophylactic use of intraocular intraoperative antibiosis in cataract surgery revealed an economically relevant decrease in direct endophthalmitis associated costs.[13] Cost and availability are important considerations in the Indian scenario.

Topical Antibiotics

Topical antibiotics are part of the typical regimen to prevent postoperative infections in patients receiving cataract surgery. These antibiotics have been shown to significantly reduce bacterial counts when given before surgery and also to alter the conjunctival flora. The degree of bacterial reduction depends on the antibiotic selected, the frequency and duration of antibiotic use, the bacterial species present, and the antibiotic sensitivities.

Gentamicin

One of the oldest antibiotics to be evaluated, gentamicin was found to be the most effective agent available for reducing the quantity of periocular organisms. Topical gentamicin can occasionally achieve significant aqueous and ocular tissue concentration, although intravitreal concentration remain variable. Fortified preparations lead to significant intraocular levels.

Trimethoprim-Polymyxin B Sulphate

Trimethoprim is synergistic when combined with polymixin B. Trimethoprim can be bacteriostatic or bactericidal depending upon its concentration and is effective against a wide variety of gram-positive and gram-negative organisms including *S. aureus* and *S. epidermidis*. Polymyxin B is effective against gram-negative organisms including *Pseudomonas*. The combination of trimethoprim and polymyxin B is effective against most of the gram-positive and gram-negative organisms.

Trimethoprim-polymyxin sulphate antibiotics have variable effect on conjunctival and lid organisms. One study by Bell et al[20] demonstrated that trimethoprim and polymyxin combination drugs have no demonstrable clinically significant antibacterial effect but another study by Osher et al[9] showed complete eradication of all organisms except *S. epidermidis* with these combination drugs. However, polymyxin-trimethoprim does not achieve significant concentration in the anterior chamber. Asley et al[21] showed that this combination is less effective than chloramphenicol or a combination of neomycin/polymyxin B/gramicidin and most effective against *Haemophilus influenzae*.

CHLORAMPHENICOL

Chloramphenicol, an antibiotic originally isolated from *Streptomyces venezuelae* but now produced synthetically was introduced into clinical practice in the year 1948. It is effective against both gram-positive and gram-negative organisms. But *Pseudomonas aeruginosa* and Mycobacteria are usually resistant. Seal et al[22] in a study involving 738 patients demonstrated 6 percent resistance to chloramphenicol, 9 percent resistance to tetracycline and around 20 percent resistance to aminoglycosides. Doona and Walsh[23] in a controversial article in British Medical Journal recommended that the use of chloramphenicol should be restricted as it may cause blood dyscrasias. However, many subsequent studies by various ophthalmologists and hematologists countered this view. Walker et al[24] reported that the reversible marrow suppression occur in dose dependant manner with serum levels greater than 25 mg/L. They found that serum lever never reached 1 mg/L when the drug was administered topically at four times daily dose and concluded that chloramphenicol did not present any risk of inducing dose related bone marrow toxicity.

It is one of the ideal drug for topical use as its ocular toxicity is low, ocular penetration is excellent and has broad spectrum of activity.

TOPICAL FLUOROQUINOLONES

Fluoroquinolone eyedrops have excellent broad-spectrum activity, minimal toxicity and desirable kinetics. These agents nowadays are the most commonly used topical antibiotics as these agents achieve more antibiotic concentration in the anterior chamber as compared to other routinely used antibiotics including tobramycin. Within the fluoroquinolone group, different quinolone drugs achieve different antibiotic concentration within the anterior chamber. Topical ofloxacin 0.3 percent applied preoperatively achieve mean aqueous humor levels of 0.338 g/ml, which is significant higher than those achieved with 0.3 percent ciprofloxacin and 0.3 percent norfloxacin.[8] Level of ofloxacin in the tear film 4 hours after topical application exceed MIC_{90} for wide range of ocular isolates. Again between ciprofloxacin and norfloxacin, ciprofloxacin has more antibacterial activity upon the ocular flora as compared to norfloxacin. Diamond et al[25] demonstrated that ciprofloxacin 0.3 percent was a patent perioperative prophylaxis of ocular infection.

Second and third generation fluoroquinolones which include ciprofloxacin and ofloxacin have broad spectrum of activity against gram-positive and gram-negative organisms. Ciprofloxacin 0.3 percent eye drugs is wide used clinically for the treatment of corneal upper and superficial infection of the eye and ocular adnexa caused by susceptible organisms. With topically used prophylacticals before cataract surgery, most of the susceptible organisms are inhibited. These drugs should be given only a few day before surgery at a dose of 4 times daily.

LOMEFLOXACIN

Lomefloxacin is specifically effective against superficial bacterial infections particularly acute bacterial conjunctivitis. Agius-Fernandez et al[26] compared the relative efficacy of lomefloxacin and chloramphenicol bacterial conjunctivitis patients and showed that both the drugs were equally well-tolerated with no serious systemic or local adverse reactions. They concluded that lomefloxacin 0.3 percent eyedrops instilled twice daily were as effective and well-tolerated as chloramphenicol 0.5 percent eyedrops instilled 5 times daily. Jauch et al[27] demonstrated that lomefloxacin eye drops used with a loading dose followed by a twice daily regimen proved as effective as other standard antibiotic drugs like gentamicin 0.3 percent, tobramycin 0.3 percent and norfloxacin 0.3 percent. Another advantage of lomefloxacin was that after the loading dose, lomefloxacin can be given in twice daily dose regimen.

Dosage: Ophthalmic solution 0.3 percent fortified drugs, 20 mg/ml subconjunctival dose, 20-30 mg/ml intravitreal, 200 mg/ml oral dose 400 mg OD.

Sparfloxacin: It has an excellent broad-spectrum activity against both gram-positive and gram-negative organisms including anaerobes especially *Bacteroides fragilis* and multidrug resistant enterococci. It is more effective than ciprofloxacin against *Streptococcus pneumoniae, Staphylococcus aureus* and *Staphylococcus epidermidis.*

Dosage: Ophthalmic solutions 0.3 percent
Intravitreal dose: 20-60 mg/ml
Fortified drugs: 20 mg/ml
Subconjunctival dose: 20-40 mg.

Ofloxacin

Ofloxacin has broad-spectrum activity against both gram-positive and gram-negative organisms. It can be effective against bacterial strains which are resistant to ciprofloxacin. It is commonly used as 0.3 percent ophthalmic solution.

FOURTH GENERATION FLUOROQUINOLONES

The fourth generation fluoroquinolones include gatifloxacin and moxifloxacin and were approved by the US Food and Drug Administration (FDA) in 2003.

Both these antibiotics bound more strongly to topoisomerase II as compared to older generation fluoroquinolones. With the addition of methoxy group on carbon 8, the newer fluoroquinolone bind more effectively to topoisomerase II and IV, giving these drugs better clinical activities against gram-positive organisms. As these drugs act at two different sites these drugs have less chance of inducing drug resistance as the susceptible bacteria has to develop two mechanisms for development of resistance.

Both gatifloxacin and moxifloxacin have a lower MIC 90 against gram-positive bacteria than the 2nd and third generation fluoroquinolones. Both these drugs are effective against coagulase-negative *Staphylococcus* and *Streptococcus viridans*, two of the most common causes of postoperative endophthalmitis. The efficacy rate against gram-negative organisms are more or less same as seen with older fluoroquinolones.

Following topical use, the concentration of both gatifloxacin and moxifloxacin in the anterior chamber reach levels in excess of the MIC_{90} for most pathogenic organisms. Solomon et al[28] investigated cataract patients who received moxifloxacin 0.5 percent, gatifloxacin 0.3 percent, or ciprofloxacin 0.3 percent four times a day for 3 days before surgery and then every 15 minutes 3 times 1 hour before surgery. Anterior chamber drug levels were significantly higher in patients receiving moxifloxacin than in patients taking gatifloxacin.

Subconjunctival Antibiotics

Most of the topically used antibiotics can be given subconjunctivally. The ocular penetration following this route is diffusion through corneal stroma rather than tear film. The therapeutic level may remain for more than 12 hours and because of longer duration of action antibiotics injected through subconjunctival route may be more effective in preventing postoperative endophthalmitis. The intravitreal concentration of most of the antibiotics given through subconjunctival route is extremely low. So once endophthalmitis has developed, subconjunctival antibiotics are of no value. Ideally the subconjunctival antibiotics should be given preoperatively so that effective concentration of antibiotic is present in the anterior chamber at the time the organisms are introduced.[8] Subconjunctival antibiotics have decreased the incidence of experimental endophthalmitis in animal models; animal models in which cataract extraction was followed by intentional inoculation of bacteria into the vitreous cavity.

Routinely the antibiotics used for subconjunctival route include gentamicin, tobramicin, cefazoline, vancomycin.

INTRACAMERAL ANTIBIOTICS

Intracameral antibiotics involve the use of antibiotics directly into anterior chamber either through direct injection into anterior chamber or through irrigating solution. Gills[28] reported low rate of postoperative endophthalmitis when the antibiotics were given through irrigating solutions. Gimbel et al[29] used 8 g/ml gentamicin in the irrigating solution and 1 mg vancomycin into the capsular bag at the end of the surgery with no cases of endophthalmitis in 11,748 procedures.

The spectrum of pathogens causing postcataract endophthalmitis changes over time, as also resistance to antibiotics used for its prophylaxis. In many instances, current routine practices of antibiotic prophylaxis reflect personal preferences, are empirical, and in a strict sense, not evidence-based. While recent studies suggest a beneficial role of antibiotic prophylaxis, such benefit is not yet unequivocally proven, the limitations being the relatively low prevalence of endophthalmitis that makes controlled studies with a large cohort difficult, and often, the non-availability of microbiological facilities where cataract surgeries are performed in large numbers. Presurgical antibiotic prophylaxis must be combined with additional measures such as topical preoperative 5 percent povidone-iodine, the use of an adhesive foil, and surgical technique. Rational antibiotics usage demands that a reserve bactericidal drug(s) be available. In the majority of situations, it is a combination of vancomycin (for gram-positive), and ceftazidime or amikacin (for gram-negative), used intravitreally for the treatment of endophthalmitis. Prevention of post-cataract surgery endophthalmitis is of utmost importance, and future prospective studies based on human clinical trials and microbiological studies will be required to continually provide updated information necessary to guide patient care.

REFERENCES

1. McCulley JP. Low acute endophthalmitis rate: Possible explanations. J Cataract Refract Surg 2005;31:1074-75.
2. Eifrig CWG, Flynn HW Jr, Scott IU, Newton J. Acute-onset postoperative endophthalmitis: Review of incidence and visual outcomes (1995-2001). Ophthalmic Surg Lasers 2002;33:37-38; erratum, 34:80.
3. Montan PG, Koranyi G, Setterquist H, et al. Endophthalmitis after cataract surgery: Risk factors relating to technique and events of the operation and patient history—A retrospective case-control study. Ophthalmology 1998;105:2171-77.
4. Ciulla TA, Starr MB, Masket S. Bacterial endophthalmitis prophylaxis for cataract surgery: An evidence-based update. Ophthalmology 2002;109:13-26.
5. Bannerman TL, Rhoden DL, McAllister SK, et al. The source of coagulase-negative staphylococci in the endophthalmitis vitrectomy study: A comparison of eyelid and intraocular isolates using pulsed-field gel electrophoresis. Arch Ophthalmol 1997;115:357-61.
6. Han DP, Wisniewski SR, Wilson LA, et al. Spectrum and susceptibilities of microbiologic isolates in the endophthalmitis vitrectomy study. Am J Ophthalmol 1996;122:1-17;erratum, 920.
7. Ariyasu RG, Nakamura T, Trousdale MD, Smith RE. Intraoperative bacterial contamination of the aqueous humor. Ophthalmic Surg 1993;24:367-73;discussion 373-74.
8. Liesegang TJ. Perioperative antibiotic prophylaxis in cataract surgery. Cornea 1999;18:383-402.
9. Osher RH, Amdahl LD, Cheetham JK. Antimicrobial efficacy and aqueous humor penetration of preoperative and postoperative topical trimethoprim/polymyxin B sulfate versus tobramycin. J Cataract Refract Surg 1994;20:3-8.
10. Allen HF, Mangiaracine AB. Bacterial endophthalmitis after cataract extraction. Arch Ophthalmol 1964;72:454-62.
11. Arantes TE, Cavalcanti RF, Diniz Mde F, Severo MS, Lins Neto J, Castro CM. Conjunctival bacterial flora and antibiotic resistance pattern in patients undergoing cataract surgery. Arq Bras Oftalmol 2006;69:33-6. Epub 2006, Feb 10.
12. Recchia FM, Busbee BG, Pearlman RB, Carvalho-Recchia CA, Ho AC. Changing trends in the microbiologic aspects of postcataract endophthalmitis. Arch Ophthalmol 2005;123:341-46.
13. Wejde G, Samolov B, Seregard S, Koranyi G, Montan PG. Risk factors for endophthalmitis following cartaract surgery: A retrospective case-control study. J Hosp Infect 2005;61:251-56.
14. Krummenauer F, Kurz S, Dick HB. Epidemiological evaluation of intraoperative antibiosis as a protective agent against endophthalmitis after cataract surgery. Pharmacoepidemiol Drug Saf 2006;15:662-66.
15. Rosha DS, Ng JQ, Morlet N, Boekelaar M, Wilson S, Hendrie D, Semmens JB. Cataract surgery practice and endophthalmitis prevention by Australian and New Zealand ophthalmologists. Clin Experiment Ophthalmol 2006;34:535-44.

16. Kim DH, Stark WJ, O'Brien TP, Dick JD. Aqueous penetration and biological activity of moxifloxacin 0.5% ophthalmic solution and gatifloxacin 0.3% solution in cataract surgery patients. Ophthalmology 2005;112:1992-96. Epub 2005 Sep 23.
17. Romero P, Mendez I, Salvat M, Fernandez J, Almena M. Intracameral cefazolin as prophylaxis against endophthalmitis in cataract surgery. J Cataract Refract Surg 2006;32:438-41.
18. Ball JL, Barrett GD. Prospective randomized controlled trial of the effect of intracameral vancomycin and gentamicin on macular retinal thickness and visual function following cataract surgery. J Cataract Refract Surg 2006;32:789-94.
19. ESCRS endophthalmitis prophylaxis clinical trial. ESCRS office at escrs@escrs.org.
20. Bell TA, Slack M, Harvey SG, Gibson JR. The effect of trimethoprim-polymyxin B sulphate ophthalmic ointment and chloramphenicol ophthalmic ointment on the bacterial flora of the eye when administered to the operated and unoperated eyes of patients undergoing cataract surgery. Eye 1988;2:324-29.
21. Ashley KC. The anti-bacterial activity of topical anti-infective eye preparations. Med Lab Sci 1986;43:157-62.
22. Seal DV, Barrett SP, McGill JI. Aetiology and treatment of acute bacterial infection of the external eye. Br J Ophthalmol 1982;66:357-60.
23. Doona M, Walsh JB. Use of chloramphenicol as topical eye medication: Time to cry halt? BMJ 1995;310:1217-18.
24. Walker S, Diaper CJM, Bowman R, Sweeney G, Seal DV, Krikness CM. Lack of evidence for systemic toxicity following systemic chloramphenicol use. Eye 1998;12:875-79.
25. Diamond JP, White L, Leeming JP, Bing Ho H, Easty DL. Topical 0.3 percent ciprofloxacin, norfloxacin, and ofloxacin in treatment of bacterial keratitis: A new method for comparative evaluation of ocular drug penetration. Br J Ophthalmol 1995;79:606-09.
26. Agius-Fernandez A, Patterson A, Fsadni M, Jauch A, Sunder Raj P. Topical lomefloxacin versus topical chloramphenicol in the treatment of acute bacterial conjunctivitis. Clin Drug Invest 1998;15:263-69.
27. Jauch A, Esadni M, Gamba G. Meta-analysis of six clinical phase III studies comparing lomefloxacin 0.3% eye drops twice daily to five standard antibiotics in patients with acute bacterial conjunctivitis. Graefes Arch Clin Exp Ophthalmol 1999;237:705-13.
28. Gills JP. Filters and antibiotics in irrigating solution for cataract surgery [Letter]. J Cataract Refract Surg 1991;17:385.
29. Gimbel HV, Sun R, DeBroff BM. Prophylactic intracameral antibiotics during cataract surgery: The incidence of endophthalmitis and corneal endothelial loss. Eur J Implant Refract Surg 1994;6:280-85.

Management of Iatrogenic Inflammation of the Eye

NR Biswas, GK Das, Vinay Gupta (India)

For the treatment of any type of inflammation including iatrogenic, both the asteroids and nonsteroidal anti-inflammatory drugs may be used.

The corticosteroids are essential drugs in ophthalmological diseases. It is a boon to the patients when it is used with proper indications. It is a two-edged sword, however, and can cause serious complications and side effects if it is used unwisely. Are we using corticosteroids judiciously? This question must always be kept in mind and answered before instituting this therapy. Before planning the corticosteroid therapy, we must keep in mind its ocular hazards. In clinical practice corticosteroids are often used as shotgun therapy or as a placebo when all is not going well. This practice must be discouraged.

TOPICAL APPLICATION

The route of administration of corticosteroids depends primarily on the site of involvement. Topical therapy is effective in anterior segment diseases, including disorders of lids, conjunctiva, cornea, iris and ciliary body. Ease of application, relatively low cost, and absence of systemic complications strongly favor local routes whenever they are effective.

The course of posterior segment disease (chorioretinitis, optic neuritis, and posterior scleritis) is not appreciably affected by topical corticosteroids and requires systemic therapy.

- *Are diluted corticosteroid drops effective in controlling intraocular inflammation?*
  It was demonstrated that diluted corticosteroids have therapeutic anti-inflammatory effect in strengths of 0.01 and 0.005 percent.
- *Corticosteroids in infective corneal diseases:* Local installation of corticosteroids in frank suppurative conditions are generally considered as contraindications to their use. In experimental studies the available 0.1 percent dexamethasone further diluted as 1:10 or 1:20 dilution had no virus or fungal replications enhancing effect when instilled 10 times a day, while 1:5 dilution or undiluted available dexamethasone drops (0.1%) enhanced virus and fungal growth. Moreover, adequately diluted corticosteroid does not increase the risk of enhancing the collagenase effect.
- *Corticosteroid therapy in vernal conjunctivitis and allergic disorders:* The use off corticosteroids locally has a beneficial

effect in vernal conjunctivitis. But prolonged use is attended by unwanted side effects like cataracts, glaucoma and secondary keratoconus.

- *Use of corticosteroids in alkali burns of cornea and conjunctiva:* The use of corticosteroids in alkali burns is obligatory and seems beneficial.
- *Use of corticosteroids in pseudophakic bullous keratopathy (PBK):* The effects of 5 percent hypertonic sodium chloride drop and detergescent drops, prepared by mixing betamethasone eyedrops (0.1%) 1 ml; glycerin, 1 ml and artificial tear drops 8 ml, achieving 10 percent glycerin and 1:0 betamethasone eye drops (0.1%), were compared in a controlled clinical trial in 50 cases of PBK. These were instilled 10 times a day. The detergescent drops were significantly superior in subjective as well as objective parameters like discomfort, foreign body sensation, corneal clarity and improvement in vision, etc. as compared to 5 percent hypertonic saline.
- *Ocular hypertensive effect of corticosteroids:* Surgical trauma causes inflammation which demands the use of corticosteroids to prevent the trabecular meshwork, corneal endothelium and other inner structures of the eye from damage by inflammatory response as well as its debris. But, ocular hypertension inducing effects restrict their wide usage. In this regard, 1:10 or 1:20 diluted steroid did not have any ocular hypertensive effect.

The use of 1:10 or 1:20 dexamethasone (0.1%) for specified periods is safe to be used in glaucoma patients after intraocular surgery or when there is an associate uveitis, as there should be negligible risk of producing hypertension.

Systemic Therapy

Prednisone has become a corticosteroid of choice because it is inexpensive, short acting, and relatively free from sodium retention. It may be used in divided doses, a single daily dose, or a single alternate day dose.

Single daily dose: For long-term low-dosage maintenance (as for chronic uveitis), a single, morning, daily dose of prednisone may be optimal.

Alternate day therapy: The undesirable side effects of systemic corticosteroid therapy can be substantially reduced by using alternate day therapy rather than divided dosage. Briefly stated, the entire total dose of corticosteroid that would have been given during a 2-day period is administered as a single dose every other morning.

Repository Injection

The ophthalmologist who wishes to administer corticosteroids by "subconjunctival" injection should consider use of the repository form of methylprednisolone acetate (Depo-Medrol). Thus suspension form of prednisolone provides a constant source of corticosteroid that lasts for 2-4 weeks.

Intravitreal Injection

Intravitreal 0.1 ml (Dose 50 mg/ml) is injected to prevent proliferation of fibroblast. It seems helpful to combat proliferative vitreoretinopathy.

Controlled Release Vehicles

Ocusert devices delivering 10 mg of hydrocortisone acetate/hour were used to treat allergic conjunctivitis.

Pulse Therapy

Slow intravenous infusion of 100 mg prednisolone daily for consecutive three days shows good response in Harada's disease. If needed, repeat dose can be given after 14 days.

Indications

In general, corticosteroid therapy may be helpful for all allergic ocular diseases, for most nonpyogenic inflammations (episcleritis, scleritis, uveitis, interstitial keratitis, optic neuritis and the like), and for the reduction of immunologic responses.

Use in Ocular Surgery

- Cataract
- Corneal graft rejection
- Glaucoma surgery
- Retinal detachment
- Vitreous surgery
- Strabismus
- Intraocular foreign body.

Contraindications and Complications

Systemic Complications

- Peptic ulceration
- Osteoporosis
- Femoral head ischemia necrosis
- Pseudotumor cerebri
- Exophthalmos.

Local Contraindications and Complications

- Superinfection
- Activation of tuberculosis
- Uveitis

- Glaucoma
- Corticosteroid mydriasis
- Corticosteroid induced cataract.

The severe scleritis associated with rheumatoid arthritis, an example of immunological disorder does respond to corticosteroid treatment but the patient may suffer structural loss of sclera up to more severe scleromalacia as a result of treatment.

Sympathetic ophthalmia is a classic example of a disease responsive to corticosteroid therapy, but requires prolonged therapy.

Nonspecific iridocyclitis and chorioretinitis, as well as herpetic keratitis do seem to benefit from corticosteroid therapy.

Posterior ocular effects require systemic administration or retrobulbar injection.

Responsive Diseases

Boeck's Sarcoid Uveitis

The response of Boeck's sarcoid uveitis to corticosteroid therapy may be very gratifying. Topical use of corticosteroids and mydriatics is often insufficient to arrest the disease. Addition of systemic corticosteroid therapy has frequently given prompt subjective relief, followed within a few weeks by considerable objective improvement. Up to 200 mg daily was used and produced a consistently favorable symptomatic effect.

Orbital Myositis

Acute inflammation of one or more extraocular muscles may be a sequel to upper respiratory infections. These painful restrictions of movement may respond promptly to corticosteroid therapy.

Ocular Pemphigoid

Although pemphigoid is characteristically a slowly progressive chronic subepithelial scarring process, episodes of acute inflammation may occur. These typically are nonresponsive to topical corticosteroid therapy. Systemic corticosteroids in dosage of 60–100 mg/day have caused remission of the disease.

Herpes-Zoster

In a small series of 11 patients with herpeszoster, very favorable results were reported from the systemic administration of cortisone or ACTH.

Neoplasms

Hemangiomas, intracranial plasmacytoma, medulloblastoma, Ewing's tumors respond well to corticosteroid therapy.

Tolosa-Hunt Syndrome

Recurrent unilateral, painful, acute ophthalmoplegia responds dramatically to corticosteroid therapy within 2-3 days. A daily dosage of 60 mg prednisone was used.

Anterior Segment Ischemia

Prednisolone 1 percent was used four times daily, with gradual clearing of the corneal edema and anterior chamber cellular reaction.

Pseudotumor Cerebri

Dexamethasone 0.5 mg is prescribed three doses daily for 3 weeks.

Toxoplasmosis

It can be treated with high corticosteroid doses (up to 100 mg prednisone per day for a prolonged period with specific antitoxoplasmic therapy).

Other Indications

Corticosteroid is found to be useful in cysticercosis.

USE OF NONSTEROIDAL ANTI-INFLAMMATORY DRUGS IN INFLAMMATION

In the treatment of ocular inflammation, the appeal of nonsteroidal anti-inflammatory drugs (NSAIDs) hinges on the complications associated with the more established therapy for ocular inflammation, i.e. corticosteroids. Although an overlap exists between the mechanisms of action of both, the use of NSAIDs may be safer than the use of corticosteroids, as the latter may produce adverse effects such as glaucoma, opportunistic infections, and posterior subcapsular cataracts. In sharp contrast, topical NSAIDs are known to cause only minor adverse effects such as burning, stinging and hyperemia of the conjunctiva.

Ocular Inflammation

A simple definition of ocular inflammation would be inflammation of any part of the eye. Intraocular inflammation can be subdivided into inflammation of the anterior and posterior segments of the eye. The cardinal signs of ocular inflammation are hyperemia, increased vascular permeability, edema, and cellular (leukocytes, mast cell, platelets, etc) infiltration into ocular fluids and tissues. In experimental anterior uveitis, miosis and a rise in intraocular pressure which is usually due to the breakdown of the blood-aqueous barrier with subsequent release of protein and fibrin into the aqueous humor, but not of cellular infiltration, is observed. Inflammation after paracentesis usually disappears within 2-3 hours.

To understand the history of NSAID use in ophthalmology, one must appreciate the relevance of prostaglandins in the eye. In 1971, Vane and Smith established the connection between the clinical effect of acetylsalicylate and inhibition of prostaglandin synthesis.[1,2] It is now well-known that aspirin and other NSAIDs produce their clinical efficacy by inhibiting cyclo-oxygenase and thus inhibiting prostaglandin synthesis (Fig. 29.1). Specific drugs belonging to each class are listed in Tables 29.1 and 29.2.

Mechanism of Action

Nonsteroidal anti-inflammatory drugs act mainly as anti-inflammatory agents by inhibiting cyclo-oxygenase and lipo-oxygenase enzymes which lead to inhibition of products like prostaglandins, thromboxane and leukotrienes which induce inflammation. Ocular actions of prostaglandins include an increase in vascular permeability, breakdown of the blood-aqueous barrier and induction of miosis.[3]

Cystoid Macular Edema

Topical NSAIDs are effective in preventing postsurgical angiographic cystoid macular edema (CME) when topical or subtenon's corticosteroid injections are given concurrently. Only one study (involving 50 patients) has demonstrated similar effect with a topical NSAID in the absence of concurrent corticosteroid

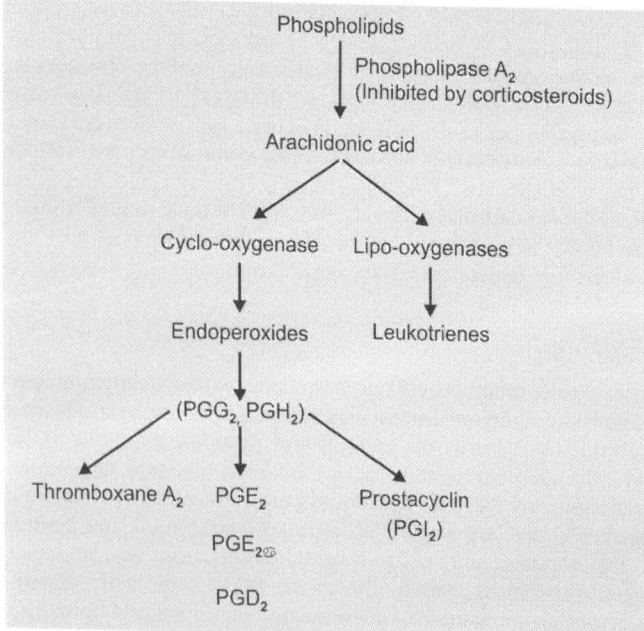

Fig. 29.1: Mechanism by which nonsteroidal anti-inflammatory drugs produce their clinical effect

TABLE 29.1: Systemic nonsteroidal anti-inflammatory agents

Drug	Drug name	How supplied (mg)	Typical adult daily dose (mg)
Salicylates	Aspirin	325–925	650 q4h
	Diflunisal	250, 500	250–500 bid
Fenamates	Mefenamate	250	250 qid
	Meclofenamate	50, 100	50–100 qid
Indoles	Indomethacin	25, 50, 75 (slow release)	25–50 tid-quid, 75 bid
	Sulindac	150, 200	150–200 bid
	Tolmetin	200, 400, 600	400 tid
Phenylacetic acids	Diclofenac	35, 50, 75	35–75 bid
Phenylalkanoic acids	Fenoprofen	200, 300, 600	300–600 tid
	Ketoprofen	25, 50, 75	75 tid–50 quid
	Piroxicam	10, 20	10 bid, 20 daily
	Flurbiprofen	50, 100	100 tid
	Ketorolac	10	10 qid
	Naproxen	250, 375, 500	250–500 bid
		275–550	275–550 bid
	Ibuprofen	200, 300, 400 600, 800	400–800 tid
Pyrazolones	Phenylbutazone	100	100 tid-qid
	Oxyphenbutazone	100	100 tid-qid
Para-aminophenols	Acetaminophen	80, 325, 500, 650	650 q4h

TABLE 29.2: Topical nonsteroidal anti-inflammatory agents

Name	Strength	Typical doses
Flurbiprofen	0.03% solution	1 drop every 30 minutes for 2 hour Preoperatively (Total dose: 4 drops)
Suprofen	1.0% solution	2 drops at 1.2 and 3 hours preoperatively or every 4 hours while awake on the day of surgery
Diclofenac	0.1% solution	qid
Ketorolac	0.5% solution	tid
Indomethacin	0.5%-1.0% suspension	qid

therapy.[4] Several studies have demonstrated that prophylactic treatment with a topical NSAID has a beneficial effect on visual function. In one study, this effect was shown even in the absence of concurrent corticosteroid therapy. Topical NSAIDs also are effective in the treatment of angiographically documented subclinical CME, and this can translate into improved visual function. Oral NSAIDs have also been shown to be effective in both the prevention and treatment of CME after cataract surgery.

However, a study demonstrating a positive effect on visual function with oral promote one NSAIDs still is lacking. There is no strong evidence to promote one NSAID over another.

Postoperative Inflammation

Fluorophotometric analysis has made available a quantitative means of studying anterior chamber inflammation. With this tool, it has been possible to evaluate, in a reproducible fashion, the effect of NSAIDs on postoperative inflammation. By using both slit lamp and fluorophotometric analysis as a part of randomized double-masked placebo-controlled studies, several topical NSAIDs like indomethacin 1.0 percent,[5] flurbiprofen 0.03 percent,[6] ketorolac 0.5 percent[7,8] and diclofenac 0.1 percent[9] have been shown to reduce postoperative inflammation. The positive effect of NSAIDs was seen in both intracapsular and extracapsular cataract surgery. It is important to note that whereas in most of the studies, corticosteroids were given concurrently, two of these studies were conducted without concurrent corticosteroid therapy.[7,8] In these studies, topical ketorolac 0.05 percent proved to be better than placebo in controlling inflammation after cataract surgery.

In the treatment of postsurgical inflammation, the superiority of NSAID over placebo has led to a comparison of NSAIDs with corticosteroid. Ketorolac 0.5 percent[10] and diclofenac[11] were compared to dexamethasone and prednisolone, respectively. In both studies, there was no significant difference in the reduction of postoperative inflammation by slit-lamp examination between patients on NSAIDs and those on corticosteroid topical therapy. However, it should be noted that in the ketorolac study, a subtenon injection of corticosteroid was given to all the patients and this may have contributed to the lack of difference between the two treatment groups. Concurrent corticosteroid therapy was not a factor in the study comparing diclofenac with prednisolone. When fluorophotometry was used in both comparative studies, it was found that control of inflammation in the topical NSAID treatment group was better achieved than in the corticosteroid groups.

Regardless of the preceding findings, it is a common practice to use topical corticosteroid alone to control post cataract surgery inflammation. Nevertheless, the US food and Drug Administration (FDA) has approved the use of the diclofenac 0.1 percent four times daily, starting 24 hours after cataract surgery for this purpose. Thus, it is possible to substitute a topical NSAID for a topical corticosteroid to control postoperative inflammation, especially in eyes with significant steroid responsive glaucoma.

Uveitis

In contrast to postsurgical inflammation, many forms of uveitis require prolonged steroid therapy to control inflammation. At times, the therapeutic effort must be escalated to the use of subtenon injections or oral administration of corticosteroid. Of course, the risk of iatrogenic glaucoma and cataract becomes substantial I these situations. Therefore, NSAIDs are gaining a more secure position in the treatment of certain forms of uveitis.

Scleritis and Episcleritis

Topical NSAIDs have no proven efficacy in the treatment of episcleritis. In fact, they appear to be less effective than topical corticosteroids in reducing episcleral injection and pain associated with episcleritis.[12] In contrast, systemic NSAIDs are the agents of choice in the treatment of nonnecrotizing simple, diffuse, and nodular scleritis.[13] One may have to proceed sequentially through several different NSAIDs until one find the one that works. Furthermore, when a steroid is needed, the duration and dose of the steroidal may be reduced with the adjunctive use of an NSAID.

Allergic and Giant Papillary Conjunctivitis

Vernal keratoconjunctivitis most commonly occurs children and young adults. It shares with contact lens-associated giant papillary conjunctivitis (GPC). The common finding of giant papillary conjunctivitis on the upper palpebral conjunctiva. The standard treatment for both is topical steroids until a topical mast cell stabilizer takes effect.

Side Effects of NSAIDs

Common adverse effects following instillation of topical NSAIDs include burning, stinging, and hyperemia of conjunctiva. Allergic and hypertensive reactions are also reported following use of topical NSAIDs. Systemic side effects following use of NSAIDs mainly include gastritis, but are unlikely to occur with topical administration.

CONCLUSION

Nonsteroidal anti-inflammatory drugs (NSAIDs) have wide potential for use in various ocular disorders, though the effects vary from one individual to another and the effect is unpredictable. More research is required to develop newer NSAIDs which can be used for various inflammatory disorders of the eye with more effective action with minimal ocular toxicities.

Currently corticosteroids are still the drugs of choice in the treatment of ocular inflammation. However, because their prolonged use may result in severe ocular side effects, it would be therapeutically beneficial to develop nonsteroidal anti-inflammatory drugs that have similar or greater efficacy than steroids but not their ocular side effects.

REFERENCES

1. Flck AJ. Cyclo-oxygenase inhibitors in Ophthalmology. Surv Ophthalmol 1992;36:259-84.

2. Gilman AG, Rall TC, Nies AS, Taylor P. The pharmacologic basis of therapeutics. Elmsford: Pergamon 1990.pp.638-81.
3. Abramson SB, Weisman G. The mechanism of nonsteroidal anti-inflammatory drugs. Arthritis Rheum 1989;32:1-9.
4. Flach AJ, Jampol LM, Weinberg D, et al. Improvement in visual acuity in chronic aphakic and pseudophakic cystoid macular edema after treatment with topical 0.5 percent ketorolac tromethamine. Am J Ophthalmol 1991;112:514-19.
5. Sanders DR, Kraff ML. Steroidal and nonsteroidal anti-inflammatory agents. Effects on postsurgical inflammation and blood-aqueous barrier breakdown. Arch. Ophthalmol 1984;102:1453-6.
6. Sabiston MB, Tessler D, Summersk H, et al. Reduction of inflammation following cataract surgery by flurbiprofen. Ophthalmic Surg 1987;18:873-7.
7. Flach AJ, Graham J, Kruger LP, et al. Quantitative assessment of postsurgical breakdown of the blood-aqueous barrier following administration of ketorolack tomethmine solution. A double-masked, paired comparison with vehicle-placebo solution study. Arch Ophthalmol 1988;106:344-7.
8. Flach AJ, Lavelle CJ, Olander KW, et al. The effect of ketorolac 0.5 percent solution in reducing postsurgical inflammation following ECCE with IOL. Double masked, parallel comparison with vehicle. Ophthalmology. 1988;95:1277-84.
9. Vickers FF, McGuigan LJB, Ford C, et al. The effect of diclofenac sodium ophthalmic drops on the treatment of postoperative inflammation. Invest Ophthalmol Vis Sci (ARVO suppl) 1991;32:793.
10. Flach AJ, Kraff MC, Sanders DR, et al. The quantitative effect of 0.5 percent ketorolac tromethamine solution and 0.1 percent dexamethasone sodium phosphate solution on postsurgical blood aqueous barrier. Arch Ophthalmol 1988;106:480-83.
11. Kraff MC, Sanders DR, McGuigan L, et al. Inhibition of blood aqueous humour barrier breakdown with diclofenac. A fluorophotometric study. Arch Ophthalmol 1990;108:380-3.
12. Lyons CH, Hakin KN, Watson PG. Topical flurbiprofen: An effective treatment for episcleritis? Eye 1990;4:521-25.
13. Vitale A, Foster CS. Nonsteroidal anti-inflammatory drugs. In: Zimmerman TJ, (Ed): Textbook of ocular pharmacology. New York: Lippincott-Raven; 1995.

Management of Postrefractive Keratitis

Eric D Donnenfeld (USA)

Laser assisted *in situ* keratomileusis (LASIK) is the most commonly performed surgical procedure to correct refractive errors and is the most common elective procedure performed in the United States. LASIK offers many benefits over photorefractive keratectomy, including increased visual rehabilitation, decreased stromal scarring, less postoperative pain, less irregular astigmatism, minimal regression, and the ability to treat a greater range of refractive disorders.[1,2] Compared to other refractive procedures, LASIK preserves the integrity of Bowman's membrane and the overlying epithelium, thus decreasing the risk of microbial keratitis. However, microbial keratitis following LASIK has become an increasingly recognized, sight-threatening complication of refractive surgery.[3-10]

The incidence of infectious keratitis following LASIK is unknown and can vary widely depending on the study. One large, retrospective study investigating the complications associated with LASIK surgery found an incidence of two infections in 1,062 eyes,[7] and another similar study found an incidence of one infection in 1,019 eyes.[8] A more recent case series of LASIK-associated infections encountered at a single institution quotes an estimated incidence between 1:1000 and 1:5000.[9] Based on a comprehensive review and analysis of the published literature on infections following LASIK, Chang and colleagues[5] also noted that the incidence of infection after LASIK can vary widely (0-1.5%). The American Society of Cataract and Refractive Surgery (ASCRS) Cornea Clinical Committee developed a post-LASIK infectious keratitis survey and conducted a survey of the organization's members in 2001 and again in 2004.[10] In the 2001 survey, there was an incidence of 1 infection for every 2919 procedures performed by physicians returning the questionnaire (116 post-LASIK infections were reported by 56 LASIK surgeons who had performed an estimated 338,550 procedures). These results are contrasted to 1 infection for every 2131 procedures performed by physicians returning the questionnaire in 2004. The increase in incidence of infections is presumably due to an increase in gram-positive resistant organisms, most likely due to methicillin resistant *Staphylococcus aureus*. Culture results revealed opportunistic infections and gram-positive bacteria as the most common organisms in 2001 (Fig. 30.1A). In contrast, as noted above, in 2004 gram-positive bacteria have increased in incidence while opportunistic infections, specifically atypical mycobacteria, have seen a marked reduction (Fig. 30.1B).

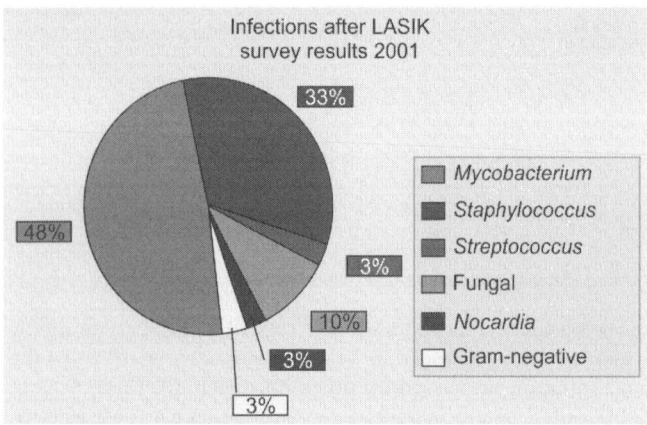

Fig. 30.1A: ASCRS 2001 culture results of post-LASIK infectious keratitis

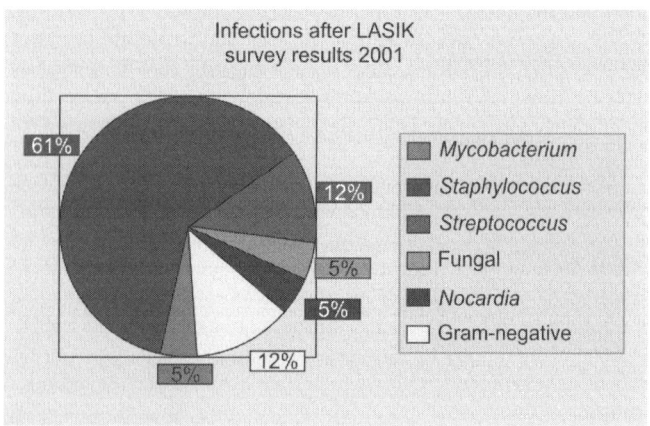

Fig. 30.1B: ASCRS 2004 culture results of post-LASIK infectious keratitis

In 2004, the epidemic of atypical mycobacteria that was seen in 2001 (Fig. 30.1B) ended. Cases from atypical mycobacteria decreased from 48 to 5 percent. This decrease is presumably due to the use of fourth generation fluoroquinolones and improved sterile technique. It was interesting to note that no patient who received a fourth generation fluoroquinolone as prophylaxis developed an atypical mycobacteria infectious keratitis in the 2004 survey. However, the overall incidence of infectious keratitis increased in 2004 from 2001.

The results of these surveys and an analysis of the trends seen in the data can help to guide prophylaxis and treatment of infections keratitis following LASIK. Infectious keratitis is a potentially devastating complication of LASIK. A high degree of suspicion coupled with a rapid diagnosis and appropriate therapy can result in visual recovery. For prophylaxis against a post-LASIK infectious keratitis, there are several steps which can be implemented.

Preoperatively, all patients considering refractive surgery should have a thorough examination of their eyelids and lacrimal apparatus. Treatment of infectious lid disease prior to LASIK with hot compresses and a topical antibiotic ointment applied three times daily to the lid margin may decrease the risk of a bacterial keratitis. A small minority of clinicians recommend performing monocular surgery or the use of separate instruments when performing bilateral surgery.[11] Some clinicians recommend the use of sterile drapes, gowns, gloves and masks by the treating physician and assisting technician. A 10 percent betadine solution lid prep prior to cataract surgery has been shown to decrease the incidence of endophthalmitis following cataract surgery and is recommend by many clinicians when performing LASIK.[12] Proper sterilization techniques can prevent the use of contaminated instruments. As several epidemics of atypical mycobacteria have been associated with the use of non-sterile water to clean instruments or the use of ice during LASIK surgery, all fluids applied to the eye before, during and after LASIK should be sterile.[13]

Antibiotic prophylaxis for LASIK should emphasize the need to provide broad-based spectrum coverage with gram-positive emphasis. The antibiotic should be non-toxic to promote epithelial healing and should provide coverage against atypical mycobacteria which is the most common opportunistic organism responsible for post-LASIK infections. Finally, the antibiotic should penetrate effectively into the cornea and achieve therapeutic levels in the mid stroma. Fourth generation fluoroquinolones (gatifloxacin 0.3% and moxifloxacin 0.5%) for antibiotic prophylaxis of LASIK and PRK are recommended as they best meet the criteria listed above.[13] We begin topical therapy 1 hour prior to surgery and at the conclusion of LASIK we dehydrate the cornea for 1-2 minutes to improve flap adherence and then apply antibiotic directly on the dehydrated flap to improve antibiotic absorption into the cornea. With PRK, we place the antibiotic directly onto the stromal bed and soak the bandage contact lens in antibiotic for 30 seconds prior to placing the contact lens on the eye. Postoperatively, patients receive a fourth generation fluoroquinolone four times a day for 5 days with LASIK and for one day after the epithelial defect has closed with PRK.

We divide infectious keratitis following LASIK into rapid onset within the first-two weeks of surgery and late onset which can occur from two weeks to three months following surgery.[13] The organisms seen in early onset infectious keratitis within the first-two weeks are common bacterial pathogens such as staphylococcal and streptococcal species. Gram-negative organisms are rare. The organisms seen in late onset infectious keratitis after two weeks are usually opportunistic such as fungi, *Nocardia* and atypical mycobacteria. The published literature review of LASIK-associated infections by Chang and colleagues supports this classification of infection.[5] Based on their study, gram-positive organisms were more likely to present within 7 days of surgery ($p = 0.001$) while mycobacterial infections were more likely to present 10 or more days after surgery ($p < 0.001$).[5]

Since, the organisms are responsible for infectious keratitis following LASIK often will not respond to empiric therapy, as with the results from the previous survey, we recommend lifting the flap, scraping, and culturing all suspicious cases, and selecting appropriate culture media including blood agar, chocolate agar, Sabouraud's agar and thioglycolate broth.[13] For infectious keratitis after two weeks, we recommend a growth media for atypical mycobacteria such as Lowenstein-Jensen or Middlebrook 7H-9 media in addition to the previous culture media. If these special media are unavailable, we recommend using blood agar as atypical mycobacteria grow quite well on these plates. At the time of culture, we also recommend scraping the infiltrate and performing a Gram stain, Gomori-methenamine silver stain, and Ziehl-Neelsen stain to rule out unusual pathogens such as *Nocardia*, atypical mycobacteria, and fungi. In cases, in which cultures are negative and the infection continues to a corneal biopsy or PCR should be considered.

For the treatment of both rapid-onset and delayed-onset infectious keratitis, it is recommended to elevate the flap and culture. Irrigation of the flap interface with an appropriate antibiotic solution (fortified vancomycin 50 mg/ml for rapid-onset keratitis and fortified amikacin 20 mg/ml for delayed-onset keratitis) may be helpful. For rapid-onset keratitis, we recommend a fourth generation topical fluoroquinolone such as gatifloxacin 0.3 percent or moxifloxacin 0.5 percent be given in a loading dose every 5 minutes for 3 doses and then every 30 minutes alternating with an antimicrobial which is rapidly bacteriocidal and has increased activity against gram-positive organisms, such as cefazolin 50 mg/ml every 30 minutes.[13] In patients who work in a hospital environment or have been exposed to a hospital surgical setting or healthcare environment, there is an added risk of methicillin-resistant *Staphylococcus aureus* (Solomon R, Donnenfeld E, Perry H, et al. Methicillin Resistant *Staphylococcus aureus* Infectious Keratitis Following Refractive Surgery. Presented as a paper at the American Society of Cataract and Refractive Surgery Symposium on Cataract, IOL, and Refractive Surgery, San Diego, Calif, 2004). In those patients, who work in a hospital environment or have had exposure to a healthcare environment, we recommend the substitution of vancomycin 50 mg/ml every 30 minutes instead of cefazolin to provide more effective therapy against MRSA. In addition, we advocate the use of oral doxycycline 100 mg twice daily (to inhibit collagenase production) and also recommend discontinuing corticosteroids.

For delayed-onset keratitis, which is commonly due to atypical mycobacteria, *Nocardia* and fungi, we recommend beginning therapy with amikacin 35 mg/ml every 30 minutes alternating with vancomycin 50 mg/ml every 30 minutes, starting oral doxycycline 100 mg BID, and discontinuing corticosteroids. Alternative therapy for delayed-onset keratitis, which would cover atypical *Mycobacteria*, includes clarithromycin and fourth generation fluoroquinolones. This treatment will not cover fungal infections, and therefore, treatment for all cases of infectious keratitis should be modified based on culture and scraping results and response to therapy.

Infectious keratitis after LASIK frequently presents with inflammation in the corneal interface, which can mimic diffuse lamellar keratitis (DLK). DLK usually occurs within the first few days following LASIK, unless there is postoperative ocular trauma.[14] The appearance of an interface inflammation more than one week following LASIK should be presumed to be infectious unless proven otherwise. Since DLK usually presents with a diffuse appearance while infectious keratitis has focal area of infiltration, any focal infiltrate surrounded by inflammation following LASIK should be considered infectious until proven otherwise.

In conclusion, infectious keratitis is a potentially devastating complication following LASIK. Culture results reveal gram-positive bacteria as the most common organisms. Infectious keratitis may present as late as months following LASIK, and its frequent misdiagnosis at initial presentation may result in significant vision loss. Antibiotic prophylaxis for LASIK should emphasize the need to provide broad-based spectrum coverage with gram-positive emphasis. For treatment, we do not recommend empiric therapy as most organisms are opportunistic and do not respond to conventional therapy. A high degree of suspicion with flap elevation and culturing should be performed on all eyes suspected of infectious keratitis following LASIK.

REFERENCES

1. Hersh PS, Brint SF, Maloney RK, et al. Photorefractive keratectomy versus laser *in situ* keratomileusis for moderate to high myopia: a randomized prospective study. Ophthalmology 1998;105:1512-23.
2. Azar DT, Farah SG. Laser *in situ* keratomileusis versus photorefractive keratectomy: an update on indications and safety. Ophthalmology 1998;105:1357-8.
3. Garg P, Bansal AK, Sharma S, et al. Bilateral infectious keratitis after laser *in situ* keratomileusis: a case report and review of the literature. Ophthalmology 2001;108:121-5.
4. Solomon A, Karp, CL, Miller D, et al. Mycobacterium interface keratitis after laser *in situ* keratomileusis. Ophthalmology 2001;108:2201-8.
5. Perry HD, Doshi SJ, Donnenfeld ED, et al. Herpes simplex reactivation following laser *in situ* keratomileusis and subsequent corneal perforation. CLAO J 2002;28:69-71.
6. Chang MA, Jain S, Azar DT. Infections following laser *in situ* keratomileusis: an integration of the published literature. Surv Ophthalmol. 2004;49:269-80. after laser *in situ* keratomileusis. J Cataract Refract Surg 2002;28:898-9.
7. Stulting RD, Carr JD, Thompson KP, et al. Complications of laser *in situ* keratomileusis for the correction of myopia. Ophthalmology 1999;106:13-20.
8. Lin RT, Maloney RK. Flap complications associated with lamellar refractive surgery. Am J Ophthalmol 1999;127:129-36.

9. Karp CL, Tuli SS, Yoo SH, et al. Infectious keratitis after LASIK. Ophthalmology 2003;110:503-10.
10. Solomon R, Donnenfeld ED, Azar DT, Holland EJ, Palmon FR, Pflugfelder SC, Rubenstein JB. Infectious keratitis after laser *in situ* keratomileusis: results of an ASCRS survey. J Cataract Refract Surg 2003;29:2001-6.
11. Kohnen T. Infections after corneal refractive surgery: can we do better? (editorial). J Cataract Refract Surg 2002;28:569-70.
12. Speaker MG, Menikoff JA. Prophylaxis of endophthalmitis with topical povidone-iodine. Ophthalmology 1991;98:1769-75.
13. Donnenfeld ED, Kim T, Holland E, et al. Management of infectious keratitis following laser *in situ* keratomileusis. J Cataract Refract Surg 2005;31:2008-11.
14. Stulting RD, Randleman JB, Couser JM, Thompson KP. The epidemiology of diffuse lamellar keratitis. Cornea 2004;23:680-8.

Ocular Pharmacotherapeutics in Corneal Refractive Surgery

Ashok Garg (India)

Every since Theo Seiler in 1987 and Marguerite McDonald in 1988 did the first corneal ablation in normal sighted eye, Excimer Laser Refractive Surgery has produced revolutionary changes in the field of ophthalmology. Refractive Surgery is certainly a high tech advancement in the field of ophthalmic surgery of the last decade of this millenium which has come as a great boon to spectacle weary patients all around the world.

Laser assisted *in situ* keratomileusis (LASIK) and Laser assisted subepithelial keratectomy (LASEK) offer a unique opportunity to provide ametropia to patients with refractive error ranging from -20.00 D of myopia to +8.00 D of hyperopia. The rapid visual recovery and decreased incidence of complications associated with LASIK and LASEK make them far superior to both excimer photoablation (PRK) and automated Lamellar Keratoplasty (ALK).

LASIK and LASEK provide an extra-ordinary accurate method of tissue removal (0.20-0.25 um tissue per pulse). The extreme pain, haze, regression and slow visual rehabilitation of PRK are absent thus the minimum use of postprocedure medications especially topical steroids and its potential adverse effects.

Although preprocedure medications are same in LASIK and LASEK as those in PRK surgery while postprocedure medications are drasticaly reduced in LASIK and LASEK surgery leading to quick visual rehabilitation of patient postoperatively.

Development of automated microkeratome Hansatome and Laser Microkeatome has make LASIK and LASEK surgery more safe even in the hand of novice Refractive Surgeon. Indeed the LASIK and LASEK surgery have come of age.

Here, now I shall discuss the ocular therapeutics used in LASIK and LASEK surgery before and after the procedure.

PREPROCEDURE THERAPEUTIC MEDICATIONS

Preoperatively patient is given broad range topical antibiotic eye drops (Preferably Gatifloxacin (0.3%) or Moxifloxacin (0.5%) at 4 hourly interval starting 24 hours prior to surgery.

A mild oral sedation (diazepam 3-10 mg) is given in all cases. Bilateral simultaneous surgery is done in all cases.

Topical Anesthesia

For LASIK/LASEK Surgery, refractive surgeon prefer to give topical anesthesia because of rapid onset of action and lesser irritation to the patient.

Two to five minutes prior to the surgery, any of the following topical anesthetic agent can be safely used.
- Proparacaine HCl - 0.5 percent
- Benoxinate HCl - 0.4 percent
- Tetracaine HCl - 0.5 percent

Proparacaine is most commonly used anesthetic agent followed by Benoxinate and tetracaine. Other topical agent like Xylocaine (4%) is less commonly used due to problems of irritation, allergy, etc.

Proparacaine, benoxinate and tetracaine have rapid onset of action and cause little tingling sensation and irritation to the patient.

Onset of anesthetic action starts with in 15-20 seconds with these agents and effects last for 15-20 minutes sufficient for the completion of LASIK/LASEK Surgery. Proparacaine or Benoxinate are given topically in the dosage of 2 drops in each eye 2-3 times repeated at the interval of one minute.

After topical anesthesia some refractive surgeon prefer to instill Pilocarpine 1 percent in the eye to aid in marking the optical axis.

Pachymetry is performed and patients is carefully centered and eyelids are cleaned with betadine solution (Iodine solution) and operative eye is given a sterile plastic ophthalmic drape to cover the eyelid margins and the cilia.

POSTPROCEDURE THERAPEUTIC MEDICATIONS

The biggest advantage of LASIK and LASEK over PRK is the minimum use of ocular therapeutic in postoperative phase. The visual recovery in LASIK and LASEK is virtually immediate owing to the preservation of the epithelium of the cornea. Typically recovery is painless and postprocedure refractions and vision are remarkably stable during the postoperative period. Postprocedure medications are quite significant for early visual rehabilitation and recovery of the patient. During the initial active postoperative phase. Refractive Surgeons prefer to give:

a. Oral antibiotic (Gatifloxacin 400 mg OD or Levofloxacin 500 mg OD for 5 days).
b. Topical Fluorometholone (FML, 0.1%) eye drops four times a day for two weeks.
c. Topical lubricant like Polyvinyl alcohol liquifilm tear drops four times a day for two weeks.
d. Topical antibiotic (Moxifloxacin 0.5%). QID for a week. Immediately after LASIK/LASEK procedure. Some surgeon prefer to give patch for 2-3 hours. While other view is to ask the patient to wear a clear eye shield nightly for a week.
e. Oral analgesic (Tab. Diclofenac 75 mg SR BD for three days if needed but not in routine).

Patient operated for LASIK/LASEK surgery is called for follow-up on:
- 2nd day postprocedure
- 1st week
- 2nd week
- 3rd week

One each follow-up following examination are done:
- Vision check up
- IOP with noncontact tonometer
- Slit Lamp Examination for Haze
- Topography to see corneal profile.

Corneal wound healing and its modulations after LASIK/LASEK surgery have multiple components. LASIK/LASEK is a refractive surgical procedure that is performed in several steps and each step involved a different structure of cornea.

Phases of Healing

Following LASIK/LASEK injury healing occurs in several phases. The earliest phase involves the healing of epithelial injury and is characterized by the migration of epithelium which occurs 12-24 hours after procedure 2.3 days after the insult, epithelial cell proliferation is evident. Six months after the surgical insult, the development of fibrous metaplasia is complete. Throughout these phases of healing the types of cytokine communication are operating to create an integrated repair of injured corneal areas.

Although LASIK/LASEK is safe and reliable procedure yet it is susceptible to all the complications noted in PRK procedure which includes overcorrection, undercorrection, decentration, infection, loss and displacement of flap, central islands and epithelial in growth.

Cornea healing following LASIK/LASEK should be considered as a combination of events involving the response to injury of the epithelium and stroma.

Understanding these events and the molecules that regulate the wound healing response should enable the refractive surgeon to induce fewer complications and aid in developing therapeutic modalities to alter would healing precisely.

Close follow-up and attention to postoperative medications and surface lubrication will enable the surgeon to achieve better results.

BIBLIOGRAPHY

1. Agarwal A. Textbook of ophthalmology, 1st edn. New Delhi: Jaypee Medical Publishers, 2002.
2. Bartlett JD. Clinical Ocular Pharmacology, 4th edn. Boston: Butterworth-Heinemann, 2001
3. Bartlett JD. Ophthalmic Drug facts: Lippincott – William and Wilkins, 2001.
4. Crick RP, Trimble RB. Textbook of clinical ophthalmology: Hodder and Stoughton, 1986.

5. Duane TD. Clinical ophthalmology, 4th edn. Butterworth–Heinemann, 1999.
6. Duvall. Ophthalmic Medications and Pharmacology: Slack Inc, 1998.
7. Ellis PP. Ocular Therapeutics and Pharmacology, 7th edn. CV Mosby, 1985.
8. Fechner. Ocular Therapeutics: Slack Inc., 1998.
9. Fraunfelder. Current Ocular Therapy, 5th edn. WB Saunders, 2000.
10. Garg A. Current Trends in ophthalmology, 1st edn. New Delhi: Jaypee Medical Publishers, 1997.
11. Garg A. Manual of Ocular Therapeutics, 1st edn. New Delhi: Jaypee Medical Publishers, 1996.
12. Garg A. Ready Reckoner of Ocular Therapeutics, 1st edn. New Delhi: 2002.
13. Goodman LS, Gilman A. Pharmacological basis of Therapeutics, 7th edn. New York: Macmillan, 1985.
14. Havener's. Ocular Pharmacology, 6th edn. CV Mosby, 1994.
15. Kanski. Clinical ophthalmology, 4th edn. Butterworth–Heineman, 1999.
16. Kershner. Ophthalmic Medications and Pharmacology: Slack. Inc., 1994.
17. Olin BR, et al. Drugs Facts and Comparisons: Facts and Comparisons, St. Louis, 1997.
18. Onofrey. The Ocular Therapeutics; Lippincott-William and Wilkins, 1997.
19. Rhee. The Wills Eye drug Guide: Lippincott – William and Wilkins, 1998.
20. Steven Podos. Textbook of ophthalmology, New Delhi: Jaypee Medical Publishers, 2001.
21. Zimmerman. Textbook of Ocular Pharmacology: Lippincott and William and Wilkins, 1997.

Antioxidants and Their Role in Ophthalmology

CS Dhull, Sumit Sachdeva, Manisha Rathi, Ashuma Sachdeva (India)

A lot of interest today is generated on the use and efficacy of antioxidants. Their use and misuse is a topic of much debate so a proper and extensive knowledge about these substances is essential for understanding their exact role in prevention of the deleterious effects of free radicals. Antioxidants by nature are substances whose presence in relatively low concentrations significantly inhibits the rate of oxidation of cells. In other words, an antioxidant is a molecule that simply inhibits the oxidation of other molecules.

They thus protect cells from the damaging effects of oxygen radicals, which are highly reactive chemicals that have been reported to have a causative role in atherosclerosis, cancer and several other diseases including ARMD and cataract in humans. Thus, it is proposed that antioxidants have a protective effect on these conditions.

Why do We Need Antioxidants?

Free radical is an atom or molecule with an unpaired electron that is chemically reactive. These occur when an atom loses an electron due to stress, toxins or even normal metabolism. This makes the atom unstable and it races around the body looking for the electron it is missing. In the process, it steals electrons from other atoms, which causes a chain reaction that injures and deforms the body's cells and ultimately causes their death. Over time, this results in symptoms such as decreased energy, a weaker immune system, memory loss, heart problems and, ultimately, a shorter life. Free radicals are believed to be involved in all chronic disorders of aging, such as age-related macular degeneration (ARMD) in the eye, cataracts, etc. There are reports to suggest that they are even responsible for Alzheimer's disease and cancer. Examples of free radicals are superoxide anion O_2, hydrogenperoxide H_2O_2 and hydroxyl radical OH. Antioxidants act by neutralizing free radicals (by donating them the missing electrons) (Fig. 32.1) and thus help remove them by converting them into less damaging and less reactive molecules.

A change in lifestyle has led to more free radicals in our daily lives, for example pollutants such as cigarette smoke and smog, smoke from automobiles and factories and last but not least junk food, which also reduces the dietary intake of natural antioxidants.

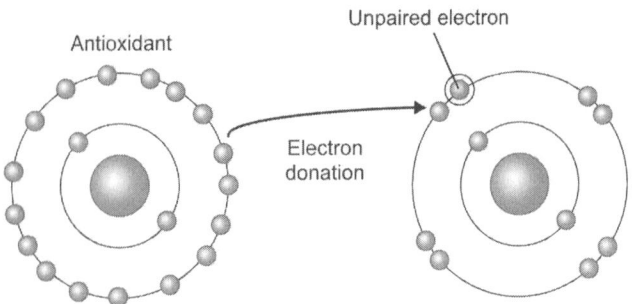

Fig. 32.1: Antioxidant action by reducing unpaired electrons

Although oxidation reactions are crucial for life, they can also be damaging. Plants and animals maintain complex systems of multiple types of antioxidants, such as glutathione, vitamin C, and vitamin E as well as enzymes such as catalase, superoxide dismutase and various peroxidases.

Antioxidants terminate chain reactions by removing free radical intermediates, and inhibit oxidation reactions. They do this by being oxidized themselves, so antioxidants are often reducing agents such as thiols, ascorbic acid, or polyphenols. Insufficient levels of antioxidants, or inhibition of the antioxidant enzymes, cause oxidative stress and may damage or kill cells.

As oxidative stress appears to be an important part of many human diseases, the use of antioxidants in pharmacology is intensively studied, particularly as treatments for stroke and neurodegenerative diseases. Moreover, oxidative stress is both the cause and the consequence of disease.

Antioxidants are widely used in dietary supplements and have been investigated for the prevention of diseases such as cancer, coronary heart disease, ARMD, cataract and even altitude sickness.

Supplemental neutraceutical antioxidants, a term used for therapeutic doses of nutrients with antioxidant properties, are used for prevention and treatment of deficiency of antioxidants. Their use is now a part of clinical practice. Studies have shown that, with rare exceptions, vitamins and minerals in the correct dosage are safe.

Specifically for the eye, lutein, zeaxanthin and astaxanthin have a vital role, as these carotenoids are essential for the eye to be well protected from developing macular degeneration and cataract. Lycopene is a carotenoid which has a special place in eye defense since it neutralizes singlet oxygen—a reactive oxygen species which causes damage particularly in the eye.

Initially, there was a lot of controversy regarding the protective effect of antioxidants for both systemic and ocular use. But in recent past, several clinical trials have suggested that their role is beneficial.

Why Does the Eye Need Antioxidants?

The eye is an organ that is relatively more exposed to the environment. The eye is affected by oxidative stress due to its physical and metabolic characteristics. All ocular tissues and fluids are susceptible to damage by oxidative stress.

Nowadays, there are more patients seeking treatment for eye diseases. The main causes of this increase can be attributed to xenobiotics caused by environmental pollution and increasing ultraviolet radiation intensity. There is a change in lifestyle with an altered dietary intake with a reduced amount of natural antioxidants due to an increase in fast food with more fats and carbohydrates, which is made worse by physical inactivity. There is an increasing number of patients with degenerative diseases such as diabetes, ARMD and cardiovascular problems.

All the above factors can generate harmful chemicals to ocular tissues called oxidant agents or free radicals. To protect against external agents, the eye has several nonspecific defense mechanisms, such as eyelids, tear film, cornea, and lens. When harmful agents overcome these barriers, the natural antioxidants in the body try to come to the rescue. It is when these antioxidants are overwhelmed, that the disease process begins to accelerate.

Macular Degeneration and Cataracts-Leading Cause of Blindness

Blindness is an increasing problem worldwide.

Age-related macular degeneration is the leading cause of blindness for people over the age of 50.
- Sixty million people suffer from ARMD worldwide, and 10 million are blind.
- Severe, irreversible vision loss affects 30 percent of people over the age of 55.
- Cataracts are another major cause of blindness, caused by lipid peroxidation of the epithelial layer of the lens. The commonest type is related to aging.

Clinical studies tell us that photic injury from the cumulative effect of repeated "photic insults" leading to a gradual loss of photoreceptors is a major cause of ARMD and antioxidants are postulated to help by reducing this damage.

CLASSIFICATION OF ANTIOXIDANTS

Preventive Antioxidants (Majority are Endogenous, Produced in the Body)

- Superoxide dismutase
- Catalase
- Glutathione peroxidase
- Ceruloplasmin
- Transferrin
- Albumin

Chain-breaking Antioxidants

Water-soluble

- Uric acid
- Ascorbate
- Thiols
- Bilirubin
- Flavanoids

Fat-soluble

- Tocopherols
- Ubiquinol-10
- Beta-carotene
- Estrogens

The most important antioxidants are the following:

Antioxidant vitamins
- Carotenoids
- Vitamin E
- Vitamin C

Antioxidant minerals
- Selenium
- Zinc
- Manganese
- Copper

Bioflavonoids and flavonoids.

Carotenoids

Carotenoids are the compounds that give fruits, vegetables and flowers their various colors. Almost all living things obtain their colors from these natural pigments, which carry out several vital biological functions. They are critical to the photosynthetic process and protect the plant or organism from damage by light and oxygen. Many animals incorporate carotenoids into their diets, which provide them with antioxidants and a source of vitamin A activity.

There are more than 600 naturally occurring carotenoids, but humans only consume about 20.

Carotenoids are classified into two groups:
1. Carotenes, which contain no oxygen atoms: lycopene (the red in tomatoes), alpha-carotene and beta-carotene (the orange in carrots) are examples.
2. Xanthophylls, which contain oxygen atoms: lutein, canthaxanthin, zeaxanthin, and astaxanthin are examples.

Carotenoids of human importance are: Lutein, zeaxanthin, lycopene, alpha carotene, beta-cryptoxanthin and astaxanthin.

The retina and choroids additionally contain lycopene, alpha- and beta-carotene. In the ciliary body, all the carotenoids taken in

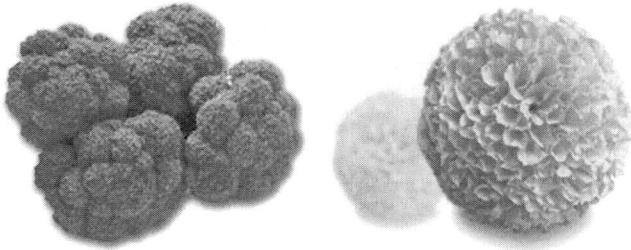

Fig. 32.2: Broccoli and marigold are considered to be two of the richest sources lutein and zeaxanthin

foodstuff or as dietary supplement get accumulated. The carotenes are obtained from tuberous vegetables, such as carrots, sweet potatoes, and yams.

The xanthophylls—lutein and its isomer zeaxanthin—are two to four times more common than are beta-carotene in foods. As far as the eye is concerned, *Lutein* and *zeaxanthin* are exclusively concentrated in the macula, lens and iris. Zeaxanthin is the most common carotenoid found in nature (peppers, marigold, maize, kiwi, grapes, oranges and squash) (Fig. 32.2). They are abundant in green leafy vegetables, such as spinach, kale, parsley, and collard greens. Lutein has been shown to an important anti-oxidant through powerful inhibition of lipid peroxidation and its chemical oxidation by free radicals. Human metabolism appears to convert lutein to the proper amount of zeaxanthin.

The xanthophylls were shown in studies performed in the 1940s and 1950s to improve night vision and adaptation to dusk. Lutein and zeaxanthin now are known to be present in the lens of the eye and have a role in cataract prevention.

Astaxanthin is the most commonly occurring red carotenoid in marine and aquatic animals, especially salmon which get it from their diets, which include zooplankton and krill. Astaxanthin is by far the most powerful carotenoid antioxidant when it comes to free radical scavenging: it is 65 times more powerful than vitamin C, 54 times more powerful than beta-carotene, and 14 times more powerful than vitamin E. It crosses the blood-brain barrier and the blood-retinal barrier, which is an advantage in protecting the eye. It is soluble in lipids, so it incorporates into cell membranes. It is a potent UVB absorber, reduces DNA damage, is a powerful natural anti-inflammatory agent.

Carotenoids are reported to protect against:
- ARMD
- Diabetic neuropathy
- CME
- Central retinal vein occlusion (CRVO)
- Glaucoma
- Inflammatory eye diseases.

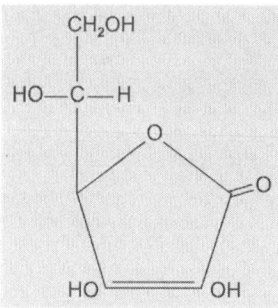

Fig. 32.3: Ascorbic acid

Ascorbic Acid

Ascorbic acid (vitamin C) is the major water-soluble extracellular antioxidant that humans are unable to synthesize (Fig. 32.3). It is an ideal scavenger due to its water solubility, stability, and mobility and the fact that it can be transported, reabsorbed, and recycled. Compared to plasma, it is highly concentrated in all ocular tissues in diurnal animals. There is evidence to show that it prevents cataract. Most fruits and vegetables are excellent sources of vitamin C, including oranges, grapefruit, strawberries and papaya, as well as green peppers and tomatoes.

Tocopherols and Tocotrienol Isomers

D-alpha-tocopherol is a lipid-soluble, membrane-bound antioxidant. Vitamin E provides protection against lipid peroxidation chain reactions in biological membranes. Randomized, controlled, masked studies indicate a beneficial effect in immunity, cardiovascular disease, diabetes, cancer, and Alzheimer's disease. Several studies suggest it to be protective in ARMD. Vitamin E and lutein appear to be major players in prevention and treatment of atrophic ARMD.

Vitamin E is more difficult to obtain from food sources alone since it is found in very small quantities in foods, such as vegetable oils, nuts and seeds. Good food sources include vegetable oils (including safflower and corn oil), almonds, pecans, wheat germ and sunflower seeds.

Zinc, Manganese and Copper

Zinc (Zn), manganese (Mn) and copper (Cu) are constituents of superoxide dismutase (SOD) antioxidant enzyme. The SOD is widely distributed in tissues as well as fluid compartments. The SOD attacks free radicals like hydroxyl radical to convert these into hydrogen peroxide.

Zn serves an important structural role, whilst Cu is necessary for functioning of another antioxidant called catalase. In the retina, SOD plays an important role to prevent the oxidative damage which plays a role in the prevention of ARMD. Catalases have been shown to protect the lens.

Selenium

Selenium (Se) is the most important indictator of glutathione peroxidase activity. Glutathione peroxidase is concentrated in various tissues, besides blood and synovial fluid. Like catalases, glutathione peroxidase breaks down hydrogen peroxide, besides reducing lipid peroxidation like vitamin E and beta-carotene.

Glutathione peroxidase and related enzymes, along with N-acetylcysteine, L-glycine, and glutamine and selenium are protective against damage to human RPE cells. Glutathione peroxidase prevents apoptosis (cell suicide) and helps prevent or treat ARMD.

Bioflavonoids

An important class of antioxidants is known as bioflavonoids. They are oligomeric proanthocynaidins, reported to be 20 and 50 times more potent than vitamin C and vitamin E respectively. They can cross the blood-brain barrier and detoxify and replenish the antioxidant effect of the ocular fluids, which help protect the eye against UV rays. They are large polyphenolic molecules derived from the peel and coverings of teas, grapes, bark, red wine, some white wines, pine bark, peanut skin and berries. They have extensive anti-inflammatory, antibacterial, and antiviral properties and potent iron-binding and antioxidant properties. They include, for example, red wine, quercitin, and pycnogenol. Green tea polyphenols (catechins) are very potent antioxidants. Bilberry has been suggested and investigated for treatment of diabetic retinopathy and night-vision abnormalities. Ginkgo biloba has been found to afford retina protection against light-induced damage and to benefit low-tension glaucoma.

Flavonoids

They have also been referred to as 'super antioxidants' due to antiviral, antiallergic, anti-inflammatory, antithrombogenic and anticarcinogenic effects (Fig. 32.4). They get rid of free radicals associated with oxygen and iron, and inhibit oxidative enzymes. They fall into four different groups which are flavones, flavanones, catechins and anthocyanins.

They are found in fruits, flowers, roots, stems, tea, wine, grains and vegetables.

Age-related Macular Degeneration

It is a complex disorder involving several factors including genetic, cardiovascular and environmental factors. It is related to exposure to long-term blue light, and nutrition. Studies indicate lutein, astaxanthin and vitamin E have a protective effect against it. The retina is fast-metabolizing. Polyunsaturated oxidation-prone

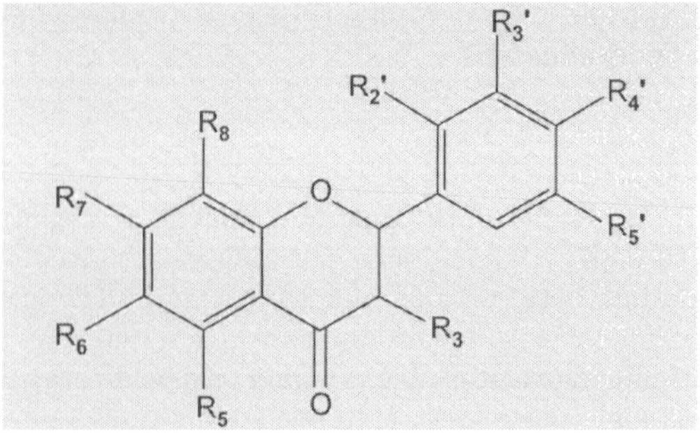

Fig. 32.4: Molecular structure of flavonoid

photoreceptor outer segments are exposed to ultraviolet photons in youth and blue visible radiation in older age. The layer of retinal pigment epithelium (RPE) cells contains a number of protective antioxidants. Melanin absorbs and dissipates radiation but decreases with age and is reduced in blue-eyed individuals.

It is seen that lutein has specific protective role in macular degeneration. In addition to antioxidant protection and blue radiation-filtering properties, retinal lutein provides biophysical structural support for the vulnerable cells. Finally, recent work by Hammond and coworker has demonstrated preservation into the seventh decade of life of visual function in patients who maintain macular pigment density.

Vitamin E increases in the retina to age 50 and then declines. Decreased xanthophyll pigment consumption (i.e. lutein), Vitamin E, and other supporting cofactor minerals and vitamins are believed to be responsible for the etiopathogenesis of ARMD. Other theories include impairment of choroidal circulation and degradation (calcification) of Bruch's membrane. These theories are ultimately related to nutritional factors.

Results from the age-related eye disease study (AREDS) showed that high levels of antioxidants and zinc significantly reduce the risk of advanced AMD and its associated vision loss. The specific daily amounts of antioxidants and zinc used by the study researchers were:
- 500 milligrams of vitamin C
- 400 International Units of vitamin E
- 15 milligrams of beta-carotene (often labeled as equivalent to 25,000 International Units of vitamin A)
- 80 milligrams of zinc as zinc oxide
- Two milligrams of copper as cupric oxide (Copper was added to the AREDS formulations containing zinc to prevent copper deficiency anemia, a condition associated with high levels of zinc intake).

Diabetic Retinopathy

Diabetic retinopathy is the major cause of blindness in adults in developed nations. The retina is highly susceptible to oxidative stress because of intense exposure to light and oxygen and its high polyunsaturated fatty acid (PUFA) content that is prone to lipid peroxidation, along with its high metabolic rate. There has been a lot of interest in oxidative stress and its potential roles in diabetogenesis and development of diabetic complications. Oxidative stress has been widely regarded as the key factor for the emergence of ocular disease as it causes increased vascular permeability, disruption of blood-retinal barrier, apoptotic loss of retinal capillary cells, microvascular abnormalities and retinal neovascularization. The oxidative stress appears to be caused by an imbalance between the increased production of reactive oxygen species and the sharp reduction in antioxidant defenses.

Dietary supplementation with antioxidants has been related with inhibition of reduction of apoptosis and partial restoration of pericytes. Administration of antioxidants to diabetic rats is reported to prevent the development of retinopathy. High doses of vitamin E, the major antioxidant in lipid phase were studied and found to restore retinal blood flow in diabetic type I patients to control levels. Superoxide production in the retina in rats was suppressed by a combination of vitamins C and E and reduction in neovascularization of the retina. Trolox is a water-soluble analog of vitamin E with potent antioxidant properties, which was shown to partially prevent the loss of pericytes in diabetic rats. Studies in humans suggested that antioxidant therapy with vitamin E might normalize diabetic retinal hemodynamics.

Green tea supplementation in diabetic rats reduced retinopathy signs as evident by reductions in acellular capillaries and pericyte ghosts . Evidences suggest that green tea significantly inhibited diabetic cataracts in streptozotocin-induced rat model of diabetes. This provides encouraging rationale for its possible therapeutic use to inhibit retinopathy in diabetic patients. Thus, supplementation with antioxidants represents an achievable adjunct therapy to help preserve vision in diabetic patients.

Cataract Prevention

There are several reports available, some of which do and some do not support the supplementation with antioxidants to prevent cataract. On a study carried out in an Indian population, supplementation with β carotene, vitamins C and E did not affect cataract progression in a population with a high prevalence of cataract whose diet was deficient in antioxidants. The AREDS study also did not find any beneficial effect of the antioxidants (that were used for ARMD) on cataract progression.

However, in another study, on lutein and zeaxanthin in women, it was found that those who ate almost 7 mg of lutein and zeaxanthin per day were 18 percent less likely to develop cataracts than those who ate only about 1 mg per day. Researchers believe that this pair of antioxidants may help build and maintain the pigment layer of the retina. Another theory is that they help filter out blue light, protecting the eye from sunlight damage. The same investigators who reported this looked at the effect of vitamins E and C and found that women who consumed the most vitamin E from food and supplements, about 262 mg a day were 14 percent less likely to develop cataracts than those who consumed only 4 mg a day. Several other studies have found similar results. Several other epidemiological studies have found a lower risk of cataracts or cataract progression in those who took high levels of vitamin C.

In another study, people with the highest blood concentrations if either beta- or alpha-carotene, lutein and lycopene were less likely to develop cataracts.

CONCLUSION

There is a lot of evidence which supports significant beneficial effects of nutritional supplementation for most degenerative conditions, especially ocular conditions.

Age-related degenerative diseases, including cataract and macular degeneration, appear to be the result of oxidative stress. As we grow older, natural inborn endogenous gene-derived enzymatic protective systems become less functional along with a decrease in the quality of nutrition. This appears to lead to a slow progressive increase in degenerative disease. Basic research studies suggest that antioxidants can protect against the effects of oxidative stress and onset and progression of these diseases. Taking supplements, specifically containing zeaxanthin, lutein and lycopene in adequate doses, is postulated to provide protection to macula and lens.

Prevention and early intervention are essential, as the damage is largely irreversible. Once diagnosed, it is important to slow further progression at any stage of development. Protection of lens and macula from the ultraviolet rays and hazard of smoking, however, along with a healthy diet and lifestyle such as avoiding smoking and inactivity must be emphasized.

SUMMARY

- The first-step is educating the public to eat a healthy diet of fresh fruits, vegetables and nuts. Eat a rainbow of all colors of food
- Stop or at least limit eating fast/ junk food
- Stop smoking
- Alcohol in moderation, preferably only red wine
- Avoid exposure to direct sunlight
- Avoid exposure to environmental pollutants
- Exercise on a daily basis
- Get annual medical baseline check-ups
- If required, supplementation of diet with antioxidants may be prescribed and monitored
- The dosage of antioxidants should be correct.

If we follow the above said rules there is a high chance that we would be protected from the harmful effects of the dreaded free radicals.

BIBLIOGRAPHY

1. Delori F, Goger D, Hammond B. Foveal lipofuscin and macular pigment. Schepens Eye Research Institute and Harvard Medical School. Poster presented at the ARVO meeting, Sarasota, FL, 1997.
2. Eye Disease Case Control Study Group. Antioxidant status and neovascular age-related macular degeneration. Arch Ophthalmol 1993;111:104-19.
3. Eye Disease Case Control Study Group. Risk factors for age related macular degeneration. Arch Ophthalmol 1992;110:1701-18.
4. Hammond B, Johnson E, Russel R, et al. Dietary modification of macular pigment density. Invest Ophthalmol 1997;38(9):1795-1801.
5. Hammond BR, Wooten BR, Snodderly DM. Preservation of visual sensitivity of older subjects: association with macular pigment density. Invest Ophthalmol Vis Sci 1998;39:397-406.
6. http://bjo.bmj.com/content/90/7/847.full.
7. http://development.aao.org/eyecare/treatment/alternative-therapies/antioxidant-cataract-prevention.cfm.
8. http://informahealthcare.com/doi/abs/10.1517/13543784.10.9.1665.
9. http://www.aoa.org/x4729.xml.
10. http://www.articlesbase.com/nutrition-articles/role-of-antioxidants-in-ophthalmology-5183922.html.
11. http://www.molvis.org/molvis/v16/a16/mv-v16-a16-izuta.pdf.
12. http://www.naturaleyecare.com/study.asp?s_num=177.
13. http://www.ncbi.nlm.nih.gov/pmc/articles/PMC3140028.
14. http://www.ncbi.nlm.nih.gov/pubmed/22065212.
15. http://www.omicsonline.org/2155-6156/2155-6156-1-111.php.
16. http://www.scribd.com/doc/50013836/6/Classification-of-Antioxidants.
17. http://www.slideshare.net/pharmastuffblogspotcom/role-of-antioxidants-in-diabetes.
18. Jakus V. The role of free radicals, oxidative stress and antioxidant systems in diabetic vascular disease. Bratisl Lek Listy 2000;101: 541-51.
19. Kuijk FV, Siems W, Sommerburg O. Carotenoid localization in human eye tissues. Poster presented at the ARVO meeting, Ft Lauderdale, FL, 1998.
20. Landrum J, Bone R, Joa H, et al. A one year study of the macular pigment: the effect of 140 days of a lutein supplement. Exp Eye Res 1997;65:57-62.
21. Meyers D, Maloley P, Weeks D. Safety of antioxidant vitamins. Arch Intern Med 1996;156:925-35.
22. Mustata GT, Rosca M, Biemel KM, Reihl O, Smith MA, et al. Paradoxical effects of green tea (Camellia sinensis) and antioxidant vitamins in diabetic rats: improved retinopathy and renal mitochondrial defects but deterioration of collagen matrix glycoxidation and cross-linking. Diabetes 2005;54: 517-26.
23. Peluffo F. Efficacia clinica degli oligomeri di antocianosidi di vitis vinifera sui disturbi visivi del paziente anziano. Int J Toxocol Pharmacol Ther 1988;9:173-91.
24. Polak M, Zagorski Z. Lipid peroxidation in diabetic retinopathy. Ann Univ Mariae Curie Sklodowska [Med] 2004; 59:434-7.[PMID: 16146026].

25. Richer S. Part I: A protocol for the evaluation and treatment of atrophic age-related macular degeneration. J Am Optom Assoc 1999;70(1):13-23.
26. Richer S. Part II: ARMD-Pilot (case series) environmental intervention data. J Am Optom Assoc 1999;70(1):24-36.
27. Sabu MC, Smitha K, Kuttan R. Anti-diabetic activity of green tea polyphenols and their role in reducing oxidative stress in experimental diabetes. J Ethnopharmacol 2002;83:109-116.
28. Sbrozzi F, Landini J, Zago M. Il comportamento della visione notturna dopo tratta- mento con antocianosidi. Farmacol Clini Minerva Oftalmol 1982;24:189-93.
29. Scharrer A, Ober M. Anthocyanoside in der behandlung von retinopathien. Klin Mbl Augenheilk 1981;178:386-9.
30. Seddon J, Ajani U, Sperduto R, et al. Dietary carotenoids, vitamins A, C, and E, and advanced age-related macular degeneration. JAMA 1994;272(18):1413-20.
31. Snodderly DM, Hammond B. *In vivo* pyschophysical assessment of nutritional and environmental influences on human ocular tissues: lens and macular pigment. In: Taylor A (ed). Nutritional and environmental influences on the eye. Boca Raton, FL: CRC Press, 1999:251-73.
32. Snodderly DM. Evidence for protection against age-related macular degeneration by carotenoids and antioxidant vitamins. Am J Clin Nutr 1995;62(suppl):1448s-1461s.
33. Taylor A, Jacques P, Dorey C. Oxidation and aging: impact on vision. J Toxicol Ind Health 1993;9:349-71.
34. Taylor A. Nutritional and environmental influences on risk for cataract. In: Taylor A (Ed). Nutritional and environmental influences in the eye. Boca Raton, FL: CRC Press.
35. Varma SD. Ascorbic acid and the eye with special reference to the lens. Ann NY Acad Sci 1987.pp.280-300.

33

Tetracyclins for Ocular Surface Diseases

Robert Latkany (USA)

The signs and symptoms of ocular rosacea, blepharitis, meibomian gland dysfunction, trachoma, recurrent corneal erosions, phlyctenular keratoconjunctivitis and ulcerative corneal thinning may all benefit from the use of an antibiotic from the tetracycline family (Fig. 33.1). The most common include tetracycline, doxycycline, and minocycline. Their benefit lies not so much in their ability to destroy bacteria but rather a plethora of mechanisms that prevent the degradation of the ocular surface.

For instance, tetracyclines block the production of matrix metalloproteinases (MMP-9), which are capable of destroying extracellular matrix proteins like collagen.[1] Its anticollagenase activity may ultimately prove to be the reason why tetracyclines prevent further tissue degradation in corneal ulcers. This same action may also explain why the use of doxycycline has proven useful in the treatment and resolution of previously unresolved recurrent corneal erosions for up to 22 months.[2] Tetracyclines also block the production of lipases by Staphylococci and alter the quality of meibum or meibomian gland secretions.[4] The enhanced functional quality of the meibum resulting from the reduction in free fatty acids and diglycerides remained 3 months after stopping a course of minocycline therapy.[4] Prolonged benefit may prove to be very useful as ongoing therapy may not be necessary and thereby limits potential side effects. The tetracycline family also works through immunomodulation[5] and by altering the ocular flora.[6] However, 3 months after stopping treatment the ocular lid flora returned almost back to baseline pretreatment levels.[6] More research is needed to determine which has greater therapeutic value, altering the quality of the meibum or reducing the ocular

> Ocular Rosacea
> Blepharitis
> Meibomian Gland Disease
> Trachoma
> Recurrent Corneal Erosions
> Phlyctenular Keratoconjunctivitis
> Corneal Ulcers
> Dry Eyes

Fig. 33.1: Diseases that can improve with tetracycline use

lid flora. Despite the obvious therapeutic value, the question still remains how often and how long should a patient be prescribed a tetracycline?

There are a wide range of suggested dosages including doxycycline 100 mg twice daily for up to 3 weeks then tapering down to 25 mg or 50 mg daily based on the therapeutic response[7] while others have had success with initial dosages of only 100 mg daily.[8] The recommended dosage of minocycline is 50 mg daily for two weeks and then increasing the dosage to 100 mg daily for up to three months.[6] The author prefers doxycycline 100 mg twice daily for three weeks and upon re-examination for therapeutic assessment will either stop treatment all together if there was no obvious improvement of clinical signs or symptoms or taper immediately down to 25 mg per day if there was an appreciable improvement for an additional month. Patients need to be made aware that dairy products can limit the absorption of tetracyclines. Tetracycline concerns, however, do not end there.

There are several side effects that warrant careful consideration as to when a patient should receive an antibiotic from the tetracycline family. Most notably, a recent article showed an increased likelihood of breast cancer with an increased number of days on systemic antibiotics.[9] Of equal importance, minocycline may induce autoimmune syndromes.[10] Other often reported side effects include scleral pigmentation and tooth discoloration.[11-13] Gastrointestinal side effects were noted in 12.5 percent of patients treated with 100 mg of doxycycline daily and 37.5 percent of patients treated with 1 gram of tetracycline daily.[14] So, it is recommended to use doxycycline in patients with sensitive gastrointestinal issues.

The true anti-inflammatory benefit of the tetracycline family will need to be clarified with future studies. Conflicting studies only shed light on the fact that we are in the very early stages of understanding the exact mechanisms of action. In some areas, where one could imagine a noticeable benefit with the use of tetracylcines none was found. Tetracycline did not show any reduction in corneal haze post photorefractive keratectomy in a study involving 30 rabbits.[15] However, other areas show more promise such as chemical injuries where tetracyclines may inhibit the collagenolytic degradation of the cornea stroma.[16] The coverage can extend even further to involve all patients with dry eye disease secondary to meibomian gland disease and/or blepharitis as one study involving 39 ocular rosacea patients showed a significant improvement in tear break-up time from 5.7 seconds to 10.8 seconds after receiving 100 mg of doxycycline for 12 weeks.[8] These types of evaluations are necessary because we cannot rely on patients symptoms alone to judge efficacy because it is well known that signs do not often correlate with symptoms in ocular surface disease.

Even a lose dose of 20 mg of doxycycline twice a day proved effective in a study involving 300 eyes of patients with chronic meibomian gland dysfunction in improving tear break-up time, schirmer test, the number of symptoms reported and the degree of improved subjective symptoms.[17] This same study, interestingly enough, showed no statistical difference in improvement of any of the above between the groups of patients receiving the low dose of 20 mg of doxycycline twice a day and the high dose of 200 mg twice a day. So, further comparative studies are necessary to assess what is the maximum dosage required to achieve a noticeable therapeutic benefit.

Other studies only highlight the early stages of our understanding of the use of tetracyclines with ocular surface disease. Sixteen patients received short-term minocycline therapy and showed an improvement of the turbidity of the meibomian gland secretions and microbial cultures; however, surprisingly, there was a decrease in aqueous tear volume and flow with increased evaporation.[18] Also equally disturbing was an *in vitro* study that showed doxycycline induced keratocyte cell death, and detachment of epithelial cells from their basement membrane.[19] It would be interesting to know if there is a therapeutic benefit with the use of a topical tetracycline cream or drop and if it shows any ocular surface toxicity. The use of a topical tetracycline may reduce systemic side effects but possibly increase surface related toxicity. And yet another concern lies in the open chronic use of this family of antibiotics and their possibility of developing resistance. Four of ten patients tested carried tetracycline resistant strains in a study involving three months of minocycline therapy.[6]

It is certain that there is a place for the anti-inflammatory properties of tetracyclines in a number of external diseases of the eye. However, it is also clear that more work is needed to clarify the exact mechanisms of action, the most effective dosage, the route of administration, and the total duration of therapy necessary with the use of these tetracyclines.

REFERENCES

1. Sadowski T, Steinmeyer J. Effects of tetracyclines on the production of matrix metalloproteinases and plasminogen activators as well as of their natural inhibitors, tissue inhibitor of metalloproteinases-1 and plasminogen activator inhibitor-1. Inflamm Res 2001;50:175-82.
2. Dursun D, Kim MC, Solomon A, et al. Treatment of recalcitrant corneal erosions with inhibitors of matrix metalloproteinases-9, doxycycline and corticosteroids. Am J Ophthalmol 2001;132(1):8-13.
3. Dougherty JM, McCulley JP, Silvany RE, Meyer DR. The role of tetracycline in chronic blepharitis. Inhibition of lipase production in staphylococci. Invest Ophthalmol Vis Sci 1991;32:2970-5.
4. Shine We, McCulley JP, Pandya AG. Minocycline effect on meibomian gland lipids in meibomianitism patients. Exp Eye Res 2003;76(4):417-20.
5. Thong YH. Immunomodulation by antimicrobial drugs. Med Hypotheses 1982;8:361-70.
6. Ta CN, Shine WE, McCulley JP, et al. Effects of minocycline on the ocular flora of patients with acne rosacea or seborrheic blepharitis. Cornea 2003;22:545-8.
7. Alvarenga LS, Mannis MJ. Ocular Rosacea. The Ocular Surface 2005;3(1):41-58.

8. Quarterman MJ, Johnson DW, Abele DC, et al. Ocular Rosacea. Signs, symptoms, and tear studies before and after treatment with doxycycline. Arch Dermatol 1997;133:49-54.
9. Velicer CM, Heckbert SR, Lampe JW, et al. Antibiotic use in relation to the risk of breast cancer. JAMA 2004;291:827-35.
10. Elkayam O, Yaron M, Caspi D. Minocycline-induced autoimmune syndromes: an overview. Semin Arthritis Rheum 1999;28:392-7.
11. Fraunfelder FT, Randall JA. Minocycline-induced scleral pigmentation. Ophthalmology 1997;104:936-8.
12. Bradfield YS, Robertson DM, Salomao DR, et al. Minocycline-induced ocular pigmentation.
13. Morrow GL, Abbott RL. Minocycline-induced scleral, dental, and dermal pigmentation. Am J Ophthalmol 1998;125:396-7.
14. Frucht-Pery J, Sagi E, Hemo I, et al. Efficacy of doxycycline and tetracycline in ocular rosacea. Am J Ophthalmol 1993;116(1):88-92.
15. Corbett MC, O'Brart DP, Patmore AL, et al. Effect of collagenase inhibitors on corneal haze after PRK. Exp Eye Res 2001;72(3):253-9.
16. Ralph RA. Tetracyclines and the treatment of corneal stromal ulceration: a review. Cornea 2000;19(3):274-7.
17. Yoo Se, Lee DC, Chang MH. The effect of low-dose doxycycline therapy in chronic meibomian gland dysfunction. Korean J Ophthalmol 2005;19(4):258-63.
18. Aronowicz JD, Shine WE, Oral D, et al. Short-term oral minocycline treatment of meibomianitis. Br J Ophthalmol 2006;90(7):856-60.
19. Smith VA, Cook SD. Doxycycline-a role in ocular surface repair. Br J Ophthalmol 2004;88(5):619-25.

34

Clinical Applications of Antimycotic Agents in the Eye

Niranjan Nayak (India)

INTRODUCTION

Fungal infections of the eye can give rise to severe ocular morbidity, often leading to blindness, if not treated early. In many tropical countries, including India, keratitis is the most frequently encountered fungal infection.[1] However, infections of the orbit, lids, lacrimal apparatus, sclera, conjunctiva and intraocular structures due to fungi are not uncommon. Early diagnosis followed by immediate therapeutic intervention may help in preventing many vision threatening complications. Thus, informations on the choice of appropriate antifungal agents and their clinical applications certainly help the ophthalmologist in the effective management of the cases. In the present review, discussion will mainly be focused on the therapeutic modalities for the most important clinical entities like Keratomycosis, Endophthalmitis, Orbital cellulitis and Dacryocystitis.

KERATOMYCOSIS

Keratomycosis or fungal infection of the cornea was described for the first time by Leber[2] in Germany in the year 1879. Since then it has been recognized as a major public health problem in the tropical parts of many developing countries.[3-5] Corneal infection of fungal etiology may represent 40–50 percent of all cases of culture proven infectious keratitis.[3,6] If not treated early, this condition may lead to corneal blindness.

Treatment of Fungal Keratitis

If direct microscopic examinations of corneal scrapes or corneal biopsies yield definite results that are consistent with the clinical picture, treatment should be initiated immediately.[5] The antifungal agents available today to combat fungal keratitis are not so well developed as those available against bacterial infections. Most of the available agents only inhibit the growth of the fungus necessitating the host defense mechanisms to eradicate the infection.[7]

The currently used antifungal agents belong to:
- Polyenes
- Azoles, including newer azoles

- Pyrimidines
- Other derivatives.

Polyenes

The polyene antibiotics bind to the ergosterol of fungal cell membrane, creating pores that disrupt the homeostatic mechanisms leading to cell death. Nystatin was the first polyene antifungal to be identified. It has been recommended for topical use (100,000 units). However, its only limitations are corneal toxicity and poor ocular penetration.[7]

Amongst all the polyenes, *Natamycin* is often the first drug of choice to be used for filamentous infections since it is commercially easily available. It is marketed as a 5 percent suspension for topical use. It has broad spectrum of acitivity against filamentous fungi. A 5 percent suspension in the eye is well tolerated. However, this drug may be ineffective in cases with deep stromal abscess because of poor corneal penetration.[7]

Amphotericin B has widely been used as a topical and systemic drug for ocular infections. Preparation of a 0.15 percent suspension of this drug, reconstituted from the 50 mg vial powder (for IV formulation) is universally adopted for topical use as the first line drug both for *Candida* keratitis as well as for keratitis due to other mycelial fungi.[8] After topical application, this drug can penetrate deep into the corneal stroma and 0.15 percent suspension is well tolerated, when instilled round the clock every 15 to 30 minutes.

Pyrimidines—5 Fluorocytosine is a synthetic pyrimidine analog. This drug is available in the form of 1 percent suspension for topical use. It can be given orally (150 mg/kg) as well. It has synergistic effect if given in combination with Amphotericin B in fungal keratitis. Its topical form is nontoxic to the eye. If given systemically, it may cause transient bone marrow depression and gastrointestinal upset. The main drawback of this drug is its limited spectrum of activity against filamentous fungi and rapid development of resistance by *Candida* species.[9,10]

Azoles—Azoles include the imidazoles and the structurally related N-substituted triazoles. These two share the same antifungal spectrum and similar mechanism of action. However, systemic triazoles have a longer half-life than imidazoles. The imidazoles include clotrimazole, miconazole and ketoconazole. The triazoles include fluconazole and itraconazole.

Clotrimazole is usually used topically for skin and genital *Candida* infections. It is marketed as a 1 percent lotion for fungal dermatitis and as 1 percent cream for *Candida* vaginitis. A 1 percent vaginal cream placed into an ophthalmic ointment container can be used for topical use in the eye for the treatment of keratomycosis.

Miconazole can be used as 1 percent eye drop, or through systemic infusion (20 mg/kg body weight).[1] The 1 percent topical application is well tolerated and is reported to be quite successful in treating keratomycosis due to *Aspergillus* and *Candida* species.[12] A perspective series from India[13] found it to be effective in 64.7 percent of the cases when administered topically every 2 hours.

It is usually reserved as a second-line drug in the management of fungal keratitis.[2]

Ketoconazole is another imidazole with pharmacological properties similar to that of miconazole. However, it is less toxic and is easily absorbable from the gastrointestinal tract. It is available as oral preparation in the form of 200 mg tablets. It can also be administered topically as 2 percent eye drops. Studies on rabbit models[14,15] of keratitis showed effective intra-ocular penetration of ketoconazole after oral administration. This drug was also shown to be quite effective both as a prophylactic and a therapeutic agent after topical administration.[16]

Fluconazole is a triazole compound, which can be administered both systemically (200-400 mg per day) and topically (0.2% eye drops). After topical application, as 0.2 percent eye drop it shows good penetration into the anterior chamber.[17] The preparation is also well tolerated in the eye.

Itraconazole is a newer triazole which has larger spectrum of activity than fluconazole against filamentous fungi.[2] However, its only drawback is its hydrophobicity, and hence tissue penetration is poor. A study from India reported an effectivity rate of 69 percent when topical or systemic itraconazole was used as the sole therapeutic agent for keratomycosis.[18]

Coad et al[19] on the basis of tube dilution minimal inhibitory concentration and minimal fungicidal concentration testing, determined that the imidazoles such as miconazole and ketoconazole consistently showed the lowest geometric mean titer for filamentus fungi. Thus, systemic azoles, in general have a good penetration and are frequently used for fungal keratitis. However, they have drug interactions and require monitoring of liver function tests.

Newer Azoles

Voriconazole is a new azole with broad spectrum efficacy for fungal keratitis and endophthalmitis. In a recent study,[20] *in vitro* susceptibility of various fungal isolates in infectious keratitis towards Voriconazole was 100 percent, towards Ketoconazole 82.4 percent, Amphotericin B 76.5 percent, Itraconazole 67 percent, Fluconazole 60 percent and 5-Fluorocytosine 60 percent. Voriconazole MIC (90) was lowest for *Candida* species (0.016 μg/ml). They concluded that Voriconazole was a better alternative for the therapeutic management of *Candida* and *Aspergillus* ocular infections, as compared to other antifungals.

Testing of topical voriconazole in a rabbit model of *Paecilomyces* induced fungal keratitis, was quite encouraging.[21] It was observed that voriconazole therapy caused lesions to decrease within 8 days. Hyphal masses were present in the control infected eyes (not treated with the drug), but absent in the treated infected eyes (as observed after sacrificing the animals and examining the sections of the eye ball). It was therefore postulated that topical voriconazole was a good and effective alternative to topical Amphotericin B, because *Paecilomyces* species were often resistant to Amphotericin B. In yet another development, Ozbek et al[22] emphasised the role of voriconazole in the management of *Alternaria* keratitis.

Other Derivatives

Echinocandins: These drugs have recently emerged as valuable antifungal agents. These are cell wall acting agents unlike Amphotericin B which acts on the cell membrane. These drugs inhibit β 1-3 glucan synthesis, and include Caspofungin and Micafungin. Recently, topical Caspofungin was tried in a rabbit model,[23] in which a 0.5 percent suspension of the drug was found to be as effective as 0.15 percent Amphotericin B, in the treatment of keratitis caused by *Candida*.

Povidone-iodine (Betadine) and Polyhexamethyl biguanide (PHMB): The effectiveness of Povodone-iodine (Betadine) and PHMB as topical antifungals was evaluated by a study group in India[24] in experimentally induced *Aspergillus fumigatus* keratitis in rabbits. Keratitis was induced by corneal intrastromal infection of spores of *A. fumigatus* in four groups of six healthy rabbits each. Drugs used were 5 percent Natamycin, 0.02 percent PHMB, 1 percent Betadine and 0.5 percent hydroxypropyl methyl cellulose (HPMC) as control. The average healing time of ulcers were 21.5 ± 3.08 days for Natamycin, 27.8 ± 2.28 days for PHMB, 36.4 ± 2.57 days for Betadine and 38.2 ± 4.7 for HPMC. While no corneal perforation occurred with Natamycin therapy, there was one perforation case with PHMB, three with Betadine and 5 with HPMC. Thus, 1 percent Betadine was not effective in fungal keratitis while 0.02 percent PHMB was moderately effective.

Silver sulfadiazine: Another antifungal agent that has been used successfully in fungal keratitis is topical silver sulfadiazine, an ointment generally used for prophylactic purpose in patients with burns.[2] In a study of a series of 110 patients from India using the ointment 5 times a day, the drug was found to be effective in 76.3 percent of the cases caused by a variety of fungi, especially by Fuarium species.[25] A randomized clinical trial, conducted by the same workers,[26] found silver sulfadiazine more effective than miconazole in a group of patients with keratomycosis (80% vs 55%). However, their view was that additional clinical trials were needed comparing silver sulfadiazine to polyenes in the treatment of mycotic keratitis.

Therefore, the overall view on the management of mycotic keratitis is that the condition responds slowly over a period of weeks to antifungal therapy. Thus, in order to evaluate the prognosis, clinical signs of improvement should carefully be noted which include diminution of pain, decrease in the size of the infiltrate, disappearance of satellite lesions, rounding of the feathery margins of the ulcer and hyperplastic masses or fibrous sheets in the region of healing fungal lesions.[3] Negative scrapings during treatment do not always indicate that fungal infection has been eradicated, since there may be active proliferation of the fungi deep in the stroma; hence therapy should be continued for at

TABLE 34.1: Antifungal regime for keratomycosis	
Yeasts	Alternatives
First Choice Amphotericin B 0.15% eye drops Fluconazole (0.5% drops, 200 mg orally)	Flucytosine (1% drops, 150 mg/kg orally) Miconazole 1% drops, subcunjunctival/injection Ketoconazole 1% drops Ketoconazole 200 mg bd orally
Filamentous fungi First Choice Natamycin 5% drops	Alternatives Amphotericin B 0.15% drops + Flucytosine Itraconazole (1% cream + 200–400 mg orally)

least 6 weeks, depending upon the antifungal agent selected (Table 34.1).

Patients with deep stromal infections and those who have received corticosteroids appear to respond poorly to medical therapy.[27] Surgery may be necessary in such cases. Every attempt is made, however, to prolong medical therapy for as long as possible, since this renders the infecting fungus nonviable, thereby improving the outcome of surgery. At the same time surgery may help medical management by increasing drug penetration. For example, in small superficial corneal fungal infections, regular surgical debridement of the base of the ulcer helps elimination of fungi and necrotic material, facilitating the penetration of antifungal drugs into the corneal stroma.[3]

ORBITAL CELLULITIS

Orbital cellulitis is an infection of the soft tissue surrounding the orbit. Orbital cellulitis of fungal origin is the most serious ocular infection with significant potential morbidity, including loss of vision, cavernous sinus thrombosis, intracranial spread of infection and occasionally death.[28,29] Therefore, it is essential that patients with periorbital infection need careful evaluation and treatment.

Treatment Modalities for Orbital Cellulitis

Systemic Amphotericin B is the drug of choice. As has been emphasised earlier, the condition being acute and fatal, clinical diagnosis and positive smear report are quite suggestive of starting systemic Amphotericin B therapy without waiting for the culture report which may take days. Conventional Amphotericin B being nephrotoxic, it is administered with gradually increasing dosage each day, starting with 0.25 mg/kg/day, increasing each day by 0.25 mg/kg/day till a dosage of 5 mg/kg/day is achieved.

The drug should be administered in the form of slow intravenous drip in 5 percent dextrose solution. During the course of therapy, constant monitoring of blood urea is recommended.

In case of development of features of renal toxicity, systemic Amphotericin B should be omited and in place of that oral itraconazole 200 mg twice daily for 4-6 weeks should be started. If there is no renal toxicity and the clinical condition of the patient improves after systemic administration of Amphotericin B, then the patient is put on itraconazole therapy, Amphotericin B being omited. Attempts have also been made to deliver Amphotericin B directly to the infected orbital tissue, in the form of daily irrigation and packing.[30]

In addition to the aforementioned modalities, several novel formulations of Amphotericin B have been tried clinically with excellent results, keeping in view the potent toxicity of the conventional drug. Such preparations include Amphotericin B colloidal dispersion and liposomal Amphotericin B.[30,31] However, controlled trials are needed to assess the efficacy of these lipid formulations and of the conventional Amphotericin B in the therapy of ophthalmic mycoses.

DACRYOCYSTITIS

Dacryocystitis is infection of the lacrimal sac. The primary lesion is the obstruction of nasolacrimal duct (NLD). As a result, there occurs obstruction to the normal flow of tears through the sac. This alongwith retained microbial contents give rise to inflammation of the sac.

Treatment of Dacryocystitis

Mycotic dacryocystitis responds well to topical administration of 5 percent Natamycin. Sometimes, alongwith the topical application, local syringing of the sac with either Amphotericin B (1.5 to 8 mg/ml) or Nystatin (100,000 units/ml) solutions may be quite helpful.[32]

ENDOPHTHALMITIS

Endophthalmitis is an inflammatory reaction of intraocular fluid or tissues. Endophthalmitis can be infectious or non-infectious. Infectious endophthalmitis is one of the most serious and vision threatening complications of ophthalmic surgery. Infectious endophthalmitis may be postoperative, post-traumatic or endogenous.

Recommended therapy for endophthalmitis.

Intravitreal Amphotericin B

The recommended dosage of intravitreal Amphotericin B is 7.5 µg in 0.1 ml (prepared from a 50 mg vial by serial dilution). Table 34.2 illustrates the details of the steps for preparation of intravitreal formulation of Amphotericin B.

TABLE 34.2: Amphotericin B (AmB) for intraocular injection (7.5 µg/ml)
• Inject 10 ml water into the bottle with 50 mg dry AmB.   – Shake until transparent (50 mg Am B)
• Take 1 ml of this into a 10 ml syringe (5 mG AmB)
• Dilute with water to 10 ml, shake well
• 1 ml of the above (500 ug AmB) is diluted with water to 6.7 ml and must be shaken (74.62 ug/ml AmB)
• Take 0.1 ml of this with an insulin syringe (7.4 ug AmB)

Systemic

Ketoconazole 200 mg tid orally is also advocated. However, intravenous Amphotericin B is quite effective. This is administered by IV infusion in 5 percent Dextrose solution, starting with 0.25 mg/kg on the 1st day, increasing by 0.25 mg/kg/day till a total dosage of 0.6 mg/kg is achieved.

Influence of Fungal Species on Therapeutic Outcome of Infection

The therapeutic implications of the above clinical entities are often influenced by the various fungal species causing the infections. For example the situation is quite alarming in cases of endophthalmitis caused by species of *Candida* other than *C. albicans*. These *Candida* species are reportedly showing *in vitro* resistance to Fluconazole. In addition, *C. tropicalis* is intrinsically resistant to many azole compounds. Thus, newer azoles like voriconazole and posaconazole are worth trying.[22]

Similarly, considering about mycotic keratitis one would surely appreciate that the most common fungi like *Fusarium* species produce very severe infection with rapid onset of perforation of the cornea. Vision may be completely lost if timely therapeutic intervention is not initiated.[33,34] The same is true for keratitis due to *Aspergillus flavus* and *Pseudallescheria boydii* Keratitis. In all the above situations the organisms give rise to severe form of keratitis with very poor clinical improvement, in spite of all possible medical therapy and may thus require surgical intervention.[35,36]

Considering the aforementioned clinical situations, therapy of such cases always remains a challenge before the treating ophthalmologist[22] and thus, testing for antifungal drug susceptibility seems to be a suitable solution to this.[28,36]

Some progress has been made in this field during the past decade with the standardization of various parameters of antifungal sensitivity testing. The methods currently recommended by Clinical and Laboratory standard Institute (CLSI) have been adopted by many laboratories for the standardization of the techniques both for filamentous fungi and yeasts and reproducibilities of the results have been claimed.[37-40]

A recent study, based upon such testing, documented the superiority of Voriconazole over Itraconazole towards Fluconazole resistant *Candida* isolates. Thus, antifungal drug sensitivity testing in a routine laboratory could help the clinician in prescribing drugs which are effective against a particular clinical isolate, rather than putting the patient on empirical therapy without knowing whether the patient is going to respond to the prescribed treatment or not. In this context, the results of a recent study[41] are noteworthy. While studying on the risk factors and treatment outcome in fungal keratitis the authors highlighted the importance of selecting the appropriate antifungal agent particularly for patients who were refractory to the primary therapy.[41] In addition to this there are scanty reports of inadequetly treated fungal keratitis (because the sensitivity pattern was not known) leading to serious complications like endophthalmitis.[42] All the above mentioned observations only point towards one thing that antifungal susceptibility testing is a prerequisite in the management of all problematic clinical situations mentioned above.

Of all the clinical conditions mentioned above, orbital cellulitis is the one the clinical outcome of which is invariably fatal unless appropriate and timely therapeutic measures are undertaken. This is especially so if there is intracranial spread, which is not unusual in an immunocompromised patient. More importantly, *Mucor* and *Rhizopus* can give rise to a fulminant and acutely fatal disease when the patient is ketoacidotic. In such cases, the prognosis is very poor.[43,44]

Although the best available therapeutic modality in such cases is intravenous Amphotericin B, problem sometimes arises in managing the cases. This is owing to the fact that fungal isolates from deep seated infections like this often show higher MICs for Amphotericin B. Thus the patient might have to be put on a high dose regime, i.e. 5 mg/kg/day of the drug, with a constant watch on blood urea and creatinine levels. In case of blood chemistry abnormality, the drug should be replaced with oral pasaconazole.[44]

Mycotic dacryocystitis, though uncommon invariably responds satisfactorily to topical antifungals mentioned above. However, if medical management fails, surgery is advocated.

In spite of the above mentioned effective antifungal regime, the clinical outcome of fungal dacryocystitis, especially those due to *Aspergilius* or *Candida* is not quite encouraging. About 40 percent of the cases managed by medical treatment alone do recur, whereas around 80 percent of those who undergo surgery alongwith medical treatment get cured.[32,45]

REFERENCES

1. Srinivasan R, Kanungo R, Goyal JL. Spectrum of oculomycosis in South India. Acta Ophthalmol 1991;69:744-9.
2. Abad JC, Foster CS. Fungal keratitis. Intl Ophthalmol Clinic 1996;36:1-15.
3. Agarwal V, Biswas J, Madhavan HN, et al. Current perspectives in infectious keratitis. Indian J Ophthalmol 1994;42:171-92.

4. Sharma S, Srinivasn M, George C. The current status of *Fusarium* species in mycotic keratitis in South India. Indian J Med Microbiol 1993;11:140-7.
5. Thomas PA. Fungal infections of the cornea. Eye 2003;17:852-62.
6. Vajpayee RB, Ray M, Panda A, Sharma N, Taylor HR, Murthy GV, Satpathy G, Pandey RM. Risk factors of pediatric presumed microbial keratitis. Ann Ophthalmol 2002;34:204-310.
7. Walsh TJ, Pizzo A. Treatment of systemic fungal infections: Recent progress and current problems. Eur Clin Microbiol Infect Dis 1988;1:460-75.
8. Tanure MA, Cohen EJ, Grewal S, Rapuano CJ, Laibson PR. Spectrum of fungal keratitis at Wills Eye Hospital, Philadelphia, Pennsylvania. Cornea 2000;19:307-12.
9. Beggs WH. Mechanism of synergistic interaction between Amphotericin B and Flucytosine. J Antimirob Chemother 1986;17:403-4.
10. Viviani MA. Flucytosine-what is its future? J Antimicrob Chemother 1995;35:241-4.
11. Pflugfelder SC, Flynn HW, Zwickey TA, et al. Exogenous fungal endophthalmitis. Ophthalmology 1988;95:19-30.
12. Fitzsimons R, Peters AI. Miconazole and ketoconazole as satisfactory first-line treatment for kerato-mycosis. Am J Ophthalmol 1986;101:605-8.
13. Mohan M, Panda A, Gupta SK. Management of human keratomycosis with miconazole. Aust N Z J Ophthalmol 1989;17: 295-7.
14. Komadina TG, Wilkes TD, Shock JP, et al. Treatment of *Aspergillus fumigatus* keratitis in rabbits with oral and topical ketoconazole. Am J Ophthalmol 1985;99:476-9.
15. Hemady RK, Foster CS. Intra-ocular penetration of ketoconazole in rabbits. Cornea 1992;11:329-33.
16. Oji EO. Ketoconazole: A new imidazole agent has both prophylactic potential and therapeutic efficacy in keratomycosis in rabbits. Int Ophthalmol 1982;5:163-7.
17. Behrens-Baumann W, Klinge R, Richel R. Topical flucanazole for experimental *Candida* keratitis in rabbits. Br J Ophthalmol 1990;74:40-2.
18. Rajasekaran J, Thomas PA, Kalavathy CM, Joseph PC, Abraham DJ. Itraconazole therapy for fungal keratitis. Indian J Ophthalmol 1987;35:157-60.
19. Coad CT, Robinson NM, Weilhelmus KR. Antifungal sensitivity testing for equine keratomycosis. Am J Vet Res 1985;46:676-8.
20. Marangon FB, Miller D, Giacore JA, Alfonso EC. *In vitro* investigation of voriconazole susceptibility for keratitis and endophthalmitis fungal pathogens. Am J Ophthalmolol 2004;137: 820-5.
21. Sponset W, Chen N, Dang D, Paris G, Graybill J, Najvar LK, Zhou L, Lam KW, Glickman R, Scribbick F. Topical voriconazole as a novel treatment for fungal keratitis Antimicrob Agents Chemother 2006;50:262-8.
22. Ozbek Z, Kang S, Sivalingam J, Rapuano CJ, Cohen EJ, Hammersmith KM. Voriconazole in the management of *Alternaria* keratitis. Cornea 2006;25:242-4.
23. Goldblum D, Fruch BE, Sarra GM, Katsoulis K, Zimmerli S. Topical Caspofungin for treatment of keratitis caused by *Candida*

albicans in a rabbit model. Antimicrob Agents Chemother 2005;49:1359-63.
24. Panda A, Ahuja R, Biswas NR, Satpathy G, Khokhar S. Role of 02 percent polyhexamethyl biguanide and 1 percent puvidone iodine in experimental *Aspergillus* keratitis. Cornea 2003;22:138-41.
25. Mohan M, Gupta SK, Kalra VK, Vajpayee RB, Sachdev MS. Silver sulphadiazene in the treatment of mycotic keratitis. Indian J Med Res 1987;85:572-5.
26. Mohan M, Gupta SK, Kalra VK, Vajpayee RB, Sachdev MS. Topial silver sulphadiazine—a new drug for ocular keratomycosis. Br J Ophthalmol 1988;72:192-5.
27. Wilhelmus KR, Jones DB. *Curvularia* keratitis. Trans Am Ophthalmol Soc 2001;99:111-32.
28. Israele V, Nelson JD. Periorbital and orbital cellulitis. Pediatr Infect Dis J 1987;6:404-10.
29. Jackson K, Barker SR. Clinical implications of orbital cellulitis. Laryngoscope 1986;96:568-74.
30. Khoo SH, Band J, Denning DW. Administering Amphotericin B – a practical approach. J Antimicrob Chemother 1994;33:203-13.
31. Walker S, Tailor SAN, Lee M, et al. Amphotericin B in lipid emulsions : stability, compatibility and *in vitro* antifungal acitiviy. Antimicrob Agents Chemother 1998;42:762-6.
32. Ghose S, Mahajan VM. Microbiology of congenital dacryocystitis: Its clinical significance. J Ocul Ther Surg 1985;4:54-7.
33. Jones BR. Principles in the management of oculomycosis. Am J Ophthalmol 1975;79:719-51.
34. Vemuganti GK, Garg P, Gopinathan U, et al. Evaluation of agent and host factors in progression of mycotic keratitis: A histologic and microbiologic study of 167 corneal buttons. Ophthalmology 2002;109:1538-46.
35. Bloom PA, Laidlaw DA, Easty DL, Warnock DW. Treatment failure in case of fungal keratitis caused by *Pseudallescheria boydii*. Br J Ophthalmol 1992;76:367-8.
36. Ozkurt Y, Oral Y, Kuleckei Z, Benzonana N, Ustaoglu R, Dogan OK. Pseudallescheria boydii keratitis. J Paed Ophthalmol Strabismus 2006;43:114-5.
37. Pujol I, Guarro J, Sala J, Riba MD. Effects of incubation temperative, inoculum size, and time of reading on broth microdilution susceptibility test results for Amphotericin B against *Fusarium*. Antimicrob Agents and Chemother 1997;41:808-11.
38. Espinel-Ingroff A, Barchiese F, Cuenca-Estrella M, et al. International and multicenter comparison of EUCAST and CLSI M27-a2 broth microdilution methods for testing susceptibility of *Candida* species to flucanazole, itraconazole, posaconazole and voriconazole. J Clin Microbiol 2005;43:3884-9.
39. Roma, Kaushal Anju, Roy P, Singh H. Antifungal susceptibility patern of non-albicans *Candida* species and distribution of species isolated form candidaemia cases over a 5 year period. Indian J Med Res 1996;106:171-6.
40. Nguyen MH, Yu CY. Influence of incubation time, inodulum size, and glucose concentration on spectrophotometric endpoint: determinants of Amphotericin B, fluconazole and itraconazole. J Clin Microbol 1999;37:141-5.

41. Lalitha P, Prajna NV, Kabra A, Mahadevan K, Srinivasan M. Risk factors and Rx outcome in fungal keratitis. Ophthalmology 2006;113:526-30.
42. Rosenberg KD, Flynn HW Jr, Alfonse EC, Miller D. Fusarium endophthalmitis following keratitis associated with contact lens. Oph Surg Laser Imaging 2006;37:310-3.
43. Lessner A, Stern GA. Preseptal and orbital cellulitis. Infect Dis Clin of North America 1972;6:933-52.
44. Rutor T, Cockerham KP. Periorbita zygomycosois (Mucormycosis) trated with posaconazole. Am J Ophthalmol 2006;142:187-8.
45. Ghose S, Jha RK, Nayak N, Satpathy G, Bajaj MS, Pushker N, Balasubramaniam ST, Prasad R. Current microbial correlates of the eye and nose in Dacryocystitis- their clinical significance. Proceedings of All India Ophthalmological Society Conference 2005.pp.437-9.

35. Recommended Antibiotic Dosages for Various Clinical Conditions of the Eye

Ashok Garg (India)

In this chapter I shall discuss important optimal antibiotic dosages in various ocular clinical conditions and surgical prophylaxis of the eye.

TABLE 35.1: Recommended non-toxic doses of antimicrobial infusion fluids for vitrectomy	
Agent	Dose (mg/ml)
Aminoglyosides	
Gentamicin	0.008
Tobramycin	0.010
Amikacin	0.010
Penicillins	
Penicillin G	0.010
Methicillin	0.020
Oxacilin	0.010
Dicloxacillin	0.010
Clindamycin	0.009
Chloramphenicol	0.010
Lincomycin	0.010
Imipenem	0.010
Ciprofloxacin	0.010
Ofloxacin	0.010
Pefloxacin	0.010
Lomefloxacin	0.010
Sparfloxacin	0.010
Gatifloxacin	0.010
Moxifloxacin	0.010
Besifloxacin	0.010
Ceftazidime	0.040
Vancomycin	0.030

TABLE 35.2: Recommended doses of intravitreal antimicrobial agents

	Agent	Dose (mg/0.1 ml)
a.	*Aminoglycosides*	
	Gentamicin	0.10
	Tobramycin	0.10
	Amikacin	0.40
	Netilmicin	0.10
	Kanamycin	0.40
b.	*Cephalosporins*	
	Cefazolin	2.25
	Cephalothin	2.0
	Cephaloridine	0.25
c.	*Penicillins*	
	Methicillin	2.0
	Oxacillin	0.50
	Carbenicillin	2.0
	Ampicillin	5.0
d.	*Fluoroquinolones*	
	Norfloxacin	0.10
	Ciprofloxacin	0.10
	Ofloxacin	0.10
	Pefloxacin	0.10
	Lomefloxacin	0.08
	Sparfloxacin	0.08
	Levofloxacin	0.10
	Gatifloxacin	0.10
	Moxifloxacin	0.10
	Besifloxacin	0.10
	Vancomycin	1.0
	Clindamycin	0.45-1.0
	Erythromycin	0.50
	Roxithromycin	0.50
	Clarithromycin	0.50
	Chloramphenicol	2.0
	Lincomycin	1.5
	Imipenem	0.50

TABLE 35.3: Preparation of intravitreal antibiotic injections

Drug	Vial size (Commercial)	Amount of initial diluent (ml)	Initial conc (per ml)	Aliquot (ml)	Vol Nos. (ml)	Final conc (ml)	Final intravitreal dose in (0.1 ml)
Amikacin	500 mg/2 ml	–	250 mg	0.1	6.15	4 mg	400 mg
Ampicillin	1 g	3.4	250 mg	0.3	1.2	50 mg	5 mg
Cefazolin	500 mg	2.0	225 mg	0.1	0.9	22.5 mg	2.25 mg
Chloramphenicol	2 mg	1 g	100 mg	0.1	0.4	20 mg	2 mg
Clindamycin	300 mg/2 ml	–	150 mg	0.1	1.4	10 mg	1 mg
Gentamicin	80 mg/2 ml	–	40 mg	0.1	1.9	2 mg	200 ug
Kanamycin	500 mg/2 ml	–	250 mg	0.1	4.9	50 mg	5 mg
Vancomycin	500 mg	10.0	50 mg	0.2	0.8	10 mg	1 mg
Tobramycin	80 mg/2 ml	–	40 mg/ml	0.5 ml	0.5 ml	2 mg/ml	0.2 mg/0.1 ml

TABLE 35.4: Various topical antibiotic preparations (Fortified and commercial with dosages)

Antibiotic preparation	Commercial drops	Fortified drops	Self life	Subconjunctival final doses
Chloramphenicol	0.4-1.0%	5-10 mg/ml	15 days	100 mg
Penicillin	100000 units/ml	0.15-0.30 lac IU/ml	24 hours	1 million units/ml
Framycetin	0.5%	NE	NE	—
Gentamicin	0.3%	20 mg/ml	30 days (RT)	20-40 mg
Tobramycin	0.3%	20 mg/ml	30 days (RT)	20-40 mg
Amikacin	3%	10-20 mg/ml	30 days (RT)	20-50 mg
Sisomicin	0.3%	20 mg/ml	30 days (RT)	20-40 mg
Neomycin	0.17%	30-40 mg/ml	7 days*	250-500 mg
Netilmycin	NE	15-20 mg/ml	7 days*	—
Kanamycin	NE	10 mg/ml	7 days*	—
Tetracycline	1	NE	NE	—
Polymixin B	0.5-1.0%	1-2 mg/ml	1 week*	10000 units/ml
Bacitracin	NE	10000 units/ml	7 days*	5000 units
Erythromycin	NE	5 mg/ml	14 days (RT)	100 mg/ml
Roxithromycin	NE	5 mg/ml	14 days (RT)	100 mg/ml
Clarithromycin	NE	5 mg/ml	14 days (RT)	100 mg/ml

Contd...

Contd...

Antibiotic preparation	Commercial drops	Fortified drops	Self life	Subconjunctival final doses
Norfloxacin	0.3%	20 mg/ml	14 days®	20-40 mg/ml
Ciprofloxacin	0.3%	20 mg/ml	14 days®	20-40 mg/ml
Ofloxacin	0.3%	20 mg/ml	14 days®	20-40 mg/ml
Pefloxacin	0.3%	20 mg/ml	14 days®	20-40 mg/ml
Lomefloxacin	0.3%	20 mg/ml	14 days®	20-40 mg/ml
Sparfloxacin	0.3%	20 mg/ml	14 days®	20-40 mg/ml
Levofloxacin	0.5%	20 mg/ml	14 days®	20-40 mg/ml
Gatifloxacin	0.3%	20 mg/ml	14 days®	20-40 mg/ml
Moxifloxacin	0.5%	20 mg/ml	14 days®	20-40 mg/ml
Besifloxacin	0.6%	20 mg/ml	14 days®	20-40 mg/ml
Cephaloridine	NE	50 mg/ml	14 days®	100 mg/ml
Cephamandole	NE	50 mg/ml	7 days®	100 mg
Cephazolin	NE	50 mg/ml	7 days®	100 mg
Cefoperazone	NE	40-50 mg/ml	7 days®	100 mg
Cefadroxyl	NE	40-50 mg/ml	7 days®	100 mg
Ceftriaxone	NE	130 mg/ml	10 days®	100 mg
Ampicillin	NE	10 mg/ml	7 days®	—
Penicillin G	NE	100000 units/ml	24 hours ®	1 million unit ml
Methicillin	NE	4 mg/ml	7 days®	—
Carbenicillin	NE	4 mg/ml	7 days®	100 mg
Vancomycin	NA	20 mg/ml	1 week®	25 mg
Clindamycin	NA	10 mg/ml	7 days®	—
Ticarcillin	NA	6 mg/ml	7 days®	—

For fortified drops use BSS or isotonic saline (For 5% fortified drops, 50 mg/ml, dissolve 500 mg of salt in 10 CC of BSS).

TABLE 35.5: Initial topical antibiotic therapy choice for external ocular infections based on Gram's stain findings

	Bacteria type	Drugs of choice (fortified)	Alternative drug (Fortified and Non-fortified)
1.	Gram-positive cocci	Cefazolin 100 mg/ml	Vancomycin 25 mg/ml Bacitracin 10000 units/ml Ciprofloxacin Lomefloxacin 20 mg/ml Gatifloxacin Besifloxacin 20 mg/ml
2.	Gram-positive bacilli	Penicillin G 100000 units/ml	Vancomycin—25-50 mg/ml Bacitracin—1000 units/ml
3.	Gram-positive rods	Gentamicin 14 mg/ml	Tobramycin—14 mg/ml
4.	Gram-negative cocci	Ceftriaxone 50 mg/ml	Ofloxacin Lomefloxacin 20 mg/ml Sparfloxacin Moxifloxacin Chloramphenicol—5 mg/ml
5.	Gram-negative bacilli	Tobramycin 14 mg/ml Amikacin 10 mg/ml Ticarcillin—6 mg/ml	Gentamicin—14 mg/ml Polymixin B-50000 units/ml Ciprofloxacin Ofloxacin 20 mg/ml Gatifloxacin Lomefloxacin
6.	Bacteria suspected (No organism seen)	Cefazolin 100 mg/ml and Tobramycin 14 mg/ml	Gentamicin—14 mg/ml or Amikacin—10 mg/ml plus Vancomycin—25 mg/ml or Lomefloxacin Sparfloxacin 20 mg/ml Moxifloxacin Besifloxacin 20 mg/ml

TABLE 35.6: Topical antibiotic therapy for culture specific bacterial ulcers

	Organism	Topical (Fortified or non-fortified)	Subconjunctival
1.	Pseudomonas	Tobramycin 14 mg/ml or Amikacin—10 mg/ml Lomefloxacin Sparfloxacin 20 mg/ml Gatifloxacin	Tobramycin 40 mg (1 ml) Amikacin 25 mg
2.	Staphylococcus	Cefazolin 100 mg/ml Vancomycin 25-50 mg/ml or Bacitracin—10000 units/ml	Cefazolin —100 mg Vancomycin—25 mg Oxacillin—100 mg
3.	Proteus	Gentamicin 14 mg/ml Tobramycin 14 mg/ml Amikacin 10 mg/ml Ceftriaxone 50 mg/ml	Gentamicin—20-40 mg Amikacin—25 mg Carbenicillin—100 mg
4.	Enterobacter E. coli Klebsiella Acinetobacter	Tobramycin 14 mg/ml Amikacin 10 mg/ml Pefloxacin Sparfloxacin 20-40 mg Lomefloxacin Gatifloxacin	Tobramycin—40 mg Amikacin—25 mg Pefloxacin Sparfloxacin Lomefloxacin Moxifloxacin Besifloxacin

TABLE 35.7: Specific antibiotics therapy for the treatment of bacterial endophthalmitis

Microorganisms	Intravitreal injection	Systemic therapy	Topical/sub-conjunctival
Staphylococcus	Vancomycin/Cefazolin	Cefazolin	Cefazolin/vancomycin
Streptococcus	Vancomycin/Cefazolin	Cefazolin and Ampicillin	Cefazolin/vancomycin
Haemophilus	Chloramphenicol	Ceftazidine/Ciprofloxacin Gatifloxacin	Lomefloxacin/Ciprofloxacin Moxifloxacin Besifloxacin
Propionibacterium	Vancomycin	Penicillin/Erythromycin Cloxithromycin	Vancomycin/Penicillin Cefazolin
Corynebacterium	Vancomycin and Cefazolin	Cefazolin	Cefazolin
Bacillus	Clindamycin and Amikacin/Vancomycin	Clindamycin and Gentamicin Ciprofloxacin Gatifloxacin	Clindamycin and Gentamicin/Cipro/Sparfloxacin Moxifloxacin Besifloxacin
Listeria	Ampicillin and Vancomycin	Ampicillin	Vancomycin
Clostridium	Clindamycin/Penicillin	Clindamycin/Penicillin	Clindamycin/Penicillin
Nocardia	Amikacin	Cotrimoxazole	Amikacin
Pseudomonas	Amikacin/Ceftazidime	Moxifloxacin/Ceftazidime	Gatifloxacin/Gentamicin/Lomefloxacin Besifloxacin
Enterobacter	Amikacin	Amikacin	Amikacin
Proteus	Sisomycin and Cefazolin	Cefazolin and Ofloxacin Moxifloxacin	Gentamicin Ofloxacin Gatifloxacin
Serratia	Amikacin	Gentamicin/Lomefloxacin Gatifloxacin	Gentamicin/Lomefloxacin Moxifloxacin Besifloxacin
Klebsiella	Amikacin	Cefazolin/Gentamicin	Cefazolin/Gentamicin

BIBLIOGRAPHY

1. Agarwal A. Textbook of Ophthalmology, 1st edn. New Delhi: Jaypee Medical Publishers, 2002.
2. Bartlett JD. Clinical Ocular Pharmacology, 4th edn. Boston: Butterworth-Heinemann, 2001.
3. Bartlett JD. Ophthalmic Drug facts. Lippincott – William and Wilkins, 2001.
4. Crick RP, Trimble RB. Textbook of Clinical Ophthalmology: Hodder and Stoughton, 1986.
5. Duane TD. Clinical Ophthalmology, 4th edn. Butterworth – Heinemann, 1999.
6. Duvall. Ophthalmic Medications and Pharmacology: Slack Inc, 1998.
7. Ellis PP. Ocular Therapeutics and Pharmacology, 7th edn. CV Mosby, 1985.
8. Fechner. Ocular Therapeutics. Slack Inc., 1998.
9. Fraunfelder. Current Ocular Therapy, 5th edn. WB Saunders, 2000.
10. Garg A. Current Trends in Ophthalmology, 1st edn. New Delhi: Jaypee Medical Publishers, 1997.
11. Garg A. Manual of Ocular Therapeutics, 1st edn. New Delhi: Jaypee Medical Publishers, 1996.
12. Garg A. Ready Reckoner of Ocular Therapeutics, 1st edn. New Delhi: 2002.
13. Goodman LS, Gilman A. Pharmacological basis of Therapeutics, 7th edn. New York: Macmillan, 1985.
14. Havener's, Ocular Pharmacology, 6th edn. CV Mosby, 1994.
15. Kanski. Clinical ophthalmology, 4th edn. Butterworth – Heineman, 1999.
16. Kershner. Ophthalmic Medications and Pharmacology: Slack. Inc., 1994.
17. Kucers A, Bennett NM. The use of Antibiotics, 4th edn. Philadelphia: JB Lippincott Company, 1987.
18. Olin BR, et al. Drugs Facts and Comparisons: Facts and Comparisons, St. Louis, 1997.
19. Onofrey. The Ocular Therapeutics; Lippincott-William and Wilkins, 1997.
20. Rhee. The Wills Eye drug Guide: Lippincott–William and Wilkins, 1998.
21. Seal. Ocular infection management and treatment: Martin – Dunitz, 1998.
22. Steven Podos. Textbook of Ophthalmology. New Delhi: Jaypee Medical Publishers, 2001.
23. Zimmerman. Textbook of Ocular Pharmacology. Lippincott-William and Wilkins, 1997.

Endophthalmitis Prevention Strategies

John D Sheppard (USA)

Perfected treatment strategies depend on a surgeon's preferences and individual patient needs.

Infectious complications following routine cataract surgery are the most feared of all ophthalmic infections, due to the high expectations for cataract operations in the 21st century. Endophthalmitis complicates approximately one in every 1,000 cataract operations. With clear corneal incisions, this rate may be rising. Risk factors cited in the peer-reviewed literature include extracapsular surgery, intracapsular surgery, clear corneal incisions, diabetes mellitus, prolonged surgical time, previous or concurrent trabeculectomy, repeated instrument entry and exit, chronic blepharitis, chronic conjunctivitis, keratitis sicca, ocular surface disease, capsular rupture, vitreous prolapse, and vitrectomy surgery. The potential for this risk may rise to one in every 100 cases with vitreous loss. Although rapid diagnosis and expeditious surgical intervention can preserve excellent visual function in many patients with endophthalmitis, preventive measures are the cornerstone of any surgical management strategy.

NEW CONCEPTS IN ENDOPHTHALMITIS TREATMENT

The landmark Endophthalmitis Vitrectomy Study (EVS), conceived by Dr Bernard Doft and completed in 1995, found that 70 percent of endophthalmitis cases were caused by coagulase-negative, gram-positive micrococci, overwhelmingly *Staphylococcus epidermidis*.[1] This study has revolutionized our treatment algorithm for postcataract surgery endophthalmitis, recognizing the essential aspects of vitreous-tap diagnosis and expeditious injection of intravitreal antibiotics, while surprisingly raising the threshold for pars plana vitrectomy for patients with light perception or worse-quality vision.

New data have extended our understanding of the pathogenesis and prevention of postoperative endophthalmitis since the completion of the EVS. Postcataract infections originate by one of three routes: (1) introduction through instrumentation at the time of surgery; (2) inoculation through the wound after cataract surgery and (3) (although extremely rarely) by endogenous spread from concurrently infected extraocular tissues, such as a tooth abscess or infected diverticulum. Material presented at the 2002

ARVO meeting in Fort Lauderdale, Florida, in particular offered insight into bacteriologic factors relevant to cataract surgery.

EXISTING LITERATURE

With experience and consideration of extensive laboratory data, most surgeons now believe that postcataract infections are introduced into the eye from the ocular surface. This belief brings into question the traditional use of topical perioperative aminoglycosides for cataract patients, especially when most endophthalmitis are gram-positive and aminoglycosides are so insoluble. In our analysis, gram-positive isolates from 163 patients with bacterial conjunctivitis were only 85 percent sensitive to tobramycin, while 97 percent were sensitive to levofloxacin, a third-generation fluoroquinolone, 83 percent to sulfasoxazole, 77 percent to ciprofloxacin, and only 75 percent to trimethoprim, commonly used in combination with the gram-negative agent, polymyxin B.[2]

Franco Recchia of Vanderbilt University and colleagues clearly showed that an increasingly higher percentage of postcataract infections are due to gram-positive organisms.[3] In a study of 493 consecutive patients with postcataract endophthalmitis, researchers cultured an organism from the vitreous in 318 cases (65%). During the last decade of the 20th century, gram-positive isolates increased from 92-97 percent. Furthermore, resistance rates to commonly used prophylactic antibiotics increased; resistance among all isolates to ciprofloxacin rose significantly (23-38%), while resistance to ciprofloxacin and cefazolin rose among coagulase-negative staphylococci (18-38%).

In his new study from Stanford University, Christopher Ta and associates compared the ability of 21 different antibiotics to cover coagulase-negative *Staphylococcus* organisms.[4] Researchers took preoperative conjunctival swabs from 66 patients prior to applying antibiotics or antiseptic. Their analysis concluded that, among the four fluoroquinolones tested, levofloxacin had the highest antistaphylococcal susceptibility (91%) compared to norfloxacin (79%), ofloxacin (75%), and ciprofloxacin (73%). Conversely, resistance patterns also favored levofloxacin at only 5 percent, whereas norfloxacin was 18 percent, ciprofloxacin 20 percent, and ofloxacin 23 percent.

PRACTICAL CLINICAL PRACTICE

Revealing *in vivo* data from Frank Bucci, MD, in Wilkes-Barre, Pennsylvania, demonstrate that levofloxacin reaches therapeutic aqueous concentrations, therefore exceeding the MIC90 for both *Staphylococcus* and *Streptococcus*.[5] Dr Bucci found that 0.5 percent levofloxacin reached 4 to 7 fold higher aqueous concentrations than 0.3 percent ciprofloxacin when administered according to identical preoperative regimens. The ciprofloxacin levels were below the established NCCLS MIC90 for both *Staphylococcus* and *Streptococcus*. Dr Bucci also noted that, higher intracameral levofloxacin concentrations could be achieved with a regimen of administering five drops every 10 minutes immediately prior to surgery, when compared to administering the drug four times per day for 2 days preoperatively. He achieved an additional 50 percent increase in aqueous levels by combining the two regimens.

Starr, Jensen and Fiscella[6] showed that, of 24 endophthalmitis cases in 9,079 patients, eyes receiving topical ofloxacin postoperatively developed endophthalmitis significantly less often than those receiving topical ciprofloxacin (P<.0009). According to these investigators, this difference in endophthalmitis rates may reflect differences in pharmacological and bioavailability properties that exist among fluoroquinolone antibiotics. Ciprofloxacin, the least soluble of available topical fluoroquinolones, achieves the lowest intraocular levels. Levofloxacin, with 3.3 times more active drug per drop than ofloxacin, might be the preferred choice at this time because of superior gram-positive coverage and solubility.

Even though some surgeons have popularized the use of antibiotic infusion through balanced saline-irrigating solutions during cataract surgery, a group of researchers in Arizona, led by Robert Snyder, MD, do not see the efficacy of this approach.[7] Dr Snyder and his colleagues noted that antibiotics chosen for infusion should be fast-acting, due to the limited time exposure to purported intracameral bacterial contaminants. The fluoroquinolones showed dose-dependent killing. On the other hand, vancomycin killing did not correlate with drug concentration relative to the MIC of *Staphylococcus* species tested. Fluoroquinolones may be more suitable for killing bacteria seeded into the anterior chamber than vancomycin. Because vancomycin concentration decreases rapidly in the anterior chamber following surgery completion, residual surviving organisms with exposure to this antibiotic of last resort could have a high likelihood of vancomycin resistance. Those who advocate aminoglycoside antibiotic infusion during routine surgery ignore both the severe potential retinal toxicity of this class, and waning gram-positive sensitivity.

MICROBIAL ANTIBIOTIC RESISTANCE

Careful clinical analysis customized to each prospective cataract patient by a knowledgeable, conscientious surgeon provides the best solution to endophthalmitis risk. There is no single agent capable of killing every microbe known to cause postoperative infections.[8] Even in this brief review of recent ARVO abstracts, epidemiologic patterns differ between hospitals, cities, and regions, a fact that renders each surgeon uniquely capable of understanding the peculiarities of their own bacteriologic environs. Although newer fourth-generation fluoroquinolones, such as moxifloxacin and gatifloxacin, may demonstrate increased potency for gram-positive bacteria over second- and third-generation drugs, the fourth-generations demonstrated no advantage for gram-negative coverage in a keratitis study conducted by Kowalski et al[9] gram-negative resistance appears to cross all fluoroquinolone generations. Thus, miniscule but significant holes have appeared in the once-invincible fluoroquinolone family's gram-negative coverage spectrum. The best protection of all may be a thorough povidone-iodine preparation,[10] including the periorbital skin, lids, lashes, and conjunctival cul-de-sac.

Consistent routines, meticulous iodine preparation and reliable surgical technique, coupled with highly effective and penetrating topical antibiotics given frequently prior to surgery, provide our patients with the best defense against infection.

REFERENCES

1. Han DP, Wisniewski SR, Wilson LA, et al. Spectrum and susceptibilities of microbiologic isolates in the Endophthalmitis Vitrectomy Study. Am J Ophthalmol 1998;122:1-17.
2. Sheppard JD, Oefinger PE, Wegerhoff PE. Susceptibility patterns of conjunctival isolates to newer and established anti-infective agents. IOVS 2002 (abstr 1588) (suppl).
3. Recchia FM, Busbee BG, Pearlman RB, et al. Changing trends in the microbiologic aspects of post-cataract endophthalmitis. Arch Ophthalmol 2005;123:341-46.
4. Ta CN, Mino de Kaspar H, Chang RT, et al. Antibiotic susceptibility pattern of coagulase-negative staphylococci in patients undergoing intraocular surgery. IOVS 2002 (abstr 4444) (suppl).
5. Bucci FA. An *in vivo* comparison of the ocular absorption of levofloxacin versus ciprofloxacin prior to phacoemulsification. IOVS 2002 (abstr 1579) (suppl).
6. Starr MB, Jensen MK, Fiscella RG. A retrospective study of endophthalmitis rates comparing quinolone antibiotics. Am J Ophthalmol 2005;140;769-71.
7. Snyder RW, Krueger T, Nix DE. Kill curves for vancomycin versus 3rd generation quinolones. IOVS 2002 (abstr 4452) (suppl).
8. Benz MS, Scott IU, Flynn HW, et al. *In vitro* susceptibilities to antimicrobials of pathogens isolated from the vitreous cavity of patients with endophthalmitis. IOVS 2002 (abstr 4428) (suppl).
9. Kowalski RP, Karenchak LM, Romanowski EG, et al. An *in vitro* comparison of 2nd, 3rd, and 4th generation fluoroquinolones against bacterial keratitis isolates. IOVS 2002 (abstr 1585) (suppl).
10. Ciulla TA, Starr MB, Masket S. Bacterial endophthalmitis prophylaxis for cataract surgery: An evidence-based update. Ophthalmology 2002;109(1):13-24.

Management of Myopic Choroidal Neovascularization

Jose M Ruiz Moreno, Javier A Montero (Spain)

Following the results of the VIP 1 trial, photodynamic therapy (PDT) was considered as the first line therapy to treat myopic subfoveal choroidal neovascularization (CNV), instead of laser photocoagulation and surgical removal.[1]

PHOTODYNAMIC THERAPY

Photodynamic therapy (PDT) has been a major advance in the management of myopic CNV after the promising results achieved by the VIP 1 study,[1,2] which concluded that PDT increased the chances of stabilization or improvement of visual acuity compared with sham treatment at one year.[1] The response of myopic CNV to PDT is considerably better than that of age-related macular degeneration (AMD), requiring less PDT sessions and resulting in better final visual acuity.[3] The difference between the results of PDT in AMD and high myopia is probably due to the more reduced activity of the choriocapillaris and lower degree of inflammation in myopic CNV.

It has demonstrated that age and spherical equivalent (SE) play a role in the outcome of myopic CNV treated by PDT, both as part of the natural history of the condition[4] and after PDT.[5] We have reported similar results in a previous series with short follow-up.[3] Best corrected visual acuity (BCVA) gain was significantly better for younger patients between months 6 and 24, though the difference was no longer significant for longer follow-up. No correlation was found between BCVA gain and SE, sex, number of PDT sessions or choriocapillaris atrophy (multiple regression analysis). Better final BCVA in younger patients and those with better initial BCVA may be associated with a better inicial chorioretinal condition. Age may play a role inducing choriocapillaris sclerosis and retinal pigment epithelium defects as has been reported for chorioretinal atrophy, which might reduce the chances for improving final BCVA.[6]

In a published series we have reported the outcome of 39 eyes from 36 highly myopic patients with subfoveal classic CNV treated by PDT which completed four years follow-up. Eighteen eyes gained two to seven lines (46%), ten eyes (26%) remained stable within one line basal BCVA, and 11 eyes (28%) lost two to six lines by the end of the follow-up period. CNV was completely inactive by the end of month 48 in 38 eyes (97%). A statistically significant correlation between BCVA gain and initial BCVA ($p < 0.002$) was found at all time intervals; a similar correlation was observed for

BCVA gain and lesion diameter (p < 0.04) and for BCVA gain and age between months 6 and 24 (p < 0.04).[7]

Iatrogenic changes have been reported following PDT on highly myopic eyes, such as lacquer cracks,[8] subretinal hemorrhage,[9] and subretinal fibrosis.[10] However, the appearance of adverse events seems to be less frequent than in patients with AMD.[11-14]

The lack of satisfaction after PDT in patients with CNV secondary to high myopia and AMD prompted the association of PDT with intravitreal steroids.[15,16] Better results were reported for combined therapy in the subgroup of patients with greater diameter of CNV and worse initial visual acuity. However, the effect of combined therapy was similar to PDT alone on the whole group of patients and on those patients with better initial BCVA and smaller CNVs. These relatively positive results were associated with a considerable risk of increased intraocular pressure and cataracts.

The use of intravitreous triamcinolone associated with PDT to treat CNV was first proposed by Spaide in a short series of AMD eyes,[17] and was later followed by different authors for varied indications such as retinal angiomatous proliferation,[19] inflammatory and idiopathic CNV [122, 123]. There is no consensus on the dosage (1–24 mg), timing (before or after PDT), and procedure for concentration or removal of the benzyl alcohol vehicle from commercial triamcinolone for any of these indications.[15,17,21-26] Neither there is consensus on the need or frequency of reinjections, nor whether they should be performed always associated with new PDT sessions, in cases of CNV reactivation or prior to intraocular surgery. Most of the authors agree on the potential risks of this adjuvant therapy: cataract formation (21–50% during the first year),[21,26,27] which may be of greater consequence among young patients as is the case for myopic or inflammatory CNV; apparition of transitory high intraocular pressure (20–83% during the first year),[15,26,28] which may occasionally need surgical therapy, or disappear during the first or the second year, depending on the amount of drug injected; less frequently and highly depending on the injecting technique, retinal detachment, vitreous hemorrhages and infectious or sterile endophthalmitis may appear.[29,30] However, the trend for associating intravitreous triamcinolone with PDT was on the rise during some years.[31,32]

Photodynamic therapy associated with intravitreous triamcinolone for myopic CNV has been reported in several series.[15,33,34] However, the use of adjuvant triamcinolone to treat myopic CNV may show several disadvantages. The appearance of cataracts after triamcinolone injection in a group of young patients implies a need to perform surgery with cessation of the accommodation capability and a higher risk of retinal detachment. Myopic eyes are known to be more sensitive to damage caused by high intraocular pressure, and glaucomatous damage is more difficult to be monitored. We should also consider a higher risk of retinal detachment associated to the injection procedure, due to the more frequent presence of degenerative lesions and peripheral vitreoretinal adhesions.[35]

Chan et al reported on their results after treating myopic CNV by PDT associated to intravitreal triamcinolone showing that the subgroup of patients with greater diameter of CNV and worse initial visual acuity is the one that shows more benefit from the association of PDT with intravitreous triamcinolone.[16] Combined therapy seemed to offer similar results to PDT alone in the whole group of patients or among those with better initial visual acuity and smaller CNVs.

INTRAVITREAL ANTI-VEGF DRUG INJECTION

The good results observed after the intravitreal injection of antiangiogenic drugs to treat myopic CNV have questioned PDT indication.[36-54] The presence of high levels of vascular endothelial growth factor (VEGF) and pigment epithelium-derived factor is suspected to be involved in the development of myopic CNV.[55]

Most of the papers reporting on the results obtained treating myopic CNV with anti-VEGF drugs, mention different schedules of treatment for intravitreal bevacizumab (IVB)[42-54,56] and a lower number of authors report other antiangiogenic drugs such as pegaptanib[36] or ranibizumab.[37-39] Good results have been reported after intravitreal ranibizumab in short series[37,38] and at one-year follow-up[39] with a therapeutical regime of one single initial injection followed by *pro re nata* treatment. Silva et al[39] reported an average visual acuity gain of 8 letters from baseline to 12-month after an average 3.6 injections and no systemic or ocular side effects.

Several papers have reported on the outcome of IVB in the short term.[40,41,45-48,50,51,57] Six papers have reported on the outcome at one year follow-up;[42-44,49,52,53] in three of them the initial therapeutic protocol was three monthly consecutive injections,[42,43,49] whereas in the remaining studies only one injection was used as initial treatment protocol.[44,52,53]

In spite of the good visual and anatomical results published, an important limitation of papers reporting on the use of intravitreal bevacizumab and ranibizumab to treat myopic CMV, is that the result was not compared with PDT, that still is the standard of care.[36-53,56,58] Five authors have performed a comparison of the outcomes obtained with PDT and IVB to treat myopic CNV.[59-63] Yoon et al retrospectively compared the results of 51 eyes with myopic CNV treated by PDT, 63 eyes treated with intravitreal antiangiogenic drugs and 28 eyes treated with a combined therapy PDT plus anti-VEGF at one-year follow-up. The authors concluded that intravitreal anti-VEGF was more effective than PDT alone or combined therapy to treat myopic CNV.[62]

Ikuno et al analyzed the results after treating 31 eyes with myopic CNV in Japanese women who received either PDT or intravitreal bevacizumab.[61] Baba et al compared 12 eyes treated with PDT with 12 eyes treated with IVB.[59] Both authors concluded that IVB was superior to PDT in myopic CNV.[59,61]

Hayashi et al performed a prospective, nonrandomized study comparing the results of 44 eyes with myopic CNV treated by PDT and 43 eyes treated by IVB. Intravitreal bevacizumab (IVB) was more effective at one year and BCVA improved from 0.68 to 0.45 (LogMAR) in the bevacizumab group vs. 0.61 to 0.54 in the PDT group.[60]

Our group[63] performed a prospective, randomized, multi-center, consecutive, masked, interventional phase III study at two years. Fifty-five highly myopic eyes from 55 patients with active subfoveal or juxtafoveal classic CNV from seven different centers from Spain were treated at baseline by PDT or IVB. PDT was performed at baseline and every three months if CNV activity was detected. IVB was performed at baseline (three consecutive monthly injections of 1.25 mg bevacizumab) and then monthly if CNV activity was detected. Best corrected visual acuity (BCVA) and macular thickness were evaluated at baseline and then during two years follow-up. Fluorescein angiography was performed at baseline, and whenever CNV activity was suspected.

Both groups were found to be similar for age, spherical equivalent, sex, ratio of pseudophakic eyes, ratio of eyes with previous PDT, LogMAR BCVA, ETDRS letters read and central foveal thickness at baseline. IVB was more effective at one year and BCVA improved from 53.0–64.2 (letters ETDS) in the bevacizumab group vs 52.8–52.5 in the PDT group.[63] The average number of letters read in the bevacizumab group was 62.4 (SD 16.1) at month 24 ($p = 0.002$). The average number of letters read in the PDT group was 49.5 (SD 18.2) at month 24 ($P = 0.84$). Sixty-four percent of eyes in the bevacizumab group gained 10 or more letters vs 25 percent in the PDT group ($P = 0.008$). Mean number of IVB during the first and second year was 3.5 and 0.6 respectively.

Our results agree with the previously reported data and are very similar to those published by Hayashi et al with statistically significant improvement of BCVA in the bevacizumab group versus no improvement in the PDT group at one year. The secondary analysis performed showed that BCVA gain was more marked among the younger patients (under 50 years) presenting initial BCVA under 65 letters in the bevacizumab group.

The appearance of chorioretinal atrophy around myopic CNV is a major complication of myopic CNV and the principal cause of BCVA loss in these patients. PDT might increase the risk of chorioretinal atrophy in eyes with myopic CNV.[60]

Previous studies showed that myopic eyes previously treated by PDT were less prone to show BCVA gain after IVB than treatment naïve eyes.[42,49,64] Yoon et al showed that simultaneous PDT may reduce the visual improvement achieved using anti-VEGF therapy.[62]

The role of PDT in the induction of chorioretinal atrophy has been explained by the closure of the choriocapillaris network following PDT which may result in RPE dysfunction and contribute to chorioretinal atrophy.[65] The better BCVA results obtained in eyes treated by IVB may be secondary to two factors: the different rate of development of chorioretinal atrophy (the area of chorioretinal atrophy surrounding the CNV was significant smaller in Group 1) and the different pattern of CNV regression.[60] Eyes treated by IVB showed a reduced CNV whereas CNV in Group 1 PDT showed a bigger area than at baseline.[60]

Our study was performed with three initial intravitreal injections per protocol as has been previously reported,[42,43,49] but new publications using one single initial IVB per protocol have shown similar results in terms of visual acuity.[44,52,53] New papers have reported on the comparative efficacy of protocols showing similar results in BCVA gain.[66]

Some papers have reported on the two years results treating myopic CNV with IVB.[56,66-70] The published outcome at two years follow-up was different for the different authors. For Hayashi et al[56] with 75 eyes treated, Iacono et al[68] treating 30 eyes, Voykov et al[67] in 11 eyes and Ruiz-Moreno et al[66] with 19 highly myopic eyes, the difference between BCVA at baseline and that at 2 years was not significant. On the contrary, Nakanishi et al[70] with 23 eyes, Gharbiya et al[71] with 20 eyes and Chen et al[69] with 26 eyes (with 2.5 µmg/0.1 ml), BCVA gain was significant by the end of the second year. Our results at the second year follow-up show a statistically significant increase in visual acuity (logMAR and letters read) in bevacizumab treated group vs. no improvement in the PDT group.

In another paper,[72] our group has performed a retrospective, nonrandomized, multicenter, interventional case series study with 108 eyes with subfoveal or juxtafoveal CNV with more than 4 years follow-up. Patients were treated by intravitreal injections (IVI) on a *pro re nata* regime. BCVA and macular thickness were evaluated at baseline and monthly afterwards. Main outcome measures were: change in number of letters read, influence of SE, type of drug and previous PDT on the visual outcome.

The average number of letters read at baseline was 49.5 (SD 18.0); at 12 months 58.3 (SD 18.9); at 24 months 57.4 (SD 20.9); at 36 months 56.2 (SD 22.0) and 54.3 (SD 22.6) at 48 months ($p < 0.0001$, between initial vs 12, 24 and 36 months and $p = 0.008$ between initial vs 48 months). Mean number of IVI was 4.6 (SD 5.1; 1–29). No systemic adverse reactions were detected during follow-up. Age, SE, drug and previous PDT had no influence on the visual outcome.

We have not found differences in our series after 4 years follow-up; the initial loading dose had no effect on the number of reinjections needed (3.6 ± 5.4 with one vs 2.0 ± 3.5 with three; $p = 0.16$, Student test).

Only one retrospective, nonrandomized paper with 4 years follow-up has been published on 21 eyes with myopic CNV treated with bevacizumab. In this series 15/21 eyes gained one or more Snellen lines, 3 eyes remained stable ± 1 line and 3 eyes lost of one or more lines.[35]

Previous papers showing results on myopic CNV treated by PDT with longer follow-up, found BCVA stabilization or improvement in 72 to 76 percent of the eyes.[7] Our group reported one series with four years follow-up,[7] in which BCVA stabilization or improvement was found in most of the patients; however, this improvement was not statistically significant. We have found a positive correlation of the number of lines gained and the initial diameter of the lesion and better final BCVA for the younger population, though the difference was not statistically significant. We have found no correlation for SE and final BCVA.[7]

Our long-term follow-up results confirm the statistically significant improvement of BCVA in myopic eyes with CNV treated with anti-VEGF drugs (mean gain 4.7 ± 18.3 letters at 4 years). It did not make any difference what drug was used (bevacizumab vs ranibizumab), or previous PDT. Correlation with SE was not statistically significant (as in PDT at four years[42]) and a low but significant correlation was found between BCVA change and age. The final status of CNV as determined by SD-OCT had a significant influence on final BCVA and change in number of letters read. BCVA gain was more marked among younger patients, than in the group of older patients; however, this difference was not statistically significant, as occurred with PDT.[42]

Bevacizumab and ranibizumab had similar clinical effects with no differences on age, SE, percent of previous PDT, initial BCVA, final BCVA, change in number of letters read, number of reinjections performed and number of total IVI needed. The total number of IVI required during the four years averaged 4.6 ± 5.1. No systemic adverse reactions were detected during follow-up.

SUMMARY

Following the recent reports comparing both PDT vs. anti-VEGF drugs, an the results with intravitreal anti-VEGF drugs to treat myopic CNV, the IVI of anti-VEGF drugs to treat CNV associated with high myopia is a useful procedure with significant BCVA gain at long-term follow-up, and must be considered as a first line therapy. Bevacizumab and ranibizumab had similar clinical effects in BCVA gain and number of IVI required.

REFERENCES

1. Photodynamic therapy of subfoveal choroidal neovascularization in pathologic myopia with verteporfin. 1-year results of a randomized clinical trial—VIP report no. 1. Ophthalmology 2001;108:841-52.
2. Verteporfin in Photodynamic Theory Study Group. Photodynamic therapy of subfoveal choroidal neovascularization in pathologic myopia with verteporfin. 1-year results of a randomized clinical trial—VIP report no. 1. Ophthalmology 2001; 108: 841-52.
3. Montero JA, Ruiz-Moreno JM. Verteporfin photodynamic therapy in highly myopic subfoveal choroidal neovascularisation. Br J Ophthalmol 2003; 87: 173-6.
4. Yoshida T, Ohno-Matsui K, Ohtake Y, et al. Long-term visual prognosis of choroidal neovascularization in high myopia: a comparison between age groups. Ophthalmology 2002; 109: 712-9.
5. Pece A, Vadala M, Isola V, Matranga D. Photodynamic therapy with verteporfin for juxtafoveal choroidal neovascularization in pathologic myopia: a long-term follow-up study. Am J Ophthalmol 2007; 143: 449-54.
6. Curcio CA, Saunders PL, Younger PW, Malek G. Peripapillary chorioretinal atrophy: Bruch's membrane changes and photoreceptor loss. Ophthalmology 2000; 107: 334-43.

7. Ruiz-Moreno JM, Amat P, Montero JA, Lugo FL. Photodynamic therapy to treat choroidal neovascularization in highly myopic patients: 4 years outcome. Br J Ophthalmol 2008; 92: 792-4.
8. Ladas ID, Moschos MM, Rouvas AA, Karagiannis DA, Kokolakis SN. Lacquer crack formation after photodynamic therapy. Eur J Ophthalmol 2003; 13: 729-33.
9. Diaz-de-Durana-Santa-Coloma E, Fernandez-Ares ML, Iturralde-Errea D, Salazar-Diez JL, Vazquez-Cruchaga E, Lopez-Garrido JA. Submacular heamorrhage following photodynamic therapy in the treatment of choroidal neovascularization. Arch Soc Esp Opthalmol 2006; 81: 685-91.
10. Ruiz-Moreno JM, Montero JA. Subretinal fibrosis after photodynamic therapy in subfoveal choroidal neovascularisation in highly myopic eyes. Br J Ophthalmol 2003; 87: 856-9.
11. Waisbourd M, Loewenstein A, Goldstein M, Leibovitch I. Targeting vascular endothelial growth factor: a promising strategy for treating age-related macular degeneration. Drugs Aging 2007; 24: 643-62.
12. Potter MJ, Szabo SM. Recurrence of choroidal neovascularisation after photodynamic therapy in patients with age-related macular degeneration. Br J Ophthalmol 2007; 91: 753-6.
13. Rogers AH, Martidis A, Greenberg PB, Puliafito CA. Optical coherence tomography findings following photodynamic therapy of choroidal neovascularization. Am J Ophthalmol 2002; 134: 566-76.
14. Moschos MN, Panayotidis D, Moschos MM, Bouros C, Theodossiadis PG, Theodossiadis GP. A preliminary assessment of macular function by MF-ERG in myopic eyes with CNV with complete response to photodynamic therapy. Eur J Ophthalmol 2003; 13: 461-7.
15. Marticorena J, Gomez-Ulla F, Fernandez M, Pazos B, Rodriguez-Cid MJ, Sanchez-Salorio M. Combined photodynamic therapy and intravitreal triamcinolone acetonide for the treatment of myopic subfoveal choroidal neovascularization. Am J Ophthalmol 2006; 142: 335-7.
16. Chan WM, Lai TY, Wong AL, Liu DT, Lam DS. Combined photodynamic therapy and intravitreal triamcinolone injection for the treatment of choroidal neovascularisation secondary to pathological myopia: a pilot study. Br J Ophthalmol 2007; 91: 174-9.
17. Spaide RF, Sorenson J, Maranan L. Combined photodynamic therapy with verteporfin and intravitreal triamcinolone acetonide for choroidal neovascularization. Ophthalmology 2003; 110: 1517-25.
18. Hunter MA, Dunbar MT, Rosenfeld PJ. Retinal angiomatous proliferation: clinical characteristics and treatment options. Optometry 2004; 75: 577-88.
19. Hogan A, Behan U, Kilmartin DJ. Outcomes after combination photodynamic therapy and immunosuppression for inflammatory subfoveal choroidal neovascularisation. Br J Ophthalmol 2005; 89:1109-11.
20. Smithen LM, Spaide RF. Photodynamic therapy and intravitreal triamcinolone for a subretinal neovascularization in bilateral idiopathic juxtafoveal telangiectasis. Am J Ophthalmol 2004;138: 884-5.

21. Rechtman E, Danis RP, Pratt LM, Harris A. Intravitreal triamcinolone with photodynamic therapy for subfoveal choroidal neovascularisation in age related macular degeneration. Br J Ophthalmol 2004; 88: 344-7.
22. Spaide RF, Sorenson J, Maranan L. Photodynamic therapy with verteporfin combined with intravitreal injection of triamcinolone acetonide for choroidal neovascularization. Ophthalmology 2005;112: 301-4.
23. Arias L, Garcia-Arumi J, Ramon JM, Badia M, Rubio M, Pujol O. Photodynamic therapy with intravitreal triamcinolone in predominantly classic choroidal neovascularization: one-year results of a randomized study. Ophthalmology 2006;113:2243-50.
24. Augustin AJ, Offermann I. Emerging drugs for age-related macular degeneration. Expert Opin Emerg Drugs 2006;11:725-40. Treatment of Choroidal Neovascularization in High Myopia Current Drug Targets, 2010;11(5):643.
25. Chan WM, Lai TY, Wong AL, Tong JP, Liu DT, Lam DS. Combined photodynamic therapy and intravitreal triamcinolone injection for the treatment of subfoveal choroidal neovascularisation in age related macular degeneration: a comparative study. Br J Ophthalmol 2006; 90: 337-41.
26. Ruiz-Moreno JM, Montero JA, de la Vega C, Alio JL, Zapater P. Macular choroidal neovascularization in myopic eyes after phakic intraocular lens implantation. J Refract Surg 2006;22:689-94.
27. Ergun E, Maar N, Ansari-Shahrezaei S, et al. Photodynamic therapy with verteporfin and intravitreal triamcinolone acetonide in the treatment of neovascular age-related macular degeneration. Am J Ophthalmol 2006;142:10-6.
28. Spaide RF, Sorenson J, Maranan L. Combined photodynamic therapy and intravitreal triamcinolone for nonsubfoveal choroidal neovascularization. Retina 2005;25:685-90.
29. Moshfeghi AA, Puliafito CA. Pegaptanib sodium for the treatment of neovascular age-related macular degeneration. Expert Opin Investig Drugs 2005; 14: 671-82.
30. Roth DB, Chieh J, Spirn MJ, Green SN, Yarian DL, Chaudhry NA. Noninfectious endophthalmitis associated with intravitreal triamcinolone injection. Arch Ophthalmol 2003; 121: 1279-82.
31. Anijeet DR, Hanson RJ, Bhagey J, Bates RA. National survey of the technique of intravitreal triamcinolone injection in the United Kingdom. Eye 2006.
32. Chakravarthy U, Adamis AP, Cunningham ET Jr, et al. Year 2 efficacy results of 2 randomized controlled clinical trials of pegaptanib for neovascular age-related macular degeneration. Ophthalmology 2006; 113: 1508 e1-25.
33. Degenring RF, Jonas JB. Photodynamic therapy in combination with intravitreal triamcinolone for myopic choroidal neovascularization. Acta Ophthalmol Scand 2005; 83: 621.
34. Potter MJ, Szabo SM, Ho T. Combined photodynamic therapy and intravitreal triamcinolone for the treatment of myopic choroidal neovascularization in a 13-year-old girl. Graefes Arch Clin Exp Ophthalmol 2006; 244: 639-41.
35. Montero JA, Ruiz-Moreno JM. Combined photodynamic therapy and intravitreal triamcinolone injection for the treatment of choroidal neovascularisation secondary to pathological myopia: a pilot study. Br J Ophthalmol 2007;91:131-3.

36. Bennett MD, Yee W. Pegaptanib for myopic choroidal neovascularization in a young patient. Graefes Arch Clin Exp Ophthalmol 2007;245:903-5.
37. Konstantinidis L, Mantel I, Pournaras JA, et al. Intravitreal ranibizumab (Lucentis) for the treatment of myopic choroidal neovascularization. Graefes Arch Clin Exp Ophthalmol 2009; 247:311-8.
38. Silva RM, Ruiz-Moreno JM, Nascimento J, et al. Short-term efficacy and safety of intravitreal ranibizumab for myopic choroidal neovascularization. Retina 2008;28:1117-23.
39. Silva RM, Ruiz-Moreno JM, Rosa P, et al. Intravitreal ranibizumab for myopic choroidal neovascularization: 12-month results. Retina 2010;30:407-12.
40. Arias L, Planas N, Prades S, et al. Intravitreal bevacizumab (Avastin) for choroidal neovascularisation secondary to pathological myopia: 6-month results. Br J Ophthalmol 2008;92:1035-9.
41. Chan WM, Lai TY, Liu DT, Lam DS. Intravitreal bevacizumab (Avastin) for myopic choroidal neovascularization: six-month results of a prospective pilot study. Ophthalmology 2007;114:2190-6.
42. Chan WM, Lai TY, Liu DT, Lam DS. Intravitreal bevacizumab (Avastin) for myopic choroidal neovascularisation: 1-year results of a prospective pilot study. Br J Ophthalmol 2009;93:150-4.
43. Gharbiya M, Allievi F, Mazzeo L, Gabrieli CB. Intravitreal bevacizumab treatment for choroidal neovascularization in pathologic myopia: 12-month results. Am J Ophthalmol 2009; 147:84-93.
44. Ikuno Y, Sayanagi K, Soga K, et al. Intravitreal bevacizumab for choroidal neovascularization attributable to pathological myopia: one-year results. Am J Ophthalmol 2009;147:94-100.
45. Laud K, Spaide RF, Freund KB, et al. Treatment of choroidal neovascularization in pathologic myopia with intravitreal bevacizumab. Retina 2006;26:960-3.
46. Mandal S, Venkatesh P, Sampangi R, Garg S. Intravitreal bevacizumab (Avastin) as primary treatment for myopic choroidal neovascularization. Eur J Ophthalmol 2007;17:620-6.
47. Nguyen QD, Shah S, Tatlipinar S, et al. Bevacizumab suppresses choroidal neovascularisation caused by pathological myopia. Br J Ophthalmol 2005;89:1368-70.
48. Ruiz-Moreno JM, Gomez-Ulla F, Montero JA, et al. Intravitreous bevacizumab to treat subfoveal choroidal neovascularization in highly myopic eyes: short-term results. Eye 2009;23:334-8.
49. Ruiz-Moreno JM, Montero JA, Gomez-Ulla F, Ares S. Intravitreal bevacizumab to treat subfoveal choroidal neovascularisation in highly myopic eyes: 1-year outcome. Br J Ophthalmol 2009;93:448-51.
50. Sakaguchi H, Ikuno Y, Gomi F, et al. Intravitreal injection of bevacizumab for choroidal neovascularisation associated with pathological myopia. Br J Ophthalmol 2007;91:161-5.
51. Tewari A, Dhalla MS, Apte RS. Intravitreal bevacizumab for treatment of choroidal neovascularization in pathologic myopia. Retina 2006;26:1093-4.
52. Wu PC, Chen YJ. Intravitreal injection of bevacizumab for myopic choroidal neovascularization: 1-year follow-up. Eye 2009;23:2042-5.

53. Ruiz-Moreno JM, Montero JA, Arias L, et al. Twelve-Month Outcome after One Intravitreal Injection of Bevacizumab to Treat Myopic Choroidal Neovascularization. Retina 2010;30:1609-15.
54. Tong JP, Chan WM, Liu DT, et al. Aqueous humor levels of vascular endothelial growth factor and pigment epithelium-derived factor in polypoidal choroidal vasculopathy and choroidal neovascularization. Am J Ophthalmol 2006;141:456-62.
55. Ruiz-Moreno JM, Montero JA, Gomez-Ulla F. Photodynamic therapy may worsen the prognosis of highly myopic choroidal neovascularisation treated by intravitreal bevacizumab. Br J Ophthalmol 2009;93:1693-4.
56. Hayashi K, Shimada N, Moriyama M, Hayashi W, Tokoro T, Ohno-Matsui K. Two-year outcomes of intravitreal bevacizumab for choroidal neovascularization in Japanese patients with pathologic myopia. Retina 2012;32:687-95.
57. Yamamoto I, Rogers AH, Reichel E, et al. Intravitreal bevacizumab (Avastin) as treatment for subfoveal choroidal neovascularisation secondary to pathological myopia. Br J Ophthalmol 2007;91:157-60.
58. Ruiz-Moreno JM, Montero JA, Arias L, et al. Three versus one intravitreal bevacizumab injections as initial protocol to treat myopic choroidal neovascularization. Acta Ophthalmol 2012; 90:e82-3.
59. Baba T, Kubota-Taniai M, Kitahashi M, et al. Two-year comparison of photodynamic therapy and intravitreal bevacizumab for treatment of myopic choroidal neovascularisation. Br J Ophthalmol 2010;94:864-70.
60. Hayashi K, Ohno-Matsui K, Teramukai S, et al. Comparison of visual outcome and regression pattern of myopic choroidal neovascularization after intravitreal bevacizumab or after photodynamic therapy. Am J Ophthalmol 2009;148:396-408.
61. Ikuno Y, Nagai Y, Matsuda S, et al. Two-Year Visual Results for Older Asian Women Treated with Photodynamic Therapy or Bevacizumab for Myopic Choroidal Neovascularization. Am J Ophthalmol 2010;149:140-6.
62. Yoon JU, Byun YJ, Koh HJ. Intravitreal anti-VEGF versus photodynamic therapy with verteporfin for treatment of myopic choroidal neovascularization. Retina 2010;30:418-24.
63. Ruiz-Moreno JM, López-Gálvez MI, Donate J, Gomez-Ulla F, García-Arumí J, García-Layana A, Sellés I, Reche J, Montero JA, Pazos B, Zapata MA, Pastor JC. Myopic choroidal neovascularization. Ophtahlmology 2011;118:2521-3.
64. Moshfeghi DM, Kaiser PK, Grossniklaus HE, et al. Clinicopathologic study after submacular removal of choroidal neovascular membranes treated with verteporfin ocular photodynamic therapy. Am J Ophthalmol 2003;135:343-50.
65. Peters S, Heiduschka P, Julien S, et al. Ultrastructural findings in the primate eye after intravitreal injection of bevacizumab. Am J Ophthalmol 2007;143:995-1002.
66. Ruiz-Moreno JM, Montero JA. Intravitreal bevacizumab to treat myopic choroidal neovascularization: 2-year outcome. Graefes Arch Clin Exp Ophthalmol 2010;248:937-41.
67. Voykov B, Gelisken F, Inhoffen W, et al. Bevacizumab for choroidal neovascularization secondary to pathologic myopia: Is there a decline of the treatment efficacy after 2 years? Graefes Arch Clin Exp Ophthalmol 2010;248:543-50.

68. Iacono P, Parodi MB, Papayannis A, Kontadakis S, Sheth S, Bandello F. Intravitreal bevacizumab therapy on an as-per-needed basis in subfoveal choroidal neovascularization secondary to pathological myopia: 2-year outcomes of a prospective case series. Retina 2011;31:1841-7.
69. Chen CH, Wu PC, Chen YJ, Liu YC, Kuo HK. Intravitreal injection of 2.5 mg bevacizumab for treatment of myopic choroidal neovascularization in treatment-naïve cases: a 2-year follow-up. J Ocul Pharmacol Ther 2011;27:395-400.
70. Nakanishi H, Tsujikawa A, Yodoi Y, Ojima Y, Otani A, Tamura H, Yamashiro K, Ooto S, Yoshimura N. Prognostic factors for visual outcomes 2-years after intravitreal bevacizumab for myopic choroidal neovascularization. Eye (Lond) 2011;25:375-81.
71. Gharbiya M, Allievi F, Conflitti S, et al. Intravitreal bevacizumab for treatment of myopic choroidal neovascularization: the second year of a prospective study. Clin Ter 2010;161:e87-93.
72. Ruiz-Moreno JM, Arias L, Montero JA, Carneiro A, Silva R. Intravitreal antivascular endothelial growth factor therapy for choroidal neovascularization secondary to pathologic myopia: four years outcome. In press.

Treatment of Central Serous Choroidopathy

Pedro Amat Peral, Francisco Lugo, Jose M Ruiz-Moreno (Spain)

INTRODUCTION

Concept and Classification

First described by Von Graefe (Von Graefe, 1866) in 1866, central serous chorioretinopathy (CSC) is characterized by the presence of a serous detachment of the neurosensory retina associated with one or more lesions in the retinal pigment epithelium (RPE) (Wang 2008). There are two main types of CSC. The most common type, the typical or classic CSC, is seen in younger patients and produces an acute localized detachment of the retina with visual acuity loss from mild-to-moderate. The second presentation, the chronic CSC is characterized by diffuse disturbance of RPE pigmentation associated with the chronic presence of a small amount of subretinal fluid. This type is common in patients with CSC associated with chronic use of corticosteroids (Carvalho-Recchia, 2002).

Epidemiology

The better understanding of the clinical manifestations of the CSC has changed considerably our knowledge about their demographics. The overall incidence in men versus women in numerous publications was about 8 or 9 to 1, but the incidence in women was twice between 31 and 40 years compared with those aged between 21 and 30 years (Klein, 1974). The male-female ratio was 2.6 to 1 without differences between the age groups. Although traditionally considered the CSC as a disease of young men, some studies have found a higher incidence than expected in women and in patients older than 50 years.

Etiology

It has been described the possible influence of psychological factors on the onset and course of the CSC (Huke, 1982). It has been observed more frequently in individuals with personality type A and with elevated levels of catecholamines (Yanuzzi, 1987). There must be a racial predisposition, with the highest incidence among Caucasians, Hispanics and possibly Asians, and an extremely low rate in African Americans (Gelber 1987, Guyer 1994A). There is no

a refractive defect associated in most cases, although there has been a slight hyperopia in some cases.

Endogenous cortisol levels are up to 50 percent higher in patients with CSC; glucocorticoid treatment also increases the risk of developing the disease, especially in a chronic type (Carvalho-Recchia, 2002).

Pregnancy has been described as a risk factor for the development of CSC, probably induced by elevated glucocorticoid levels (Quillen, 1996).

Symptoms

Many patients complain of blurred vision at the beginning, followed by varying degrees of metamorphopsia, micropsia, dyschromatopsia, central scotoma, loss of contrast sensitivity and increased of hyperopia. In some patients the onset of symptoms precedes or accompanies headaches similar to migraine (Gass, 1970).

Typically, the area of metamorphopsia is reproducible in the Amsler grid test. Visual acuity in the acute phase is between 20/20 and 20/200. The vision can be improved with a small hyperopic correction (Klais, 2009).

Clinical Forms and Natural History

Acute CSC

The typical acute CSC is characterized by spontaneous resolution of neurosensory detachment in less than 6 months, recovering in most cases the basal visual acuity (VA). Recurrences may affect a third or half of the cases after the first episode, half of which occurs in the first year and less frequent until 10 years later and 10 percent have three or more recurrences (Ficker, 1988).

Chronic CSC

When the neurosensory detachment persists for more than six months, it is considered a chronic form of the disease, also called diffuse retinal pigment epitheliopathy (Cohen, 1983). In these patients can remain a relative scotoma, metamorphopsia, dyschromatopsia and decreased contrast sensitivity (Klais, 2009). A small percentage may develop CNV, perifoveal RPE atrophy or cystic macular degeneration with serious or irreversible loss of visual function.

Diagnosis

Biomicroscopy

On examination of the fundus is observed in the form of neurosensory detachment transparent blister well-defined at the posterior pole, therefore the fovea luminous reflection is absent. The subretinal fluid is usually clear. According to the duration of symptoms, fluid can be transformed into granular or fibrinous (Ie 1993, Wang 2005). Occasionally, fovea xanthophyll pigment appears more intense. The PED are seen frequently in the fundus examination, there are often two or more, which are located in areas above neurosensory detachment, are round or oval (van Velthoven 2005, Mitarai 2006). The longstanding chronic DEP can appear with pigment migration or atrophy.

The diagnosis of CSC is supported by CSC-compatible RPE changes in the fellow eye.

Complementary Test

Fluorescein Angiography (FA)

Before the advent of optical coherence tomography (OCT), the FA was an essential tool in the diagnosis of CSC, currently remains primarily useful in the differential diagnosis of CNV and treatment planning. The angiographic finding is more characteristic of one or several points in contrast leakage of ink spot shape under neurosensory detachment absence of choroidal neovascularization (CNV). The leakage spots are hypopigmented transmission by choroidal fluorescence. Most of the leakage spots are located 0.5 to 1.5 mm from the foveal center and the most common site is the superonasal quadrant (Spitznas, 1987). In 10 percent of cases staining neurosensory detachment amounts within funnel-shaped and extends laterally mushroom-shaped or umbrella until the upper limit of detachment.

Fundus Autofluorescence Imaging

In the acute phase of the CSC, background autofluorescence hypofluorescence characterized by a level of the leakage spots (Eandi, 2005), if the neuroretinal detachment persists over time, the detachment area is displayed with a pattern of granular or confluent hyperfluorescence (Sekiryu, 2010). In chronic forms of the disease can be displayed a mixed pattern of hypo and hyperfluorescence (Frame 2005, von Rückmann 2002). After detachment resolution the autofluorescent subretinal deposits disappear over a few weeks. The irregular pattern of autofluorescence may be due to the elongation of the outer segments and is observed at the level of the neurosensory retina detachment area (Matsumoto, 2011). Recently it has been established that the pattern of background fluorescence can be a good predictor of visual function in patients with CSC (Imamura, 2011). The autofluorescence may be a complementary tool in the diagnosis and differentiation of the CSC of acute or chronic phase (Dinc, 2011).

Indocyanine Green Angiography

The Indocyanine green (ICG) angiography has demonstrated hyperpermeability of the choroid which is part of the pathogenesis of the disease. This feature results in the staining of ICG inner choroidal vessels, which are best viewed in the intermediate stages of the angiogram. As the study proceeds is an image feature of hyperfluorescence patches in the choroid with negative staining of large vessels in the late phases of the angiogram (Spaide, 1996). These areas of choroidal hyperfluorescence centrifugally increase in the later stages and does not reflect only the leakage spots observed with FA, also seen in clinically normal areas and unaffected contralateral eyes. Choroidal veins may appear congested. Findings on ICG may also be useful for predicting the outcome of treatment with photodynamic therapy (PDT) (Inoue, 2010).

Optical Coherence Tomography

Optical Coherence tomography (OCT) is a fundamental tool for the diagnosis and monitoring of macular pathology in general and in particular CSC. It is useful for the diagnosis of very shallow serous that are difficult to diagnose in the slit lamp examination and also to distinguish them from DEP. It is also essential to monitor the disease, to see if the treatment is objectively beneficial in achieving the resolution of the detachment and to reduce the frequency of FA.

Modern equipment SD-OCT have identified an increased choroidal thickness in patients with CSC. CT in patients with CSC does not usually decrease with age, unlike healthy patients (Imamura, 2009).

The enhanced depth imaging-OCT (EDI-OCT) using "swept-source" increases the depth resolution of the tomographic image, in practice can achieve much lower sensitivity with increasing imaging deep as compared with convencional SD-OCT, which is useful in the study of the choroid. With this tool has also been studied the CT in patients with CSC and found a significant difference between the affected and contralateral eye almost 100 microns, and the unaffected eyes of patients with CSC have almost 250 microns thicker the choroid than patients without the disease (Maruko 2011, Kim 2011).

Microperimetry

In patients with CSC macular microperimetry shows a decreased macular sensitivity (Ozdemir, 2008). It may be useful to determine the benefit of treatment with PDT. Studies have shown that visual acuity can be a parameter to underestimate the improvement after treatment with PDT. It has been determined that the macular function is improving progressively between 3 and 6 months after treatment although the VA does not change in that time (Ehrlich, 2012).

Electrophysiology

The electroretinogram (ERG) in CSC has demostrated reduction photoreceptor function of the neurosensory detachment level [decreased amplitude and increased latencies of the B-wave, decreased oscillatory potential (Miyake, 1988)]. Meanwhile, the multifocal ERG has demostrated variable negrees of dysfunction outsider the area of detachment (Marmor, 1999). It also found multifocal ERG amplitudes in the contralateral eyes abnormally low in subclinical CSC.

DIFFERENTIAL DIAGNOSIS

Although the clinical diagnosis of CSC is usually confirmed by FAG and OCT, there are many entities that should be considered in the differential diagnosis:
- Age macular degeneration (AMD)
- Polypoidal choroidal vasculopathy
- Tumors (choroidal hemangioma, choroidal melanoma, choroidal metastasis, choroidal osteoma, choroidal leukemic infiltrates)
- Vascular diseases (lupus erythematosus, polyarteritis nodosa, scleroderma, dermatomyositis and relapsing polychondritis, malignant hypertension, toxemia of pregnancy)
- Optic nerve pit with serous macular detachment
- Inflammatory and infectious diseases (Presumed histoplasmosis syndrome, Harada's disease, posterior scleritis, multifocal choroiditis, hypertensive retinopathy, sympathetic ophthalmia and uveal effusion syndrome).

TREATMENT

Observation

In about 90 percent of patients with CSC, is appreciated the resolution of neurosensory retinal detachment in the first six weeks with conservative measures (Sharma, 2004), as advice about lifestyle or suspension in the administration of corticosteroids, which making reasonable initial conservative treatment.

Some controversy exists about the precise time before starting a more aggressive treatment such as photodynamic therapy or laser photocoagulation, although it was observed that a neurosensory retinal detachment exceed 4 months induces some degree of retinal atrophy (Wang, 2002), so that time can be considered reasonable to administer treatment.

In cases of: visual loss in patients for occupational reasons require a quick recovery, permanent visual loss in untreated cotralateral eye in a patient experiencing an outbreak of CSC with visual loss the healthy eye or in cases of multiple RPE detachment or bullous subretinal fluid, may bring forward the treatment. (Reche-Frutos, 2010).

Pharmacological Treatment

Antiangiogenic Drugs

Bevacizumab: Small case series have shown a potential benefit in the treatment of CSC with bevacizumab (Lee 2011, Inouea 2011).

However, another cases series showed no beneficial effect of bevacizumab in CSC (Lim, 2010).

Semeraro et al compare the efficacy of treatment with bevacizumab versus low fluence PDT in patients with chronic central serous chorioretinopathy. Twenty-two patients were divided into two groups, observing that there are no statistically significant differences in the results of both groups but appreciate better results in bevacizumab group (Semeraro 2012).

Benefit has been observed with bevacizumab treatment for choroidal neovascularization secondary to photodynamic therapy applied for the CSC (Montero, 2011).

Ranibizumab: Konstantinidis et al conclude that intravitreal ranibizumab can be effective in the treatment of CNV secondary to chronic CSC, however, persists intraretinal or subretinal fluid and residual choroidal permeability increased (Konstantinidis 2010).

SH Bae et al perform a comparative study of 6 months to evaluate the efficacy of low fluence PDT versus ranibizumab injections for the treatment of chronic CSC. At 3 months there was no improvement in BCVA statistically significant in group of L-PDT compared to the ranibizumab group. However, this tendency does not hold. Concludes that, in anatomical terms, the effect of ranibizumab injections is not promising compared with L-PDT (Bae, 2011).

Glucocorticoids Inhibiting Drugs

Since glucocorticoids are involved in the development of CSC, it has been observed that certain drugs that suppress glucocorticoid production promote the resolution of CSC.

Rifampicin produces glucocorticoid inhibition because it increases metabolism of endogenous steroids through its induction of cytochrome *P450 3A4* (Jampol, 2002) Should be taken into account the implementation of a control liver enzymes and platelet count in blood analysis. It has been used in a small series of patients to treat chronic CSC successfully (Steinle, 2012).

Mifepristone is an antagonist of the glucocorticoid and progesterone receptor, has a antiandrogen action peak. It was observed favorable response to treatment in a group of 16 patients with chronic CSC treated with 200 mg of mifepristone daily for 12 weeks (Nielsen, 2011).

Ketoconazole prospective exerts its effects in the treatment of CSC by decreased levels of cortisol, aldosterone and androgen and in elevation of progesterone (Caccavale, 2011). A study showed a treatment response at eight weeks when given a dose of 600 mg daily administered for four weeks. (Meyerle, 2007).

Other Drugs

Finasteride (inhibitor of dihydrotestosterone synthesis) with a regimen of 5 mg daily, was observed in a small number of patients with chronic CSC that caused a positive response although exudation relapsed after discontinuation (Forooghian, 2011).

Acetylsalicylic acid (aspirin), at doses of 75-100 mg, has been shown in one study to be beneficial to allow resolution of CSC (Caccavale, 2010). The effect of therapy may be associated with anti-inflammatory and antiplatelet effects of aspirin and their ability to reduce serum levels of plasminogen activator-1, and its action on the inhibition of the overaction of hypothalamic pituitary adrenal axis.

In a small cases series were used metronidazole and omeprazole as a regimen for eradication of *H.pylori* in patients with CSC. Compared to a control group that did not receive this treatment, patients experienced greater absorption of subretinal fluid (Bagher, 2011).

Several clinical trials have used beta blockers in patients with CSC, with promising short-term results (Avci, 2005), although there is no long-term evidence of the possible effectiveness of them.

The administration of acetazolamide can reduce subretinal fluid although it has not been proven to be effective in improving visual acuity or reduce long-term recurrence rate (Gonzalez, 1992).

Furthermore, it has been observed that poor sleep quality is often interrupted in patients with obstructive sleep apnea syndrome, induces an overactivation of the hypothalamic-pituitary-adrenal and sympathetic nervous system, which may contribute to development of CSC. A case report highlighted the potential importance of the identification and treatment of obstructive sleep apnea to allow resolution of CSC in some patients (Kim, 2011).

Argon Laser Photocoagulation

Laser photocoagulation reduces the duration of neurosensory retinal detachment compared to conservative treatment (Burumcek, 1997). While reducing the time of neurosensory retinal detachment may induce lower RPE degeneration, there is no conclusive data about whether laser photocoagulation improves visual prognosis (Ticker, 1988).

There is also disagreement about whether laser photocoagulation reduces the recurrence rate or not (Yap 1996, Brancato 1987).

The argon laser is applied directly to the leakage spot, in order to produce a limited alteration in RPE and a secondary subretinal fluid resorption. Under normal conditions, fluid reabsorption occurs from two to six weeks from the administration of the laser, while the visual recovery tends to be completed in 12 weeks.

Laser photocoagulation involves some potential complications such as damage to the EPR in the impact zone, so it can not be applied to subfoveal level.

Photodynamic Therapy

Several uncontrolled case series have employed treatment with verteporfin (Visudyne®, Novartis, Basel, Switzerland) in acute CSC (Ober, 2005) and chronic (Cardillo, 2003), with resolution of subretinal fluid and increased visual acuity. Visual recovery is, in many cases of chronic CSC, limited by EPR damage (Reche-Frutos, 2008).

In contrast to argon laser used guided by FA, PDT is given according to the findings of the IGC.

It has been suggested that PDT cause choroidal hypoperfusion in short-term and long-term remodeling choroidal circulations, inducing an improvement in the choroidal congestion and hyperpermeability (Schmidt-Erfurth, 2002).

The observation of threatening complications secondary to PDT treatment, as CNV (Coluccielo, 2006), persistent choroidal hypoperfusion or chronic changes in the RPE (Cardillo, 2003), secondary to excessive radiation on healthy tissue, has justified the appearance of modified protocols of PDT regarding dose reduction (Stewart, 2006) or fluence (Reibaldi, 2009).

For wet AMD the parameters of Photodynamic therapy may be given in the "standard" fluence and dose (83 seconds of 689 nm light wavelength spot at an exposure of 600 mW/cm^2, five minutes after a 10-minute infusión of verteporfin dose 6 mg/m^2, fielding 50 J/cm^2 fluence).

Half-fluence PDT (6 mg/m^2, 25 J/cm^2)

The observation of complications secondary to PDT treatment, has justified its change in terms of dose reduction (Inouea, 2011) or fluence (Lim, 2010). New protocols may be safer for eyes with CSC.

A multicenter, retrospective study indicates that half-fluence PDT was as effective as convencional PDT, while minimizing PDT's adverse effects on choriocapilaris perfusion and retinal thickness (Shin, 2011).

The results of a recent and prospective study evaluating microperimetry data on chronic CSC patients treated with standard-fluence vs low-fluence PDT indicated a significant improvement in macular sensitivity after PDT in eyes with chronic CSC, with greater efficacy in low-fluence-treated eyes (Reibaldi, 2011).

A retrospective review showed that ICG angiography-guided half-fluence PDT with verteporfin is effective in treating acute symptomatic CSC, resulting in visual improvement and complete resolution of exudative macular detachment (Smretschnig, 2012).

Half-dose PDT (3 mg/m^2)

The modified protocol of PDT using a half-dose of verteporfin to treat CSC showed no RPE atrophy developed (Chan, 2003).

Half-dose verteporfin PDT in case of CSC induced significant increases in central 10°, 20°, and paracentral 10° to 20° sensitivity, as well as PDT laser spot area retinal sensitivity over six months (Senturk, 2011).

A recent retrospective series demonstrated that subfoveal choroidal thickness significantly decreased after half-dose PDT treatment of central serous chorioretinopathy (Maruko, 2010).

In CSC patients after treatment with half-dose verteporfin, PDT was demonstrated multifocal electroretinography improved retinal function at the central macula (Wu, 2011).

Reibaldi et al in a prospective, non-randomized, comparative study between standard fluence PDT and reduced fluence PDT have been observed similar results in terms of improvement in visual acuity and retinal thickness reduction with increased frequency of choroidal hypoperfusion at 12 months in eyes treated with a standard fluence PDT (Reibaldi, 2010).

PATHOGENESIS

Despite advances in diagnostic testing and treatment of CSC, the precise cause of the disease remains controversial. It is known that the origin of the disease is located on the choroid with RPE affectation.

Clinical findings and abnormal choroidal circulation in patients with CSC obtained by indocyanine green (ICG) angiography have demonstrated a choroidal vascular leakage in these patients.

The increased hydrostatic pressure in the choroid, an alteration of the RPE mechanical barrier, with consequent damage to the RPE cells and the accumulation of fluid under the retina. Disruption of RPE in contiguous areas causes accumulation of fluid in the subretinal space producing the neurosensory detachment.

Indocyanine green (ICG) in patients with CSC has demonstrated evidence of choroidal lobular ischemia and choroidal venous congestion (Hayashi 1986, Prünte 1995, 1996). The late choroidal hyperpermeability areas show a delay in filling, which is attributed to the decrease of the perfusion pressure or venous outflow.

The cause of choroidal venous dilatation may be a response to ischemia and delayed arterial filling or a consequence of outflow obstruction.

The impact of these anatomical alterations produces microvascular decompensation, RPE detachment and finally, neuroepithelial detachment.

Despite the widely studied and documented relation of the CSC with corticosteroids and catecholamines and the highest incidence of the disease in young patients with type A personality is not yet established the real role of these substances in the pathogenesis of CSC, but several considerations were established. Adrenergic agonists cause vasoconstriction and impaired blood flow in the choroidal vasculature. Corticosteroids reduce the production of nitric oxide, a autoregulatory vasodilator controlling local blood flow. The high levels of corticosteroids may also cause capillary fragility and hyperpermeability decompensation producing choroidal circulation and leak of fluid into the subretinal space. Corticosteroids may also cause delayed in healing of RPE defects, slowing reparative process of the damaged cells. It has also been shown that increased levels of catecholamines and corticosteroids alters choriocapillaris blood flow autoregulation (Klais, 2009).

It has been established that people infected with the *Helicobacter pylori* have increased risk of CSC, the interaction between the bacteria and the vascular endothelium determines the choroidal ischemia mechanism that can precipitate disease (Rahbani-Nobar, 2011). The urease of *H. Pylori* also produces an activation of platelets, which would start at choroidal congestion and choroidal vascular ischemia leading to the CSC (Wassermann, 2010).

Prolonged alteration of choroidal microcirculation specifically in the choriocapillaris leads to a fluid gradient sub-RPE space, initially RPE cells are able to maintain balance and pump the fluid in correct direction, however, prolonged effect produce failure and loss of this function of the RPE. Both, choroidal hyperpermeability processes and maintained damage RPE function lead to accumulation of fluid in the sub-RPE space with eventual subretinal space leak.

The spontaneous repair and fluid reabsorption occur during the procces resolution, however, if microvascular alteration remains at time, the recurrence and chronicity of disease occurs (Klais, 2009).

CASE REPORT (FIGURES 38.1 TO 38.9)

A 42-year-old male who has a base diabetic retinopathy and multifocal central serous chorioretinopathy of 1-year evolution. He had previously been treated with argon laser photocoagulation for extrafoveal lesion. After relapse, visual acuity decreases to 20/32. Treatment is performed using photodynamic therapy presenting the resolution of the clinical.

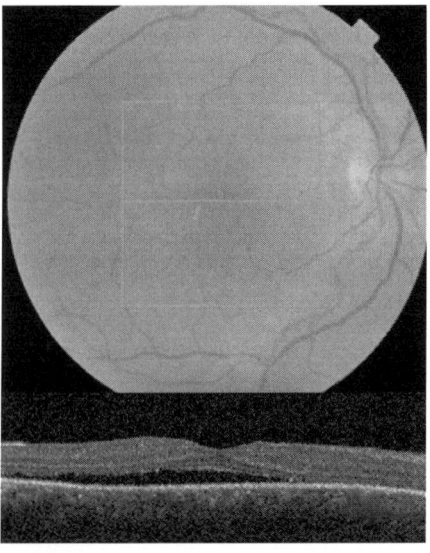

Fig. 38.1: Posterior pole color fundus and OCT of the patient showing a serous detachment of the neurosensory retina

Treatment of Central Serous Choroidopathy

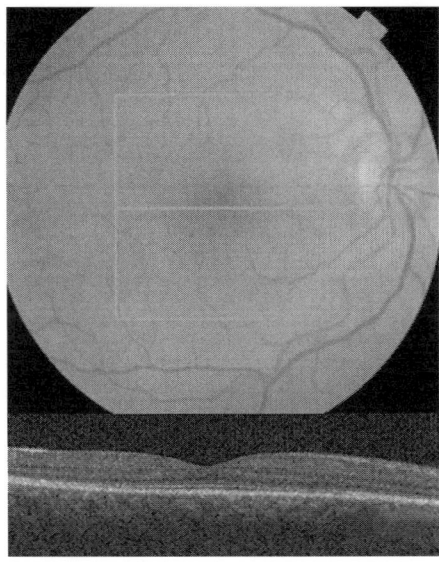

Fig. 38.2: Posterior pole color fundus and OCT of the patient showing the resolution of a serous detachment of the neurosensory retina

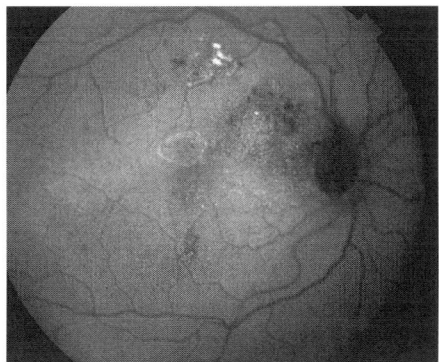

Fig. 38.3: Patient fundus autofluorescence imaging

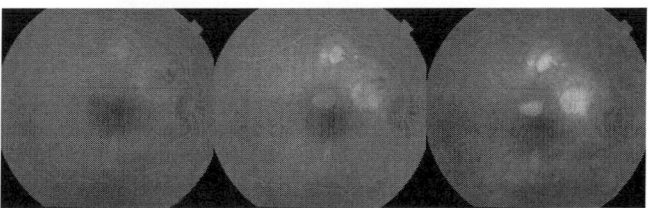

Fig. 38.4: Fluorescein angiography (FA) of the patient showing leakage spots placed in superonasal quadrant of posterior pole

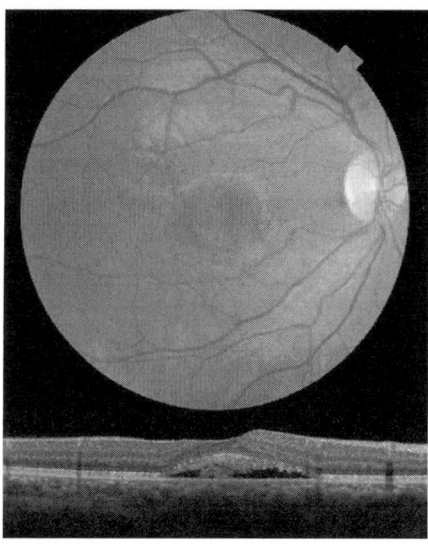

Fig. 38.5: Posterior pole color fundus and OCT showing CSC activity as a serous detachment of the neurosensory retina

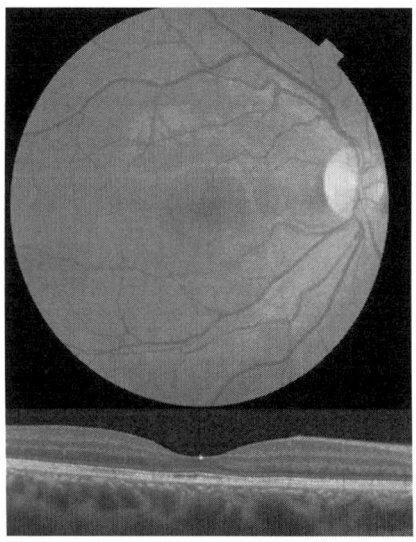

Fig. 38.6: Posterior pole color fundus and OCT showing CSC inactivity. The serous detachment of the neurosensory retina has disappeared

Treatment of Central Serous Choroidopathy

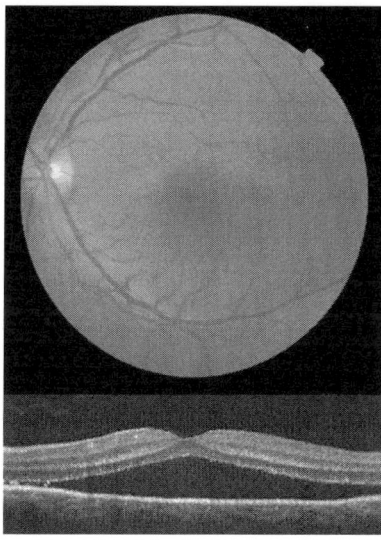

Fig. 38.7: Posterior pole color fundus and OCT showing a serous detachment of the neurosensory retina affecting the entire posterior pole has disappeared

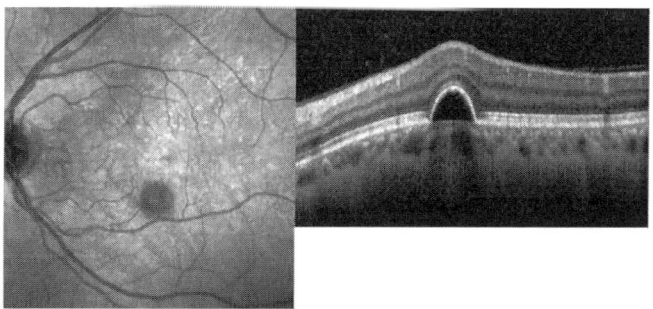

Fig. 38.8: Fundus autofluorescence imaging and OCT showing a retinal pigment epithelium (RPE) detachment

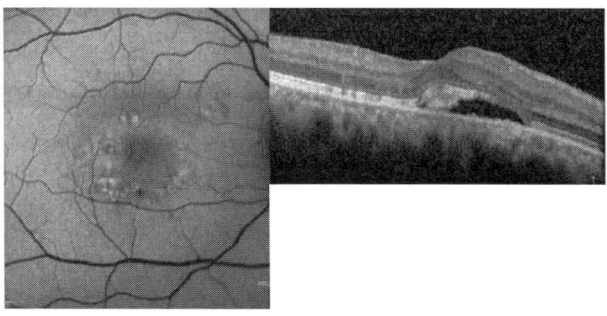

Fig. 38.9: Fundus autofluorescence imaging and OCT showing a serous detachment of the neurosensory retina. OCT shows the prolongation of outer segments of photoreceptors

BIBLIOGRAPHY

1. Bae SH, Heo JW, Kim C, Kim TW, et al. A randomized pilot study of low-fluence photodynamic therapy versus intravitreal ranibizumab for chronic central serous chorioretinopathy. Am J Ophthalmol 2011;152:784-92.
2. Bagher M, Rahbani-Nobar R, Alireza Javadzadeh A, et al. The effect of *Helicobacter pylori* treatment on remission of idiopathic central serous chorioretinopathy. Mol Vis 2011;17:99-103.
3. Caccavale A, Romanazzi F, Imparato M, et al. Low-dose aspirin as treatment for central serous chorioretinopathy. Clin Ophthalmol 2010;4:899-903.
4. Caccavale A, Romanazzi F, Imparato M, Negri A, Morano A, Ferentini F. Central serous chorioretinopathy: A pathogenetic model. Clin Ophthalmol 2011;5:239-43.
5. Cardillo PF, Eandi CM Ventre L, et al. Photodynamic therapy for chronic central serous chorioretinopathy. Retina 2003;23:752-63.
6. Carvalho-Recchia CA, Yanuzzi LA, Negrao S, et al. Corticosteroids and central serous chorioretinopathy. Ophthalmology 2002; 109:1834-7.
7. Cohen D, Gaudric A, Coscas G, Quentel G, Binaghi M. Diffuse retinal epitheliopathy and central serous chorioretinopathy. J Fr Ophthalmol 1983;6:339-49.
8. Chan WM, Lam DS, Lai TY, et al. Choroidal vascular remodelling in central serous chorioretinopathy after indocyanine green guided photodynamic therapy with verteprofin: A novel treatment at the primary disease level. Br J Ophthalmol 2003;87:1453-8.
9. Dinc UA, Tatlipinar S, Yenerel M, Görgün E, Ciftci F. Fundus autofluorescence in acute and chronic central serous chorioretinopathy. Clin Exp Optom 2011;94:452-7.
10. Eandi CM, Ober M, Iranmanesh R, Peiretti E, Yannuzzi LA. Acute central serous chorioretinopathy and fundus autofluorescence. Retina 2005;25:989-93.
11. Ehrlich R, Mawer NP, Mody CH, Brand CS, Squirrell D. Visual function following photodynamic therapy for central serous chorioretinopathy: A comparison of automated macular microperimetry versus best-corrected visual acuity. Clin Experiment Ophthalmol 2012;40:e32-9.
12. Ficker L, Vafidis G, While A, Leaver P. Long-term follow-up of a prospective trial of argon laser photocoagulation in the treatment of central serous retinopathy. Br J Ophthalmol 1988;72:829-34.
13. Forooghian F, Meleth AD, Cukras C, et al. Finasteride for chronic central serous chorioretinopathy. Retina 2011;31:766-71.
14. Framme C, Walter A, Gabler B, Roider J, Sachs HG, Gabel VP. Fundus autofluorescence in acute and chronic-recurrent central serous chorioretinopathy. Acta Ophthalmol Scand 2005;83:161-7.
15. Gass JDM. Pathogenesis of disciform detachment of the neuroepithelium. I. General concepts and classification. Am J Ophthalmol 1967;63:573-85.
16. Gass JDM. Pathogenesis of disciform detachment of the neuroepithelium. II. Idiopathic central serous choroidopathy. Am J Ophthalmol 1967;63:587-615.
17. Gass JDM. Stereoscopic atlas of macular diseases. Mosby: St Louis, 1970.
18. Gelber GS, Schatz H. Loss of vision due to central serous choroidopathy following psychological stress. Am J Psychiatry 1987;144:46-50.

19. Guyer DR, Gragoudas ES. Central serous chorioretinopathy. In: Albert DM, Jakobiec FA (Eds). Principles and practice of ophthalmology, vol 2, Philadelphia: WB Saunders, 1994.
20. Hayashi K, Hasegawa Y, Tokoro T. Indocyanine green angiography of central serous chorioretinopathy. Int Ophthalmol 1986;9:37-41.
21. Huke J. Retinopathia centralis serosa, disertation, Bonn, 1982
22. Ie D, Yannuzzi LA, Spaide RF, Rabb MF, Blair NP, Daily MJ. Subretinal exudative deposits in central serous chorioretinopathy. Br J Ophthalmol 1993;77:349-53.
23. Imamura Y, Fujiwara T, Margolis R, Spaide RF. Enhanced depth imaging optical coherence tomography of the choroid in central serous chorioretinopathy. Retina 2009; 29:1469-73.
24. Imamura Y, Fujiwara T, Spaide RF. Fundus autofluorescence and visual acuity in central serous chorioretinopathy. Ophthalmology 2011;118:700-5.
25. Inouea M, Kadonosonoa K, Watanabea Y, et al. Results of one-year follow-up examinations after intravitreal bevacizumab administration for chronic central serous chorioretinopathy. Ophthalmologica 2011;225:37-40.
26. Inoue R, Sawa M, Tsujikawa M, Gomi F. Association between the efficacy of photodynamic therapy and indocyanine green angiography findings for central serous chorioretinopathy. Am J Ophthalmol 2010;149:441-6.
27. Jampol LM, Weinreb R, Yannuzzi L. Involvement of corticosteroids and catecholamines in the patogénesis of central serous chorioretinopathy: A rationale for new treatment strategies. Ophthalmology 2002;109:1765-6.
28. Kim, JT, Eichiling, PS, Wang, M. Central serous chorioretinopathy associated with narcolepsy. Retin Cases Brief Rep 2011;5:302-5.
29. Kim YT, Kang SW, Bai KH. Choroidal thickness in both eyes of patients with unilaterally active central serous chorioretinopathy. Eye (Lond) 2011;25:1635-40.
30. Kim SW, Oh J, Kwon SS, Yoo J, Huh K. Comparison of choroidal thickness among patients with healthy eyes, early age-related maculopathy, neovascular age-related macular degeneration, central serous chorioretinopathy, and polypoidal choroidal vasculopathy. Retina 2011;31:1904-11.
31. Klais CM, Ober MD, Ciardella AP, Yanuzzi LA. Choriorretinopatía serosa central. Ryan SJ, Schachat AP (Eds). En Ryan RETINA 2009;63:1021-45.
32. Klein ML, Van Buskirk EM, Friedman E, Gragoudas E, Chandra S. Experience with nontreatment of central serous choroidopathy. Arch Ophthalmol 1974;91:247-50.
33. Konstantinidis L, Mantel I, Zografos L, Ambresin A. Intravitreal ranibizumab in the treatment of choroidal neovascularization associated with idiopathic central serous chorioretinopathy. Eur J Ophthalmol 2010;20:955-8.
34. Marmor MF, Tan F. Central serous chorioretinopathy: Bilateral multifocal electroretinographic abnormalities. Arch Ophthalmol 1999;117:184-8.
35. Maruko I, Iida T, Sugano Y, et al. Subfoveal choroidal thickness after treatment of central serous chorioretinopathy. Ophthalmology 2010;117:1792-9.
36. Maruko I, Iida T, Sugano Y, Ojima A, Sekiryu T. Subfoveal choroidal thickness in fellow eyes of patients with central serous chorioretinopathy. Retina 2011;31:1603-8.

37. Matsumoto H, Kishi S, Sato T, Mukai R. Fundus autofluorescence of elongated photoreceptor outer segments in central serous chorioretinopathy. Am J Ophthalmol. 2011;151:617-23.
38. Meyerle CB, Freund KB, Bhatnagar P, et al. Ketoconazole in the treatment of chronic idiopathic central serous chorioretinopathy. Retina. 2007;27:943-6.
39. Mitarai K, Gomi F, Tano Y. Three-dimensional optical coherence tomographic findings in central serous chorioretinopathy. Graefes Arch Clin Exp Ophthalmol. 2006;244:1415-20.
40. Miyake Y, Shiroyama N, Ota I, Horiguchi M. Local macular electroretinographic responses in idiopathic central serous chorioretinopathy. Am J Ophthalmol. 1988;106:546-50.
41. Montero JA, Ruiz-Moreno JM, Fernandez-Muñoz M. Intravitreal bevacizumab to treat choroidal neovascularization following photodynamic therapy in central serous choroidopathy. Eur J Ophthalmol. 2011;21:503-5.
42. Nielsen JS, Jampol LM. Oral mifepristone for chronic central serous chorioretinopathy. Retina. 2011;31:1928-36.
43. Ober MD, Yanuzzi LA, Do DV, et al. Photodynamic therapy for focal retinal pigmentoepithelial leaks secondary to central serous chorioretinopathy. Ophthalmology. 2005;112:2088-94.
44. Ozdemir H, Senturk F, Karacorlu M, Arf Karacorlu S, Uysal O. Macular sensitivity in eyes with central serous chorioretinopathy. Eur J Ophthalmol. 2008;18:799-804.
45. Prünte C. Indocyanine green angiographic findings in central serous chorioretinopathy. Int Ophthalmol. 1995;19:77-82.
46. Prünte C, Flammer J. Choroidal capillary and venous congestion in central serous chorioretinopathy. Am J Ophthalmol. 1996;121:26-34.
47. Quillen DA, Gass DM, Brod RD, et al. Central serous chorioretinopathy in women. Ophthalmology. 1996;103:72-9.
48. Rahbani-Nobar MB, Javadzadeh A, Ghojazadeh L, Rafeey M, Ghorbanihaghjo A. The effect of *Helicobacter pylori* treatment on remission of idiopathic central serous chorioretinopathy. Mol Vis. 2011;17:99-103.
49. Reche-Frutos J, Calvo-Gonzalez C, Donate-López J, et al. Photodynamic therapy in severe chronic central serous chorioretinopathy. Arch Soc Esp Oftalmol. 2008;83: 9-14.
50. Reche-Frutos J, Calvo-Gonzalez C. Coriorretinopatía serosa central. En Patología y Cirugía de la Mácula. Ponencia de la SEO 2010;V5:273-8.
51. Reibaldi M, Boscia F, Avitabile, et al. Low-fluence photodynamic therapy in long-standing chronic central chorioretinopathy with foveal and gravitacional atrophy. Eur J Ophthalmol 2009;19:154-8.
52. Reibaldi M, Cardascia N, Longo A, et al. Standar-fluence versus low-fluence photodynamic therapy in chronic central serous chorioretinopathy: a non-randomized clinical trial. Am J Ophthalmol. 2010;149:307-15.
53. Reibaldi M, Boscia F, Avitabile T, et al. Functional retinal changes measured by microperimetry in standard-fluence photodynamic therapy in chronic central serous chorioretinopathy. Am J Ophthalmol. 2011;151:953-60.
54. von Rückmann A, Fitzke FW, Fan J, Halfyard A, Bird AC. Abnormalities of fundus autofluorescence in central serous retinopathy. Am J Ophthalmol. 2002;133:780-6.
55. Sekiryu T, Lida T, Maruko I, Saito K, Kondo T. Infrared fundus autofluorescence and central serous chorioretinopathy. Invest Ophthalmol Vis Sci. 2010;51:4956-62.

56. Semeraro F, Romano MR, Danzi P, Morescalchi F, Costagliola C. Intravitreal bevacizumab versus low-fluence photodynamic therapy for treatment of chronic central serous chorioretinopathy. Jpn J Ophthalmol, 2012.
57. Senturk F, Karacorlu M, Ozdemir H, et al. Microperimetric changes after photodynamic therapy for central serous chorioretinopathy. Am J Ophthalmol 2001;151:303-9.
58. Sharma T, Shah N, Rao M, et al. Visual outcome after discontinuation of corticosteroids in atypical severe central serous chorioretinopathy. Ophthalmology 2004;111:1708-14.
59. Shin JY, Woo SJ, Yu HG, et al. Comparison of efficacy and safety between half-fluence and full-fluence photodynamic therapy for chronic central serous chorioretinopathy. Retina 2011;31:119-26.
60. Smretschnig E, Ansari-Shahrezaei S, et al. Half-fluence photodynamic therapy in acute central serous chorioretinopathy. Retina 2012;10:1-6.
61. Spaide RF, Hall L, Haas A, Campeas L, Yannuzzi LA, Fisher YL, Guyer DR, Slakter JS, Sorenson JA, Orlock DA. Indocyanine green videoangiography of older patients with central serous chorioretinopathy. Retina 1996;16:203-13.
62. Spaide RF, Klancnik JM Jr. Fundus autofluorescence and central serous chorioretinopathy. Ophthalmology 2005;112:825-33.
63. Spitznas M, Huke J. Number, shape, and topography of leakage points in acute type I central serous retinopathy. Graefes Arch Clin Exp Ophthalmol 1987;225:437-40.
64. Steinle NC, Gupta N, Yuan A, et al. Oral rifampin utilisation for the treatment of chronic multifocal central serous retinopathy. Br J Ophthalmol 2012;96:10-13.
65. Stewart JM. Half dose verteporfin PDT for central serous chorioretinopathy. Br J Ophthalmol 2006;90:805-6.
66. Von Graefe A. Ueber centrale recidivierende Retinitis, Graefes Arch Clin Exp Ophthalmol 1866;12:211-5.
67. Van Velthoven ME, Verbraak FD, Garcia PM, Schlingemann RO, Rosen RB, de Smet MD. Evaluation of central serous retinopathy with en face optical coherence tomography. Br J Ophthalmol 2005;89:1483-8.
68. Wang MS, Sander B, Larsen M. Retinal atrophy in idiopathic central serous chorioretinopathy. Am J Ophthalmol 2002;133:787-93.
69. Wang M, Sander B, la Cour M, Larsen M. Clinical characteristics of subretinal deposits in central serous chorioretinopathy. Acta Ophthalmol Scand 2005;83:691-6.
70. Wang M, Munch IC, Hasler PW, Prünte C, Larsen M. Central serous chorioretinopathy. Acta Ophthalmol 2008;86:126-45.
71. Wu ZH, Lai RY, Yip YW, et al. Improvement in multifocal electroretinography after half-dose verteporfin photodynamic therapy for central serous chorioretinopathy: A randomized placebo-controlled trial. Retina 2011;31:1378-86.
72. Wassermann GE, Olivera-Severo D, Uberti AF, Carlini CR. *Helicobacter pylori* urease activates blood platelets through a lipoxygenase-mediated pathway. J Cell Mol Med 2010;14:2025-34.
73. Yanuzzi LA. Type A behavior and central serous chorioretinopathy. Retina 1987;7:111-31.
74. Yannuzzi LA, Slakter JS, Gross NE, et al. Indocyanine green angiography-guided photodynamic therapy for treatment of chronic central serous chorioretinopathy: A pilot study. Retina 2003;23:288-98.

Treatment of Retinal Angiomatous Proliferation

Javier A Montero, Jose M Ruiz-Moreno, Jorge Ruiz-Medrano (Spain)

Retinal angiomatous proliferation (RAP) was first described by Yannuzzi et al in 2001[1] as a distinct form of neovascular age-related macular degeneration (AMD) characterized by an angiomatous proliferation originated from the retinal vascularization extending posteriorly into the subretinal space and eventually communicating with choroidal neovascularization (CNV). In this specific entity the initial neovascular event is the retinal angiomatous proliferation that extends into the deep retina and subretinal space, surrounded by pre, intra and subretinal hemorrhages and hard exudates. Fluorescein angiography (FA) usually shows an unspecific pattern with indistinct staining simulating occult CNV. Indocyanine green angiography (ICG) reveals a focal area of intense hyperfluorescence corresponding to the neovascularization.

Three distinct vasogenic stages can be defined in RAP. Stage I is characterized by proliferation of intraretinal capillaries (intraretinal neovascularization). Stage II is defined by the growth of the retinal vessels into the subretinal space (subretinal neovascularization). Eyes in stage III show a well-defined CNV.

Freund et al dubbed RAP as a type 3 CNV (following the previous classification of type I CNV for occult CNV and type II for classic CNV) when they observed that the neovascularization in RAP might originate from deep retinal capillaries as well as from the choroid.[2]

Even though it is generally accepted that RAPs are a part of the clinical spectrum of neovascular AMD, the management is frequently disappointing and the frequency of recurrences is high. Once the vascular complex is well-established, anatomical closure is rarely achieved. In 2005, Bottoni et al reported on the management of RAP in a retrospective study in which they revised 99 eyes from 101 patients with different stages of RAP, treated by laser photocoagulation, photodynamic therapy (PDT), and transpupillary thermotherapy. Complete obliteration of RAP was achieved in almost 60 percent of the stage 1 lesions, 26 percent of the stage 2 lesions and 15 percent of stage 3 lesions.[3] To make things worse, RAPs are frequently bilateral, the risk of neovascular involvement of the fellow eye is higher than in other exudative forms of AMD and the form affecting the fellow eye is almost always RAP, as was reported by Gross et al (Figs 39.1 to 39.3).[4]

One registered phase I/II open label interventional case series sponsored by the National Retina Institute (and several more

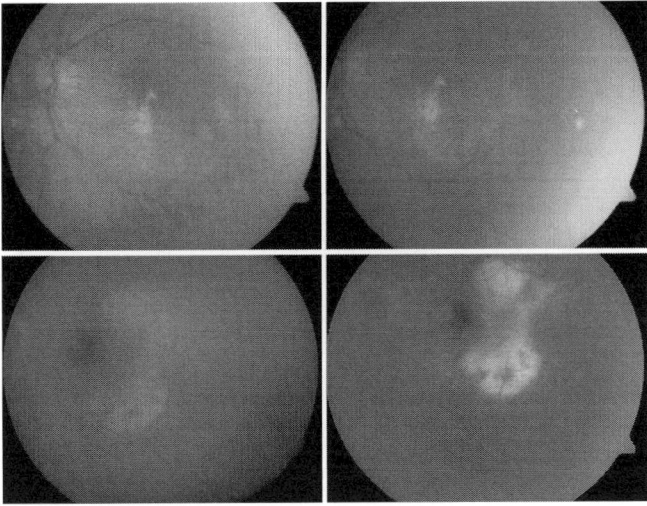

Fig. 39.1: Color retinography, red free retinography, and early and late phase fluorescein angiography in a patient with RAP stage III

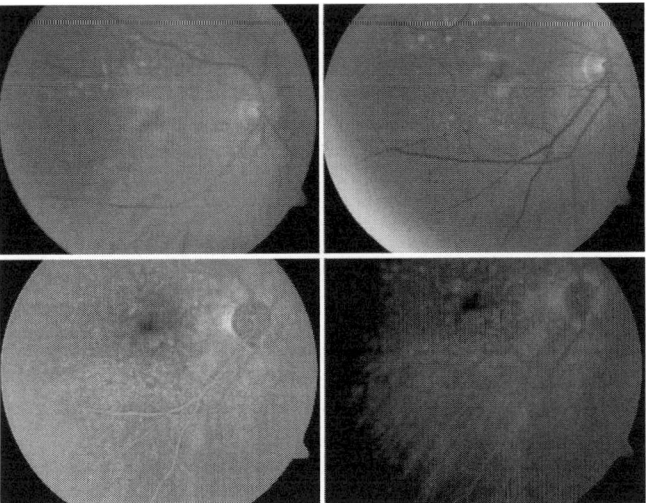

Fig. 39.2: Color retinography, red free retinography, and early and late phase fluorescein angiography of the fellow eye in the same patient as Figure 39.1. This eye presents drusen and a drusenoid foveal detachment without neovascular changes

unregistered trials) (http://clinicaltrials.gov) have been performed using different concentrations of monthly intravitreal ranibizumab (RAP study to determine safety/efficacy of lucentis for treatment of retinal angiomatous proliferation secondary to age-related

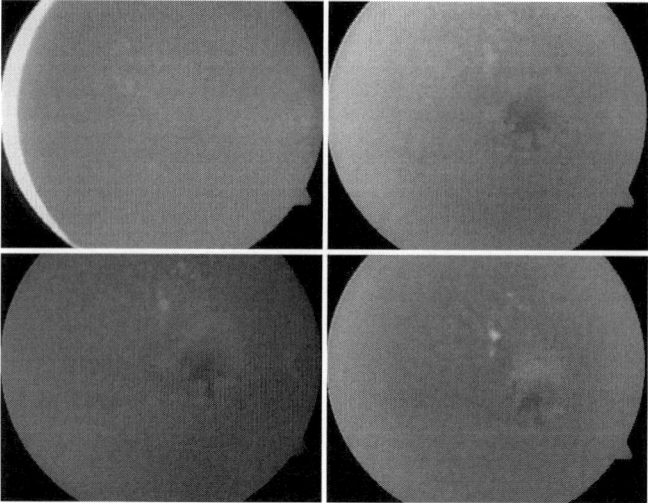

Fig. 39.3: The same eye as in Figure 39.2, six months later. The macula presents retinal hemorrhages and fluorescein leakage corresponding to RAP stage I

macular degeneration, NCT00395707). The trial was initiated in 2006 and last updated in February 2009 and tried to establish the proportion of patients with stabilization of visual acuity, vision loss of <15 letters, the proportion of subjects who gained at least 15 letters at 6 and 12 months and the incidence of ocular and systemic adverse events. However, the results of these trials have not been reported.

In this chapter, we shall summarize the most relevant facts about RAP treatment.

NATURAL HISTORY

The natural history of RAPs is heterogeneous. Viola et al reported in 2009 on the natural history and visual outcome of untreated RAP lesions on 14 consecutive patients (16 eyes) who were prospectively evaluated for a mean of 20 months. Mean visual acuity was 0.48 at baseline, decreased to 0.23 after 6 months, and was 0.19 at the final examination (mean decrease of 6 lines). By the time of the final examination, visual acuity was 0.1 or worse in 11 eyes, 10 eyes showed subretinal fibrosis and 9 eyes showed a retinal choroidal anastomosis (Fig. 39.4).[5] RPE and choriocapillaris atrophy are also a frequent finding in advanced forms of RAP.[6] Scott et al analyzed the data of the eyes with subfoveal occult CNV within the placebo arm of the verteporfin in photodynamic therapy (VIP) trial and their findings suggested that the true natural history of RAP lesion might be highly variable and similar to that of other CNV lesions.[7] Spontaneous resolution of RAP lesions is infrequent, but it has been reported at least by one group[2] and many more cases have probably not been reported.

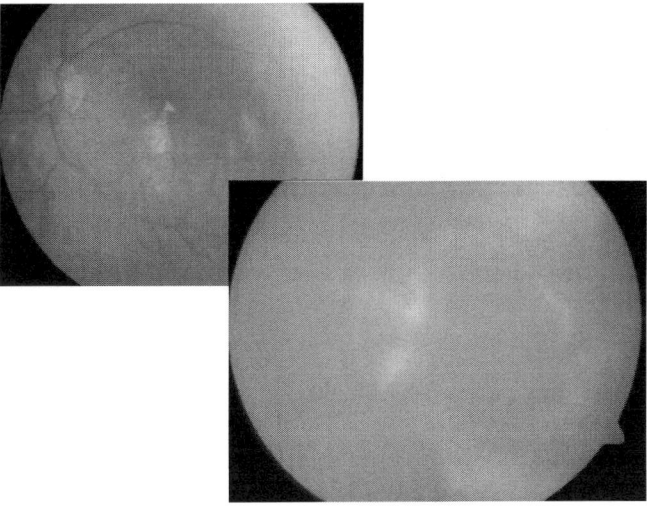

Fig. 39.4: Natural history of the eye in Figure 39.1. Notice the exudative macular detachment

Laser Photocoagulation

Laser photocoagulation has been performed in RAP as in other forms of exudative AMD. However, the reported outcomes have been irregular and highly dependent of the stage and the personal technique and skill of the treating physician. Borrillo et al reported good results through specific lysis of the feeding arteriole and draining venule of an RAP lesion that was followed by visual acuity gain and resolution of intraretinal edema and flattening of associated pigment epithelial detachment.[8] In a later series reported by Bottoni et al complete obliteration of RAP was achieved in about 73 percent of the stage 1 lesions by direct laser photocoagulation of the vascular lesion. Only 38 percent of the stage 2 lesions treated by scatter "grid-like" laser photocoagulation and 17 percent of those managed by direct laser photocoagulation of the vascular lesion succeeded.[3]

Johnson and Glaser[9] treated 16 eyes with stage I or II RAP lesions with green or yellow laser, applied to completely ablate the intraretinal component of the lesion with an average of 1.9 treatment sessions. After a mean follow-up of 15.5 months, 94 percent of eyes had stable or improved visual acuity. During the same year, Krieglstein et al[10] reported on a series of 13 patients with extrafoveal RAP stage I lesions treated by laser photocoagulation that was combined with the intravitreal injection of 4 mg triamcinolone before laser treatment in cases with marked macular edema. Visual acuity improved in five cases (2-5 lines), and stabilized in four cases (-1 to +1 line change), while exudation on fluorescein angiography was stopped in 11 cases.

More series with combined laser photocoagulation and intravitreal triamcinolone followed during the triamcinolone-rush years like those reported by Roth with micropulsed laser[11] and Mendis.[12] Triamcinolone acetonide injection preceded laser treatment by a median duration of 7 days, was simultaneous or followed laser treatment by a median duration of 7 days. Eyes were followed a median of 18 months after treatment. Visual acuity at 12 months and the last follow-up examination was stable or improved in almost 80 percent of the eyes. The median visual acuity before treatment was 20/200 compared with 20/80 at 3 months after treatment and 20/200 at 12 months. Elevated intraocular pressure occurred in 2 eyes and 7of 9 phakic eyes had cataract progression.[11]

Transpupillary Thermotherapy

Transpupillary thermotherapy (TTT) is based on the effect of low energy, near infrared diode laser (810 nm) delivered to the retina during one minute through a dilated pupil. This treatment raises the temperature of the tissue by 10°C inducing apoptosis and the appearance of heat shock proteins.[13]

Few reports appear in the literature regarding the use of TTT in RAP lesions, but the authors agree in the poor visual outcome in these cases, with the occasional appearance of retinal scars.[3,14,15]

Photodynamic Therapy with Visudyne

The retrospective analysis of the VIP trial[7] revealed the presence of RAP lesions among the patients with subfoveal occult forms of exudative AMD.

Treatment of RAP with quarterly PDT initially revealed successful in lesions with small pigment epithelium detachments (PED). Timely, PDT in the early stages and small lesions showed a potential for a beneficial effect on vision.[16] However, the visual outcome was poor in most of the cases.[17] Treated eyes show occlusion of RAP and PED flattening, persistence of PED or disciform lesions or hemorrhagic PEDs. Lesions with large PEDs exceeding 50 percent of lesion area eventually develop RPE tears.[18]

Combined surgical ablation of the inflow and outflow vessels and PDT was also unsuccessful and a high frequency of reperfusion from retinal inflow vessels was reported.[19]

Combined PDT and triamcinolone therapy showed a potential benefit in stage 2 RAP without large PED lesions[20] with up to 40 percent of the eyes showing short-term visual acuity improvement.[21-24] However, other authors did not find significant benefits in combined treatment.[25]

Our group performed a retrospective analysis of the relative efficacy of PDT, PDT associated with intravitreal triamcinolone and PDT associated with periocular triamcinolone in stage III lesions. Our findings suggested that combined PDT-intravitreal triamcinolone might offer better results than PDT monotherapy or PDT associated with periocular triamcinolone (Figs 39.5 to 39.7).[24] Intravitreal triamcinolone combined with PDT showed potential adverse effects, as in other intravitreal triamcinolone treatments (high intraocular pressure, cataracts), as well as macular atrophy that might lead to further visual loss.[26]

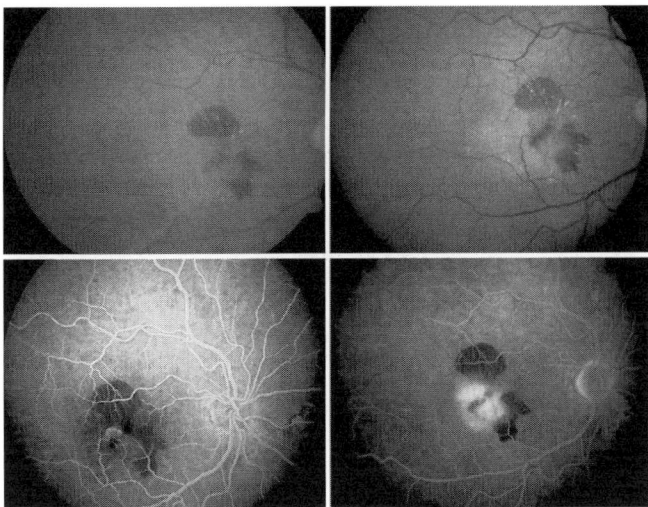

Fig. 39.5: Color retinography, red free retinography, and early and late phase fluorescein angiography of one patient with RAP II

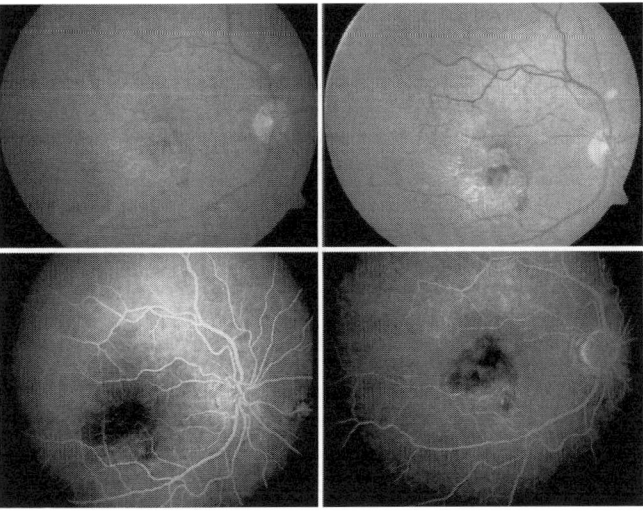

Fig. 39.6: Color retinography, red free retinography, and early and late phase fluorescein angiography of the same patient as in Figure 39.5, after treatment with intravitreal 20 mg triamcinolone and PDT. Notice the choriocapillaris ischemia in the treated area

High dose intravitreal triamcinolone combined with PDT leads to a marked resolution of the exudative lesion, even if a high incidence of recurrences was observed at 6 months,[27] supporting the hypothesis that these changes were caused by the effect of the intravitreal steroid rather than by PDT. In this regard, periocular

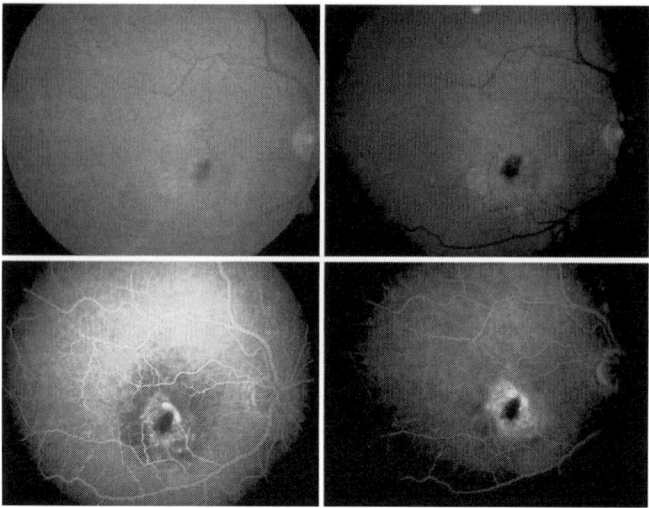

Fig. 39.7: Color retinography, red free retinography, and early and late phase fluorescein angiography of the same patient as in Figures 39.5 and 39.6. Reactivation of the treated lesion 8 months after treatment

and sub-tenon triamcinolone not combined with PDT showed a similar effect, delaying moderate to severe vision loss.[28]

Intravitreal Antiangiogenic Drugs

The use of intravitreal pegaptanib to treat RAP lesions has been seldom reported. Lommatzsch[29] performed a retrospective study on 7 eyes treated by intravitreal pegaptanib with disappointing results.

Systemic bevacizumab was initially used in the management of RAP lesions with good anatomical and visual outcome (7 letters gain) at three months.[30]

This treatment gave way to intravitreal injections of lower doses of bevacizumab with similarly good results. Costagliola et al performed intravitreal bevacizumab injections in eyes with RAP lesions refractory to PDT and observed a good visual response in stage I and II lesions with morphologic benefits in all RAP stages.[31] Other authors followed this line of treatment with similarly good results,[32-35] but soon it was clear that even if antiangiogenic treatment improved visual acuity and macular edema, it did not achieve a complete occlusion of feeder vessels.[36]

Our group reported on the effect on intravitreal bevacizumab on RAP lesions stages II and III.[37] In this paper, 26 eyes from 24 patients were treated by intravitreal bevacizumab with an average 3.3 injections. In this series intravitreal bevacizumab stabilized visual acuity during the first year, even though the visual outcome was better in RAP II lesions (Figs 39.8 and 39.9).

A short time after the first report on intravitreal bevacizumab for RAP, the results of intravitreal ranibizumab were reported.

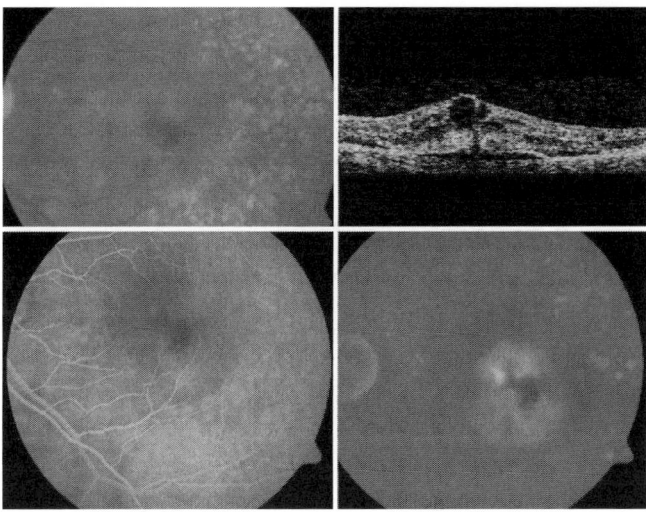

Fig. 39.8: Color retinography and optical coherence tomography in a patient with RAP stage II

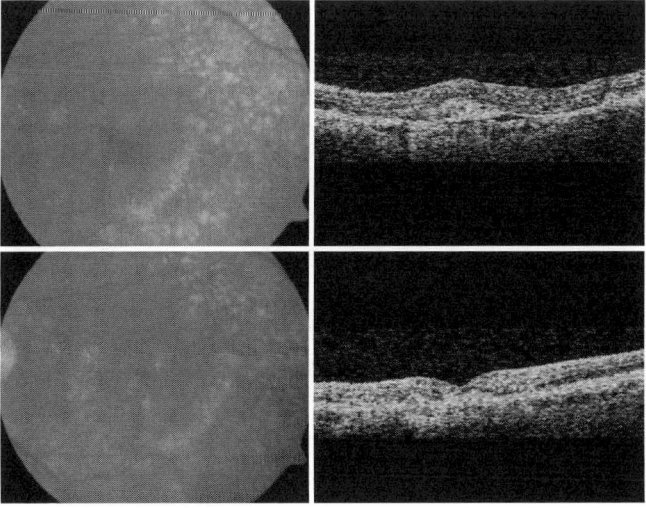

Fig. 39.9: Color retinography and optical coherence tomography in the same patient as Figure 39.8 after 1 (top) and 2 (bottom) intravitreal injections of bevacizumab

Lai et al reported on 4 cases who received 3 consecutive monthly injections. All four patients had visual improvement (mean, 3.0 lines) and complete resolution of subretinal fluid. However, and as in bevacizumab-treated cases, recurrences appeared months after commencement of treatment.[38] Konstantinidis[39] and Amani[40] performed an evaluation of visual and anatomic outcomes of patients with RAP treated by intravitreal ranibizumab during one year, finding that ranibizumab seemed to be an effective treatment for RAP, allowing stabilization of visual acuity and reduction of macular thickness.

Hemeida et al performed a retrospective evaluation of 20 eyes from 15 patients with RAP lesions, who had been treated by anti-VEGF injections (ranibizumab and bevacizumab) as monotherapy during more than two years. Sixty-two percent of the patients had stable or improved visual acuity at 2 years (not statistically significant beyond 3 months). Most of the cases (75%) required repeated treatments.[41]

In an attempt to adapt the current dosing regimes of AMD to RAP lesions, Engelbert et al performed a treat and extend regime to patients with RAP.[42] The treatment schedule was 3 initial monthly consecutive injections of ranibizumab, followed by continued treatment at intervals increasing by 2 weeks per visit, to a maximum of 10 weeks. In this group of patients the mean number of injections was 7 in the first year, 6 in the second year, and 7 in the third year, with an average gain of 3 lines (from 20/80 to 20/40) that was maintained during 3 years.

A recent study performed by Yamazaki et al revealed that the effect of intravitreal ranibizumab extends beyond the retina affecting the choroid. Subfoveal choroidal thickness decreased after the intravitreal injection during the subsequent months after the injection. The amount of choroidal thickness reduction was independent from the number of injections performed. The implications and consequences of this reduction of choroidal thickness are still unknown.[43]

Combined Therapies

As occurred with PDT and intravitreal triamcinolone, new attempts have been made to improve the results of intravitreal antiangiogenic drugs on RAP. A possible synergistic effect may arise from the combination of intravitreal bevacizumab and PDT for the treatment of RAP, as well as a possible benefit of combo therapy in the rate of intravitreal re-injections.

The timing of both treatments has not been properly established. PDT has been performed 0–1[44] or 1–2[45] days after intravitreal injection of bevacizumab, followed by 3 consecutive injections of bevacizumab. Saito et al observed a significant improvement in the mean BCVA, 1, 3 and 6 months after intravitreal bevacizumab injection and PDT. No patient had a decrease in the BCVA of 3 or more lines during any 6 months.[45] The authors also observed a significant decrease of central retinal thickness at 6 months. The treatment was effective during at least 6 months after the last sessions and no patients required retreatment during this period.

Viola et al performed a prospective study using PDT 7 days after the intravitreal bevacizumab injection on 21 eyes of 18 patients with RAP.[46] Seventy percent of the eyes had improved or stabilized visual acuity and foveal thickness decreased significantly at 9 months.

Intravitreal bevacizumab combined with PDT is significantly more effective than intravitreal triamcinolone with PDT in maintaining and improving visual acuity and in reducing the number of treatment for patients with RAP (Fig. 39.10).[47]

Intravitreal bevacizumab has also been combined with posterior subtenon injection of triamcinolone acetonide and reduced laser fluence photodynamic therapy as a triple therapy in RAP lesions.[48] Shirakata retrospectively evaluated the effects of this triple therapy on 15 eyes with RAP. The triple therapy was repeated if recurrences of retinal-retinal anastomosis or retinal-choroidal anastomosis and marked leakage from subretinal neovascularization were observed, whereas intravitreal bevacizumab as monotherapy was performed if only intraretinal exudative and/or hemorrhagic changes occurred. Visual acuity improved significantly in most of the cases (90%). The mean number of triple therapy performed during the 12-month study period was 1.2, and the mean number of bevacizumab monotherapy treatments was 1.4.

Treatment with intravitreal triamcinolone plus PDT may result in stabilization of the disease with better results than ranibizumab plus PDT in terms of functional and anatomical features according to one series. Rouvas et al compared the 3 years outcome of intravitreal ranibizumab (Group 1), intravitreal ranibizumab plus PDT (Group 2), and intravitreal triamcinolone plus PDT (Group 3) in 37 eyes with RAP.[6] Visual acuity remained stable or improved in most of the patients (60% in Group 1, 50% in Group 2, and 90% in Group 3). Patients in Group 3 received on average the lowest number of injections. However, geographic atrophy was detected in 0 percent in Group 1, 25 percent in Group 2, and 56 percent in Group 3.

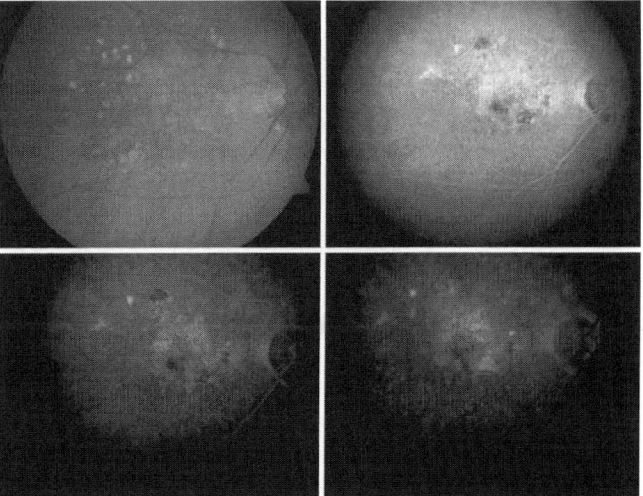

Fig. 39.10: The same eye as in Figure 39.2, 4 years after successful treatment with one single session of low fluence PDT combined with intravitreal triamcinolone the RAP remains silent. However, a progressive atrophy of the RPE can be observed

However, the simultaneous combination of PDT with bevacizumab or triamcinolone in patients with RAP may increase the hypofluorescent post-photodynamic therapy treatment spot due to an enhanced photochemical stress and ischemia in the normal choriocapillaris.[49] The consequences of these ischemic changes are still unknown.

CONCLUSION

Proper prospective, randomized trials are required since most of the results presented in this chapter are referred to retrospective and a few prospective case series.

At present, RAP is still a challenging condition within the spectrum of neovascular AMD. Different therapeutical approaches have been tried. Most of the authors agree that, even though the visual outcome seems to be better and better with the new therapeutical approaches, the main limitations are the frequent recurrences and the progressive atrophic changes in the choriocapillaris and RPE.

REFERENCES

1. Yannuzzi LA, Negrao S, Iida T, et al. Retinal angiomatous proliferation in age-related macular degeneration. Retina 2001;21:416-34.
2. Freund KB, Ho IV, Barbazetto IA, et al. Type 3 neovascularization: the expanded spectrum of retinal angiomatous proliferation. Retina 2008;28:201-11.
3. Bottoni F, Massacesi A, Cigada M, et al. Treatment of retinal angiomatous proliferation in age-related macular degeneration: a series of 104 cases of retinal angiomatous proliferation. Arch Ophthalmol 2005;123:1644-50.
4. Gross NE, Aizman A, Brucker A, et al. Nature and risk of neovascularization in the fellow eye of patients with unilateral retinal angiomatous proliferation. Retina 2005;25:713-8.
5. Viola F, Massacesi A, Orzalesi N, et al. Retinal angiomatous proliferation: natural history and progression of visual loss. Retina 2009;29:732-9.
6. Rouvas AA, Chatziralli IP, Theodossiadis PG, et al. Long-term results of intravitreal ranibizumab, intravitreal ranibizumab with photodynamic therapy, and intravitreal triamcinolone with photodynamic therapy for the treatment of retinal angiomatous proliferation. Retina 2012;32:1181-9.
7. Scott AW, Bressler SB. Retinal angiomatous proliferation or retinal anastomosis to the lesion. Eye (Lond) 2010;24:491-6.
8. Borrillo JL, Sivalingam A, Martidis A, Federman JL. Surgical ablation of retinal angiomatous proliferation. Arch Ophthalmol 2003;121:558-61.
9. Johnson TM, Glaser BM. Focal laser ablation of retinal angiomatous proliferation. Retina 2006;26:765-72.
10. Krieglstein TR, Kampik A, Ulbig M. Intravitreal triamcinolone and laser photocoagulation for retinal angiomatous proliferation. Br J Ophthalmol 2006;90:1357-60.

11. Roth DB, Scott IU, Gloth JM, et al. Micropulsed laser photocoagulation and intravitreal triamcinolone acetonide injection for the treatment of retinal angiomatous proliferation. Retina 2007;27:1201-4.
12. Mendis R, Leslie T, McBain V, Lois N. Combined therapy for retinal angiomatous proliferation with intravitreal triamcinolone and argon laser photocoagulation. Br J Ophthalmol 2008;92:1154-6.
13. Mainster MA, Reichel E. Transpupillary thermotherapy for age-related macular degeneration: principles and techniques. Semin Ophthalmol 2001;16:55-9.
14. Kuroiwa S, Arai J, Gaun S, et al. Rapidly progressive scar formation after transpupillary thermotherapy in retinal angiomatous proliferation. Retina 2003;23:417-20.
15. Olea JL, Sastre M, Aragon JA, et al. [Treatment of retinal angiomatous proliferation (RAP). A retrospective study]. Arch Soc Esp Oftalmol 2007;82:27-35.
16. Boscia F, Parodi MB, Furino C, et al. Photodynamic therapy with verteporfin for retinal angiomatous proliferation. Graefes Arch Clin Exp Ophthalmol 2006;244:1224-32.
17. Panagiotidis D, Karagiannis DA, Baltatzis S. Photodynamic therapy in retinal angiomatous proliferation stage I. Eur J Ophthalmol 2006;16:326-9.
18. Boscia F, Furino C, Sborgia L, et al. Photodynamic therapy for retinal angiomatous proliferations and pigment epithelium detachment. Am J Ophthalmol 2004;138:1077-9.
19. Nakata M, Yuzawa M, Kawamura A, Shimada H. Combining surgical ablation of retinal inflow and outflow vessels with photodynamic therapy for retinal angiomatous proliferation. Am J Ophthalmol 2006;141:968-70.
20. Mantel I, Ambresin A, Zografos L. Retinal angiomatous proliferation treated with a combination of intravitreal triamcinolone acetonide and photodynamic therapy with verteporfin. Eur J Ophthalmol 2006;16:705-10.
21. Nicolo M, Ghiglione D, Lai S, Calabria G. Retinal angiomatous proliferation treated by intravitreal triamcinolone and photodynamic therapy with verteporfin. Graefes Arch Clin Exp Ophthalmol 2006;244:1336-8.
22. Van de Moere A, Kak R, Sandhu SS, Talks SJ. Anatomical and visual outcome of retinal angiomatous proliferation treated with photodynamic therapy and intravitreal triamcinolone. Am J Ophthalmol 2007;143:701-4.
23. Hikichi T, Ohtsuka H, Higuchi M, et al. Combined intravitreal triamcinolone and photodynamic therapy for retinal angiomatous proliferation after photodynamic therapy. Nihon Ganka Gakkai Zasshi 2008;112:361-70.
24. Montero JA, Ruiz-Moreno JM, Sanabria MR, Fernandez-Munoz M. Efficacy of intravitreal and periocular triamcinolone associated with photodynamic therapy for treatment of retinal angiomatous proliferation. Br J Ophthalmol 2009;93:166-70.
25. Krebs I, Krepler K, Stolba U, et al. Retinal angiomatous proliferation: combined therapy of intravitreal triamcinolone acetonide and PDT versus PDT alone. Graefes Arch Clin Exp Ophthalmol 2008;246:237-43.
26. Sutter FK, Kurz-Levin MM, Fleischhauer J, et al. Macular atrophy after combined intravitreal triamcinolone acetonide (IVTA)

and photodynamic therapy (PDT) for retinal angiomatous proliferation (RAP). Klin Monbl Augenheilkd 2006;223:376-8.
27. Reche-Frutos J, Calvo-Gonzalez C, Donate-Lopez J, et al. Retinal angiomatous proliferation reactivation 6 months after high-dose intravitreal acetonide triamcinolone and photodynamic therapy. Eur J Ophthalmol 2007;17:979-82.
28. Rutishauser-Arnold Y, Tholen AM. Periocular sub-tenon triamcinolone acetonide injections for the treatment of retinal angiomatous proliferation (RAP) and occult choroidal neovascularisation. Klin Monbl Augenheilkd 2007;224:269-73.
29. Lommatzsch AP, Heimes B, Gutfleisch M, et al. Treatment of vascularised serous pigment epithelium detachment in AMD-observations after changing the intravitreal agent due to lack of response. Klin Monbl Augenheilkd 2008;225:874-9.
30. Abi-Ayad N, Mauget-Faysse M, Amara-Allieu S, Ardisson P. Systemic bevacizumab for retinal angiomatous proliferation associated with retinal pigment epithelial detachment. Eur J Ophthalmol 2007;17:987-91.
31. Costagliola C, Romano MR, dell'Omo R, et al. Intravitreal bevacizumab for the treatment of retinal angiomatous proliferation. Am J Ophthalmol 2007;144:449-51.
32. Kang JH, Park KA, Chung SE, Kang SW. Retinal angiomatous proliferation and intravitreal bevacizumab injection. Korean J Ophthalmol 2007;21:213-5.
33. Meyerle CB, Freund KB, Iturralde D, et al. Intravitreal bevacizumab (Avastin) for retinal angiomatous proliferation. Retina 2007;27:451-7.
34. Pedersen R, Soliman W, Lund-Andersen H, Larsen M. Treatment of choroidal neovascularization using intravitreal bevacizumab. Acta Ophthalmol Scand 2007;85:526-33.
35. Amselem L, Diaz-Llopis M, Cervera E, et al. Intravitreal injection of bevacizumab (Avastin) for retinal angiomatous proliferation. Arch Soc Esp Oftalmol 2008;83:53-6.
36. Joeres S, Heussen FM, Treziak T, et al. Bevacizumab (Avastin) treatment in patients with retinal angiomatous proliferation. Graefes Arch Clin Exp Ophthalmol 2007;245:1597-602.
37. Montero JA, Fernandez MI, Gomez-Ulla F, Ruiz-Moreno JM. Efficacy of intravitreal bevacizumab to treat retinal angiomatous proliferation stage II and III. Eur J Ophthalmol 2009;19:448-51.
38. Lai TY, Chan WM, Liu DT, Lam DS. Ranibizumab for retinal angiomatous proliferation in neovascular age-related macular degeneration. Graefes Arch Clin Exp Ophthalmol 2007;245:1877-80.
39. Konstantinidis L, Mameletzi E, Mantel I, et al. Intravitreal ranibizumab (Lucentis) in the treatment of retinal angiomatous proliferation (RAP). Graefes Arch Clin Exp Ophthalmol 2009;247:1165-71.
40. Atmani K, Voigt M, Le Tien V, et al. Ranibizumab for retinal angiomatous proliferation in age-related macular degeneration. Eye (Lond) 2010;24:1193-8.
41. Hemeida TS, Keane PA, Dustin L, et al. Long-term visual and anatomical outcomes following anti-VEGF monotherapy for retinal angiomatous proliferation. Br J Ophthalmol 2010;94:701-5.
42. Engelbert M, Zweifel SA, Freund KB. "Treat and extend" dosing of intravitreal antivascular endothelial growth factor therapy for type 3 neovascularization/retinal angiomatous proliferation. Retina 2009;29:1424-31.

43. Yamazaki T, Koizumi H, Yamagishi T, Kinoshita S. Subfoveal Choroidal Thickness after Ranibizumab Therapy for Neovascular Age-related Macular Degeneration: 12-Month Results. Ophthalmology 2012;119:1621-7.
44. Lo Giudice G, Gismondi M, De Belvis V, et al. Single-session photodynamic therapy combined with intravitreal bevacizumab for retinal angiomatous proliferation. Retina 2009;29:949-55.
45. Saito M, Shiragami C, Shiraga F, et al. Combined intravitreal bevacizumab and photodynamic therapy for retinal angiomatous proliferation. Am J Ophthalmol 2008;146:935-41 e1.
46. Viola F, Mapelli C, Villani E, et al. Sequential combined treatment with intravitreal bevacizumab and photodynamic therapy for retinal angiomatous proliferation. Eye (Lond) 2010;24:1344-51.
47. Saito M, Shiragami C, Shiraga F, et al. Comparison of intravitreal triamcinolone acetonide with photodynamic therapy and intravitreal bevacizumab with photodynamic therapy for retinal angiomatous proliferation. Am J Ophthalmol 2010;149:472-81 e1.
48. Shirakata Y, Shiragami C, Yamashita A, et al. One-year results of bevacizumab intravitreal and posterior sub-Tenon injection of triamcinolone acetonide with reduced laser fluence photodynamic therapy for retinal angiomatous proliferation. Jpn J Ophthalmol, 2012.
49. Rouvas AA, Papakostas TD, Ladas ID, Vergados I. Enlargement of the hypofluorescent post photodynamic therapy treatment spot after a combination of photodynamic therapy with an intravitreal injection of bevacizumab for retinal angiomatous proliferation. Graefes Arch Clin Exp Ophthalmol 2008;246:315-8.

Conjunctival Allergen Challenge for Evaluating Anti-inflammatory Therapy

Mitchell Friedlaender, Daphne Bresheaus (USA)

ABSTRACT

Background: Ocular allergic reactions are typically evaluated subjectively for erythema, edema and itching. Objective measurements may have greater accuracy and reproducibility than subjective methods.

Objective: To apply objective measurements of erythema, edema, and ocular surface sensation (the EES method) to ocular allergic reactions induced by conjunctival allergen challenge (CAC).

Method: Twenty allergic subjects were evaluated 5 minutes before and 5 minutes after CAC for objective and subjective signs of conjunctival erythema, edema, and sensation. Objective evaluations were determined by spectroradiometry (erythema), a fractional millimeter reticule in a slit lamp microscope eyepiece (edema), and esthesiometry (ocular surface sensation). Subjective evaluations were performed by observation (erythema and chemosis), and questioning the subject (itching). Repeat measurements were made after instillation of a vasoconstrictor/antihistamine eyedrop.

Result: Objective measurements of erythema and eyelid edema increased significantly after CAC ($p < 0.001$). Subjective measurements of erythema, chemosis, and itching also increased significantly after CAC ($p < 0.001$). The objective measurement of sensation decreased after CAC, but the change was not statistically significant. After treatment with a vasoconstrictor/antihistamine eyedrop, a significant decrease in erythema (but, not edema or sensation) could be measured objectively and subjectively ($p < 0.001$). There was a correlation between objective and subjective measurements of erythema and edema following CAC ($r_s = 0.838$ and 0.893, respectively), and for the reduction of erythema after treatment with a vasoconstrictor/antihistamine eyedrop ($r_s = 0.822$).

Conclusion: Ocular allergic reactions and the effects of antiallergic treatment can be measured objectively by the EES (erythema, edema, sensation) method, and subjectively, by observation and questioning.

INTRODUCTION

Conjunctival allergen challenge (CAC) has been used for over one hundred years to confirm the diagnosis of systemic allergy,[1] study the ocular features of the allergic reaction,[2-5] and evaluate antiallergic therapy.[6-9] Conjunctival reactions are typically graded subjectively on the basis of severity. Conjunctival erythema and conjunctival edema, or chemosis, are usually graded by observation on a 0-4 scale. Itching is graded on a 0-4 scale by questioning the subject. While subjective methods are useful for documenting large differences in allergic signs and symptoms, they are less useful for documenting small differences. In addition, a reaction may be graded differently when viewed by multiple examiners, and even a single examiner may grade two identical reactions differently.

Attempts have been made previously to evaluate ocular allergic reactions objectively by measuring ocular surface temperature,[2] chemical mediators in the tear film,[2,5,10-12] and cellular responses after CAC.[4,13,14] Such objective measurements are, for the most part, cumbersome, time consuming, expensive, and imprecise. For objective measurements to be useful in studies with multiple evaluations of large numbers of allergic patients, they must be quick, accurate, and easy to record.

Recently, we have found that allergic and toxic conjunctival reactions can be evaluated objectively with simple, accurate, and reproducible methods. Conjunctival erythema can be measured with a spectroradiometer, a device for measuring the color of reflected light.[15] Eyelid edema can be measured using a fractional millimeter reticule in the eyepiece of a slit lamp microscope. Ocular surface sensation can be measured with a esthesiometry.

The purpose of this study is to determine if conjunctival erythema, edema, and ocular surface sensation can be measured before and after allergen challenge, and after administration of vasoconstrictor-antihistamine eyedrops. We also sought to determine whether there is a correlation between erythema, edema, and sensation when measured objectively and subjectively.

METHODS

Conjunctival Allergen Challenge

Twenty subjects with allergy to either cat dander, grass, or ragweed were recruited. All subjects had participated in previous CAC studies, and all had positive skin and conjunctival tests to specific allergens when previously tested. The study was approved by the Scripps Clinic Human Subjects Committee, and all subjects signed approved consent forms. Thirty microliters of allergen were instilled in the inferior conjunctival cul-de-sac of both eyes beginning with a low dose (Table 40.1). If necessary, medium and high doses of allergen were instilled at 5-minute intervals until a moderate, subjective allergic reaction (itching = 2, and redness = 2) was achieved.

TABLE 40.1: Allergen concentrations used for conjunctival allergen challenge			
	Low	Medium	High
Cat dander	2,500 AU/ml	5,000 AU/ml	10,000 AU/ml
Grass	10,000 PNU/ml	20,000 PNU/ml	40,000 PNU/ml
Ragweed	10,000 PNU/ml	20,000 PNU/ml	40,000 PNU/ml

Objective Measurements

Erythema

Conjunctival erythema was measured using a PR-650 Spectrascan spectroradiometer (Photo Research Inc., Chatsworth, CA), 5 minutes before and 5 minutes after CAC. Using consistent room illumination and subject positioning, the spectroradiometer was placed on an adjustable tripod 18 inches from the subject's eye. With the subject looking up, a 5 mm focusing spot was positioned on the inferior bulbar conjunctiva. Using the u' measurement of the 1976 Commission Internationale d'Eclairage (CIE), a mean of three consecutive readings was calculated.

Edema

Anterior to posterior width of the lower eyelid margin was measured using a fractional millimeter reticule in the eyepiece of a slit lamp microscope (Haag-Streit, Bern, Switzerland). The measurement was made posteriorly from the gray line (the junction of the skin and conjunctiva at the lid margin) to the posterior most central eyelash.

Sensation

Ocular surface sensation was measured using the esthesiometer of Cochet and Bonnet (Luneau, Chartres, France). This device has an adjustable nylon filament which can be extended from 0 to 6 cm. With the filament fully extended, sensation was tested on the conjunctival side of the 6 o'clock limbus (the junction of the cornea and conjunctiva), one millimeter from the cornea. The filament was shortened by 0.5 cm increments until the subject perceived the sensation of touch. The shorter the filament, the more force is delivered to the eye, and the easier it is for the subject to perceive the sensation of touch. The filament length which first produced a threshold sensation of touch was recorded.

Subjective Measurements

Conjunctival erythema, chemosis, and itching were graded 5 minutes before and 5 minutes after CAC by observation at the slit lamp microscope, using a 0–4 scale (Table 40.2).

TABLE 40.2: Subjective grading of erythema, chemosis, and itching	
0	None
1	Mild
2	Moderate
3	Moderately severe
4	Severe

Instillation of Vasoconstrictor/Antihistamine Eyedrops

Fifteen minutes after CAC, eyes were randomized so that one eye of each subject received one drop containing 30 microliters of a solution of naphazoline hydrochloride 0.025 percent and pheniramine maleate 0.3 percent, and the fellow eye received 30 microliters of normal saline.

Repeat Measurements

All objective and subjective measurements were repeated 5 minutes before, and 5 minutes after instillation of eyedrops.

Statistical Analysis

Data were analyzed using a paired sample t-test. A probability value of 0.05 was considered statistically significant, and data are presented as means ± the standard deviation. Spearman rank-correlation coefficients were calculated to determine if there was a correlation between objective and subjective measurements.

RESULTS

Conjunctival Allergen Challenge

All 40 eyes had an onset of conjunctival allergic reactions within 5 minutes of allergen challenge, and all reactions achieved at least moderate intensity (redness = 2, itching = 2). Ten subjects required low dose allergen (6 cat dander, 3 grass, 1 ragweed), and 10 subjects required medium dose allergen (5 cat dander, 3 grass, and 2 ragweed). Both eyes of each subject required the same allergen dose in all cases, and reactions of the two eyes were of similar intensity.

Objective Measurements

Erythema

Conjunctival erythema increased after CAC (Fig. 40.1). The mean u' value for erythema before CAC was 0.280 ± 0.01, and the mean u' value 5 minutes after CAC was 0.293 ± 0.01 ($p < 0.001$).

Edema

Mean lower lid edema increased after CAC (Fig. 40.2). Mean lid edema before CAC was 1.10 mm ± 0.08 mm, and 1.31 mm ± 0.04 mm after CAC ($p < 0.001$).

Sensation

Ocular surface sensation decreased after CAC (Fig. 40.3). Mean ocular surface sensation before CAC was 3.2 ± 2.2 mm, and

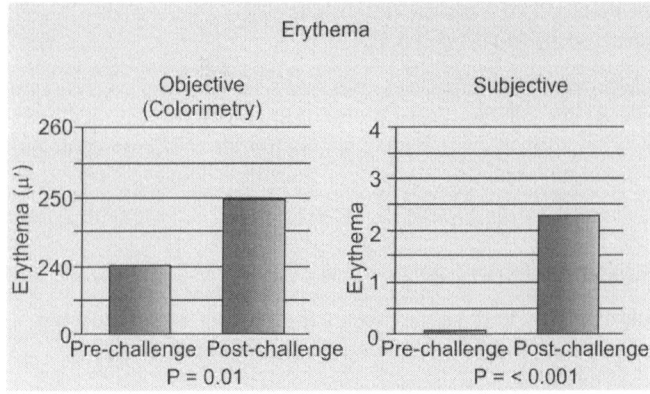

Fig. 40.1: Objective and subjective measurements of conjunctival erythema before and after conjunctival allergen challenge

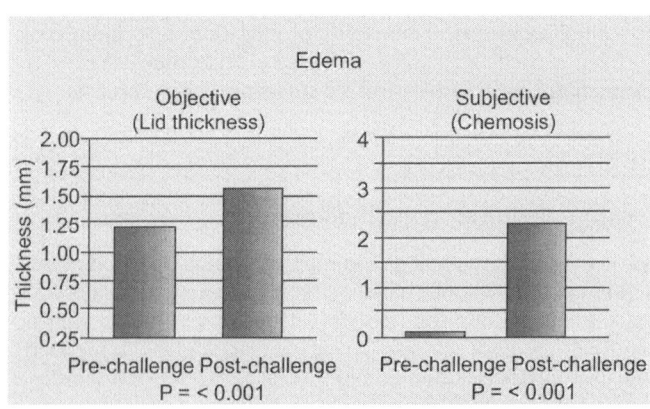

Fig. 40.2: Objective measurement of lower eyelid edema and subjective measurement of chemosis before and after conjunctival allergen challenge

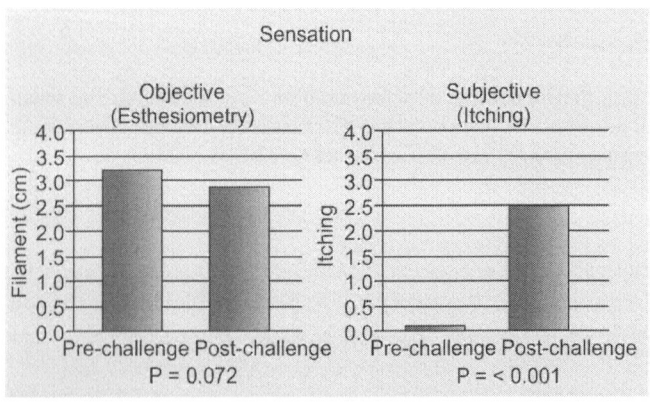

Fig. 40.3: Objective measurement of ocular surface sensation and subjective measurement of itching before and after conjunctival allergen challenge

3.1 ± 1.8 mm after CAC. This difference was not statistically significant (p = 0.72).

Subjective Measurements

Erythema

Erythema increased significantly after CAC (Fig. 40.1). Mean erythema before CAC was 0, and 2.0 ± 0.39 after CAC (p < 0.001).

Edema

Chemosis increased after CAC (Fig. 40.2). Mean chemosis was 0 before CAC, and 2.0 ± 0.42 after CAC (p < 0.001).

Itching

Itching increased after CAC (Fig. 40.3). Mean itching before CAC was 0, and 2.0 ± 1.2 after CAC (p < 0.001).

Statistical Analysis

Following CAC, Spearman rank-correlation analysis showed a correlation between objective and subjective measurements of conjunctival erythema (r_s – 0.838), and between lower lid edema and chemosis (r_s = 0.893).

SUMMARY

The results of objective and subjective testing are summarized in Table 40.3.

Repeat Measurements After Instillation of Vasoconstrictor/Antihistamine Eyedrops

In eyes receiving naphazoline/pheniramine eyedrops, objective erythema diminished from a mean u' value of 0.290 ± 0.02 to 0.278 ± 0.02 (p < 0.001) (Fig. 40.4). Objective evaluation of eyelid edema and ocular surface sensation did not change significantly. Subjective erythema decreased from 1.8 ± 0.02 to 0.08 ± 0.02 (p < 0.001), but itching, and chemosis, did not change significantly. There was a correlation between objective and subjective measurements of conjunctival erythema (r_s = 0.822).

In eyes receiving saline eyedrops, objective and subjective measurements of erythema, edema, itching and ocular surface sensation did not change significantly.

DISCUSSION

Objective measurements have the advantage of being highly reproducible, and free of subjective influences.[16,17] If objective measurements can be made quickly and accurately, they should be useful in CAC. Objective measurements would not be expected

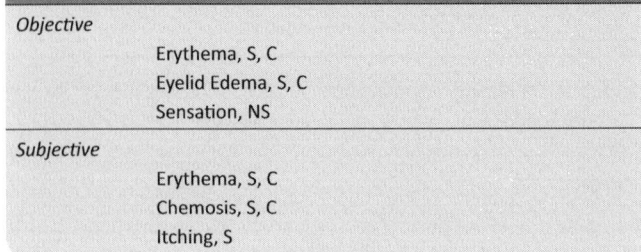

TABLE 40.3: Comparison of objective and subjective measurements of ocular allergic reactions before and after conjunctival allergen challenge indicating significant (S), or not significant (NS) changes and correlation (C) between objective and subjective methods

Objective	
	Erythema, S, C
	Eyelid Edema, S, C
	Sensation, NS
Subjective	
	Erythema, S, C
	Chemosis, S, C
	Itching, S

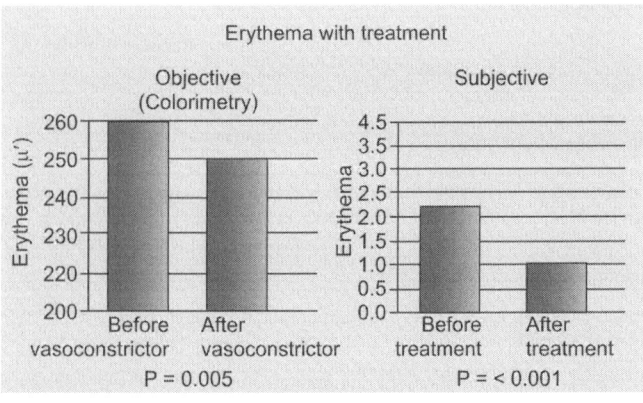

Fig. 40.4: Objective and subjective measurements of conjunctival erythema before and after treatment of ocular allergic reactions with one drop of a vasoconstrictor/antihistamine eyedrop

to vary from one study to another, or from one examiner to another. Erythema and edema measurements should be graded consistently on any given day by any given examiner.

Attempts have been made in the past to objectively quantify ocular inflammation after CAC.[2,11,12] These attempts have been cumbersome, variable, and sometimes expensive. Mediator studies are usually difficult to perform, and require highly precise collection techniques.[11] These studies involve lengthy and costly techniques which must be performed in a laboratory setting.

Ideally, objective measurements of ocular inflammation should be rapid and easy to perform. They should be standardized and adaptable from one center to another. Spectroradiometry, fractional millimeter measurements, and esthesiometry, the EES (erythema, edema, sensation) Method seem to fulfill the criteria for desirable objective measurements of ocular inflammation.

Spectroradiometry measures the color coordinates that describe any color in the visible spectrum. Color can be measured in several ways. We have chosen the u' coordinate of the 1976

Commission Internationale d'Eclairage. This measurement is easily obtainable, since it can be read directly from the display of the colorimeter, and it increases proportionally with increasing intensity of conjunctival erythema.

Eyelid edema can be easily measured with a fractional millimeter reticule in the eyepiece of a slit lamp microscope. Increased lid edema most likely reflects edema of the palpebral conjunctiva in response to mast cell degranulation following allergen challenge. We have chosen to measure the width of the lower eyelid centrally from the gray line posteriorly to the posterior most central eyelash. This direct measurement of lid thickness is straightforward and reproducible.

Esthesiometry is a technique for measuring corneal sensation.[18-20] The esthesiometer of Cochet and Bonnet is commercially available and easy to use. Our impression is that ocular surface sensation is slightly reduced after CAC, and the amount of reduction may be proportional to the intensity of inflammation. Although this study showed a mild reduction of ocular surface sensation following CAC, the reduction of ocular surface sensation from baseline levels was not statistically significant. We anticipate that further studies with larger numbers of subjects will help clarify the relationship of ocular surface sensation to the ocular allergic reaction.

These studies demonstrate that objective measurements of erythema, but not edema or ocular surface sensation, can be documented following treatment with a vasoconstrictor/ antihistamine eyedrop. A similar reduction in conjunctival erythema was reported following the use of vasoconstrictor/ antihistamine eyedrops in normal subjects.[21] This is not surprising, since these eyedrops are known to be highly effective in reducing conjunctival erythema. These drops are less effective in reversing edema and altering ocular surface sensation.

It remains unclear whether objective measurements are superior to subjective measurements for evaluating ocular allergic reactions. Subjective measurements showed greater differences in erythema, conjunctival edema, and itching from baseline evaluation to postchallenge evaluations. On the other hand, the small standard deviation of objective measurements suggests a certain precision and repeatability of objective measurements.

We believe objective measurements of the ocular allergic reaction provide new ways in which allergic reactions can be quantified. We believe that further study and refinement of objective measurements of ocular allergic reactions will improve our ability to measure these reactions with less variability and greater objectivity.

REFERENCES

1. Blackley CH. Experimental researches on the cause and nature of catarrhous acativas. In: Hay Fever or Hay Asthma. London: Bailliere, Tindal, Cox, Ltd; 1873.
2. Friedlaender MH. Conjunctival provocation tests: A model of human ocular allergy. Trans Am Ophthalmol Soc 1989;87:577-97.

3. Allansmith MR, Baird RS, Greiner JV, Bloch KJ. Late-phase reactions in ocular anaphylaxis in the rat. J Allergy Clin Immunol 1984;76:49-55.
4. Leonardi A, Secchi AG, Briggs R, Allansmith MR. Conjunctival mast cells and the allergic late phase reaction. Ophthalmic Res 1992;24:234-42.
5. Leonardi A, Borghesan F, Faggian D, et al. Tear and serum soluble leukocyte activation markers in conjunctival allergic diseases. Am J Ophthalmol 2000;129:151-8.
6. Friedlaender MH, Harris J, LaVallee N, et al. Evaluation of the onset and duration of effect of azelastine eyedrops (0.05%) versus placebo in patients with allergic conjunctivitis using an allergen challenge model. Ophthalmology 2000;107:2152-7.
7. Abelson MB, Allansmith MR, Friedlaender MH. Effects of topically applied ocular decongestant and antihistamine. Am J Ophthalmol 1980:90:254-7.
8. Ciprandi G, Cerqueti P, Sacca S, et al. Levocabastine versus cromolyn sodium in the treatment of pollen-induced conjunctivitis. Ann Allergy 1990;65:156-8.
9. Emmi L, Rossi O. A new H1-blocking antihistamine. Critical review of pharmacological and clinical studies [Italian]. Minerva Medica 2002;79:219-27.
10. Kari O, Salo OP, Halmepuro L, Suvilehto K. Tear histamine during allergic conjunctivitis challenge. Graefes Arch Clin Exp Ophthalmol 1985;223:60-2.
11. Proud D, Sweet J, Stein P, et al. Inflammatory mediator release on conjunctival provocation of allergic subjects with allergen. J Allergy Clin Immunol 1990;85:896-905.
12. Margrini L, Bonini S, Centofanti M, et al. Tear tryptase levels and allergic conjunctivitis. Allergy 1996;51:577-81.
13. Abelson M, Chambers WA, Smith LM. Conjunctival allergen challenge. A clinical approach to studying allergic conjunctivitis. Arch Ophthalmol 1990;108:84-8.
14. Bonini S, Magrini L, Rotiroti G, et al. The eosinophil and the eye. Allergy 1997;52:44-7.
15. Simpson T, Chan A, Fonn D. Measuring ocular redness: First and second order (luminance and chromaticity) measurements proved more informative than second order (spatial structure) measurements. Optom Vis Sci 1998;75 (Suppl):125.
16. Fieguth P, Simpson T. Automated measurement of bulbar redness. Invest Ophthalmol Vis Sci 2002;43:340-7.
17. Efron N, Morgan PB, Katsara SS. Validation of grading scales for contact lens complications. Ophthalmic Physiol Opt 2001;21: 17-29.
18. Beuerman RW, McCulley JP. Comparative clinical assessment of corneal sensation with a new esthesiometer. Am J Ophthalmol 1978;85:812-5.
19. Lawrenson JG, Corbett MC, O'Brart DPS, Marshall J. Effect of beam variables on corneal sensitivity after excimer laser photorefractive keratectomy. Br J Ophthalmol 1997; 81:686-90.
20. Barequet IS, Soriano ES, Green WR, O'Brien TP. Provision of anesthesia with single application of lidocaine 2% gel. J Cataract Refract Surg 1999;25:626-31.
21. Simpson TL, Sin T. The effect of topical vasoconstriction on bulbar redness measured objectively. ARVO Abstract, May 8, 2002.

Steroid Therapy for Allergic Ocular Disease

John D Sheppard (USA)

NEW CONCEPTS IN TOPICAL STEROID THERAPY

Ophthalmic use of steroids has been a balancing act for many years. Therapeutically the clinician must balance the benefits of steroids against the risks. Nevertheless, by avoiding steroids in the past, patients may not have received the optimal treatment for certain diseases. As a result, patients with ocular surface and corneal diseases can develop unnecessary pain, surface damage, and internal ocular cicatrization. As a student of ophthalmology, the astute clinician follows the lessons and embraces the ideas of respected mentors. But as the science has grown and changed, therapeutic options change as well. Now with more experience utilizing newer steroid molecules and more aggressive approaches to ocular inflammatory diseases including allergy, ophthalmology and optometry see a clear picture of appropriate steroid use, acknowledging the low incidence of side effects and embracing the potent therapeutic effects.

Treatment wisdom dictates that it is far better to utilize a potent agent infrequently as opposed to prescribing a weaker agent frequently. The more potent agent can be used as infrequently as once per day, thus improving compliance, reducing costs to the patient, and also reducing exposure of the ocular surface to preservatives found in most topical ocular anti-inflammatory agents. Steroids certainly fulfill this billet.

The True Risk to Benefit Profile for Allergic and Ocular Surface Disease

Years ago, instructors told soon-to-be-ophthalmologists that steroids were not a first-choice treatment because they carried serious risks.

Considerations include cataracts, 'steroid dependence,' IOP response, delayed wound healing and opportunistic infections made us fear corticosteroids. This fear was rooted in the strong corticosteroid molecules such as prednisolone acetate, which had serious potential side effects, particularly with chronic use. These agents controlled inflammation, but they were stronger than they typically needed to be, unlike modulated designer corticosteroids we can use today. Previously clinicians either avoided steroids completely except for severe blinding diseases, or discontinued treatment before it was effective or reduced the concentration to an ineffective level. Only by treating hundreds of external disease patients does the corneal external disease specialist as well as the comprehensive ophthalmologist learn that a little tincture of steroid is one of the most effective ways to control many types of ocular surface disease, including chronic dry eye, allergy and blepharitis. These 3 conditions represent the bulk of external diseases, and a significant percentage of emergency presentations to the eye care practitioner.

Another lingering idea is so-called steroid dependence. 'Steroid dependence' is not really dependence. Certainly, we have not seen addiction or classic withdrawal reactions from steroids. There is clearly a rebound in inflammation, however, when steroids are withdrawn too rapidly or without any weaning or tapering process whatsoever. There are two likely reasons for this misconception. First, some patients need steroids to manage chronic diseases where the blood-aqueous barrier has broken down. And second, patients might appear to need more steroids because they have not received enough steroids. They seem to rebound or develop new problems, but it is really a return of an inadequately treated condition.

Some patients develop chronic irreversible breakdown of the blood aqueous barrier due to severe disease, inadequately treated disease, misdiagnosed inflammatory disease, or poor compliance. It can be virtually impossible to control uveitis or eliminate flare in these patients. Similarly, chronic ocular surface inflammation due to atopic conditions can produce irreversible vascular changes in the lids and conjunctiva that remain perpetually inflamed or red despite massive regular doses of seemingly appropriate topical anti-inflammatory medications.

Insufficient Steroid Treatment Adversely Impacts Outcomes

Early intervention with corticosteroids can help save a patient's vision, although clinicians do not always seize this opportunity. One of the biggest problems in corneal external disease referral practices is under-utilization of topical steroids by referring physicians. By sparing the steroids early, they may be creating far worse outcomes for patients down the road. The sequelae to inflammation may be irreversible damage to the ocular surface, or even the retina and the eye itself. In the case of allergy, ocular surface scarring can occur in a number of locations, including the bulbar and tarsal conjunctiva, the lacrimal ductules, the cornea, and even the lids and adnexae. We can prevent this irreversible damage, and corticosteroids are usually the answer. Nervously withholding steroids will hurt patients in many ways. Withholding topical steroids in severe ocular surface disease or allergy are not beneficial in either the short-term or long-term for patient care. This decision to prescribe steroids hinges on a clinician's basic understanding of their role in treating inflammatory disease. Although it is compassionate to give a corticosteroid to control inflammation and make patients feel better, the most important goal is to interrupt the inflammatory and subsequent cicatricial process. If we see a reversible process, we can intervene early with corticosteroids and control the inflammation enough to return the patient's anatomy to normal. Topical steroids work wonders when begun early.

THE NATURE OF ALLERGIC DISEASE

Molecular Biology Allows Better Understanding of Ocular Allergic Diseases

Recent decades have seen an explosion of knowledge about the nature of allergic ocular disease. No longer accepted as part of aging or a necessary evil for the unfortunate, the disease is recognized as inflammatory in nature—and controllable. Remarkably, the basic mechanism of inflammatory ocular surface tissue damage is highly similar in patients with a wide variety of disease processes, including dry eye, allergy and blepharitis. Thus, adequate therapy for one disease may assist in control of concomitant disease. Similarly, the correct treatment for the wrong diagnosis may still produce patient satisfaction.

Reversible Inflammation

The inflammatory, reversible nature of allergic ocular surface disease is widely accepted today. If a patient has herpes and significant stromal inflammation, we prescribe steroids to prevent irreversible scarring and avoid a corneal transplant. Ocular allergy is the same type disease, and early anti-inflammatory therapy can achieve the same beneficial result. The target tissue here is generally the tarsal and bulbar conjunctiva, where severe protracted cases can produce sub-conjunctival scarring, eyelid deformity, trichiasis and entropion, and progressive gradual obliteration of the lacrimal ductules leading to dry eye.

Experience also has taught that ocular allergy sometimes has a systemic trigger. There is no doubt that ocular allergy is a biphasic inflammatory disorder, with an early phase histamine release and mast cell degranulation, followed by late phase reactants, vasodilation, leukocyte diapedesis, and long-term vascular permeability alterations. These changes can eventually lead to scarring, particularly with the onset of eosinophil major basic protein release, a highly toxic degratory protein responsible for the rapid corneal tissue loss seen in vernal ulcers among other processes. Systemic allergy, such as an exacerbation of rhinitis, sinusitis, eczema or asthma can trigger ocular allergy flares. Similarly, Stern and colleagues showed that dry eye also a true inflammatory disease, and in many patients, inflammation gradually progresses and tear production decreases. But some patients have a history of an acute episode of a systemic, sometimes infectious, disease followed quickly by an acute episode of severe dry eye. This is a systemic autoimmune phenomenon.

Thus, patients with inflammatory insult, from acute allergic conjunctivitis, to chronic vernal, to epidemic keratoconjunctivitis may develop cicatricial changes leading to lid disease or dry eye. These patients become contact lens intolerant and highly symptomatic around classic dry eye stimuli. The inflammatory stimulus triggers a mechanism that goes beyond the disease process and damages the entire ocular surface unit, from corneal nerves, to conjunctiva, to lids to lacrimal gland.

The cardinal aspect of ocular surface disease is that the underling etiology is many times driven by some sort of T-cell malfunction and therefore immunomodulation may be required. As cornea specialists, many clinicians have certainly realized that even a small dose of topical steroids does wonders for patients that have dry eye. As a rule, steroids reduce ocular surface inflammation and further normalize goblet cell numbers, for example, and reduce surface T-cell surface markers just as topical cyclosporine might. A number of companies are working on a lower dose, even lower yet than the concentrations that you might see in loteprednol as Lotemax 0.5 percent or Alrex 0.2 percent (Bausch & Lomb), Pred Forte (prednisolone acetate 1%), or FML (fluorometholone 0.1%, both Allergan), or a topical steroid that would reduce ocular surface inflammation as a primary treatment for the underlying etiology of the dry eye. Rimexolone (Alcon) in very low concentrations may be a useful agent for this strategy, and is currently in Phase III clinical trials.

COMBINED SURFACE DISEASES PRESENT DIAGNOSTIC CHALLENGES

Rapid Diagnosis of Dry Eye, Blepharitis and Allergy

Classic allergic disease is readily diagnosed, particularly when itching or systemic manifestations are obvious. Concomitant ocular disease is another story. A multifaceted phenomenon, dry eye disease can present as an amalgamation of different processes. Simultaneously, these conditions may include any combination of keratitis sicca, allergy, blepharitis, eyelid deformity, neurotrophic keratitis, nutritional deficiencies and previous eye surgery.

One of the most difficult aspects of managing dry eye is diagnosing it. First, patients do not always recognize their symptoms, describe them inaccurately or offer insufficient detail. Blepharitis or environmental changes can cloud the diagnosis as well. But once a clinician suspects dry eye disease, proper testing — in particular, supravital staining with fluorescein, lissamine and Rose Bengal—can clarify the diagnosis quickly. Once blepharitis is suspected, eversion of the superior tarsus similarly reveals the greatest amount of potentially diagnostic information.

Clarify Concomitant Ocular Surface Disease

Dry eye patient questionnaires include important questions like: Do your eyes feel dry? Itchy? Does it feel like you have something in your eye? When do your eyes bother you? What other medical conditions do you have? Thus it is possible to quantify not only the signs but also the symptoms of dry eye—redness, burning, itch, foreign body sensation. Although only some patients complain about these, others are stoic and do not mention them. It is very important to know what to look for and how to look. Patients often do not volunteer their history, especially if they have had a problem for years and see it as a normal part of getting older or common to everyone in their own age group. If we can train our staff to obtain a good history, we can diagnose patients early. Patients present with various combinations of dry eye signs and symptoms. Some patients feel bad and look good, and other patients look bad and feel good. Patients who look bad may have a neurotropic component so they just do not feel what they should, and neurotropic ocular surface disease can be extremely serious in its advanced stages.

It is important to caution against diagnosing allergy alone, advising further dry eye testing or tarsal eversion to rule out concomitant disease. Many corneal experts note that ocular allergies are over-diagnosed, and dry eye is very under-diagnosed, True itching is a symptom of allergic eye disease, along with burning, discomfort and other complaints, but the term 'itching' frequently sends us off on the wrong course. Patients often use 'itching' to describe foreign body sensation. Then we start looking for allergic eye disease and may prescribe anti-allergy medications to manage what is really dry eye. Conversely, patients treated with lubricants alone for dry eye will fare far better when treated for allergy utilizing a standard, aggressive anti-allergy regimen.

Tear Film and Schirmer Testing

If symptoms indicate dry eye disease, the next step is to administer standard tests. Measure the volume of the tear meniscus, look for debris and possibly check tear film break-up time using fluorescein. The gold standard in ophthalmology has been Schirmer testing with and without anesthesia. The Schirmer's test is important in diagnosing Sjögren syndrome. A score of 0—no wetting whatsoever—is a diagnosis of true Sjögren syndrome. Such a patient likely suffers from a systemic autoimmune disease and faces a risk of epithelial erosion or stromal melt, and should be observed and treated aggressively. Rose Bengal or lissamine green will show significant abnormal tear film disruption that fluorescein will not show, and are especially useful for delineating the degree of conjunctival surface diseases. These supravital stains are essential to ocular surface disease evaluations. Thus, with highly depressed Schirmer's tests or severe staining patterns, begin anti-inflammatory therapy that very day and send every such patient for a collagen vascular work-up to look for systemic disease. With fluorescein alone, we can detect dry eye only in its advanced stage. Rose Bengal or lissamine green will show significant abnormal tear film disruption that fluorescein will not show. By using either of these stains, we can detect conjunctival pathology in the interpalpebral area that we would certainly miss with fluorescein. Lissamine green staining is a key factor in diagnosing dry eye. Thus with supravital staining, physicians can better recognize dry eye disease. Improved understanding of the disease, combined with better treatment regimens, put reversal of this inflammatory disease within easy reach. The astute clinician understands and addresses the interaction of dry eye, allergy, blepharitis, environmental factors, and systemic disease when treating ocular surface inflammation.

Sjögren's Syndrome can Accompany Allergic Disease

Dry eye disease encompasses aqueous tear deficiency, mucin deficiency, lipid layer abnormalities and exposure due to eyelid abnormalities. In terms of aqueous tear deficiency, clinicians often differentiate between patients with Sjögren syndrome, which damages the lacrimal glands, and non-Sjögren patients.

This differentiation is intellectually important, however, the treatment for the two types of patients is the same today. Sjögren patients have more severe dry eye and are at risk for stromal inflammation and necrosis. In the past, we classified Sjögren patients as actively inflamed, in contradistinction to age-related acquired tear deficiency. Now, with awareness that all dry eye patients have inflammation in the conjunctiva and the lacrimal gland, our concept of the disease spectrum has changed our approach. Instead of using anti-inflammatories to treat only Sjögren syndrome, we use them to treat all aqueous deficient patients: it is just a matter of degree. The histopathology is identical for Sjögren and non-Sjögren dry eye. The FDA clinical studies of cyclosporine ophthalmic emulsion 0.05 percent (Restasis) showed the conjunctival biopsy proven histopathogenesis of ocular surface disease was the same among Sjögren and non-Sjögren patients, but the former had systemic problems that warranted action.

Sjögren-related uveitis, scleritis, keratitis or vasculitis may be the first presentation of extra synovial inflammatory disease. Early intervention is essential, before systemic problems develop, and referral to primary physicians or a rheumatologist may interrupt an otherwise devastating systemic illness.

INNOVATIVE STRATEGIES FOR OCULAR SURFACE DISEASES

Dry Eye and Ocular Allergy have Overlapping Therapeutic Profiles

Clinicians have finally started to think that other eye diseases might contribute to allergy. For instance, posterior blepharitis is one major disease category that clearly occurs concomitantly with dry eye and allergy.

As a result, clinicians would apply blepharitis treatments like topical steroids, oral doxycycline and warm compresses to dry eye, and the dry eye would improve as the lid disease improved. Similarly, allergy affects the entire conjunctival surface. With a chronically inflamed tarsus, the patient bathes the corneal epithelium with inflammatory cells and cytokines. Thus, allergy patients may have seasonal or environmental exacerbations of dry eye symptoms and vice versa.

Now, that we understand that inflammation is the key component of dry eye as well as allergy, we have entered a new era of formulating concomitant therapy for the condition. The intention is to simplify the regimen while reducing toxicity from topical medications. Substituting an aqueous replacement simply washes the problem away temporarily. What really needed is better endogenous tear production, both in quality and quantity.

At first, encounter with a moderate to severe dry eye patient, an anti-inflammatory agent prescription is clearly indicated instead of punctal occlusion. The prescription form of cyclosporine ophthalmic 0.05 percent emulsion (Restasis) in low concentration, with high bioavailability and a specially formulated micelle lipid base, gives us an agent that replaces the aqueous component and lipid component of tears. By replacing the essential oil and mucin tear layers while providing an ideal delivery strategy for the cyclosporine the 0.05 percent topical cyclosporine emulsion is biochemically designed and formulated to control ocular surface inflammation. Restasis compared to much higher but less bioavailable concentrations of cyclosporine that were used in the past clearly has less better tissue penetration with lower toxicity. Restasis has been effectively utilized for patients with concomitant allergy and dry eye, as well as vernal and atopic disease.

Newer agents are under investigation to eliminate safely the tear film deficiency and surface inflammation of dry eye disease. These include, FK-506 or tacrolimus (Sucampo), pimecrolimus (Novartis), Ecabet sodium (Ista), and the P2Y2 agonist diquafasol tetrasodium (Prolacria, Inspire), a secretagogue. Pimecrolimus (Elidel cream dermatologic) and Tacrolimus (Protopic ointment dermatologic) have been tainted by recent reports of a potential link with cancer. Topical ocular investigations of tacrolimus have as a result been terminated.

Clinicians have also begun to link dry eye with systemic medications, such as antihistamines, antidepressants, diuretics and such HMG Co-A reductase inhibitors as Mevacor, Zocor and Lipitor. But no one until recently realized the importance of inflammation to the condition. Thus a strong common link to allergic ocular surface disease.

In the past, a diagnosis of dry eye prompted a therapy regimen that usually included: treatment of aggravating factors, such as blepharitis; tear supplementation; lid hygiene; and finally, punctal occlusion. Many patients were not well served. Tear substitutes are still address aggravating factors, but inflammation control is still central to improvement.

Punctal Occlusion, Past and Present

Prior to modern punctual plug technology, dry eye patients received punctual occlusion through cautery or pre-cut cat-gut or collagen dissolving temporary plugs. Prior to the advent our understanding of inflammation as the underlying etiology of dry eye, punctal occlusion was a primary therapeutic intervention. This approach has changed drastically as both the literature and clinical experience revealed problems with early punctal occlusion. Now the paradigm has really changed because we know plugs can trap 'bad tears.' Pflugfelder and colleagues have shown that punctal occlusion can worsen a Schirmer test score, and premature occlusion can harm the biofeedback loop to the ocular surface enervation. In the old paradigm, we gave dry eye patients some artificial tears and occluded their puncta. The eyes looked moist, but they were still red and painful. The patient had more tears and maybe even a better Schirmer's test, but often was not content. Using a bathtub analogy to describe the situation, one would obviously drain the dirty water and refill it before the next bath. The same applies to punctal plugs: in an eye with inflammatory mediators like cytokines, interleukin and neutrophils, punctual plugs trap these inflammatory cells on the ocular surface. With the new anti-inflammatory approach, treatment improves not only the quantity of tears, but also the quality of the tear film on the ocular surface.

In this approach, physicians start by improving the quality of the tear film, eliminating the cytokines, down-regulating the T-cell activation on the ocular surface and improving goblet cell production and the mucin layer of the tear film by reducing ocular surface inflammation. If anti-inflammatory therapy does not work or it does not work completely—and that often happens in moderate and severe cases—then follow with punctal occlusion 4 to 6 weeks after starting anti-inflammatory therapy. The occlusion therapy can be trialed with properly sized collagen plugs, then after a month of no epiphora, a silicone plug inserted.

By prescribing an anti-inflammatory first, physicians have greater success with punctal occlusion. The anti-inflammatory makes a big difference because we mitigate pro-inflammatory mediators of the pain seen in allergy and dry eye. If a new patient already has punctal plugs, anti-inflammatory therapy is still recommended, although not the preferred order.

Therapy for Every Allergy Level

The first line of treatment for ocular allergy depends on the degree of disease severity. Many patients already are using some type of over-the-counter artificial tears or vasoconstrictor. If a patient presents with mild allergy, it is best to continue with a tear replacement, with preference to preservative-free or vanishing preservative preparations, such as Refresh (Allergan), Systane (Alcon) or GenTeal (Novartis). These generally produce a less toxic effect on the ocular surface.

Physicians also must consider patients' other medications or practices that may exacerbate pre-existing allergic and dry eye disease and interfere with therapy. Many of these patients need better contact lens-wearing regimens, or they should stop wearing their contact lenses, particularly if there is concomitant dry eye and allergy. Patients with superior tarsal disease are also prone to more severe contact lens intolerance. Some can also taken off oral diuretics because they were taking them unnecessarily for underlying hypertension or resolved fluid retention. It is incumbent upon clinicians to help patients identify and control environmental situations that aggravate their dry eye and allergic disease. Patients might stay up late at night and not use their artificial tears, or sleep upon dust mite infested or down pillows. They might have terrible humidity control in the winter, or an adverse work environment laden.

Nutrition is also an important topic for discussion. Some patients have a soda-and-potato-chips diet, which robs their mucus membranes of essential dietary components, including essential fatty acids like gamma linoleic acid (GLA) and omega-3 fatty acids, which are very good for dry eye as well as allergy. Similarly, poor diets are laden with pro-inflammatory omega-6 fatty acids, saturated fats, and trans fats, all of which upregulate inflammatory pathways that worsen allergic disease.

Basic education about dry eye disease, allergic environmental factors, and proper contact lens care are an essential element of early therapy. Patients often arrive in our offices dissatisfied because they have not had anti-inflammatory treatment, and they demand a cure. Allergy, dry eye and blepharitis are not curable. This is a lifelong process, and the disease can progress with age or repeated insult.

Treating Moderate to Severe Disease

Moderate to severe allergic disease is easy to detect. Severe itching, redness, papillary tarsal conjunctivitis, discharge, limbal hyperemia, and even chronic follicles betray the underlying allergic etiology. On the other hand, patients with moderate to severe dry eye can be challenging to detect. Regardless, early diagnosis is essential for their ocular health.

We need to examine high-risk dry eye patients carefully. This group includes people who take medications that dry their eyes, have collagen vascular disease, are postmenopausal, abuse contact lenses or work in a very dry environment. They may have severe, rapid disease progression without even feeling the symptoms.

Once diagnosed with moderate to severe dry eye, anti-inflammatory therapy should be started immediately. When patients are using transiently preserved tears but are still breaking through on this therapy and showing dry eye signs and symptoms, they always need anti-inflammatory therapy. Signs may be minimal with subtle fluorescein, lissamine green or Rose Bengal staining, and minimal depression of the tear meniscus. Many of the most severely affected patients receive two medications, cyclosporine ophthalmic emulsion 0.05 percent (Restasis) bid and loteprednol etabonate ophthalmic suspension (Lotemax or Alrex) bid. The loteprednol induces an initial rapid response with increased comfort; and the cyclosporine provides preservative-free immunomodulation in the long-term. Patients can use the loteprednol during the day and the cyclosporine before and after sleeping. Those who have stinging trouble with cyclosporine may go on qid loteprednol. Those who do not tolerate loteprednol can use chilled cyclosporine tid to start.

Dosages can be titrated to individual needs. For example, increase the dosage and frequency of loteprednol with the severity of dry eye disease—low for mild to moderate patients, higher for severe patients and highest for patients with concomitant ocular surface disease. One might prefer the lower concentration of loteprednol found in Alrex for mild cases.

Combining agents produces many favorable results. Not only do patients have a better experience with this approach, but they also have better outcomes with this combination. The loteprednol and the cyclosporine both have anti-inflammatory effects, but they use different mechanisms of action on different stages of the inflammatory process. Together, the dual-action mechanism and the synergy between the two drops deliver better outcomes faster. It is desirable to bring the ocular surface to homeostasis at about 4-6 months, and then see patients less frequently—enough to pick up any changes.

Tapering and Titration

In severe or chronic cases, better judgment warns against tapering steroids early, even when patients feel better. Instead, strive to eliminate every last cell in a uveitic patient, every last papillae in an allergic patient, and every last punctuate corneal stain in a dry eye patient. If absolute control is not established, then as dosage of steroids is decreased, the patient will show a rejuvenated response and have an increased risk of developing terrible consequences, such as chronic inflammation, cicatrization, chronic cystoid macular edema with cystic edema, and even epiretinal membrane formation in severe atopic patients or complex postoperative cases. Patients with advanced uveitic disease, for example, may develop hypotony as the ciliary body shuts down. Similarly, we do not want to allow permanent structural changes in the lacrimal gland, limbal stem cells or conjunctival mucosa. Allergic patients can exhibit prolonged post cataract cystoid macular edema, presumably because the choroid, and not the conjunctiva, contains the highest concentration of mast cells in the body.

Regardless of the etiology of ocular surface inflammation, begin tapering anti-inflammatory medications for patients who are feeling well at about the 6-month mark. However, they still need to use the medications to treat any acute episodes that arise. Patients will have episodes of discomfort, so they must use loteprednol 0.5 percent one to four times a day on those days. There is no standard for tapering loteprednol in dry eye patients because the disease is so individual. It is necessary to titrate the medication to the disease. Patients with concomitant ocular surface disease—perhaps blepharitis or severe periocular cutaneous allergy, vernal or tarsal conjunctival changes or concomitant rosacea—receive a higher initial dose and maintenance dose of loteprednol or other steroid. Exacerbations may be more frequent and require pulse-dosing at a higher frequency and intensity. With loteprednol it is possible to titrate to the patient, the disease and the response. In the long run, it enables minimization of the cumulative dose. Loteprednol's markedly reduced risk of glaucoma and cataract enables this facility.

Perspective on Risks

Because ketone steroids, loteprednol and cyclosporine work so differently and cyclosporine performs well as a constant bid medication, it is not usually necessary to taper cyclosporine in patients on both drugs. In the Ilyas study, patients on loteprednol 0.2 percent for years had insignificant risks for glaucoma. Part of the individualized approach to tapering anti-inflammatory medications is thus to lower the dosage. The 0.2 percent (Alrex) dose is lower, and the safety profile is even better than that of loteprednol 0.5 percent (Lotemax).

Far from ignoring the possibility of steroid-related risks, clinicians should choose to put them in perspective. Although steroids are less risky with close observation and newer formulations, we still have to remember the risks and the benefits. We can fix cataracts, but we can not fix permanent cicatrization of the ocular surface, obliteration of the lacrimal ductules or changes in corneal clarity. Corneal ectasia and opacification are irreversible changes, often necessitating a $25,000 corneal transplant. Many severe corneal problems, including severe scarring from vernal corneal ulceration, can be eliminated or controlled rapidly with topical steroids.

Environmental Control

In addition to sophisticated topical anti-inflammatory medications, environmental control is key to the control of ocular surface diseases. For the allergy patient, even on aggressive topical therapy, simple removal of antigens through intelligent management of the sleep and work space can provide tremendous relief and thereby a reduction in required medications. For the dry eye patient, removal of convection currents from fans and open window or convertible automobiles can make a huge difference. For both diseases, hand washing and avoidance of eye rubbing behavior is important to reduce mast cell degranulation and itching, and to avoid secondary bacterial infections and lash deformities associated with excessive lid manipulation.

One of the worst challenges is air travel where the relative humidity is below 20 percent. Thus, always forewarning patients prior to airline travel is judicious. Occasionally patients with known pre-existing dry eye return from dry climates with corneal ulcers because of the unfamiliar low humidity in that environment. Such an environmental change warrants patient education and increased lubrication. Many seaside locations on the other hand are blessed with year-round natural humidification.

BLEPHARITIS EXACERBATES DRY EYES AND ALLERGY

Cornea specialists see a great deal of blepharitis or chronic meibomian gland dysfunction. These patients experience significant discomfort and often take time to receive a diagnosis. As with dry eye disease, clinical findings for blepharitis point to inflammation as the basis of pain and discomfort. Fortunately, with accurate diagnosis and proper treatment, these patients can get much-needed relief.

Blepharitis Diagnosis

Blepharitis, also called meibomianitis or meibomitis for posterior lamellar lid disease, is caused by inspisation of the meibomian glands. Normal lipid secretions do not melt at body temperature, so they become saturated fats effectively cloggin the meibomian gland orifices. Bacteria grow in these lipids and secrete degratory enzymes such as lipases and collagenases, sequentially leading to lid ocular surface inflammation. Ocular surface stability breaks down because the lipids degrade into soaps and fatty acids. The tear film becomes inflammatory, which is a good reason not to put plugs in these eyes as a first line treatment. Plugs actually trap unhealthy tears on the ocular surface, exacerbating symptoms. This situation is often unrecognized clinically.

Tear film break-up time in these patients is generally shortened. The tear film has lost its lipid layer over the surface, so the diagnosis is readily apparent. When bubbly tiny soap suds appear in the meniscus and along the lower lid margin, normal lipid is breaking down into soaps and fatty acids: classic meibomian gland dysfunction.

Schirmer test results may be normal or even high for these patients because this blepharitis causes an evaporative dry eye. Blepharitis can have serious long-term effects, so fast diagnosis and effective treatment are important. Chronic inflammation can cause corneal scarring, so these patients are at high risk for eventual costly corneal transplantation. Whenever corneal neovascularization (KNV) and corneal scarring are findings, aggressive therapy is indicated. Patients with blepharitis also may have no corneal symptoms, but their conjunctiva may be minimally injected. One characteristic of all blepharitis patients is discomfort, whether it is pain, burning, ache, or photophobia.

Patients with blepharitis frequently have rosacea, regardless of their race, so secondary infections are common. Treatment with both systemic and topical medications, as well as lid scrubs and dietary changes is indicated.

Topical Ointments: Bacitracin and Erythromycin

Meibomian gland dysfunction often results in secondary infections. The most likely culprit is *staphylococcus*, so a rotation between erythromycin and bacitracin provides good gram-positive coverage. After a short-term trial with bacitracin ointment for a month or two, a switch to erythromycin helps because prolonged use of a single antibiotic will create resistance. Many staphylococcal organisms are already resistant, particularly to Erythromycin, but much higher levels can be obtained with surface application than with systemic drugs, the standard upon which MIC data are based. Thus the surface concentration afforded by drops and ointments may sufficiently surpass standard MIC levels utilized in all microbiology laboratories.

Systemic Therapy

Blepharitis is a chronic disease, so patients require continuous treatment. The centerpiece is anti-inflammatory therapy. Blepharitis patients are at risk for KNV, which can progress to opacification, so aggressive first-line therapy wtih oral doxycycline, hot compresses and dietary supplements containing flaxseed and fish oils is recommended. Among the tetracyclines, doxycycline has a greater anti-inflammatory, anti-collagenolytic effect than tetracycline or minocycline. For patients with gastrointestinal intolerance, minocycline may be preferred.

With blepharitis, it is important to start the patient on a preservative-free topical solution, and then when they are comfortable, one can have the luxury of switching to a transiently preserved artificial tear solution. Topical steroids are also very helpful in the initial and long-term strategic picture. Above all, however, the oral agents have proven efficacious, particularly for posterior lamellar disease. Patients can start with doxycycline, 50 mg four times a day, or 100 mg bid, always with food. High-dose tetracycline is less effective and far less well tolerated: only 50 percent of patients can continue high doses because of gastrointestinal side effects and photosensitivity. A lower 20 mg doxycycline preparation (Periostat) given bid is also acceptable anti-inflammatory, anti-lipid drug therapy.

Many patients, especially those with rosacea, may need to take doxycycline for a prolonged period. There is generally little difficulty in prescribing male patients with nearly continuous doxycycline therapy when indicated, giving perhaps a 1 month hiatus every summer when the sun is highest. Some have been successfully treated with low dose doxycycline for decades. After 2–4 months of treatment, patients can initially stop the medication if they get better. If symptoms come right back, they must necessarily resume therapy. A significant number of patients take doxycycline for 3 or 4 months, stop it for a few months, and then go back. Some patients can learn to titrate their own medication.

Tetracyclines have been in use for a long time for meibomitis, a very comfortable method of treatment. However, a February 2004 issue of The Journal of the American Medical Association looked at antibiotic risk and antibiotic use in relation to the risk of breast cancer. The investigators found that with the tetracyclines, those women who cumulatively were on tetracycline for longer than seven weeks doubled their risk of getting breast cancer and doubled their risk of dying from breast cancer. The effect was related specifically to cumulative dose. Currently there is a one in eight risk that a woman will get breast cancer anyway: therefore with chronic tetracyclines we are potentially doubling that risk to one in four. This is a major clinical, psychological and medico-legal concern.

As a result of that keynote publication, therapeutic recommendations have to be altered for women who might require chronic oral doxycycline therapy. For patients with mild to moderate meibomitis or posterior blepharitis on omega-3 supplementation alone, oral antibiotic therapy is not necessary. Those severe blepharitis sufferers with severe disease can be kept on low-dose doxycycline, 20 mg or 50 mg a day, along with omega-3 supplementation, with informed consent regarding the breast cancer risk of course. In more severe patients, simply stop the doxycycline at four weeks and then maintain on omega-3 supplementation alone. Unfortunately, no alternative regimen exists for these severely affected female patients. On the horizon is a topical doxycycline preparation (Alacrity) which may revolutionize the treatment of ocular rosacea, but will not benefit patients with facial cutaneous disease.

Loteprednol, Metronidazole, Topical Doxycycline, and Cyclosporine

For particularly challenging patients with significant conjunctival injection and corneal findings, long-term topical anti-inflammatory therapy becomes mandatory. Newer agents such as loteprednol 0.5 percent (Lotemax) are indicated. Loteprednol has a well-documented dual safety and efficacy profile resulting from its retro-metabolic engineered ester biochemistry. This allows for breakdown of all free steroid molecules into bio-inactive compounds if not initially bound to the glucocorticoid receptor. Other topical ketone steroids such as prednisolone acetate, dexamethasone or rimexolone can be prescribed, but with closer attention to the potential for secondary steroid induced glaucoma. Many of these patients are truly members of the "steroid for life club," which includes severe blepharitis, severe chronic dry eye, ocular cicatricial pemphigoid, post chemical burn, Stevens-Johnson, severe Vernal, atopic keratoconjunctivitis, corneal allograft patients, and uveitis sufferers.

Patients respond quickly to topical steroids like loteprednol 0.5 percent. Some patients have chronic pain without corneal pathology. They utilize lid hygiene with preferred products such as Ocusoft (Cynacon) or Eye Scrub (Novartis) and take doxycycline, yet the eye remains uncomfortable. For these topical steroids provide rapid relief. A starting dose of four times a day with subsequent taper, either to intermittent use or twice a day long-term to control inflammation and discomfort.

Several other topical and systemic compounds have useful secondary anti-inflammatory effects. These include metronidazole, which is available in oral or topical form from a compounding pharmacy. Some patients with rosacea find it helpful to use the ointment on their eyelids. Many with concomitant oculo-facial disease respond to topical therapy to the skin on the nose, cheeks, or chin. This is accomplished with metronidazole 1 percent gel (Galderma) or metronidazole 0.75 percent lotion or cream.

Steroids also can work well in combination with cyclosporine ophthalmic emulsion 0.05 percent (Restasis). Cyclosporine is helpful for chronic blepharitis. Steroids control the inflammation better than cyclosporine, but there is a synergy between the two. The cyclosporine in effect becomes a steroid sparing agent, similar in philosophy to the use of multiple chemotherapeutic agents to arrest cancer. Together, steroids and cyclosporine alter the deleterious milieu of an inflamed ocular surface by improving tear quality and quantity, increasing goblet cell density, and producing more and better mucin. In addition, steroids combined with cyclosporine also treat lid disease, reducing inflammation and creating a better lipid layer on the tear film surface. Thus, combination anti-inflammatory therapy treats and improves every component of the tear film. The 0.05 percent cyclosporine preparation from Allergan is also preservative free, further enhancing the integrity of the inflamed ocular surface on chronic therapy.

Off-label studies of cyclosporine reveal that it works well for allergic eye diseases, such as vernal keratoconjunctivitis and giant papillary conjunctivitis. Milder forms of allergic eye disease, such as seasonal allergic conjunctivitis, also may benefit. But these milder forms tend to be more transient and not necessarily matched to cyclosporine as a first-line therapy. On the other hand, if a patient has allergy and dry eye, concomitant chronic use of cyclosporine significantly attenuates the seasonal exacerbation of eye disease.

It is also necessary to work with patients' internists, allergists, oncologists, hematologists or rheumatologists to prescribe the simplest, most cost-effective repertoire of medications. By juggling the patients' systemic medications, we can significantly improve, simplify and reduce the cost of therapy.

Nutrition for Blepharitis and Ocular Allergy

Dietary changes may help resolve meibomian gland dysfunction and reduce the time patients need to use doxycycline. Nutritional supplementation with omega-3 fatty acids clearly has a salutary effect for all forms of ocular surface disease. A therapeutic dose of supplements includes iso-pentanoic acid, eicosa-pentaenoic acid, cod liver oil, other fish oils, flaxseed oil, and black currant seed oil, an excellent source of gamma linoleic acid (GLA). These oral supplemental agents taken commensurate with doxycycline and minocycline help limit the time patients need to take the prescription component of their regimen, thus reducing side effects. This multi-faceted approach focuses on the root problem of inflammation and the effects of meibomian gland dysfunction, ocular surface cytokine and T cell activiation, and mast cell degranulation.

The currently available commercial sources of omega fatty acids now available to ophthalmologists in the United States are flaxseed oil, which is predominantly omega-3, Hydroeye (ScienceBased Health, Corte Madera, Calif.), which is a mixture of omega-3 and omega-6, and BioTears (Biosyntryx, Lexington, SC), which is very similar. There are a few additives to these formulations, but they are basically a combination of omega-6 and omega-3. The Science Based Health formulation is continuously updated to most accurately reflect current nutritional research, and contains only fresh natural ingredients. TheraTears Nutrition (Advanced Vision Research, Woburn, Mass.), is more predominantly omega-3s. Tears Again Hydrate (Cynacon) contains primarily flaxseed oil with evening primrose oil as a source of GLA.

These are five choices among others, or one may recommend a simple trip to the health food store for the flaxseed oil, Omega-3, or black currant seed oil alone or in combination. Hydroeye and BioTears are a combination of black currant seed oil and cod liver oil, so there is a plant source of omega fatty acid and a fish source of omega fatty acid, again combining omega-6 and omega-3. Although a combination of omega-3 and beneficial omega-6s is preferred, it is better to have the patient use the flaxseed oil instead of nothing. The omega-3 in flaxseed oil is generally less bioavailable than that of fish oil, but some patients also have a seafood allergy precluding the most common supplemental source of omega-3.

STEROIDS FOR CONTACT LENS WEARERS AND REFRACTIVE SURGERY PATIENTS

Awareness of Ocular Surface Disease

Another point to be aware of is the constellation of ocular surface disease that creates discontent with contact lenses in the younger LASIK population, including allergy and blepharitis. There are many perturbations of overlapping presentations, including the itch that you see in dry eye that may be partially allergy, and the tear film break-up time acceleration you might see with concomitant blepharitis. This all comes into play with a therapeutic approach. There is overlap in the dry eye success story of the therapy of omega-3s with blepharitis, and certainly Restasis (Allergan, Irvine, Calif.) and topical steroids are effective against allergy as well.

Steroids can be effectively utilized for both difficult contact lens patients and those with upcoming refractive surgery. The same therapeutic tenets apply: close observation, titration of dosage to the individual patient's needs, and maximum utilization of all therapeutic options available.

In a landmark Wisconsin retrospective study of 360 myopic LASIK patients by Boorstein in 2003, pre-emptive treatment with an oral antihistamine in an allergic patient population reduced the risk of developing DLK. Atopy is therefore a patient-specific risk factor for the development of DLK after primary bilateral LASIK for either myopia or myopic astigmatism. Atopic individuals benefited from preoperative treatment to minimize the incidence of DLK and the potential for visual loss. The lessons of the study can be furthered by evaluation of topical rather than drying systemic antihistamines to reduce potential DLK in allergic patients, as well as prophylactic topical steroids prior to LASIK in allergic individuals. Thus, with the entire ocular surface milieu in mind, preventive therapy is essential. Surgeons must consider not just the etiology of dry eye or the tarsal surface changes seen in chronic allergy, since these conditions are clearly interrelated, but also medication use, both topically and systemically.

Challenging Refractive Patients and Informed Consent

In clinical practice, every surgeon sees problem patients—the ones whose dry eye and allergy are unidentified, ignored, or become dry following refractive surgery. Many troubled patients travel from doctor to doctor, disgruntled with their primary surgeon, and they are the last patient you want to see on a busy day because they complain, they have other psychosomatic problems, they are extremely disgruntled with the other doctor whose lawyer you are trying to bypass altogether if humanly possible, and they eat up a lot of chair time with really minimal problems, and minimal findings, and maximal symptoms. Thus, we know that dry eye and allergy, which predispose to poor outcomes and unpredictable refractive surgery results, are so important to the informed consent process. These shattered hopes are often a result of falsely high expectations for elective surgery.

The most highly effective way to minimize the deleterious effects that allergy and dry eye can have on LASIK outcomes is to take proactive preventive steps. Placing patients into a routine that manages allergy or any existing irritation due to dry eye is invaluable.

With a dry eye prior to LASIK, the primary goal leading up to surgery is to achieve a healthy ocular surface. More frequent artificial tears will help and can be continued postoperatively. Familiarizing patients with this rigorous schedule as early as possible before surgery is helpful not only in preparing the ocular surface for LASIK, but in developing the discipline to use the drops with enough frequency to avoid complications.

The best approach for ocular allergic LASIK candidates is the same as that for all ocular allergic patients: topical therapy. New generation anti-allergic agents prevent the release of histamine, cytokines and other pro-inflammatory and proliferative mediators such as those involved in corneal trauma and healing, including IL-8, ICAM-1. Generally these patients are better treated with topical anti-allergic agents such as mast-cell stabilizer/antihistaminic solutions that will not compromise, and may even enhance, corneal wound healing. For example, agents such as olopatadine have been shown to decrease the release of tryptase from mast cells *in vitro*. In human clinical study, these agents stabilize the conjunctival mast cells.

Parallel to the routine of artificial tears for dry eye, a regular regimen of anti-allergy eye drops before LASIK can get patients out of the habit of rubbing their eyes, decreasing the risk of their continuing to do so after LASIK and dislocating their flaps.

Careful diagnosis of allergy and dry eye is naturally an important step in optimizing the success of LASIK. A specific medication history concerning the use of oral antihistamines, over-the-counter ocular allergy drops, nasal sprays, diuretics, anti-depressants and other drying agents or anti-pruritic agents is essential for identifying allergy. Also, the anatomic location and severity of allergic symptoms should be identified, including sinusitis, rhinitis, pharyngitis, dermatitis, eczema, asthma, food intolerance, and of course conjunctivitis.

Accurate assessment of tear-film status may also be predictive of postoperative dry-eye symptoms. Since allergy and dry eye can sometimes be confused with one another, tear film quantification would allow for a precise differential diagnosis in ambiguous cases. You can optimize ocular surface health by discontinuing oral antihistamines in the preoperative period and begin supplementing a typical LASIK medication regimen with potent topical anti-allergy therapy or preservative free artificial tears.

Recognition of allergy and dry eye as risk factors for LASIK complications is something that takes little time or effort, but may have profound effects upon the surgical outcome. Recognition allows for the identification of a patient category that may benefit from preoperative prophylactic therapy and closer postoperative observation. It is always better to treat the eye than to not treat it and run the risk of complications.

Certainly, the astute clinician can offer an allergic or dry eye patient PRK where the risk is lower, and now there is a conglomerate of other alternative procedures, including clear lens extraction, phakic IOLs, the Crystalens (Eyeonics, Aliso Viejo, Calif.), and the recently approved ReSTOR lens (Alcon) and ReZoom lens (AMO). So the informed consent process becomes even more complex when presented with an ocular surface disease patient, when they really need to know about these alternative therapies. LASIK patients complain bitterly when they have not effectively anticipated going from being healthy to past the reserve and into a dry eye. Likely their biggest complaint is fluctuating, or decreased vision, often ahead of symptoms of irritation. Visual disturbance postoperative LASIK secondary to manifestations of dry eyes and severe ocular allergies are common yet avoidable. Nevertheless, all potential refractive patients should be made aware of the potential for interference by ocular surface diseases and the need for continued vigilance, particularly during the perioperative period.

BIBLIOGRAPHY

1. Armaly MF. Statistical attributes of the steroid hypertensive response in the clinically normal eye. I. The demonstration of three levels of response. Invest Ophthalmol 1965;4:187-97.
2. Asano-Kato N, Toda I, Hori-Komai Y, Tsubota K. Allergic conjunctivitis as a risk factor for laser *in situ* keratomileusis. J Cataract Refract Surg 2001;27:1469-72.
3. Bartlett JD, Horwitz B, Leibovitz R, et al. Intraocular pressure response to loteprednol etabonate in known steroid responders. J Ocul Pharmacol 1993;9:157-65.
4. Bartlett JD, Woollery TW, Adams, CM. Identification of high intraocular pressure responders to topical ophthalmic corticosteroids. J Ocul Pharmacol 1993;9:35-45.
5. Biswas J, Ganeshbabu TM, Raghavendran SR, et al. Efficacy and safety of 1 percent rimexolone versus 1 percent prednisolone acetate in the treatment of anterior uveitis—a randomized triple masked study. Int Ophthalmol 2004;25:147-53.
6. Boorstein SM, Henk HJ, Elner VM. Atopy: a patient specific risk factor for diffuse lamellar keratitis. Ophthalmology 2003;110:131-7.
7. Brown NA, Bron A, Hardin JJ, Dewar HM. Nutrition supplements and the eye. Eye. 1998;12(Pt. 1):127-133. Review.
8. Christine M Velicer, Susan R Heckbert, Johanna W Lampe, John D Potter, Carol A Robertson, Stephen H Taplin. Antibiotic Use in Relation to the Risk of Breast Cancer; JAMA. 2004;291:827-35.

9. Ilyas H, Slonim CB, Braswell GR, et al. Long-term safety of loteprednol etabonate 0.2 percent in the treatment of seasonal and perennial allergic conjunctivitis. Eye Contact Lens 2004;30:10-3.
10. Leibowitz HM, Kupferman A. Antiinflammatory Medications. In Clinical Pharmacology of the Anterior Segment. Holly FJ (Ed). Int Ophthalmol Clinics 1980;20(3):117-34.
11. Leibowitz HW, Bartlett JD, Rich D, et al. Intraocular pressure-raising potential of 1.0 percent rimexolone in patients responding to corticosteroids. Arch Ophthalmol 1996;114:933-7.
12. McCluskey P, Powell RJ. The eye in systemic inflammatory diseases. Lancet 2004;364:2125-33.
13. Pflugfelder SC, Maskin SL, Anderson B, et al. A randomized, double-masked, placebo-controlled, multicenter comparison of loteprednol etabonate ophthalmic suspension, 0.5 percent, and placebo for treatment of keratoconjunctivitis sicca in patients with delayed tear clearance. Am J Ophthalmol 2004;138:444-57.
14. Pflugfelder SC, Solomon A, Dursun D, Li DQ. Dry eye and delayed tear clearance: A call to arms. Adv Exp Med Biol. 2002;506(Pt B):739-43. Review.
15. Pflugfelder SC. Antiinflammatory therapy for dry eye. Am J Ophthalmol 2004;137:337-42.
16. Ramamurthy NS, Rifkin BR, Greenwald RA, et al. Inhibition of matrix metalloproteinase-mediated periodontal bone loss in rats: A comparison of 6 chemically modified tetracyclines. J Periodontol. 2002;73:726-34.
17. Restasis package insert.
18. Sheppard J, Alison N, Martin D, et al. Diquafosol tetrasodium is effective in a broad spectrum of patients with dry eye. Poster presented at The Association for Research in Vision and Ophthalmology (ARVO) 2004 Annual Meeting. 2004 April 25-9; Fort Lauderdale, Florida, USA.
19. Stern ME, Beuerman RW, Fox RI, et al. A unified theory of the role of the ocular surface in dry eye. Adv Exp Med Biol. 1998;438:643-51.
20. Stern ME, Beuerman RW, Fox RI, et al. The pathology of dry eye: The interaction between the ocular surface and lacrimal glands. Cornea 1998;17:584-9.
21. The loteprednol etabonate US uveitis study group. Controlled evaluation of loteprednol and prednisolone acetate in the treatment of uveitis. Am J Ophthalmol 1999;127:537-44.
22. Yang H-Y, Fujishima H, Toda I, et al. Allergic conjunctivitis as a risk factor for regression and haze after photorefractive keratectomy. Am J Ophthalmol 1998;125:54-8.
23. Yolton DP. Use of Topical Steroids for the Treatment of Anterior Segment Ocular Disease, Pacific University College of Optometry, 2006.

Optimizing Visual Outcomes with NSAIDs Therapy in Cataract and Refractive Surgeries

Eric D Donnenfeld, Henry D Perry (USA)

Ophthalmic nonsteroidal anti-inflammatory drugs (NSAIDs) are becoming a cornerstone for the management of ocular pain and inflammation. Their well-characterized anti-inflammatory activity, analgesic property, and established safety record have also made NSAIDs an important tool to optimize surgical outcomes. Ophthalmic NSAIDs currently play four principle roles in ophthalmic surgery including the prevention of intraoperative miosis during cataract surgery, management of postoperative inflammation, the reduction of pain and discomfort following cataract and refractive surgery, and the prevention and treatment of cystoid macular edema following cataract surgery.

Ocular inflammation is characterized by redness, swelling, and/or pain associated with irritation or trauma to the eye. Common triggers of ocular inflammation include allergies, meibomian gland dysfunction, ocular diseases (traumatic iritis, peripheral corneal inflammatory keratitis, episcleritis, and unilateral nongranulomatous idiopathic iritis), and most importantly ophthalmic surgical procedures.

The strict regulation of inflammatory reactions within the eye is vital in maintaining both anatomical integrity and visual function. Left unregulated, inflammation within the eye may lead to extensive ocular damage, resulting in impaired vision.

Ocular inflammatory pathways commence with the triggering of the arachidonic acid cascade. The cascade is triggered either by mechanical stimuli (such as the case of surgically-inflicted trauma) or by chemical stimuli (such as foreign substances or allergens). Prostaglandins are generated in most tissues by activation of the arachidonic acid pathway. Phospholipids in the cell membrane are the substrate for the enzyme phospholipase A to cause generation of arachidonic acid and, in turn, the enzymes cyclooxygenases and lipoxygenases act on arachidonic acid to produce a family of chemically distinct prostaglandins, and leukotrienes (McColgin). Clinical symptoms of prostaglandin production include hyperemi, miosis, poor vision, pain, and cystoid macular edema (CME).

It is well accepted that inhibition of prostaglandin synthesis and release reduces the inflammatory response induced by surgery and allergies, thereby reducing the clinical symptoms of prostaglandin production (McColgin). Prostaglandin synthesis can be suppressed by inhibiting phospholipase A2, which inhibits the release of arachidonic acid from the intracellular stores, or by inhibiting the conversion of arachidonic acid to prostaglandin via the cyclooxygenase pathway. Multiple portions of this pathway can be blocked and different classes of anti-inflammatory medications have differing effects on this pathway. For example, corticosteroids interfere with the activity of phospholipase A2, thereby inhibiting the release of arachidonic acid and the production of all arachidonic acid metabolites including prostaglandins (Polansky and Weinreb, 1984).

In contrast, the nonsteroidal anti-inflammatory drugs (NSAIDs) specifically and irreversibly inhibit the synthesis of prostaglandins by interfering with the activity of cyclooxygenases (COX-1 and COX-2). (Polansky and Weinreb, 1984).

RATIONALE FOR TREATING OCULAR INFLAMMATION

Reducing ocular inflammation is critical because failure to do so may cause patients discomfort, pain, visual loss, and increase the risk for the development of CME.

Cystoid macular edema (CME) is potentially the most adverse ocular outcome of prostaglandin production. CME is caused by cystic accumulation of intraretinal fluid in the outer plexiform and inner nuclear layers of the retina, as a result of breakdown of the blood-retinal barrier. It is most common following intraocular surgery, and in patients with venous occlusive disease, diabetic retinopathy, and posterior segment inflammatory conditions (Quin). However, CME can develop in surgeries with no obvious complications. The condition is often asymptomatic and may only be detected with fluorescein angiography or optical coherence tomography (Quin, Roberts). Although, the exact incidence of CME is still unclear, CME is a frequent cause of visual loss following even uncomplicated cataract surgery. Studies suggest that the rate of clinical CME ranges from 1–2 percent (Ray), while

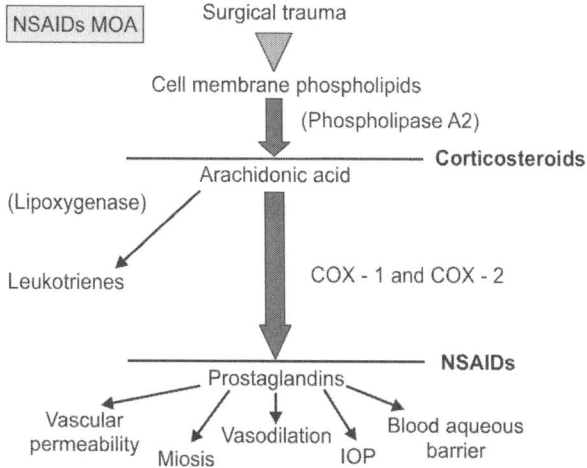

Fig. 42.1: Prostaglandin synthesis

the incidence of angiographic CME may be as high as 9-19 percent (Ursell, Mentes). In a recent study, patients using ketorolac tromethamine 0.4 percent preoperatively 1-3 days prior to surgery had no instances of CME, whereas the steroid-only group and the group that got the NSAID just one hour prior for antimiosis had a rate of 12 percent CME as detected by OCT (Donnenfeld). CME frequently has a late onset, occurring 4-6 weeks postoperatively. CME often presents with blurred or decreased central vision or painless retinal inflammation or swelling. Visual loss is usually temporary but may be irreversible in refractory to conservative treatment. In high risk patients such as diabetics the risk of CME and permanent vision loss is even greater.

NSAIDs are also frequently used to inhibit intraoperative miosis during cataract surgery. Miosis may restrict the surgeon's field of view during cataract surgery, thereby hindering the progression of the procedure, and increasing the risk of complications and posterior capsule rupture (Guzek, Stewart). The NSAIDs prevent miosis by limiting prostaglandin synthesis within the tissues by inhibiting cyclooxygenase and reducing inflammation. They also help to maintain increased pupillary size during the surgical procedure thereby helping to reduce complications.

PHARMACOLOGIC THERAPY FOR OCULAR INFLAMMATION

Ocular inflammation is currently treated with either topical corticosteroids or NSAIDs. The corticosteroids, considered the gold standard for the treatment of ocular inflammation, are associated with an increased incidence of adverse events that warrant their judicious use. These adverse events include cataract formation, a

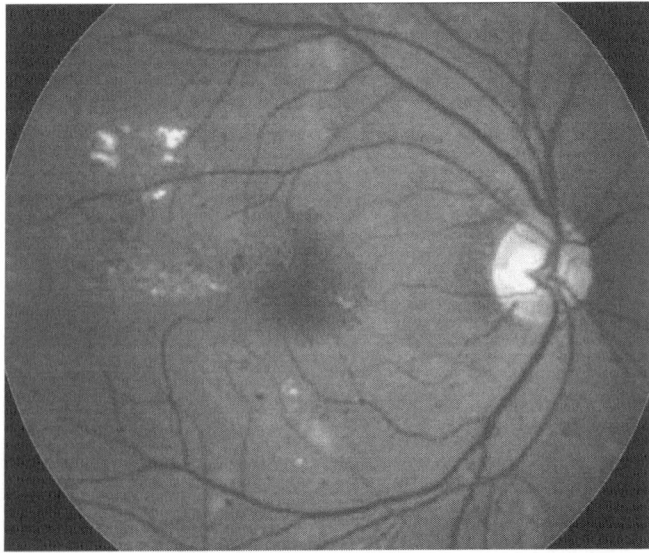

Fig. 42.2: Background diabetic retinopathy increases the risk of CME

rise in intraocular pressure, increased susceptibility to microbial infections due to a suppressed host immune-response, retardation in corneal epithelial and stromal wound healing. Steroids are not safe for periods of extended use as prolonged use is associated with development of glaucoma, visual acuity defects and loss of visual field, and posterior subcapsular cataract formation.

A safer alternative to corticosteroids for the treatment of ocular inflammation are the NSAIDs. There are four classes of NSAIDs available for topical ophthalmic use: indoles, phenylacetic acids, an arylacetic acid prodrug, and phenylalkanoic acids. Indomethacin 1 percent aqueous suspension is an indole derivative that is available outside of the United States (O'Brien). Diclofenac 1 percent is a water-soluble phenylacetic derivative approved by the FDA as a treatment to minimize inflammation related to cataract surgery and as a therapeutic option for the reduction of pain and photophobia after cataract surgery. Bromfenac 0.09 percent is a recently approved twice-daily topical phenylacetic compound indicated for the treatment of postoperative cataract inflammation. Originally available as a systemic medication, the product was removed from the market in the United States because of potentially fatal liver toxicity but has been available as an ophthalmic agent in Japan for several years. Nepafenac 0.1 percent is approved as a three times a day treatment for pain and inflammation associated with cataract surgery. This agent is an arylacetic acid prodrug. Flurbiprofen 0.03 percent and suprofen 1 percent are water-soluble phenylalkanoic acids approved by the FDA for intraoperative use during cataract surgery for inhibition of excessive miosis during cataract surgery. Ketorolac tromethamine 0.4 percent is also a water-soluble phenylalkanoic acid and is approved for the treatment of for the reduction of ocular pain and burning/stinging following corneal refractive surgery.

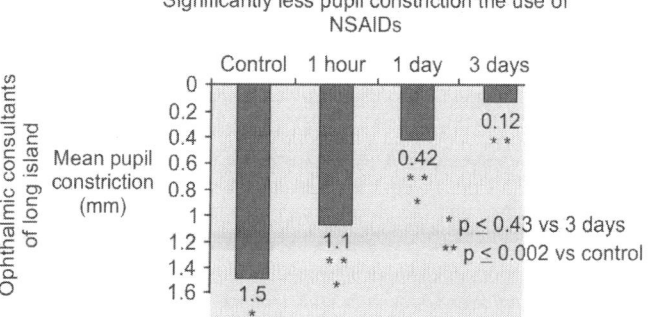

- 1 pupil contraction was dose-dependent
- 3 days of ketorolac 0.4% resulted in significantly less contraction than 1 day, 1 hour, or placebo, $p \leq 0.043$
- 1 day of ketorolac 0.4% resulted in significantly less contraction than, 1 hour, or placebo, $p \leq 0.001$

Fig. 42.3: Preoperative NSAIDs reduce pupil constriction during cataract surgery (Donnenfeld)

NSAIDs for Control of Pain Following Photorefractive Keratectomy

The recently reported pooled analysis of two multicenter, randomized, double-masked, vehicle-controlled, parallel-group studies of 313 patients with unilateral photorefractive keratectomy (PRK) evaluated the safety and analgesic efficacy of ketorolac tromethamine 0.4 percent ophthalmic solution in postoperative patients (Solomon). After surgery, patients were treated with one drop of ketorolac tromethamine 0.4 percent ophthalmic solution (n = 156) or vehicle (n = 157) four times daily for up to four days. Pain intensity, pain relief, use of escape medication, and severity of ocular symptoms were assessed and adverse events, epithelial healing, and visual acuity recorded. Patients in the ketorolac group reported significantly less pain intensity than patients in the vehicle group ($P < 0.001$). During the first 12 hours post PRK, 50 percent fewer patients in the ketorolac group than in the vehicle group had severe to intolerable pain (41.6 percent [64/154] and 84.5 percent [131/155], respectively). The median time to no pain was 30 hours in the ketorolac group and 54 hours in the vehicle group ($P < 0.001$). Ketorolac patients reported significantly greater pain relief than vehicle patients throughout the study ($P < 0.001$) and used significantly less escape medication than vehicle patients for 48 hours post PRK ($P < 0.008$). The authors concluded that ketorolac 0.4 percent ophthalmic solution is safe and effective in reducing ocular pain when used four times daily for up to four days post-PRK.

NSAIDs vs Steroids

A recent study compared the efficacy, safety and patient comfort of two topical steroids (prednisolone 1% and rimexolone 1%) with ketorolac tromethamine 0.5 percent after extracapsular cataract extraction in a prospective, randomized, double-masked study of 45 patients. Patients were assigned to receive topical treatment with prednisolone, rimexolone or ketorolac tromethamine ophthalmic solution after phacoemulsification for cataract extraction. Although there were no significant between-group differences in inflammatory cell counts ($P = 0.165$), flare readings in the anterior chamber were lowest ($P = 0.008$) in the ketorolac group. One patient in the prednisolone group experienced elevated IOP and had to be excluded. The authors concluded that ketorolac tromethamine provides good control of intraocular inflammation after cataract extraction without the risk of a steroidal IOP increase (Herneiss).

Holzer and associates reported that ketorolac tromethamine ophthalmic solution 0.5 percent was is effective as loteprednol etabonate ophthalmic suspension 0.5 percent in reducing inflammation after routine phacoemulsification and IOL implantation, suggesting that ketorolac tromethamine 0.5 percent is a safe and effective anti-inflammatory alternative to steroids after cataract extraction.

Similarly, Solomon and associates reported ketorolac tromethamine 0.5 percent is a safe and effective anti-inflammatory alternative to steroids after cataract extraction. In that study, ketorolac tromethamine 0.5 percent was as effective as rimexolone 1 percent in reducing inflammation after cataract surgery. There were no between-group differences in signs and symptoms of inflammation, intraocular pressure, or Kowa cell and flare measurements in this double-masked, prospective evaluation of 36 patients (Solomon and Vroman, 2001).

NSAIDs for the Inhibition of Miosis

Srinivisin and associates reported that topical ketorolac was a more effective inhibitor of miosis than topical diclofenac during extracapsular cataract extraction and IOL implantation. Ketorolac also provided a more stable mydriatic effect throughout surgery. In a study of 51 patients who were prospectively randomized to receive ketorolac 0.5 percent or diclofenac 0.1 percent at three intervals preoperatively. In this study, the ketorolac group showed a consistent trend toward larger pupil diameters at subsequent surgical intervals as well as greater inhibition of miosis in the ketorolac group.

Similarly, Snyder and associates reported that the use of ketorolac as a single agent negated the need for use of a combination of preoperative NSAID (flurbiprofen) and postoperative corticosteroid for the prevention of intraoperative miosis and postoperative inflammation in cataract surgery. In their study of 26 patients, there were no statistically significant differences in dilation (preoperative versus postoperative) or cell and flare postoperatively. The authors concluded that the use of ketorolac as a single agent could eliminate the expense of using separate anti-inflammatory and antimiotic preparations preoperatively and postoperatively, thereby enhancing surgeon convenience and patient convenience and compliance (Snyder).

Recently, a large study (n = 118) compared the effects of topical ketorolac with topical 0.03 percent flurbiprofen on the inhibition of surgically induced miosis during phacoemulsification cataract surgery. Mean horizontal pupillary diameter measurements for both medications were similar at the start of surgery. However, a consistent trend of larger pupillary diameter was seen in all subsequent surgical intervals in the ketorolac-treated group. Changes from baseline measurements also indicated a more significant inhibition of miosis at all subsequent intervals, and a more stable mydriasis throughout the procedure in the ketorolac-treated group (Solomon, 1997).

NSAIDs and Topical Steroids

It is well accepted that combination topical therapy with a corticosteroid and a NSAID is more effective than either agent dosed individually for treatment of CME following cataract surgery, and a recent study by Rho and associates supports this paradigm. The authors compared combination therapies of diclofenac sodium 0.1 percent and prednisolone acetate 1 percent, with ketorolac tromethamine 0.5 percent and prednisolone acetate 1 percent, for treatment of CME in 68 patients following uncomplicated cataract surgery. Complete resolution of CME was noted in 28 percent of diclofenac patients and in 25 percent of ketorolac patients. Final vision improved three or more lines in 58 and 53 percent of patients, respectively. None of the patients showed signs of corneal toxicity or significant intraocular pressure rise during the treatment period. The authors concluded that combination therapy with NSAIDs and steroids was effective in reducing the severity of pseudophakic CME and in improving final vision.

The findings of Rho and associates are supported by another recent study by Heier and associates (Heier, 2000). That study evaluated the efficacy of ketorolac, prednisolone acetate 1.0 percent, and ketorolac and prednisolone combination therapy in the treatment of acute, visually significant, clinical CME following cataract extraction surgery in a randomized, double-masked, prospective trial of 28 patients. Treatment was continued until CME resolved or for three months, whichever occurred first and then tapered over three weeks. The average improvements in Snellen visual acuity were 1.6 lines with ketorolac monotherapy, 1.1 lines with steroid monotherapy, and 3.8 lines with combination therapy. More patients in the combination group achieved at least a two-line improvement (89% of combination patients versus 67% of ketorolac and 50% of steroid patients). Moreover, these patients improved faster with combination therapy than with monotherapy with either agent (1.33 months for combination therapy compared with 1.43 months for ketorolac patients and 2.75 months for steroid patients). Improvements in contrast sensitivity and leakage on fluorescein angiography tended to mirror improvements in Snellen acuity. The authors concluded that treatment of acute, visually significant pseudophakic CME with ketorolac and prednisolone combination therapy appears to offer benefits over monotherapy with either agent alone.

A study by Arshinoff et al evaluated postoperative pain in 97 PRK patients using different topical NSAID protocols. In their study, treatment with topical homatropine hydrobromide, either diclofenac sodium or ketorolac tromethamine, and a soft contact lens was most effective in achieving post-PRK analgesia. They also found that NSAIDs added to topical steroid protocols had a significantly greater effect than steroids alone on reducing myopic regression for one year postoperatively (Arshinoff, 1994).

Prevention of CME

All available evidence demonstrates that ketorolac is an effective treatment for acute and chronic CME. Several studies, however, suggest that ketorolac is also able to prevent CME in postoperative patients. A study by Flach and associates (1990) suggested that ketorolac prevents CME without the risks associated with concomitant topical steroid treatment. In that study, 50 patients with bilateral cataracts were enrolled in a placebo-controlled, paired-comparison, double-masked study. Eleven patients had evidence of angiographic (angiographic aphakic CME) ACME on postoperative day 40. Two of these patients demonstrated bilateral ACME, one patient had ACME in the NSAID-treated eye, and eight patients had ACME in the placebo-treated eye. This was a statistically significant difference favoring drug treatment. In addition, the signs of anterior ocular inflammation were greater in the eyes with ACME.

Roberts presented data from a clinical study at the 2005 meeting of ASCRS that demonstrated that patients using preoperative and postoperative NSAIDs had less postoperative increase in macular thickness than those who did not use NSAIDs. In that study, 200 patients undergoing phacoemulsification were randomized to two pharmaceutical treatment regimens, differing only by the inclusion/exclusion of ketorolac 0.4 percent into the standard treatment regimen. Outcome measures included macular thickness by OCT at preoperative and four weeks post-operative, contrast sensitivity by FACT, and Snellen visual acuity. After four weeks, the change in macular thickness was substantially greater without NSAIDs than with NSAIDs (10.4 µm compared with 4.2 µm, respectively). There were no differences in visual acuity. The author concluded that macular edema decreases the quality of postoperative vision and that the use of preoperative and postoperative NSAIDs decreases the amount of postoperative macular edema.

Many clinicians are hesitant to prescribe topical NSAIDs for long-term use because of prior reports of corneal melting associated with topical NSAIDs (Flach, Gaynes). However, analysis of NSAID-associated corneal events implicates the now defunct generic diclofenac product, diclofenac sodium ophthalmic solution as the agent primarily responsible (Gaynes). The demonstrated safety of ketorolac throughout numerous studies, some as long as six weeks duration, suggests that this drug is safe for extended use. In fact ketorolac has actually been recommended for the treatment of postcataract inflammation in a patient with systemic steroid treated rheumatoid arthritis postphacoemulsification. In this patient the fear of "melting" led the physician to avoid topical NSAIDs. However, the severe reaction postoperatively led him to using it successfully in the second eye with excellent results (Caronia).

The available evidence demonstrates that NSAIDs are highly effective analgesics for pain associated with cataract and refractive procedures. The ability to provide relief of patient pain is critical because patients have high expectations and expect almost no pain with ophthalmic surgeries. Patients who experience ocular pain or discomfort may therefore believe that their surgeon may have substandard surgical skills and the resulting patient dissatisfaction and potential for negative word of mouth to the patient's colleagues and friends may have adverse consequences for a surgical practice. Choosing the most effective topical agent for relief of ocular inflammation and pain postoperatively is therefore.

The adjunctive use of NSAIDs with steroids optimizes surgical outcomes as numerous studies have demonstrated that the combination of an NSAID and steroid is more effective for the treatment of postoperative inflammation, CME, and improving visual acuity than either NSAID or steroid monotherapy.

Perhaps the most important effect to surgeons is the increased amount of dilation preoperatively and the tendency for the dilation to remain for the entire procedure. Some surgeons have likened this effect as like having a third hand during surgery. Other studies point out the direct relationship between pupil size and rate of surgical complications (Donnenfeld).

In recent years, there has been a substantially amount of debate in the ophthalmic community regarding the use of NSAIDs prior to surgery to prevent the formation of CME. We understand and accept that increased inflammation postoperatively is associated with an increased risk of developing CME. In fact, a study by Ursell and associates reported that patients who had angiographic CME at day 60 were more likely to have had more postoperative inflammation than patients who did not develop CME (Ursell). It follows, therefore, that preventing inflammation with prophylactic dosing would decrease the risk of developing CME. A recent study by Donnenfeld and associates (Donnenfeld) does provide us with evidence supporting the use of ketorolac 0.4 percent as surgical prophylaxis against CME. The study was a prospective evaluation of 100 patients randomized in a double-masked fashion prior to phacoemulsification into four groups: one group received preoperative ketorolac tromethamine 0.4 percent four times daily for three days and three doses every 15 minutes immediately preceding surgery, another received four doses on the day before surgery ketorolac 0.4 percent and three doses every 15 minutes immediately preceding surgery, another received ketorolac only three times (every 15 minutes) in the hour immediately preceding surgery, and the fourth group was randomized to control. In that study, use of ketorolac for one or three days reduced the incidence of CME. No patients in these groups had CME at week 2, compared with 12 percent (3/25) of control patients and 4 percent (1/25) of patients in the one hour group. This study suggests that three days preoperative dosing with ketorolac effectively prevents CME. Other findings of that study demonstrated that ketorolac maintained pupil size, reduced discomfort, limited reductions in epithelial cell counts, and reduced patient need for additional anesthesia. Ketorolac also provided substantial reductions in the amount of time needed to perform surgery, making it a cost-effective pharmaceutical for cataract surgery. Most of these data followed a clear dose-response pattern, suggesting that maximum prophylaxis can be expected with the three days dosing regimen, though even one day of ketorolac was consistently superior to one hour of ketorolac or to control. This study further confirms the previous work by Flach and Roberts that ketorolac is an effective prophylaxis against CME.

If a three-day dosing regimen of ketorolac is effective surgical prophylaxis, what is the most appropriate postoperative dosing regimen? In my experience, four weeks of QID dosing with ketorolac 0.4 percent is optimal for most patients, in patients with diabetes mellitus we use at least six weeks of therapy and most important in patients with diabetic retinopathy we use ketorolac 0.4 percent for at least three months to help protect this most susceptible group from developing CME.

BIBLIOGRAPHY

1. Arshinoff S, D'Addario D, Sadler C, Bilotta R, Johnson TM. Use of topical nonsteroidal anti-inflammatory drugs in excimer laser photorefractive keratectomy. J Cataract Refract Surg 1994;20:216-22.
2. Caronia RM, Perry HD, Donnenfeld ED. J Cataract and Refractive Surg 2002;28:1880-1.
3. Donnenfeld ED, Perry HD, Wittpenn JR, Solomon R, Nattis A, Chou T. Preoperative ketorolac tromethamine 0.4 percent in phacoemulsification outcomes: Pharmacokinetic-response Curve. J Cataract Refract Surg 2006;32(9):1474-82.
4. Evans RE, Bucci FA Jr, Amico LM. Efficacy of Ketorolac 0.5 percent versus Ketorolac 0.4 percent Following Cataract Surgery. Presented at ARVO, 2005.
5. Flach AJ. Corneal melts associated with topically applied nonsteroidal anti-inflammatory drugs. Trans Am Ophthalmol Soc. 2001;99:205-10; discussion 210-2.
6. Flach AJ, Stegman RC, Graham J, Kruger LP. Prophylaxis of aphakic cystoid macular edema without corticosteroids. A paired-comparison, placebo-controlled double-masked study. Ophthalmology 1990;97:1253-8.
7. Gaynes BI, Fiscella R. Topical nonsteroidal anti-inflammatory drugs for ophthalmic use: a safety review. Drug Saf 2002;25:233-50.
8. Goyal R, Shankar J, Fone DL, Hughes DS. Randomized controlled trial of ketorolac in the management of corneal abrasions. Acta Ophthalmol Scand 2001;79(2):177-9.
9. Guzek JP, Holm M, Cotter JB, et al. Risk factors for intraoperative complications in 1000 extracapsular cataract cases. Ophthalmology 1987;94:461-6.
10. Heier J, Cheetham JK, Degryse R, et al. Ketorolac tromethamine 0.5 percent ophthalmic solution in the treatment of moderate to severe ocular inflammation after cataract surgery: a randomized, vehicle-controlled clinical trial. Am J Ophthalmol 1999;127:253-9.
11. Hirneiss C, Neubauer AS, Kampik A, Schonfeld CL. Comparison of prednisolone 1 percent, rimexolone 1 percent and ketorolac tromethamine 0.5 percent after cataract extraction. A prospective, randomized, double-masked study. Graefes. Arch Clin Exp Ophthalmol. 2005; 9 [Epub ahead of print].
12. Kaiser PK, Pineda R 2nd. A study of topical nonsteroidal anti-inflammatory drugs and no pressure patching in the treatment of corneal abrasions. Corneal Abrasion Patching Study Group. Ophthalmology 1997;104:1353-9.
13. McColgin AZ, Heier JS. Control of intraocular inflammation associated with cataract surgery. Curr Opin Ophthalmol 2000;11(1):3-6.
14. Mentes J, Erakgun T, Afrashi F, Kerci G. Incidence of cystoid macular edema after uncomplicated phacoemulsification. Ophthalmology 2003;217(6):408-12.
15. O'brien TP. Emerging guidelines for use of NSAID therapy to optimize cataract surgery patient care. Curr Med Res Opin 2005; 21(7):1131-8.
16. Polansky JR, Weinreb RN. Steroids as anti-inflammatory agents. In: Sears ML, (Ed). Pharmacology of the Eye. New York, NY: Springer-Verlag 1984;460-538.

17. Price FW Jr, Price MO, Zeh W, Dobbins K. Pain reduction after laser *in situ* keratomileusis with ketorolac tromethamine ophthalmic solution 0.5 percent: a randomized, double-masked, placebo-controlled trial. J Refract Surg 2002;18(2):140-4.
18. Price FW, Tonon E, van Denburgh AM, Stern K, Cheetham JK, Schiffman RM. Safety and efficacy of reformulated ketorolac tromethamine 0.4 percent ophthalmic solution in post-photorefractive keratectomy patients. Presented at ARVO, 2003.
19. Price MO, Price FW. Efficacy of topical ketorolac tromethamine 0.4 percent for control of pain or discomfort associated with cataract surgery. Curr Med Res Opin 2004;20(12):2015-9.
20. Quinn CJ. Cystoid macular edema. Optom Clin. 1996;5(1):111-30.
21. Ray S. D'Amico DJ. Pseudophakic macular edema. Semin Ophthalmol 2002;17:167-80.
22. Rho DS. Treatment of acute pseudophakic cystoid macular edema: Diclofenac versus ketorolac. J Cataract Refract Surg 2003;29(12):2378-84.
23. Rho DS, Soll SM. Combination therapy for pseudophakic cystoid macular edema: diclofenac sodium 0.1 percent and prednisolone acetate 1 percent vs ketorolac tromethamine 0.5 percent and prednisolone acetate 1 percent. Presented at ARVO 2004.
24. Roberts CW. Comparison of the ocular comfort of acular LS with acular pf in healthy volunteers. Presented at ARVO 2004.
25. Roberts CW. Pretreatment with topical diclofenac sodium to decrease postoperative inflammation. Ophthalmology 1996;103:636-9.
26. Rossetti L, Autelitano A. Cystoid macular edema following cataract surgery. Curr Opin Ophthalmol 2000;11:65-72.
27. Sandoval HP, Fernandez de Castro LE, Vroman DT, Solomon KD. Comparison of 0.4 percent ketorolac tromethamine ophthalmic solution vs 0.5 percent ketorolac tromethamine ophthalmic solution to prevent inflammation after phacoemulsification and intraocular lens implantation: A Prospective, Randomized, Double-Masked, Clinical Trial. Presented at ARVO 2005.
28. Schechter BA, Wittpenn JR. Evaluation of ketorolac (Acular LS) during the induction phase of cyclosporine a (Restasis) therapy to improve patient comfort. Presented at ARVO 2005.
29. Singal N, Hopkins J. Pseudophakic cystoid macular edema: ketorolac alone vs ketorolac plus prednisolone. Can J Ophthalmol 2004;39(3):245-50.
30. Snyder RW, Siekert RW, Schwiegerling J, Donnenfeld E, Thompson P. Acular as a single agent for use as an antimiotic and anti-inflammatory in cataract surgery. J Cataract Refract Surg 2000;26:1225-7.
31. Solomon KD, Donnenfeld ED, Raizman M, et al. Safety and efficacy of ketorolac tromethamine 0.4 percent ophthalmic solution in post-photorefractive keratectomy patients. J Cataract Refract Surg 2004;30(8):1653-60.
32. Solomon KD, Vroman DT, Barker D, Gehlken J. Comparison of ketorolac tromethamine 0.5 percent and rimexolone 1 percent to control inflammation after cataract extraction. Prospective randomized double-masked study. J Cataract Refract Surg 2001; 27(8):1232-7.
33. Srinivasan R, Madhavaranga. Topical ketorolac tromethamine 0.5 percent versus diclofenac sodium 0.1 percent to inhibit miosis during cataract surgery. J Cataract Refract Surg 2002;28(3): 517-20.

34. Stewart R, Grosserode R, Cheetham JK, et al. Efficacy and safety profile of ketorolac 0.5 percent ophthalmic solution in the prevention of surgically induced miosis during cataract surgery. Clin Ther 1999;21:723-32.
35. Ursell PG, Spalton DJ, Whitcup SM, Nussenblatt RB. Cystoid macular edema after phacoemulsification: relationship to blood-aqueous barrier damage and visual acuity. J Cataract Refract Surg 1999;25(11):1492-7.
36. Waterbury LD, Flach AJ. Efficacy of low concentrations of ketorolac tromethamine in animal models of ocular inflammation. J Ocul Pharmacol Ther 2004;20:345-52.

Immunosuppressive Drugs in Ophthalmology

Ashok Garg (India)

INTRODUCTION

Immunosuppressive drugs should be prescribed by ophthalmologist preferably with greater caution and in concert with an oncologist.

Till date there appears to have been very low incidence of severe complications from the combined regimen of corticosteroids and immunosuppressive agents probably because of lower dosage use and better general health of ophthalmic patients receiving them. Patients should be fully informed as to potential risks and benefits.

SELECTION OF PATIENTS

- Selection involves those patients who have progressive, usually bilateral vision threatening disease.
- Failed to respond to conventional corticosteroid therapy or have unacceptable side effects from them.
- Have Wegener's granulomatosis, polyarteritis nodosa or Behcet's disease (Drugs of first choice).
- Have adequate follow-up.
- Good compliance about following instructions.
- Are ready to undergo therapy voluntarily with knowledge of potential side effects.
- May benefit certainly from the use of the drugs.
- Have no primary contraindication like active tuberculosis, toxoplasmosis or other infectious process.

Immunosuppressive agents used in ocular inflammatory diseases are classified into three groups:
1. Alkylating agents
2. Antimetabolites
3. Antibiotics.

ALKYLATING AGENTS

Common alkylating agents used in ophthalmic conditions are cyclophosphamide and chlorambucil. They work by suppression of lymphocyte T cell (cell mediated immunity) and to lesser extent B cell (antibodies) function.

Clinical Indications

Behcet's disease, sympathetic ophthalmia, rheumatoid arthiritis, polyarteritis nodosa, Wegner's granulomatosis, relapsing poly chondritis, Bullous pemphigoid and Malignancy.

Dosage

Cyclophosphamide

In adult patients start at 150-200 mg/day (1-2 mg/kg/day) taken empty stomach. A white blood count (WBC) is taken at day 1 and after every 2-3 days until at about 7 days. At this point dosage is reduced by 25-50 mg to stabilize the WBC at about 3000 cells/ul. WBC and complete blood count (CBC) with differential are than followed weekly and fortnightly once stabilized.

Chlorambucil Dosage

In adult patients start at 0.1-0.2 mg/kg/day and increased every 3-4 days to total dosage of 10-12 mg/day if there is no idiosyncratic reaction. The WBC and CBC with differential leukocyte count (DLC) are followed as for cyclophosphamide.

Adverse Reactions

Adverse side effects of alkylating agents include:
- Thrombocytopenia
- Anemia and oppurtunistic infections
- GIT disturbances
- Alopecia, Jaundice
- Pulmonary interstitial fibrosis
- Renal toxicity and testicular atrophy
- Hemorrhagic cystitis is an indication for discontinuing the medication. There is report of increased incidence of myeloproliferative and lymphoproliferative malignancy in patients on these drugs.

ANTIMETABOLITES

The antimetabolites used in ophthalmology are:
- Azathioprine which interfers with purine metabolism.
- Methotrexate which interfers with folate action.
  Both functions are essential for nucleic acid synthesis.

Clinical Indications

- In rheumatoid arthritis, pemphigoid and regional ileitis.
- Sympathetic ophthalmia and VKH syndrome.
- Pars planitis and Behcet's disease.
- Recalcitrant cases of intermediate uveitis.

Dosage

Azathioprine

Azathioprine dosage starts at 1–2 mg/kg/day gradually increasing to 2.5 mg/kg/day. The usual dose range is 100–200 mg/day in one or divided doses. Patient WBC, CBC with differential are taken at regular intervals.

Adverse Reaction
- Uncontrolled leukopenia
- Thrombocytopenia
- Hyperuricemia
- GIT disturbances.

Methotrexate Dosage

Methotrexate dosage is variable due to high drug toxicity. Generally for 1–4 weeks oral, IM or IV dose of 2.5–15 mg is given over 36–48 hours until a therapeutic response is noted and then maintained as per hematologic (weekly) and renal and hepatic (monthly) monitoring.

Adverse Effects of Methotrexate
- Leukopenia and thrombocytopenia
- Hepatic and renal toxicity
- GIT disturbances
- Interstitial pneumonitis
- CNS toxicity and sterility.

Hematological monitoring (WBC, CBC with differential) is similar to that of cyclophosphamide.

ANTIBIOTIC CYCLOSPORIN A

It probably interfers with T cell lymphocyte activation and interleukin activity and dapsone may work by lysosomal stabilization.

Indications

Clinical Indications

- Behcet's disease (for which corticosteroids are contraindicated).
- Birdshot chorioretinopathy
- Sarcoid, VKH and sympathetic ophthalmia.

Relative Indications

All noninfectious cases of uveitis unresponsive to maximum tolerated steroid therapy.
- Eales disease
- Retinal vasculitis (noninfectious)
- Serpiginous choroiditis.

- Anterior segment diseases include Pemphigoid, Mooren's ulcer, high risk corneal transplant rejection and cataract surgery in uveitis patients.

Dosage

2.5–5 mg/kg/day given orally in an olive oil—ethanol solution with milk or juice. Maximum dose is 10 mg/kg/day.

Adverse Effects

- Systemic hypertension
- Partially reversible renal toxicity
- Opportunistic infections
- Hyperuricemia
- Hepatotoxicity

Monthly and if required weekly blood tests (CBC with differential and WBC) should monitor these effects.

- A combination of steroid and cyclosporin A therapy augment each other such that addition of prednisone (10-20 mg/day) or short-term 1 mg/kg/day may allow a lowering of the cyclosporin A dosage (4-6 mg/kg/day) with no loss of therapeutic efficacy).
- Chlorambucil or cyclophosphamide and steroid management module

It involves initial treatment with prednisone 1 mg/kg/day along with cytotoxic drug at an appropriate dose. This treatment should be continued for 4 weeks until the disease is suppressed than steroids are tapered and stopped over 2 months. The cytotoxic drug dose is adjusted to keep the WBC at 3000-4000/ul and continued for one year to induce remission before being stopped. Monitor the CBC and urine analysis weekly until stable than at every 2 weeks.

OCULAR DRUG TOXICITY OF IMMUNOSUPPRESSIVE AGENTS USED IN OPHTHALMIC CONDITIONS

- Decrease in vision
- Visual hallucinations
- Lids or conjunctiva—redness, conjunctivitis, subconjunctival hemorrhage and hypertrichosis
- Eyelashes or brow losses
- Retinal hemorrhages
- Retinal pigment epithelium disturbances
- Cortical blindness (cyclosporin).

RECENT ADVANCES IN IMMUNOSUPPRESSIVE THERAPY

- Active research is going on competitive inhibition of IgE binding to effector cells using Fc fragments from human IgE. Isolation of the specific binding site and fragment production

with recombinant DNA technology may allow selective inhibition of mast cells or eosinophils in ocular allergic disorders.
- Adhesion molecules are proteins that allow cells to interact with one another. In patients of SAC and VKC there is a marked increase in conjunctival expression of ICAM-1, ICAM-3 and other adhesion molecules when compared to normal.

  Intensive efforts are going on in developing specific therapeutic agents that can modulate these adhesion molecule (proteins) and diminish the allergic response.
- Clinical trials are going on in development of suitable therapeutic agents that could modulate the actions of cytokines such as IL-3, IL-5 and GM-CSF suppressing aspects of the immune response that are not strongly affected by current available medications. A better clinical understanding of the role of specific cytokines in the different ocular allergic disorders shall stimulate the development of tailoring therapeutic agents to each of these entities.

Liposomes

New drug delivery systems may offer advantages in future therapy for ocular allergic disorders. Liposomes are vesicles consisting of lipid bilayers alternating with aqueous compartments. They may provide several advantages over current therapeutic modalities in ocular diseases.
- These allow prolonged contact between the medication and ocular tissue by preventing excessive rapid drug removal via tears.
- Changes in lipid composition and liposome structure can alter the amount of intraocular drug absorption.
- Incorporation of monoclonal antibodies into outer lipid bilayer of the liposome would transport the liposome to the target tissue or cell type where the drug is required.

A safe liposome system is now available for ocular use. Cationic lipids such as BDSA can be added to the outer surface of liposomes thereby increasing the contact time of medication with ocular tissues. This liposome system cause minimal eye irritation and may prove valuable in clinical treatment of ocular allergy.

BIBLIOGRAPHY

1. Agarwal A. Textbook of Ophthalmology, 1st edn. New Delhi: Jaypee Brothers Medical Publishers, 2002.
2. Bartlett JD. Clinical Ocular Pharmacology, 4th edn. Boston: Butterworth-Heinemann, 2001.
3. Bartlett JD. Ophthalmic Drug Facts, Lippincott–William and Wilkins, 2001.
4. Bartlett JD, Ross RN. Primary Care of Ocular Allergy J Am. Optom Assoc. 1990;61:S3-46.
5. Ciprandi G, et al. Drug Treatment Allergic Conjunctivitis: Drugs. 1992;43:154.
6. Crick RP, Trimble RB. Textbook of Clinical Ophthalmology, Hodder and Stoughton, 1986.

7. Duane TD. Clinical Ophthalmology, 4th edn. Butterworth-Heinemann, 1999.
8. Duvall. Ophthalmic Medications and Pharmacology, Slack Inc, 1998.
9. Ellis PP. Ocular Therapeutics and Pharmacology, 7th edn. CV Mosby, 1985.
10. Fechner. Ocular Therapeutics, Slack Inc, 1998.
11. Fraunfelder. Current Ocular Therapy, 5th edn. WB Saunders, 2000.
12. Garg A. Current Trends in Ophthalmology, 1st edn. New Delhi: Jaypee Brothers Medical Publishers, 1997.
13. Garg A. Manual of Ocular Therapeutics, 1st edn. New Delhi: Jaypee Brothers Medical Publishers, 1996.
14. Garg A. Ready Reckoner of Ocular Therapeutics, 1st edn. New Delhi, 2002.
15. Goodman LS, Gilman A. Pharmacological Basis of Therapeutics, 7th edn. New York: Macmillan, 1985.
16. Havener's. Ocular Pharmacology, 6th edn. CV Mosby, 1994.
17. Kanski. Clinical Ophthalmology, 4th edn. Butterworth-Heinemann, 1999.
18. Kershner. Ophthalmic Medications and Pharmacology, Slack. Inc, 1994.
19. Olin BR, et al. Drugs Facts and Comparisons: Facts and Comparisons, St. Louis, 1997.
20. Onofrey. The Ocular Therapeutics; Lippincott-William and Wilkins, 1997.
21. Rhee. The Wills Eye Drug Guide, Lippincott-William and Wilkins, 1998.
22. Steven Podos. Textbook of Ophthalmology, New Delhi: Jaypee Brothers Medical Publishers, 2001.
23. Zimmerman. Textbook of Ocular Pharmacology, Lippincott-William and Wilkins, 1997.

Management of Cystoid Macular Edema

Arturo Pérez Arteaga, René-Cano Hidalgo (Mexico)

INTRODUCTION

Cystoid macular edema (CME) is an inflammatory condition of the central retina that can be produced for many causes, since drugs for other ophthalmic diseases until surgical intervention of the eye. If well the initial descriptions of the disease can be found as a surgical complication, now we know much more conditions that can produce these clinical and para-clinical findings, so that we can talk about a multifactorial disease.

Many drugs are involved in the treatment of this condition. The choose of each one is according the etiology of the inflammatory process, preference of the physician, response of the patient, underlying disease, severity of visual loss and anatomic findings. Even surgical treatment has been described, and so the use of specifical drugs during and after the procedure; so it is a very good way to review the drugs involved in the treatment of this pathologic condition according to the philosophy of this book, the use of anti-inflammatory drugs in ophthalmology. In fact several proven treatment modalities are available and so on new therapies are continuing to expand our horizons.

First the reader will find in this chapter a brief description of CME definition, etiology, clinical findings and diagnostic strategies. Then the drugs that are involved in the treatment of this condition, including those used in the surgical treatment will be described.

DEFINITION

The CME is a pathologic condition of the macula with swelling where multiple cyst-like (cystoid) areas of fluid appear in the central retina, mostly in the outer plexiform layer. It is a painless disorder that according to the cause and severity can be fully reversed or can cause permanent visual loss. Sometimes this condition has clinical manifestations from low to severe, but also can occur in the sub-clinic plane.

ETIOLOGY

Postsurgical, Primary or Secondary (Capsulotomy)

It was first described as the Irving-Gass syndrome; a pathologic condition where Irving in 1953 mentioned a decrease in the visual acuity with vitreoretinal alterations after the intracapsular surgery of the lens, and Gass and Norton described the typical fluoroangiographic changes of this condition. At that time 77 percent of the eyes operated with intracapsular cataract surgery developed some degree of CME, even sometimes sub-clinical.

During the days of the extracapsular cataract extraction the incidence decreased because the preservation of the posterior capsule and the decrease of vitreous loss. Even so, this incidence increase when there is posterior capsule rupture in an extracapsular technique. With the entrance of phacoemulsification techniques for cataract surgery the incidence was even less, but again, it was demostrated that the main goal to decrease this condition is the conservation of the posterior capsule and to avoid the vitreous loss. It is still to be proved that the newest technologies of minimally invasive cataract surgery can produce a statistical significative reduction of postcataract surgery CME.

The posterior capsulotomy is also a very well-known procedure that can lead to CME, and it is also related to the rupture of the retinal and aqueous barriers; so in this field new technologies and evolution of intraocular lenses that can reduce the incidence of posterior capsule opacification are very important.

Any kind of intraocular surgery can produce sometime some degree of CME. At the end the cascade of events become from the rupture of the intraocular barriers. The initial trauma (damage, surgery, etc.) produce the liberation of the chemical mediators of the inflammation to the aqueous and vitreous; mainly prostraglandins are produced by the damaged tissue and the traumatized epithelial cells, but many other factors like the complement, the platelet activation factor, lysosomal enzymes, cytoquines, nitric oxide, endothelin and interleuki. We can conclude that any factor that contributes to the rupture of the barriers blood-aqueous and blood-retinal is going to increase the possibility to develope CME.

Microvascular Damage

This is commonly found in diabetic retinopathy, occlusive diseases like retinal vein occlusions, and other less commonly diseases like idiopathic juxtafoveal capillary telangiectasia. The main factor is again the rupture of the intraocular barriers that this vascular alterations produce and the liberation of the mentioned mediators during the acute vascular event. Some other factors like the VEGF and IGF-1 liberated by the ischemic tissues, have been involved in the rupture of the intraocular barriers and so in the production of CME. Any syndrome associated with sub-retinal neovascularization can have the same effect.

Inflammatory Diseases

The most well-known form of uveitis that can produce CME is pars planitis; in fact CME is the main cause of visual loss in this inflammatory process, but many other forms of uveitis like Behçet´s disease, Crohn´s disease, rheumatoid arthritis, sarcoidosis and some other forms of non-specificual uveitis can produce some degree of CME. The cause is as mentioned before, the liberation of the inflammatory mediators.

Postmedication (Antiglaucoma Drugs and Preservatives)

The first reference about the relation between an anti-glaucoma medication and the development of CME was described by Becker in 1967 and was with the use of epinephrine; was noted years after, that this incidence was more in the aphakic patient. It is well known at this time, that the topical epinephrine increase the prostraglandins in the eye, in particular in the aphakic one, and so the rupture of the intraocular barriers.

Some other medications were described to produce this effect like dipivalil epinephrine, timolol and benzalkonium chloride. Recently with the arise of new pharmacologic groups of anti-glaucomatous medication, in particular prostraglandins, the incidence of post-medication CME has increase. A lot of studies have been conducted in this field and what we know currently is that latanoprost, travoprost, bimatoprost and unoprostone can produce some degree of CME and that this incidence can increase with the association of risk factors like cataract surgery, uveitis, posterior capsulotomy and diabetic retinopathy.

This concepts must be taken in count by the physician at the time to prescribe this medications in particular if some risk factors are present in some patient. If the therapy can be done with another medication it will be better, but if it must be continued for some reason, the utilization of nonsteroidal anti-inflammatory drugs can avoid the development of CME without loss of the hypotensor effect of the anti-glaucoma drugs. Also a constant follow up with the explanation to the patient of specific symptoms of macular disease and Amsler test in each visit for glaucoma control, are mandatory.

Peripheral Retinal Lesions

A peripheral lesion, can lead by itself, to the rupture of the intraocular barriers and so the development of CME. It is a good behavior to explore the periphery of the retina in a case when we find CME and we are trying to know the cause.

Tumoral Diseases

Because of acummulation of leakage and rupture of the barriers, many ocular tumors, like malignant melanomas, peripheral capillary hemangiomas and Coat's disease can be also cause of CME.

Eye Hypotony

It can be post-traumatic, with or without rupture of the globe, it can be followed cataract surgery, glaucoma procedures or choroidal effusions of any cause. At the end, the low intraocular pressure is the cause for the rupture of the intraocular barriers and so the liberation of mediators.

Optic Nerve Diseases

Optic nerve inflammations like true papilledema, neuropathy or some ischemic diseases can produce CME.

Retinal Traction

Peripheral traction, macular traction, epiretinal membranes, and traction produced by diabetic retinopathy (even without direct macular traction) are common entities that can produce CME.

Final Common Pathway of Underlying Diseases

Ischemic, tractional, inflammatory, toxic and genetic.

HISTOPATHOLOGY

The breakdown of the inner blood retinal barrier due to vasogenic and/or cytotoxic causes is the initial event in CME. There is a leaking of the perifoveal capillaries leading the formation of edema. The fluid collects in the loosely arranged outer plexiform layer of Henle; in this layer the fibers are arranged in an horizontal pattern. This is the cause of the petaloid flower appearance that is seen as characteristic of this disease in the angiogram (cystic pattern) (Fig. 44.1). Electronic microscopy has shown acummulation of intracellular fluid within expanded Müller cell processes.

CLINICAL FINDINGS

There is always an history of previous ocular disease, surgery, medication, vitreous pathology or another condition in the patient that develops CME. Sometimes it can be very easy to obtain, like

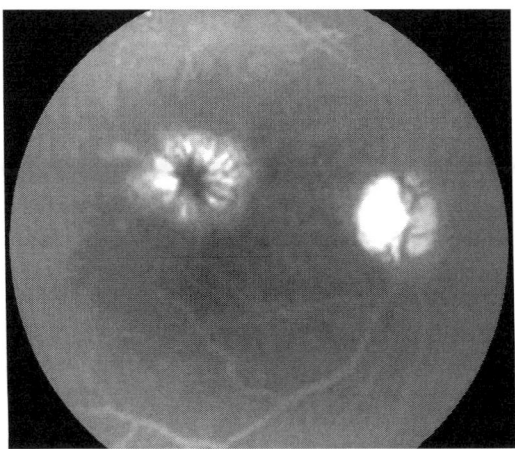

Fig. 44.1. Cystic pattern

previous cataract surgery or posterior capsulotomy, but in some others, the physician must be very accurate like in glaucoma medications, posterior vitreous detachment or peripheral tears that may lead to the break of the inner blood retinal barrier.

The main symptom of CME is the reduction of visual acuity, even so, here are many forms of CME that goes free of visual symptoms. Many patients that undergo a cataract surgery can develop some degree of sub-clinical CME, and the only one evidence can be found in a retinal fluorogram. The degree of the disease and so the severity of symptoms frequently correlates with the degree of complications during the cataract surgery, if this is the case. So, the reduction of visual acuity may undergo from a minimal degree, like 20/25 and be not notice by the patient, until very poor visuality like 20/400 or less in severe cases. Like some others macular diseases the patients can experience some degree of metamorphopsia.

At the clinical examination the evidence of surgery, trauma, vascular retinal diseases and others like glaucoma diseases must be achieved. Of course, the main study is the fundoscopy where the macular thickening and/or swelling can be found. It also can be found in many degrees depending upon the severity of the disease, and can go since a loss of foveolar reflex without clinical evidence of edema, to a characteristic cystic appearance. This is the typical clinical finding in the ophthalmoscopy, radiating cystic spaces emanating from the macula. Of course, in these cases, there is a complete loss of the red reflex. The red free light examination is mandatory, where a "honeycombed" appearance is seen, and it corresponds to the fluid filled cyst (Fig. 44.2). In severe cases, these cyst may coalesce into a macular cyst and then form a hole.

PARACLINICAL APPROACH

No laboratory studies are necessary to establish the diagnosis of CME. The main study in the establishment of this diagnosis is the fluorescein angiogram (FA).

In the FA, parafoveal retinal capillary leakage is seen in the early and mid phases. These phases are not characteristic of CME, because the acummulation of fluid in certain conditions is delayed,

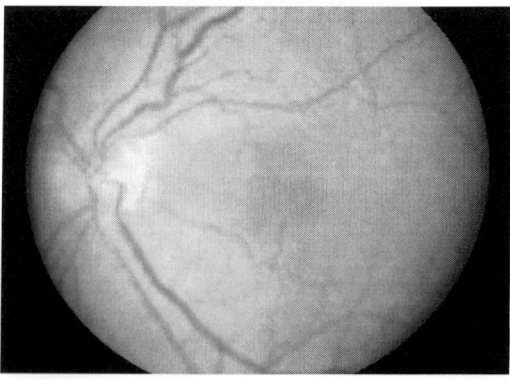

Fig. 44.2. Loss of red reflex

so, the late phase has a particular importance, and it is about 20 minutes and sometimes can be more, to find the characteristic petaloid pattern of leakage in the macula.

Another related conditions can be seen in the FA according the underlying disease: if leakage microaneurisms are present, diabetic retinopathy can be the cause; vascular collaterals can be due to retinal occlusion; optic nerve findings are also useful in the final etiologic diagnosis establishment.

Optical coherence tomography (OCT) is a non-invasive method also very useful in the final diagnosis of CME because the fluid-filled spaces in the retina are easily seen. This cross-sectional image of the retina can also be helpful in the monitoring over time of the disease by quantifying the amount of fluid inside the retina in serial studies. A non-invasive study can be the ideal modality in monitoring the response to treatment.

In particular cases an electroretinogram can also be helpful but not mandatory.

TREATMENT

The treatment of CME can be divided in two approaches that finally in the practice are combined, but in the theory, we are going to describe separately.

Nonsurgical Approach

Many drugs have been involved for the treatment of CME during the time. Some of them are used as a traditional fashion and some others are emerging as new therapeutic resources.

Nonsteroidal Anti-inflammatory Drugs

The main effect of this group of drugs is to stabilize the blood-retinal barrier. This effect is because they inhibit the enzyme cyclooxygenase. They can be used by systemic way and also in the form of eyedrops. The main examples of this group of medications are:
- Indomethacin
- Ketorolac
- Diclofenac.

They inhibit the prostaglandin synthesis by decreasing the activity of the enzyme cyclooxygenase. These drugs in the topical form must be used as a medication in the preoperative and postoperative period of some intraocular procedures like cataract surgery, posterior capsulotomy and peripheral iridectomy for example, to reduce the incidence of CME. This profilactic form also helps to reduce the postoperative inflammatory process. As has been said before, the development of CME in some way correlates with the degree of manipulation during the ocular surgery and some factors have been demonstrated in the development of CME like the time of light microscope exposure, posterior capsule rupture and vitreous manipulation. Of course, a real "clean" surgery can decrease the incidence of CME, but anyway, the use of

NSAIDs is mandatory. New operative devices that avoid the use of direct light exposure during the ocular surgery are promising in the near future to decrease the incidence of CME in uncomplicated surgery cases.

The use of systemic NSAIDs is only reserve for the cases of complete diagnosis of CME; even so some surgeons are using them as a profilactic medication. There is not a recomended time for the use of systemic NSAIDs for the treatment of CME; the time of use will depend upon the response of each patient in particular according the follow-up.

Because sometimes it is a long-term medication, secondary effects of NSAIDs must be always taken in count. In the systemic medication, gastric effects should be monitoring during the visits of the patient. A history of gastric diseases including ulcerative disease and bleeding is mandatory when oral indometacine is in use. If some of these effects are present the therapeutic must be suspended and replaced by other medication.

Local NSAIDs have also some secondary effects; long-term use may delay wound healing and has been reported cases of corneal stromal thinning or melting in some particular patients receiving diclofenac eyedrops for extended period of time. If symptoms like blurred or diminished vision and signs of corneal deposits, retinal changes and scotoma are present, the medication must be suspended.

Corticosteroids

Steroidal medication is very useful in the treatment of CME and also in the prevention of it. The routine use of steroids in the eyedrops form before and after surgical procedures, has decrease the incidence of postsurgical CME, even in complicated cases.

The most frequent form of steroid medication for CME is topical, in the form of prednisolone acetate; it is indicated in several conditions of steroid-responsive intraocular inflammation. The presentation is at 1 percent solution and can be used several times in a day according to the severity of the inflammation. The amount and time of administration must be measured according to the response of the disease to the treatment. Monitoring of the side effects of topical steroids like, raise in the intraocular pressure and an increased risk of secondary ocular infections, must be evaluating during the time of therapy and this should be discontinued if some of these effects are found. Not all patients have the same response to steroids according to the rise in the intraocular pressure; some patients can tolerate large periods of time without changes in the pressure, but some others can not tolerate too much medication. If the topical steroid therapy is really needed in these cases, the physician can add some glaucoma therapy; medications that can increase the CME, should be avoided (e.g. latanoprost, travoprost, epinephrine); the best adjunctive anti-glaucoma medication is dorzolamide that also can have some benefit effect in the macula. Other side effects of long-term topical steroids like subcapsular cataract formation must be addressed.

The use of injections of long acting depot-steroids (e.g. triamcinolone) into the sub-Tenon space has also a role in the treatment of CME. This external way of administration that can have more penetration to the retina; the drug delivery to the retina is superior by this route in comparison to peribulbar. In some cases of uveitic CME refractory to conventional treatment, the triamcinolone has been used in intravitreous injection alone or in combination with some other drugs. Triamcinolone alone has been effectively in reducing CME and improving vision; some studies are currently underway in the combination of this steroidal drug with other drugs, like bevacizumab (avastin).

Oral steroids play also an important role in the treatment of CME because the effect in the stabilization of the blood-ocular barrier. They can be useful in some forms of uveitic CME. Nevertheless, the secondary effects of systemic corticoid medication must be avoided, and this is why recently the medication of CME is trying to move to the ocular space instead the systemic route.

Carbonic Anhydrase Inhibitors

Carbonic anhydrase is an enzyme present in the apical and basal surfaces of the retinal pigment epithelium cell membrane. It´s action is to pump and produce a change in the ion flux. CAIs enhance this pumping action of these cells, and help to improve this ion flux that affects the cellular environment of the retina.

Carbonic anhydrase inhibitors (CAIs) are commonly used in ophthalmology, in particular in the glaucoma cases, where the topical medication is not enough to control the intraocular pressure, so it is a well-known resource. Also, the physician is close to side effects of the CAIs, like the alteration in the ionic composition of blood, increase in urine excretion, and in large doses hepatic and metabolic problems. So, it is known that it is not a chronic medication, it has to be used according the severity and response to treatment of CME and the physician has to advice the patient the side effects, the mode to contrarest them and the total communication they both have to maintain in order to manage the dose in good response, but also in good levels of side effects. This medication should be suspended as soon as possible according the evolution of CME.

The presentation of acetazolamide is in tablets of 250 mg and can be given until three to four times a day. Close monitoring of anti-inflammatory and side effects is mandatory.

Intravitreal Medication

Recently new drugs are appearing in the retinal medication field for intravitreal injection, like bevacizumab (avastin) and pegaptanib, also called macugen. These drugs are promising results in many retinal vascular disorders like occlusive diseases and diabetic retinopathy. The side effects are not completely known, and many trials around the world are in progress at this time to achieve consistent results.

The apparently positive action seen in some vascular disorders lead the possibility to use them in CME. Some of them are including only diabetic patients, some others only postoperative cataract patients and some others are combining the avastin with triamcinolone.

Surgical Approach and Drugs Related

The surgical treatment is not the first choice in the treatment of CME; nevertheless, some particular situations can lead to the indication of pars plana vitrectomy (PPV):
- Cases of uveitis related CME.
- Remove of vitreous strands that can have an effect of "pull the retina", from anterior and posterior segment structures.
- Remove inflammatory mediators from the vitreous (e.g. memory cells, cytokines), that can be maintaining an inflammatory response.
- Remove of retained lens fragments.
- Remove of epiretinal membrane.

Because the rupture of the blood-retinal barrier, after the PPV there is an increase in the penetration of topical and oral steroids. Also some surgeons are happy with the use of triamcinolone during the surgical approach, achieving so the benefit effect of both, vitrectomy and intravitreal medication. We believe at this time, that the PPV by itself is not enough for the treatment of CME; we agree that it must be accompanied by intravitreal medication.

The side effects of steroids in the vitreous cavity must be addressed continuously because the possibility of changes in IOP; in this particular case sometimes it is very difficult to achieve a good IOP because the deposit effect of the steroid. Even so, sometimes without steroid medication in the vitreous cavity, PPV itself, is able to produce an increase in IOP of difficult control.

The final decision to perform a PPV must be carefully evaluated and consented between the surgeon and patient, because of the possible side effects.

CONCLUSION

At the end of the day a lot of factors are going to influence the prognosis of a patient who develops CME. The main factor of all is the inherent cause of the disease; it will not be the same a patient who develops CME because of a glaucoma treatment (in this case the suspension of the prostaglandin and the medical treatment with NSAIDs can be enough to reverse by complete the disease without any permanent loss of vision), that a CME caused by a chronic pars planitis of difficult treatment (in this case a chronic CME can lead to severe decrease of vision).

Patients, who are going to be operated, in particular anterior segment procedures, must be medicated since the preoperative period, through the operation and during the postoperative time, with drugs that can decrease the development of CME, like steroids and NSAIDs according the case. After all, we know about this disease, prevention and treatment we believe this should be mandatory. Also in patients with glaucoma control with prostaglandines, this therapy should be avoided and the control must be followed with another anti-glaucoma medication, during the pre, trans and postoperative period. It is not possible to eliminate the prostaglandin and NSAIDs should be started in addition.

Of particular importance is the glaucoma patient, who is receiving medication that can produce CME; the physician must be alert to any kind of sign that can advice the presentation of CME. The adjunctive NSAIDs therapy can be helpful in cases where is impossible to avoid prostaglandins.

New medications are promising good results, even alone or in combination, for the treatment of refractory CME. Like all new products, we are expecting some new non-reported adverse effects; the test of time, like always, will lead us to the complete knowledge of their specific indications.

BIBLIOGRAPHY

1. Antcliff RJ, Standorf MR, Chauhan DS, et al. Comparison between optical coherence tomography and fundus fluorescein angiography for detection of cystoid macular edema in patients with uveitis. Ophthalmology 2000;107:593-9.
2. Ayyala RS, Cruz DA, Margo CE, et al. Cystoid macular edema associated with latanoprost in aphakic and pseudophakic eyes. Am J Ophthalmol 1998;126:602-4.
3. Becker B. Topical epinephrine in the treatment of the glaucomas. In New Orleans Glaucoma Symposium: 152-159. The CV Mosby Company. St Louis, 1967.
4. Bhattacherjee P, Kulkarny PS, Eakins KE. Metabolism of arachidonic acid in rabbit ocular tissues. Invest Ophthalmol Vis Sci 1979;18:172-8.
5. Callanan D, Fellmann RL, Savage JA. Latanoprost associated cystoid macular edema. Am J Ophthalmol 1998;126:134-5.
6. Clinical Trials Gov. US National Institutes of Healt. Effect of Prophylactic Ketorolac on CME after cataract surgery. Queens University. May, 2006. Trial ongoing.
7. Clinical Trials Gov. US National Institutes of Healt. The Effect of Macugen in Patients with chronic, Post-Operative Cystoid Macular Edema. John Hopkins University. July, 2006. Trial ongoing.
8. Clinical Trials Gov. US National Institutes of Healt. To compare Therapeutic effect of Intravitreal Bevacizumab and Triamcinolone in Resistant Uveitic Cystoid Macular Edema. Shaheed Beheshti Medical University. September, 2006. Trial ongoing.
9. Flach AJ, Jampol LM, Weinberg D, et al. Improvement in visual acuity in chronic aphakic and pseudophakic cystoid macular edema after treatment with topical 0.5 percent ketorolac tromethamine. Am J Ophthtalmol 1991;112:514-9.
10. Furuichi M, Chiba T, Abe K, Kogure S, Iijima H, Tsukahara S, Kashiwagi K. Cistoid macular edema associated with topical Latanoprost in glaucomatous eyes with a normal functioning blood-ocular barrier. J Glaucoma 2001;10:233-6.
11. Gass JDM, Norton EDW. Cystoid macular edema and papilledema following cataract extraction. A fluorescein, funduscopic and angiografic study. Arch Ophthalmol 1966;76:646-61.

12. Handa J, Henry JC, Krupìn T, et al. Extracapsular cataract extraction with posterior chamber lens implantation in patients with glaucoma. Arch Ophthalmol 1987;105:765-9.
13. Hanna C, Sharp JD. Ocular absorption of indomethacin by the rabbit. Arc Ophthalmol 1972;88:196-8.
14. Heier JS, Steinert RF, Frederick AR. Cystoid macular edema associated with latanoprost use. Arch Ophthalmol. 1998;116:680-2.
15. Irvine SR. A new defined vitreous syndrome following cataract surgery interpreted according to recent concepts of the structure of the vitreous. Am J Ophthalmol 1954;36:599-619.
16. Jaffe NS, Clayman HM, Jaffe MS. Cystoid macular edema after intracapsular and extracapsular cataract extraction with and without an intraocular lens. Ophthalmology 1982;89:25-9.
17. Jampol LM, Sanders DR, Kraff MC. Prophylaxis and therapy of aphakic cystoid macular edema. Suv Ophthalmol 1984;28:535-9.
18. Kass MA, Holmberg NJ. Prostaglandin and thronboxane synthesis by microsomes of rabbit ocular tissues. Invest Ophthalmol Vis Sci 1979;18:166-71.
19. Kent D, Vinores SA, Campochiaro PA. Macular oedema: the role of soluble mediators. Br J Ophthalmol 2000;84:542-5.
20. Kolker AE, Becker B. Epinephrine maculopaty. Ach Ophthal 1968;79:552-62.
21. Liesegang TJ, Bourne WJ, Ilstrup DM. Secondary surgical and neodimium: YAG laser discussions. Am J Ophthalmol 1985;100:164-8.
22. Lima MC, Paranhos A, Salam S, et al. Visually significant cystoid macular edema in pseudophakic and aphakic patients with glaucoma receiving Latanoprost. J of Glaucoma 2000;9:317-24.
23. Malecaze F, Chollet P, Cavrois E, et al. Role of interleuquin 6 in the inflammatory response after cataract surgery. An experimental and clinical study. Arch Ophthalmol 1991;109:1681-3.
24. Mehelas TJ, Kollarits CR, Martin WG. Cystoid macular edema presumably induced by dipivefrin hydrochloride (Propine). Am J Ophthalmol 1982;94:682.
25. Meredith TA, Kenyon KR, Singerman LJ, et al. Perifoveal vascular leakage and macular edema after intracapsular cataract extraction. Br J Ophthalmol 1976;60:765-76.
26. Michels RG, Maumenne AE. Cystoid macular edema associated with topically applied epinephrine in aphakic eyes. Am J Ophthalmol 1975;80:379-88.
27. Miyake K, Ibaraki N, Goto Y, Oogiya S, Ishigaki J, Ota I, Miyake S. ESCRS Binkhorst lecture 2002: Pseudophakic preservative maculopathy. J Cataract Refract Surg 2003;29:1800-10.
28. Miyake K, Ibaraki N. Prostaglandins and cystoid macular edema. Surv Ophthalmol 2002; 47(Suppl 1): S203-S218.
29. Miyake K, Kayazawa F, Manabe R, et al. Indomethacin and the epinephrine-induced breakdown of the blood-ocular barrier in rabbits. Invest Ophthalmol Vis Sci 1988;29:332-4.
30. Miyake K, Mibu H, Horiguchi M, et al. Inflammatory mediators in postoperative aphakic and pseudophakic baboon eyes. Arch Ophthalmol 1990;108:1764-7.
31. Miyake K, Miyake Y, Kuratomi R. Long-term effects of topically applied epinephrine on the blood-ocular barrier in humans. Arch Ophthalmol 1987;105:1360-3.

32. Miyake K, Miyake Y, Maekubo K, et al. Incidence of cystoid macular edema after retinal detachment surgery and the use of topical indomethacin. Am J Ophthalmol 1985;100:510-9.
33. Miyake K, Ota I, Ibaraki N, et al. Enhanced disruptionof the blood-ocular barrier and the incidente of angiographic cystoid macular edema by topical timolol and its preservative in early posoperative pseudophakia. Arch Ophthalmol 2001;119:387-94.
34. Miyake K, Ota I, Maekubo K, Ichihashi S, Miyake S. Latanoprost accelerates disruption of the blood-aqueous barrier and the incidence of angiographic cystoid macular edema in early postoperative pseudophakias. Arch Ophthalmol 1999;117:34-40.
35. Miyake K, Shirasawa E, Hikita M, et al. Síntesis of prostaglandin E in rabbit eyes with topically applied epinephrine. Invest Ophthalmol Vis Sci 1988;29:332-4.
36. Miyake K, Sugiyama S, Norimatsu I, et al. Prevention of cystoid macular edema after lens extraction by topical indomethacin. Albrecht von Graefes Arch Klin Exp Ophthalmol 1978;209:83-8.
37. Miyake K. Prevention of cystoid macular edema after lens extraction by topical indomethacin. A preliminary report. Albrecht Von Graefes Arch Klin Exp Ophthalmol 1977;203:81-8.
38. Mondino BJ, Nagata S, Glovsky MM. Activation of the alternative complement pathway by intraocular lenses. Invest Ophthalmol Vis Sci 1985;26:905-8.
39. Nishi O, Nishi K, Imanishi M. Synthesis of interleukin-1 and prostaglandin E2 by lens epithelial cells of human cataracts. Br J Ophthalmol 1992;76:338-41.
40. Ohrloff C, Schalnus R, Rothe R, et al. Role of the posterior capsule in the aqueous-vitreous barrier in aphakic and pseudophakic eyes. J Cataract Refract Surg 1990;16:198-201.
41. Ozaki H, Hayasi H, Vinores SA, et al. Intravitreal sustained release of VEGF causes retinal neovascularization in rabbits and breakdown of the blood-retinal barrier in rabbits and primates. Exp Eye Res 1997;64:505-17.
42. Pollack A, Leiba H, Bukelman A, et al. Cystoid macula oedema following cataract extraction in patients with diabetes. Br J Ophthalmol 1992;76:221-4.
43. Rossetti L, Chaudhuri J, Diickersin K. Medical profilaxis and trteatment of cystoid macular edema after cataract sugery. The results of a meta-analysis. Ophthalmology 1998;105:397-405.
44. Schumer RA, Camras CB, Mandahl AG. Putative side effects of prostaglandin analogs. Sur Ophthalmol 2002;47 (Suppl 1): S219-S230.
45. Schumer RA, Camras CB, Mandalh AK. Latanoprost and cystoid macular edema: is there a causal relation? Current Opin Ophthalmol 2000.pp.94-100.
46. Sjoquist B, Almegard B, Khalilef V, et al. The bioavailability of Xalatan in the human eye. Invest Ophthalmol Vis Sci 1997;38:S248.
47. Solomon LD. Efficacy of topical flubriprofen and indomethacin in preventing pseudophakic cystoid macular edema. Flubiprofen-CME Study Group I. J Cataract Refract Surg 1995;21:73-81.
48. Thomas JV, Gragoudas ES, Blair NP, et al. Correlation of epinephrine use and macular edema in aphakic glaucomatous eyes. Arch Ophthalmol 1978;96:625-8.
49. Ursell PG, Spalton DJ, Withcup SM, et al. Cystoid macular edema after phacoemulsification: Relationship to blood-aqueous barrier damage and visual acuity. J Cataract Refract Surg 1999;25:1492-7.

50. Vinores SA, Sen H, Campochiaro PA. An adenosine agonist and prostaglandin E1 cause breakdown of the blood-retinal barrier by opening tigth junctions between vascular endothelial cells. Invest Ophthalmol Vis Sci 1992;33:1870-8.
51. Wand M, Gaudio AR, Shields MB. Latanoprost and cystoid macular edema in high risk aphakic or pseudophakic eyes. J Cat Refract Surgery 2001;27:1397-1401.
52. Wand M, Gaudio AR. Cystoid macular edema associated with ocular hypotensive lipids. Am J Ophthalmol 2002;133:403-5.
53. Wand M, Shields BM. Cystoid macular edema in the era of ocular hypotensive lipids. Am J Ophthalmol 2002;133:393-7.
54. Warwar RE, Bullock JD, Deepti B. Cystoid macular edema and anterior uveitis associated with latanoprost use. Experience and incidence in a retrospective review of 94 patients. Ophthalmology 1998;105:263-8.
55. Weisz JM, Bressler NM, Bressler SB, et al. Ketorolac treatment of pseudophakic cystoid macular edema identified more than 24 months after cataract extraction. Ophthalmology 1999;106:1656-9.
56. Yousufzai SYK, Abdel-Latif AA. Prostaglandin F2α and its analogs induce release of endogenous prostaglandins in iris and ciliary muscles isolated from cat and other mammalian species. Ex Eye Res 1996;63:305-10.

Blepharitis

Mitchell H Friedlaender (USA)

Blepharitis is a classic example of a chronic condition with infectious and inflammatory components. It is one of the most common conditions seen in ophthalmic practice, and probably represents the leading cause of "red eyes". Curiously, blepharitis has received little attention from ophthalmologists and from the pharmaceutical industry.

CLASSIFICATION

Blepharitis may be defined as an inflammation of the eyelids. There are a variety of causes: genetic, infectious, and allergic being the most common. There are three main anatomic patterns of blepharitis:
1. Anterior, affecting the eye lashes and surrounding tissues,
2. Posterior, affecting the meibomian oil glands, and
3. Mixed, a combination of anterior and posterior blepharitis.

Anterior blepharitis (Fig. 45.1) is characterized by seborrheic scales, known as "scurf", adhering to the eye lashes (Fig. 45.2). Fibrin deposits may be lifted from the surface of the lid margins as the lashes grow, forming rings around the lashes, known as "collarettes". Inflammatory material around the base of the shaft may create the appearance of "sleeves" surrounding the eyelashes.

GENETICS

Genetic factors play a role in both anterior and posterior blepharitis. People with a tendency toward seborrhea, and dandruff, will often

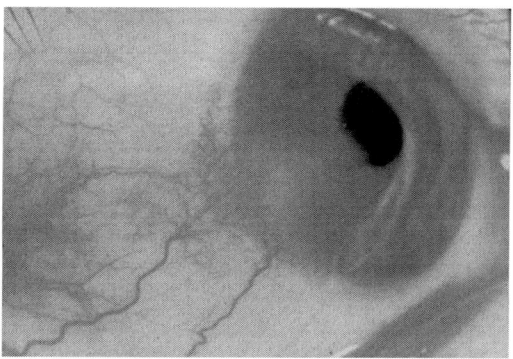

Fig. 45.1: Anterior blepharitis

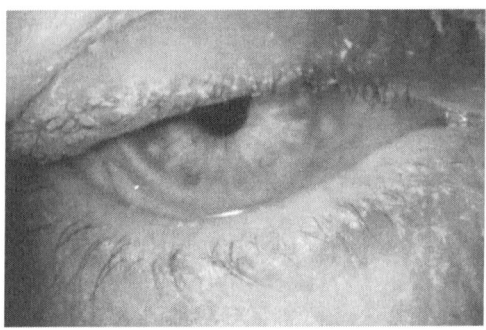

Fig. 45.2: Dandruff, or scurf adhering to the eyelashes

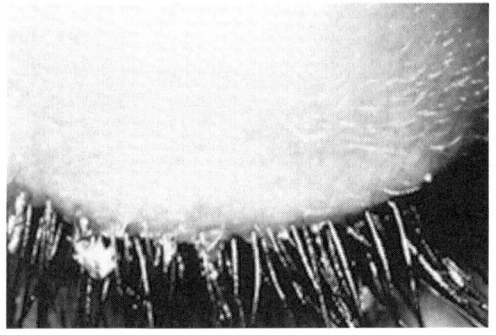

Fig. 45.3: Rosacea

have scales adhering to the eyelashes. Individuals with roscaea have plugging of the oil glands of the nose, cheeks, and forehead (Fig. 45.3). They also have plugging of the meibomian glands (Fig. 45.4), and sluggish secretions. Complete obstruction may lead to the formation of styes, or chalazia.

INFECTION

Bacteria, particularly staphylococci, have an affinity for the eyelids. It is common to culture *Staphylococcus aureus* from the lid margins of patients with blepharitis (Fig. 45.5). Other gram-positive and gram-negative organisms have also been recovered. Although swabs from the lid margins often show confluent growth of bacteria, conjunctival cutures from the same patients are often sterile. This may represent antibacterial factors in the tear film, or in the conjunctiva itself, and a resistance of conjunctival tissue to bacterial colonization.

Staphylococcus aureus can frequently be cultured from the eyelids of blepharitis patients.[1] It is widely acknowledged that *Staphylococcus* is capable of colonizing the eyelid margins, creating a chronic, low grade infection. Staphylococcal toxins probably enter the tear film and produce symptoms such as burning, stinging, redness, and discharge. Toxins may cause

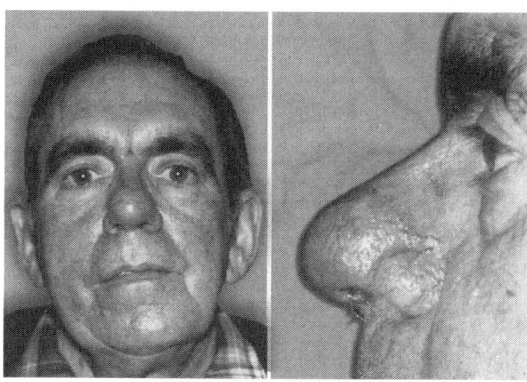

Fig. 45.4: Meibomian gland plugging

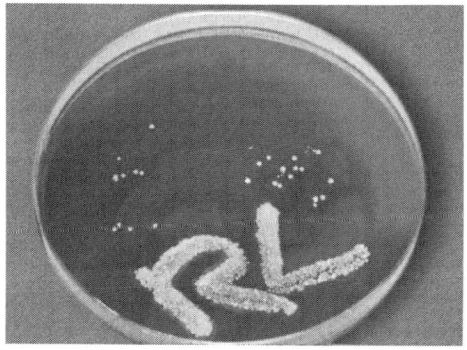

Fig. 45.5: *Staphylococcus* cultured from the lid margins

inflammation and breakdown of the delicate skin of the eyelids (Fig. 45.6). Other organisms have been implicated in blepharitis. For example, the parasite *Demodex folliculorum* has been found in about one-third of blepharitis cases.[2] No clear pathologic role has been established for *Demodex* in blepharitis, and the organism's presence may be an incidental finding. More recently, *Helicobacter pylori*, the bacteria associated with peptic ulcers, gastritis, gastric cancer, and possibly gastric lymphoma, has been found in 76 percent of blepharitis cases.[3] Again, a causal role for this organism has not been established. We have cultured *Serratia marscesans*, along with *Staphylococcus aureus* from the eyelids of a child with a congenital immunodeficiency syndrome.

Blepharitis is common with viral infections, particularly herpes simplex, and herpes zoster. These conditions are readily identified by the characteristic appearance and distribution of vesicles and pustules on the eyelids.

ALLERGY

Allergy, particularly contact allergy, can produce inflammation of the eyelids (Fig. 45.7). Cosmetics, soaps, and shampoos, often

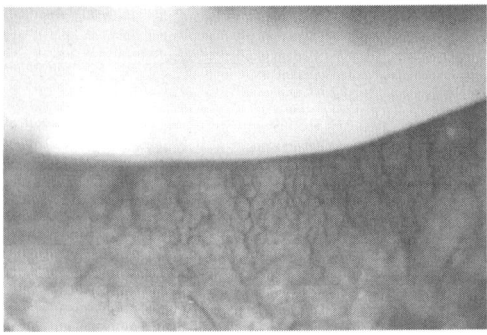

Fig. 45.6: Skin toxicity from staphylococcal blepharitis

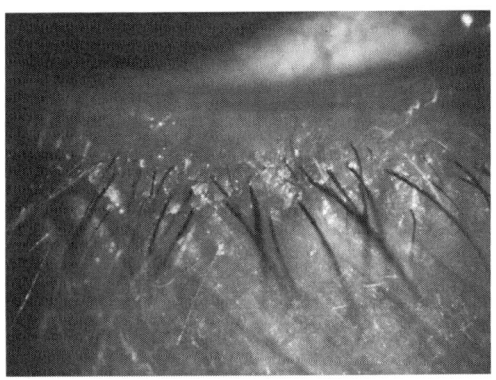

Fig. 45.7: Contact allergy

contain allergenic substances which can cause a cell-mediated, or delayed, hypersensitivity reaction, of the eyelids. Eyedrops containing neomycin, or sulfa, are frequent causes of contact allergic blepharits. Typically, contact blepharitis reactions begin one to three days after exposure to the offending agent. The eyelids become inflamed and itchy. The proper treatment involves the identification of the allergenic substance, and withdrawal of the offending agent. Corticosteroids, usually in cream or ointment form, will help relieve symptoms of itching, swelling, and discomfort. Blepharitis can also be seen in IgE-mediated allergy, especially severe types, such as atopic keratoconjunctivitis, and vernal keratoconjunctivitis. It is believed that allergic mediators, produced by mast cells, eosinophils, and other inflammatory cells have a toxic effect on the delicate skin of the eyelids.

CORNEAL MANIFESTATIONS

Corneal complications are often associated with chronic blepharitis. Catarrhal infiltrates occur in the peripheral cornea at the 2, 4, 8, and 10 o'clock positions (Fig. 45.8). They usually appear as white, or translucent, infiltrated, but sometimes they are confluent

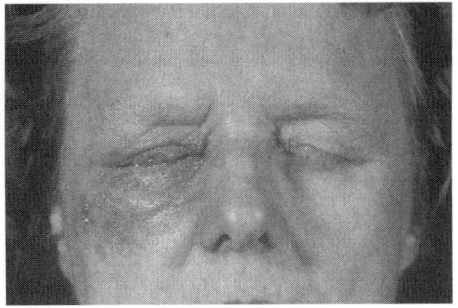

Fig. 45.8: Phlyctenule

and may form a complete, or incomplete, ring around the cornea, approximately 1 mm central to the limbus. Catarrhal infiltrates may leave spade-shaped scars near the limbus. Sometimes, these contain a leash of blood vessels, extending in from the limbus. The appearance of these characteristic corneal scars is often a clue to the diagnosis of blepharitis. Phlyctenules, are much less common than catarrhal infiltrates, but they can be associated with staphylococcal blepharitis, particularly in children.[4]

CHEMISTRY

Considerable work has been done on the chemistry of the lipids and proteins in the meibomian oil gland secretions of patients with blepharitis. McCulley[5] has demonstrated a defect in polar lipids, and suggested this may produce an unstable tear film, and abnormally rapid tear evaporation, and a resultant dry eye. Gilbard[6] has suggested that abnormal meibomian lipids may alter tear film osmolarity, and lead to, or aggravate, a dry eye condition. The profile of tear proteins, analyzed by mass spectroscopy, is different in blepharitis patients, than in normal controls.[7]

TREATMENT

Treatment of blepharitis usually consists of a combination of lid scrubs and topical or systemic treatment. Lid scrubs, using baby shampoo are highly effective, and should be recommended on a daily basis. When patients include lid hygiene in their daily routine, especially during a bath or shower, they minimize symptoms, as well as periodic flare-ups. An illustrated hand out, or instruction sheet is frequently beneficial (Fig. 45.9).

Topical treatment with a broad spectrum antibiotic ointment, such as erythromycin, bacitracin, or a combination of bacitracin and polymyxin B is often useful. Antibiotic-corticosteroid combination ointments are particularly beneficial. These include tobramycin-dexamethasone combinations (Tobradex®, Alcon, Ft. Worth), and sulfacetamide sodium-prednisolone acetate (Blephamide®, Allergan, Irvine).

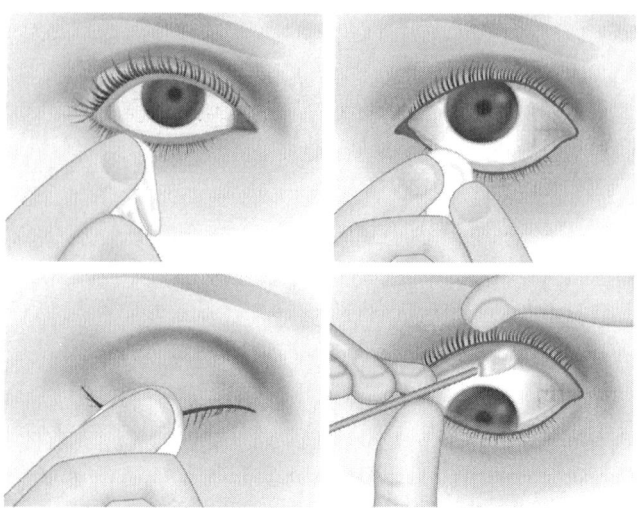

Fig. 45.9: Lid scrub instructions

More recently, cyclosporine suspension,[8] and tacrolimus ointment[9] have been advocated.

Oral antibiotics may be used in the treatment of blepharitis. Most popular are tetracycline, doxycycline, minocycline, and erythromycin.[10] Often a course of a few weeks to a few months is necessary to achieve the desired effect. Patients should be made aware of the possible side effects of long-term oral antibiotics, such as photosensitivity, and opportunistic infections, such as *Candida*.

For the treatment of allergic contact dermatitis, the treatment is identification, withdrawal, and avoidance of the offending allergen. For atopic and vernal keratoconjunctivitis, a corticosteroid cream or ointment may be applied to the affected area of the eyelids.

Herpetic viral infections may be self-limited, however, oral antivirals, such as acyclovir, famcyclovir, and valacyclovir, may lead to more rapid resolution. Patients should be aware of the triggers for herpetic disease, particularly ultraviolet radiation, fever, stress, menstruation, and immunosuppression. UV radiation can be minimized by wearing a hat with a brim, sun block, and sunglasses. Fever can be treated with aspirin or nonsteroidal anti-inflammatory agents to minimize the possibility of an outbreak of skin lesions.

SUMMARY

Blepharitis has a number of causes. The most common cause is a combination of hereditary factors, particularly a tendency toward rosacea, and staphylococcal bacteria. Other infectious causes, such as viral infections, are amenable to antimicrobial treatment. Allergic blepharitis requires avoidance of the offending allergen, and treatment of the allergic process.

REFERENCES

1. Smolin G, Okumoto M. Staphylococcal blepharitis. Archives of Ophthalmology 1977;95(5):812-6.
2. Kemal M, Sumer Z, Toker MI, Erdogan H, Topalkara A, Akbulut M. The prevalence of Demodex folliculorum in blepharities patients and the normal population. Ophthalmic Epidemiology 2005;12(4):287-90.
3. Sacca SC, Pascotto A, Venturino GM, Prigione G, Mastromarino A, Baldi F, Bilardi C, Savarino V, Brusati C, Rebora A. Prevalence and treatment of *Helicobacter pylori* in patients with blepharitis. Investigative Ophthalmology and Visual Science 2006;47(2):501-8.
4. Suzuki T, Mitsuishi Y, Sano Y. Phlyctenular keratitis associated with meibomitis in young patients. American Journal of Ophthalmology 2005;140(1):77-82.
5. McCulley JP, Shine WE. Changing concepts in the diagnosis and management of blepharitis. Cornea 2000;19(5):650-8.
6. Gilbard JP. Dry eye, blepharitis and chronic eye irritation: Divide and conquer. Journal of Ophthalmic Nursing and Technology 1999;18(3):109-15.
7. Koo B, Lee Do-Yeon, Ha H, Kim J, Kim C. Comparative analysis of the tear protein expression in blepharitis patients using two-dimensional electrophoresis, J Proteome Res 2005;4(3):664.
8. Rubin M, Rao S. Efficacy of topical cyclosporin 0.05 percent in the treatment of posterior blepharitis. Journal of Ocular Pharmacology and Therapeutics 2006;22(1):47-53.
9. Joseph MA, Kaufman HE, Insler M. Topical tacrolimus ointment for treatment of refractory anterior segment inflammatory disorders. Cornea 2005;24(4):417-20.
10. Hammersmith KM, Cohen EJ, Blake TD, Laibson PR, Rapuano CJ. Blepharokeratoconjunctivitis in children. Archives of Ophthalmology 2005;123(12):1667-70.

Trypan Blue in the Management of Mature Cataract

Amar Agarwal, Athiya Agarwal, Sunita Agarwal (India)

INTRODUCTION

One of the biggest bugbears for a phaco surgeon is to perform a rhexis in a mature cataract. Once one performs rhexis in mature and hypermature cataracts, then phaco can be done in these cases and a foldable IOL implanted.

RHEXIS IN MATURE CATARACTS

Various techniques are present which can help one perform rhexis in mature cataracts.
1. One should use a good operating microscope. If the operating microscope is good one can faintly see the outline of the rhexis.
2. Use of an endoilluminator. While one is performing the rhexis with the right hand (Dominant hand), in the left hand (non-dominant hand) one can hold an endoilluminator. By adjusting the endoilluminator in various positions, one can complete the rhexis as the edge of the rhexis can be seen.
3. Use of a forceps. A forceps is easier to use than a needle especially in mature cataracts. One can use a good rhexis forceps to complete the rhexis.
4. Use of paraxial light.

But with all these techniques, still one is not very sure of completing a rhexis in all cases. Many times if the rhexis is incomplete, one might have to convert to an extracapsular cataract extraction (ECCE) to prevent a posterior capsular rupture or nucleus drop.

TRYPAN BLUE

The solution to this problem is to have a dye, which stains the anterior capsule. This dye is trypan blue. It is marketed as Blurex made by Dr Agarwal Pharma Ltd. Each ml of Blurex contains 0.6 mg trypan blue 1.9 mg of sodium monohydrogen orthophosphate, 0.3 mg of sodium dihydrogen orthophosphate, 8.2 mg of sodium chloride, sodium hydroxide for adjusting the pH and water for injection.

TECHNIQUE

We always tend to perform a temporal clear-corneal incision. If the astigmatism is plus at 90 degrees then the incision is made superiorly. First of all, a needle with viscoelastic is injected inside the eye in the area where the second site is made (Fig. 46.1). This will distend the eye so that when you make a clear-corneal incision, the eye will be tense and one can create a good valve. Now use a straight rod to stabilize the eye with the left hand. With the right hand make the clear corneal incision (Fig. 46.2).

Now inject air into the anterior chamber (Fig. 46.3). This prevents water-like dilution of the trypan blue. Then the trypan blue is withdrawn from the vial into a syringe. This is then injected by a cannula into the anterior chamber between the air-bubble and the lens capsule (Fig. 46.4). It is kept like that for a minute or two for staining of the anterior capsule to occur. Next viscoelastic is injected into the anterior chamber (Fig. 46.5) to remove the air-bubble and the trypan blue.

Now, rhexis is started with a needle (Fig. 46.6). One can use a forceps also. We prefer to use a needle as it gives better control on the size of the rhexis. Note the left hand holding a rod stabilizing

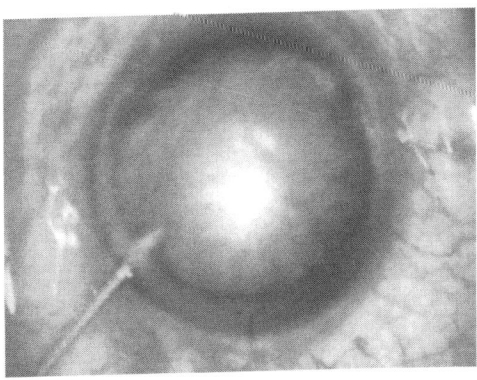

Fig. 46.1: Left hand injects viscoelastic using a 26 gauge needle

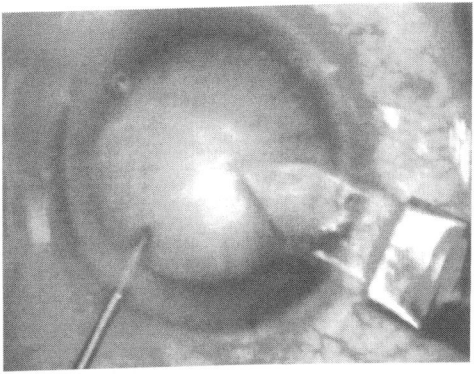

Fig. 46.2: Clear-corneal incision

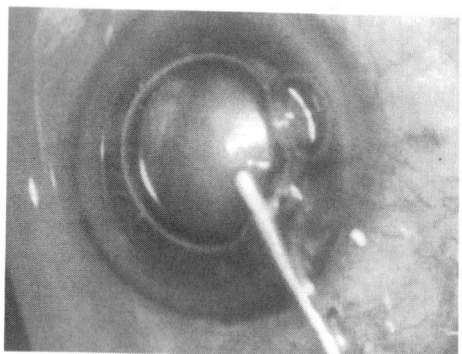

Fig. 46.3: Air injected inside the anterior chamber

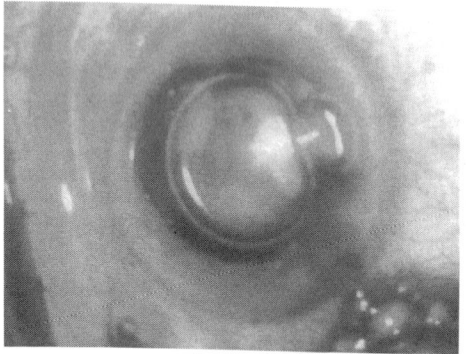

Fig. 46.4: Trypan blue injected between the air-bubble and the anterior lens capsule

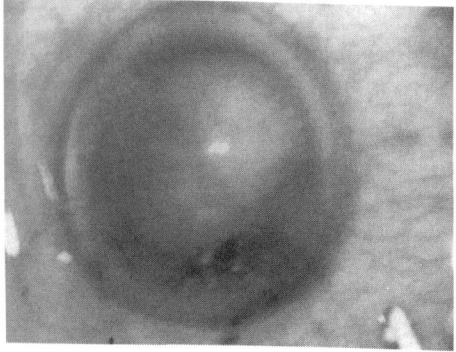

Fig. 46.5: Viscoelastic injected to remove the air bubble and the trypan blue

the eye while the rhexis is being performed. The rhexis is continued with the needle (Fig. 46.7). Note the contrast between the capsule, which has been stained, and the cortex, which is not stained. The

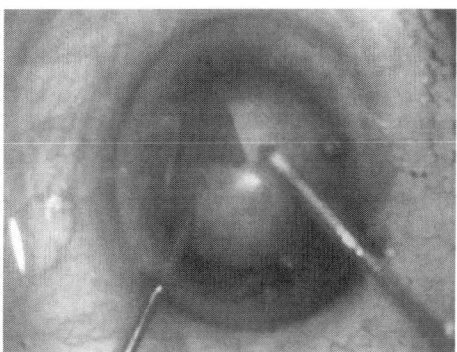

Fig. 46.6: Rhexis started with the needle. Note a straight rod in the left hand to stabilize the eye

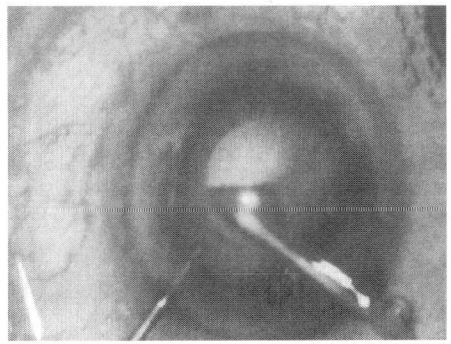

Fig. 46.7: Rhexis continued. Note the contrast between the stained anterior capsule and the unstained cortex

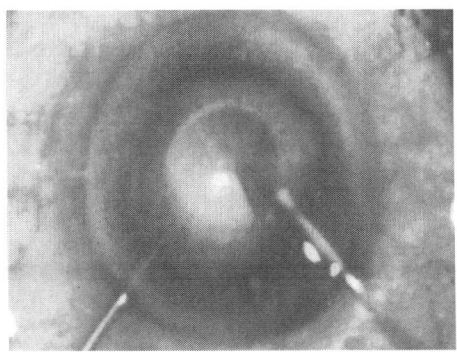

Fig. 46.8: Rhexis nearing completion

rhexis is continued (Fig. 46.8) and finally completed (Fig. 46.9). When the rhexis is complete, we can see the stained anterior capsule lying in the anterior chamber (Fig. 46.10).

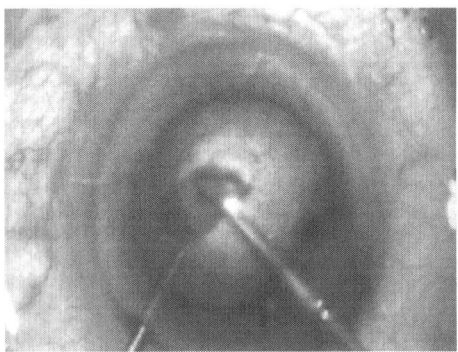

Fig. 46.9: Rhexis completed

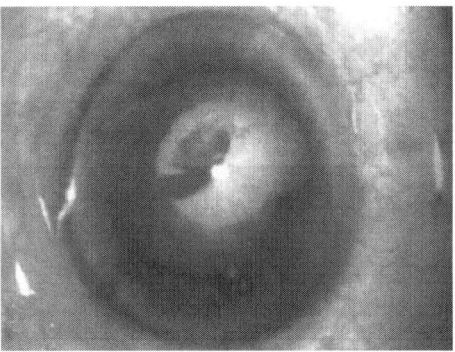

Fig. 46.10: Note the stained anterior capsule lying in the anterior chamber

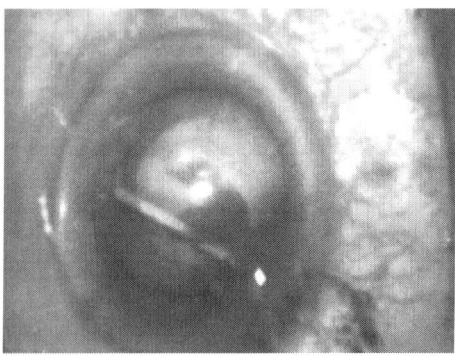

Fig. 46.11: Hydrodissection

Hydrodissection is then done (Fig. 46.11). One will not be able to see the fluid wave in such cases as the cataract is very dense. In such cases a simple way is to see if the lens comes up anteriorly a little bit. This will indicate hydrodissection being completed. One can also test this by rotating the nucleus before starting phaco.

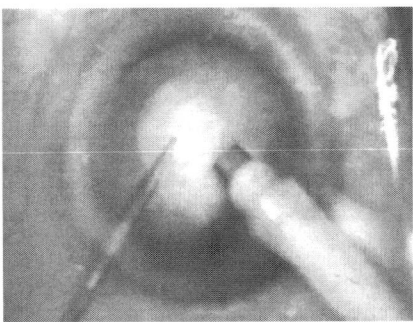

Fig. 46.12: Phaco probe at the superior end of the rhexis. Left hand holds the chopper

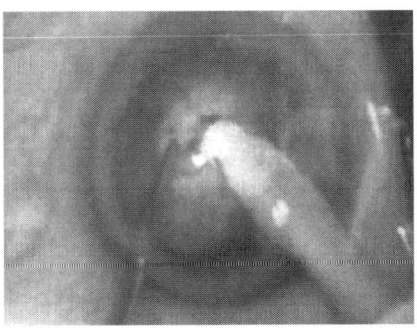

Fig. 46.13: Phaco probe embedded in the nucleus

We then insert the phaco probe through the incision slightly superior to the center of the nucleus (Fig. 46.12). At that point apply ultrasound and see that the phaco tip gets embedded in the nucleus (Fig. 46.13). The direction of the phaco probe should be obliquely downwards toward the vitreous and not horizontally towards the iris. Then only the nucleus will get embedded. The settings at this stage are 80 percent phaco power, 24 ml/minute flow rate and 101 mm of Hg suction. By the time the phaco tip gets embedded in the nucleus the tip would have reached the middle of the nucleus. Now, with the chopper cut the nucleus with a straight downward motion (Fig. 46.14) and then move the chopper to the left when you reach the center of the nucleus. In other words, your left hand moves the chopper like an inverted L. Do not go to the periphery for chopping but do it at the center. Once you have created a crack, split the nucleus till the center (Fig. 46.15). Then rotate the nucleus 180 degrees and crack again so that you get two halves of the nucleus.

Now that you have two halves, you have a shelf to embed the probe. So, now place the probe with ultrasound into one-half of the nucleus (Fig. 46.16) and chop. Like this create three quadrants in one-half of the nucleus. Then make another three halves with the second half of the nucleus. Thus, you now have 6 quadrants or pie-shaped fragments.

788 Applied Ocular Therapeutics in Ophthalmic Surgery

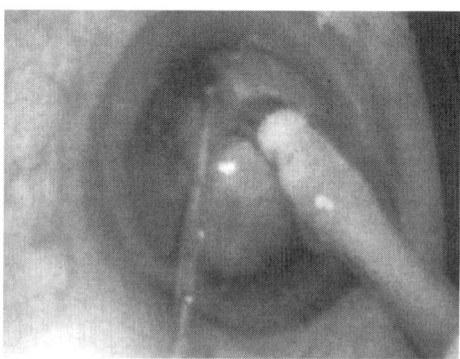

Fig. 46.14: Left hand holding the chopper chops the nucleus

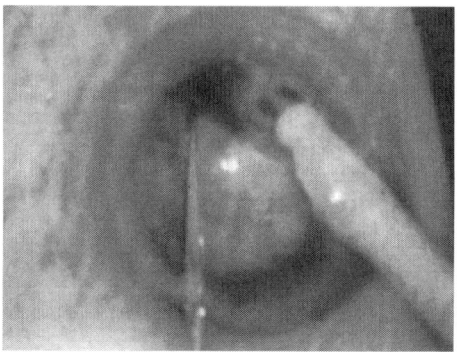

Fig. 46.15: The two halves of the nucleus are split

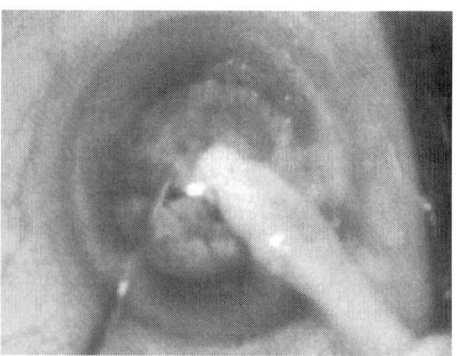

Fig. 46.16: Embed the probe in one-half of the nucleus. Go horizontally and not vertically as you have now a shelf of nucleus to embed

Once all the pieces have been chopped, take out each piece one by one and in pulse phaco mode (Figs 46.17 and 46.18) aspirate the pieces at the level of the iris. Do not work in the bag unless the cornea is preoperatively bad or the patient is very elderly.

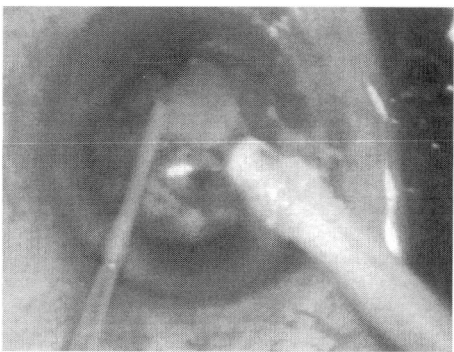

Fig. 46.17: Using pulse phaco the pieces of nuclei are emulsified

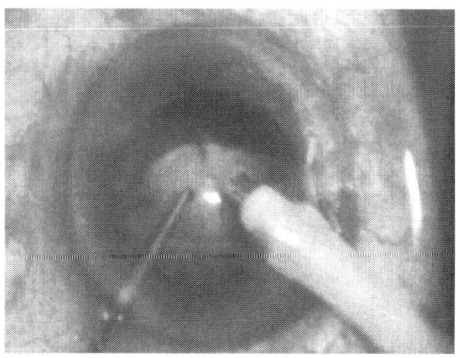

Fig. 46.18: Final bits of nucleus being removed

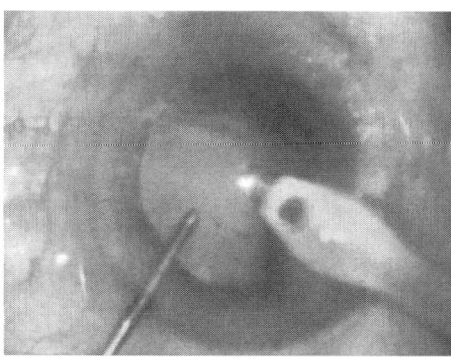

Fig. 46.19: Cortical aspiration done

The next step is to do cortical washing (Fig. 46.19). Always try to remove the subincisional cortex first, as that is the most difficult. Note that everytime the left hand has the straight rod controlling the movements of the eye. If necessary use a bimanual irrigation-aspiration technique. Then inject viscoelastic and implant the IOL (Fig. 46.20). At the end of the procedure, inject the BSS inside the lips of the clear-corneal incision. This will create a stromal hydration at the wound. This will create a whiteness, which will

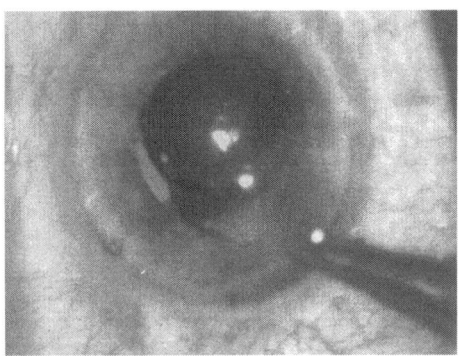

Fig. 46.20: IOL being implanted

disappear after 4–5 hours. The advantage of this is that the wound gets sealed better.

ADVERSE EFFECTS

1. One is still not sure if extended contact of trypan blue with the corneal endothelium produces corneal damage. At present, no cases have been reported as the trypan blue is washed off with the viscoelastic and the BSS fluid.
2. Postsurgical inflammatory reactions and some bullous keratopathy have been known to occur after using vital staining agents.
3. Extreme care must be taken when using trypan blue on patients who are hypersensitive to any of its components.
4. During animal experiments, a teratogenic and/or mutagenic effect has been reported after repeated and/or high dose intraperitoneal or intravenous injections with trypan blue. So, one should not use trypan blue in pregnant women.

STERILIZATION

Sterilization is done by autoclave.

INDOCYANINE GREEN DYE

Indocyanine green (ICG) dye has also been tried for staining of the anterior capsule. It does not have any mutagenic effects but it is costlier.

SUMMARY

Trypan blue can make life much easier for the phaco surgeon, especially in cases of mature and hypermature cataracts by staining the anterior capsule. Another dye, which has been tried, is ICG, which is much costlier.

Trypan Blue Assisted Epiretinal Membrane Removal

Amar Agarwal, Athiya Agarwal, Sunita Agarwal, Saurabh Choudhry, Reena M Choudhry (India)

INTRODUCTION

Epiretinal membranes can form in various proliferative retinopathies and cause complications like decreased visual acuity directly by involving the macula itself or indirectly by causing tractional retinal detachments, combined retinal detachments or macular detachments. It can also occur in cases of epimacular proliferation. Epiretinal membrane removal has been a challenging procedure in posterior segment surgery. Various methods like peeling, segmentation, delaminating and en bloc removal have been described in the literature. Identifying the translucent epiretinal membranes can be a major challenge and differentiating them from retinal tissue can prevent iatrogenic retinal tears.

We have successfully used Blurhex (trypan blue manufactured by Dr Agarwal's Pharma, Chennai, India) to stain epiretinal membranes thus making their removal easier. Blurhex solution is being widely used in the anterior segment surgery for staining anterior capsule in white cataracts1 to perform capsulorhexis (Fig. 47.1). It has been proved to be safe and nontoxic to the ocular tissue at low concentration.

PATIENTS AND TECHNIQUE

Ten cases who had proliferative retinopathies with vitreous hemorrhage underwent conventional three port pars plana vitrectomy (PPV) and epiretinal membrane removal under peribulbar anesthesia by the same surgeon at Agarwal's eye hospital, Chennai. All the patients included in this study underwent detailed preoperative investigations including indirect ophthalmoscopy, B scan and IOP measurement. All cases with increased IOP, signs of rubeosis iridis and fresh vitreous hemorrhage were excluded from the study.

Patients with significant amount of cataract were taken up for combined phacoemulsification with IOL and pars plana vitrectomy (PPV). Phacoemulsification was performed prior to PPV but the IOL was implanted at the end of the surgery. The removal of vitreous in the meridians of the instrument sclerotomy sites and in the vitreous cavity was first performed. In cases where the posterior hyaloid was not detached completely it was carefully removed with the vitrectomy probe. About 0.2 ml of Blurhex (trypan blue) was

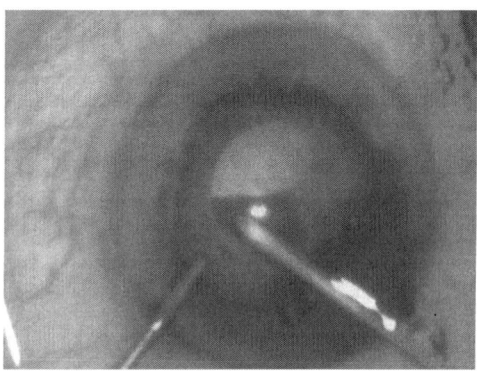

Fig. 47.1: Capsulorhexis in a white cataract using Blurhex to stain the anterior capsule

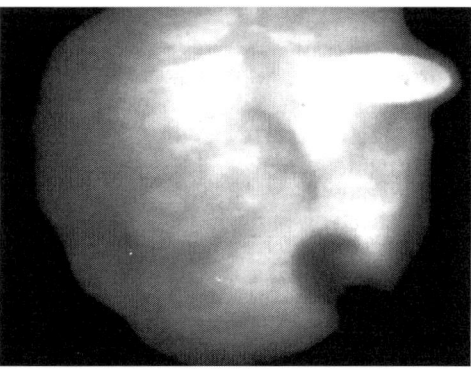

Fig. 47.2: Epiretinal membrane stained with Blurhex. 0.2 ml of Blurhex was injected inside the vitreous cavity over the epiretinal membranes and the excess Blurhex removed with the vitrectomy probe

slowly injected into the vitreous cavity over the optic nerve head and epiretinal membranes. All epiretinal membranes stain light blue in color (Fig. 47.2). The internal limiting membrane does not stain hence increasing the contrast between the underlining retina and epiretinal membranes facilitating precise removal of the tissue.

The membranes were either peeled, segmented or delaminated depending on the nature of the membranes. Using the Sutherland scissors (Fig. 47.3) the attachments between the epiretinal membranes and the retina were cut (Fig. 47.4). Gradually, the membrane is lifted off the retina (Fig. 47.5) till the entire traction has been released (Fig. 47.6) and the membrane is then removed with the vitrectomy probe (Fig. 47.7). In all the cases successful epiretinal membrane removal could be achieved without any iatrogenic retinal breaks.

Eyes with pre-existing retinal breaks underwent fluid-air exchange (FAE) and focal endolaser photocoagulation. The IOL was implanted after the completion of vitrectomy in cases which underwent a combined cataract surgery.

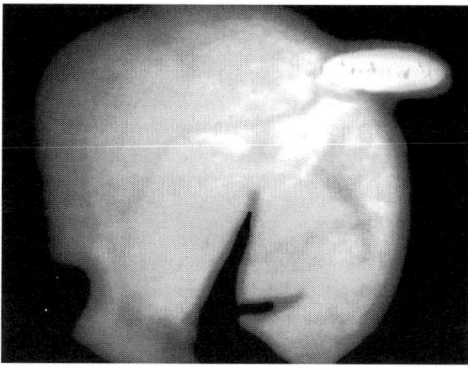

Fig. 47.3: Segmentation of the epiretinal membrane started using the Sutherland scissors

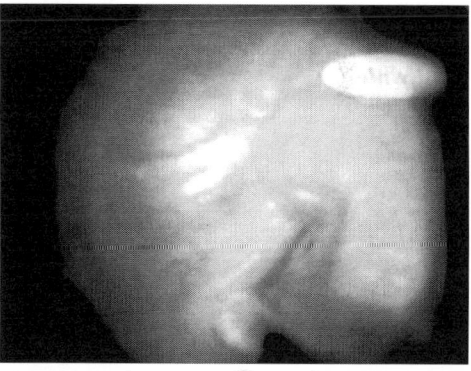

Fig. 47.4: The membrane which is colored blue is lifted using the Sutherland scissors after the attachments between the membrane and the retina have been cut. Note the blue coloration of the epiretinal membrane and the normal color of the retina behind it

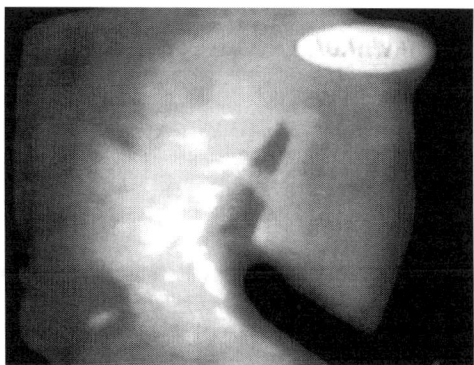

Fig. 47.5: Stained epiretinal membranes being removed

RESULTS

None of the 10 cases had intraoperative or postoperative complications. Marked improvement in the visual acuity compared

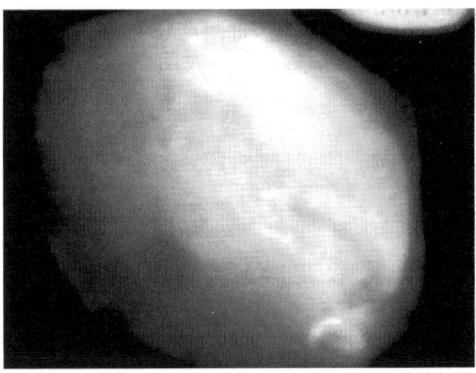

Fig. 47.6: The epiretinal membrane has been removed from its attachment to the retina and is now lying free in the vitreous cavity near the peripheral retina. It can be removed easily now with the vitrectomy probe without a risk of a retinotomy

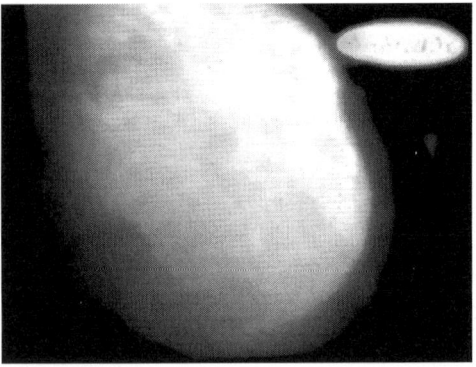

Fig. 47.7: The retina is seen without any epiretinal membranes. Note the blue colored epiretinal membrane is not present as it has been removed

to the preoperative levels was observed in all the eyes. The patients were followed up on the first, seventh, fourteenth days and one month postoperative. There was no evidence of residual stain in all the cases postoperatively.

CONCLUSION

In conclusion, Blurhex (trypan blue) assisted pars plana vitrectomy is a safe and effective adjunct for epiretinal membrane removal and can minimize intra- and postoperative complications.

BIBLIOGRAPHY

1. Agarwal, et al. Trypan blue in management of mature cataracts. In: Agarwal A, Agarwal S, Agarwal A, et al. (Eds): Phacoemulsification, Laser Cataract Surgery and Foldable IOLs, 2nd edn. Jaypee Brothers: New Delhi; 2000.pp.618-23.

Perfluorocarbon Liquids in Vitreoretinal Surgery

Amar Agarwal (India)

INTRODUCTION

Since long vitreoretinal surgeons have been using "lighter-than-water" liquids for tamponading the retina. It was Dr Stanley Chang from USA who introduced a "heavier-than-water" liquid. This was used to flatten the retina and was an N-perfluorocarbon amine. The basic idea of these liquids is that as they are heavier than water liquids, they would flatten the retina or unfold a giant tear.

TYPES

There are four types of perfluorocarbon liquids used at present.
1. Perfluoro-N-octane
2. Perfluoro-tributylamine
3. Perfluoro-decaline
4. Perfluoro-phenanthrene.

The differences in the physical properties between these liquids are shown in Table 48.1.

PHYSICAL PROPERTIES

The question which we should ask ourselves is—why perfluorocarbons? In other words, what is so good about perfluorocarbons that they can unfold giant tears or make an IOL float on it.[2-5] To answer[2-5] this question, we should understand some basics on physics and also understand the physical properties of these liquids.

Density

Liquids and gases have no definite shape of their own and are capable of flowing freely around places. Hence, liquids and gases are called fluids. The study of fluids at rest is called hydrostatics. Now, we say that perfluorocarbons are heavier than water liquids. This means that their density is more than water. The density of a substance is calculated by dividing its mass by its volume.

Density = Mass/Volume

(The difference between mass and weight is that mass is the same everywhere, whereas weight depends on the gravitational force).

TABLE 48.1: Properties of perfluorocarbon liquids

Characteristics	Perfluoro-N-octane	Perfluoro-tributylamine	Perfluoro-decaline	Perfluoro-phenanthrene
Chemical formula	C_8F_{18}	$C_{12}F_{27}N$	$C_{10}F_{18}$	$C_{14}F_{24}$
Molecular weight	438	671	462	624
Specific gravity	1.76	1.89	1.94	2.03
Refractive index	1.27	1.29	1.31	1.33
Surface tension (dyne/cm at 25°C)	14	16	16	16
Viscosity (Centistokes at 25°C)	0.8	2.6	2.7	8.03
Vapor pressure (mm Hg at 37°C)	50	1.14	13.5	<1

If you take your weight on the earth and also take your weight on the moon, then the values will be different as the gravitational force in both the places is different, whereas your mass will be the same in both the places.

So, when we say, Density = Mass/Volume, and we take water as an example, it means the density of water is 1 gm/cc because 1 cc of water weighs 1 gm. In other words, when we say that perfluorocarbons are heavier than water liquids, it means that their density is more than water, i.e. if we take 1 cc of perfluorocarbon, it weighs 1.76–2.03 gm.

Relative Density or Specific Gravity

As water has a density of 1 gm/cc, it is taken as a standard. If you would compare the density of any other substance, you should compare it with water and that gives us the relative density of that substance or the specific gravity of that substance.

Relative Density = Density of the substance/Density of water

As relative density or specific gravity is only a mere number, it has no units. When we say that perfluorocarbons have a specific gravity from 1.76 to 2.03 depending on the type of perfluorocarbon, it means its density is 1.76–2.03 gm/cc and as the density of water is 1 gm/cc, the relative density of perfluorocarbon is 1.76/1 or 2.03/1 which is 1.76 or 2.03. For example, let us take the example of perfluoro-octane.

Density of perfluoro-octane = 1.76 gm/cc
Density of water = 1 gm/cc
Relative density or specific
 gravity of perfluoro-octane = 1.76/1
 = 1.76

The application of this specific gravity is that as the perfluorocarbons are heavy and have a higher specific gravity compared to water, when they are injected into the vitreous cavity, the liquid flattens the retina, displacing subretinal fluid anteriorly through the peripheral retinal breaks. The flattening force exerted by perfluorocarbon is approximately 3 times greater than an equivalent volume of fluorosilicone oil and more than 100 times greater than that exerted by sodium hyaluronate 1 percent.

Refractive Index

To understand refractive index, we should first understand refraction. In a homogeneous transparent medium, light travels in straight lines. But, if a ray of light travels from one homogeneous medium to another, a change in direction of the ray takes place at the surface of separation between the two media. This bending of the rays of light is called refraction (Fig. 48.1).

Laws of Refraction

Law I The incident ray, refracted ray and the normal to the surface at the point of incidence lie in the same plane.

Law II For a given color of light passing from one medium to another, the ratio of the sine of the angle of incidence to the sine of the angle of refraction is a constant. This is called the refractive index of the second medium and is denoted by the letter m.

Refractive Index = Sine angle of incidence/Sine angle of refraction

The refractive index of water for instance is 1.33. The refractive index of the perfluorocarbons varies from 1.27 to 1.33 depending on the type of perfluorocarbon. From this, we realize that the index of refraction of the perfluorocarbons is slightly dissimilar to saline. Optically, the liquids are clear, and as the index of refraction of the perfluorocarbons is different from that of saline, the perfluorocarbon bubble interface with saline is visible when it is injected into the vitreous cavity. As the difference in refraction between saline is most with perfluoro-N-octane (1.27), it has the most visible interface when compared to perfluoro-phenanthrene (1.33) which has the least visible interface.

Another point about the refractive index is that though the refractive index between perfluorocarbons and saline is dissimilar it is only slightly dissimilar, so optical aberrations during membrane

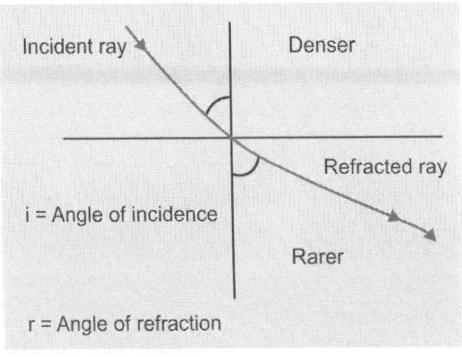

Fig. 48.1: Refraction of light

dissection are not induced. If there was a lot of difference in the refractive index between saline and perfluorocarbons, all the instruments which are passed into the vitreous cavity when perfluorocarbons are in the vitreous cavity, will appear distorted. This can be understood if we pass a stick in a swimming pool. The stick appears to be broken and bent at the water surface. This is because in this case, there is a lot of difference between the refractive index of air and water (Fig. 48.2).

The perfluorocarbons are also immiscible with silicone oil, and the optical interface is well seen during perfluorocarbon-silicone oil exchange as the refractive index between the two is different.

Surface Tension

When water is in a liquid form, its water molecules are connected to each other by hydrogen bonds (Fig. 48.3). One water molecule connects with four other immediate neighboring water molecules by the hydrogen bonds. An exception is at the level of the water surface, where the water molecule connects with the other water molecules below and at the sides but not above as there is no water above. It is these bonds that pull water surface into a taut sheet, and this phenomenon is known as surface tension. When water is in the form of ice, these bonds hold the molecules in a more or less rigid pattern. When water is heated, then the molecules break-off from each other and vaporize as gas.

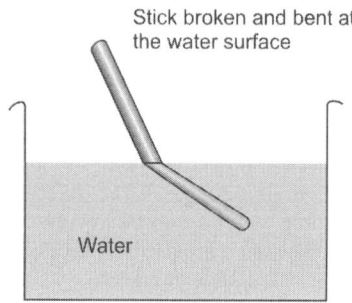

Fig. 48.2: Refraction—a stick in water appears broken and bent

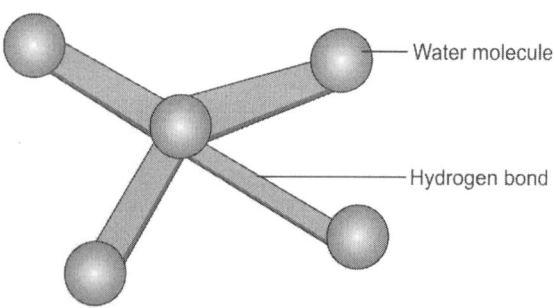

Fig. 48.3: Surface tension water molecule in a liquid state

The surface of water can support amazing weight due to surface tension if the object is flat enough to take advantage of surface tension. Imagine a round object of 1 gm. It will sink in water, but if the same object of 1 gm is made flat as much as possible and placed on the surface of water it will float, because it has taken advantage of surface tension of water (Figs 48.4 and 48.5).

If a needle is floating on the surface of the water, the surface film behaves like an elastic membrane. As soon as, any deformation is produced in the film by the weight of the object, it is opposed by the surface tension. This is measured by force per unit length and is expressed in dynes per cm (Fig. 48.6).

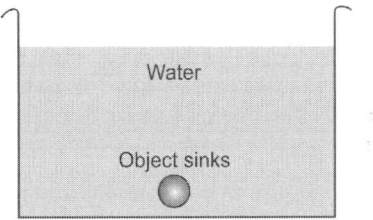

Fig. 48.4: Surface tension—round object sinks in water

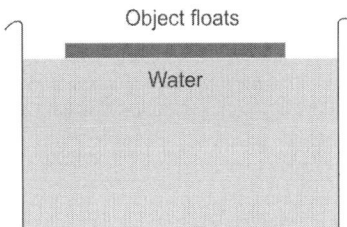

Fig. 48.5: Surface tension—same object made flat floats in water

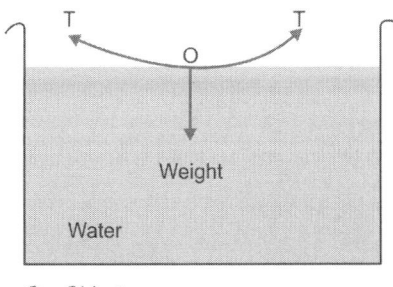

O = Object
T = Surface tension

Fig. 48.6: Surface tension—expressed as force per unit length

The application of surface tension in regard to perfluorocarbons is that perfluorocarbons have a surface tension ranging from 14 to 16 dynes/cm at 25 degree centigrade. It is because of this surface tension that an IOL can float on the surface of the perfluorocarbon. Similarly, a lens can also float on the surface of the perfluorocarbon. This property of the surface tension of the perfluorocarbon is used when removing a lens or IOL from the retinal surface by the vitreoretinal surgeon.

It is because of surface tension that a waterdrop is formed. What happens is that the cohesive force between the water molecules keeps the water molecules together and so a drop is formed. Once again this has a clinical application with perfluorocarbons. As they have a high surface tension, the molecules between the perfluorocarbons have a strong bond and keep the molecules of perfluorocarbons together. This helps the perfluorocarbons to remain in one large bubble (Fig. 48.7). This helps the vitreoretinal surgeon while operating and also while removing the perfluorocarbon.

Viscosity

There is a certain amount of attraction between molecules of a liquid. The more the molecules are drawn together the greater the internal friction in the liquid. In other words, the greater the resistance to the flow of the liquid. This resistance is called viscosity or fluid friction (Fig. 48.8). So, if we want the fluid to flow fast, then its molecules should not be firmly attracted to each other

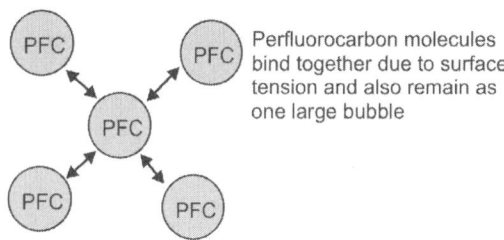

Fig. 48.7: Surface tension—perfluorocarbon molecules

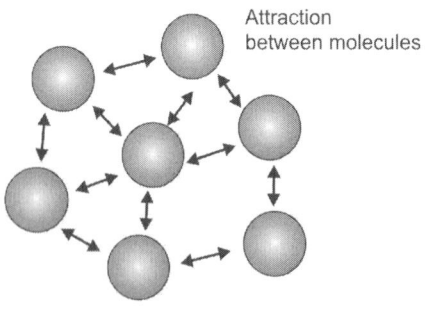

Fig. 48.8: Viscosity

or in other words the fluid should be less viscous like water. If the fluid is more viscous like silicone oil, then it flows less smoothly.

The perfluorocarbon liquids used are of low viscosity ranging from 0.8 to 8.0 centistokes at 25 degree centigrade. These are useful to use intraoperatively because they can be easily injected and aspirated while using small gauge microsurgical instruments. The low viscosity also allows perfluorocarbon liquids to be injected for diagnostic determination of areas of residual traction and can be easily removed if further membrane dissection is required. Perfluoro-N-octane is the least viscous, and the problem is that if there is a posterior break it can go through the break into the subretinal space. As perfluoro-phenanthrene has a higher viscosity it has the advantage of not flowing through a posterior retinal break or through the zonules into the anterior chamber.

Vapor Pressure

When a liquid is lying on the surface, part of the liquid turns into vapor, i.e. gas. This is due to evaporation. The vapor formed above a liquid has its own kind of pressure known as vapor pressure which is measured in mm of Hg at 37 degree centigrade (Fig. 48.9). The vapor pressure of the perfluorocarbons varies from 50 to less than 1 mm of Hg at 37 degree centigrade. Perfluoro-N-octane has the highest vapor pressure. This is advantageous because a thin layer of liquid will always remain on the surface of the retina during fluid-air exchange and with perfluoro-N-octane, this layer will evaporate quickly as the infusion system flushes air through the eye.

Boiling Point

As the temperature of the liquid is raised, its vapor pressure rises. When it equals the prevailing atmospheric pressure, the liquid reaches its boiling point. In evaporation, only the surface of the liquid turns to gas, whereas in boiling all the liquid turns to gas. Thus, boiling is an extreme case of evaporation. When the liquid reaches its boiling point, bubbles of vapor form in its interior,

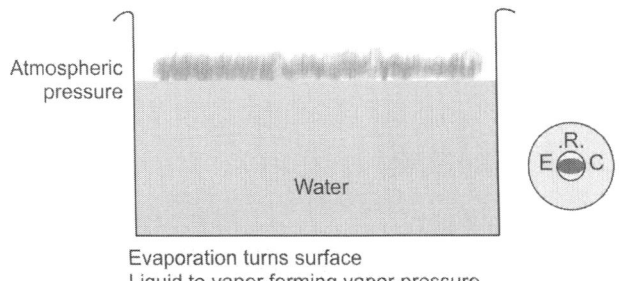

Fig. 48.9: Vapor pressure

growing larger and larger and violently agitate the entire liquid causing it to boil away (Fig. 48.10). For instance, water boils at 100 degree centigrade.

Perfluorophenanthrene has a boiling point of 215°C. Thus, we realize that perfluorocarbons has a boiling point which exceeds that of saline so that endophotocoagulation can be applied through the fluid without intraocular vaporization.

INDICATIONS

There are various indications in which perfluorocarbons are[6-13] used (Fig. 48.11).

Giant Tears

Perfluorocarbon liquids offer the greatest advantages in the management of giant retinal tears. First of all, a vitrectomy is done and the epiretinal membranes are removed. When the tear is inverted, then perfluorocarbon is injected over the disk to

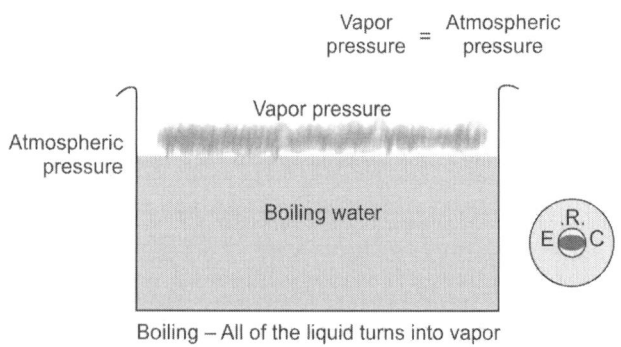

Fig. 48.10: Boiling

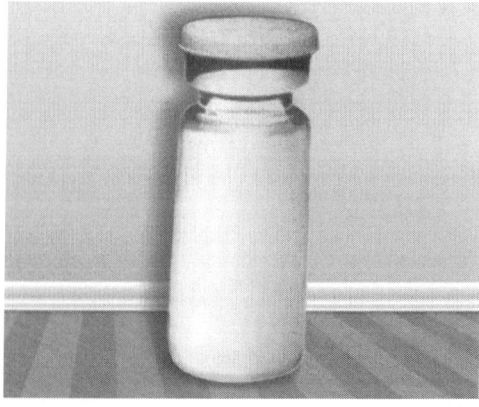

Fig. 48.11: Vitreon (perfluorophenanthrene)

stabilize the posterior flap (Fig. 48.12). Additional membranes causing the edge of the tear to curl are then removed. Finally, more perfluorocarbon liquid is injected till the edge of the tear, flattening the retina to the periphery (Fig. 48.13). Endophotocoagulation is applied through the perfluorocarbon along the edge of the tear.

Care should be taken to see that the perfluorocarbon does not cross the edge of the tear as it can seep into the subretinal space. Further, one should avoid letting the anterior meniscus of perfluorocarbon being disturbed by a forceful stream of balanced salt solution (BSS) otherwise the result is the creation of numerous small bubbles of perfluorocarbon that are difficult to remove (Fig. 48.14A). One should also be careful that the anterior meniscus of perfluorocarbon must not come in direct contact with the tip of the infusion cannula where the concentrated stream of BSS will stir up numerous small bubbles of perfluorocarbons that are difficult to remove later (Fig. 48.14B).

Once the endophotocoagulation is completed, a slow and deliberate fluid-air exchange is done, stopping frequently to allow the edges of torn retina to dry as much as possible. This should be done to prevent the posterior flap of the giant retinal tear from

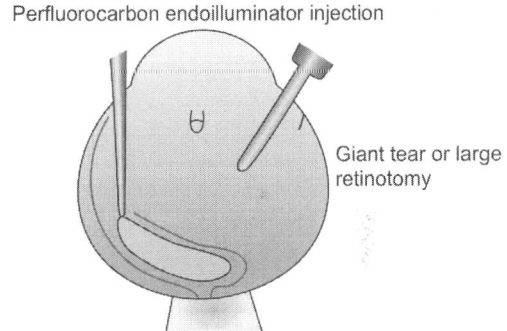

Fig. 48.12: Surgery for giant retinal tears—perfluorocarbon liquids injected to unfold the giant retinal tear

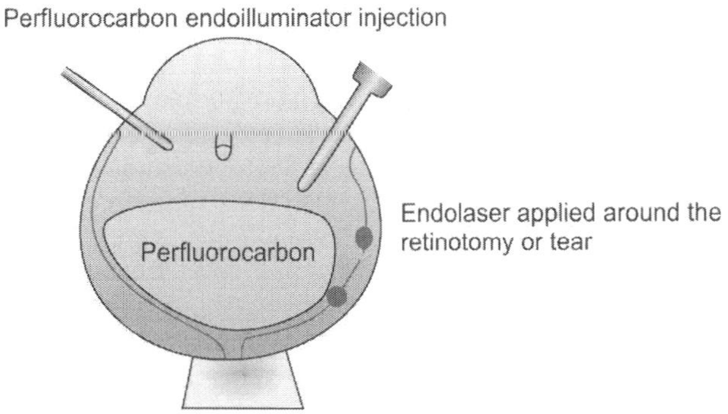

Fig. 48.13: Surgery for giant retinal tear unfolded followed by endolaser photocoagulation

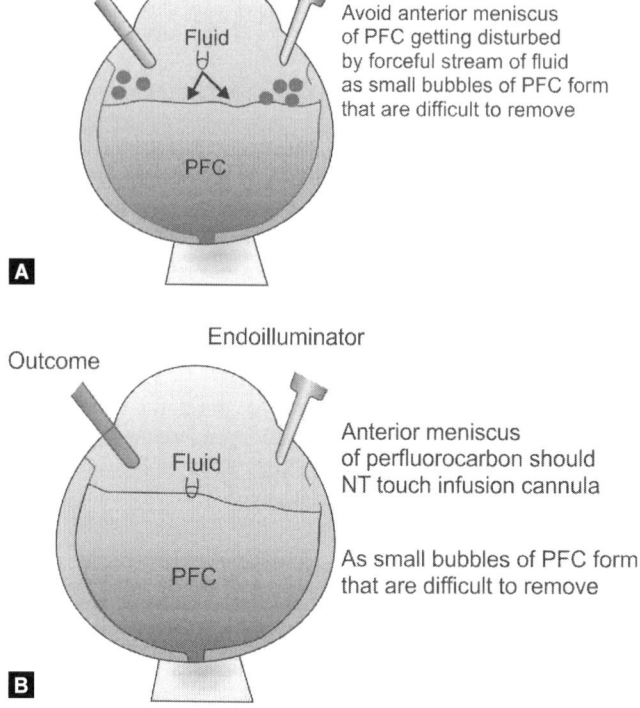

Figs 48.14A and B: Precautions when injected perfluorocarbon liquids

slipping posteriorly. When the edge of the posterior flap of the giant retinal tear is within the air-bubble, and relatively dry, it does not slip posteriorly due to the capillary attraction generated by having only a microscopic layer of fluid remaining between the retina and the pigment epithelium. Once the edges of the giant, retinal tear are within the air-bubble, the fluid-air exchange is continued replacing all the perfluorocarbon and saline with the air-bubble.

For long-term tamponade, one can use perfluoropropane gas or silicone oil. Sometimes, the case might redetach postoperatively and so another alternative is to use perfluorophenanthrene which can be left in the eye for 5 to 30 days. Then at that time, the endolaser reactions would have set in and the perfluorophenanthrene can be removed and replaced once again by some long-term tamponade.

Proliferative Vitreoretinopathy

In these cases, perfluorocarbons are used to assist with membrane dissection. If the case is a bad case, where the tunnel is closed (Fig. 48.15) and the disk is not seen, a little bit of perfluorocarbon

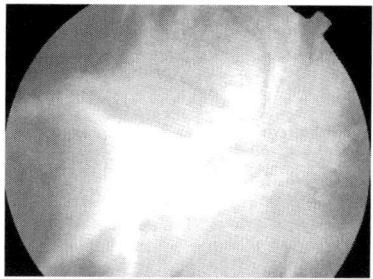

Fig. 48.15: Proliferative vitreoretinopathy

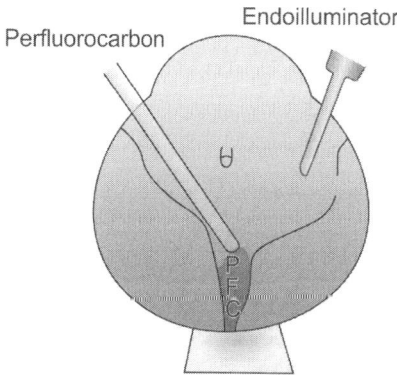

Fig. 48.16: Perfluorocarbon liquids injected to settle proliferative vitreoretinopathy

is injected over the disk after a vitrectomy (Fig. 48.16). When the tunnel of retina opens and the disk becomes visible, membrane dissection is continued using either delamination, segmentation or peeling. Then some more perfluorocarbon is injected (Fig. 48.17) flattening the retina more. The subretinal fluid will flow out through the anterior break in the retina. The peripheral retina can be flattened by a partial fluid-air exchange. Once the retina is flattened, endolaser photocoagulation is done over the retinal breaks (Fig. 48.18). The perfluorocarbon can then be replaced by some long-term tamponade. This technique avoids creating a posterior retinotomy to drain the subretinal fluid and also assist in membrane dissection.

Proliferative Diabetic Retinopathy

Perfluorocarbons can be used for managing proliferative diabetic retinopathies with tractional retinal detachments by stabilizing the retina and assisting in membrane dissection. Further, it also helps like a traction test to tell the surgeon where the traction is.

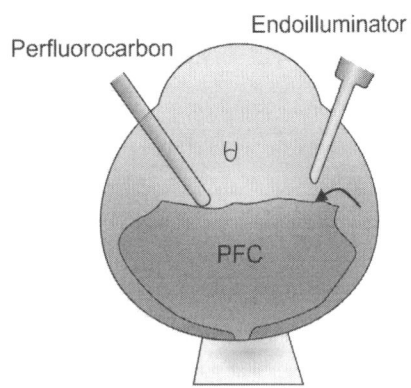

Fig. 48.17: Perfluorocarbon liquids injected to settle proliferative vitreoretinopathy. Part of retina settled

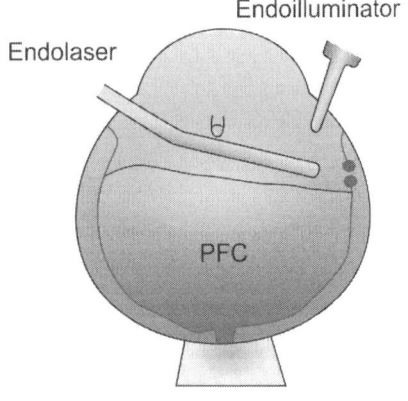

Fig. 48.18: Perfluorocarbon liquids injected to settle proliferative vitreoretinopathy. Endolaser now done once the retina is flat

Dislocated Crystalline Lenses or Intraocular Lenses

Due to the quality of surface tension, crystalline lenses or IOL float on the surface of the perfluorocarbons. When there is a crystalline lens or IOL on the surface of the retina, a vitrectomy is done and the perfluorocarbon injected under the crystalline lens or IOL. Gradually, the crystalline lens or IOL (Fig. 48.19) floats up to the pupil as the perfluorocarbons are continuously injected. Once in the anterior chamber, the crystalline lens can be removed or the IOL if necessary be sutured onto the sclera.

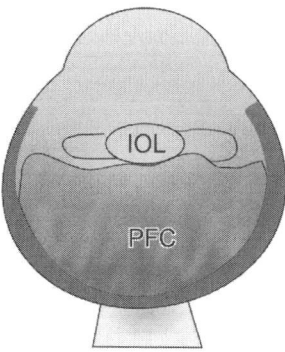

Fig. 48.19: Dislocated IOL floating on perfluorocarbon liquids

MISCELLANEOUS

Other indications in which perfluorocarbons are used are as follows:
1. Management of choroidal or expulsive hemorrhage to assist with drainage of serous or hemorrhagic fluid.
2. Removal of subretinal macular hemorrhage in patients with subretinal neovascularization. In these cases, a retinotomy is made temporal to the hemorrhage and the perfluorocarbon injected. Due to their heaviness, they push out the hemorrhage through the retinotomy.
3. Rhegmatogenous retinal detachment with a peripheral break to avoid a posterior retinotomy.
4. Retinal incarceration to the pars plana sclerotomy to reposition the retina.
5. Traumatic vitreous hemorrhage associated with retinal detachment, to assist in mechanical separation of the posterior hyaloid and stabilization of the retina during the vitrectomy.
6. Retinal detachment in patients with a permanent keratoprosthesis to reattach the posterior retina.
7. Retinal detachment resulting from a macular hole can be assisted by injection of a small amount of perfluorocarbon liquid over the posterior pole. The macular hole will flatten against the pigment epithelium so that endophotocoagulation can be applied. The liquid is then removed, and a fluid-air exchange done. Diagnostically, also the perfluorocarbons can be used to rule out any coexistent peripheral retinal breaks. When only the macular hole is present, the subretinal fluid will be displaced peripherally, resulting in a more bullous configuration around the bubble. However, if a peripheral retinal break is also present, the retinal detachment will be less elevated around the perfluorocarbon bubble, and the schlieren of subretinal fluid will be seen in the vitreous.
8. Removal of subretinal gas

9. When the retinal breaks are not found in a rhegmatogenous retinal detachment, vitrectomy with perfluorocarbons can be helpful in flattening the retina and localizing the retinal break. After vitrectomy, the perfluorocarbon liquid is injected to flatten the retina. The subretinal fluid will be pushed through the retinal break, exhibiting schlieren, seen when two liquids of differing refractive indices are mixed. The retinal breaks can be located by observing the direction of schlieren flow.

OTHER MEDICAL APPLICATIONS

Perfluorocarbon liquids have been used as:
  i. Artificial blood replacements
  ii. Sensitizers during radiotherapy for malignant tumors.

COMPLICATIONS

One should be careful that the perfluorocarbon is not left so that it touches the corneal endothelium. Perfluorophenanthrene can be left in the eye up to 30 days. Sometimes, the residual perfluorocarbon is encountered as small gas bubbles might inadvertently be left behind. Increased intraocular pressure has also been encountered. Due to the mechanical effects of the perfluorocarbon, there can be narrowing of the outer plexiform layer and degenerative thinning of the outer nuclear layer of the retina.

REFERENCES

1. Chang S. Perfluorocarbon liquids in vitreoretinal surgery. International Ophthalmology Clinics: New Approaches to Vitreoretinal Surgery 1992;32(2):153-63.
2. Lakshminarayanan K, Venkataraman M. Physics. Chennai: KCS Desikan and Co, 1992.
3. Leopold LB, Davis KS. Life Science Library Matter. USA: Time Life International BV, 1974.
4. Lapp RE. Life Science Library Matter. USA: Time Life International BV, 1974.
5. Subramanyam N, Lal B. A Textbook of BSc Physics. New Delhi: S Chand and Co, 1985.
6. Glasser BM, Carter JB, Kuppermann BD, et al. Perfluoro-octane in the treatment of giant retinal tears with proliferative vitreo-retinopathy. International Ophthalmology Clinics: New Approaches to Vitreo-retinal Surgery 1992;32(2):1-14.
7. Nabin M, Peyman GA, Clark Jr LC, et al. Experimental evaluation of perfluorophenanthrene as a high specific gravity vitreous substitute: A preliminary report. Ophthalmic Surgery 1989;20: 286-93.
8. Blinder KJ, Peyman GA, Paris CL, et al. Vitreon: A new perfluorocarbon. Br J Ophthalmol 1991;75:240-44.
9. Liu Kwan-Rong, Peyman GA, Chen Muh-Shy, et al. Use of high density vitreous substitutes in the removal of posteriorly dislocated lenses or intraocular lenses. Ophthalmic Surgery 1991; 22: 503-07.

10. Paris CL, Peyman GA, Blinder KJ, et al. Surgical technique for managing rhegmatogenous retinal detachment following prosthokeratoplasty. Retina 1991;11: 301-4.
11. Peyman GA, Conway MD, Soike KF, et al. Long-term vitreous replacement in primates with intravitreal vitreon or vitreon plus silicone. Ophthalmic Surgery 1991;22:657-64.
12. Peyman GA, Blinder KJ, Paris CL, et al. Vitreon: A new perfluorocarbon vitreous substitute. Afro-Asian J Ophthalmol 1991;10:48-57.
13. Blinder KJ, Peyman GA, Desai UR, et al. Vitreon: A short-term vitreoretinal tamponade. Br J Ophthalmol 1992;76:525-28.

Use of Tissue Adhesives in Ophthalmology

Prateek Gujar, Purendra Bhasin, Priyamvada Bhasin (India)

Tissue adhesives have been used in ophthalmology since long.[1-3] The role of tissue adhesives in ophthalmology revolves around:
- As a structural filler or support instead of donor tissue.
- As an adhesive in lieu of sutures to minimize operating time.
- As a barrier to facilitate epithelial healing and prevent collagen breakdown.

Tissue adhesives can be subdivided into:
- Synthetic adhesives (e.g. cyanoacrylate derivatives)
- Biologic adhesives (e.g. fibrin-based adhesives).

Cyanoacrylate derivatives are synthetic and non-biodegradable. These are compounds with very high tensile strength that rapidly polymerize on contact with basic substances such as water or blood to form a strong bond. These adhesives are known to induce an inflammatory foreign body reaction, including neovascularization and tissue necrosis (Fig. 49.1). They are usually used on an external surface like in the management of corneal perforations and severe thinning.[4,5]

Fibrin-based adhesives are biologic and biodegradable. They induce minimal inflammation. They have been used in ophthalmology for indications including pterygium autografting, lamellar keratoplasty, glaucoma surgery, and strabismus wound closure.[6-9] As fibrin glues use human thrombin, this blood product still carries a small risk of infection from a contaminated donor

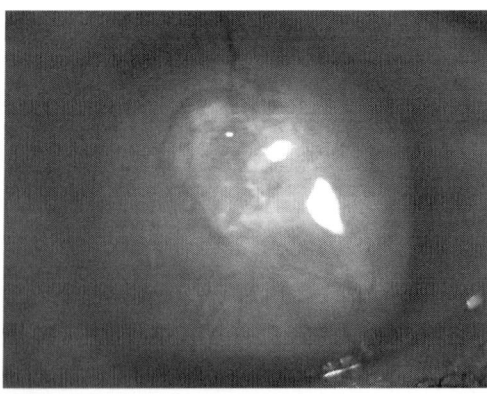

Fig. 49.1: Cyanoacrylate glue attracting corneal neovascularization

pool. In addition, the preparation and application of fibrin-based glues is significantly more complex as compared to synthetic glues.

CYANOACRYLATE TISSUE ADHESIVES

Many forms of cyanoacrylate glues have been developed. Methyl 2-cyanoacrylate was the first to be tested experimentally in the eye, which was followed by n-butyl and n-heptyl derivatives.[1,2] Octyl derivatives are the latest CTA to be developed, and are more flexible then butyl derivatives when dry; however, with less tensile strength.

Uses in Ophthalmology

- *Corneal perforations and corneal thinning/melting*: Studies have shown the benefits of CTAs in the setting of corneal perforation or progressive thinning, with lower rates of penetrating keratoplasty, conjunctival flap surgery, and enucleation.[10,11] use of antibiotic prophylaxis has been recommended while the CTA is in place, to avoid development of infectious infiltrates.[10]
- Besides corneal perforations, it has also been tried in cataract surgery wound closure, scleral buckle attachment in retinal detachment repair, postoperative leaking wounds, temporary tarsorrhaphy, strabismus surgery, scleral reinforcement in patients with thin sclera, and punctal occlusion.[4]

Mechanism of Bonding

Rapid polymerization of liquid monomers into solid polymers occurs in the presence of anions, with thin layers of adhesive polymerizing faster than thick layers.[4] In presence of water, polymerization is too rapid for tissue adhesion to occur. Thus, in practice, a minimal amount of CTA usually works best on a surface dried immediately before application.

Cyanoacrylate tissue adhesives (CTA) are used to treat corneal perforations and thinning. This can be done in office setting at the slit lamp, although a complex perforation where air, viscoelastic, or tissue patch may be used to separate iris or lens from the perforation site and to prevent intraocular spread of glue can be done in the operation room.

For application, a small drop of CTA is placed onto the dry aspect of a small round disk of plastic stuck to a wooden applicator stick (e.g. by ointment), which is then applied onto the perforation site that has just been dried and debrided of epithelium or necrotic tissue to promote adhesion. A soft bandage contact lens is then applied.[2]

Another technique of application is using a needle. A minimal amount of CTA may be placed at the tip of a needle, and gently wiped across the thinned or perforated surface.

The reported duration of cyanoacrylate glue adherence is 1–940 days (mean 45–72 days).[12]

HUMAN FIBRIN GLUES

Fibrin adhesives have undergone several modifications to improve the quality, consistency, and safety. Significant modification included the addition of aprotinin to slow the lysis of the fibrin clot and the use of human derived thrombin as opposed to bovine-derived thrombin to decrease the potential for allergic reactions and cross-reactivity to human clotting factors.[13]

Mechanism of Bonding

Human fibrin glues (HFGs) produce a biocompatible fibrin matrix similar to a natural plasma clot, simulating the final stage of the coagulation cascade. The commercial Tisseel Kit VH (Baxter AG, Vienna, Austria)contains freeze-dried powders and diluents that are combined to form a two component system:
1. A sealant protein solution, composed of human fibrinogen, plasminogen, fibronectin, and factor XIII in a bovine aprotinin solution.
2. A sealant setting solution, composed of human thrombin reconstituted in a calcium chloride solution. The two components are mixed immediately before application, the fibrinogen is converted to fibrin by thrombin, and factor XIII crosslinks the fibrin monomers to form a semirigid fibrin clot. Fibrin and fibronectin crosslink with the collagen in tissues, which explains the high adherence of HFG to collagen-rich corneal stroma.[14]

Glue Preparation and Application

Prior to surgery, the Tisseel Kit VH vials are first heated to 37ºC using a proprietary device (Fibrinotherm) provided by Baxter. Lyophilized fibrinogen is reconstituted with aprotinin 3000 KIU/ml solution, and thrombin 4 IU/ml is reconstituted with calcium chloride solution. The respective constituents are mixed and stirred in the Fibrinotherm.[15] The two components are then applied simultaneously using a dual syringe system with a common plunger (Duploject) that ensures the feeding of equal volumes of the two components into a common joining piece.

Any tissue that is to be placed over top of the HFG (e.g. conjunctival flap, amniotic membrane, lamellar corneal graft) must be prepared in advance and be of correct dimension. When ready, the base of the area to be glued is dried with a cellulose sponge and the HFG is applied using the double syringe system, followed by placement of additional overlying tissue if planned. Excess HFG may be squeezed out from under the tissue using a gentle sweeping pressure from a blunt instrument or cellulose sponge.[7] If applied to the cornea without overlying tissue, then a bandage contact lens is recommended after the HFG has set to slow the disintegration of the fibrin clot from repeated mechanical action from the eyelids.

The degradation of HFG occurs in days to several weeks, as compared to CTA.[13] This degradation of a fibrin clot yields no toxic metabolites, as in the case of CTA.

Although no documented cases of viral transmission have occurred from the use of commercial HFGs till now, human viral contamination of blood-derived products with hepatitis (especially hepatitis A), HIV, and parvovirus B19 continues to be a theoretic risk despite viral inactivation techniques.[16]

Uses in Ophthalmology

- *Corneal perforations and thinning*: HFGs can be used for corneal perforations either alone or in combination with amniotic membrane or conjunctival flap.[17] Study comparing the efficacy of HGFs and CTA has found that HFG provide a similar success rate, more physiologic healing, and significantly less corneal vascularization as compared to CTA.[12]
- Sutureless conjunctival autograting or amniotic membrane transplant (Fig. 49.2)
- Conjunctival closure during strabismus surgery
- Conjunctival wound closure in trabeculectomy surgery and to repair bleb leaks
- Sutureless lamellar keratoplasty
- Glued scleral fix intraocular lens implant.

RECENT ADVANCES IN TISSUE ADHESIVES IN OPHTHALMOLOGY

Both HFGs and CTA have there limitations, owing to which there is significant interest in the development of improved sealants for ophthalmic use. Goins et al and Khadem et al have reported on the use of laser-activated biologic tissue glue composed of 18 percent fibrinogen and 0.3 percent riboflavin-5-phosphate in corneal incisions and penetrating keratoplasty wounds in human cadaveric eyes.[18,19] Miki et al have reported success in closing

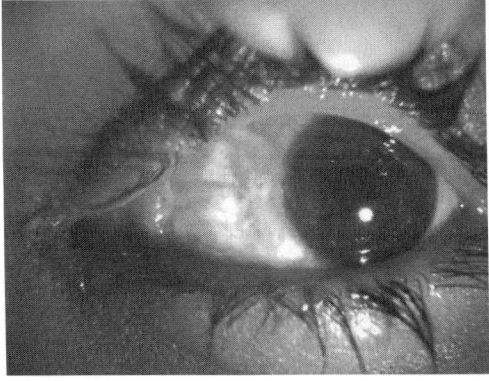

Fig. 49.2: Pterygium excision with amniotic membrane transplant using fibrin glue

various corneal lacerations in animal eyes using a novel polymer made from hyaluronic acid modified with methacrylate groups that may be crosslinked using laser activation.[20] Kalayci et al has reported using a hydrogel compound which polymerize when mixed together to form a hydrogel layer to seal corneal incisions.[21]

To summarize, the main indication for CTA is in the treatment of progressive corneal thinning and small, uncomplicated corneal perforations of ≤ 2 mm size. Alternately, human fibrin glues may be used to treat such conditions, potentially resulting in less corneal and conjunctival inflammatory reaction. In addition to this, HFGs is biocompatible. This allows application over a larger surface area and the use of a superficial covering layer such as amniotic membrane or conjunctiva to further reinforce the site of perforation or thinning and to promote rapid re-epithelialization. In addition to this HFGs can be used in various ophthalmic surgery to avoid the use of sutures. This reduces the surgical time and avoids suture related complications. The principal limitations with HFGs are the theoretic risk of viral transmission and the complexity in preparation and application when compared with CTA.

REFERENCES

1. Bloomfield S, Barnert AH, Kanter PD. The use of Eastman 910 monomer as an adhesive in ocular surgery: I. Biologic effects on ocular tissues. Am J Ophthalmol 1963;55:742-8.
2. Refojo MF, Dohlman CH, Ahmad B, et al. Evaluation of adhesives for corneal surgery. Arch Ophthalmol 1968;80:645-56.
3. Webster RG Jr, Slansky HH, Refojo MF, et al. The use of adhesive for the closure of corneal perforations: report of two cases. Arch Ophthalmol 1968;80:705-9.
4. Khodadoust AA. Tissue adhesives in ophthalmology. In: Sears ML, Tarkkanen A (Eds). Surgical Pharmacology of the Eye. New York: Raven Press 1985:223-34.
5. Gilbert C. Adhesives in retinal detachment surgery. Br J Ophthalmol 1991;75:309-10.
6. Biedner B, Rosenthal G. Conjunctival closure in strabismus surgery: Vicryl versus fibrin glue. Ophthalmic Surg Lasers 1996;27:967.
7. Kaufman HE, Insler MS, Ibrahim-Elzembely HA, et al. Human fibrin tissue adhesive for sutureless lamellar keratoplasty and scleral patch adhesion: a pilot study. Ophthalmology 2003;110:2168-72.
8. O'Sullivan F, Dalton R, Rostron CK. Fibrin glue: an alternative method of wound closure in glaucoma surgery. J Glaucoma 1996;5:367-70.
9. Cohen RA, McDonald MB. Fixation of conjunctival autografts with an organic tissue adhesive [letter]. Arch Ophthalmol 1993;111:1167-8.
10. Weiss JL, Williams P, Lindstrom RL, et al. The use of tissue adhesives incorneal perforations. Ophthalmology 1983;90:610-5.
11. Hirst LW, Smiddy WE, Stark WJ. Corneal perforations: changing methods of treatment 1960–1980. Ophthalmology 1982;89:630-5.
12. Sharma A, Kaur R, Kumar S, et al. Fibrin glue versus N-butyl-2-cyanoacrylate in corneal perforations. Ophthalmology 2003;110: 291-8.

13. Radosevich M, Goubran HA, Burnouf T. Fibrin sealant: scientific rationale, production methods, properties, and current clinical use. Vox Sang. 1997;72:133-43.
14. Papatheofanis FJ, Barmada R. The principles and applications of surgical adhesives. Surg Annu. 1993;25:49-81.
15. Tisseel Package Insert. Available at www.adcock.co.za/Resources/ProductDocs/TISSEEL%20KIT%20PACKAGE%20INSERT.pdf. Accessed April 2008;14.
16. Atrah HI. Fibrin glue. Br Med J. 1994;308:933-4.
17. Duchesne B, Tahi H, Galand A. Use of fibrin glue and amniotic membrane transplant in corneal perforation. Cornea. 2001;20:230-2.
18. Goins KM, Khadem J, Majmudar PA. Relative strength of photodynamic biologic tissue glue in penetrating keratoplasty in cadaver eyes. J Cataract Refract Surg. 1998;24:1566-70.
19. Khadem J, Truong T, Ernest JT. Photodynamic biologic tissue glue. Cornea. 1994;13:406-10.
20. Miki D, Dastgheib K, Kim T, et al. A photopolymerized sealant for corneal lacerations. Cornea. 2002;21:393-9.
21. Bloom JN, Duffy MT, Davis JB, et al. A light-activated surgical adhesive technique for sutureless ophthalmic surgery. Arch Ophthalmol. 2003;121:1591-5.

50

Photodynamic Therapy (Verteporfin) in Age-related Macular Degeneration

S Natarajan, Anand Bagmar (India)

INTRODUCTION

Age-related macular degeneration (ARMD) is the major cause of blindness in elderly people.[1] Ten percent those affected patients retain usable vision.[2] Out of these, 25 percent are caused by retinal pigment epithelium (RPE), choriocapillaris and neurosensory retina atrophy also called dry ARMD.[3] Currently there is no treatment available for these patients. Remaining 75 percent of patients have wet or exudative ARMD. They experience severe visual loss. The disease process includes choroidal neovascularization (CNV), disciform scarring, vitreous hemorrhage, pigment epithelial detachment and tears.[3]

There are various modalities of treatments like laser treatment, radiation therapy, vitamin supplements, surgical excision of neovascular membranes, macular translocation, and transpupillary thermotherapy and photodynamic therapy.[4-9]

Macular photocoagulation study (MPS) showed 50 percent recurrence of treated vessels and scotoma following the treatment. Submacular surgery and fovea translocation did not show magnificent visual benefit due to RPE atrophy.[4-9] Photodynamic therapy (PDT) is an emerging technology for the treatment of neovascular process affecting eye and other parts of the body especially treatment of CNV in wet ARMD.[10]

The basic principle of PDT is the activation of a dye by low power laser light to induce coagulation of the neovascular vessels. The dye particles absorb the photons and move to a higher energy state which results in the creation of an excited oxygen which damages cell membranes, mitochondria and vascular endothelial cells.[11,12] This can be performed with safety with regard to the surrounding normal neurosensory retina. In photocoagulation therapy, pigments present in a neovascular as well as surrounding normal tissue absorb thermal energy, which results in unintended but unavoidable bystander effect on the normal tissue. This lack of specificity limits the usefulness of photocoagulation for CNV especially in subfoveal and juxtafoveal region.

In contrast to photocoagulation, in PDT due to nonthermal and photodynamic properties of verteporfin where drug is activated by laser to induce regression of CNV, we achieve its therapeutic effect. Although a large area of retina is exposed to energy, there is no thermal effect exerted on the neurosensory tissue. Instead a laser

Photodynamic Therapy (Verteporfin) in Age-related Macular Degeneration

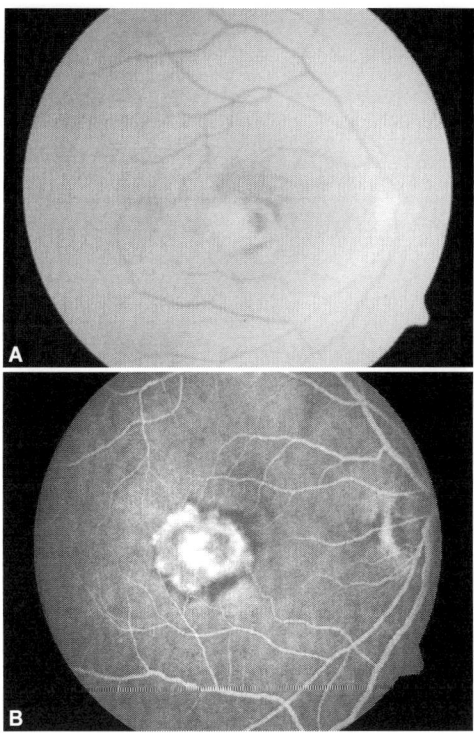

Figs 50.1A and B: Fundus photograph and FFA of right eye shows subfoveal CNV. Visual acuity – 6/60. Patient underwent PDT

light acts as a catalyst to activate the photoactive dye within the neurosensory vessels, inducing occlusion of the vessel and sparing the normal surrounding tissue.

TECHNIQUE

Photodynamic therapy (PDT) is done by an IV infusion of (1–2 mg/kg) of the verteporfin into the antecubital vein.

After administration for IV infusion of a drug for 10 minutes, laser energy is then applied 15 minutes from the time of infusion to the area of interest with the help of fundus contact lens. The patient is advised to sit in a light restricted room for one hour after treatment to minimize the possibility of photo toxicity from the dye.

Verteporfin

Visudyne is administered in liposomal form as an IV infusion over 10 min. It binds to circulating low-density lipoprotein (LDL) in the bloodstream. Prolioferative endothelial cells in CNV have higher levels of LDL receptors than normal vascular tissue. Verteporfin-LDL complexes are rapidly absorbed by CNV. Nonthermal red laser light at 689 nm, 50 J/cm^2, 600 mW/cm^2) for 83 seconds.[13] Fifteen

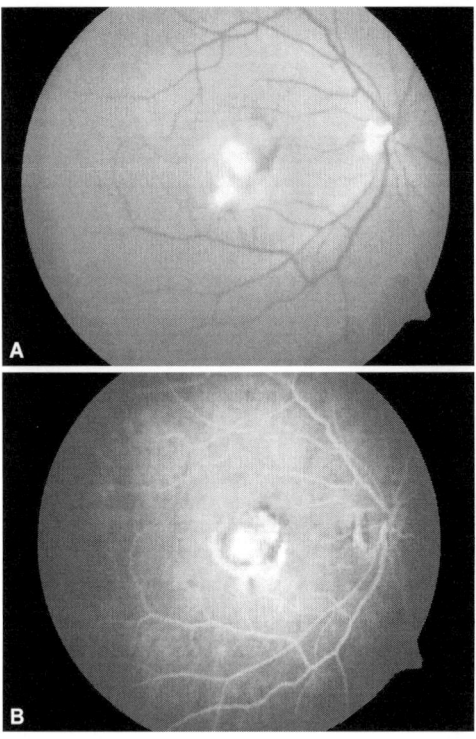

Figs 50.2A and B: At 3 months follow-up after 1st treatment, FFA showed leakage. Visual acuity –6/24. Patient underwent 1st retreatment

minutes after the start of the visudyne infusion. Activation causes release of oxygen free redials. Endothelial damage and throbs formation occurs due to it. It leads to an occlusion of abnormal vessels.

The treatment effect of PDT is not immediately visible to examine but the lesion develops over a period of hours after the appreciation of laser energy to the fundus.

Various drugs available for PDT like ethyl etiopurpurin, Lutein texaphyrin, Verteporfin. Verteporfin (VisudyneTM) is most widely used.

Post-treatment Regime

- Completely avoid exposure to sunlight for 48 hours
- Avoid halogen light
- To wear ANSI approved 100 percent UV protecting glasses
- To wear clothes that completely cover the body.

PREPARATION OF THE PATIENT FOR PDT

For the correct diagnosis of CNV, eligible for treatment with Visudyne, FFA and ICG angiography associated with stereoscopic color fundus photography have to be performed.

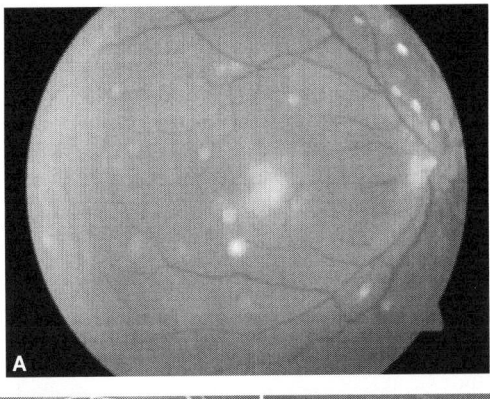

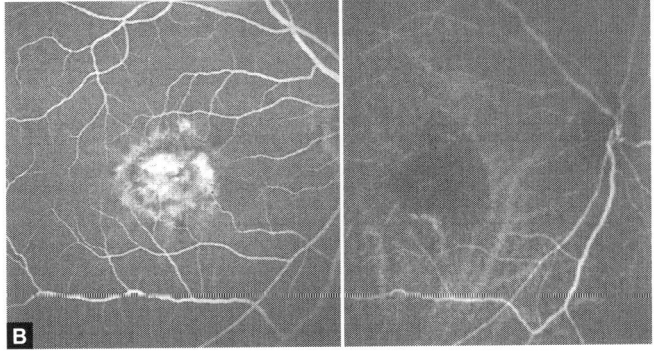

Figs 50.3A and B: At 6 months follow-up, FFA and ICG showed healed CNV. Visual acuity stabilized to 6/9

The angiogram should not be taken more than 7 days before treatment with Visudyne.

Define eligibility of the patient based on the lesion, components—classic and occult CNV, their proportions, size and closeness to the optic disk.

CALCULATION OF THE TREATMENT SPOT SIZE REQUIRED COVERING THE CNV

- Determine the GLD (greatest linear dimension) on the photographic image (It should include additional 1000 mm to allow margin of 500 mm to ensure the coverage of the lesion)
- Divide GLD/ magnification of the image (2.5)—Actual GLD on the retina
- Treatment spot size—GLD on the retina +1000 mm.

Procedure

Dilution—15 mg/7.5 ml vials reconstituted by dilution with 5 percent D to make 30 ml of 6 mg/ml. Syringe is loaded into infusion pump. Time is set to 15 minutes to begin laser. Start infusion pump for 10 minutes. Start laser 15 minutes after start of infusion for 83 sec.

Results

Results of TAP (Treatment of ARMD with PDT study) -13, 246 (61%) of 402 eyes lost < 15 letters of visual acuity from baseline, compared to 96 (47%) of 207 placebo eye (P< 0.001).

Subgroup Analysis

Sixty-seven percent classic (>50% classic lesion) vs 39 percent occult eyes lost < 15 letters of visual acuity.

Results of VIP Study[14]

- VIP Study Group
- High Myopia Group

	1 year follow-up	
	Control	PDT
VA gain 1 line or more	15 percent	32 percent
VA no gain or loss	28 percent	30 percent
VA loss 3 lines or more	33 percent	14 percent

CONCLUSION

Photodynamic therapy (PDT) is a promising treatment modality for the treatment of SRNV in ARMD. Though there is a high rate of recurrence of CNV following treatment with PDT, retreatment is possible.

REFERENCES

1. Abdelsalam A, Del Priorel, Zarbin MA. Drusens in ARMD, Pathogenesis, natural courses and laser photocoagulation induced regression. Surv Ophthalmol 1999;44:1-29.
2. Elman NJ, Fine SZ. Exudative ARMD. Retina. Mosby: Ryan SJ, 1994.pp.1103-41.
3. Klein R, Klein BE, Jensen SC, Meuer SM. The 5 years incidence and progression of age related maculopathy: The Beaver-Dam eye Study. Ophthalmology 1997;104:7-12.
4. Macular photocoagulation study group: 5-year. follow-up of fellow eyes of patients with ARMD and unilateral extrafoveal choroidal neovascularization. Arch Ophthalmol 1993;111:1189-99.
5. Devis H, Kaiser PK, Lewis S, Estafanous M. Macular translocation for subfoveal CNV in ARMD: A prospective study. Am J Ophthalmol 1999;128:135-46.
6. Mauget Faysee M, Chiquet C, Mileu D, et al. Long term results of radiotherapy for subfoveal NV in ARMD. Br J Ophthalmol 1999; 83:923-8.
7. Smith W, Mitchell P, Webb K, Leader SR. Dietary antioxidants and age related maculopathy: The blue mountains eye study. Ophthalmology 1999;106:761-7.
8. Meril PT, Loruso FJ, Lomeo MD, et al. Surgical removal of subfoveal SRNV in ARMD. Ophthalmology 1999;106:782-9.

9. Chong TA, Bird AC. Alternative therapies in exudative ARMD. Br J Ophthalmol 1998;82:1441-3.
10. Bressler NM. TAP study group. PDT with vertiporfin of subfoveal SRNV in ARMD.
11. Henderson BW, Dougherty TJ. How does PDT work? Photochem Photobiol 1992;55:145-57.
12. Moshfeghi DM, Peyman GA, Moshfeghi AA, et al. Ocular vascular Thrombosis following Tinethyl etiopurpurin (SnET2) PDT: Time dependencies. Oph Surg Lasers 1998;29:663-8.
13. Treatment of ARMD with PDT (TAP) study group. PDT of subfoveal CNV in ARMD with Verteporfin: One year results of 2 randomized clinical trials: TAP report. Arch Ophthalmol 1999;117:1329-45.
14. Mones J. VIP Study Group. PDT with verteporfin of subfoveal CNV in ARMD study–design and baseline VIP randomized clinical trial. Invest Ophthalmol Vis Sci 1999;40:S321.

Indocyanine Green Angiography

S Natarajan, Anand Bagmar (India)

INTRODUCTION

In the last few decades there have been major advancements in procedures for retinal evaluation. Fluorescein angiography revolutionized the diagnosis of retinal disorders but had some inherent limitations which could be overcome to a large extent by indocyanine green (ICG) angiography.

ADVANTAGES OF ICG

Indocyanine green (ICG) dye is a large molecule, highly protein bound and does not escape from the choroidal vasculature. The dye remains largely within the choriocapillaris. Its activity is in the infrared range, absorbing at 790-805 nm and emitting maximally at 835 nm. The retinal pigment epithelium and choroid absorb only 21-38 percent of near infrared light as compared to 55-75 percent of blue green light used in fluorescein angiography (FA).[1] These properties allow enhanced visualization of the deeper lying choroid and its associated abnormalities. Overlying hemorrhages, serous fluid, lipid and pigment that block view of fluorescein angiography, however, allow visualization of ICG.

HISTORY

Kogure and associates[2] performed the first choroidal absorption angiography in monkeys in 1970. David performed the first ICG angiograms in humans during carotid angiography.[3] In 1971 Hochheimer[4] described choroidal absorption angiography in cats using ICG injections. One year later, Flower and Hochheimer[5,6] performed intravenous absorption ICG angiography for the first-time in humans. The same group then described the superior technique of ICG fluorescein angiography.[7,8] However, since the fluorescence efficacy of ICG is only 4 percent of that of sodium fluorescein, it was difficult to produce high resolution images of clinical relevance. This was achieved with the advent of digital imaging systems coupled to infrared cameras[9,10] as well as scanning laser ophthalmoscopes (SLO) for ICG videoangiography. The use of 1024 line digital imaging system produces high resolution and enhanced ICG images.[10]

Realtime ICG Angiography

Realtime ICG angiography uses a fundus camera with a diode laser illumination system that has an output at 805 nm which can produce images at 30 frames per second acquired either as a videotape or as a single image at a frequency of 30 images per second.

Wide Angle Image

Wide angle image can be obtained with the aid of wide angle contact lenses with the fundus camera set on positions for aphakia (A) or hypermetrophia (+).

Digital Subtraction

Digital subtraction uses digital subtraction techniques and allows imaging in greater detail and in a shorter period of time.

PHARMACOLOGY

Indocyanine green (ICG) is tricarbocyanine dye which has been used to measure cardiac output since 1957.[11,12] It is water soluble with an empiric formula of $C_{43}H_{47}NaO_6S_2$. The dye is an anhydro-3, 3, 3, 3-tetramethyl 1-1,1-di (4-sulfobutyl)-4, 5, 4, 5, dibenzoindo tricarbocyanine hydroxide sodium salt. It has a molecular weight of 775 daltons. It is highly protein bound to globulins such as a1 lipoproteins. It is excreted by the liver via bile. It is not detected in cerebrospinal fluid[13,14] and does not cross the placenta.[15]

TOXICITY

The dye is relatively safe and appears to be safer than fluorescein. Nausea and vomiting are extremely uncommon. However, it should not be performed on patients allergic to iodine since it contains approximately 5 percent iodide by weight. Also it should not be performed on patients who are uremic or who have liver disease. Appropriate emergency equipment should be readily available.

TECHNIQUE

Indocyanine green (ICG) can be performed before or after fluorescein angiography. Usually 25 ml of ICG dissolved in 2 ml solvent is used (Fig. 51.1). Alternatively 50 mg dissolved in 3 ml of aqueous solvent is used in poorly dilated or darkly pigmented patients. Images are taken up to 30 minutes.

VARIOUS PHASES OF ICG ANGIOGRAPHY

Early phase A: Seen in the first two seconds. There is rapid filling of choroidal arteries and choriocapillaris and an early filling of choroidal veins. Major retinal blood vessels are not filled and are

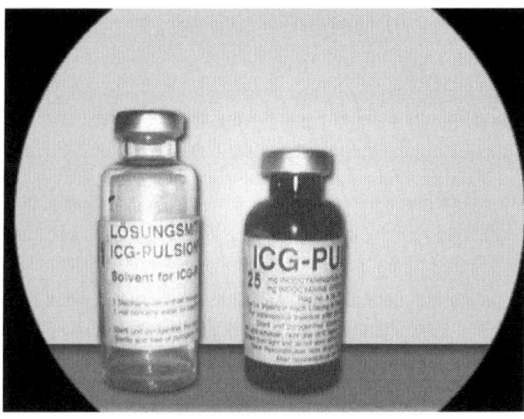

Fig. 51.1: Photograph of the indocyanine green dye (25 mg vial) in the dark bottle and its solvent

silhouetted as dark structures. A water shed zone is seen running vertically adjacent to the optic nerve head.

Early phase B: Seen between 2 to 5 seconds. There is a complete filling of the large choroidal veins and an early filling of the retinal arterioles.

Early phase C: Seen between 5 seconds to 3 minutes. There is a gradual filling of the choroidal arterioles. The large choroidal veins are still seen and the water shed zone is filled.

Middle phase: Seen between 3 to 15 minutes. There is a fading of the choroidal and retinal vasculature.

Late phase: Seen between 15 to 60 minutes. There is a background hyperfluorescence resulting from the staining of extrachoroidal tissue. The hypofluorescent choroidal vasculature is silhouetted against the background. The retinal vasculature is not visible.

ICG IN AGE RELATED MACULAR DEGENERATION

By fluorescein angiography about 13 percent of patients with wet ARMD are found to have a well-defined or classic neovascular membrane that are amenable to treatment.[16] ICG angiography improves the visualization of the neovascular complex and thus allows potential treatment of more patients. Yanuzzi and associates reported that in 39 percent of choroidal neovascular membranes, seen as occult by fluorescein angiography, they were able to differentiate into well-defined CNVMs using ICG angiography. Conducting a study on 1000 consecutive eyes with occult neovascular membranes, they were able to identify 3 morphological types using ICG angiography.[17] These lesions include focal spots (29%), plaques (61%) and combination lesions (8%) with both focal spots and plaques. There are three subtypes of combination lesions based on the location of the hot spot relative to the plaque, i.e marginal spot (focal spot at edge of plaque) (3%); overlying spot (hot spot overlying the plaque) (4%) and remote spot (hot spot remote from the plaque) (1%). In some, however, a mixture of these lesions were noted whereas in a few no hyperfluorescence was noted. The authors found that patients tended to develop the same morphologic type of CNVM in the fellow eye.

Focal spots: Appear as hyperfluorescent lesions less than 1 disk area in size. They are often seen outside the foveal avascular zone and thus potentially treatable by ICG guided/enhanced laser photocoagulation.

Plaque: The most common pattern of neovascularization seen. It is seen as a hyperfluorescent area greater than 1 disk area in size. These lesions are usually subfoveal. Hayashi and coworkers showed that leakage of ICG from CNV was slow compared to fluorescein.[18]

Chang et al[19] reported on the clinicopathologic correlation of ARMD with CNV detected by ICG angiography. Histopathologic examination of the lesion revealed a thick subretinal pigment epithelium CNVM corresponding to the plaque like lesion seen with ICG angiography. Yanuzzi and coworkers10 also reported the contribution of videoangiography in converting cases of serous and vascularized pigment epithelial detachments with occult CNVM into well-defined classic CNVMs.

ICG Dye Enhanced Diode Laser Photocoagulation

The peak absorption of ICG is at a similar wavelength as the peak emission of the diode laser. Thus, dye enhanced laser photocoagulation may allow selective ablation of the ICG containing CNVM with relative sparing of the normal neighboring retina. This is specially useful in subfoveal CNVMs.

Feeder Vessel Treatment

Figures 51.2A to C is a new modality of treatment where high speed ICG angiography is used to detect extrafoveal feeder vessels supplying any choroidal neovascular membranes, specially in cases of subfoveal CNVM. They are seen in early phase of ICG angiography. The two patterns noted are the racquet and umbrella. Racquet patterns are favorable for treatment.

ICG angiography has enhanced the understanding of several pathologies occurring primarily at the choroidal level.

Idiopathic Polypoidal Choroidal Vasculopathy

Idiopathic polypoidal choroidal vasculopathy (IPCV) is an anomaly of the choroidal vasculature wherein some vessels of the inner choroidal vascular network of vessels end in an aneurysmal bulge or polyp like structure. These appear as reddish orange, spheroidal structures and are associated with multiple, recurrent

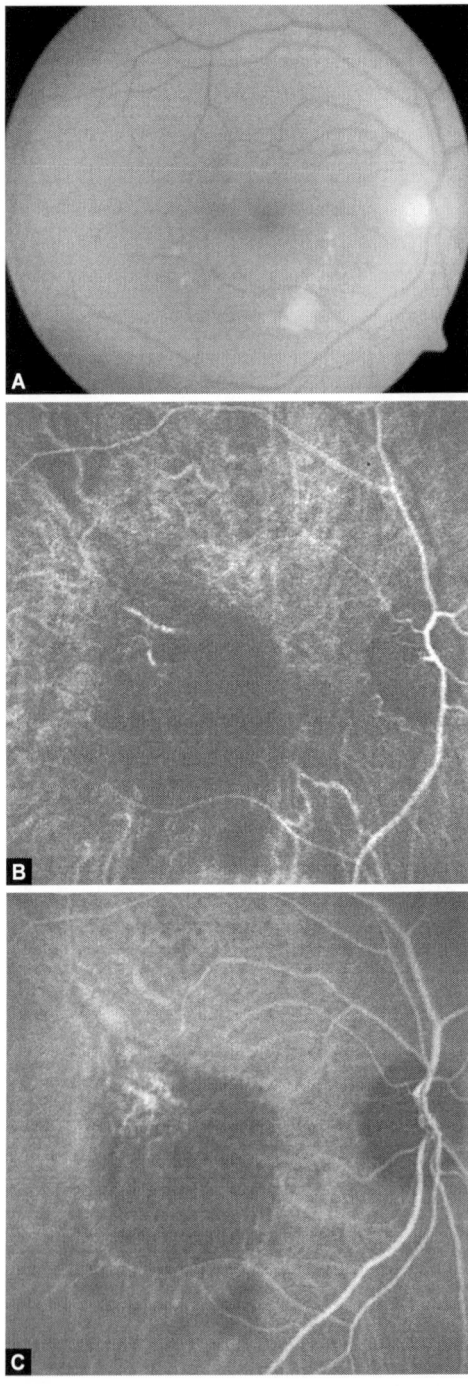

Figs 51.2A to C: (A) Fundus photograph of a patient with a pigment epithelial detachment and exudative age related macular degeneration; (B) Early and middle phase; (C) ICG angiograms showing a pigment epithelial detachment and a feeder vessel supplying the occult plaque

serosanguinous detachments of the RPE and neurosensory retina following bleeding from these polyps.[20]

During ICG the larger vessels of the network start to fill before the retinal vessels. Shortly afterwards, small hyperfluorescent "polyps" become visible. They appear to leak slowly and the surrounding hypofluorescent. In late phases there is a 'washout' or disappearance of the dye and the characteristic late staining of an occult CNVMs absent (Figs 51.3A to D).

Central Serous Chorioretinopathy

The early phase of ICG may show diffuse or multifocal areas of choroidal hyperpermeability. In the late phases there is dispersion of the fluorescence and a silhouetting of the larger choroidal vessels.

Intraocular Tumors

Certain tumors have characteristic ICG patterns.[21] Pigmented choroidal melanomas block ICG fluorescence and are differentiated from hemangiomas and osteomas. Choroidal hemangiomas show a marked progressive hyperfluorescence due to the vascularity, which can be visualized even through overlying hemorrhages.

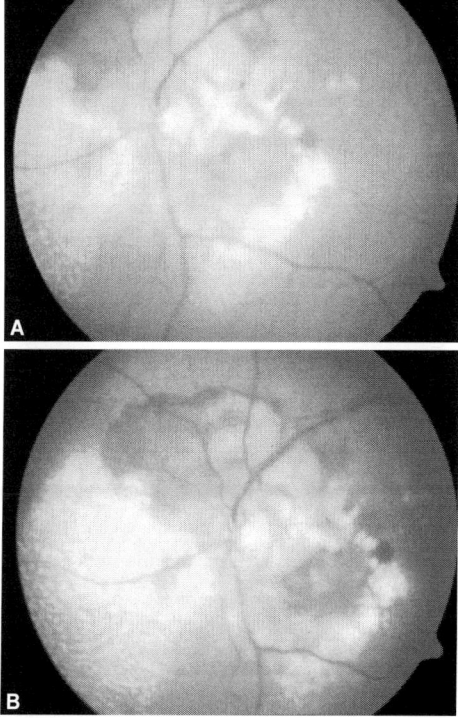

Figs 51.3A and B: (A and B) Fundus photographs of a patient with idiopathic polypoidal choroidal vasculopathy

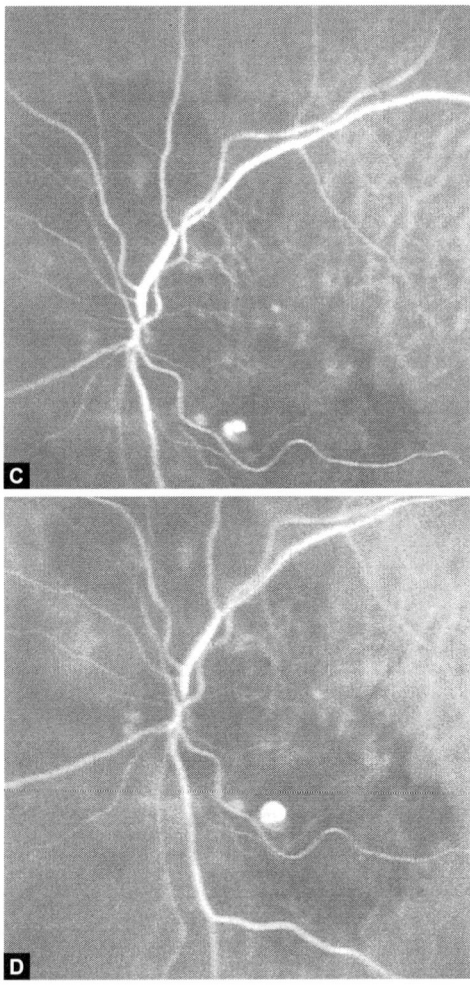

Figs 51.3C and D: (C) Early and middle phase; (D) ICG angiograms of the patient in Figure showing filling of the polypoidal lesions with surrounding hypofluorescence due to subretinal hemorrhage and exudation

Choroidal osteomas show characteristic small vessels and variable blockage in bony areas.

Choroiditis

Indocyanine green (ICG) is useful in the diagnosis and monitoring of patients with posterior uveitis.

Bird Shot Retinochoroidopathy

The creamy lesions seen clinically are seen as multiple hypofluorescent lesions resembling 'holes' in the fluorescence of the choriocapillaris. They are seen along larger choroidal vessels.[22]

Serpiginous Choroiditis[23]

The acute lesions show blockage of fluorescence on ICG, which reappears after resolution (Figs 51.4A to D).

Multifocal Choroiditis

Multifocal choroiditis patches block fluorescence on ICG angiography. Some hyperfluorescent spots seen appear to be subclinical foci of choroiditis.

Acute Multifocal Placoid Pigment Epitheliopathy[24]

Acute multifocal placoid pigment epitheliopathy (AMPPE)[24] lesions are hypofluorescent in both the early and late phases and suggest the pathogenesis of choroidal vascular occlusion secondary to occlusive vasculitis.

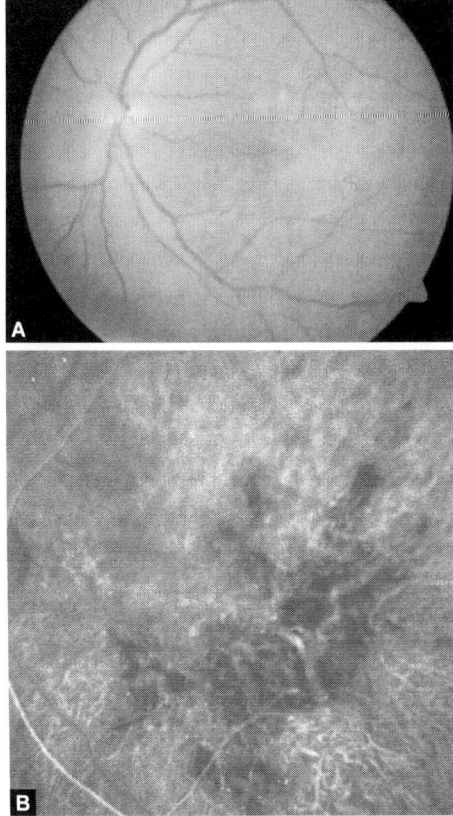

Figs 51.4A and B: (A) Fundus photograph of a patient with healed serpiginous choroiditis; (B) Photograph early phase indocyanine green angiogram of the patient showing areas of hypofluorescence with larger choroidal vessels seen

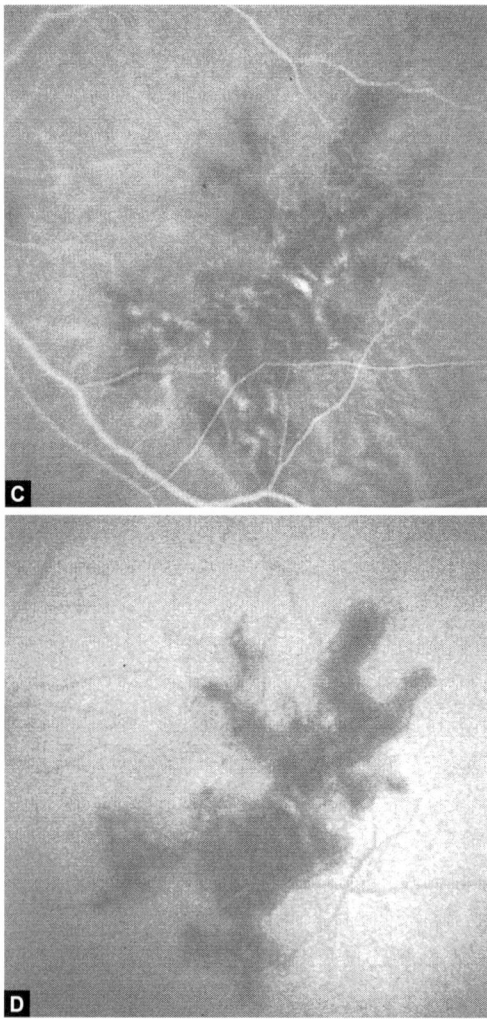

Figs 51.4C and D: (C) Photograph middle and late; (D) Phase indocyanine green angiogram of the patient showing areas of hypofluorescence with larger choroidal vessels seen

Multiple Evanescent White Dot Syndrome[25]

Multiple evanescent white dot syndrome (MEWDS)[25] has a characteristic pattern of hypofluorescent spots throughout the posterior pole and peripheral retina, which appear 10 minutes after dye injection and then persists.

Vogt Koyanagi Harada Disease

The ICG shows signs of choroidal inflammatory vasculopathy such as delayed choriocapillaris perfusion, perivascular leakage and diffuse choroidal hyperfluorescence. Hypofluorescent dark dots seen in intermediate stages, represent granulomas. Areas of exudative retinal detachment may show hyperfluorescent pinpoint areas. In cases of severe papillitis disk hyperfluorescence is seen.[26]

SUMMARY

Indocyanine green (ICG) is an investigational tool to study the choroidal anatomy and pathology. Used as an adjunct to fluorescein angiography it has greatly enhanced our understanding of hitherto ill-understood lesions. It is specially useful in cases of occult and recurrent choroidal neovascular membranes. It has been used to detect and characterize the IPCV abnormality. Various types of choroiditis and choroidal tumors can be differentiated. ICG videoangiography is being used to study the choroidal blood flow. The clinical usefulness of this relatively new technique will become apparent with greater experience.

REFERENCES

1. Geerates WJ, Berry ER. Ocular spectral characteristics as related to hazards from lasers and other light sources. Am J Ophthalmol 1968;66:15-20.
2. Kogure K, David NJ, Yamanouchi U, Choromokos E. Arch Ophthalmol 1970;83:209-14.
3. David NJ. Infrared absorption fundus angiography. In Proceedings of International Symposium on Fluorescein Angiography, Albi, France, 1969, Basel, 1971, Karger.
4. Hochheimer BF. Angiography of the retina with indocyanine green. Arch Ophthalmol 1971;86:564-5.
5. Flower RW. Infrared absorption angiography of the choroid and some observations on the effects of high intraocular pressures. Am J Ophthalmol 1972;74:600-14.
6. Flower RW, Hochheimer BF. Clinical infrared absorption angiography of the choroid. Am J Ophthalmol 1972;73:458-9 (letter).
7. Flower RW, Hochheimer BF. A Clinical technique and choroidal circulation. Invest Ophthalmol 1973;2:248-61.
8. Flower RW, Hochheimer BF. Indocyanine green dye fluorescence and infrared absorption choroidal. Johns Hopkins Med J 1976; 138:3-42.
9. Guyer DR, Puliafito CA, Mones JM, Friedman E, Chang W, Verdooner SR. Digital indocyanine green angiography in chorioretinal disorders. Ophthalmology 1992;99:287-90.
10. Yannuzzi LA, Slakter JS, Sorenson, JS, Guyer, DR, Orlock DA. Digital indocyanine green videoangiography and choroidal neovascularization. Retina 1992;12:191-223.
11. Guyer DR, Yannuzzi LA, Slakter JS, Sorenson JA, Hope-Ross M, Orlock DR. Digital indocyanine green videoangiography of occult choroidal neovascularization. Ophthalmology 1994;101:1727-37.
12. Fox IJ, Wodd EH. Applications of dilution curves recorded from the right side of the heart or venous circulation with the aid of a new indicator dye. Mayo Clin Proc 1957;32:541.
13. Ketterer SG, Wiengand BD. The excretion of indocyanine green its use in the estimation of hepatic blood flow. Clin Res 1959;7:71.

14. Ketterer SG, Wiengand BD. Hepatic clearance of indocyanine green. Clin Res 1959;7:289.
15. Probst P, Paumgartner G, Caucig H, Fruohlich H, Grabner G. Studies on clearance and placental transfer of indocyanine green during labor. Clin Chim Acta 1970;29:157.
16. Freund KB, Yanuzzi LA, Sorenson JA, et al. Age related macular degeneration and choroidal neovascularization. Am J Ophthalmol 1993;115:786-91.
17. Guyer DR, Yannuzi LA, Slakter JS, et al. Classification of choroidal neovascularization by digital indocyanine angiography. Ophthalmology 1996;103:2054-60.
18. Hayashi K, DeLaey JJ. Indocyanine green angiography of neovascular membranes. Ophthamologica 1985;190:30-9.
19. Chang TS, Freund KB, de la Cruz Z, et al. Clinicopathologic correlation of choroidal neovascularization demonstrated by indocyanine green angiography in a patient with retention of good vision for almost four years. Retina 1994;14:114-24.
20. Kleiner RC, Brucker, AJ, Johnston, RL. The posterior uveal bleeding syndrome. Retina 1990;10:9-17.
21. Guyer DR, Yanuzzi LA, Krupsky S, Slakter JS, et al. Digital indocyanine green angiography of intraocular tumours, Semin. Ophthalmol 1993;8:224-9.
22. Krupsky S, Foster S, Guyer DR, Gragoudas ES, Friedman E. Digital indocyanine green angiography of choroidal inflammatory disorders. Invest Ophthalmology (suppl); 1999. p.33.
23. Giovannini A, Ripa E, Scasellati-Sforzolini B, et al. Indocyanine green angiography in serpiginous choroidopathy. Eur J Ophthalmol 1996;6:299-306.
24. Howe LJ, Woon H, Graham EM, et al. Choroidal hypoperfusion in acute multifocal posterior placoid pigment epitheliopathy: an indocyanine green angiography study. Ophthamology 1995;102:790-8.
25. Ie D, Glaser BM, Murphy RP, et al. Indocyanine green angiography in multiple evanescent white-dot syndrome. Am J Ophthalmol 1994;117:7-12.
26. Bouchenaki N, Herbert CP. The contribution to the appraisal and management of Vogt Koyanagi Harada disease. Ophthalmology 2001;108(1):54-64.

Management of Dry Eye—Current Trends and Recent Advances

Anthony Vipin Das, Virender Sangwan (India)

The ecosystem of the ocular surface depends on the dynamic interactions of healthy adnexa (eyelid margins), adequate blink rate, normal tear production, and ocular surface tissue, consisting of cornea and conjunctiva. The management of Dry eye ranges from a variety of modalities depending on the severity of the disease and the extent of complications secondary to the disease itself. Consultation with the physician in treating the systemic diseases also is vital in efficient management. The various approaches can be broadly categorized into the following:

Medical management:
- Tear substitutes
- Autologous serum
- Secretagogues
- Anti-inflammatory agents
- Eyelid integrity
- Systemic disease

MEDICAL MANAGEMENT

Tear Substitutes

Artificial Tears used either alone or in combination with other medications form the mainstay of treatment in dry eye disease. Their primary action is lubrication but also includes other actions such as replacement of deficient tear constituents, dilution of proinflammatory substances, reduction of tear osmolarity,[1] and protection against osmotic stress.[2] The electrolyte composition, osmolarity/osmolality, viscosity, preservatives, and compatible solutes vary between different medications.

Potassium and bicarbonate appear to be the most important of the solutes.[1] Dry eye patients have higher-than-normal tear film osmolarity (i.e. crystalloid osmolarity, which relates to the concentration of small dissolved particles, such as ions). Colloid osmolality (which relates to macromolecule concentration) influences water transport across the ocular surface epithelium. Higher artificial tear viscosity increases tear retention time and may help protect the ocular surface. Viscosity agents used in artificial tears include carboxymethylcellulose (CMC), polyvinyl alcohol, polyethylene glycol, propylene glycol, hydroxypropyl-guar (HP-guar), and lipids such as castor oil or mineral oil.[1]

Carboxymethylcellulose

Carboxymethylcellulose (CMC) is a cellulose derivative with carboxymethyl groups ($-CH_2-COOH$) bound to some of the hydroxyl groups of the glucopyranose monomers that make up the cellulose backbone. It is often used as its sodium salt, sodium carboxymethylcellulose. The Ophthalmic solution concentration is 1 percent or 0.5 percent w/v. The common preservatives used along with CMC are Stabilized Oxychloro Complex 0.0075 percent w/v and Benzalkonium Chloride. The indications include for temporary relief from burning irritation and discomfort due to dryness of the eye or due to exposure to wind or sun. It may also be used as a protectant against further irritation. The contraindications include hypersensitivity to any components of this medication.

$R = H$ or CH_2CO_2H

Hydroxypropyl Methylcellulose

Hypromellose solutions were patented as a semisynthetic substitute for tear-film. Its molecular structure is predicated upon a base celluloid compound that is highly water-soluble. Postapplication, celluloid attributes of good water solubility reportedly aids in visual clarity. When applied, a hypromellose solution acts to swell and absorb water, thereby expanding the thickness of the tear-film. Hypromellose augmentation therefore results in extended lubricant time presence on the cornea, which theoretically results in decreased eye irritation, especially in dry climates, home, or work environments. On a molecular level, this polymer contains beta-linked D-glucose units that remain metabolically intact for days to weeks.[3]

$R = H$ or CH_3 or $CH_2CH(OH)CH_3$

The ophthalmic solution is available as 0.3, 0.7 and 2 percent solutions. In another preparation combined with Dextran 70

(1 mg), the polymers mimic the action of conjunctival mucin, helping mucin-deficient states and increasing the ocular retention time in aqueous-deficient states through the adsorption action of the polymers attaching to the ocular surface. The adsorption effect is independent of the viscosity thus ensuring a prolonged wetting action with a low viscosity. It increases precorneal tear-film stability evidenced by tear-film break-up studies. Eye discomfort/irritation/redness, tearing, eye sensitivity to light, sticky eyelashes, or temporary blurred vision may occur after instillation but an allergic reaction to these drops is rare.

Polyvinyl Alcohol

Polyvinyl alcohol (PVOH, PVA, or PVAl) is a water-soluble synthetic polymer. Used in eye drops and hard contact lens solution as a lubricant. Polyvinyl alcohol, a nonionic surfactant, is used as a stabilizing agent, lubricant and as an agent to increase viscosity in pharmaceutical manufacturing. In eye preparations, polyvinyl alcohol is used to increase the viscosity and thereby prolonging contact time of the active ingredient with the eye. It is often found in artificial tears preparations for dry eye and in contact lens solutions. It is used as a 0.5–3 percent solution with or without povidone-iodine. The common preparations are 14 mg or 30 mg per mL, amounts to 1.4 percent and 3 percent of the solution. There might be side effects like mild stinging/burning/irritation in the eye; temporary blurred vision.

Polyethylene Glycol

PEG refers to an oligomer or polymer of ethylene oxide. It is used in Lubricating eye drops. One of the most popular combination includes Polyethylene Glycol 400 0.4 percent and Propylene Glycol 0.3 percent. In a study conducted comparing PEG and HP Guar, the biphasic mechanism of action of *in situ* PEG/PG gellable lubricant eye drops, afforded by their unique structure, renders them more effective at reducing the signs and symptoms of dry eye.[4]

Propylene Glycol

Propylene glycol is an organic compound with formula $C_3H_8O_2$ or $HO\text{-}CH_2\text{-}CHOH\text{-}CH_3$. It is a colorless, nearly odorless, clear, viscous liquid. It is commonly used in combination with Polyethylene Glycol as Lubricating Eye drops in the concentration of 0.3 percent. Other concentrations include 0.55 percent, 0.6 percent, 0.95 percent and 1.0 percent.

HP-Guar

HP-guar is believed to form a bioadhesive gel when exposed to ocular pH, increasing aqueous retention and protecting the ocular surface by mimicking the mucous layer of the tear film.[4,5]

Hyaluronic Acid

Hyaluronic acid is a naturally occurring viscoelastic substance[6] that may also have anti-inflammatory activity.[7] High-viscosity agents tend to cause visual blurring; therefore, lower-viscosity agents are generally preferred for mild to moderate Dry Eye Disease. A study compared the efficacy and safety of a 0.1 percent solution of hyaluronan with 0.9 percent saline, when administered topically to the eye, in the treatment of symptoms of severe dry eye syndrome and found significant improvements in Schirmer's and rose Bengal staining score.[8]

Ophthalmic gels and ointments have higher viscosity than liquids; they are also associated with more visual blurring than liquids and, therefore, are usually prescribed for overnight use.[9] Gels containing carbomers cause less blurring than petrolatum-based ointments, because carbomer viscosity decreases rapidly on exposure to tear salts.[10]

Preservative Concerns

Preservatives are added to artificial tears to reduce the risk of bacterial contamination in multidose containers, and to prolong shelf life and are of 2 main types: detergent and oxidative.

Detergent preservatives act by altering bacterial cell membrane permeability. Detergents have toxic effects on the ocular surface epithelium and, with frequent use, can cause epithelial irritation and damage. Patients with a compromised tear film are at higher risk. Benzalkonium chloride, the most widely used preservative in topical ophthalmic preparations, is an example of a detergent preservative. Oxidative preservatives penetrate the bacterial cell membrane and act by interfering with intracellular processes. They are sometimes referred to as "vanishing" preservatives because they dissipate on contact with the eye and, therefore, are less likely than detergents to cause ocular damage. Stabilized oxychloro complex is an example of an oxidative preservative.

Preserved tears are usually well tolerated in mild DED, when used no more than 4 to 6 times daily.[1] Unpreserved tear substitutes need to be considered if the management is expected to be long-term.[9]

The corneal epithelium is exposed to hyperosmolar tears and is subject to osmotic stress in dry eye disease and tend to lose water. They compensate by increasing their internal electrolyte concentration to stabilize their volume. However, elevated electrolyte concentrations can eventually lead to cellular damage.[2] Compatible solutes are small nonionic molecules (e.g. glycerin 0.9% or 1%) that can be taken up by cells, increasing intracellular osmolarity without disrupting cellular metabolism.

Autologous Serum Tears

Autologous serum eye drops have been recommended for the treatment of several ocular surface disturbances, such as Sjögren's syndrome-related tear deficiency, non-Sjögren's tear deficiency associated with graft-versus-host disease, neurotrophic keratitis, persistent epithelial defects, superior limbic keratoconjunctivitis. Human serum contains substances such as epidermal growth factor, vitamin A, transforming growth factor-β, fibronectin, and cytokines normally found in tears.[12] These factors are important for maintaining a healthy corneal and conjunctival epithelium. Fox et al[13] initially described the benefits of autologous serum application in dry eyes in patients with Sjögren's syndrome followed by Tsubota et al.[14] who evaluated the efficacy of autologous serum drops diluted with saline in the treatment of 12 patients with Sjögren's syndrome. They are unpreserved but can be stored frozen for 3 to 6 months[15,16] and the frequency to prepare it from the patient's blood is about 2 to 4 times a year. Their constitution is similar to the tear film as described in the Table 52.1. The serum can be prepared in the following dilutions of 20 percent, 33 percent, 50 percent, or 100 percent and the diluents include 0.9 percent NaCl, BSS, 0.5 percent chloramphenicol eye drops.

The drawbacks associated with the autologous serum is its ability to transmit infections.[17] It requires frequent blood extractions, mainly in the groups requiring prolonged treatment. Autologous serum contains no preservatives, which avoids the risk of preservative toxicity, however, microbial contamination of the dropper bottle can occur.[18] Leite et al.[19] analyzed 11 autologous serum samples after 30 days of use by the patients, in which 6 of them were contaminated by single or multiple microorganisms such as: *Klebsiella pneumoniae* (4/6), *Streptococcus viridans* (3/6), *Micrococcus* sp (1/6), *Pseudomonas aeruginosa* (1/6), *Candida* sp (1/6), *Bacillus sp* (1/6) and *Staphylococcus aureus* (1/6), Autologous serum treatment is usually well tolerated and most patients report improvement of discomfort sensation. Although

TABLE 52.1: Comparison of the biochemical properties of normal human tears and serum[2,5]

	Tears	Serum
pH	7.4	7.4
Osmolarity	298	296
EGF (ng/ml)	0.2-3.0	0.5
TGF-β (ng/ml)	2-10	6-33
Vitamin A (mg/ml)	0.02	46
Lysozyme (mg/ml)	1.4	6
IgA (µg/ml)	1190	2
Fibronectin (µg/ml)	21	205

EGF = Epithelial growth factor; TGF = Transforming growth factor

uncommon, some patients may experience increased discomfort, slight epitheliopathy, bacterial conjunctivitis or eyelid eczema.[20]

Secretagogues

Cholinergic agents (i.e. muscarinic acetylcholine receptor agonists) are given orally to treat aqueous-deficient Dry eye disease. Two agents, pilocarpine and cevimeline, have been used for treatment of dry eye associated with Sjögren syndrome.[21] Pilocarpine significantly improved global assessment of dry eye disease symptoms at doses of 5.0 to 7.5 mg QID.[22-24] Pilocarpine also significantly decreased the use of artificial tears and improved salivary flow (measured by 5-minute saliva sample collection).[22] The most common drug-related Adverse Event was sweating.[22-24] Other adverse events include urinary frequency, flushing, headache, nausea, rhinitis, dizziness and hypersalivation.[24]

Both cevimeline doses of 20 or 30 mg improved subjective symptoms, tear dynamics, ocular surface condition, and global assessment; however, statistical significance was not reached for all parameters at all time points in the initial trials. The 20 mg dose demonstrated the most consistent improvements at 4 weeks. The most common AEs were gastrointestinal symptoms (including nausea and diarrhea) and increased sweating which were mild to moderate.[25]

Anti-inflammatory Agents

Several randomized trials have demonstrated that short-term topical corticosteroid use (as long as 4 weeks) improves signs and symptoms of Dry eye disease.[1] Although topical corticosteroids are effective, they are generally recommended only for short-term use because prolonged use may result in ocular complications that include ocular infection, glaucoma, and cataract.

Oral tetracyclines have been used primarily in Dry Eye Disease associated with ocular rosacea. Tetracyclines are used in DED primarily for their anti-inflammatory rather than antibacterial actions. Mechanisms may include decreased matrix metalloproteinase activity, and decreased production of proinflammatory cytokines such as interleukin (IL)-1 and tumor necrosis factor-alpha.[1]

Cyclosporine ophthalmic emulsion 0.05 percent is indicated to increase tear production in patients whose tear production is presumed to be suppressed due to ocular inflammation associated with keratoconjunctivitis sicca. Evidence suggests that cyclosporine is disease modifying rather than merely palliative. In studies of Dry Eye Disease patients, cyclosporine reduced conjunctival IL-6 levels,[26] decreased activated lymphocytes in the conjunctiva,[27] reduced conjunctival inflammatory and apoptotic markers[28,29] and increased conjunctival goblet cell numbers.[30]

Nutritional Supplements

Essential fatty acids (EFAs) may, theoretically, benefit DED in 2 ways: by reducing inflammation and by altering the composition of meibomian lipids. Omega-3 and omega-6 EFAs are the precursors of eicosanoids, locally acting hormones involved in mediating inflammatory processes. It is largely via the production of these eicosanoids that the essential fatty acids influence human health and disease. In general, the omega-3 derived eicosanoids are anti-inflammatory while the n-6 pathway eicosanoids promote inflammation.[31] Omega-3 EFA's include alpha linoleic acid (ALA), eicosapentaenoic acid (EPA), and docosahexaenoic acid (DHA). Typical omega-3 fish oil preparations contain 300 mg of EPA and DHA per 1000 mg capsule.[32] Comparative data regarding the benefit of EFAs is limited in literature.

Mucolytics

Topical acetylcysteine was mentioned in the literature as a Dry Eye Disease treatment as early as the 1960s,[33] and is still sometimes used in Dry Eye Disease patients with dense mucus accumulation,[34] for example, in filamentary keratitis.[35]

Topical Vitamin A (Retinol)

Vitamin A deficiency is a known cause of xerophthalmia; however, most patients are not vitamin A deficient. Based on the hypothesis of local retinol deficiency at the ocular surface, topical retinol has been used to treat various forms of DED, with variable results.[34] Limited data suggest a possible role in reversing squamous metaplasia and keratinization of the ocular surface in severe DED, for example, in cicatrizing conjunctivitis or graft-versus-host disease.[36-38] However, the use of topical retinol in Dry Eye Disease remains controversial.[34]

Eyelid Integrity

Meibomian gland disease if any, must be treated first before addressing the aqueous component. Washing the eyelid margin with a gentle soap decreases bacterial colonization. Bacterial colonization is believed to inhibit conjunctival goblet cell proliferation[39] and may also increase the breakdown of meibomian lipid, thereby improving both the mucous and lipid layers of the tear film.[1] Warm compresses may reduce evaporative loss by temporarily thickening the lipid layer. Manual expression of the meibomian glands has been shown to increase lipid layer thickness and tear film stability in normal subjects.[40] The use of Blephagel which is a colorless, aqueous gel comprising carbomer, poloxamer 188, macrogol 4000, sodium hydroxy methyl glycinate, sodium hydroxyde 1 N, and purified water applied twice a day for 3 weeks has been published. It has shown to be well tolerated and accepted by the patients.[41]

A daily regimen of eyelid scrubbing and warm compresses, plus meibomian gland expression performed as an office procedure every 6 weeks, resulted in less-solidified meibomian secretions and significantly increased lipid layer thickness in patients with meibomian gland dysfunction (MGD) with improvement of dry eye symptoms.[42]

Systemic Disease

New and possible biologic agents in the treatment of Sjögren's Disease include:[43]

B-cell-targeted therapies
- Rituximab (anti-CD20)
- Ocrelizumab (humanized anti-CD20)
- Epratuzumab (anti-CD22)
- Belimumab (anti-BAFF)

T-cell-targeted therapies
- Efalizumab (anti-CD11a)
- Alefacept (anti-CD2)
- Abatacept (anti-CD80/86)

Cytokine-targeted therapies
- Infliximab (anti-TNF)
- Etanercept (anti-TNF)
- Tocilizumab (anti-IL6r)
- Anti-IL10
- Anti-IL17
- Anti-IFN

Complement-targeted therapies
- Eculizumab (anti-C5a/C5b-9)

ONGOING CLINICAL TRIALS

Thymosin Beta 4 (Tβ4)[44]

Thymosin Beta 4 (Tβ4) is a synthetic copy of the naturally-occurring 43-amino acid peptide that is found in a variety of tissues. Tβ4 promotes wound repair and regeneration in various tissues. In the eye, it promotes corneal epithelial cell migration, decreases inflammation and has antiapoptotic activities. It up-regulates the gene expression of laminin-5, a major subepithelial adhesion protein, located in the basement membrane region of the cornea, conjunctiva, and important in wound healing. In compassionate-use cases, Tβ4 has demonstrated efficacy in repairing non-healing neurotrophic corneal ulcers and other corneal epithelial wounds. In twenty-four nonclinical toxicology and safety pharmacology studies, the safety of Tβ4 has been demonstrated for its current and planned uses in man.

Hydroxypropyl Guar Galactomannan[45]

The efficacy of 0.25 percent (HPGG) Ophthalmic Gel compared to Vehicle for the treatment of dry eye is being studied. Primary Outcome Measures includes Mean change from baseline in sodium fluorescein corneal staining score and the Secondary Outcome measures Mean change from baseline in Dry Eye Symptom Questionnaire score.

Lotemax[50]

Lotemax, an ophthalmic corticosteroid, targets inflammation with a unique, site-active mechanism of action. Structural modifications associated with an ester ophthalmic steroid make Lotemax highly lipid soluble, enhancing penetration into cells and enabling Lotemax to exert anti-inflammatory activity within the eye. Lotemax is indicated for the treatment of steroid responsive inflammatory conditions associated with the palpebral and bulbar conjunctiva, cornea, and anterior segment of the globe. It is hypothesized that the anti-inflammatory activity of Lotemax may help mitigate the stinging with cyclosporine administration and the dry eye signs and symptoms experienced during the initiation of therapy. Restasis is indicated to increase tear production in patients whose tear production is presumed to be suppressed due to ocular inflammation associated with a condition called keratoconjunctivitis sicca. The relief of dry eye signs and symptoms with Restasis therapy is often delayed by 1-6 months from the initiation of therapy. Stinging on installation, particularly when initiating therapy, has been reported.

Dexamethasone Phosphate (Ocular Iontophoresis)[54]

Safety and efficacy of EGP-437 at two different dose levels: Ocular Iontophoresis with EGP-437 4.0 mA-min at 1.5 mA and Ocular Iontophoresis with EGP-437 6.5 mA-min at 2.5 mA compared to

Ocular Iontophoresis with placebo (sodium citrate buffer solution) for the treatment of the signs and symptoms of dry eye is also being evaluated.

Other durgs that are being tested for use in dry eye syndrome include Rimexolone (FID 109980),[46] RX-10045,[47] T-cell inhibhitors like SAR 1118,[48] Rebamipide 2 percent solution,[49] 2 percent diquafosol tetrasodium ophthalmic solution / INS365 Ophthalmic Solution.[51,52] Intravenous administration of AIN457 (10 mg/kg) or ACZ885 (10 mg/kg),[53] KLS-0611,[55] KCT-0809,[56] KCT-0809,[57] 3 percent or 5 percent DA-6034 eye drops.[58]

Guidelines for Treatment Selection

International Task Force (ITF) guidelines, published in 2006, propose a classification of DED severity based on clinical signs and symptoms. The ITF also developed treatment algorithms according to severity classification and the presence or absence of lid margin disease.

TABLE 52.2: DEWS dry eye severity grading scheme[2]				
Dry eye severity Level	1	2	3	4*
Discomfort severity and frequency	Mild and/or episodic; occurs under environmental stress	Moderate episodic or chronic, stress or no stress	Severe frequent or constant without stress	Severe and/or disabling and constant
Visual symptoms	None or episodic mild fatigue	Annoying and/or activity-limiting episodic	Annoying, chronic and/or constant, limiting activity	Constant and/or possibly disabling
Conjunctival injection	None to mild	None to mild	+/−	+/++
Conjunctival staining	None to mild	Variable	Moderate to marked	Marked
Corneal staining (severity/location)	None to mild	Variable	Marked central	Severe puncture erosions
Corneal/tear signs	None to mild	Mild debris, ↓meniscus	Filamentary keratitis, mucus clumping, ↑ tear debris	Filamentary keratitis, mucus clumping, ↑ tear debris, ulceration
Lid/meibomian glands	MGD variably present	MGD variably present	Frequent	Trichiasis, keratinization, symblepharon
TBUT (sec)	Variable	≤ 10	≤ 5	Immediate
Schirmer score (mm/5 min)	Variable	≤ 10	≤ 5	≤ 2

*Must have signs and symptoms.
DEWS; Dry Eye WorkShop; TBUT, tear breakup time; MGD, meibomian gland dysfunction. Modified from International Task force guidance for the classification of dry eye disease.[32]

Level 1:
Education and counseling
Environmental management
Elimination of offending systemic medications
Preserved tear substitutes, allergy eye drops
Level 2:
If level 1 treatments are inadequate, add:
Unpreserved tears, gels, ointments
Steroids
Cyclosporine A
Secretagogues
Nutritional supplements
Level 3:
If Level 2 treatments are inadequate, add:
Tetracyclines
Autologous serum tears
Punctal plugs (after control of inflammation)
Level 4:
If Level 3 treatments are inadequate, add:
Topical vitamin A
Contact lenses
Acetylcysteine
Moisture goggles
Surgery

Modified from International Task Force dysfunctional tear syndrome treatment algorithm.[32]

In 2007 the Management and Therapy Subcommittee of the International Dry Eye WorkShop (DEWS) adopted a modified form of the ITF severity grading, as shown in Table above. The DEWS treatment recommendations were based on the modified severity grading.

REFERENCES

1. Management and therapy of dry eye disease: report of the Management and Therapy Subcommittee of the International Dry Eye WorkShop. Ocul Surf 2007;5:163-78.
2. McDonald M. Latest trends in dry eye treatments (advertorial). Cornea Society News. Spring 2007;3:7-8.
3. Koroloff N, Boots R, Lipman J, Thomas P, Rickard C, Coyer F. "A randomised controlled study of the efficacy of hypromellose and Lacri-Lube combination versus polyethylene/Cling wrap to prevent corneal epithelial breakdown in the semiconscious intensive care patient". Intensive Care Med 2004;30(6):1122-6.
4. Drugs Today (Barc). Clinical evaluation of the efficacy of PEG/PG lubricant eye drops with gelling agent (HP-Guar) for the relief of the signs and symptoms of dry eye disease: a review. Foulks GN 2007;43(12):887-96.
5. Gifford P, Evans BJ, Morris J. A clinical evaluation of Systane. Cont Lens Anterior Eye 2006;29:31-40.

6. Prabhasawat P, Tesavibul N, Kasetsuwan N. Performance profile of sodium hyaluronate in patients with lipid tear deficiency: randomised, double-blind, controlled, exploratory study. Br J Ophthalmol 2007;91:47-50.
7. Moon JW, Lee HJ, Shin KC,Wee WR, Lee JH, Kim MK. Short term effects of topical cyclosporine and viscoelastic on the ocular surfaces in patients with dry eye. Korean J Ophthalmol 2007;21:189-94.
8. Double blind, randomised, placebo controlled, crossover, multicentre study to determine the efficacy of a 0.1 percent (w/v) sodium hyaluronate solution (Fermavisc) in the treatment of dry eye syndrome. Patrick I Condon, Charles G McEwen, Mark Wright, Graeme Mackintosh, Robin J Prescott, Carolyn McDonald. Br J Ophthalmol 1999;83:1121-4.
9. Asbell PA. Increasing importance of dry eye syndrome and the ideal artificial tear: consensus views from a roundtable discussion. Curr Med Res Opin 2006;22:2149-57.
10. Vehige JG, Simmons PA. Ocular lubrication vs. viscosity of ophthalmic products. Contact Lens Spectrum; December 2004.
11. Harvey B. Five days in Denver (conference report). Optician 2007 Jan 12;233:15-6.
12. Koffler BH. Autologous serum therapy of the ocular surface with novel delivery by platelet concentrate gel. Ocul Surf 2006;4(4): 188-95.
13. Fox RI, Chan R, Michelson JB, Belmont JB, Michelson PE. Beneficial effect of artificial tears made with autologous serum in patients with keratoconjunctivitis sicca. Arthritis Rheum 1984;27(4):459-61.
14. Tsubota K, Goto E, Fujita H, Ono M, Inoue H, Saito I, Shimmura S. Treatment of dry eye by autologous serum application in Sjögren's syndrome. Br J Ophthalmol 1999;83(4):390-5.
15. Geerling G, MacLennan S, Hartwig D. Autologous serum eye drops for ocular surface disorders. Br J Ophthalmol 2004;88:1467-74.
16. Noble BA, Loh RS, MacLennan S, et al. Comparison of autologous serum eye drops with conventional therapy in a randomised controlled crossover trial for ocular surface disease. Br J Ophthalmol 2004;88:647-52.
17. Geerling G, Maclennan S, Hartwig D. Autologous serum eye drops for ocular surface disorders. Br J Ophthalmology 2004;88(11):1467-74.
18. Lee GA, Chen SX. Autologous serum in the management of recalcitrant dry eye syndrome. Clin Experiment Ophthalmol 2008;36(2):119-22.
19. Leite SC, de Castro RS, Alves M, Cunha DA, Correa ME, da Silveira LA, et al. Risk factors and characteristics of ocular complications, and efficacy of autologous serum tears after haematopoietic progenitor cell transplantation. Bone Marrow Transplant 2006;38(3):223-7.
20. López-García JS, García-Lozano I, Rivas L, Martínez-Garchitorena J. Use of autologous serum in ophthalmic practice. Arch Soc Esp Oftalmol 2007;82(1):9-20.
21. Management of Dry Eyes. Michael Lemp. Am J Manag Care 2008;14:S88-S101.
22. Nelson JD, Friedlaender M,Yeatts RP, et al; and MGI Pharma. Sjögren's Syndrome Study Group. Oral pilocarpine for

symptomatic relief of keratoconjunctivitis sicca in patients with Sjögren's syndrome. Adv Exp Med Biol 1998;438:979-83.
23. Papas AS, Fernandez MM, Castano RA, Gallagher SC, Trivedi M, Shrotriya RC. Oral pilocarpine for symptomatic relief of dry mouth and dry eyes in patients with Sjögren's syndrome. Adv Exp Med Biol 1998;438:973-8.
24. Vivino FB, Al-Hashimi I, Khan Z, et al, for the P92-01 Study Group. Pilocarpine tablets for the treatment of dry mouth and dry eye symptoms in patients with Sjögren syndrome: a randomized, placebo-controlled, fixed-dose, multicenter trial. Arch Intern Med 1999;159:174-81.
25. Ono M, Takamura E, Shinozaki K, et al. Therapeutic effect of cevimeline on dry eye in patients with Sjögren's syndrome: a randomized, double-blind clinical study. Am J Ophthalmol 2004;138:6-17.
26. Turner K, Pflugfelder SC, Ji Z, Fener WJ, Stern M, Reis BL. Interleukin-6 levels in the conjunctival epithelium of patients with dry eye disease treated with cyclosporine ophthalmic emulsion. Cornea 2000;19:492-6.
27. Kunert KS, Tisdale AS, Stern ME, Smith JA, Gipson IK. Analysis of topical cyclosporine treatment of patients with dry eye syndrome: effect on conjunctival lymphocytes. Arch Ophthalmol 2000;118:1489-96.
28. Brignole F, Pisella PJ, De Saint Jean M, Goldschild M, Goguel A, Baudouin C. Flow cytometric analysis of inflammatory markers in KCS: 6-month treatment with topical cyclosporine A. Invest Ophthalmol Vis Sci 2001;42:90-95.
29. Baudouin C, Brignole F, Pisella PJ, De Saint Jean MS, Goguel A. Flow cytometric analysis of the inflammatory marker HLA DR in dry eye syndrome: results from 12 months of randomized treatment with topical cyclosporine A. Adv Exp Med Biol 2002;506(Pt B):761-9.
30. Kunert KS, Tisdale AS, Gipson IK. Goblet cell numbers and epithelial proliferation in the conjunctiva of patients with dry eye syndrome treated with cyclosporine. Arch Ophthalmol. 2002;120:330-337. Erratum in: Arch Ophthalmol 2002;120:1099.
31. Essential fatty acids in the treatment of dry eye. Rosenberg ES, Asbell PA. Ocular Surface 2010;8(1):18-28.
32. Nutritional supplements for dry eye syndrome. Rand AL, Asbell PA. Curr Opin Ophthalmol 2011;22(4):279-82.
33. Absolon MJ, Brown CA. Acetylcysteine in keratoconjunctivitis sicca. Br J Ophthalmol 1968;52:310-16.
34. Calonge M. The treatment of dry eye. Surv Ophthalmol 2001;45:S227-S239.
35. Albietz J, Sanfilippo P, Troutbeck R, Lenton LM. Management of filamentary keratitis associated with aqueous- deficient dry eye. Optom Vis Sci 2003;80:420-30.
36. Murphy PT, Sivakumaran M, Fahy G, Hutchinson RM. Successful use of topical retinoic acid in severe dry eye due to chronic graft-versus-host disease. Bone Marrow Transplant 1996;18:641-2.
37. Tseng SC, Maumenee AE, Stark WJ, et al. Topical retinoid treatment for various dry-eye disorders. Ophthalmology 1985;92:717-27.
38. Herbort CP, Zografos L, Zwingli M, Schoeneich M. Topical retinoic acid in dysplastic and metaplastic keratinization of corneoconjunctival epithelium. Graefes Arch Clin Exp Ophthalmol 1988;226:22-6.

39. Gilbard JP. The diagnosis and management of dry eyes. Otolaryngol Clin North Am 2005;38:871-85.
40. Craig JP, Blades K, Patel S. Tear lipid layer structure and stability following expression of the meibomian glands. Ophthalmic Physiol Opt 1995;15:569-74.
41. Tolerability and acceptability of Blephagel: a novel eyelid hygiene aqueous gel. Serge Doan. Clinical Ophthalmology 2012;6:71-7.
42. Korb DR, Greiner JV. Increase in tear film lipid layer thickness following treatment of meibomian gland dysfunction. Adv Exp Med Biol 1994;350:293-8.
43. Review. Emerging biological therapies in primary Sjögren's syndrome. M. Ramos-Casals and P. Brito-Zero´n. Rheumatology 2007;46:1389-96.
44. Safety and Efficacy of Thymosin Beta 4 Ophthalmic Solution in Patients With Dry Eye. NCT01387347.
45. A Study of Hydroxypropyl Guar Galactomannan 0.25 percent (HPGG) Versus Vehicle in Dry Eye Patients. NCT00840268.
46. Phase II Study of AL-2178 (FID 109980) in the Treatment of Dry Eye. NCT00471419.
47. Safety and Efficacy Study of RX-10045 on the Signs and Symptoms of Dry Eye. NCT00799552.
48. Safety and Efficacy Study of SAR 1118 to Treat Dry Eye (OPUS-1). NCT01421498.
49. Safety and Efficacy Study of Rebamipide 2 percent Ophthalmic Suspension in Subjects With Dry Eye - Effects on Central Cornea. NCT01057147.
50. Multicenter, Randomized, Controlled Study of the Effect of Lotemax on Initiation of Dry Eye Treatment With Restasis. NCT00407043.
51. Study of Diquafosol Tetrasodium Ophthalmic Solution in Subjects with Dry Eye Disease. NCT00403975.
52. Study of INS365 Ophthalmic Solution in Subjects with Dry Eye Disease. NCT00404131.
53. The Effects of a Single Intravenous Administration of AIN457 or ACZ885 in Dry Eye Patients. NCT01250171.
54. Safety and Efficacy Study of EGP-437 (Dexamethasone Phosphate Formulated for Ocular Iontophoresis) to Treat Dry Eye. NCT01129856.
55. Phase 2 Study of KLS-0611 in Patients With Dry Eye Syndromes. NCT00721656.
56. A Phase II Study of KCT-0809 in Patients With Dry Eye Syndrome. NCT01427816.
57. A Study of KCT-0809 in Patients With Dry Eye Syndromes. NCT01211951.
58. Phase II Study of DA-6034 Eye Drops in Dry Eye Syndrome (DES). NCT01670357.

53
Management of Endophthalmitis: Antibiotic Schedule and Dosages

Pei-Chang Wu, Hsi-Kung Kuo (Taiwan)

Endophthalmitis is defined by marked inflammation of intraocular fluids and tissues. When caused by microorganisms, endophthalmitis often results in severe visual loss. The broad categories of endophthalmitis include postoperative (acute-onset, chronic or delayed onset, bleb-associated), post-traumatic, endogenous and miscellaneous, such as intravitreous triamcinolone associated endophthalmitis, microbial keratitis and suture removal (Table 53.1). These categories are important in predicting the causative organism and guiding therapeutic decisions before microbiological confirmation.

ACUTE POSTOPERATIVE ENDOPHTHALMITIS

Acute postoperative endophthalmitis is defined as the occurrence of intraocular infection within six weeks after surgery by the Endophthalmitis Vitrectomy Study (EVS).

Prophylaxis

In recent evidence-based literature, Cillua et al found preoperative irrigation with povidone-iodine (PI) to be a most strongly recommended technique based on the current clinical evidence

---

TABLE 53.1: Classification of endophthalmitis and most frequent organisms

- Postoperative
  - *Acute-onset*: Coagulase (-) staphylococci *(Staphylococcus epidermidis)*, *Staphylococcus aureus, Enterococcus* species, *Streptococcus* species, gram-negative bacteria (Pseudomonas)
  - *Chronic*: P. acnes, coagulase (-) staphylococci, fungi
  - *Bleb-associated*: *Streptococcus* species, Hemophilus influenza, *Staphylococcus* species
- *Post-traumatic*: *Bacillus* species, Staphylococci
- *Endogenous*: *Candida* species, gram-negative bacteria *(Klebsiella pneumoniae)*, S. aureus
- Miscellaneous
  - *Corneal ulcer perforation*: *Pseudomonas, Staphylococcus* species
  - Intravitreous triamcinolone associated
  - Suture removal associated

(Table 53.2).[1] PI is a potent antiseptic with a wide-spectrum of activity against both gram-positive and gram-negative bacteria, fungi and viruses. Antimicrobial activity contributes to the 1 percent free iodine released that occurs after contact with the skin for 30 seconds to 1 minute, and this effect will last for 1 hour.[2,3] Iodine penetrates the cell wall and reacts with aminoacids and nucleotides, which ultimately disrupt the cell's protein synthesis. Despite the wide use of PI solutions as disinfectants in hospitals, these solution have been reported to be susceptible to contamination with *Pseudomonas cepacia*, which could be passed on to the patient.[4]

Preoperative preparation with 5 percent PI solution dropped into the conjunctival sac followed by a skin preparation of 10 percent PI solution has been recommended.[5] Our retrospective, case-controlled study found that patients who received 10 percent PI skin disinfection combined with 5 percent PI conjunctival disinfection had significantly less risk of developing post-cataract surgery endophthalmitis. However, a modified preparation method of 5 percent PI on both the skin and conjunctiva has been used in many institutes and for simple ocular surgery, such as intravitreous injection.[6,7] Caution should be taken to avoid touching the lid margin and lashes when the needle is inserted into the eye.

Grade 'A' is considered very important or crucial to clinical outcome, grade 'B' as moderately important, and grade 'C' is of questionable use.

Intraocular Antibiotics

Intravitreal antibiotic therapy could reach far greater intraocular antibiotic concentration than any other method of administration. It is the main stay of treatment for infective endophthalmitis. In instances of instant and prompt treatment required in order to save the vision, inaccuracies of gram-staining results and unavailable culture results, broad-spectrum intravitreal antibiotics covering almost all the gram-positive and gram-negative bacteria

TABLE 53.2: Prophylactic methods to prevent bacterial endophthalmitis after cataract surgery[1]

Prophylactic intervention	Clinical recommended
Postoperative subconjunctival antibiotics	C
Preoperative lash trimming	C
Preoperative saline irrigation	C
Preoperative povidone-iodine antisepsis	B
Preoperative topical antibiotic therapy	C
Irrigating solutions containing antibiotics	C
Intraoperative heparin	C

are necessary. A few selected drugs are currently recommended, including vancomycin, ceftazidime and amikacin. In the EVS, the antimicrobial sensitivity profile of amikacin and ceftazidime was similar at 89 percent against gram-negative organism, and all gram-positive cocci were sensitive to vancomycin.[8]

Vancomycin

Vancomycin is the drug of choice for gram-positive bacteria in acute postoperative endophthalmitis. It is a bactericidal drug whose primary mode of action is inhibiting synthesis and assembly of the bacterial cell wall. It has a strong antimicrobial effect against gram-positive bacteria, especially *Staphylococcus aureus, Staphylococcus* epidermidis and *Enterococcus*, including methicillin-resistant *Staphylococcus aureus*. In intraocular use, concentrations of up to 2 mg/0.1 ml have been demonstrated to be nontoxic to the retina.[9] The EVS recommended a dose of 1.0 mg/0.1 ml.[10] The half-life of the drug is reduced in inflamed eyes and prolonged in normal vitreous.[11] Even in inflamed eyes, therapeutic levels are still detected up to 72-84 hours after injection. Vancomycin is also cleared more rapidly in aphakic, vitrectomized eyes.[9, 11]

Ceftazidime

Ceftazidime is a third-generation cephalosporin that has a bactericidal effect by disrupting cell wall synthesis. Third-generation cephalosporins have strong antibacterial effects against gram-negative bacilli. They also have an added effect against *Streptococcus pneumonia, pyogenes* and other streptococci. Cephalosporins have little effect against *Staphylococcus aureus* but a strong effect against *Pseudomonas aeruginosa*. In contrast to the aminoglycosides, ceftazidime carries a lower risk of retinal toxicity and a broader therapeutic index. However, intravitreous ceftazidime was not evaluated in the EVS and it has been shown that *in vitro* ceftazidime precipitates in vitreous humor at body temperature, irrespective of the presence of vancomycin.[12] In clinical studies, ceftazidime has been demonstrated to precipitate in inflamed eyes resulting in possible subtherapeutic concentration. Reconstitution with normal saline as opposed to balanced salt solution produced less precipitation. Intravitreous ceftazidime is typically injected at a concentration of 2.25 mg/0.1 ml.[13] Like vancomycin, half-life is decreased in aphakic, vitrectomized and inflamed eyes.

Aminoglycosides

Aminoglycosides have a bactericidal effect through ionic interaction with the cell surface, energy dependent uptake phases and binding to ribosomes. Amikacin has a strong bactericidal effect against aerobic and facultative gram-negative bacilli. It has a synergistic effect with vancomycin and other cell wall active antimicrobials (penicillins and cephalosporins). Aminoglycosides such as amikacin and gentamicin have been used for intravitreous injection. Gentamicin has been reported to cause macular toxicity.[14] Aminoglycoside-induced macular infarction is thought to result from an increased concentration by the gravity-induced accumulation of drugs on the macula in a supine patient. Although animal experiments[15] have shown that amikacin is safer than gentamicin, a potential for macular toxicity might still exist. Amikacin has been shown to cause macular infarction with loss of macular capillaries and preretinal hemorrhage.[16-18]

The standard intravitreous dose of amikacin is 0.4 mg/0.1 ml. This is the dose used in the EVS. Pharmacokinetic studies in animals were similar to vancomycin pharmacokinetics in the vitreous cavity. However, levels measured 24 hours after injection were equal to or less than the minimal inhibitory concentration (MIC) for most organisms sensitive to amikacin.[19] Lower concentrations in the vitreous may necessitate the need for repeat injections of amikacin if there is no response. No toxicity has been contributed to a single injection but repeated injections should be undertaken with caution due to the possible risk of macular infarction.[18, 19] Nasal side recumbency for about 30 minutes might be suggested after intravitreous injection of amikacin.

Repeated vitreous tapping and injection of antibiotics, together with pars plana vitrectomy, should be consider if there is no clinical improvement or if the condition deteriorates within 48–72 hours.[20]

Systemic Antibiotics

The systemic antibiotics that cross the blood retinal barrier include cefazolin, ceftazidime and ciprofloxacin.[21-23] In the EVS, intravenous ceftazidime and amikacin were evaluated, and it was concluded that these antibiotics did not alter final visual acuity or media clarity.[10] However, subsequent to the publication, this conclusion has come under question. First, these two drugs did not cover the most common microorganisms of gram-positive bacteria in postoperative endophthalmitis. Second, intravenous amikacin has little intraocular penetration. The recommendation against intravenous antibiotic use was not warranted and might be based on inadequate data.

Intravenous vancomycin has been suggested as an alternative therapy to systemic ceftazidime and amikacin because of its superior gram-positive coverage. However, vancomycin penetrates poorly into the vitreous yielding an inadequate antibacterial effect.[24,25]

Oral ciprofloxacin might be an effective drug against many common infecting organisms causing endophthalmitis.[26] However, older-generation fluoroquinolones (ciprofloxacin, ofloxacin and levofloxacin) are increasingly ineffective against some of the pathogens most commonly responsible for postoperative endophthalmitis. In contrast, the newer-generation fluoroquinolones (gatifloxacin and moxifloxacin) show promising results; they not only display effective activity against gram-negative bacteria, as do the older-generation fluoroquinolones, but also demonstrate enhanced potencies against gram-positive bacteria.[27] Orally administered gatifloxacin was able to penetrate into the noninflamed human eye, and reach therapeutic levels in the aqueous and vitreous humors.[28] Gatifloxacin has a broad-spectrum of coverage over the bacteria involved in endophthalmitis. It also has a low MIC of 90, good tolerability and excellent bioavailability after oral administration. Oral gatifloxacin has the ability to achieve rapid, effective levels in the aqueous and vitreous, with the notable exceptions of not achieving effective levels against *Enterococcus* or *Pseudomonas*. Gatifloxacin may thus represent a good adjunctive treatment for certain types of endophthalmitis.

Subconjunctival and Topical Antibiotic Therapy

Subconjunctival and topical antibiotics are often used to supplement intravitreal injections in attempt to increase the concentration of antibiotics within the anterior segment of the eye. Subconjunctival administration can reach therapeutic concentrations in the eye, especially in the aqueous humor. However, conflicting data regarding the intravitreal penetration after periocular antibiotic injection have been reported.[29] In addition, subconjunctival injection is more painful and could not be as frequently administered as topical antibiotics. A risk of macular infarction when using gentamicin has also been reported.[14] Of the currently used antibiotics, the third-generation cephalosporins (ceftazidime and ceftriaxone) achieve the highest vitreous levels.

Topical application is associated with very poor vitreous penetration. However, significant intraocular levels of antibiotics can be achieved with frequent administration of highly concentrated solutions,[30] especially if the corneal epithelium has been damaged. For acute-onset postoperative endophthalmitis, topical vancomycin (50 mg/ml) with amikacin (20 mg/ml) or ceftazidime (50 mg/ml) administered hourly is recommended. This regimen can then be adjusted for the specific organism after culture and sensitivity results are available.

Steroid Treatment

The early use of corticosteroids, in addition to antibiotics, reduces inflammation and subsequent retinal damage in endophthalmitis. Corticosteroid therapy may be administered topically, intravitreally or systemically. In the EVS, oral prednisone was used at a dose of 30 mg orally twice a day for 5–10 days.

Intravitreous dexamethasone has been increasingly employed as an alternative to systemic therapy. Dexamethasone sodium phosphate is typically used in an intravitreous concentration of 0.4 mg/0.1 ml. This is equivalent to 40 mg of oral prednisone. Experimental studies have shown that intravitreal dexamethasone has a large safety window and that it prolongs the half-life of intravitreal vancomycin.[31,32] Triamcinolone acetonide (4 mg/0.1 ml) is more potent and equivalent to 50 mg of oral prednisone. Recently, it has been reported that intravitreal triamcinolone combined with intravitreal antibiotics appear to have a safety profile similar to current modalities, with a favorable effect on visual recovery and function in acute postoperative endophthalmitis.[33]

Vitrectomy

Vitrectomy debulks the vitreous cavity, reduces the load of bacteria and toxins, and makes space for intravitreous antibiotics. Only core vitrectomy is recommended, due to fear of causing retinal break as the vitrector is near to the fragile, inflamed retina in a cloudy vitreous. In addition, it is always combined with intravitreous antibiotic injection. The EVS concluded that immediate vitrectomy was not beneficial for patients with an initial visual acuity of hand movement or better.[10] Among patients with initial light-perception-only vision, it was three times more likely that a visual acuity of 20/40 or better would be achieved after vitrectomy. Complications of pars plana vitrectomy include infection, bleeding, cataract, glaucoma and retinal detachment.

In summary, the authors recommend the following for management of acute postoperative endophthalmitis. Noting the patient's unusual symptoms, carefully examining signs associated with infection and a highly alert mind in the physician are important in early intervention, especially for immunocompromised and diabetic patients. It is good to initiate topical antibiotics and cycloplegics immediately during close follow-up when there is suspicion of infection. The current choice of drugs is ciprofloxacin 0.3 percent or ofloxacin 0.3 percent. If infection is strongly suspected, the presenting vision is important in deciding between a vitreous tap and vitrectomy in conjunction with intraocular antibiotic injection. Culture of vitreous fluid from a vitreous tap or vitrectomy is essential for microbiology sensitivity patterns. The flow chart for management of acute endophthalmitis is shown in Flow chart 53.1. For intravitreous antibiotic injection, we prefer intravitreal vancomycin (1 mg) and ceftazidime (2.25 mg) or

TABLE 53.3: Recommended doses of initial management of infective postoperative endophthalmitis

Route	Drug	Dose
Intravitreal	Vancomycin	1 mg in 0.1 ml
	Ceftazidime	2.25 mg in 0.1 ml
	Amikacin	0.4 mg in 0.1 ml
	Dexamethasone	0.4 mg in 0.1 ml
Subconjunctival	Vancomycin	25 mg in 0.5 ml
	Ceftazidime	100 mg in 0.5 ml
Topical	Vancomycin	50 mg/ml drop q1h
	Amikacin	20 mg/ml drops q1h
Systemic	Fluoroquinolones (oral)	
	Gatifloxacin	400 mg bid

Flow chart 53.1: Flow chart for the manage of acute postoperative endophthalmitis

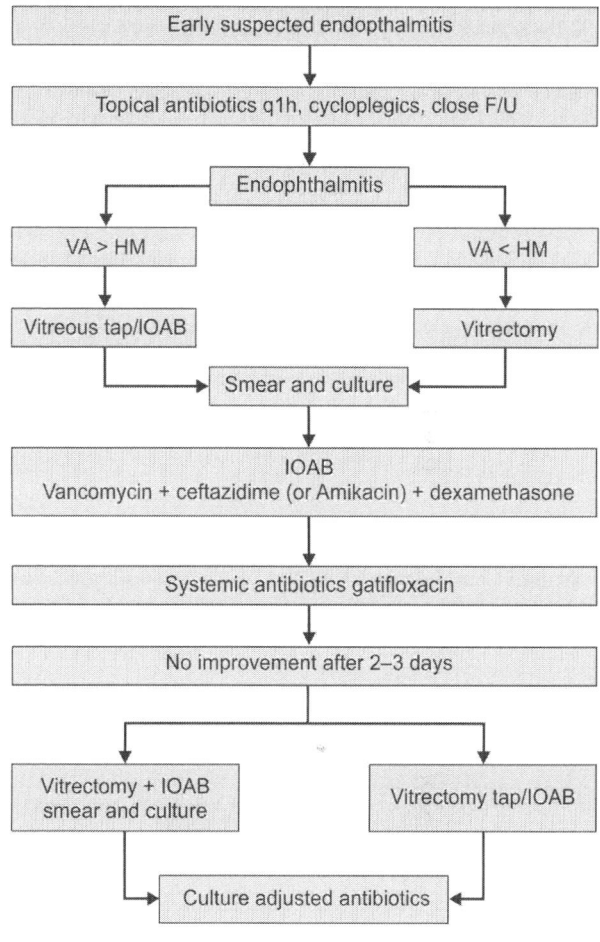

IOAB: intraocular antibiotics

amikacin (0.4 mg) combined with intravitreal dexamethasone (0.4 mg). The rationale and choice of systemic antibiotics is best left to the treating physician. Systemic fluoroquinolone is suggested.

Chronic Postoperative Endophthalmitis

There are two different types of chronic postoperative endophthalmitis, one is caused by *Propionibacterium acnes* and the other is caused by fungus. These microorganisms should be considered especially when the initial culture result is negative. The culture plates should be investigated for at least two weeks. However, the culture rate is very low. Polymerase chain reaction (PCR) detection of bacterial DNA with specific primers from vitreous samples may prove a useful means of diagnosing delayed postoperative endophthalmitis.[34]

There are two important retrospective studies by Aldave et al[35] and Clark et al[36] on *P. acnes* induced postoperative endophthalmitis. The choice for intravitreous antibiotic injection is vancomycin (1 mg in 0.1 ml). However, intravitreous injection of antibiotics alone is associated with a very high rate recurrence. Pars plana vitrectomy, partial capsulectomy and intravitreous antibiotic injection without intraocular lens (IOL) exchange are usually successful on long-term follow-up. For patients with recurrent intraocular inflammation, pars plana vitrectomy, total capsular bag removal, intravitreous antibiotic injection and IOL exchange or removal is a uniformly successful strategy.

Recommended treatment for chronic fungal endophthalmitis is pars plana vitrectomy and intravitreal injection of amphotericin B (5-10 mg in 0.1 ml).[37] Effective systemic amphotericin concentration is still unknown. In cases of yeast endophthalmitis (i.e. *Candida* species), high doses of oral fluconazole (400-600 mg/day) are recommended.[38]

Bleb-associated Endophthalmitis

It is important to distinguish between a localized bleb infection (blebitis) and true bleb-associated endophthalmitis. In cases of blebitis, topical antibiotics and subconjunctival antibiotics, such as vancomycin and ceftazidime, can usually be given in an out-

TABLE 53.4: Antimicrobial agents: dosages for ophthalmic use

Drug	Topical	Subconjunctival (in 0.5 ml)	Intravitreal (in 0.1 ml)	Intravenous dose	Oral dosage
Aminoglycosides					
Gentamicin	14 mg/ml	20 mg	0.1 mg	1.4 mg/kg q8-12 hr	
Tobramycin	14 mg/ml	20 mg	0.1 mg	1.4 mg/kg IV, IV, q8-12 hr	
Amikacin	20 mg/ml	25-50 mg	0.4 mg	7.5 mg/kg q12 hr	
Cephalosporins					
Cefazolin	50 mg/ml	50 mg	2.0 mg	1 g q8h	
Cefotetan			3.0 mg	1 g q12h	
Ceftrixone			2.0 mg	1-2 g q8h	
Ceftazidime	50 mg/ml	100 mg	2.25 mg	1-2 g q8h	
Penicillins					
Oxacillin	50 mg/ml		0.5 mg	2 g q4h	500 mg qid
Miscellaneous					
Clindamycin	20 mg/ml	15-40 mg	1 mg	600 mg q8h	150-450 mg qid
Ciprofloxacin	0.3%		0.1 mg	400 mg q12h	500-75 mg bid 400 mg bid
Gatifloxacin					
Chloramphenicol	5 mg/ml	2 mg		750 mg q6h	250-750 mg qid
Erythromycin	10 mg/ml		0.5 mg	500-1000 mg q6h	250-500 mg qid
Vancomycin	50 mg/ml	25 mg	1-2 mg	1 g q12h	

TABLE 53.5: Antifungal dosages in ophthalmic use

Drug	Topical	Subconjunctival (in 0.5 ml)	Intravitreal (in 0.1 ml)	Usual Intravenous dose	Oral dosage
Polyenes					
Amphotericin B	2.5–10 mg/ml	300 mg	5–10 mg/ml	1 mg/kg/day	
Natamycin	5%				
Nystatin	100,000 U/g ointment				
Imidazoles					
Fluconazole	2%				400 mg/day
Clotrimazole	1%	5–10 mg			60–150 mg/kg/day
Econazole	1%			30 mg/kg/day	200 mg tid
Ketoconazole	1–5%				200–400 mg/day
Miconazole	1%	5–10 mg	0.25 mg	25 mg/kg/day in 2–3 divided doses	
Thiabendazole	4%				25 mg/kg/day
Pyrimidines					
Flucytosine	1%				50–150 mg/kg/day

patient setting.[39] Bleb-associated endophthalmitis is typically characterized by a delayed onset, more virulent pathogens and poor visual prognosis. Due to the more virulent microorganisms (*Streptococcus species* and *Haemophilus influenzae*) and resulting poor visual prognosis, immediate pars plana vitrectomy, and intravitreal injection of vancomycin and ceftazidime are recommended.[40] Topical and systemic antibiotics (vancomycin and ceftazidime) should be used.

Post-traumatic Endophthalmitis

Due to the initial injury, delay in primary wound repair and more virulent organisms (*Bacillus* or *Staphylococcus* species), post-traumatic endophthalmitis generally has a worse visual outcome than other categories. Endophthalmitis caused by *Bacillus* species is characterized by a rapidly progressive course, ring corneal infiltrates and, generally, a poor visual outcome, even with prompt therapy.[41] Prophylactic intravitreal broad spectrum antibiotic injection decreases the risk of post-traumatic endophthalmitis.[42] In addition, systemic antibiotics are usually administered.[43]

Endogenous Endophthalmitis

Endogenous endophthalmitis is more commonly diagnosed in immunocompromised and debilitated patients. Once the diagnosis of endophthalmitis is suspected, blood or urine cultures should be obtained and other organ involvement must be sought by consultation with an infectious disease specialist or internist. The use of systemic antibiotics is also usually undertaken.

Candida albicans is the most common organism causing endogenous fungal endophthalmitis and *Aspergillus* species is the second most common fungal cause.[44] The management of endogenous *Candida* endophthalmitis is generally tailored to the clinical situation. When chorioretinal infiltrates are present with no or minimal vitreous involvement, systemic therapy alone is recommended. With moderate or severe vitritis, or deterioration in spite of systemic therapy, vitrectomy and intraocular amphotericin B are recommended.

Endogenous bacterial endophthalmitis often is an initial finding leading to the diagnosis of bacterial endocarditis, sepsis and liver abscess in Asians. In patients with diabetes and liver abscess, endogenous *Klebsiella pneumoniae* endophthalmitis is endemic in the Chinese population.[45] It is a very fulminant infection and often results in poor visual outcome. Prompt diagnosis and vigorous treatment with intravitreous injections of vancomycin, amikacin and dexamethasone within 24 hours can save the patient's eyes and vision.[46] Systemic antibiotics and intraocular antibiotics are recommended. Early vitrectomy for endogenous *Klebsiella pneumoniae* endophthalmitis might be beneficial.[47] However, debilitation and confinement in bed because of the sickness in these patients often results in it being unlikely that anesthesia and surgery can be performed in the operating room.

Intravitreous Triamcinolone-associated Endophthalmitis

Triamcinolone injection has become popular for treating macula edema in many diseases. Although some patients appear to have an infectious endophthalmitis, many reports detail a "pseudoendophthalmitis" that resolves without invasive treatment, which might be caused by triamcinolone crystal in the anterior chamber or an inflammatory reaction to the solvent toxin. Infectious endophthalmitis usually manifests acutely or subacutely with pain. It was concluded that in certain eyes injected with triamcinolone, the differential diagnosis should include a sterile, toxic endophthalmitis and it may be appropriate to observe the patient closely every 8–12 hours to determine if the inflammation is worsening or improving. However, if new symptoms develop more than several days after injection, infectious endophthalmitis should be presumed and treatment initiated immediately.[48]

CONCLUSION

Early recognition of endophthalmitis, together with appropriate and timely treatment, can often reduce visual loss.

REFERENCES

1. Ciulla TA, Starr MB, Masket S. Bacterial endophthalmitis prophylaxis for cataract surgery: an evidence-based update. Ophthalmology 2002;109(1):13-24.

2. Saggers BA, Stewart GT. Polyvinyl-Pyrrolidone-Iodine: An Assessment of Antibacterial Activity. J Hyg (Lond) 1964;62:509-18.
3. Connell JF, Jr, Rousselot LM. Povidone-Iodine. Extensive Surgical Evaluation of a New Antiseptic Agent. Am J Surg 1964;108:849-55.
4. Berkelman RL, Lewin S, Allen JR, et al. Pseudobacteremia attributed to contamination of povidone-iodine with *Pseudomonas cepacia*. Ann Intern Med 1981;95(1):32-6.
5. Johns KJ, Feder RS, Hamill MB, Miller-Meeks MJ. Surgery for Cataract. In: Johns KJ, Feder RS, Hamill MB, Miller-Meeks MJ (Eds). Basic and Clinical Science Course Section 11: Lens and Cataract: American Academy of Ophthalmology 2003-2004.
6. Ferguson AW, Scott JA, McGavigan J, et al. Comparison of 5 percent povidone-iodine solution against 1 percent povidone-iodine solution in preoperative cataract surgery antisepsis: a prospective randomised double blind study. Br J Ophthalmol 2003;87(2):163-7.
7. Ta CN. Minimizing the risk of endophthalmitis following intravitreous injections. Retina 2004;24(5):699-705.
8. Han DP, Wisniewski SR, Wilson LA, et al. Spectrum and susceptibilities of microbiologic isolates in the Endophthalmitis Vitrectomy Study. Am J Ophthalmol 1996;122(1):1-17.
9. Pflugfelder SC, Hernandez E, Fliesler SJ, et al. Intravitreal vancomycin. Retinal toxicity, clearance, and interaction with gentamicin. Arch Ophthalmol 1987;105(6):831-7.
10. Results of the Endophthalmitis Vitrectomy Study. A randomized trial of immediate vitrectomy and of intravenous antibiotics for the treatment of postoperative bacterial endophthalmitis. Endophthalmitis Vitrectomy Study Group. Arch Ophthalmol 1995;113(12):1479-96.
11. Coco RM, Lopez MI, Pastor JC, Nozal MJ. Pharmacokinetics of intravitreal vancomycin in normal and infected rabbit eyes. J Ocul Pharmacol Ther 1998;14(6):555-63.
12. Kwok AK, Hui M, Pang CP, et al. An *in vitro* study of ceftazidime and vancomycin concentrations in various fluid media: implications for use in treating endophthalmitis. Invest Ophthalmol Vis Sci 2002;43(4):1182-8.
13. Tanabe J, Kitano K, Suzuki T, et al. Nontoxic concentration of ceftazidime and flomoxef sodium for intravitreal use—evaluated by *in vitro* ERG. Lens Eye Toxic Res 1990;7(3-4):677-83.
14. Campochiaro PA, Conway BP. Aminoglycoside toxicity—a survey of retinal specialists. Implications for ocular use. Arch Ophthalmol 1991;109(7):946-50.
15. D'Amico DJ, Caspers-Velu L, Libert J, et al. Comparative toxicity of intravitreal aminoglycoside antibiotics. Am J Ophthalmol 1985;100(2):264-75.
16. Campochiaro PA, Lim JI. Aminoglycoside toxicity in the treatment of endophthalmitis. The Aminoglycoside Toxicity Study Group. Arch Ophthalmol 1994;112(1):48-53.
17. Kumar A, Dada T. Preretinal haemorrhages: an unusual manifestation of intravitreal amikacin toxicity. Aust N Z J Ophthalmol 1999;27(6):435-6.
18. Seawright AA, Bourke RD, Cooling RJ. Macula toxicity after intravitreal amikacin. Aust N Z J Ophthalmol 1996;24(2):143-6.
19. Mandell BA, Meredith TA, Aguilar E, et al. Effects of inflammation and surgery on amikacin levels in the vitreous cavity. Am J Ophthalmol 1993;115(6):770-4.

20. Shaarawy A, Grand MG, Meredith TA, Ibanez HE. Persistent endophthalmitis after intravitreal antimicrobial therapy. Ophthalmology 1995;102(3):382-7.
21. Aguilar HE, Meredith TA, Shaarawy A, et al. Vitreous cavity penetration of ceftazidime after intravenous administration. Retina 1995;15(2):154-9.
22. Keren G, Alhalel A, Bartov E, et al. The intravitreal penetration of orally administered ciprofloxacin in humans. Invest Ophthalmol Vis Sci 1991;32(8):2388-92.
23. Martin DF, Ficker LA, Aguilar HA, et al. Vitreous cefazolin levels after intravenous injection. Effects of inflammation, repeated antibiotic doses, and surgery. Arch Ophthalmol 1990;108(3):411-4.
24. Ferencz JR, Assia EI, Diamantstein L, Rubinstein E. Vancomycin concentration in the vitreous after intravenous and intravitreal administration for postoperative endophthalmitis. Arch Ophthalmol 1999;117(8):1023-7.
25. Souli M, Kopsinis G, Kavouklis E, et al. Vancomycin levels in human aqueous humour after intravenous and subconjunctival administration. Int J Antimicrob Agents 2001;18(3):239-43.
26. Das T, Sharma S. Current management strategies of acute postoperative endophthalmitis. Semin Ophthalmol 2003;18(3):109-15.
27. Mather R, Karenchak LM, Romanowski EG, Kowalski RP. Fourth generation fluoroquinolones: new weapons in the arsenal of ophthalmic antibiotics. Am J Ophthalmol 2002;133(4):463-6.
28. Hariprasad SM, Mieler WF, Holz ER. Vitreous and aqueous penetration of orally administered gatifloxacin in humans. Arch Ophthalmol 2003;121(3):345-50.
29. Foster RE, Rubsamen PE, Joondeph BC, et al. Concurrent endophthalmitis and retinal detachment. Ophthalmology 1994;101(3):490-8.
30. Barza M. Antibacterial agents in the treatment of ocular infections. Infect Dis Clin North Am 1989;3(3):533-51.
31. Kwak HW, D'Amico DJ. Evaluation of the retinal toxicity and pharmacokinetics of dexamethasone after intravitreal injection. Arch Ophthalmol 1992;110(2):259-66.
32. Park SS, Vallar RV, Hong CH, et al. Intravitreal dexamethasone effect on intravitreal vancomycin elimination in endophthalmitis. Arch Ophthalmol 1999;117(8):1058-62.
33. Falk NS, Beer PM, Peters GB, 3rd. Role of intravitreal triamcinolone acetonide in the treatment of postoperative endophthalmitis. Retina 2006;26(5):545-8.
34. Hykin PG, Tobal K, McIntyre G, et al. The diagnosis of delayed postoperative endophthalmitis by polymerase chain reaction of bacterial DNA in vitreous samples. J Med Microbiol 1994;40(6):408-15.
35. Aldave AJ, Stein JD, Deramo VA, et al. Treatment strategies for postoperative *Propionibacterium acnes* endophthalmitis. Ophthalmology 1999;106(12):2395-401.
36. Clark WL, Kaiser PK, Flynn HW, Jr, et al. Treatment strategies and visual acuity outcomes in chronic postoperative *Propionibacterium acnes* endophthalmitis. Ophthalmology 1999;106(9):1665-70.
37. Ciulla TA. Update on acute and chronic endophthalmitis. Ophthalmology 1999;106(12):2237-8.

38. Luttrull JK, Wan WL, Kubak BM, et al. Treatment of ocular fungal infections with oral fluconazole. Am J Ophthalmol 1995;119(4):477-81.
39. Chen PP, Gedde SJ, Budenz DL, Parrish RK, 2nd. Outpatient treatment of bleb infection. Arch Ophthalmol 1997;115(9):1124-8.
40. Kangas TA, Greenfield DS, Flynn HW, Jr., et al. Delayed-onset endophthalmitis associated with conjunctival filtering blebs. Ophthalmology 1997;104(5):746-52.
41. Foster RE, Martinez JA, Murray TG, et al. Useful visual outcomes after treatment of *Bacillus cereus* endophthalmitis. Ophthalmology 1996;103(3):390-7.
42. Narang S, Gupta V, Gupta A, et al. Role of prophylactic intravitreal antibiotics in open globe injuries. Indian J Ophthalmol 2003;51(1):39-44.
43. Reynolds DS, Flynn HW, Jr. Endophthalmitis after penetrating ocular trauma. Curr Opin Ophthalmol 1997;8(3):32-8.
44. Weishaar PD, Flynn HW, Jr, Murray TG, et al. Endogenous *Aspergillus* endophthalmitis. Clinical features and treatment outcomes. Ophthalmology 1998;105(1):57-65.
45. Chen YJ, Kuo HK, Wu PC, et al. A 10-year comparison of endogenous endophthalmitis outcomes: an east Asian experiene with *Klebsiella pneumoniae* infection. Retina 2004;24(3):383-90.
46. Chou FF, Kou HK. Endogenous endophthalmitis associated with pyogenic hepatic abscess. J Am Coll Surg 1996;182(1):33-6.
47. Yoon YH, Lee SU, Sohn JH, Lee SE. Result of early vitrectomy for endogenous *Klebsiella pneumoniae* endophthalmitis. Retina 2003;23(3):366-70.
48. Roth DB, Chieh J, Spirn MJ, et al. Noninfectious endophthalmitis associated with intravitreal triamcinolone injection. Arch Ophthalmol 2003;121(9):1279-82.

Surgical Techniques of Glued IOL

Ashvin Agarwal, Amar Agarwal (India)

INTRODUCTION

We devised a new surgical technique for implantation of a posterior chamber intraocular lens (IOL) in eyes with deficient or absent posterior capsule with the use of biological glue. We used a quick acting surgical fibrin sealant derived from human blood plasma, with both hemostatic and adhesive properties.

SCLERAL FIXATED IOL

Intraocular lens (IOL) implantation in eyes that lack posterior capsular support has been accomplished in the past, by means of iris fixated IOL,[1,2] anterior chamber intraocular lens and transscleral IOL fixation,[3-12] through the ciliary sulcus or pars plana. Surgical expertise, prolonged surgical time, suture induced inflammation, suture degradation, and delayed IOL subluxation or dislocation due to broken suture are some of the limitations in sutured scleral fixated intraocular lenses (SFIOL). It is also difficult and time consuming requiring minute and perfect adjustment of suture length and tension to ensure good centration of SFIOL.

FIBRIN GLUE

Fibrin glue[13-15] has been used previously in various medical specialties as a hemostatic agent to arrest bleeding, seal tissues and as an adjunct to wound healing. The fibrin kit we used was ReliSeal™ (Reliseal, Reliance Life Sciences, India). It is available in a sealed pack, which contains freeze dried human fibrinogen (20 mg/0.5 ml), freeze dried human thrombin (250 IU/0.5 ml), aprotinin solution (1500 kIU in 0.5 ml), one ampule of sterile water, four 21G needles, two 20G blunt application needles and an applicator with two mixing chambers and one plunger guide.

SURGICAL TECHNIQUE

After inserting the infusion cannula or anterior chamber maintainer, localized peritomy is done. Two partial thickness limbal based scleral flaps about 4 mm × 4 mm are created exactly 180 degrees diagonally apart (Fig. 54.1) and about 1.5 mm from the limbus. This is followed by vitrectomy via pars plana or anterior

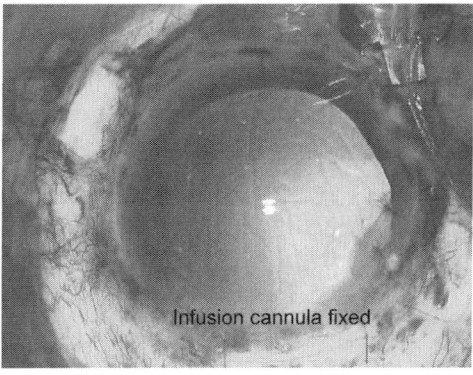

Fig. 54.1: Scleral flaps prepared 180 degrees diagonally apart. Note the infusion cannula fixed in and eye without any capsule

route to remove all vitreous traction. Two straight sclerotomies with a 22G needle are made about 1.5 mm from the limbus under the existing scleral flaps. The sclerotomies are positioned such a way that the superior one lies close to the upper edge of the flap and the inferior one close to the lower edge of the flap. A scleral tunnel incision is then prepared about 2 mm from the limbus for introducing the IOL. While the IOL is being introduced with the left hand of the surgeon using a McPherson forceps, an end gripping 25G micro rhexis forceps (Micro Surgical Technology, USA) is passed through the inferior sclerotomy. The tip of the leading haptic is then grasped with the micro rhexis forceps, pulled through the inferior sclerotomy following the curve of the haptic (Fig. 54.2) and is externalized under the inferior scleral flap. Similarly, the trailing haptic is also externalized through the superior sclerotomy under the scleral flap (Fig. 54.3). Then, the reconstituted fibrin glue thus prepared is injected through the cannula of the double syringe delivery system under the superior (Fig. 54.4) and inferior scleral flaps. Local pressure is given over the flaps for about 10 to 20 seconds for the formation of fibrin polypeptides (Fig. 54.5). The anterior chamber maintainer or the infusion cannula is removed. Conjunctiva is also closed with the same fibrin glue.

In case of those patients who had a luxated IOL, similar lamellar scleral flaps as described earlier were made and the luxated IOL haptic was then grasped with the 25 gauge rhexis forceps and exteriorized and glued under the scleral flaps (Figs 54.6A to E). The haptic of the IOL if protruding beyond the scleral flap can be tucked in a tunnel created in the sclera. (Fig. 54.7). Our follow-up anterior segment OCT (Figs 54.8A and B) showed postoperative perfect scleral flap adhesion as early as day one and continues to remain well maintained at one week and one month.

DISCUSSION

This fibrin glue assisted sutureless PC-IOL implantation technique as described by us would be useful in a myriad of clinical situations

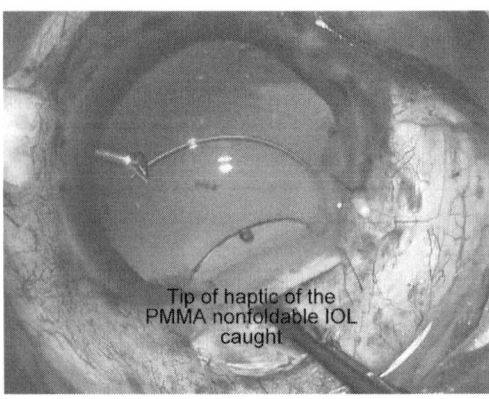

Fig. 54.2: Tip of the haptic grabbed by the 25 gauge micro-rhexis forceps (MST, USA) and then that haptic is externalized under the scleral flap

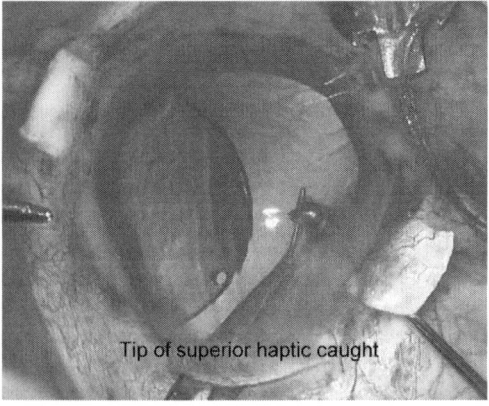

Fig. 54.3: Superior haptic grabbed by the 25 gauge micro-rhexis forceps (MST, USA) and then externalized under the scleral flap

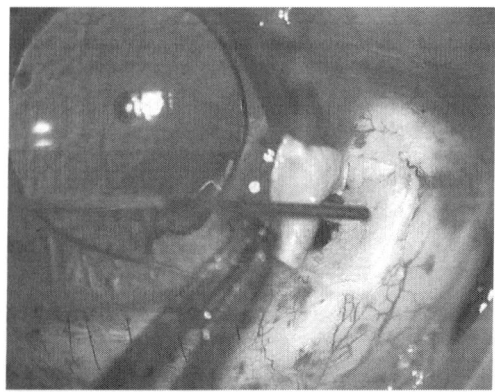

Fig. 54.4: Fibrin glue applied. Note the haptic which is externalized

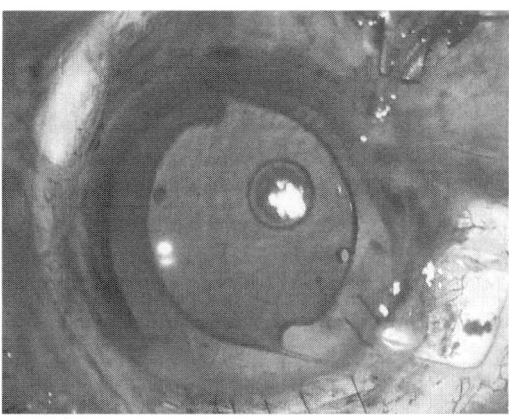

Fig. 54.5: PC-IOL well positioned and centered

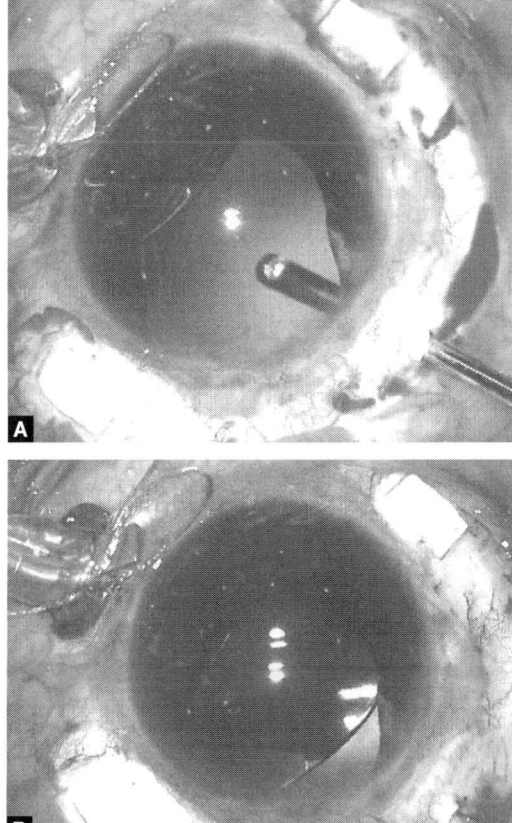

Figs 54.6A and B: (A) Subluxated IOL. Note the infusion cannula fixed and scleral flaps prepared. Vitrectomy being done; (B) Haptics externalized under the scleral flaps and IOL well centered

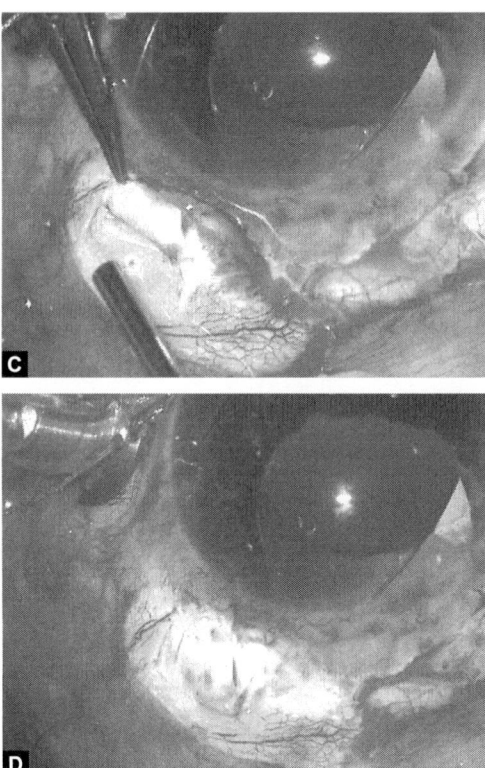

Figs 54.6C and D: (C) Fibrin glue applied and scleral flaps seal the haptic of the IOL; (D) IOL haptic now glued by the fibrin glue

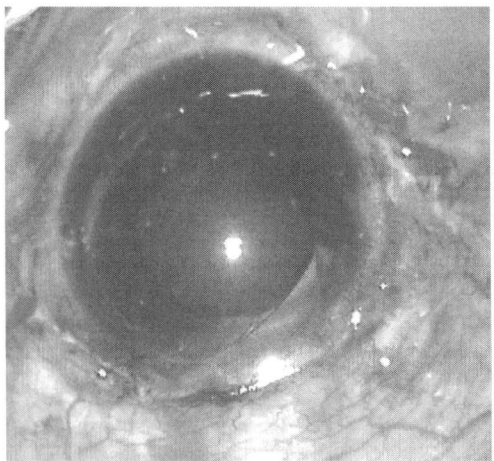

Fig. 54.6E: Fibrin glue seals the conjunctiva

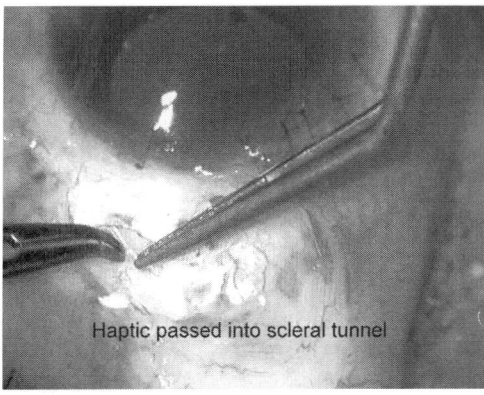

Fig. 54.7: IOL haptic tucked through a scleral tunnel

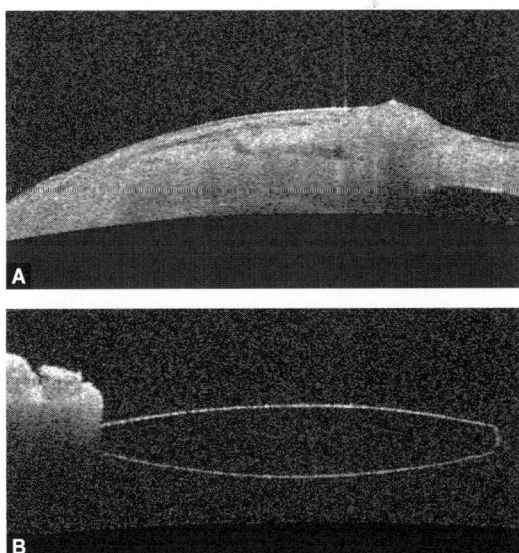

Figs 54.8A and B: (A) Anterior segment OCT of scleral flap; (B) Anterior segment OCT of the IOL. Note IOL well centered

where scleral fixated IOLs are indicated, such as, luxated IOL, dislocated IOL, zonulopathy or secondary IOL implantation. In dislocated posterior chamber PMMA-IOL, the same IOL can be repositioned thereby reducing the need for further manipulation. Externalization of the greater part of the haptics along its curvature stabilizes the axial positioning of the IOL and thereby prevents any IOL tilt.[16] In the 12 eyes of our 12 patients, no complications like postoperative inflammation, hyphema, decentration, glaucoma or corneal edema were seen after a regular follow-up till now. We expect less incidence of UGH syndrome in fibrin glue-assisted IOL implantation as compared to sutured scleral fixated IOL. This is because, in the former the IOL is well stabilized and stuck onto the scleral bed and thereby, has decreased intraocular mobility whereas in the latter, there is increased possibilty of IOL movement or persistent rub over the ciliary body. Visually significant complications due to late subluxation[17] which has been known to occur in sutured scleral fixated IOL may also be prevented as sutures are totally avoided in this technique. Moreover, the frequent complications[18] of secondary IOL implantation like secondary glaucoma, cystoid macular edema or bullous keratopathy were not seen in any of our patients. Another important advantage of this technique is the prevention of suture related complications[19-21] like suture erosion, suture knot exposure or dislocation of IOL after suture disintegration or broken suture. Chances of scleral melt[22-24] and haptic exposure is not increased by this technique except possibly, in high-risk patients like rheumatoid arthritis.

The other advantage of this technique is the rapidity and ease of surgery. Since all the steps of tying the difficult to handle 10-0 Prolene suture to the IOL haptic eyelets, the time required to ensure good centration before tying down the knots as well as time for suturing scleral flaps and closing conjunctiva are done away with, the total surgical time is significantly reduced. It is also easier and does not require much surgical expertise to use the 25 gauge forceps to grasp and exteriorize the haptic. Fibrin glue takes only 20 seconds to act in the scleral bed and it helps in adhesion as well as hemostasis. Fibrin glue has been shown to provide airtight closure and by the time the fibrin starts degrading, surgical adhesions would have already occurred in the scleral bed. This is well shown in Figure 54.6E.

The commercially available fibrin glue that we used is virus inactivated and is checked for viral antigen with polymerase chain reaction, hence the chances of transmission of infection is very low. But with tissue derivatives, there is always a theoretical possibility of transmission of viral infections,[25] therefore it is mandatory to get informed consent from the patient before the procedure. Though the use of fibrin glue in ophthalmology is considered off-label, it has been successfully used in the eye since long. Its various uses in the eye include repair of lacerated canaliculi[28] to seal full thickness macular holes,[26,27] to seal cataract incisions,[32-35] corneal perforations, and traumatic lens capsule perforations,[29] It has also been used for temporary closure of scleral flaps[31] after trabeculectomy in eyes with hypotony, conjunctival fistula closure,[30] conjunctival autografts,[31] and amniotic membrane transplantation.[36,37]

Gabor et al[38] have shown sutureless scleral IOL fixation by placing the IOL haptic in a scleral tunnel. Our technique differed from other sutureless methods[38,39] by use of the fibrin glue which enhances the rate of adhesion with hemostasis. We also used scleral flaps as in conventional sutured SFIOLs and this makes the learning curve very simple. There is also no danger of intra-ocular infection gaining entry through the tunnel as the fibrin glue hermetically seals the flaps leaving behind no possible entry route for microbes. There was no glue induced intraocular inflammation in any of our patients and all 12 eyes had clear media on the postoperative visits. Scleral indentation performed in the operated eyes showed no change in the axial positioning of the IOL. After one month of follow-up, we found no IOL decentration or any other complications in any of the operated 12 eyes.

SUMMARY

Fibrin glue-assisted sutureless PC IOL implantation is appropriate for eyes with deficient or absent posterior capsule and this can be performed easily with the available IOL designs, instruments and with less surgical time. However, a longer duration follow-up might be necessary to judge the long-term functional and anatomical results of the procedure.

REFERENCES

1. Zeh WG, Price FW. Iris fixation of posterior chamber intraocular lenses. J Cataract Refract Surg 2000;26:1028-34.
2. Lorencova V, Rozsival P, Urminsky J. Clinical results of the aphakia correction by means of secondary implantation of the iris-fixated anterior chamber intraocular lens. Cesk Slov Oftalmol 2007;63(4):285-91.
3. Bleckmann H, Kaczmarek U. Functional results of posterior chamber lens implantation with scleral fixation. J Cataract Refract Surg 1994;20:321-6.
4. Holland EJ, Djalilian AR, Pederson J. Gonioscopic evaluation of haptic position in trans-sclerally sutured posterior chamber lenses. Am J Ophthalmol 1997;123:411-3.
5. Lee JG, Lee JH, Chung H. Factors contributing to retinal detachment after transscleral fixation of posterior chamber intraocular lenses. J Cataract Refract Surg 1998;24:697-702.
6. Solomon K, Gussler JP, Gussler C, Van Meter WS. Incidence and management of complications of transsclerally sutured posterior chamber lenses. J Cataract Refract Surg 1993;19:488-93.
7. Teichmann KD, Teichmann IAM. Haptic design for continuous-loop, scleral fixation of posterior chamber lens. J Cataract Refract Surg 1998;24:889-92.
8. Chang S, Coll GE. Surgical techniques for repositioning a dislocated intraocular lens, repair of iridodialysis, and secondary intraocular lens implantation using innovative 25-gauge forceps. AJO 1995;120:126.
9. Mensiz E, Avtulner E, Ozerturk Y. Scleral fixation suture technique without lens removal for posteriorly dislocated intraocular lenses. Can J Ophthalmol 2002; 37(5):290-4.
10. Mittelviefhaus H, Witschel H. Transscleral suture fixation of posterior-chamber lenses after cataract extraction associated with vitreous loss. Ger Jr Ophthalmol 1995;4(2):80-5.
11. Koh HJ, Kim CY, Lim SJ, Kwon OW. Scleral fixation technique using 2 corneal tunnels for a dislocated intraocular lens. J Cataract Refract Surg 2000;26(10):1439-41.
12. Oh H, Chu Y, Woong known O. Surgical technique for suture fixation of a single-piece hydrophilic acrylic intraocular lens in the absence of capsule support. J Cataract Refract Surg 2007;33:962-5.

13. Fink D, Klein JJ, Kang H, et al. Application of biological glue in repair of intracardiac structural defects. The ann of thoraxic surg 2004;77(2):506-11.
14. AF Matar, JG Hill, W Duncan, et al. Use of biological glue to control pulmonary air leaks. Thorax 1990;45(9):670-4.
15. PD Mintz, L Mayers, N Avery H, et al. Fibrin Sealant: Clinical Use and the Development of the University of Virginia Tissue Adhesive Center. Ann Clin Lab Sci 2001;31(1):108-18.
16. Teichmann KD, Teichmann IAM. The torque and tilt gamble. J Cataract Refract Surg 1997;23:413-8.
17. McCluskey P, Harrisberg B. Long-term results using scleral-fixated posterior chamber intraocular lenses. J Cataract Refract Surg 1994;20:34-9.
18. Biro Z. Results and complications of secondary intraocular lens implantation. J Cataract Refract Surg 1993;19:64-7.
19. Heilskov T, Joondeph BC, Olsen KR, Blankenship GW. Late endophthalmitis after transscleral fixation of a posterior chamber intraocular lens. Arch Ophthalmol 1989;107:1427.
20. Mowbray SL, Chang S-H, Casella JF. Estimation of the useful lifetime of polypropylene fiber in the anterior chamber. Am Intra-Ocular Implant Soc J 1983;9:143-7.
21. Jongebloed WL, Worst JFG. Degradation of polypropylene in the human eye: a SEM-study. Doc Ophthalmol 1986;64:143-52.
22. Ahmed TY, Carrim ZI, Diaper CJM, Wykes WN. Spontaneous\ intraocular lens extrusion in a patient with scleromalacia secondary to herpes zoster ophthalmicus. J Cataract Refract Surg 2007;33:925-6.
23. Mamalis N, Johnson MD, Haines JM, et al. Corneal-scleral melt in association with cataract surgery and intraocular lenses: A report of four cases. J Cataract Refract Surg 1990;16:108-15.
24. Watson PG, Hayreh SS. Scleritis and episcleritis. Br J Ophthalmol 1976;60:163-91.
25. Schlegel A, Immelmann A, Kempf C. Virus inactivation of plasma-derived proteins by pasteurization in the presence of guanidine hydrochloride. Transfusion 2001;41:382-9.
26. Tilanus MAD, Deutman T, Deutman AF. Full-thickness macular holes treated with vitrectomy and tissue glue. Int Ophthalmol 1994-1995;18:355-8.
27. Olsen TW, Sternberg P Jr, Capone A Jr, et al. Macular hole surgery using thrombin-activated fibrinogen and selective removal of the internal limiting membrane. Retina 1998;18:322-9.
28. Steinkogler FJ. Fibrin tissue adhesive for the repair of lacerated canaliculi lacrimales. In: Schlag G, Redl H (Eds). Fibrin Sealant in Operative Medicine, vol 2: Ophthalmology-Neurosurgery. Berlin: Springer;1986.pp.92-4.
29. Buschmann W. Progress in fibrin sealing of eye lens and conjunctiva. In: Schlag G, Ascher PW, Steinkogler F Stammberger H (Eds). Fibrin Sealing in Surgical and Nonsurgical Fields, vol 5: Neurosurgery, Ophthalmic Surgery, ENT. Berlin: Springer-Verlag; 1994. pp.97-106.
30. Grewing R, Mester U. Fibrin sealant in the management of complicated hypotony after trabeculectomy. Ophthalmic Surg Lasers 1997;28:124-7.
31. Cohen RA, McDonald MB. Fixation of conjunctival autografts with an organic tissue adhesive [letter]. Arch Ophthalmol 1993;111:1167-8.

32. Grewing R, Mester U. Radial suture stabilized by fibrin glue to correct preoperative against-the-rule astigmatism during cataract surgery. Ophthalmic Surg 1994;25:446-8.
33. Mester U. Wound closure with fibrin adhesive in cataract surgery. In: Schlag G, Ascher PW, Steinkogler FJ, Stammberger H (Eds). Fibrin Sealing in Surgical and Nonsurgical Fields, vol 5: Neurosurgery, Ophthalmic Surgery, ENT. Berlin: Springer-Verlag; 1994.pp.123-32.
34. Rauber M, Mester U, Zuche M. Fibrin adhesive for wound closure in small-incision cataract surgery. In: Schlag G, Ascher PW, Steinkogler FJ, Stammberger H (Eds). Fibrin Sealing in Surgical and Nonsurgical Fields, vol 5: Neurosurgery, Ophthalmic Surgery, ENT. Berlin: Springer-Verlag;1994.pp.116-22.
35. Henrick A, Kalpakian B, Gaster RN, Vanley C. Organic tissue glue in the closure of cataract incisions in rabbit eyes. J Cataract Refract Surg 1991;17:551-5.
36. Lagoutte FM, Gauthier L, Comte PRM. A fibrin sealant for perforated and preperforated corneal ulcers. Br J Ophthalmol 1989;73:757-61.
37. Duchesne B, Tahi H, Galand A. Use of human fibrin glue and amniotic membrane transplant in corneal perforation. Cornea 2001;20:230-3.
38. Gabor SG, Pavilidis MM. Sutureless intrascleral posterior chamber intraocular lens fixation. J Cataract Refract Surg 2007;33(11):1851-4.
39. Maggi R, Maggi C. Sutureless scleral fixation of intraocular lenses. J Cataract Refract Surg 1997;23(9):1289-94.

55

Intraocular Gases

S Natarajan, Pandurang Kulkarni, Navendu Rai, Shachi Desai,
Vinay Prasad, Rishi Bhardwaj, Anoop Sivaraman (India)

PHYSICAL PROPERTIES OF GASES

It is important to understand the physical properties of expansile gases in order to understand the principles of usage in vitreoretinal surgery. It is difficult to describe the detailed physics and geometry associated with these, we have still tried to compile in a short and lucid manner. The properties worth mentioning are surface tension and its importance, intraocular tamponade achieved and the buoyancy or flotation force. A brief knowledge about these properties gives an understanding of the indications of use for these gases.

A gas bubble provides tamponading effect thereby flattening the retinal break against retinal pigment epithelium. This tamponade prevents liquid vitreous from entering the vitreous cavity, helping the existing subretinal fluid to get absorbed.[1]

Surface tension occurs at the interface of a liquid and liquid or a liquid and gas, if the two are immiscible. It is due to the van der Walls forces and other forces like intermolecular polar bonding forces in water. These forces cause a net inward force ate the surface tending the bubble to assume a spherical shape.[2] This force along with size of retinal break and the distance between break and retinal pigment epithelium influence prolapse of bubble and migration into the subretinal space. Bubbles of size larger than the retinal break do not prolapse through and migrate into subretinal space. Similarly if the distance between break and retinal pigment epithelium is larger than the radius of the break, more force is required to spread the bubble in subretinal space than to prolapse it through the break. This prolapse also depends upon the flexibility of retina, the bubble can push a mobile retina better against the retinal pigment epithelium than prolapsing through it.[3]

The force exerted by the bubble tending to prolapse it through the retinal break is the flotation force or buoyancy. The bubble is affected by three forces, two causing it to sink (force of water pressure on upper surface and the weight of the bubble) and one causing it to rise (water pressure on the lower surface of bubble). Weight being negligible, the flotation force is difference between the pressure at upper and lower surfaces of the bubble. Largest flotation force occurs when the bubble fills the eyeball completely. This force is the greatest at the apex (there lies the importance of correct positioning) and when the bubble is near retinal pigment epithelium.[1]

INTRAOCULAR GAS GEOMETRY

Surface Tension, Buoyancy and Arc of Contact

Purpose of using gas in cases of retinal detachment is to provide functional closure of the retinal break and to displace the retina outward. Closure of the retinal break will prevent flow of vitreous fluid in the subretinal space. Remaining fluid in subretinal space is pumped out by retinal pigment epithelium attaching the retinal break. During this process, due to surface tension of the gas, it does not pass through the break unless gas size is small compared to large break. Surface tension occurs at the interface of a liquid with another liquid or gas, if the two substances are immiscible.[1]

Intraocular tamponade also depends on buoyancy or floatation force which is dependent of volume of the gas injected. Volume of the intraocular gas is estimated if height of the bubble is known with help of equations. Clinical estimation of height of the bubble is determined by viewing inferior meniscus of bubble in the reference with corneal limbus. Superior limbus corresponds to 25 percent of gas bubble and inferior limbus corresponds to 75 percent of gas bubble. More the height of the bubble, higher the floatation force pushing the retina on its place. Maximum force is at the apex of the bubble explaining the importance of positioning in the postoperative period. Position in which retinal break remains superiorly is advised to the patient.

Arc of contact is another clinically important feature determined by volume of the gas. Formulas are available to measure arc of contact from the amount of gas inside the eye. Usually gas bubble larger than 50 percent of the volume provides arc of contact of 180 degree.

INTRAOCULAR GAS KINETICS

Intraocular gas kinetics includes partial pressure gradient, diffusion, expansion and absorption of gas, half life and longevity of gas. Partial pressure gradient that is difference in the concentration of gases in blood stream and in bubble determines rate of diffusion of gas and accordingly expansion and absorption of gases determining half life and longevity of gas in the vitreous cavity.

Diffusion, Expansion and Absorption

Gases injected in the vitreous cavity gradually dissolves in the intraocular fluids and are ultimately absorbed in the blood stream. Diffusion of gases occurs through thin barrier where bubble touches eye wall and is dependent on partial pressure of gases on both the sides of barrier that is bubble in vitreous cavity and blood stream. According to Fick's diffusion equation, diffusion is directly proportionate to difference of pressure gradient across the barrier and gas solubility in fluid and area of the barrier and inversely related to thickness of barrier. Eye wall thickness being more or less same (approximately 100 microns), diffusion is more with higher pressure gradient, more gas solubility and larger area of contact between gas and the wall.

Gas diffusion and expansion depends on differential exchange of nitrogen and also on long acting gas used. When pure gas is injected in the vitreous cavity at the end of surgery, in immediate postoperative period partial pressure of Nitrogen (N_2) in the blood stream is more than in gas bubble leading to its diffusion in the gas bubble causing expansion of the gas. After this initial stage, expansion stops once the equilibrium of nitrogen is achieved along with slow reduction in volume of gas. Gradually the pressure gradient of long acting gas is developed between the bubble and blood stream overcoming its low diffusibility leading to efflux of gases in blood stream.

Timing and amount of expansion of gas depends on the concentration and type of gas used. Most commonly used gases for intraocular tamponades are Sulfur hexafluoride (SF_6) and Perfluoropropane (C_3F_8). SF6 can expand up to the double the amount injected and C_3F_8 can expands up to 4 times its volume.[4,5] Gas bubble does most of its expansion in 8 hours but it may expand slowly up to 96 hours.[6]

Nonexpansile Concentration

Sclera being inelastic IOP may increase with postoperative expansion of gas. Aqueous outflow increases slowly to compensate increase in the volume of gas bubble which normalizes the IOP in most cases. If larger amount of pure gas is injected, then normal aqueous outflow facility cannot compensate for increase in the volume leading to rise in intraocular pressure. If larger amount of gas bubble is to be injected to fill the cavity with the bubble then it is better to inject nonexpansile concentration of the gas. Maximum nonexpansile concentration for SF_6 is 20 percent with 80 percent air and for C_3F_8 is 12 percent with 88 percent of air.[7]

Longevity and Half Life

Longevity of the gas bubble inside the eye depends on various factors like amount of the gas injected, concentration of the gas, type of the gas and status of the lens. Longevity can be determined in two ways: One the time taken for complete absorption and the other is half life. Half life is determined as time taken for reduction in the amount of the gas to half of its volume from its maximum expansion. Different gases have different half lives:[6]

Gas mixture	Half life (days)	Maximum effective duration of tamponade (days)
Air	1.3	4
20% SF_6	2.6	8
15% C_3F_8	8.0	24

EFFECT OF ANESTHETIC GASES AND ATMOSPHERIC DEPRESSURIZATION

During the surgery under general anesthesia due consideration should be given while injecting gas for tamponade. Nitrous oxide is commonly used gas for general anesthesia. It is highly soluble in water and diffuses rapidly into intraocular gas bubble causing expansion of the gas bubble intraoperatively leading to rapid and dangerous rise in intraocular pressure. To prevent such sequence of events flow of nitrous oxide should be stopped 15 minutes prior to injecting gas inside the eye or other gases should be used for general anesthesia. Nitrous oxide flow once stopped is rapidly exhaled out of the body through breathing.[6]

During the travelling by air plane at the height of 5000–8000 feet, expansion of gas may occur increasing the IOP. Normally after take-off cabin pressure is adjusted to the atmospheric pressure controlling the effects of depressurization. But in situations with no or less compensatory mechanisms, normal eye does not develop rise in IOP as it is filled with liquid as minimal expansion is required to lower the IOP. If gas bubble is inside the eye, it expands with decrease in the atmospheric pressure requiring good amount of aqueous outflow leading to rise in IOP with normal aqueous outflow. Patient should not be allowed to fly with 0.6–1.0 ml of gas bubble which corresponds to more than 20 percent of the volume.[6]

CLINICAL CONSIDERATIONS

The search for an ideal vitreous substitute that is transparent, elastic and biocompatible like the vitreous itself is still on. Over a period of time, various compounds have been used.[8]

Four different intraocular gases are commonly used in vitreoretinal surgery: air, sulfur hexafluoride (SF_6), perfluoroethane (C_2F_6) and perfluoropropane (C_3F_8). In the vitreous cavity, these gases are colorless, odorless and inert. When injected into the vitreous cavity, air does not expand, whereas pure SF_6, C_2F_6 and C_3F_8 gases do.[9]

CHOICE OF GAS

The intraocular gas bubble is one of the most useful surgical adjuncts in vitreoretinal surgery. A thorough understanding of its properties, indications and potential complications of intraocular gases is essential to optimizing the outcomes of vitreoretinal surgery.[10]

Air

It is easily available and inexpensive and non-expansile but intraocular time is only 2–3 days. Additionally, the refractive index of the air (1.0008) is incompatible with the optically important tissues (~1.33). So cannot be used as long-term tamponade. As a result, air has a somewhat limited use as a vitreous substitute.

Mainly used intraoperatively during fluid air exchange facilitating retinal reattachment. It is used in pneumatic retinopexy, at the end of vitrectomy surgery, and as an emergency option when other substitutes are unavailable.

Expansile Gases

The most commonly used gases are sulfur hexafluoride (SF_6), which is five times heavier than air, and perfluoropropane (C_3F_8), which is six times heavier than air. Both gases are colorless, odorless, and nontoxic. Both SF_6 and C_3F_8 have been used commonly in pneumatic retinopexy and in non expansile concentrations for postoperative endotamponade. Gases have highest surface tension of 70 dynes/cm^2 which allows them to maintain good tamponading effect. Depending on the percentage of gas injected its intraocular stay ranges from 6 to 8 days. It is eventually replaced by aqueous avoiding the need for another surgery. Gases cannot be used for long-term tamponade in complicated cases as well as inferior tamponade in case of inferior breaks.

Advantages

Gas has the highest surface tension of all vitreous fluid replacements at approximately 70 dynes/cm. High surface tension and diffusion of other gases from the bloodstream into these gases allow them to be expansile and to maintain a tamponade effect. They also have a good success rate, exceeding 90 percent for retinopexy. Expansile gases last longer than air, but will resorb spontaneously in 6–80 days depending on perfluoropropane percentage and will be replaced with aqueous humor, avoiding a second surgery to remove them.

Disadvantages

Although the expansile nature of gas allows for maintenance of the endotamponade effect, a sudden increase in intraocular pressure could in severe cases cause central retinal artery occlusion. Similarly, patients need to avoid higher altitudes in order to prevent dangerous gas expansion. With a density less than vitreous, perfluorocarbon gas does not effectively tamponade the inferior retina. Additionally, as with air, the refractive indices of the gases are lower (~1.17) compared to that of the cornea, anterior chamber fluid, and the lens.[8,10]

Clinical Settings

- A pure SF_6 bubble expands to about double the volume injected within 24–48 hours, and exerts an effect for 1–2 weeks.
- A pure C_3F_8 bubble expands to about 4 times of its original volume within 72–96 hours and persists in the vitreous cavity for 6–8 weeks.

- The maximum effective duration of the tamponade is approximately equal to 3 half-lives.
- Intraocular gases can be used in office or in operative settings.
- Following vitrectomy for retinal detachment, most vitreoretinal surgeons use a nonexpansile gas fill that allows placement of a large gas bubble to tamponade a large area of the retina.
- In contrast, pneumatic retinopexy involves the injection of a small, usually pure, expansile intraocular gas bubble in a nonvitrectomized eye; the objective being to provide focal tamponade over a retinal break.
- Intraocular gas may also be used as an adjunct in scleral buckling procedures, and are known as 'pneumaticbuckles'.
- Superior tears with retinal detachment without proliferative vitreoretinopathy (PVR) can be treated with air or short-acting gases such as SF_6.
- A longer-acting gas such as C_3F_8 can be used for retinal detachment with inferior tears, giant retinal tears, or more complex rhegmatogenous and tractional retinal detachment cases result in PVR, except when silicone oil is preferred.
- After vitrectomy for retinal detachments, a nonexpansile long-term gas fill of C_3F_8 allows the formation of chorioretinal adhesions while minimizing the positioning requirements for the patient.
- For macular hole surgery with epiretinal membrane peel, SF_6 is used for initial procedures and the longer acting C_3F_8 in repeat attempts of closure.
- For cases of tractional retinal tears in diabetic retinopathy and proliferative vitreoretinopathy (PVR) repair, the longer-chained perfluorocarbon gases C_2F_6 or C_3F_8 are the common choices, unless the severity requires use of silicone oil.[9]

Choice of gases: Sulfur hexafluoride (SF_6) is the gas most frequently used for pneumatic retinopexy, followed by perfluoropropane (C_3F_8).

In selecting a gas, it is important to understand the longevity and expansion characteristics of the gases. SF_6 doubles in volume within the eye, reaching its maximum size at about 36 hours. It will generally disappear within 10–14 days, depending on the amount injected. C_3F_8 quadruples in volume, reaching maximum size in about three days. The bubble will last 30–45 days in the eye. Room air does not expand but immediately starts to be absorbed. The air bubble will be gone within just a few days. The choice of type and amount of gas depends on two factors:

What Size Gas Bubble is Needed?

One must usually plan for a gas bubble large enough to cover all detached breaks, simultaneously or alternately, and keep them covered for three to five days, with some extra volume as a margin of safety. In the human eye, a 0.3 ml gas bubble covers almost 60 degrees of arc of the retina, but it takes approximately a 1.2 ml bubble to cover 80–90 degrees. A very large eyeball (myopic) will require a larger volume of gas than an emmetropia eye to cover the same arc of the retina. Usually, 0.3–0.5 ml of gas is injected into the eye. If it is desired to inject more than 0.5 ml into the eye, multiple injections are usually planned, allowing return of intraocular pressure toward normal between injections. Alternatively, paracentesis of the anterior chamber may be performed prior to injecting a larger volume of gas, which may be followed by a second paracentesis five to ten minutes after the gas injection.

What Length of Time the Bubble should Stay in the Eye?

It is optimal for the gas bubble to cover the break(s) for four to five days and then disappear as soon as possible. In most cases, the prolonged longevity of a C_3F_8 bubble is a disadvantage, although it may also eliminate the need to reinject gas if a new break develops. Because of its greater expansion, C_3F_8 allows the injection of a smaller amount of gas initially, thereby eliminating the need for paracentesis. The longevity of air is probably sufficient for most cases. Air forfeits the advantage of post-injection expansion within the eye. Gas of choice in most cases is SF_6. Usually 0.5 ml of 100 percent SF_6 is injected.

For Pneumatic Retinopexy

Characteristics of gases: Two characteristics account for their efficacy in reattaching the retina.
1. Surface tension allows the gas bubble to occlude a retinal break instead of passing into the subretinal space. The surface tension of any gas is much higher than that of other substances in the eye. Once the break is occluded, the retinal pigment epithelial pump can absorb the subretinal fluid.
2. Buoyancy provides the force which pushes the uppermost retina back against the wall of the eye. Apposition of the retina against the retinal pigment epithelium is necessary in order that chorioretinal adhesion can occur.[12]

NONEXPANSILE CONCENTRATION

Nonexpansile concentration for SF_6 (molecular weight = 146) is 20 percent gas in 80 percent air, and for C_3F_8 (molecular weight = 188) is 12 percent gas in 88 percent air.

TECHNIQUES OF FLUID-AIR EXCHANGE AND INTRAOCULAR GAS INJECTION

Following vitrectomy, intraocular gases are usually injected via the pars plana infusion line after any fluid (e.g. balanced salt solution) in the vitreous cavity is replaced by air. This fluid-air exchange may be performed by passive or active aspiration under direct visualization. With passive aspiration, a silicone tip or flute needle is used and the force of air entering the vitreous cavity through the infusion cannula causes the vitreous fluid to egress through the lumen of the aspiration needle, which is vented to the atmosphere. Fluid-air exchange with active aspiration into the vitrectomy cassette is more rapid but may result in hypotony if the aspiration of fluid is faster than the inflow of air. Subretinal fluid in eyes with a retinal detachment is usually removed during the surgery via the retinal break or a drainage retinotomy.

When preparing the gas for injection, a sterile filter (e.g. 0.22 μmmillipore) is recommended to prevent microbial contamination of the gas. A 50 ml syringe is flushed several times with the pure gas to avoid dilution of the desired concentration with residual air. The gas should not be left in the syringe for a prolonged period prior to injection, as diffusion will alter the effective gas concentration. For a traditional 20-gauge vitrectomy, one sclerotomy site is closed and the second site is sutured without tying the knot. The temporary closure of the second sclerotomy site involves clamping the infusion tubing to maintain the eye at a constant pressure. The gas syringe is then attached to the infusion tubing and the clamp is removed with gentle opening of the sclerotomy. Approximately 35–40 ml of the gas mixture is gently lavaged through the eye as air in the vitreous cavity is expelled through the open sclerotomy. The suture is then tied to close the second sclerotomy site. Finally, the infusion cannula is removed and a suture is used to close the final infusion line sclerotomy site. For a 23- or 25-gauge vitrectomy, gas can be injected via the infusion cannula while the trocars are in place. The trocars can then be removed after injection of 35–40 ml of the gas mixture and the integrity of the wound can be assessed.

Another technique of injecting gas following vitrectomy is to close the second sclerotomy site completely, and follow-up by lavage of gas into the eye via the infusion cannula while allowing air expulsion using a 25-gauge needle inserted through the pars plana. If the eye becomes soft during closure of the third sclerotomy site, additional gas can be injected at the pars plana via a 30-gauge needle attached to a smaller 3 ml syringe containing the gas mixture.[9]

For Pneumatic Retinopexy

Pneumatic retinopexy involves injection of 0.4–0.6 ml of pure gas (usually SF_6).

Preparation of the Gas

A pressure reducing system is attached to the gas cylinder to allow drawing the gas from a low pressure system. High pressure can blow out the millipore filter and render it useless in sterilizing the gas. A condom catheter can be attached to the cylinder, or a step down valve system can be used. Alternatively the gas may be drawn into a large syringe and then transferred to a small syringe.

The selected gas is drawn through a millipore filter into a 3 ml syringe in sterile fashion. The tube connecting the gas cylinder with the syringe including the filter, is flushed through with gas to insure no dilution with room air. The first withdrawal of the gas is discarded and approximately 1 ml of gas is withdrawn. A disposable 30 gauge one-half inch (12 mm) needle is then placed tightly on the syringe and excess gas is expelled to leave the exact amount intended for injection. The gas should not be stored in the syringe for more than a few minutes prior to injection because of the high-risk of gas leakage.

Injection of Gas

An injection site is selected 4 mm posterior to the limbus. The selected site is ideally away from large open retinal breaks, highly detached retina, or detached pars plana epithelium. The head of the supine patient is turned 45 degrees to one side to make the injection site uppermost. The needle is then passed into the eye perpendicular to the sclera. The needle is pushed 6-8 mm into the eye to ensure that the tip is well into the vitreous, directing the tip away from areas of highly bullous detachment. Then it is withdrawn until 3 mm of the needle remains in the eye. This will ensure that the tip remains in the vitreous but is shallow enough to prevent multiple small bubbles (fish eggs).

With the needle in the correct position, a moderately brisk injection of the entire volume of gas is performed. This facilitates formation of a single bubble at the needle tip. The injection should not be so brisk as to force bubbles of gas deep into the vitreous before their buoyancy can make them rise. It requires to inject smoothly and quickly but not with excessive force and one should hold the plunger down until the needle is withdrawn to prevent escape of gas back into the syringe.[11]

CLINICAL USES

The first reported use of intraocular gas was in 1911 by Ohm,[12] using air for treating retinal detachment. In 1938 Rosengren[13] popularized the technique of internal gas tamponade. Common uses of intraocular gases are:
- Air in anterior chamber
- Pneumatic retinopexy
- Macular hole surgery
- Pneumatic displacement of submacular hemorrhage
- Unrolling giant retinal tear
- Temporary vitreous replacement in conjunction with vitrectomy for vitreous hemorrhage

Pneumatic retinopexy is a procedure for simple detachments with breaks in superior 8'O hours.[14] In this gas is injected after or before retinopexy and then a position is given so as to support the break. In macular hole surgery the gas does waterproofing of the macular hole through surface tension and also provides a template for development of nascent membrane over the hole.[15] Submacular hemorrhage due to CNVM, PCV, trauma, macroaneurysm can cause visual deficit which may be treated with injecting anti-VEGF agent with pure gas and strict prone positioning for 5–7 days.[16,17] Unrolling of GRTs has become a history due to advent of PFCL, which made the job easier and convenient.

POSTOPERATIVE MANAGEMENT

Postoperative Visits and Postoperative Care

The operated eye needs to be patched after applying topical antibiotic and cycloplegics. Maintaining the correct head posture corresponding to the axis of the retinal break need to explained to the patient. Marking an arrow on the eye patch surface will be helpful in reminding the patient about the appropriate tilt for the required postoperative period. Reports show that even three day of proper head positioning may be sufficient.[12,18,19] for optimal results. However, 7–14 days are needed for optimal scar with after retinopexy.[20,21] Hence to obtain the best outcome the patients can be asked to maintain the correct head posture for atleast a week.

It should be reminded not to assume a supine position, which can lead to contact with lens and anterior chamber shallowing.[12,17]

Close monitoring is required to watch for desired improvement, modification of the management and to ensure for minimal complications. After immediate postoperative evaluation and ensuring that the arterial perfusion is adequate, the patient can be examined the next day of surgery. Subsequent follow ups can be at 1 week later, 2–3 weeks, and monthly for the next few months. Some cases which are having associated complications need frequent examinations. If the surgeon is planning laser therapy, it can be done as soon as the retinal breaks are flattened. Laser therapy is usually done 24–48 hours after gas injection. Most of the subretinal fluid absorbs within 72 hours after adequate closure of retinal breaks.[12,18,19]

Postoperative Intraocular Pressure Management

Mild-to-moderate rise in intraocular pressure after intraocular gas injection is common and is well-tolerated by most eyes without any treatment. The perfusion of the central retinal artery should not be compromised at the end of surgery.[17,18] Corrective treatment for elevated intraocular pressure should be given for eyes with risk of deficient perfusion of arteries and those with significant glaucoma after surgery. Applanation tonometry is the preferred method for monitoring intraocular pressure after gas injection.[22] Reading with Schiotz tonometry provide falsely low IOP readings.[23] Treatment with topical and oral hypotensive agents can be given in simple cases.[17,18] However, additional corrective measures may be taken if intraocular pressure remains high. An additional paracentesis may be required after gas injection, if central retinal artery perfusion is compromised even for few minutes and if excessive intraocular pressure is not lowered.

TOXICITY AND COMPLICATIONS

No studies have proven chemical or pharmacological toxicity of the gases used for intraocular tamponade.[25] The complications associated are due to the physical effects of these gases and the technique of injection.
- Raised intraocular pressure
- Lens opacities
- Damage to corneal endothelium
- Inadvertent injection into suprachoroidal space
- Inadvertent injection in space of petit
- Subretinal 'Fish eggs'
- New breaks formation
- Detachment of previously uninvolved macula
- Endophthalmitis.

Marked elevation of IOP is the most common and most serious complication[24] leading to central retinal artery occlusion (CRAO) and blindness. IOP can be controlled by antiglaucoma medications. If uncontrolled on antiglaucoma medications, titrated amount of gas needs to be removed through pars plana route. This can be minimized by proper calculation of amount of gas to be injected and use of proper nonexpansile mixture of gases.

Effect of gases on corneal endothelium and lens are mainly due to the interference with nutrition and the drying effect of the gases. Endothelium shows proliferative changes which are usually reversible and do not cause metabolic damage.[27] Subcapsular lens cortex shows vacuolar or feathery changes which are reversible initially but if the contact of gas with posterior lens surface is prolonged, it may lead to posterior subcapsular cataract.[26] Visual field defects have been reported in long-term gas temponade. Especially damage to the superonasal retina postvitrectomy using conventional inferotemporal infusion line has been reported.

Gas can be injected into the space of petit if the anterior hyaloids face is not pierced before injecting. This shows a 'sausage sign' and usually breaks through anterior hyaloids face to enter vitreous cavity. If this does not happen for 24–48 hours, gas can be removed in a controlled manner.[27] If while injecting multiple 'fish eggs' form, the gas can enter subretinal space through the break. If subretinal gas is small and break well covered with rest of gas, it may be left and gets absorbed with time. Otherwise attempts should be made to massage the gas back into the vitreous cavity through the break.[28] Endophthalmitis and CRAO are rare complications.

REFERENCES

1. Wilkinson CP, Rice TA, Michels RG. Retinal Detachment. Mosby: St Louis 1990;pp.412-28.
2. White FM. Fluid Mechanics, 2nd edn. New York: WH Freeman and Co, 1986;p. 30.
3. de Juan E Jr, McCuen B, Teedman J. Intraocular Tamponade and surface tension. Surv Ophthalmol 1985;30:47.

4. Killey FP, Edelhauser HF, Aaberg TM. Intraocular sulfur hexafluoride and octofluorocyclobutane. Effects on intraocular pressure and vitreous volume. Arch Ophthalmol 1978;96:511.
5. Lincoff H, Coleman J, Kreissig I, et al. The perfluorocarbon gases in the treatment of retinal detachment. Ophthalmology 1983;90:546.
6. Peyman GA, Meffert SA, Conway MD. Vitreoretinal Surgical Techniques. UK Informa. 2008;pp. 153-6.
7. Peters MA, Abrams GW, Hamilton LH, et al. The nonexpansile equilibrated concentration of perfluoropropane gas in the eye. Am J Ophthalmol 1985;100:831-9.
8. Azad SV, Mahajan D, Sain S, Jain A, Brijesh Takkar, Azad R. Vitreous Substitutes. DJO 2012;23(1): 9-13.
9. Shaheeda Mohamed, Timothy YY Lai. Intraocular gas in vitreoretinal Surgery. HKJ Ophthalmol 2010;14(1):8-13.
10. Teri T Kleinberg, Radouil T Tzekov, Linda Stein, Nathan Ravi, Shalesh Kaushal. Vitreous Substitutes: A Comprehensive Review. Survey of Ophthalmology 2011;56(4):300-22.
11. Hilton GF, Das T, Majji AB, Jalali S. Pneumatic retinopexy: principles and practice. Indian J Ophthalmol 1996;44:131-43.
12. Olm J. Über die Behandlung der Netzhautablösung durch operative Entleerung der Subretinalen Flüssigkeit und Einspritzung von Luft in den Glaskörper. Albrecht von Graefes Arch Ophthalmol 1911;79:442-65.
13. Rosengren B. Results of treatment of detachment of the retina with diathermy and injection of air into the vitreous. Acta Ophthalmol 1938;16:573-9.
14. Chan CK, Lin SG, Nuthi AS, Salib DM. Pneumatic retinopexy for the repair of retinal detachments: A comprehensive review (1986-2007). Surv Ophthalmol 2008;53:443-78.
15. Kelly NE, Wendel RT. Vitreous surgery for idiopathic macular holes. Results of a pilot study. Arch Ophthalmol 1991;109:654-9.
16. Ohji M, Saito Y, Hayashi A, Lewis JM, Tano Y. Pneumatic displacement of subretinal hemorrhage without tissue plasminogen activator. Arch Ophthalmol 1998;116:1326-32.
17. Chawla S, Misra V, Khemchandani M. Pneumatic displacement and intravitreal bevacizumab: A new approach for management of submacular hemorrhage in choroidal neovascular membrane. Indian J Ophthalmol 2009;57:155-7.
18. Brinton DA, Hilton GF. Pneumatic retinopexy and alternative retinal detachment techniques, in Ryan SJ,Wilkinson CP (Eds): Retina, vol. 3. St Louis, MO, Mosby Inc, 3rd edn. 2001. pp. 2047-62.
19. Tornambe PE. Pneumatic retinopexy. Surv Ophthalmol 1988;32: 270-81.
20. Kwon OW, Kim SY. Changes in adhesive force between the retina and the retinal pigment epithelium by laser photocoagulation in rabbits. Yonsei Med J 1995;36:243-50.
21. Kita M, Negi A, Kawano SI, Honda Y. Photothermal cryogenic, and diathermic effects on retinal adhesive force *in vivo*. Retina 1991;11:441-4.
22. Poliner LS, Schoch LH. Intraocular pressure assessment in gas-filled eyes following vitrectomy. Arch Ophthalmol 1987;105:200-2.
23. Moses RA. Schiotz tonometry with an air bubble in the eye. Am J Ophthalmol 1966;62:281-2.

24. Abrams GW, Swanson DE, Sabates WL, et al. The result of a sulfur hexafluoride gas in vitreous surgery. Am J Ophthalmol 1982;94:165.
25. Van Horn DL, Edelhauser HF, Aaberg TM. *In vivo* effects of air and sulfur hexafluoride gas on rabbit corneal endothelium. Invest Ophthalmol 1972;11:1028.
26. Fineberg E, Machemer R, Sullivan P, et al. Sulfur hexafluoride in owl monkey vitreous cavity. Am J Ophthalmol 1975;79:67.
27. Lincoff H, Kressig I, Jacobiec F. The inadvertent injection of gas beneath the retina in a pseudophakic eye. Ophthalmology 1986;93:408.
28. Lowe MA, McDonald HR, Campo RV, et al. Pneumatic retinopexy: Surgical results. Arch Ophthalmol 1988;106:1672.

Pharmacology of Anti-VEGF Therapy

T Mark Johnson (USA)

VASCULAR ENDOTHELIAL GROWTH FACTOR AND ANGIOGENESIS

The development of abnormal blood vessels in ocular tissues can lead to significant visual loss. Pathologic neovascularization can lead to edema, hemorrhage and, ultimately, cicatricial changes that damages ocular structures including the cornea, trabecular meshwork, retina and choroid. Neovascularization is the central pathological process in exudative wet macular degeneration and other forms of choroidal neovascularization, diabetic macular edema, proliferative diabetic retinopathy, retinal venous occlusive disease, retinopathy of prematurity and sickle cell retinopathy.

Angiogenesis results in the proliferation of new vessels from the pre-existing vascular bed. Over the last several years many of the factors that promote and inhibit angiogenesis have been identified. Vascular endothelial growth factor (VEGF) has been shown to be a major promoter of neovascularization in the diabetic eye.[1,2] The VEGF has been isolated in surgically excised choroidal neovascular membranes (CNVM) in age-related macular degeneration (AMD).[3]

The VEGF is a mitogen for vascular endothelial cell proliferation. The VEGF also increases vascular permeability. The biological effects of VEGF are mediated by two tyrosine kinase receptors: VEGFR1 and VEGFR2. Several isoforms of VEGF result from alternative splicing of exons. The VEGF 121 is weakly acidic and has low affinity for heparin binding. The VEGF 165 is basic and has a high affinity for heparin binding. Both forms are freely diffusible. The VEGF 189 and VEGF 206 are sequestered in the extracellular matrix.[4] The properties of these isoforms may play a role in pathogenesis of different disorders.

The development of agents to inhibit VEGF has marked a major advance in ocular therapeutics.

Pharmacology of Anti-VEGF Agents

Pegaptanib

Pegaptanib is a RNA aptamer directed against the VEGF 165 isoform. Aptamers are oligonucleotide ligands that bind to the target molecule with high affinity. The complex secondary and tertiary structure of RNA aptamers increases their specificity for the target molecule. Pegaptanib is an oligonucleotide of 28 nucleotides in length that terminates in a pentylamino linker to which two 20 kilodalton monomethoxyl polyethelene glycol units are covalently attached. It has a molecular weight of 50 kilodaltons. A single dose is equivalent to 1.6 mg of pegaptanib sodium. Its mechanism of action is binding extracellular VEGF. It selectively blocks VEGF 165.

Pharmacokinetics: After intravitreal injection pegaptanib is absorbed into the systemic circulation with a peak plasma level occurring approximately 1 to 4 days post injection. Peak serum levels are measured at 80 ng/ml. The vitreous half-life of pegaptanib is approximately 10 days.[5]

Bevacizumab

Bevacizumab is a recombinant, humanized, monoclonal IgG1 antibody directed against all isoforms of VEGF. It blocks the interaction of VEGF with its receptor. It has a molecular weight of 149 kilodaltons. It is produced in mammalian Chinese hamster ovary (CHO) cells.

Pharmacokinetics: In animal models, the half-life of bevacizumab is approximately 4 days.[6] Serum levels following intravitreal injection of bevacizumab in animal models was approximately 5 ng/ml.[7] There is little data in humans.

Ranibizumab

Ranibizumab is a recombinant, humanized Fab fragment of the anti-VEGF antibody and is directed against all isoforms of VEGF. The molecule lacks an Fc region. The molecular weight is 48 kilodaltons. It is produced by an *E. coli* expression system. It is supplied in a preservative free sterile solution and is available in a 0.5 mg dose vial (0.05 ml of 10 mg/ml) or 0.3 mg dose vial (0.05 ml of 6 mg/ml). Its mechanism of action is binding to the receptor site of the active form of VEGF-A and prevents interaction of VEGF-A with the VEGF 1 and VEGF 2 receptors on the surface of endothelial cells.[8]

Pharmacokinetics: In animal models, the vitreous half-life of ranibizumab is 3 days. In human subjects administered monthly intravitreal doses the serum concentrations of ranibizumab were low, ranging from 0.3 ng/ml to 27 ng/ml. These levels are considered to be less that than the amount required to inhibit the biological activity of VEGF-A by 50 percent.[9]

Aflibercept

Aflibercept is a high affinity antagonist of VEGF that is produced by fusing the immunoglobulin domain 2 of human VEGF receptor 1 (VEGFR1) and domain 3 of human VEGF receptor 2 (VEGFR2) to the Fc fragment of IgG. It blocks VEGF in tissues and in the circulation and also binds placental growth factor (PlGF). It is administered as a 2 mg/0.05 ml injection. It has a molecular weight of 115 kDa. It is produced in recombinant Chinese hamster ovary (CHO) cells.

Pharmacokinetics: In human subjects, the serum concentration of aflibercept following 2 mg injections was 0.02 mcg/ml after 1 to 3 days. No accumulation with cumulative dosing has been observed. The serum concentrations are below the levels necessary for 50 percent inactivation of serum VEGF activity.

ADMINISTRATION OF ANTI-VEGF THERAPY

Intravitreal injections of anti-VEGF agents are typically administered in a clinic setting with little difficulty.

Local anesthesia is administered prior to injection. There is some debate as to whether a preferred method of anesthesia exists. The most common methods include: topical drops; viscous anesthetic drops; anesthetic applied with cotton tip applicator of pledget; and subconjunctival anesthetic. Overall there appears to be little difference in experienced pain with the overall procedure between the 4 techniques. Topical drops are associated with the least amount of pain during administration but higher levels of pain when the injection is performed.[10] In a randomized study of 24 patients subconjunctival lidocaine was found to have the lowest amount of pain at the time of the injection, however, the finding was not statistically significant. Subconjunctival anesthesia may be complicated by subconjunctival hemorrhage.[11]

The precise techniques of injection are highly variable. Most practitioners routinely use a sterile eyelid speculum and povidone-iodine prep on the ocular surface prior to injection. Most injections are administered directly into the vitreous cavity with a small percentage of practitioners displacing the conjunctiva prior to injection. Seventy-two percent of practitioners grossly assess visual acuity post injection to confirm perfusion of the optic nerve. 46 percent perform simultaneous bilateral injections.[12] Two thirds of practitioners used post injection antibiotics.

The use of antibiotics before and after intravitreal injections is controversial. Topical antibiotic use prior to injection was found to produce a similar decrease in bacterial colonies and species compared to topical povidone-iodine prep, however, when used together the greatest reduction in bacterial colonies was observed.[13] The DRCR network protocol for intravitreal injection did not incorporate a topical antibiotic and found a low rate of endophthalmitis.[14]

The high preponderance of streptococcal species isolated from post injection endophthalmitis has caused some authors to postulate that the primary source of infection is oral dispersion of organisms contaminating the field at the time of injection.[15] This has led some practitioners to consider the use of face masks at the time of injection or using a 'no talk' technique during injection. To date the use of face masks at the time of injection has not been shown to be clearly beneficial in the prevention of endophthalmitis.[16]

SIDE EFFECTS OF ANTI-VEGF THERAPY

Intravitreal injections of anti-VEGF agents have been associated with a remarkably high degree of safety. Safety concerns can be divided into local and systemic adverse events.

The most significant risk associated with intravitreal injection is endophthalmitis. A number of large, prospective case series have demonstrated a very low rate of injection ranging from 0.19 to 0.29 percent.[17,18] The microbial spectrum observed in endophthalmitis following intravitreal injection differs from that of post cataract surgery endophthalmitis. Specifically *Streptococcus* species seem to be the predominant pathogen. In a meta-analysis of post injection endophthalmitis *Streptococcus* species were found to represent 30.8 percent of culture positive isolates.[19]

Uveitis has been reported following intravitreal injection of anti-VEGF agents. In the FOCUS trial of ranibizumab of PDT alone or in combination with ranibizumab at 12.4 percent 2 year incidence of inflammation was reported. This formulation of ranibizumab was different than the commercially available form.[20] Bevacizumab has been associated with a 0.1 to 0.4 percent incidence of uveitis.[21,22] Sporadic lot specific inflammatory outbreaks have also been reported.

RPE tears have been described in macular degeneration patients receiving anti-VEGF therapy. It is difficult to determine whether these RPE tears represent a complication of therapy or part of the underlying pathology as they are known to occur spontaneously in AMD patients. The relatively low rate of RPE tears observed in the clinical trials of anti-VEGF agents likely reflects the exclusion of patients with pre-existing RPE detachments. The rate of RPE tears in one study of bevacizumab therapy demonstrated a 17 percent rate of RPE rip in patients with vascularized RPE detachments at initiation of therapy.[23]

Minor and transient side effects from intravitreal injection including pain, foreign body sensation, irritation, tearing and blurred vision are common but not serious.

Concerns regarding the systemic safety of anti-VEGF agents have been expressed due to the potential effects on systemic circulating VEGF. Serious cardiovascular adverse events are classified according to the Antiplatelet Trialists' Collaboration (ATC) and including nonfatal myocardial infarction, nonfatal ischemic stroke, nonfatal hemorrhagic stroke or death owing to vascular or unknown cause.[24] The rates of these events in the ANCHOR trial (PDT versus ranibizumab) at 2 years was 4.9 percent in the PDT group, 4.4 percent in the 0.3 mg ranibizumab group and 5.0 percent in the 0.5 mg ranibizumab group.[25] No statistical difference was observed in ATC outcomes in the MARINA trial (ranibizumab versus placebo in occult CNV).[26] Cardiovascular complications were shown to be low and equally distributed in the CATT trial (bevacizumab versus ranibizumab for AMD) at 2 years.[27] In the VIEW1 and VIEW2 trials of afibercept versus ranibizumab the ATC outcome rate was 2.2 percent without significant differences between treatment groups.

CONCLUSION

The advent of anti-VEGF therapy has revolutionized the care of patients with blinding retinal disorders. These agents are now first-line therapy for exudative macular degeneration, retinal venous occlusive disease and increasingly diabetic retinopathy. Their efficacy is well demonstrated as is their excellent safety profile.

REFERENCES

1. Aiello LP, Avery RL, Arrigg PG, et al. Vascular endothelial growth factor in ocular fluid of patients with diabetic retinopathy and other retinal disorders. N Engl J Med 1994;331:1480-7.
2. Miller JW, Adamis AP, Shima DT, et al. Vascular endothelial growth factor/vascular permeability factor is temporally and spatially correlated with ocular angiogenesis in a primate model. Am J Pathol 1994;145:574-84.
3. Lopez PF, Sippy BD, Lambert HM, et al. Transdifferentiated retinal pigment epithelial cells are immunoreactive for vascular endothelial growth factor in surgically excised age-related macular degeneration-related choroidal neovascular membranes. Invest Ophthalmol Vis Sci 1996;37:855-68.
4. Ferrera N. Role of vascular endothelial growth factor in regulation of physiological angiogenesis. Am J Physiol Cell Physiol 2001; 280(6):C1358-66.
5. Patel M, Whitfield L, Hutmacher M, et al. Population pharmacokinetics/pharmacodynamics (PK/PD) of pegaptanib sodium (Macugen) in patients with age-related macular degeneration (AMD). Assoc for Research in Vision and Ophthalmology, 2006. Program #2623.
6. Bakri SJ, Snyder MR, Reid JM, et al. Pharmacokinetics of intravitreal bevacizumab. Ophthalmol 2007;114:855-9.
7. Chuan L, Wu W, Yeung L, et al. Serum concentration of bevacizumab after intravitreal injection in experimental branch retinal vein occlusion. Ophthalmic Research 2011;45(1):31-5.
8. Prescribing information (package insert): Lucentis™ (ranibizumab injection), Genentech, Inc., South San Francisco, CA, June 2006.
9. Gaudreault J, Fei D, Rusit J, Suboc P, Shiu V. Preclinical pharmacokinetics of Ranibizumab (rhuFabV2) after a single intravitreal administration. Invest Ophthalmol Vis Sci 2005;46(2):726-33.
10. Kaderli B, Avci R. Comparison of topical and subconjunctival anesthesia in intravitreal injection administrations. Eur J Ophthalmol 2006;16:718-21.
11. Blaha GR, Tilton EP, Barouch FC, et al. Randomized trial of anesthetic methods for intravitreal injections. Retina 2011;31:535-9.
12. Green-Sims AE, Ekdai NS, Bakri S. Survey of intravitreal injection techniques among retinal specialists in the United States. Am J Ophthalmol 2011;151:329-32.
13. Isenberg SJ, Apt L, Yoshimori R, khwarg S. Chemical preparation of the eye in ophthalmic surgery. IV. Comparison of povidone-iodine on the conjunctiva with a prophylactic antibiotic. Arch Ophthalmol 1985;103:1340-1.
14. Bhavsar AR, Googe JM Jr, Stockdale CR, et al. Risk of endophthalmitis after intravitreal drug injection when topical antibiotics are not required: The diabetic retinopathy clinical research network laser-ranibizumab-triamcinolone clinical trials. Arch Ophthalmol 2009;127:1581-3.
15. Wen JC, McCannel CA, Mochon AB, Garner OB. Bacterial dispersal associated with speech in the setting of intravitreous injections. Arch Ophthalmol 2011;129(12):1551-4.

16. Schimel AM, Scott IU, Flynn HW. Endophthalmitis after intravitreal injections: Should the use of face masks be standard of care? Arch Ophthalmol 2011;129:1607-9.
17. Mason JO, White MF, Feist RM, et al. Incidence of acute onset endophthalmitis following intravitreal bevacizumab (Avastin) injection. Retina 2008;28(4):564-7.
18. Pilli S, Kotsolis A, Spaide RF, et al. Endophthalmitis associated with intravitreal anti-vascular endothelial growth factor therapy injections in an office setting. Am J Ophthalmol 2008;145(5):879-82.
19. McCannel CA. Meta-analysis of endophthalmitis after intravitreal injection of anti-vascular endothelial growth factor agents: causative organisms and possible prevention strategies. Retina 2011;31(4):654-61.
20. Heier JS, Boyer DS, Ciulla TA, et al. Ranibizumab combined with verteporfin photodynamic therapy in neovascular age related macular degeneration: year 1 results of the FOCUS Study. Arch Ophthalmol 2006;124(11):1532-42.
21. Wu L, Martinez-Castellanos MA, Quiroz-Mercado H, et al. Twelve-month safety of intravitreal injections of bevacizumab (Avastin): results of the Pan-American Collaborative Retina Study Group (PACORES). Graefes Arch Clin Exp Ophthalmol 2008;246(1):81-7.
22. Fung AE, Rosenfeld PJ, Reichel E. The International Intravitreal Bevacizumab Safety Survey: using the Internet to assess drug safety worldwide. Br J Ophthalmol 2006;90(11):1344-9.
23. Chan CK, Abraham P, Meyer CH, et al. Optical coherence tomography-measured pigment epithelial detachment height as a predictor for retinal pigment epithelial tears associated with intravitreal bevacizumab injections. Retina 2010;30(2):203-11.
24. Antiplatelet Trialists' Collaboration. Collaborative overview of randomised trials of antiplatelet therapy-I: Prevention of death, myocardial infarction, and stroke by prolonged antiplatelet therapy in various categories of patients. BMJ 1994;308(6921):81-106.
25. Brown DM, Michels M, Kaiser PK, et al. Ranibizumab versus verteporfin photodynamic therapy for neovascular age related macular degeneration: two-year results of the ANCHOR study. Ophthalmology 2009;116(1):57-65.
26. Rosenfeld PJ, Brown DM, Heier JS, et al. For the MARINA Study Group. Ranibizumab for neovascular age-related macular degeneration. N Engl J Med 2006;355(14):1419-31.
27. Complications of Macular Degeneration Treatments Trials Research Group. Ranibizumab and bevacizumab for treatment of neovascular age related macular degeneration: two year results. Ophthalmol 2012;119:1388-98.

Section 3

Recent Advances in Ocular Therapeutics

# Toxic Anterior Segment Syndrome

*Simon P Holland, Douglas W Morck, Richard Mathias,
Tracy L Lee, Gina Chavez, Yumi G Ohashi (Canada)*

INTRODUCTION

Toxic anterior segment syndrome (TASS) is increasingly recognized and reported as an early complication of cataract surgery.[1-9] Postoperative inflammation of unknown cause was previously considered as a sterile endophthalmitis although vitritis is uncommon. Multiple outbreaks have recently been reported stimulating extensive research and the creation of a task force. The understanding of TASS is thus rapidly evolving and will likely lead to improved prevention and management of outbreaks.

Diagnosis and Clinical Features

Toxic anterior segment syndrome presents as early and severe postoperative inflammation following anterior segment surgery. Symptoms include fibrin formation, corneal edema, minimal or no pain, and the absence of vitreous involvement.[10] Differentiation from conditions such as infectious endophthalmitis (IE) is critical. Table 57.1 summarizes the key differences between TASS and IE. TASS usually presents on the day of surgery or the first day postoperatively, whereas IE presents later, usually day 3 to 7, accompanied by pain and vitreal involvement.[10-13] Figure 57.1 shows a case of TASS with characteristic features presenting on the day of surgery, and Figure 57.2 shows a case of IE. Rarely low grade vitritis may be seen in severe cases of TASS probably from some spillover from the anterior segment. In such cases the vitritis is a result of culture-negative or sterile endophthalmitis rather than infectious endophthalmitis.[10,11] Vitreous taps and more recently PCR can be used to differentiate the two conditions.[14] When the diagnosis is unclear the practitioner should treat as IE due to the severity of its sequelae.[15,16]

Diagnosis
Postoperative
Anterior segment inflammation
Unknown cause

Differential diagnosis
Pain and/or vitritis usually indicates infectious endophthalmitis

TABLE 57.1: Differential diagnosis TASS vs. infectious endophthalmitis

Presentation	TASS	Infectious endophthalmitis
Onset (usual)	6 to 24 hours postoperatively	3 to 7 days postoperatively
Symptoms	Blurred vision	Pain, blurred vision
Cornea	Edema	Edema
Anterior chamber	Cells Fibrin, membranes Hypopyon	Cells Fibrin variable Hypopyon
External findings	None	Variable Lid swelling Discharge Conjunctival chemosis
Vitreous	Clear, rarely vitritis (culture negative)	Vitritis (primarily culture positive)
Response to topical steroids	Rapid improvement to resolution within days	No improvement

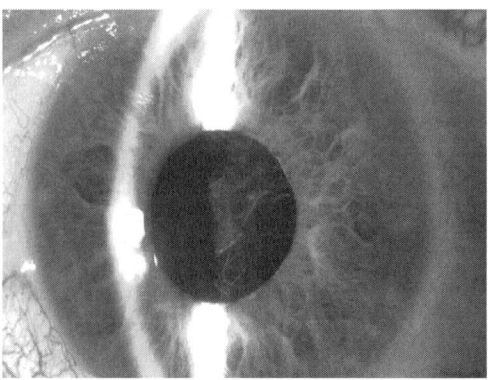

Fig. 57.1: Toxic anterior segment syndrome on the first postoperative day (*Courtesy:* SLACK Inc)[10]

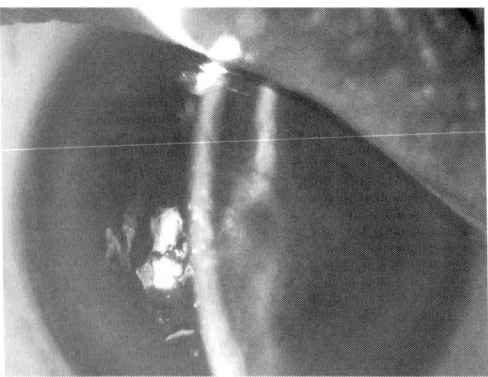

Fig. 57.2: Early endophthalmitis presenting on the day of surgery (*Courtesy:* SLACK Inc)[10]

Toxic endothelial cell destruction syndrome (TECDS) is a related syndrome that specifically indicates localized corneal endothelial damage and is considered to be within the continuum of TASS.[2,5,7,17]

The clinical features of TASS have been well described in previous literature.[1,2,5,7,10,11] Most patients are asymptomatic but may have blurred vision and redness within 24 hours of surgery. Pain is almost never a feature although there may be mild discomfort. Characteristic clinical features include a severe anterior chamber cellular response with fibrin, membrane formation and the occasional hypopyon. Corneal edema, described as limbus to limbus, is frequently present.[10,11,18] When patients present predominantly with corneal edema and less marked anterior chamber inflammation the cause is more likely to be toxic agents (e.g. preservatives, ointments).

Features
- Within 48 hours
- Cellular reaction 2-4+
- Fibrin/membranes
- Corneal edema
- No or minimal pain

Pathology

Changes to the pH and osmolality or the inadvertent introduction of an antigen can initiate a cellular response. The histological exams of corneal buttons taken from patients with TASS showed an almost absent endothelial cell layer, with the epithelium thinned and the stroma diffusely thickened.[8] The massive damage to the endothelial layer is a result of its sensitivity to toxic agents.[11]

Epidemiology and Etiology

The epidemic in the United States prompted the American Society of Cataract and Refractive Surgery (ASCRS) to assemble a special task force to deal with the growing problem.[19] The task force reported that over 100 centers experienced an outbreak of TASS prior to May 2006 and this only included clinics that chose to self report.[20] Many outbreaks may be unreported given the potential for poor publicity, and regulatory and liability issues. The increasing incidence of TASS is likely due to an actual rise in numbers rather than simply an increased awareness. Growing interest in TASS is resulting in the rapid expansion of knowledge regarding the cause and therefore the management and prevention of the condition.

The etiology of TASS is speculative, although there is increasing acceptance of its multifactorial causation. The ASCRS task force, and several other researchers have complied a list of possible risk factors and potential causes of TASS.[3,5-8,20-23] These potential etiology factors are listed in Table 57.2.[10] It is likely that individual TASS cases not occurring in an outbreak are due to complications during surgery such as iris stretching, retained cortex and a prolonged surgery.[10] Multiple factors have been associated with

> **TABLE 57.2: Potential etiology factors associated with TASS (previously published: SLACK Inc)[10]**
>
> *Intraocular causes*
> - Incomplete cortex removal, pupil stretching, and possible immunological differences (as with DLK in atopic patients).
>
> *Intraocular medication*
> - Dosing errors with antibiotics, preservatives, ointments,[8] and pH imbalance.
>
> *Instrument contamination*
> - Bacterial endotoxins, dried debris, e.g. inadequate cleaning of cannulas, persistence of detergents, irrigating solutions, endotoxins in irrigating fluids (Endosol),[10,24] incorrect pH or composition of irrigating fluids.

TASS outbreaks ranging from inappropriate chemical composition of irrigating solutions to the presence of endotoxins on poorly sterilized instruments.[13]

Intraocular medications, irrigating solutions and balanced salt solution. Many TASS outbreaks have been attributed to contaminants, endotoxins and preservatives gaining access to the anterior chamber during or following surgery.[5,7,12] Outbreaks have been linked to external eye rinses, such as eye Stream (Alcon, Ft. Worth, Texas) due to the preservative content.[5] Ointments applied postoperatively also have the potential to gain access to the anterior chamber. One study described a TASS outbreak following the application of postoperative ointments and tight eye patching.[8] The use of contaminated balanced salt solution (BSS) has also been associated with TASS outbreaks. Endotoxin was discovered in balanced salt solution (BSS) manufactured by Cytosol Laboratories (Lenoir, NC).[10,24]

Instrument Contamination

Detergent residues left on reusable instruments have the potential to cause corneal toxicity.[2,21] Prolonged cycle sterilization is needed to deactivate enzymes and other active ingredients in detergents.[11] TASS outbreaks have been associated with the dried residue on reusable cannulas.[10]

Impurities can also be present in sterilizer steam.[9,22] An outbreak of TASS was associated with inadequate maintenance of steam sterilizer systems with resulting copper, zinc, nickel, sulfate and silica impurities.[9] Instruments can also become contaminated with endotoxin following short cycle steam sterilization.[25] The sterilization process kills bacteria but does not inactivate endotoxin, which can be a potent initiator of an inflammatory immune response and has been associated with TASS outbreaks.[10,11,22,26]

Ultrasound baths may also be a source of contamination. Klebsiella pneumonia and bacterial endotoxin were identified in the ultrasonic cleaning bath during one TASS outbreak.[3]

TASS is often associated with IOL implantation, but more recently has also been observed following placement of phakic

IOL.[18] It is important to consider IOL polishing compounds, as well as the chemical structure of the lens as possible causes of TASS.[6,23]

> *Etiology*
> - Edema—toxic, e.g. preservatives
> - Inflammation—endotoxin

> *Causation*
> - Sterilization issues most common
> - Beware of reusable cannulas

Treatment

Conventional treatment is focused on the suppression of the inflammatory immune response and includes topical steroids given every half-hour to hour for the first three days followed by gradual tapering.[10] During this acute period the patient should be monitored closely for anterior segment inflammation, corneal edema, and intraocular pressure (IOP). In particular monitor for an IOP increase several days following the initial presentation due to damage to the trabecular meshwork.[11] Improvements are generally seen within the first 24 to 48 hours of steroid commencement.

Anterior chamber washout has been reported but outcomes are uncertain and it is not generally recommended.[10,11] When there is corneal and endothelial toxicity a penetrating keratoplasty may be necessary.

> *Treatment points*
> Rapid response to frequent steroid drops

Outcomes

Early diagnosis and treatment usually result in an excellent outcome. Most mild cases clear within several days to weeks.[21] Glaucoma is a potential complication due to either initial trabeculitis or fibrin membrane formation.[10] Severe TASS can result in permanent endothelial damage, cystoid macular edema and permanently dilated pupil requiring corrective surgery.[21]

> *Complications*
> - Misdiagnosis
> - Glaucoma
> - Corneal edema
> - Cystoid macular edema

Investigation and Reporting

Outbreak investigation is difficult with the multifactorial etiology although sterilization issues usually predominate. Consequences to an affected clinic may be severe with voluntary or mandated closure. Proactive reporting to local regulatory authorities and seeking support from colleagues, as well as academic and public health resources is advisable.[10,27]

Case and Outbreak Definition

Postoperative anterior segment inflammation of unknown cause occurring within 48 hours of surgery with one or more of the following features: anterior chamber response 2+ or greater, fibrin, membranes, corneal edema without significant vitritis.[10] Criteria for a TASS outbreak have not been established as they have for conditions such as DLK.[28] However, any occurrence of more than two affected patients should raise concerns and merit investigation since this may rapidly escalate.

Data Collection

Suggested data include; demographics, VA before and after surgery, symptoms, clinical features, day of surgery, day of onset and diagnosis, any associated conditions, subsequent management and outcome. It is important to record details of the surgical procedure including instrument preparation and specifically any staffing or procedural changes made prior to the onset. Retrospective collection of data is difficult and it is recommended to collect data and note changes as they happen making the creation of an epidemic curve less problematic.

Microbial Investigations

Bacterial culturing, biofilm sampling and analysis of steam distillate and BSS for endotoxin may help determine the cause of the outbreak. The sterilizer reservoir, internal tubing of the sterilizer, ultrasound baths, cannulas and air and water supplies have proved to be useful sampling areas.[10,12,13]

Toxic anterior segment syndrome investigations are often difficult and require careful planning. It is usually best to designate one staff member to manage the outbreak, including data collection and media consultation. Another important issue to consider is the disclosure of TASS as a further risk of cataract surgery, particularly during a TASS outbreak.

Once an investigation has been concluded dissemination of the findings will help other practitioners solve their TASS outbreaks or hopefully avoid them. The TASS task force is one example of how this sharing of knowledge has likely reduced the risk of further outbreaks.

> Investigation
> Suspect everything

CONCLUSION

Toxic anterior segment syndrome outbreaks have become of major concern in the ophthalmology community. The assembly of the TASS task force and the numerous recent studies on the subject has assisted in controlling TASS outbreaks. The final task force report concluded that there was no one factor attributable to TASS outbreaks but rather multiple potential etiological factors.

It appeared that cleaning and sterilization of instruments for cataract surgery was the most important of the identified factors. It is recommended that all reusable cannulas and instruments be thoroughly flushed with sterile, deionized/distilled water after cleaning at the conclusion of each case.[29]

Although TASS outbreak reports, at least in the United States, now appear to be declining it is important to constantly monitor and improve cleaning and sterilization protocols. Growing awareness resulting in early diagnosis and treatment, with prompt dissemination of new information will hopefully eliminate TASS as a significant complication of modern cataract surgery.

REFERENCES

1. Monson MC, Mamalis N, Olson RJ. Toxic anterior segment inflammation following cataract surgery. J Cataract Refract Surg 1992;18:184-9.
2. Breebaart AC, Nuyts RMMA, Pels E, et al. Toxic endothelial destruction of the cornea after routine extracapsular cataract surgery. Arch Ophthalmol 1990; 108:1121-5.
3. Kreisler KR, Martin SS, Young CW, et al. Postoperative inflammation following cataract extraction caused by bacterial contamination of the cleaning bath detergent. J Cataract Refract Surg 1992;18:106-10.
4. Nelson DB, Donnenfeld ED, Perry HD. Sterile endophthalmitis after sutureless cataract surgery. Ophthalmolgy 1992;99:1655-7.
5. Liu H, Routley I, Teichmann KD. Toxic endothelial cell destruction from intraocular benzalkonium chloride. J Cataract Refract Surg 2001;27:1746-50.
6. Jehan FS, Mamalis N, Spencer TS, et al. Postoperative sterile endophthalmitis (TASS) with the MemoryLens. J Cataract Refract Surg 2000;26:1773-7.
7. Eleftheriadis H, Cheong M, Saneman S, et al. Corneal toxicity secondary to inadvertent use of benzalkonium chloride preserved viscoelastic material in cataract surgery. Br J Ophthalmol 2002;86:299-305.
8. Werner L, Sher JH, Taylor JR, et al. Toxic anterior segment syndrome and possible association with ointment in the anterior chamber following cataract surgery. J Cataract Refract Surg 2006;32:227-35.
9. Hellinger WC, Hasan SA, Bacalis LP, et al. Outbreak of toxic anterior chamber syndrome following cataract surgery associated with impurities of autoclave steam moisture. Infect Control Hosp Epidemiol 2006;27(13):294-8.
10. Holland SP, Morck DW, Chavez G, Lee TL. Toxic anterior segment syndrome. In: Agarwal A, (Ed). Refractive Surgery Nightmares: Conquering Refractive Surgery Catastrophes. Thorofare, NJ: SLACK Incorporated. In press.
11. Mamalis N, Edelhauser HF, Dawson DG, et al. Toxic anterior segment syndrome. Review/update. J Cataract Refract Surg 2006;32:324-33.
12. Holland SP, Chavex G, Morck D, Mathias. Toxic Anterior Segment Syndrome After Cataract Surgery Associated with Short-Cycle Sterilization presented at the ASCRS Symposium on Cataract, IOL and Refractive Surgery, San Francisco, USA, March 17-22, 2006. Available at www.ascrs.org. Accessed June 12, 2006.

13. Holland SP, Morck D, Lee T. Update on toxic anterior segment syndrome. Current Opinion in Ophthalmology. In press.
14. Van Gelder RN. Applications of the polymerase chain reaction to diagnosis of ophthalmic disease. Surv Ophthalmol 2001;45(3):248-58.
15. West ES, Behrens A, McDonnell PJ, et al. The incidence of endophthalmitis after cataract surgery among the US medicare population increased between 1994 and 2001. Ophthalmology 2005;112:1388-95.
16. Wallin T, Parker J, Jin Y, et al. Cohort study of 27 cases of endophthalmitis at a single institution. J Cataract Refract Surg 2005;31:735-41.
17. Duffy RE, Brown SE, Caldwell KL, et al. An epidemic of corneal destruction caused by plasma gas sterilization; the Toxic Endothelial Cell Destruction Syndrome Team. Arch Ophthalmology 2000;118:1167-76.
18. Moshirfar M, Whitehead G, Beutler BC, et al. Toxic anterior segment syndrome after Verisyse iris-supported phakic intraocular lens implantation. J Cataract Refract Surg 2006;32(7):1233-7.
19. The American Society of Cataract and Refractive Surgery (ASCRS). (2005). Press release June 22, 2006: TASS task force. Retrieved August 15, 2006, from http://www.ascrs.org/press_releases/Toxic-Anterior-Segment-Syndrome-Outbreak-Preliminary-Report.cfm.
20. The American Society of Cataract and Refractive Surgery (ASCRS). (2005). Press release May 22, 2006: TASS Outbreak Update. Retrieved June 1, 2006, from http://www.ascrs.org/press_releases/upload/UpdateBriefing.doc.
21. Parikh C, Sippy BD, Martin DF, Edelhauser HF. Effects of enzymatic sterilization detergents on the corneal endothelium. Arch Ophthalmol 2002;120:165-72.
22. Whitby JL, Hitchins VM. Endotoxin levels in steam and reservoirs of table-top steam sterilzers. J Cataract Refract Surg 2002;18:51-2.
23. Meltzer, DW. Sterile hypopyon following intraocular lens surgery. Arch Ophthalmol 1980;98:100-4.
24. US Food and Drug Administration. Patient advisory Feb 13th 2006; FDA-Requested Recall - Cytosol Laboratories, Inc. Product Contains Dangerous Levels of Endotoxin. Retrieved Feb. 14, 2006, from http://www.fda.gov/bbs/topics/news/2006/NEW01315.html.
25. Holland SP, Mathias RG, Morck DW, et al. Diffuse lamellar keratitis related to endotoxins released from sterilizer reservoir biofilms. Ophthalmol 2000; 107(7):1227-33.
26. Rietschel ET, Brade H. Bacterial endotoxins. Sci Am 1992;267:54-61.
27. Mamalis, N. 2006. TASS outbreaks: What should we do? Cataract and Refractive Surgery Today, July 2006;53-5.
28. Bigham M, Enns CL, Holland SP, et al. Diffuse lamellar keratitis complicating laser *in situ* keratomileusis; Post-marketing surveillance of an emerging disease in British Columbia, Canada, 2000-2002. J Cataract Refract Surg 2005;31:2340-4.
29. The American Society of Cataract and Refractive Surgery (ASCRS). (2005). Press release September 22, 2006: Toxic Anterior Segment Syndrome (TASS) Outbreak Final Report. Retrieved September 22, 2006, from http://www.ascrs.org/press_releases/Final-TASS-Report.cfm.

# 58

Anesthesia Trends in Ophthalmology

Arbisser Lisa (USA)

HISTORY

Historically ophthalmic anesthesia trends recapitulate modern trends in reverse. Cocaine as a topical cataract surgery anesthetic preceded general anesthesia's invention. General anesthesia for intracapsular cataract extractions transitioned to local or regional anesthetics as surgery evolved to extracapsular techniques with smaller incisions facilitating more rapid recovery. The topical anesthetic approach steadily gained favor in modern times along with smaller self sealing incisions and outpatient cataract surgery.[1,2]

PERIOPERATIVE WORKUP

Traditionally the presence of an anesthesiologist working in concert with the ophthalmic surgeon provided a means of handling unforeseen systemic emergencies without compromising the safety of the eye as well as offering sedation and analgesia as needed intraoperatively. Economic conditions occasionally challenge payment however the vast majority of American ophthalmologists still work in collaboration with anesthesia professionals or surrogates. Intravenous access by IV or saline lock is most commonly employed for medication or emergency intervention but there is some trend towards its elimination with the use of sublingual sedation. Conscious sedation and anxiety relief enabling the patient's cooperation rather than true hypnosis and amnesia is often obtained with minute doses of versed and alfentanil or fentanyl intraoperatively.[3] If regional anesthesia is indicated, briefly obtunding the patient with propofol preceding the orbital injection is commonly but not uniformly practiced. Regardless, upwards of 90 percent of patients are monitored perioperatively for pulse rate and oxygen saturation. Blood pressure is monitored in 80 percent of cases and just over 60 percent with electrocardiogram. Regional anesthesia, most often provided by the ophthalmologist, is sometimes delegated for efficiency to specially trained and experienced anesthesiologists.[4]

The practice of obtaining blood work and chest X-ray demonstrated a poor cost/benefit ratio with the possible exception of cases requiring general anesthesia which is currently limited mostly to pediatric cataract, dementia and mentally handicapped patients or open globe injury. Getting an INR for patients on anticoagulants remains valued by some if injected regional anesthesia is considered; it is irrelevant to topical anesthesia and clear corneal incisional cataract surgery; the majority of cases today.

TRENDS IN TOPICAL ANESTHESIA

Relevant recent studies of trends[4-7] all reveal the increasing preponderance of topical anesthesia as a primary choice for cataract surgery over regional blocks producing akinesia. The use of topical grew from 7 percent in 1995 to 30 percent in 1997 to 62 percent in 2000 and has continued to climb in the US. Of those, 80 percent used 0.5 cc of intracameral preservative and preferably bisulfite free 1 percent lidocaine as well. Higher volume surgeons tended more towards the use of topical anesthesia.

The value of intracameral supplementation to topical anesthesia has been controversial however a meta-analysis of the literature showed significantly lower intraoperative pain perception. With topical technique only the trigeminal nerve endings in the cornea and conjunctiva are blocked and not intraocular structures. Pressure or pain on manipulation of the iris or stretching of the ciliary nerves can still be perceived. No significant difference in intraoperative adverse events, corneal toxicity, or the need for supplemental anesthesia was identified in one study. Another more recent randomized trail resulted in outcomes that justify its use as well.[8,9]

Over the last decade the agent for topical anesthesia trended towards lidocaine 2 percent gel. It demonstrates relatively low epithelial toxicity. This necessitates another agent, in drop rather than gel form such as tetracaine 0.5 percent or proparacaine be used in addition, as preoperative sterilization of the ocular surface with betadine 5 percent (the standard of care for endophthalmitis prophylaxis) stings on instillation and is not effective after gel is used on the ocular surface. In accordance with the results of a randomized trail comparing both the gel vs tetracaine alone showing no significant difference in analgesic effort, and for the sake of cost, the gel is less frequently used today.[10]

If complications during topical anesthetic cataract surgery arise requiring a sclerotomy for vitrectomy it is necessary to inject a subconjunctival bleb of lidocaine over the area of the intended incision prior to incising the sclera to avoid pain on penetration.

TRENDS IN REGIONAL ANESTHESIA

Regional anesthesia, the standard of care in past decades, provides akinesia as well as anesthesia. It was practiced as the primary means of anesthesia for cataract surgery by less than 20 percent of respondents to the ASCRS 2003 survey and by 26 percent at the VA in 2012 (probably owing to resident training at those facilities). This percentage is falling. A meta-analysis showed that intraoperative and postoperative pain perception was significantly higher with topical anesthesia ($P < 0.05$), resulted in more frequent inadvertent ocular movement ($P < 0.05$) and greater intraoperative need for supplementary anesthesia (P = 0.03). Never the less there was no statistically significant difference between TA and retrobulbar/peribulbar anesthesia (RBA/PBA) in intraoperative difficulties as assessed by the surgeons (P > 0.05). Despite the increased discomfort patients significantly preferred TA (P < 0.00001). The RBA/PBA group demonstrates more frequent anesthesia-related complications, such as chemosis, periorbital hematoma, and subconjunctival hemorrhage (P < 0.05). There was no statistically significant difference in surgery-related complications (P > 0.05).[11] Though not encountered in that study, complications of injection anesthesia can be vision threatening including intrasheath, intravascular, and intraocular injection and perforation as well as retrobulbar hemorrhage, strabismus and ptosis; TA eliminated those complications so the trend is understandable. Of particular note is the 60-fold higher probability of ocular penetration or perforation in eyes with staphylomas most likely seen in longer myopic eyes. These patients should be identified and considered high-risk for regional anesthesia.[12] There has been a trend towards the use of blunt rather than sharp needles for regional anesthesia though it is not clear this significantly affects the complication rate.[13]

Injection techniques other than RBA/PBA such as facial nerve block and sub-Tenon's injection (parabulbar) are rarely employed today. The former is unnecessary with the advent of hyaluronidase as an adjuvant in the anesthetic mixture. This speeds the onset of action, helps distribute the bolus through the tissues and minimizes anesthetic toxicity to extraocular muscles. Epinephrine is often added to lidocaine to prolong its effect. Bupivacaine is sometimes employed in combination with lidocaine or alone for surgeries other than cataract such as retinal detachment repair when a longer intervention is anticipated. Sub-Tenon's injection avoids the risks of sharp needles but requires a cut down to sclera often resulting in subconjunctival hemorrhage and chemosis and is rarely employed. This however is the best technique in the rare event that akenesia is required intraoperatively with an open eye.

The trend through the 1990's to now has been an increase in the use of peribulbar techniques (extraconal) over retrobulbar (intraconal) technique. This may reduce some of the risks and allows the patient to avoid amaurosis in the vast majority of cases.[14]

With minimal anesthesia and sedation patients go about their business with as little disability from their systemic side effects as from their miraculously rapid recovery of vision after cataract surgery.

AUTHOR'S TECHNIQUE

I offer my technique as a possible template. I choose the method of anesthesia at the preoperative exam based on each patient's ability to follow direction and tolerate the light of the indirect ophthalmoscope. Extreme photophobia, involuntary blepharospasm, and poor central fixation bode poorly for topical anesthesia. Cases that require suturing of iris or preoperative zonular network pathology requiring suturing of the bag or lens are also poor candidates. Those with extreme fears or anxiety after counseling may also require perbulbar injection. As I do not suspend anticoagulant therapy I consider coumadin to be a relative contraindication for PBA. Other relative contraindications include strabismus patients or those with orbital disorders such as Grave's disease or prior orbital surgery or trauma. Patients who are hard to position or have claustrophobia can usually tolerate TA with appropriate sedation, padding, and taping of the drape to the microscope off the face. These principles result in a 95 percent rate of TA. General anesthesia is reserved for the pediatric and mentally handicapped patients and the rare monocular patient who is a very poor candidate for TA for the reasons outlined above. Planning ahead reduces to nil the need to convert to akinesia or to obtund patients intraoperatively.

I still have the luxury of working with an anesthesiologist, one who has worked with me for well over two decades. When patients arrive at the surgical facility they receive an intravenous saline lock. We monitor pulse, oxygen saturation and blood pressure. In the OR after positioning, just before prep, most patients receive 1 mg Versed (range 0.5 mg to 2 mg). For TA, patients receive one drop of proparacaine prior to the betadine and another just before draping. For tense patients and lid squeezers during prep and drape we administer 125 mg alfentanil (which is diluted 8 times so final concentration is 2 cc = 125 mg, else the volume is too small to push without having to flush with saline). Intraoperatively, if the patient is uncomfortable or at the surgeon's request, alfentanil is repeated once. If still uncomfortable or for a prolonged procedure we add 10 mg of propofol with the alfentanil in the same syringe ("pinacolada"). Medications for nausea are virtually never required.

If PBA is required, after monitoring is established, either propofol 30–60 mg (if available) or versed 2–4 mg is administered appropriate to patient size to obtain brief hypnosis and retrograde amnesia in the holding area while the injection is performed. According to the original teaching of Roy Hamilton in Calgary at the Gimbel Eye Cener,[15] a single injection is given percutaneously at the junction of the medial two-thirds and the lateral third of the lower orbital margin with the eye open and held in the neutral position. With the index finger of the anesthesiologist's spare hand pushing the globe superiorly, the needle is directed posteriorly and slightly medially parallel to the floor of the orbit to avoid entering the cone. The plunger is withdrawn to confirm extravascular position. Next, 4–5 ml of a mixture of, lidocaine, epinephrine, and hyaluronidase is injected. We apply manual digital massage followed by Honan balloon within the green zone on the gauge. The patient motility is checked. The block is never supplemented as any blunting of motility of the lids and extraocular muscles is acceptable for my surgery. The patient is then transported to the operating room for prep and drape.

Postoperatively we splint PBA patients' lids shut with a piece of one inch plastic tape placed between the superior orbital rim and the lid margin. It is folded in the center to permit a tab by which to lift the lid to apply postoperative eyedrops. This method prevents occult ocular exposure unseen under a patch. This remains in place for five hours to prevent diplopia due to akinesia. Other than rare echymosis or very rare transient diplopia from inferior rectus hematoma we noted no anesthetic related complications in many thousands of injections for years.

All TA and PBA patients require and deserve "vocal local": an explanation of what to expect from their visual experience during surgery. Assurances such as: "You will be aware of my presence but should feel no pain and if anything bothers you, tell me and we will do something about it right away" empower the patient. Other established patter include: "The light is bright but your eye will rapidly adjust.", "You will see light and motion and color but nothing distinct or disturbing." "The light might come and go or change color and that is normal during surgery." These instructions reduce anxiety and the expectation of pain. Often patients can simply enjoy the "light show". Sometimes patience is required with the occasional patient who has difficulty holding the eye steady. I will grasp the globe with an instrument during the capsulorhexis in these cases and repeatedly remind the patient to hold their eye steady. I have yet to encounter a visually significant complication as a result of patient movement. In about 0.5 percent of patients TA is a sufficient challenge with the first eye to recommend PBA for the second. Risks and benefits are carefully explained.[16]

SUMMARY

According to the preferred practice patterns of AAO: "given the lack of evidence for a single optimal anesthesia strategy for cataract surgery, the type of anesthesia management should be determined according to the patient's needs and the preference of the patient, the anesthesia professionals, and the surgeon".[17] This chapter describes both the trends in ophthalmic anesthesia which are becoming ever more minimalistic and safe as well as the author's personal technique.

NOTE

The author has no financial interest to disclose. She is in private practice with Eye Surgeons Associates in the Iowa and Illinois Quad Cities and is an adjunct associate professor at the University of Utah John A Moran Eye Center.

REFERENCES

1. G Barry Smith, Robert C Hamilton, Caroline A Carr. Ophthalmic Anaesthesia. A Practical Handbook, 2nd edn. Oxford University Press Inc 1996.
2. Bryant JS, Busbee BG, Reichel E. Overview of ocular anesthesia: past and present. Curr Opin Ophthalmol 2011;22(3):180-4.
3. Ahmad S. Sedation techniques in ophthalmic anesthesia. Ophthalmol Clin North Am 2006;19(2):193-202.
4. Learning DV. Practice styles and preferences of ASCRS members—2003 survey. J Cataract Refract Surg 2004;30:892-900.

5. Ong-Tone L, Bell A, Tan YY. Practice patterns of Canadian Ophthalmological Society members in cataract surgery: 2011 survey. Can J Ophthalmol 2012;47(2):124-30.
6. Cataract surgery practice patterns in the United States Veterans Health Administration Paul B. Greenburg, Annika Havnaer, Thomas A. Oetting, m Francisco J. Garcia-Ferrer Journal of Cataract and Refractive Surgery 2012;38(4):705-9.
7. Bryant JS, Busbee BG, Reichel E. Overview of ocular anesthesia: past and Present. Curr Opin Ophthalmol 2011;22(3):180-4.
8. Ezra DG, Nambiar A, Allan BD. Supplementary intracameral lidocaine for phacoemulsification under topical anesthesia. A meta-analysis of randomized controlled trials. Ophthalmology 2008;115(3):455-87.
9. Crandall AS, Zabriskie NA, Patel BC, Burns TA, Mamalis N, Malmquist-Carter LA, Yee R. A comparison of patient comfort during cataract surgery with topical anesthesia versus topical anesthesia and intracameral lidocaine. Ophthalmology 1999;106(1):60-6.
10. Tsoumani AT, Asproudis IC, Damigos D. Tetracaine 0.5 percent eyedrops with or without Lidocaine 2 percent gel in topical anesthesia for cataract surgery. Clin Ophthalmol 2010;4:967-70.
11. Zhao LQ, Zhu H, Zhao PQ, Wu QR, Hu YQ. Topical anesthesia versus regional anesthesia for cataract surgery: a meta-analysis of randomized controlled trials. Ophthalmology 2012;119(4):659-67.
12. Scleral perforation during retrobulbar and peribulbar anesthesia: Risk factors and Outcome in 50,000 consecutive injections Roger Edge, MB, BCH, FFA, Sam Navon, MD, PhD. J Cataract Refract Surg 1999;25:1237-44.
13. Schrader WF, Schargus M, Schneider E, Josifova T. Risks and sequelae of scleral perforation during peribulbar or retrobulbar anesthesia. J Cataract Refract Surg 2010;36(6):885-9.
14. Adeela Malik, Emily C Fletcher, Victor Chong, Jay Dasan. Local anesthesia for cataract surgery. Journal of Cataract and Refractive Surgery 2010;36(1):133-52.
15. Hamilton RC. Techniques of orbital regional anaesthesia. Br J Anaesth 1995; 75:88-92. Available at: http://bja.oxfordjournals.org/cgi/reprint/75/1/88.pdf. Accessed October 3, 2009 161.
16. Sang: Protocol by Sang Sapthavie, MD (anesthesiologist).
17. American Academy Ophthalmology. Cataract in the Adult Eye; Preferred Practice Patterns. San Francisco, CA, American Academy of Ophthalmology, 2006. Available at:http://one.aao.org/CE/PracticeGuidelines/PPP_Content.aspx?cidZa80a87ce-9042-4677-85d7-4b876deed276. Accessed December 9, 2011.

Azithromycin in Ophthalmology: A New Therapy

Eric Donnenfeld, Mitchell Friedlaender (USA)

TOPICAL AZITHROMYCIN EYEDROP (AZASITE)

Topical ocular antibiotics are used to treat a variety of acute and chronic ocular surface infections such as bacterial conjunctivitis, blepharitis, keratitis and external hordeola. Topical eyedrops are often used in acute self-limiting infectious disease to speed recovery and reduce the spread of pathogens through the community. In addition, antibiotic prophylaxis is needed after ocular trauma or prior to and following ophthalmic surgery to reduce the risk of infection and improve outcomes. Despite the range of commercially available topical ocular antibiotics available, ophthalmologists frequently request topical formulations of other antibiotics to fulfill the unmet clinical need for broad spectrum activity, convenient dosing, and reduced treatment failure. Azithromycin is a well-known, convenient, and safe antibiotic with a favorable bacterial spectrum for the treatment of ocular surface infections. Its safety and efficacy as a topical eyedrop was recently evaluated in clinical trials.

Chemical Characteristics

Azithromycin was patented for systemic use in 1981 and commercialized 10 years later in the United States. Commonly known as Zithromax® (Pfizer,USA), azithromycin is a semi-synthetic molecule derived from the macrolide erythromycin. The potential use in topical ocular anti-infective therapy has been quite limited until now, largely because of its chemical instability in an aqueous medium. In contrast, the parent compound, erythromycin is frequently employed in an ointment base as topical therapy for infections caused by gram-positive organisms or in combination with systemic tetracycline to treat *Chlamydia* (Morrow GL and Abbott RL, 1998). Classified as an azalide, azithromycin differs from erythromycin by having a 15 member ring with an aza- methyl-substituted nitrogen in the aglycone ring (See arrow, Figs 59.1A and B). The development of azithromycin expanded the indications for which macrolides could be used.

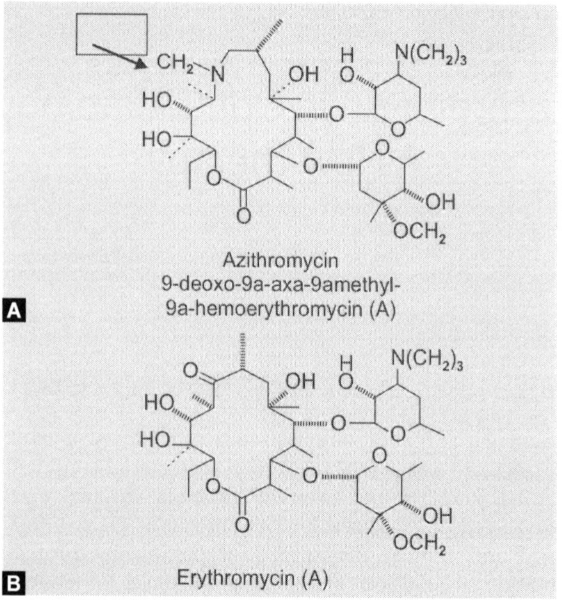

Figs 59.1A and B: Chemical Structures: (A) Azithromycin, (B) Erythromycin (Adapted from Retsema et al, antimicrobial agents and chemo 1987;31:1939)

CHEMICAL STRUCTURES OF AZITHROMYCIN AND ERYTHROMYCIN

Pharmacokinetics

Azithromycin has a broader efficacy and better pharmacokinetics than erythromycin. The antibacterial spectra as measured *in vitro* are similar, although azithromycin has superior activity against *Hemophilus influenzae*, gram-negative, and some atypical organisms (Retsema J, Girard A, Schelkly W, et al. 1987; Williams JD and Sefton AM 1993; Bryskier A and Labro MT, 1994). Compared to erythromycin, the oral and intravenous delivery forms of azithromycin are characterized by improved oral bioavailability, increased tissue penetration and persistence, and longer elimination half-lives (Rodvold KA and Piscitelli SC, 1993; Girard D, Bergeron JM, Millisen WB, et al. 1993).

The pharmacokinetics of azithromycin makes it an attractive candidate for development into a once-a-day azalide-class eyedrop therapy. In rabbits that were dosed with either 2 mg/ml or 4 mg/ml azithromycin that was prepared from an intravenous solution, the corneal concentrations of azithromycin increased with drug concentration and duration of application for up to 48 hours (Fig. 59.2). Rabbits treated with azithromycin tolerated the drug well without signs of irritation (Kuehne JJ, Yu AL, Holland GN et al. 2004). In order to expand the properties of azithromycin in a topical ocular solution, the ideal formulation would have to be comfortable, stable, and as effective or preferable more effective than oral azithromycin.

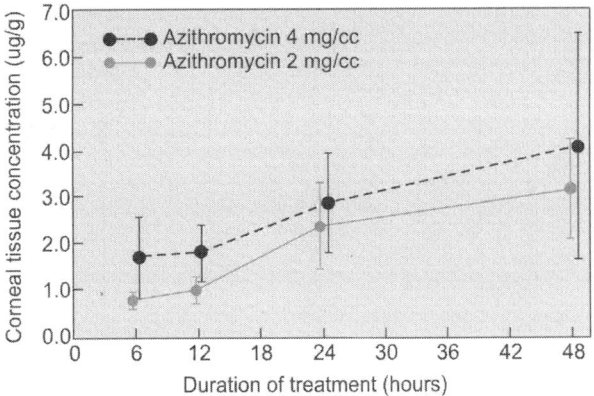

Fig. 59.2: Corneal concentrations of an azithromycin (Adapted from Kuehne et al. Am J Ophthalmol 2004:38)

DuraSite Drug Delivery System

DuraSite® (InSite Vision, Alameda, CA) is a proprietary drug delivery vehicle that stabilizes small molecules like azithromycin. The DuraSite solution of azithromycin is a polymeric mucoadhesive matrix that solubilizes and stabilizes the molecule at a pH that is comfortable for topical delivery. The 1 percent (10 mg/ml) topical solution of azithromycin in DuraSite (AzaSite™, InSite Vision, Alameda, CA) is a gel forming drop which can be instilled like traditional eyedrops but adhere longer to the ocular surface. Modeling of the concentrations achieved based on once-a-day topical dosing indicated peak (200 µg/g) and trough (40 µg/g) concentrations in the conjunctiva. This suggests that the drops could have efficacy against the majority of gram-negative, gram-positive and atypical organisms that cause ocular surface infections with once-a-day dosing. These concentrations are also, significantly higher than previous tear film concentrations of antibiotics obtained with topical dosing (Fig. 59.3).

MODELED BIOAVAILABILITY OF AZITHROMYCIN FROM AZASITE

Specifically, DuraSite is a polymer of acrylic acid. The polymer entraps water and the active drug product in a bioadhesive matrix. The viscosity of the matrix is controlled by pH. The bioavailabilty and release characteristics of the drug can be adjusted by altering the chemical environment. The 1 percent formulation of azithromycin was solubilized and stabilized under these chemical conditions at room temperature up to 12 months.

Clinical Trials

Phase three clinical trials of AzaSite were recently completed with participants who had laboratory confirmed bacterial conjunctivitis and symptoms for three days or less. Participants were randomized

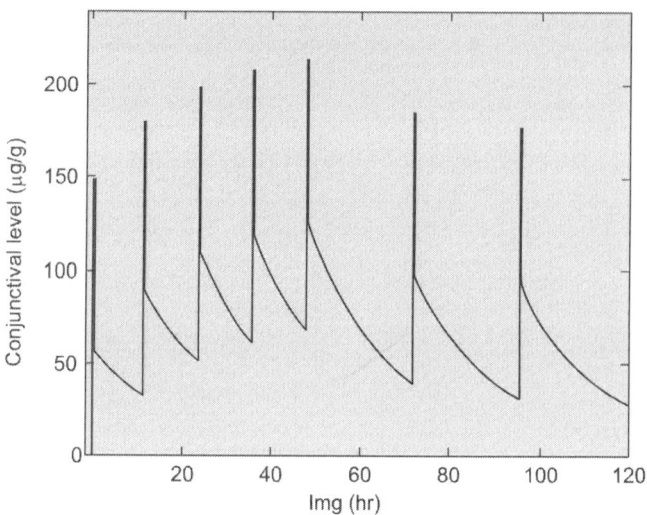

Fig. 59.3: Bioavailability model (By permission, Insite Vision, Alameda, CA, 2006)

to receive either 0.3 percent tobramycin or 1 percent azithromycin for five days. Participants in both arms were given masked drugs four times a day (q.i.d). However, participants in the AzaSite group were dosed with active drug twice-a-day on days one and two, and once-a-day on days three through five. At the test-of-cure visit on day six, the data demonstrated that a five day regimen of AzaSite comprised of seven drops was equally as effective as 20 drops of tobramycin. The AzaSite regimen required 65 percent fewer drops than tobramycin. This represents a significant reduction in dosing as compared to conventional drops that require anywhere from 3–8 doses per day.

The rate of ocular adverse events was 1.9 percent in the tobramycin comparison study (Protzko, et al. 2006). The most frequently observed ocular adverse events in the overall study population were eye irritation (1.9%), conjunctival hyperemia (1.1%) and, worsening conjunctivitis (1.1%), which compares favorably with that of tobramycin and the topical fluoroquinolone, gatifloxacin (Zymar full prescribing information).

In a parallel study, participants were randomized to receive AzaSite or a vehicle that contained DuraSite and the preservative benzylkonium hydrochloride. The same five days treatment regimen was employed. The results demonstrated that microbiological and clinical outcomes were superior in participants who used AzaSite rather than vehicle. At the test-of-cure visit on day six, treatment with AzaSite achieved clinical resolution in 63.1 percent (82/130) of participants compared to treatment with vehicle which achieved clinical resolution in 49.7 percent (74/149). The difference in resolution rate was 13.4 percent (95% CI:1.9 to 25%) and statistically significant ($P = 0.030$) in favor of AzaSite.

Expanded Killing Profile

In vitro studies that supported the phase three clinical trials, indicated that clinical isolates that showed resistance to azithromycin *in vitro* were eradicated on the ocular surface by 1 percent solution of azithromycin in DuraSite. Clinical Laboratory and Standards Institute (CLSI) breakpoints were used to identify resistant bacteria. Most strains of *Enterococcus faecalis* and methicillin resistant staphylococci are resistant to azithromycin. Although strains of *Hemophilus influenzae* and *Streptococcus pneumoniae* with decreased susceptibility to azithromycin are rare, isolated reports have appeared in literature (Cerquettu M, Cardines R, Giufre M, et al. 2004; Thornsberry C, Olgive PT, Holly HP, et al. 1999). In the phase 3 studies, AzaSite eradicated 72.4 percent (21/29) of azithromycin-resistant *Staphylococcus* and *Streptococcus* strains isolated from the patient population. In addition, although the total number was small, AzaSite eradicated all of the oxacillin (methicillin) resistant strains (2/2) that were isolated from the patient population (Abelson M, et al. 2006). The efficacy of AzaSite against resistant organisms is almost certainly due to the extremely high tear film concentrations of azithromycin which were obtained.

CONCLUSION

Azithromycin is a semi-synthetic azalide derived from erythromycin. Favorable pharmacokinetics and bacterial spectrum make azithromycin an excellent candidate for the treatment of ocular surface infections. Significant milestones in formulation technology involving mucoadhesive polymers permitted the development of a stable eyedrop with a high safety and tolerability profile and convenient once-a-day dosing. AzaSite is a significant improvement on the azithromycin molecule. The addition of the DuraSite drug delivery vehicle imparts stability and increased contact time with the ocular surface, which allows AzaSite to sustain high bactericidal tear film and conjunctival concentrations of azithromycin.

BIBLIOGRAPHY

1. Abelson M, Protzko EE, Shapiro AM. AzaSite Clinical Study Group. A randomized trial assessing microbial eradication and clinical efficacy of AzaSite (1.0% azithromycin ophthalmic solution) vs. tobramycin in adult subjects with bacterial conjunctivitis.
2. Bryskier A, Labro MT. Macrolides: New therapeutic prospects. Presse 1994;23(38):1762-66.
3. Cerquetti M, Cardines R, Giufre M, Mastrantonio P. HI Study Group. Antimicrobial susceptibility of *Haemophilus influenzae* strains isolated from invasive disease in Italy. J Antimicrob Chemo 2004;54:1139-46.
4. Girard D, Bergeron JM, Millisen WB, et al. Comparison of azithromycin, roxithromycin, and cephalexin penetration kinetics in early and mature abscesses. J Antimicrob Chemother 1993;Suppl E:17-28.

5. Kuehne JJ, Yu AL, Holland GN, et al. Corneal pharmacokinetics of topically applied azithromycin and clarithromycin. Am J Ophthalmol 2004;138:547-53.
6. Morrow GL, Abbott RL. Conjunctivitis. Am Family Physician 1998, 57 accessed at http://www.aafp.org/afp/980215ap/morrow.html, November 6, 2006.
7. Neu HC. Clinical microbiology of azithromycin. Am J Med 1991;91(3A):12S-18S.
8. Protzko E, et al. A randomized trial assessing the safety and tolerability of 1.0 percent azithromycin ophthalmic solution vs. tobramycin in pediatric and adult subjects with bacterial conjunctivitis. Invest Ophthalmol Vis Sci 2003. E-abstract@arvo.org. E-abstract 4958.
9. Retsema J, Girard A, Schelkly W, et al. Spectrum and mode of action of azithromycin (CP-62,993), a new 15-membered-ring macrolide with improved potency against gram-negative organisms. Antimicrobial Agents and Chemo 1987;31:1939-47.
10. Rodvold KA, Piscitelli SC. 1993 New oral macrolide and fluoroquinolone antibiotics: An overview of pharmacokinetics, interactions and safety. Clin Infect Dis 1993;Suppl 1:S192-9.
11. Thornsberry C, Olgive PT, Holly HP, Sahm DF. Survey of susceptibilities of *Streptococcus pneumoniae, Haemophilus influenzae,* and *Moraxella catarrhalis* isolates to 26 antimicrobial agents: a prospective U.S. study. Antimicrob Agents Chemother 1999;43:2612-23.
12. Williams JD, Sefton AM. Comparison of macrolide antibiotics. J Antimicrobi Chemother 1993;Suppl C:11-26.
13. Zymar [package insert]. Allergan, Inc; Irvine, Calif, 2004.

60

Use of Beta-adrenergic Blockers in Ocular Vascular Diseases

Javier A Montero, Jose M Ruiz-Moreno, Eugenia Sanchis-Merino (Spain)

INTRODUCTION

Chorioretinal conditions related to neovascularization are the most frequent causes of blindness in the developed world. Diabetic retinopathy, exudative age related macular degeneration (AMD), neovascular myopic maculopathy and retinopathy of the prematurity (ROP) are leading causes of blindness in their respective age groups.[1-3] During the past years new therapies have been developed to treat retinal[4,5] and choroidal[6-8] neovascularization, most of them based in ablation of pathologic tissue. More recently, new drugs with antiangiogenic effect have aided in a more conservative management of these conditions.[9-12]

Choroidal vascularization is regulated by sympathetic and parasympathetic nerves from the ipsilateral superior cervical ganglion and the pterygopalatine ganglion, respectively. Sympathetic nerves maintain structural integrity of the adult choroidal vessels as was demonstrated by Steinle et al,[13] who performed superior cervical ganglionectomy in adult rats and observed an increase in choroidal thickness and vascularity as well as a 4.5-fold increase in blood flow, that appeared to be caused by the absence of sympathetic nerve activity. Long-term administration of a beta-adrenergic receptor antagonist (propranolol) produces changes in adult rat choroidal vasculature very much like those observed following sympathectomy.[14] Choroidal vascular remodeling after beta adrenoceptor blockade does not seem to be related to nonspecific effects of propranolol on vascular resistance.

The role of norepinephrine (NE) inducing cellular expression of VEGF in brown adipocytes and cardiac myocytes and its inhibition by propranolol was described in the early 2000's. NE has growth-promoting effects in cardiac myocytes and stimulates the expression of vascular endothelial growth factor (VEGF) in cultured neonatal rat cardiac myocytes that can be blocked by antibodies neutralizing transforming growth factor (TGF) beta.[15] NE induces 3-fold VEGF expression in a dose- and time-dependent manner in mouse brown adipocytes in primary culture. The hypoxia-mimicking agent cobalt also induces VEGF expression, but the effect of NE is additive to this factor, implying a separate signaling mechanism. The effect of NE is abolished by propranolol (mediated via beta-adrenoreceptors, beta-ARs) and the induction of VEGF expression is mediated by cAMP and dependent on protein kinase A activity. Norepinephrine does not prolong VEGF mRNA half-life and its effect is transcriptional and independent of protein synthesis.[16]

The antitumor,[17-19] anti-inflammatory[20] and antiangiogenic effects[20] of propranolol have been reported. Hajighasemi showed that propranolol inhibits VEGF and metaloproteinase-2 (MMP-2) expression in two human leukemic T (Molt-4 and Jurkat) and one monocyte (U937) cell lines *in vitro*. Propranolol decreases VEGF production and MMP-2 activity in activated human leukemic cell lines Molt-4, Jurkat and U937 compared to untreated control cells.[21]

Pathogenic angiogenesis, a condition that is common to many hypoxic/ischemic vision-threatening retinal diseases, is related (at least in part) to beta(2)-AR activity and beta(2)-AR blockade can be effective against retinal angiogenesis.[23]

Oxygen-induced retinopathy (OIR) (similar to human ROP) can be produced in newborn rats by exposure to 80 percent oxygen for the first 5 days of life, with subsequent recovery for 7 days in a room air environment. In the latter phase VEGF is produced by astrocytes, or in their absence by the neurons of the inner retina. In a recent paper Ristori et al verified that blockade of beta-ARs with subcutaneous propranolol reduced up regulated VEGF in a mouse model of OIR, ameliorating the retinopathy score and reducing hypoxia-induced plasma extravasation. In their study, hypoxia did not influence beta-AR expression and up regulated VEGF, IGF-1 and their receptors. Propranolol reduced up regulated VEGF and decreased hypoxic levels of IGF-1 mRNA in a dose-dependent manner. Increased vascular permeability induced by intravitreal injection of VEGF was not affected by propranolol.[22]

In a later paper these authors used the same model to investigate the role of distinct beta-ARs on retinal proangiogenic factors and pathogenic neovascularization showing that beta(2)-AR blockade decreased retinal levels of proangiogenic factors reducing pathogenic neovascularization.[23] The presence of beta(2)-ARs has been demonstrated in several retinal cells, particularly in Müller cells, suggesting the possibility that beta(2)-ARs might play a role in regulating vascular endothelial growth factor production.[24,25]

Topical beta-blockers apparently show a similar effect on ocular neovascularization. Ricci et al. reported on the inhibitory effect of topical timolol maleate on retinal neovascularization in an animal model of OIR associated with an almost complete cessation of VEGF expression. OIR was less severe in eyes treated with timolol that in untreated rats and retinas from timolol-treated animals expressed VEGF protein though the level was inferior to that of untreated rats. The authors considered that this effect was secondary to a reduction of intraocular pressure induced by topical timolol, thus improving ocular perfusion pressure.[26]

Beta-adrenergic blocking agents have been used to treat many cardiovascular diseases such as arterial hypertension, ischemic heart failure, cardiac arrhythmia, migraine and hyperthyroidism among other conditions. Propranolol has been recently used to treat neovascular conditions such as infantile capillary hemangiomas (ICH)[27-37] and ROP;[38] clinical trials are under way to elucidate the effect of these therapies.

Infantile Capillary Hemangioma

Infantile capillary hemangioma (ICH) is infancy's most common vascular tumor and most frequent benign neoplasm. ICH affects one in every 10-20 Caucasian infants with a 3:1-5:1 predilection for females. Its incidence is higher among premature infants, newborns with low birth weight, placentary anomalies and in neonates from mothers with multiple pregnancies.

In 1996 the "International Society for the Study of Vascular Anomalies" defined the guidelines for the diagnosis and treatment of vascular anomalies such as ICH.[39] ICH presents well-defined characteristics and a natural history divided into three phases: a proliferative phase (initial growth phase through hyperplasia and hypertrophy), spontaneous regression (involuting phase) and an involuted phase (end of biological activity). ICH is composed of a complex mixture of clonal endothelial cells associated with pericytes, dendritic cells, and mast cells. Regulators of ICH growth and involution are poorly understood. During the growth phase, two major proangiogenic factors are involved: basic fibroblast growth factor (bFGF) and VEGF; histologic studies have shown that both endothelial and interstitial cells are actively dividing in this phase.

Infantile capillary hemangioma (ICH) may reach considerable dimensions in the proliferative phase and may result in the obstruction or invasion of organs causing functional problems and even threatening infant's life. The incidence of local (necrosis, repetitive ulcerations, bleeding and infections) and systemic (coagulopathy, high output cardiac failure) complications is variable. ICH may eventually leave scars or deformities with eventual psychological damage.

Treatment is indicated in 10-20 percent of the cases, especially in function—or life-threatening situations such as obstruction of airways, obstruction of vision, congestive heart failure, and hepatic and coagulation problems. Other indications are esthetical (large and disfiguring facial hemangiomas, locations that can result in a deformity and/or permanent scar such as nose, ear, lip, or glabellar area, extensive facial hemangiomas, local complications and small hemangiomas in exposed areas. Treatment may vary according to the extension, location, presence of complications and the evolutional phase.

Surgical treatment is mostly indicated for lesions in growing areas with disfiguring potential. Otherwise, pharmacological therapy is the routine, most frequently with oral prednisone. The therapeutic response is variable and the effectiveness rates may vary between 30-84 percent ranging from clearly effective responses to a mere reduction in the lesion's growth rate. The effective response usually occurs one week after the beginning of medical treatment. Among the most frequent side effects, Cushing syndrome is the most frequent with personality disorders, high blood pressure, gastrointestinal disorders, weight gain and reduced growth speed and head circumference.

The most frequent, second-line treatment drug in non-responders is subcutaneous alpha-interferon 2b.[40,41] This treatment is very effective, albeit with a higher rate of side effects such as spastic diplegia. Other drugs used in this situation are chemotherapeutic and immunomodulators;[42-44] however the reported series are short and without long follow-up to justify its routine use.

In 2008 Leaute-Labreze et al reported on the effect of propranolol on ICH.[45] Two children who presented infantile capillary hemangiomas and were on treatment with propranolol for other systemic conditions such as hypertrophic myocardiopathy and increased cardiac output secondary to corticosteroid therapy showed a marked softening, reduction and flattening of the angiomatous lesions with stable results. Nine further children who had severe or disfiguring ICH were treated at a dose of 2 mg per kilogram of body weight per day following this finding after obtaining written informed consents from their parents with similar results. Since June 2008, systemic propranolol has been used in problematic ICH, decreasing dependence on systemic corticosteroids with minimal short-term side effects.[46-62]

Topical beta blockers have been tried such as topical 0.5 percent timolol gel[63-65] or 1 percent propranolol ointment[66] with good therapeutical results.

Potential explanations for the therapeutic effect of beta-blockers on ICH include vasoconstriction (immediately visible as a change in color with a palpable softening of the hemangioma), decreased expression of VEGF and bFGF genes through the down-regulation of the RAF–mitogen-activated protein kinase pathway (showed by the progressive improvement of the hemangioma), and the triggering of apoptosis of capillary endothelial cells.

In an attempt to add scientific evidence to clinical series, clinical trials are presently under way to elucidate the efficacy of propranolol in ICH. One clinical trial has been terminated (registered at http://clinicaltrials.gov/ as NCT00744185) and six further trials are presently under way to elucidate the effect of systemic (NCT00967226, NCT01211080, NCT01056341, NCT01072045) or topical propranolol (NCT01512173), or the association of systemic propranolol and oral prednisolone (NCT01074437).

Nadolol is a systemic beta-blocker with long lasting effect that seems to be safer and more efficacious than propranolol in children, with better dosing schedules and less central nervous system penetration. The comparative efficacy of propranolol/nadolol in ICH treatment is being tried, in order to quantify its effectiveness and safety comparing it to the use of oral corticosteroid (NCT01010308).

The primary outcome measures of these trials are the variation of hemangioma thickness measured by ultrasonography from the basal state after 1 month-treatment and the proportion of subjects with at least 75 percent improvement in the extent of the hemangioma at 6 months. The secondary outcome measures are the variation of hemangioma size measured clinically and with photography after 1 month-treatment, the proportion of subjects with at least 50 percent improvement in the extent of the hemangiomas at 6 months, the correlation between the changes in the levels of angiogenesis markers and clinical response to treatment at 6 months.

Retinopathy of Prematurity

Retinopathy of prematurity (ROP) is still a major cause of blindness in children in developed countries around the world, and an increasing cause of blindness in developing countries. The ablation of the retina with photocoagulation by laser or cryotherapy reduces the incidence of blindness by suppressing the neovascular phase of ROP, frequently with poor visual outcomes after treatment.

Retinopathy of prematurity (ROP) affects the retinal microvasculature, mostly of premature infants <1500 g, and is a significant complication of extreme prematurity leading sometimes to devastating consequences. ROP may be aggressive causing neovascularization in the immature retina that may eventually progress to severe fibrovascular proliferation, retinal detachment and blindness. Laser photocoagulation of the ischemic retina is the first line therapy for moderate to severe ROP.

Retinopathy of prematurity and ICH may share the same pathogenetic role of angiogenic factors such as VEGF. Praveen et al. have reported a possible association between ROP and ICH in premature infants weighing <1250 g.[67] ICH was independently associated with any stage of ROP and was present in 16.8 percent of neonates with ROP vs. 6.7 percent of those without ROP. The number and size of ICH was not associated with the severity of ROP.

Major risk factors for ROP are low gestational age, low birth weight, hyperoxia, respiratory distress syndrome (RDS) and intraventricular hemorrhage (IVH) as well as postnatal steroid therapy. The prenatal use of beta-blockers by the mother has been reported to be associated with the development of ROP.[68] However, so far no one has reported a similar effect of the postnatal use of beta-blockers on ROP.

Two main pathogenetic theories have been proposed for the pathogenesis of ROP:
A. *One-phase theory:* Mesenchymal spindle cells exposed to extra uterine hyperoxia develop gap junctions that interfere with normal vascular formation and trigger a neovascular response.[69]
B. *Two-phase theory:* Retinal vasoconstriction and irreversible capillary endothelial cell damage occur in a first, hyperoxic phase. The retinal area affected becomes ischemic leading to an over expression of proangiogenic factors such as VEGF causing neovascularization (second phase).[70]

Vascular endothelial growth factor (VEGF) seems to play a key role in the pathogenesis of ROP by down regulation in the vasoobliterative phase and up regulation in the vasoproliferative phase. In animal models of OIR, most of the newborn rats exposed to 75–100 percent O_2 for 5 days starting at day 7 of life usually develop ROP.[71]

Sato et al evaluated the expression of 94 genes selected by microarray analyses in a murine animal model of OIR. Many genes associated with inflammation were up regulated at days 12 and

13 when both central avascular area and central vasoconstriction were maximal, and continued until day 21. Genes associated with angiogenesis such as VEGF-A and angiopoietin-2 were most up regulated at days 16 and 17 when extraretinal neovascularization became most noticeable.[72]

Sympathomimetic agents also upregulate VEGF. NE stimulates myocardial angiogenesis in rats[15] and *in vitro* protein levels of VEGF, PEDF and Ang1 were significantly increased following stimulation with isoproterenol, suggesting that beta-adrenergic receptor agonists are likely upstream of growth factors implicated in ocular vasculogenesis and may have multiple effects on choroidal endothelial cells.[73] NE and epinephrine induce an increase of VEGF expression *in vitro* in cultivated cancer cells that is blocked by propranolol.[74]

Recent studies have shown that beta-blockers can down regulate VEGF and mitigate neovascularization. Topical timolol prevented the development of OIR in 40 percent of rats and mitigated the severity of OIR in the remaining 60 percent of rats, playing a protective effect reducing the appearance of neovascularization from 100 percent to 65 percent of the timolol-treated animals.[26,75,76] VEGF expression was lower in timolol-treated rats than in controls.

The above-mentioned findings point to a VEGF-mediated pathogenesis of both ROP and infantile hemangiomas, wherein VEGF expression is reportedly upregulated by sympathomimetic agents and blocked by beta-blockers.

One clinical trial has been completed (NCT01238471) and one is presently under way (NCT01079715) to verify the safety and efficacy of propranolol in newborns with ROP (PROP-ROP). The hypothesis is that in premature infants, propranolol might suppress neovascularization and decelerate the progression of ROP towards its severe stages (III-V), avoiding the need of interventions and preventing severe ocular sequels. This study is controlled with placebo in infants with ROP stage 1 (zone I), with stage 2 or higher (any zone) or with Plus disease.

Primary outcome measure is the safety of propranolol administration. As secondary outcome measure the authors have defined the efficacy of treatment with propranolol for reducing blindness and retinal detachment in newborns with ROP six months from the beginning of treatment, compared to a control group receiving conventional laser therapy.

Propranolol is orally administered at a dosage of 0.5 mg/Kg every 6 hours and the study will be discontinued immediately in the presence of serious adverse effects attributable to the pharmacological actions of propranolol such as severe hypotension, bradycardia or bronchospasm. The study could be re started afterwards with half dose (0.25 mg/Kg oral, every 6 hours) after notification to the Ethics Committee.

Diabetic Retinopathy

The effect of topical or systemic beta-blockers to reduce the severity or progression of vasculoproliferative changes in diabetic retinopathy might become an interesting application of the previously described findings. In 1991 Newsom et al evaluated the effect of systemic beta-blockers on retinal blood flow in patients with diabetic retinopathy, trying to demonstrate a range of beta-receptor activity.[77] These authors studied the effect of a single oral dose of propranolol 80 mg, dilevalol 200 mg, salbutamol 4 mg, and placebo on retinal vessel diameter, blood velocity and volumetric retinal blood flow at baseline, 90 minutes and three hours after administration in normotensive diabetic volunteers. None of these treatments had any significant effect on retinal perfusion pressure, vessel diameter and volumetric flow. Zheng et al evaluated the effect of angiotensin-converting enzyme inhibitors and beta-adrenergic blockers on retinal vascular endothelial growth factor expression in a murine model of diabetic retinopathy.[78] They observed no significant difference in VEGF levels in diabetic rats and propranolol-treated diabetic rats. However, there was a significant difference in VEGF protein and mRNA expression in propranolol-treated diabetic rats and angiotensin-converting enzyme inhibitors-treated diabetic rats.

A clinical trial has been initiated in an attempt to evaluate if propranolol can induce regression of retinal neovascularization associated with proliferative diabetic retinopathy (NCT01535495). In this trial oral propranolol 120 mg daily will be given to 10 patients who have had complete panretinal photocoagulation laser treatment and active proliferative diabetic retinopathy, and patients with active retinal neovascularization without so called "high-risk" characteristics who have not had panretinal photocoagulation laser treatment, over a 12 weeks period to evaluate its effect on retinal neovascularization.

Primary outcome measure for this trial will be the area of retinal neovascularization on fundus photography. Secondary outcome measures will be retinopathy level in fellow eye, OCT macular thickness of treated and fellow eye, amount of fluorescein leakage on angiography and ETDRS visual acuity in study and fellow eye.

Choroidal Neovascularization in Age-related Macular Degeneration

Choroidal neovascularization (CNV) related to age-related macular degeneration (AMD) is the leading cause of severe permanent visual loss among elderly patients in developed countries. Presently the main goal of antiangiogenic therapy in patients with exudative AMD is VEGF. However, treatment of exudative AMD has become a sanitary problem with saturation of retinal units due to the frequent recurrences and the need for monthly or bimonthly controls and repeated treatments.

Inter individual variations in the response to anti-VEGF treatments has been observed and attributed to undetermined factors such as tachyphylaxis and underlying genetic differences.

In a recent paper our group evaluated the effect of systemic concomitant therapies on the antiangiogenic effect of intravitreal bevacizumab.[79] The files, optical coherence tomography scans and fluorescein angiographies of 46 eyes from 46 patients with exudative AMD that were on treatment by monthly intravitreal injections of bevacizumab were retrospectively revised and special care was taken in registering concomitant medications. The patients were treated by 3 consecutive intravitreal injections of 1.25 mg bevacizumab and followed monthly. Further intravitreal injections were performed on a pro re nata schedule. Bevacizumab treatment was performed whenever intraretinal or subretinal fluid or blood was observed in spectral domain optical coherence tomography or fundoscopy.

The primary aim of the study was to evaluate changes in BCVA and OCT central foveal thickness (CFT), as well as the number of injections required to achieve inactivation of the neovascular lesions.

The most frequent indication for treatment among the studied population was arterial hypertension (32 patients). 19 patients were on treatment with angiotensin-converting-enzyme inhibitors, 18 with beta-adrenergic blockers, 16 with diuretics and 14 with calcium channel blockers. 17 patients were on nonsteroidal anti-inflammatory drugs, mainly for arthrosis, 11 with sleep disorders with benzodiazepines, 9 with proton-pump inhibitors (mostly as gastric prophylaxis) and 8 with statins for hypercholesterolemia. 7 patients received antiaggregants and 5 patients were on treatment with acenocoumarol.

The most frequently used beta-blocker was bisoprolol (11 patients), followed by atenolol (4 patients), and propranolol, carvedilol and levobunolol with one patient each.

Multiple linear regression analysis was performed to evaluate the effect of systemic beta-blockers on visual acuity gain and final visual acuity, OCT changes and the number of intravitreal injections.

Comparing the group of patients on treatment with systemic beta-blockers and the rest of the patients, both groups were similar at baseline for age, sex, visual acuity and CFT. Both groups remained similar by the end of the 24-month follow-up in terms of final visual acuity, number of letters gained, and CFT improvement. However, the number of injections during this 2-year period was significantly lower for the group of patients receiving systemic beta-blockers (mean 6.7, standard deviation SD 3.3 for the whole group; mean 5.2 SD 2.5 for the group on systemic beta-blockers Vs. mean 8.1 SD 4.9 for the rest of the patients; $p = 0.027$, Student t-test for unpaired data). These results suggest that even though systemic beta-blockers may not prevent the appearance of choroidal neovascularization in exudative AMD, or improve visual acuity outcome, the number of required intravitreal injections in a pro re nata regime might be lower.

Propranolol, carvedilol, and levobunolol are nonselective beta-blockers, whereas bisoprolol and atenolol are considered selective beta-1-blockers. Bisoprolol shows a 19-fold higher affinity for the beta-1 receptor than for the beta-2 receptor. This residual beta-2 blocking affinity might explain the less frequent presence of intraretinal and subretinal fluid among patients on treatment with beta-blockers.

Among the limitations of this study, the most important is the low number of patients included. An evaluation of the effects of systemic concomitant beta-blockers among the patients included in other pro re nata series such as the PrONTO trial with ranibizumab or the CATT and IVAN trials with bevacizumab might increase our knowledge of the effect of beta-blockers on exudative AMD, and verify the feasibility of clinical trials on AMD patients.

Beta blocking therapy may soon become a cheap and effective tool in the management of neovascular conditions, with a wide therapeutic range, reducing the need of performing chorioretinal ablation and the number of intravitreal injections of antiangiogenic agents. However, much work is still to be done to complete the ongoing clinical trials and elaborate new ones as well as to revise the effect of concomitant medications in the previously performed trials to find out the most appropriate therapeutical regime for each condition.

REFERENCES

1. Boonstra N, Limburg H, Tijmes N, et al. Changes in causes of low vision between 1988 and 2009 in a Dutch population of children. Acta Ophthalmol 2012;90:277-86.
2. Claessen H, Genz J, Bertram B, et al. Evidence for a considerable decrease in total and cause-specific incidences of blindness in Germany. Eur J Epidemiol 2012;27:519-24.
3. Wu L, Sun X, Zhou X, Weng C. Causes and 3-year-incidence of blindness in Jing-An District, Shanghai, China 2001-2009. BMC Ophthalmol 2011;11:10.
4. Fine SL, Patz A. Ten years after the Diabetic Retinopathy Study. Ophthalmology 1987;94:739-40.
5. Mechoulam H, Pierce EA. Retinopathy of prematurity: molecular pathology and therapeutic strategies. Am J Pharmacogenomics 2003;3:261-77.
6. Mensher JH. Laser therapy for eye disorders. Postgrad Med 1984;76:51-6.
7. Lin SC, Lin CP, Feld JR, et al. The photodynamic occlusion of choroidal vessels using benzoporphyrin derivative. Curr Eye Res 1994;13:513-22.
8. Finger PT, Berson A, Sherr D, et al. Radiation therapy for subretinal neovascularization. Ophthalmology 1996;103:878-89.
9. Doggrell SA. Pegaptanib: the first antiangiogenic agent approved for neovascular macular degeneration. Expert Opin Pharmacother 2005;6:1421-3.
10. Michels S, Schmidt-Erfurth U, Rosenfeld PJ. Promising new treatments for neovascular age-related macular degeneration. Expert Opin Investig Drugs 2006;15:779-93.
11. Lin RC, Rosenfeld PJ. Antiangiogenic therapy in neovascular age-related macular degeneration. Int Ophthalmol Clin 2007;47:117-37.
12. Maloney SC, Godeiro KD, Odashiro AN, Burnier MN, Jr. Current and emerging concepts in the management of neovascular age-related macular degeneration. Cardiovasc Hematol Agents Med Chem 2007;5:147-54.

13. Steinle JJ, Pierce JD, Clancy RL, P GS. Increased ocular blood vessel numbers and sizes following chronic sympathectomy in rat. Exp Eye Res 2002;74:761-8.
14. Steinle JJ, Smith PG. Role of adrenergic receptors in vascular remodelling of the rat choroid. Br J Pharmacol 2002;136:730-4.
15. Weil J, Benndorf R, Fredersdorf S, et al. Norepinephrine upregulates vascular endothelial growth factor in rat cardiac myocytes by a paracrine mechanism. Angiogenesis 2003;6:303-9.
16. Fredriksson JM, Lindquist JM, Bronnikov GE, Nedergaard J. Norepinephrine induces vascular endothelial growth factor gene expression in brown adipocytes through a beta-adrenoreceptor/cAMP/protein kinase A pathway involving Src but independently of Erk1/2. J Biol Chem 2000;275:13802-11.
17. Zink-Lorenz A, Komitowska J, Raue F. Norepinephrine induced calcitonin secretion in rat medullary thyroid carcinoma 6-23 cells: interaction between intracellular calcium and cAMP. Exp Clin Endocrinol Diabetes 1996;104:43-9.
18. Nakamura A, Johns EJ, Imaizumi A, et al. beta(2)-adrenoceptor agonist suppresses renal tumour necrosis factor and enhances interleukin-6 gene expression induced by endotoxin. Nephrol Dial Transplant 2000;15:1928-34.
19. Zimmermann AP, Wiegand S, Werner JA, Eivazi B. Propranolol therapy for infantile haemangiomas: review of the literature. Int J Pediatr Otorhinolaryngol 2010;74:338-42.
20. Gerdin B, Svensjo E. Inhibitory effect of the flavonoid O-(beta-hydroxyethyl)-rutoside on increased microvascular permeability induced by various agents in rat skin. Int J Microcirc Clin Exp 1983;2:39-46.
21. Hajighasemi F, Hajighasemi S. Effect of propranolol on angiogenic factors in human hematopoietic cell lines *in vitro*. Iran Biomed J 2009;13:223-8.
22. Ristori C, Filippi L, Dal Monte M, et al. Role of the adrenergic system in a mouse model of oxygen-induced retinopathy: antiangiogenic effects of beta-adrenoreceptor blockade. Invest Ophthalmol Vis Sci 2011;52:155-70.
23. Martini D, Monte MD, Ristori C, et al. Antiangiogenic effects of beta2 -adrenergic receptor blockade in a mouse model of oxygen-induced retinopathy. J Neurochem 2011;119:1317-29.
24. Lashbrook BL, Steinle JJ. Beta-adrenergic receptor regulation of pigment epithelial-derived factor expression in rat retina. Auton Neurosci 2005;121:33-9.
25. Dal Monte M, Martini D, Latina V, et al. Beta-adrenoreceptor (beta-AR) agonism influences retinal responses to hypoxia in a mouse model of retinopathy of prematurity. Invest Ophthalmol Vis Sci, 2012.
26. Ricci B, Ricci F, Maggiano N. Oxygen-induced retinopathy in the newborn rat: morphological and immunohistological findings in animals treated with topical timolol maleate. Ophthalmologica 2000;214:136-9.
27. Wester ST, Johnson TE. Echographic evidence of regression of a periocular infantile capillary hemangioma treated with systemic propranolol. Ophthalmic Surg Lasers Imaging 2011;42 Online:e18-21.
28. Fabian ID, Ben-Zion I, Samuel C, Spierer A. Reduction in astigmatism using propranolol as first-line therapy for periocular capillary hemangioma. Am J Ophthalmol 2011;151:53-8.

29. Al Dhaybi R, Superstein R, Milet A, et al. Treatment of Periocular Infantile Hemangiomas with Propranolol: Case Series of 18 Children. Ophthalmology 2011.
30. Sidbury R. Update on vascular tumors of infancy. Curr Opin Pediatr 2010;22:432-7.
31. Mishra A, Holmes WJ, Gorst C, Liew SH. Role of propranolol in the management of periocular hemangiomas. Plast Reconstr Surg 2010;126:671.
32. Maturo S, Hartnick C. Initial experience using propranolol as the sole treatment for infantile airway hemangiomas. Int J Pediatr Otorhinolaryngol 2010;74:323-5.
33. Li YC, McCahon E, Rowe NA, et al. Successful treatment of infantile haemangiomas of the orbit with propranolol. Clin Experiment Ophthalmol 2010;38:554-9.
34. Jadhav VM, Tolat SN. Dramatic response of propranolol in hemangioma: report of two cases. Indian J Dermatol Venereol Leprol 2010;76:691-4.
35. Haider KM, Plager DA, Neely DE, et al. Outpatient treatment of periocular infantile hemangiomas with oral propranolol. J AAPOS 2010;14:251-6.
36. Nguyen J, Fay A. Pharmacologic therapy for periocular infantile hemangiomas: a review of the literature. Semin Ophthalmol 2009;24:178-84.
37. Loffler H, Kosel C, Cremer H, Kachel W. Die Propranolol-Therapie in der Behandlung problematischer Hämangiome. Eine neue Standardtherapie kündigt sich an. Hautarzt 2009;60:1013-6.
38. Filippi L, Cavallaro G, Fiorini P, et al. Study protocol: safety and efficacy of propranolol in newborns with Retinopathy of Prematurity (PROP-ROP): ISRCTN18523491. BMC Pediatr 2010;10:83.
39. Vanwijck R. [Vascular abnormalities]. Bull Mem Acad R Med Belg 1996;151:315-21; discussion 21-3.
40. Chang E, Boyd A, Nelson CC, et al. Successful treatment of infantile hemangiomas with interferon-alpha-2b. J Pediatr Hematol Oncol 1997;19:237-44.
41. Mortureux P, Pedespan JM, Greselle JF, et al. [Treatment of severe cervicofacial hemangioma with interferon alpha-2b]. Arch Pediatr 1995;2:237-40.
42. Yang Y, Sun M, Cheng X, et al. Bleomycin A5 plus dexamethasone for control of growth in infantile parotid hemangiomas. Oral Surg Oral Med Oral Pathol Oral Radiol Endod 2009;108:62-9.
43. Perez J, Pardo J, Gomez C. Vincristine—an effective treatment of corticoid-resistant life-threatening infantile hemangiomas. Acta Oncol 2002;41:197-9.
44. Perez Payarols J, Pardo Masferrer J, Gomez Bellvert C. Treatment of life-threatening infantile hemangiomas with vincristine. N Engl J Med 1995;333:69.
45. Leaute-Labreze C, Dumas de la Roque E, Hubiche T, et al. Propranolol for severe hemangiomas of infancy. N Engl J Med 2008;358:2649-51.
46. Sciveres M, Marrone G, Pipitone S, et al. Successful first-line treatment with propranolol of multifocal infantile hepatic hemangioma with high-flow cardiac overload. J Pediatr Gastroenterol Nutr 2011;53:693-5.
47. Shayan YR, Prendiville JS, Goldman RD. Use of propranolol in treating hemangiomas. Can Fam Physician 2011;57:302-3.

48. Solomon T, Ninnis J, Deming D, et al. Use of propranolol for treatment of hemangiomas in PHACE syndrome. J Perinatol 2011;31:739-41.
49. Spiteri Cornish K, Reddy AR. The use of propranolol in the management of periocular capillary haemangioma—a systematic review. Eye (Lond) 2011;25:1277-83.
50. Tan ST, Itinteang T, Leadbitter P. Low-dose propranolol for multiple hepatic and cutaneous hemangiomas with deranged liver function. Pediatrics 2011;127:e772-6.
51. Tan ST, Itinteang T, Leadbitter P. Low-dose propranolol for infantile haemangioma. J Plast Reconstr Aesthet Surg 2011;64:292-9.
52. Zaher H, Rasheed H, Hegazy RA, et al. Oral propranolol: an effective, safe treatment for infantile hemangiomas. Eur J Dermatol 2011;21:558-63.
53. Zhao ZF, Lu RR, Zhang J, et al. [Oral propranolol in the management of periorbital proliferating phase infantile hemangioma]. Zhonghua Zheng Xing Wai Ke Za Zhi 2011;27:174-7.
54. Zvulunov A, McCuaig C, Frieden IJ, et al. Oral propranolol therapy for infantile hemangiomas beyond the proliferation phase: a multicenter retrospective study. Pediatr Dermatol 2011;28:94-8.
55. Balma-Mena A, Chakkittakandiyil A, Weinstein M, et al. Propranolol in the management of infantile hemangiomas: clinical response and predictors. J Cutan Med Surg 2012;16:169-73.
56. Bertrand J, Sammour R, McCuaig C, et al. Propranolol in the treatment of problematic infantile hemangioma: review of 35 consecutive patients from a vascular anomalies clinic. J Cutan Med Surg 2012;16:115-21.
57. Chim H, Armijo BS, Miller E, et al. Propranolol induces regression of hemangioma cells through HIF-1alpha-mediated inhibition of VEGF-A. Ann Surg 2012;256:146-56.
58. Hsu TC, Wang JD, Chen CH, et al. Treatment with propranolol for infantile hemangioma in 13 Taiwanese newborns and young infants. Pediatr Neonatol 2012;53:125-32.
59. Kupeli S. Use of propranolol for infantile hemangiomas. Pediatr Hematol Oncol 2012;29:293-8.
60. Maguiness SM, Frieden IJ. Management of difficult infantile haemangiomas. Arch Dis Child 2012;97:266-71.
61. Prashanth GP. How "unsafe" is propranolol when used in the treatment of infantile hemangioma? J Am Acad Dermatol 2012;66:854-5; author reply 5-6.
62. Talaat AA, Elbasiouny MS, Elgendy DS, Elwakil TF. Propranolol treatment of infantile hemangioma: clinical and radiologic evaluations. J Pediatr Surg 2012;47:707-14.
63. Pope E, Chakkittakandiyil A. Topical timolol gel for infantile hemangiomas: a pilot study. Arch Dermatol 2010;146:564-5.
64. McMahon P, Oza V, Frieden IJ. Topical timolol for infantile hemangiomas: putting a note of caution in "cautiously optimistic". Pediatr Dermatol 2012;29:127-30.
65. Weissenstein A, Straeter A, Villalon G, Bittmann S. Topical timolol for small infantile hemangioma: a new therapy option. Turk J Pediatr 2012;54:156-8.
66. Kunzi-Rapp K. Topical propranolol therapy for infantile hemangiomas. Pediatr Dermatol 2012;29:154-9.

67. Praveen V, Vidavalur R, Rosenkrantz TS, Hussain N. Infantile hemangiomas and retinopathy of prematurity: possible association. Pediatrics 2009;123:e484-9.
68. Gallo JE, Jacobson L, Broberger U. Perinatal factors associated with retinopathy of prematurity. Acta Paediatr 1993;82:829-34.
69. Hittner HM, Rudolph AJ, Kretzer FL. Suppression of severe retinopathy of prematurity with vitamin E supplementation. Ultrastructural mechanism of clinical efficacy. Ophthalmology 1984;91:1512-23.
70. Zaniolo K, Sapieha P, Shao Z, et al. Ghrelin modulates physiologic and pathologic retinal angiogenesis through GHSR-1a. Invest Ophthalmol Vis Sci 2011;52:5376-86.
71. Ricci B. Oxygen-induced retinopathy in the rat model. Doc Ophthalmol 1990;74:171-7.
72. Sato T, Kusaka S, Hashida N, et al. Comprehensive gene-expression profile in murine oxygen-induced retinopathy. Br J Ophthalmol 2009;93:96-103.
73. Steinle JJ, Cappocia FC, Jr., Jiang Y. Beta-adrenergic receptor regulation of growth factor protein levels in human choroidal endothelial cells. Growth Factors 2008;26:325-30.
74. Guo K, Ma Q, Wang L, et al. Norepinephrine-induced invasion by pancreatic cancer cells is inhibited by propranolol. Oncol Rep 2009;22:825-30.
75. Ricci B, Calogero G, Caprilli A, Quaranta-Leoni FM. Reduced severity of oxygen-induced retinopathy in the newborn rat after topical administration of timolol maleate. A preliminary study. Doc Ophthalmol 1991;77:47-56.
76. Ricci B, Minicucci G, Manfredi A, Santo A. Oxygen-induced retinopathy in the newborn rat: effects of hyperbarism and topical administration of timolol maleate. Graefes Arch Clin Exp Ophthalmol 1995;233:226-30.
77. Newsom RS, Rassam SM, Kohner EM. The effect of beta blockers on retinal blood flow in diabetic patients. Eur J Ophthalmol 1991;1:131-6.
78. Zheng Z, Chen H, Xu X, et al. Effects of angiotensin-converting enzyme inhibitors and beta-adrenergic blockers on retinal vascular endothelial growth factor expression in rat diabetic retinopathy. Exp Eye Res 2007;84:745-52.
79. Montero JA, Ruiz-Moreno JM, Sanchis-Merino ME, Perez-Martin S. Systemic beta-blockers may reduce the need for repeated intravitreal injections in patients with wet age-related macular degeneration treated by bevacizumab. Retina 2012;In press.

61
Clinical Applications of Anti-inflammatory and Anti-protease Effects of Tetracyclines in Ocular Surface Disease

Stephen C Pflugfelder, Cintia S De Paiva, De-Quan Li (USA)

The first tetracycline, chlortetracycline, was produced as a fermentation product of *Streptomyces aureofaciens* in 1948. Since then, several tetracycline molecules have been synthesized from chlortetracycline, including tetracycline, doxycycline and minocycline that differ in their absorption, lipophilicity and duration of action (Fig. 61.1). In addition to their antimicrobial effects, tetracyclines have been found to have potent antiprotease and anti-inflammatory effects. Tetracycline derivatives lacking the dimethylamino group at position 4 on the tetracycline ring structure (asterisk in Fig. 61.1) lose their antibiotic properties but retain these nonantimicrobial activities.[1]

Anti-inflammatory and Antiprotease Properties of Tetracyclines

Our group has extensively investigated the effects of doxycycline on stimulated production of inflammatory cytokines and matrix

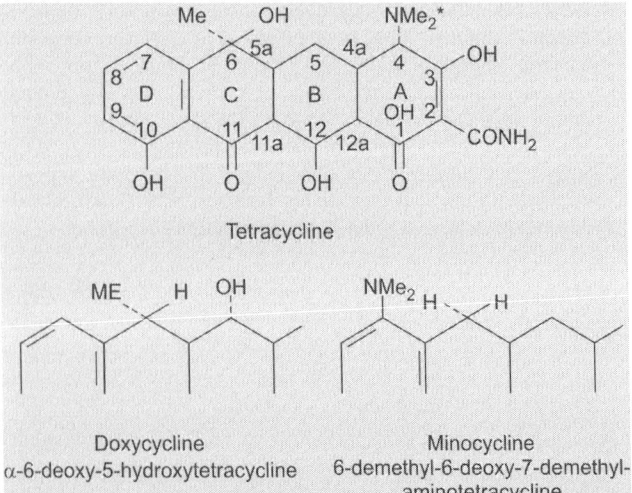

Fig. 61.1: Chemical structures of tetracycline (short-acting, top) and two long-acting derivatives, doxycycline (lower left) and minocycline (lower right). Tetracycline derivatives lacking the dimethylamino group at position 4 on the tetracycline ring structure (asterisk) loose their antibiotic properties

metalloproteinases by the corneal epithelium. Doxycycline was found to inhibit lipopolysaccharide (LPS)-induced production of IL-1β by the corneal epithelium and to stimulate expression of IL-1 receptor antagonist (IL-1 RA), the anti-inflammatory form of this cytokine.[2] Furthermore, doxycycline reduced the steady state level of cellular interleukin 1 converting enzyme (ICE), an enzyme that converts precursor IL-1β to its mature biologically active form. As anticipated, doxycycline significantly decreased IL-1 bioactivity in supernatants from LPS treated corneal epithelial cultures. These anti-inflammatory effects were of comparable magnitude to corticosteroids. Doxycycline also markedly suppressed production of IL-1β, TNF-α and IL-8 by osmotically stressed cultured corneal epithelia (Fig. 61.2).[3] This activity was found to be due in part to doxycycline's ability to block activation of JNK and ERK mitogen activated protein kinase (MAPK) pathways (Figs 61.3A and B).

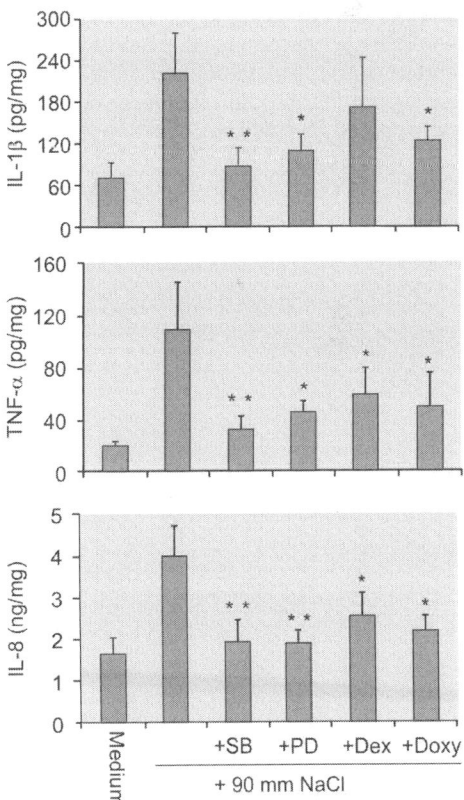

Fig. 61.2: Exposure of cultured human corneal epithelial cells to osmotic stress by adding 90 mm NaCl to their media stimulated production of IL-1β, TNF-α and IL-8. This was blocked by addition of ERK (PD) and JNK (SP) MAPK kinase inhibitors and doxycycline. The corticosteroid dexamethasone inhibited TNF-α and IL-8; *p < 0.05, **p < 0.01 (reprinted from Li DQ et al. Exp Eye Res. 2006;82:588-96)

Doxycycline in concentrations of 1 and 10 micrograms/ml was found to inhibit production of several matrix metalloproteinase (MMP) enzymes by the corneal epithelium, including MMP-1, -3, -9 and -13 in response to IL-1 or osmotic stress (Figs 61.4A and B).[4-7] This activity appeared to be related to its inhibition of the stress activated protein kinase JNK.[6] The tetracycline analog minocycline was also found to inhibit stress activated protein kinase pathways in the brain and in cultured microglial cells.[8,9] Taken together these laboratory research studies indicate that tetracyclines have potent inhibitory effects on production of MMPs and inflammatory mediators by the corneal epithelium. With regard to MMPs, the inhibitory activity of tetracyclines surpasses that of corticosteroids.

Clinical Applications of Nonantimicrobial Properties of Tetracyclines for Treatment of Ocular Surface Diseases

Tetracycline antibiotics have been recognized for years as effective therapies for improving signs and symptoms of ocular surface diseases. These salutary effects are most likely due to their nonantimicrobial anti-inflammatory and antiprotease activities. The evidence supporting the clinical efficacy of tetracyclines, as well as their proposed mechanisms of action for ocular surface diseases including: persistent corneal epithelial defects, recurrent corneal epithelial erosion, corneal stromal ulceration, mucous membrane pemphigoid, phlyctenular keratitis, ocular rosacea and keratitis sicca are provided below.

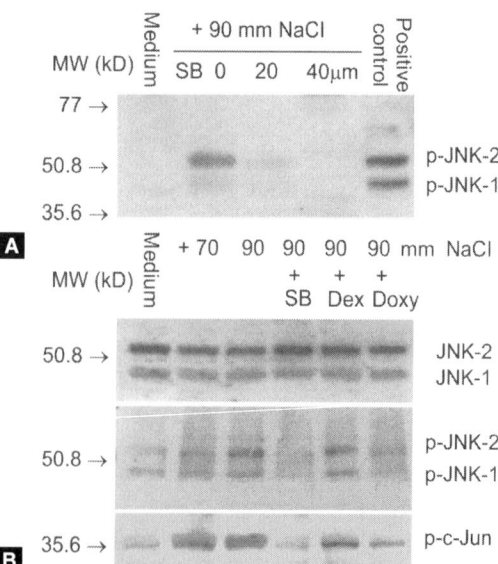

Figs 61.3A and B: Western blot showing the activated (phosphorylated) forms of JNK-1, JNK 2 and transcription factor c-jun activated by hyperosmolar media (90 mm NaCl added to media) and inhibited by SB202190 (A,B) and doxycycline, (B) in cultured human corneal epithelial cells

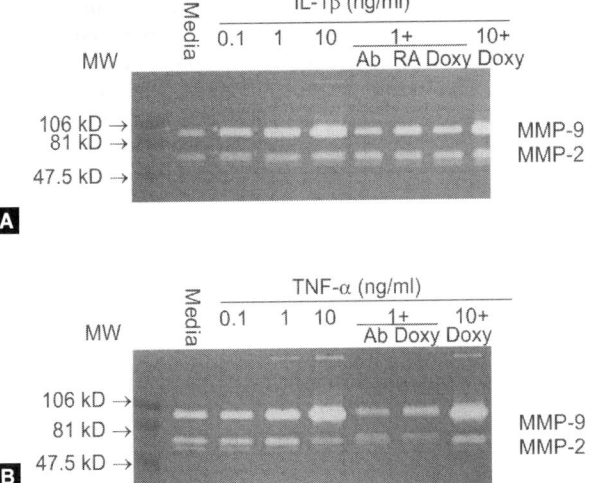

Figs 61.4A and B: (A) Gelatin zymogram evaluating regulation of MMP-9 production by IL-1β. Primary human corneal epithelial cultures were grown to subconfluence and switched to serum-free media before treatment with IL-1β at 0.1, 1.0 and 10 ng ml with or without neutralizing antibody (Ab), IL-1 receptor antagonist (IL-1 RA) or doxycycline (Doxy) 1 or 10 microgram/ml for 24 hours. The conditioned media were collected for gelatin zymography; (B) Gelatin zymogram evaluating the regulation of MMP-9 production by TNF-α. Primary human corneal epithelial cultures were grown to subconfluence and switched to serum-free media before treatment with TNF-α at 0.1, 1.0 and 10 ng/ml with or without neutralizing antibody (Ab) or doxycycline (Doxy) or 10 microgram/ml for 24 hours (reprinted from Li D-Q et al. Exp Eye Res 2001;73:449-59)

Treatment of Persistent Corneal Epithelial Defects and Recurrent Corneal Epithelial Erosion

Systemically administered tetracycline (1 gram/day) was found to promote healing of persistent corneal epithelial defects that had been present for 10 days or greater and were unresponsive to conventional treatments, including bandage contact lenses.[10] The most common causes for these epithelial defects were herpetic keratitis, recurrent erosion and dry eye. The corneal epithelial defects healed in 14 of 18 patients, with half of the defects healing within 48 hours.

Doxycycline has been reported to be effective in treating recurrent corneal epithelial erosions in two additional studies. Hope-Ross and associates performed a prospective, randomized, controlled 24 weeks trial comparing three treatment groups: standard therapies (lubricants, hypertonic saline), oral tetracycline (250 mg twice daily) and oral tetracycline and topical prednisolone for recalcitrant recurrent corneal epithelial erosions.[11] The tetracycline and tetracycline plus topical corticosteroid groups both showed significant reductions in the number of recurrent erosions compared to standard therapy during the study period. Furthermore, the tetracycline treated groups had significantly faster healing of epithelial defects than the standard group. Dursun and colleagues reported a series of 7 patients with a history of 1 to 7 prior recurrent erosions that had failed to respond to conventional therapies (artificial tears, hypertonic saline, patching, bandage contact lenses, epithelial debridement) who had resolution of their condition with oral doxycyline (50 mg twice a day) for 3 months and topical corticosteroid (methylprednisolone, prednisolone acetate or fluorometholone) two or three times daily for 3 weeks.[12] Corneal epithelial defects healed in 2-10 days when present. No recurrence was observed during a mean follow-up period of 21.9 months.

In a rabbit model of superficial alkali corneal injury, oral doxycycline at a dose of 5 mg/kg/day was noted to significantly speed healing of the corneal epithelial defects.[13]

Prevention of Sterile Corneal Stromal Ulceration and Neovascularization

In 1895, Perry and Golub initially reported the use of oral tetracycline for treatment of sterile corneal ulceration.[14] This was complimented with a study that evaluated the effects of two doses of tetracycline (10 mg/kg/day and 50 mg/kg/day) in a rabbit model of alkali-induced corneal injury. Both doses of tetracycline were effective in preventing ulceration compared to the untreated control group with the highest dose being the most effective.[15] The tetracycline treated rabbits had a marked reduction in inflammatory cell infiltration of the corneal stroma. Levy and Katz noted that systemic tetracycline decreased corneal performation in a rabbit model of *Pseudomonas* keratitis by approximately 50 percent.[16] Treatment of two human patients with severe *pseudomonas* keratitis with oral doxycycline (100 mg BID) arrested stromal ulceration in these patients.[17]

Tetracycline derivatives have also been observed to have potent inhibitory activity for corneal neovascularization in several animal models. A minocycline controlled release polymer implanted into the cornea stroma of rabbits was noted to completely inhibit tumor induced angiogenesis.[18] Doxycycline (2%) administered topically significantly inhibited development of corneal neovascularization after chemical cauterization of the rabbit cornea with silver nitrate.[19] This effect was greatly potentiated when topical doxycycline was used in combination with topical flurbiprofen or low molecular weight heparin.[20]

Ocular Rosacea

Oral tetracyclines have been recognized as highly effective therapy for the skin lesions of rosacea for decades.[21,22] Tetracyclines have also been reported to be efficacious in treating the ocular manifestations of rosacea (Fig. 61.5). Jenkins and colleagues reported that symptoms and signs of ocular rosacea improved in 36 of 37 patients treated with tetracycline 250 mg orally QID

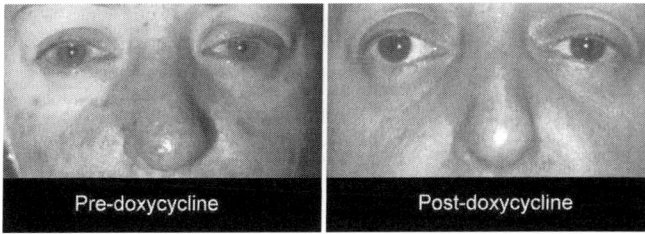

Fig. 61.5: Patient with facial and ocular rosacea before and after treatment with oral doxycycline 50 mg/ml for 6 months

for 3 weeks, followed by one week off therapy.[23] This cycle was repeated until maximum improvement was reached. Symptom improvement was noted from 4 days to 3 weeks after starting the therapy. Keratitis improved within 28 days in all patients and no chalazia recurred during the treatment period. Forty-one percent of patients had a recurrence within 5–28 months after cessation of therapy over the follow-up period that ranged from 5 to 28 months.

Bartholomew and associates performed a double-masked, placebo controlled crossover trial of oxytetracycline (250 mg BID for 6 weeks) in 35 patients with ocular rosacea.[24] Seventeen patients received oxytetracycline and 11 experienced partial or total remission of the condition. Disease signs that responded to treatment included lid swelling and redness, chalazia, conjunctival redness, corneal infiltrates, marginal ulcers and punctate epithelial erosions. No changes were noted in corneal neovascularization or scarring. Patients generally responded within 2 weeks and some patients experienced a recurrence within 2 to 3 weeks of discontinuing therapy. Frucht-Pery et al compared the effectiveness of two tetracycline regimens for treatment of ocular rosacea (tetracycline 250 mg QID or doxycycline 100 mg once daily).[25] The study was undertaken because tetracycline should not be taken with milk or dairy products, while these foods have minimal effects on absorption of doxycycline. Both regimens showed improvement in total symptoms, foreign body sensation and conjunctival hyperemia. After 6 weeks of treatment, all patients but one had symptomatic improvement. Slightly greater symptomatic relief was noted in the tetracycline group after 6 weeks; however, there was no difference between the two groups after 3 months of treatment.

In a series of 131 patients with ocular rosacea reported by Akpek and associates, 86 percent were treated with oral tetracycline derivatives (tetracycline 250 mg four times daily or doxycycline 100 mg per day).[26] All patients but 2 showed dramatic improvement in signs and symptoms in 2–6 weeks. Seven patients who had cicatrizing conjunctivitis had no further complications and remained stable on tetracycline therapy. Adverse effects, notably nausea and photosensitivity, were reported by 25 percent of tetracycline treated patients. Zengin et al performed a randomized trial comparing tetracycline (250 mg QID for 4 weeks and BID for 5 months) with meibomian gland expression therapy in 28 patients with ocular rosacea.[27] Both groups showed significant improvement in meibomian gland signs (plugging, volume and thickness of expressed meibum); however, the tetracycline treatment group also had a significant increase in tear break-up time.

With the realization that the therapeutic effect of tetracyclines for rosacea is due in large part to their antimicrobial effects, there has been a trend towards use of lower doses of oral tetracyclines for both skin and ocular disease.[28] Our current regimen is doxycycline 20 mg orally twice a day for a month. If the condition recurs after the therapy is stopped, it may be continued for several months.

Phlyctenular Disease

In 1981, Zaidman and Brown reported that oral tetracycline arrested progression of corneal scarring and vascularization in a series of 6 patients with nontuberculous phlyctenular keratoconjunctivitis.[29] Oral tetracycline was also noted to produce long-lasting remission of another series of 17 patients with phlyctenular keratoconjunctivitis.[30]

Mucous Membrane Pemphigoid

Cicatricial pemphigoid, now generally referred to as mucous membrane pemphigoid (MMP), is a rare and potentially blinding ocular surface disease. A number of inflammatory mediators including circulating autoantibodies, complement, T cells and cytokines have been implicated in its pathogenesis.[31] A number of immunomodulators have been found to be effective in treating this condition, including tetracyclines (tetracycline or minocycline), alone or in combination with nicotinamide (niacin 500 mg–3 per day) or mycophenolate mofetil (up to 2 per day).[31-35] These case reports or small nonrandomized clinical series have reported marked improvement or remission of mucosal disease, including the conjunctiva, in patients with MMP following tetracycline therapy. This therapy had minimal side effects and it has been recommended for elderly patients who are prone to develop severe complications from more potent agents such as cyclophosphamide.

Keratoconjunctivitis Sicca

Because of the increasing recognition that inflammation plays a key role in the pathogenesis of keratoconjunctivitis sicca (KCS), as well as well-documented improvement in the corneal epithelial disease of ocular rosacea following tetracycline treatment, we have utilized oral (20–50 mg/day) or topical doxycycline (0.025% formulated in saline administered QID) to treat the ocular surface epithelial disease of dry eye. In general, tetracycline alone or in combination with other topical anti-inflammatory agents (i.e. cyclosporin A or corticosteroids) has improved the severity of corneal fluorescein staining and filamentary keratitis as demonstrated by the patient with Sjögren's syndrome KCS in Figure 61.6. These clinical observations served as the basis for evaluating the effectiveness of topical doxycycline in treating experimental dry eye.

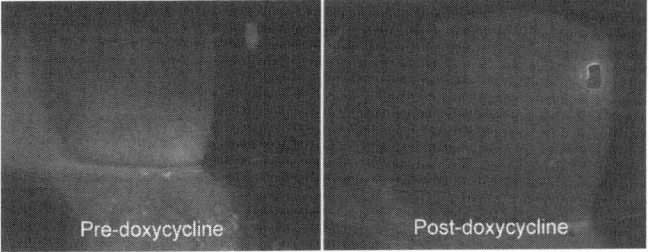

Fig. 61.6: Patient with Sjögren's syndrome keratoconjunctivitis sicca before and after treatment with topical doxycycline 0.025 percent QID for 3 weeks

Experimental dry eye was created in mice by subcutaneous scopolamine injection and continuous exposure to an air draft and low humidity environment (≤ 35% ambient humidity). Mice were treated topically treated with three different agents: balanced salt solution (BSS), methylprednisolone 1 percent or doxycycline 0.025 percent, all four times daily for five days. Corneal epithelial disease was evaluated by grading the severity of corneal staining with oregon green dextran (OGD) 70 kDa. Experimentally induced dry eye increased corneal permeability to OGD. There was no improvement in corneal staining with this dye with BSS, but significant improvement was observed with methylprednisolone and doxycycline (Fig. 61.7A).[36] Corneal smoothness was also evaluated by reflection of a white ring light. Doxycycline corneas were found to be significantly smoother than untreated or saline treated dry eyes (Fig. 61.7B).

To determine the possible cellular basis for the increased corneal permeability in response to dry eye, the integrity of corneal epithelial tight junctions which maintain the corneal barrier was evaluated by confocal fluorescent microscopy using an antibody specific to the tight junction protein occludin. Compared to untreated eyes, there was a marked increase in cytoplasmic occludin staining and focal loss of cell membrane staining in response to experimental dry eye. There was also a marked increase in desquamation of the superficial corneal epithelia in dry eye, while apical epithelial cells remained intact in eyes that were treated with methylprednisolone or doxycycline (Fig. 61.7C). A concurrent study showed that MMP-9 protein in the corneal epithelium dramatically increased in experimental dry eye and this was prevented by topical treatment with the methylprednisolone or doxycycline 0.025 percent QID.[37] Gelatinase activity in the corneal epithelium and tears also markedly decreased with these therapies.

SUMMARY

The role of inflammation and increased protease activity in the pathogenesis of ocular surface disease has become evident over the past 2 decades. There is overwhelming evidence indicating

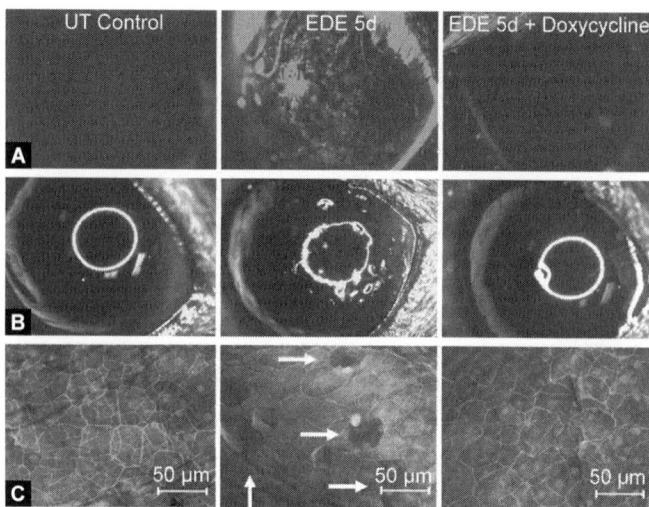

Figs 61.7A to C: (A) Corneal epithelial staining with fluorescent probe oregon green dextran (OGD) in untreated control (UT control), after 5 days of experimental dry eye (EDE 5d) and after 5d of EDE treated with topical doxycycline 0.025 percent; (B) Corneal smoothness evaluated by reflection of white ring light in the 3 groups; (C) Confocal microscopy of occludin staining in the 3 groups. Arrows in the EDE 5d group indicate areas where the superficial cells have detached (desquamation holes)

that tetracyclines have potent anti-inflammatory and antiprotease effects in treating a variety of ocular surface diseases. They are often effective in low concentrations that minimize systemic side effects and they are synergistic with other commonly utilized immunomodulatory agents. Animal studies and preliminary human experience indicate that tetracyclines, such as doxycycline may be effective when applied topically in subantimicrobial doses that would eliminate the systemic side effects that commonly accompany oral tetracycline therapy.

REFERENCES

1. Curci JA, Petrinec D, Liao S, Golub LM, Thompson RW. Pharmacological suppression of abdominal aortic aneurysms: a comparison of doxycycline and four chemically modified tetracyclines. J Vasc Surg 1998;28:1082-93.
2. Solomon A, Monroy D, Rosenblatt M, Ji Z, Lokeshwar BL, Pflugfelder SC. Doxycycline inhibition of interleukin-1 in the corneal epithelium. Invest Ophthalmol Vis Sci 2000;41:2544-57.
3. Li DQ, Luo L, Chen Z, Kim HS, Song XJ, Pflugfelder SC. JNK and ERK MAP kinases mediate induction of IL-1α, TNF-α and IL-8 following hyperosmolar stress in human limbal epithelial cells. Exp Eye Res 2006;82:588-96.
4. Li D-Q, Lokeshwar BL, Solomon A, Monroy D, Ji Z, Pflugfelder SC. Regulation of MMP-9 in human corneal epithelial cells. Exp Eye Res 2001;73:449-59.

5. Li de Q, Shang TY, Kim HS, Solomon A, Lokeshwar BL, Pflugfelder SC. Regulated Expression of Collagenases MMP-1, -8, and -13 and Stromelysins MMP-3, -10, and -11 by Human Corneal Epithelial Cells. Invest Ophthalmol Vis Sci 2003;44:2928-36.
6. Li DQ, Chen Z, Song XJ, Luo L, Pflugfelder SC. Stimulation of Matrix Metalloproteinases by Hyperosmolarity via a JNK Pathway in Human Corneal Epithelial Cells. Invest Ophthalmol Vis Sci 2004;45:4302-11.
7. Kim HS, Luo L, Pflugfelder SC, Li DQ. Doxycycline inhibits TGF-beta1-induced MMP-9 via Smad and MAPK pathways in human corneal epithelial cells. Invest Ophthalmol Vis Sci 2005;46:840-8.
8. Zhu S, Stavrovskaya IG, Drozda M, et al. Minocycline inhibits cytochrome C release and delays progression of amyotrophic lateral sclerosis in mice. Nature 2002;417:74-8.
9. Suk K. Minocycline suppresses hypoxic activation of rodent microglia in culture. Neurosci Letters 2004;366:167-71.
10. Perry HD, Kenyon KR, Lamberts DW, Foulks GN, Seedor JA, Golub LM. Systemic tetracycline hydrochloride as adjunctive therapy in the treatment of persistent epithelial defects. Ophthalmology. 1986;93:1320-2.
11. Hope-Ross MW, Chell PB, Kervick GN, McDonnell PJ, Jones HS Oral tetracycline in the treatment of recurrent corneal erosions. Eye 1994;8 (Pt 4):384-8.
12. Dursun D, Kim MC, Solomon A, Pflugfelder SC. Treatment of recalcitrant recurrent corneal epithelial erosions with inhibitors of matrix metalloproteinases-9, doxycycline and corticosteroids. Am J Ophthalmol. 2001;132:8-13.
13. Perry HD, Hodes LW, Seedor JA, Donnenfeld ED, McNamara TF, Golub LM. Effect of doxycycline hyclate on corneal epithelial wound healing in the rabbit alkali-burn model. Preliminary observations. Cornea 1993;12:379-82.
14. Perry HD, Golub LM. Systemic tetracyclines in the treatment of non-infected corneal ulcers: a case report and proposed new mechanism of action. Ann Ophthalmol 1985;17:742-44.
15. Seedor JA, Perry HD, McNamara TF, Golub LM, Buxton DF, Guthrie DS. Systemic tetracycline treatment of alkali-induces corneal ulceration in rabbits, Arch Ophthalmol 1987;105:268-71.
16. Levy JH, Katz HR. Effect of systemic tetracycline on progression os *Pseudomonas aeruginosa* keratitis in the rabbit. Ann Ophthalmol 1990;22:179-82.
17. McElvanney AM. Doxycycline in the management of pseudomonas corneal melting: Two case reports and a review of the literature. Eye Contact Lens 2003;29:258-61.
18. Riazi-Esfahani M, Peyman GA, Aydin E, Kazi AA, Kivilcim M, Sanders DR. Prevention of corneal neovascularization: Evaluation of various commercially available compounds in an experimental rat model. Cornea 2006;25:801-5.
19. Tamargo RJ, Bok RA, Brem H. Angiogenesis inhibition by minocycline. Cancer Res 1991;51:672-5.
20. Peyman GA, Kazi AA, Riazi-Esfahani M, Aydin E, Kivilcim M, Sanders DR. The effect of combinations of flurbiprofen, low molecular weight heparin, and doxycycline on the inhibition of corneal neovascularization. Cornea 2006;25:582-5.
21. Marks R, Ellis J. Comparative effectiveness of tetracycline and ampicillin in rosacea. A controlled trial. Lancet 1971;2(7733):1049-52.

22. Sneedon IB. A clinical trial of tetracycline in rosacea. Br J Dermatol 1966;78:649-52.
23. Jenkins MS, Brown SI, Lempert SL, Weinberg RJ. Ocular rosacea. Am J Ophthalmol 1979;88:618-22.
24. Bartholomew RS, Reid BJ, Cheesbrough MJ, Macdonald M, Galloway NR. Oxytetracycline in the treatment of ocular rosacea: a double-blind trial. Br J Ophthalmol 1982;66:386-8.
25. Frucht-Pery J, Sagi E, Hemo I, Ever-Hadani P. Efficacy of doxycycline and tetracycline in ocular rosacea. Am J Ophthalmol 1993;116:88-92.
26. Akpek EK, Merchant A, Pinar V, Foster CS. Ocular rosacea: Patient characteristics and follow-up. Ophthalmology 1997;104:1863-7.
27. Zengin N, Tol H, Gunduz K, Okudan S, Balevi S, Endogru H. Meibomian gland dysfunction and tear film abnormalities in rosacea. Cornea 1995;14:144-6.
28. Berman B, Zell D. Subantimicrobial dose doxycycline: A unique treatment for rosacea. Cutis 2005;75(4 Suppl):19-24.
29. Zaidman GW, Brown SI. Orally administered tetracycline for phlyctenular keratoconjunctivitis. Am J Ophthalmol 1981;92:178-82.
30. Culbertson WW, Huang AJ, Mandelbaum SH, Pflugfelder SC, Boozalis GT, Miller D. Effective treatment of phlyctenular keratoconjunctivitis with oral tetracycline. Ophthalmology 1993;100:1358-66.
31. Ahmed M, Zein G, Khawaja F, Foster CS. Ocular cicatricial pemphigoid: pathogenesis, diagnosis and treatment. Prog Retin Eye Res 2004;23:579-92.
32. Reiche L, Wojnarowska F, Mallon E. Combination therapy with nicotinamide and tetracyclines for cicatricial pemphigoid: Further support for its efficacy. Clin Exp Dermatol 1998;23:254-7.
33. Kreyden OP, Borradori L, Trueb RM, Burg G, Nestle FO [Successful therapy with tetracycline and nicotinamide in cicatricial pemphigoid] Hautarzt 2001;52:247-50.
34. Dragan L, Eng AM, Lam S, Persson T. Tetracycline and niacinamide: treatment alternatives in ocular cicatricial pemphigoid. Cutis 1999;63:181-3.
35. Sacher C, Hunzelmann N. Cicatricial pemphigoid (mucous membrane pemphigoid): Current and emerging therapeutic approaches. Am J Clin Dermatol 2005;6:93-103.
36. De Paiva CS, Corrales RM, Villarreal AL, Farley W, Li DQ, Stern ME, Pflugfelder SC. Apical corneal barrier disruption in experimental murine dry eye is abrogated by methylprednisolone and doxycycline Invest. Ophthalmol Vis Sci 2006;47:2847-56.
37. De Paiva CS, Corrales RM, Villarreal AL, Farley W, Li DQ, Stern ME, Pflugfelder SC. Corticosteroid and doxycycline suppress MMP-9 and inflammatory cytokine expression, MAPK activation in the corneal epithelium in experimental dry eye. Exp Eye Res 2006;83:526-35.

Optimized NSAIDs and Antibacterial Regimen is Key to Ocular Surgical Prophylaxis

Ashok Garg (India), Ian Bell (USA)

Cataract surgery is one of the most commonly performed ocular surgery in the world. Given the ability of ocular surface flora to enter the eye during surgery, many of the prophylactic techniques aim is to suppress their number and to limit the growth of those organisms that do enter the eye during intraocular surgery. Antimicrobial prophylaxis is an essential component of both cataract and refractive surgeries. Choosing an antibiotic for surgical prophylaxis in the clinical setting can also be challenging.

The key surgical prophylaxis paradigm shift in recent years for long practicing ophthalmologists is the growing evidence for preoperative use of both topical antibiotics and anti-inflammatory drops. The second shift is the realization that we should discontinue antibiotics more quickly and ensure use of anti-inflammatory for the full course of therapy. These changes are key for limiting postcataract (iatrogenic) inflammation and infection while they prevent the development of antibiotic resistance in patients. In the preoperative a fourth-generation fluoroquinolone such as moxifloxacin 0.5 percent solution, a nonsteroidal anti-inflammatory such as topical nepafence 0.1 percent, suspension, and a topical steroid such as prednisolone acetate 1 percent should all be administered.

Loading the eye with an antibiotic prior to the surgical insult reduces the risk of endophthalmitis. Furthermore studies have shown that the nonsteroidal, anti-inflammatory drugs (NSAIDs) and the steroids are synergistic and both work better if the eye is loaded preoperative.

There are two basic ways to approach the preoperative loading. One approach provides the drops within the three-to-four doses delating regimen in the surgical induction area. We can add neosynephrine 10 percent cyclogyl solution (1% Cyclopentolate HCl), an antibiotic, steroid, nonsteroidal, so actually they get loaded up with five different drops. Our preoperative routine is three doses of drops starting 30–60 minutes before surgery.

Some surgeons prefer to start the drops 24 hours preoperative while others start the drops three days preoperative.

There are select indications where anti-inflammatory drug dosing should begin a week preoperative including high-risk cases for inflammation and secondary macular edema. Such patients includes those with a long-term, history of chronic uveitis and diabetes mellitus and patients with pigmentary retinopathy and macular edema, and those who developed macular edema in the first eye after cataract surgery.

With high-risk patients such as those who are immunocompromised or prone to infection, we can start the antibiotic three days preoperative rather than just on the table.

In our routine cases, I load the entire drop regimen in the eye in the operating room, but the high-risk cases you may start, three to seven days preoperative. There is not yet a consensus, but you may want to go a little longer and by more intense on the high-risk patients.

The research evidence does not clearly identify whether drug delivery shortly preoperative or several days preoperative is better. However, as the patients become higher risk, we tend to have a slightly longer and more intense course of antibiotic and anti-inflammatory drops.

Routine patients that never had a problem generally start to receive the drug in the operating room prior to surgery because it is easiler on the patient.

POSTOPERATIVE SCHEDULE FOR CATARACT PATIENTS

The major changes in recent years from previous antibiotic experience is the perioperative and short postoperative course of the drugs. We now limit antibiotic use because the risk of endophthalmitis drops within a week when the wound seals. It is the long-term, low-dose use of these drugs that leads to resistant organisms.

Our approach is to administer antibiotics and anti-inflammatory drops (steroid and NSAID) at the end of the case. My staff administer them again in the recovery area before the patient goes home.

We have patients use the antibiotic drops three times a day for one week. Other surgeons have them take the antibiotic for as few as five days.

However, the anti-inflammatory drug is required for longer use. Evidence suggests the blood aqueous barrier breakdown that occurs after cataract surgery persists for four to eight weeks. Because the average breakdown lasts about six weeks, we should treat with anti-inflammatory drops for one to two months in routine cases. This will prevent any rebound of inflammation or other secondary issues.

We need to have patients use the anti-inflammatory drops a big longer than some surgeons think is necessary because often the eyes are quiet and comfortable by two to three weeks after surgery, but there is still some risk for cystoid macular edema up to six weeks postoperative.

For example, for at-risk patients preoperative dosing is recommended for one week and postoperative dosing is recommended for one week and postoperative dosing is recommended for four weeks to several months.

Drug Dosages

The dosing regimen we use instillation of the topical nevanac, which is a TID drop, a three-times daily drop. We use moxifloxacin, Nepafenac, and a topical steroid, which seems more than adequate, as these drugs have demonstrated efficacy in contributing to good surgical outcomes.

Ophthalmologists should be aware of adding NSAID to their regimen. Most patients recover without complications when surgeons only use an antibiotic and a steroid. However, there are indications that over 10 percent of patients will develop a very mild macular edema without an NSAID. That's a risk that NSAIDs can eliminate.

We have pretty minimally invasive cataract surgery today, and people work really hard at their surgical technique, but probably the one thing that could have the greatest impact on their outcomes would be to add an NSAID to their regimen.

The incidence of very mild macular edema without an NSAID, even in a good surgeon's hands, is about 12 percent and adding as NSAID takes it down to less than 1 percent so you get a hug reduction in one of the most common sight threatening complications of cataract surgery just by adding an NSAID and using it properly.

Proper dosing of antibiotics, NSAIDs, and steroid plays a very important role in preventing complications such as infection or CME.

Minimizing these complications with effective agents and proper therapeutic dosing regimens will improve our surgical outcomes.

Surgeons can greatly improve their chances of a successful surgical outcome if they keep in mind three key criteria in selecting antibiotics: potency, penetration, and safety. A good balance of these aspects—especially potency and penetration—provides the best patient protection.

An antibiotic that is highly potent and effective at killing infections at lower concentrations would lose much of its efficacy if it was unable to penetrate the tissue. Conversely, a medication that penetrates extremely well but lacks potency also would not be very functional.

Clinicians are best served by an effective combination of penetration and potency.

Although researchers are frequently asked whether potency or penetration is more important, the only clear answer is the most effective approach is to combine these factors.

MEASURING POTENCY

Identifying an antibiotics strength in penetration and potency is important, but surgeons should be aware that potency definitions vary. The most common assessment of an antibiotics potency, the minimum inhibitory concentration (MIC), traces whether organisms growth has been stopped. However, the definition still allows viable organisms to remain. This most common term may not be the most important. Another standard, minimum bactericidal concentration (MBC), tracks whether 99.9 percent of the organism is killed (MBC is approximately 4x the MIC). The final measurement, mutant prevention concentration (MPC), gauges whether the organism was killed with mutations prevented (MPC is approximately 8x the MIC).

Drugs with the lowest potency numbers in MIC, MBC or MPC are among the most potent. With postoperative infections being potentially sight threatening, it is ideal to exceed these levels with the antibiotic concentrations in the target tissues.

PENETRATION TRACKING

Antibiotic tissue penetration plays a key role in protecting against infection.

This issue arises when examining the research on various antibiotics; some may have good potency statistics *in vitro*, but we fail to identify the *in vivo* performance of the antibiotic. The latter will tell ophthalmologists what levels of the drug our patients actually will get in the cornea, the anterior chamber, and the vitreous. Our research administering fluoroquinolones to a cornea transplant model prior to corneal transplant and then examining the antibiotic levels in the cornea showed moxifloxacin had three times the concentration of gatifloxacin.

Similar research at various international research centers on aqueous concentrations of antibiotic applied a series of drops preoperative and measured aqueous concentration at the time of cataract surgery. Those researchers identified the same three-fold greater penetration of moxifloxacin. Protection can be defined by overlaying these concentrations with the MICs for potential pathogens.

In vivo potency after tissue penetration is a better measure of antibiotic efficacy than speed of kill *in vitro*. The latter removes all of the factors that determine how the antibiotic performs in human tissue. These studies disregard the reality of penetration of the antibiotic through human tissue. For these reasons *in vivo* potency and penetration studies will always have more real-world resonance than *in vitro* speed of kill research. The aqueous humor concentrations achieved in the International Research Centers were tested against a *S. aureus* ocular isolate using disk-diffusion analysis. The moxifloxacin achieve a 24 mm zone of inhibition, and gatifloxacin had no zone of inhibition. This surrogate model accounts for tissue penetration and potency at the potential site of infection, thus defining protection.

SAFETY EVALUATION

In addition to potency and penetration, a solid evaluation of antibiotics for surgical prophylaxis should assess whether the drug is nontoxic. Efforts to prevent the use of nontoxic medication should look for epithelial problems or endothelial problems.

As a class of drugs, the fluoroquinolones have proven to by very safe and nontoxic.

Our experience with all fourth-generation fluoroquinolones has found that they are very safe. Research comparing corneal epithelial healing postoperative when moxifloxacin or gatifloxacin are used have found very similar would healing rates. In fact, an independent well-controlled study evaluating wound healing post-PRK for moxifloxacin and gatifloxacin were conducted in USA. The conclusion was that both the drugs are safe. Generally, they found that eyes treated with moxifloxacin healed faster and had smaller defects than those treated with gatifloxacin.

Rabbit model studies that created epithelial defects and tracked healing when the two antibiotics are used found similar results. Clinical trials looking at healing after PRK also identified similar healing. Both fluoroquinolones are safe and nontoxic.

Ophthalmic Medications in Pediatric Age Group

Rami Pai, Kirit Mody (India)

INTRODUCTION

Many ocular medications are prescribed and used in the pediatric age group. The data regarding their safety in this group of patients are sparse. Considering that the systemic absorption of the ocular drugs in pediatric patients is much greater, it is important that we evaluate the optimum dose with the minimum effective concentration as well as the potential systemic side effects of the various groups of drugs. This will give us a clearer picture of the risk versus benefit of using such drugs in the population.

Most of the commercially available medications have not been well studied in pediatric age group; hence these are prescribed empirically. Great caution is required in using the topical ophthalmic drugs in children especially infants in whom systemic absorption carries a much greater risk. This is because of the following reasons:

- *Average blood volume*: The average blood volume is smaller in children and to a higher serum concentration of the drug up to 20 folds more.
- *Absorption*: In children the absorption of drug from the conjunctiva, nasal mucosa and skin contributes significantly. Up to 90 percent of the drop may be absorbed through the nasal mucosa. Besides this the thin keratin on the skin, reduced tear production and increased incidence of nasolacrimal duct obstruction are factors, which increase systemic absorption.
- *Drug clearance*: Immature enzymatic pathways and a reduced renal function in neonates slow down elimination of the drug from the blood.
- *Free drug*: Reduced plasma protein binding and relatively less adipose tissue results in greater amount of free drug available especially in the neonate.

PRECAUTIONS

Instructions can be given to guardians regarding technique of instillation so that the systemic absorption can be reduced significantly.

- Only one drop to be instilled at a time
- Punctal occlusion with finger for 3 to 4 minutes after instillation
- Wipe the excess overflow of drops immediately

- In uncooperative subjects, one to two drops at the medial canthus to be instilled in the supine position. When the eyes open, some of it enters the conjunctival sac, rest is to be wiped with a tissue.

As a general rule it has been suggested that the estimated required topical dosage is as follows:

Birth to two years: One-half the adult dose.
- 2–3 years : Two-thirds the adult dose
- >3 years : Adult dose.

MYDRIATIC AGENTS

These are frequently used for retinal examination and refraction besides treatment of inflammatory conditions of the iris. They are either sympathomimetics or parasympatholytics. *One has to remember when using these drugs that lighter irides requires much less concentration of the drug than dark irides.*

Adrenergic Agonist

Phenylephrine Hydrochloride

Indications: It is often used with parasympatholytics to cause maximal rapid dilatation of the pupil, especially to examine peripheral retina or preoperatively. Its action lasts for only 6 hours.

Dosage: Diagnostic purpose 1 drop twice at an interval of 5–10 minutes.

Toxicity: As an alpha-adrenergic agent, it can cause hypertension, tachycardia and arrhythmias, besides dry mouth/skin due to systemic absorption. *It should be used with caution in children especially those with hyperthyroidism or tachy-arrhythmias. In children with pheochromocytoma, it might cause sudden and precipitating rise in blood pressure and hypertensive encephalopathy.*

The preparations available in the market are with a concentration of 10 percent (Drosyn – trade name) or 5 percent as a combination with tropicamide 0.8 percent. A case of acute gastric dilatation in a preterm infant after two drops each of cyclopentolate 0.5 percent and phenylephrine 2.5 percent has been reported. Using phenylephrine in the concentration of 2.5 percent or less can significantly reduce such type of severe side effects.

The 10 percent solution should be avoided in children. As 2.5 percent soln is not available in the market, we can consider dilution of the phenylephrine 5 percent - tropicamide 0.8 percent combination for use especially in preterm infants where retinal examination is frequently carried out to rule out or assess retinopathy of prematurity (ROP).

Cycloplegic Agents/Parasympatholytics

Indications in Children

- Retinal examination with cycloplegic refraction
- Treatment of amblyopia
- Postoperative cycloplegia
- Prevent postoperative synechiae formation and relieve pain due to ciliary spasm in uveitis.

This group of drugs being parasympatholytics result if both mydriasis as well as cycloplegia. The relative cycloplegia caused by these drugs is compared below:

Drugs	Percent efficiency of cycloplegia
1% Atropine	100%
1% Cyclopentolate	92%
1% Tropicamide	80%
5% Homatropine	54%

Table 63.1 shows the pharmacokinetics of the various mydriatic eyedrops.

Atropine Sulfate

It is a potent anticholinergic used in children for complete cycloplegia.

Dosage

- *Cycloplegic refraction*: One percent eyedrop twice a day or one centimeter of 1 percent ointment once daily for 1–3 days before examination.
- *Amblyopia*: One percent once daily or twice weekly in the sound eye.
- *Uveitis*: 0.5 percent eyedrop can be instilled three times a day.

Toxicity: The general signs and symptoms include dryness of mouth, skin, fever, delirium, tachycardia and sometime even death. In children toxicity might occur with as little as one drop of 0.5 percent soln bilaterally. Lightly pigmented individuals, patients of Down's syndrome and brain damage are more susceptible.

Dose related side effects of atropine are given below::

Dose of 1 percent soln	Side effects
1–4 drops	Tachycardia, dry mouth
10 drops	Restlessness, confusion, speech disturbance, hot/dry skin. Decreased GI motility and urinary retention
20 drops	Besides above, hyperexcitability, ataxia, hallucination coma, convulsion and death

Antidote: Severe anticholinergic toxicity is treated with physostigmine 0.05 percent injected intravenously (0.02 mg/kg.) every 5 minutes up to a maximum of 2 mg.

TABLE 63.1: Comparative pharmacokinetics of various dilating agents (mydriatics)

Generic name	Trade name	Concentration	Mydriasis		Cycloplegia		
			Max. effect (Min.)	Full recovery	Max.	Full recovery	
Phenylephrine	Drosyn	10% ed			–	–	
	Drosyn T	5% ed	20–30	6 hr	–	–	
Atropine	Belpinoatrin	1% ed/eo	40	10+ days	6 hr	14 days	
Homatropine	Homide	2% ed	60	3 days	60 min	3 days	
Cyclopentolate	Cyclogil Cyclopent	1% ed 0.5% ed	60	1 day	60 min	1 day	
Tropicamide	Tropicamide	1% ed	40	6 hr	30 min	6 hr	
Tropicamide + Phenylephrine	Drosyn T Tropicalyl plus	0.8% 5%	20–30		6 hr	30 hr	6 hr

Heading: Comparative Pharmacokinetics of various Dilating Agents

Homatropine

Similar to atropine except that it acts more quickly. It has a shorter duration of action and recovery is also faster (Table 63.1).

Cyclopentolate

In view of the toxic side effects of atropine this drug is ideal for refraction in children.

Dosage: One drop once/twice at 5 minutes interval and cycloplegic refraction being done 40 minutes later. About 0.5 to 0.75 D hypermetropia might go undetected.

Toxicity
- *Gastrointestinal disturbances:* Paralytic ileus, gastric dilatation and necrotizing enterocolitis in infants.
- *Seizures and behavioral changes:* A case of seizure has been reported in cerebral palsy child after instillation of 1 percent cyclopentolate.
- Increased anterior chamber cellular infiltration has been reported. Hence to be used cautiously in case of uveitis.

Tropicamide

This is a short acting anticholinergic agent producing rapid mydriasis and incomplete cycloplegia. In combination with phenylephrine it results in rapid mydriasis with a persistant effect making it an ideal drug for fundus examination and preoperative dilatation.

Dosage

- *Cycloplegic refraction:* 1 to 2 drops twice at 5 minutes interval.
- *Preoperative mydriasis:* 1 to 2 drops at 15 minutes interval 1–2 hours prior to surgery.

Toxicity: A relatively safe drug but not ideal where cycloplegic refraction is the primary goal especially in infants and young children.

The combination of cyclopentolate hydrochloride 0.2 percent with phenylephrine hydrochloride 0.1 percent delivers optimal concentrations desirable for examining premature infants. It offers the advantage of rapid onset and short duration with minimal side effects.

GLAUCOMA MEDICATIONS

Medical treatment of glaucoma in infants is a temporary measure until surgery can be performed. Medications are often inadequate to control intraocular pressure, side effects are concern and compliance can be a challenge, while in the older age group with glaucoma medications play a greater role than surgery. The fact that these medications can cause serious systemic side effects has to be kept in mind as no controlled human studies have been done in children.

Beta-blockers

Mechanism

They decrease aqueous production in the ciliary body by blocking the beta-adrenergic receptor sites.

Advantages
- They are among the least expensive class of agents
- They reduce IOP with little or no effect on pupil size or accommodation.

Potential Side Effects

The ubiquity of beta-adrenergic receptor sites in the body can lead to a variety of systemic side effects.
- *Cardiovascular*: Bradycardia, hypotension, arrhythmias and heart block.
- *Respiratory*: Bronchospasm and apnea.
- *Central nervous system*: Behavioral changes, depression, dizziness, and cerebral ischemia.
- *Others*: Marked hypoglycemia in diabetes.

Contraindications and Toxicity

Due to the above systemic side effects, it is contraindicated in children with cardiac arrhythmias, bronchospasm, asthma and should be used in the lowest possible dose in healthy children.

One drop of 0.5 percent timolol can cause cardiac block in infants less than two years of age. One neonate developed Cheyne-Stokes breathing and apneic spells lasting up to 30 seconds, that resolved after timolol 0.25 percent was discontinued.

TABLE 63.2: Beta-blockers

Generic name	Trade name	Concentration	Dosage	Side effects	Remarks
Timolol maleate	Iotim, Glucomol Ocupress	0.25–0.5% eye drops	12 Hourly	CI – Asthma, bronchitis heart disease	Good response in children over 10 yrs 0.25% eye drop/gel preferred in pediatric age group
	Timolet GFS	0.5% gel	Once a day		
Betaxolol hydrochloride	Iobet Optipress Betoptic Optipress-S	0.5% ed 0.25% (suspension)	12 Hourly	Decreased corneal sensitivity	Greater safety in asthmatics as it is cardioselective
Carteolol hydrochloride	Ocupress	1% ed	12 Hourly	Cardio-pulmonary	Non-selective beta-blocker
Levobunolol	Betagan	0.25% ed 0.5% ed	12 Hourly	Cardio-pulmonary Dendritic keratopathy	Membrane stabilizing Longer duration

Note: The 0.25% sustained release preparation is the preferred agent in pediatric glaucoma due to the lower concentration, decreased systemic absorption and once daily dosing.

Table 63.2 shows relative pharmacokinetics of various beta-blockers for glaucoma treatment.

Carbonic Anhydrase Inhibitors

Mechanism of Action

They are sulfonamide derivatives used topically and systemically to inhibit aqueous humor production by slowing the formation of bicarbonate ions with subsequent reduction in sodium and fluid transport.

Dosage and Preparations

Generic name	Trade name	Concentration	Dose
Acetazolamide	Diamox	250 mg tab	8–30 mg/kg/day
		250 mg/ 5 ml	
Dorzolamide	Dorzox	2% ed	8–12 hourly

Systemic forms are used as adjunctives to topical glaucoma therapy. Acetazolamide is administered orally as a liquid suspension at a pediatric dose of 8–30 (generally 10–15) mg/kg/day. It is available in strength of 250 mg/5 ml.

Though not as effective as oral acetazolamide, topical dorzolamide can be used for short-term treatment. A study reported significant intraocular pressure reductions in one group of 11 pediatric glaucoma patients and was well tolerated. It is available as a 2 percent eyedrop prescribed 8–12 hourly (Dorzox). In a fixed combination with timolol 0.5 percent (Dorzox – T) it is reported to be more effective than when the two drops are used separately.

Potential Side Effects

As they are sulfonamide derivatives they are contraindicated in patients allergic to this group.

Gastrointestinal symptoms of nausea and anorexia are common and can be minimized by administering the dose with meals.

Genitourinary symptoms may present as urinary frequency. They are contraindicated in patients with kidney or liver disease or adrenal failure. Occasionally renal calculi are seen.

Other side effects are paraesthesias blood dyscrasias, Steven Johnson's syndrome and metabolic acidosis.

In view of the multiple side effects of systemic CAI, they are not the preferred drug of choice in pediatric age group.

Alpha-adrenergic Agonists

Mechanism of Action

They decrease aqueous production and may increase uveoscleral outflow.

Dosage and Preparation

Generic name	Trade name	Concentration	Dose	Remarks
Apraclonidine	Alpha drops	0.5 percent	8 hrly	Short-term use in adults only
	Alpha drops DS	1 percent		
Brimonidine	Alphagan Iobrim	0.2 percent	8–12 hrly	More selective than above

Potential Side Effects

These drugs cross the blood-brain barrier and are relatively contraindicated in children due to side effects of somnolence and fatigue secondary to CNS depression.

Local allergic reactions are common after prolonged use. Apraclonidine can cause tachyphylaxis within 3 months. Apnea, lethargy, hypotension, hypothermia, hypotonia have been reported after one drop of brimonidine in each eye of infants less than 2 months old. Two young children were unarousable and five others experienced extreme fatigue in another study. Reports of syncopal episodes in two 10-year-old are also known. These symptoms resolved after brimonidine was discontinued.

Apraclonidine should not be used in children. Brimonidine should not be used in children less than 2 years and with great caution in less than 6 years of age.

Adrenergic Agonist (Sympathomimetic)

Mechanism of Action

They decrease aqueous production by vasoconstriction in the ciliary body with prolonged use they improve aqueous outflow and uveoscleral output.

Dosage and Preparation

Generic name	Trade name	Concentration	Dosage
Epinephrine	Eppy	0.5–2 percent	8 hourly
Dipivalyl	Propine	0.1 percent	12 hourly
Epinephrine	DPE		

Potential Side Effects

Ocular side effects include allergy and cystoid macular edema especially in aphakic and pseudaphakic glaucoma patients. Hence, they are contraindicated in these patients. They can also cause conjunctival deposits.

Systemic side effects include sympathetic overactivity like palpitations, tachycardia, hypertension and sweating.

Dipivefrin causes less adverse reactions than epinephrine.

Contraindication: Narrow angle glaucoma and hypersensitivity.

As these drugs cause significant side effects and lower IOP only after prolonged use, they are not the preferred drugs of choice in children.

Parasympathomimetics

Mechanism of Action

Enhances aqueous outflow by ciliary muscle contraction, pull on the scleral spur and trabecular meshwork by acting on the acetylcholine receptors.

They are of two types:
1. Direct acting cholinergics.
2. Cholinesterase inhibitors.

Both these group of drugs cause miosis and ciliary muscle contraction.

Indications

- Chronic open angle glaucoma
- Acute angle closure glaucoma—only pilocarpine
- Preoperatively to glaucoma surgery—only pilocarpine
- Chronic synechial angle closure glaucoma—pilocarpine and physiostigmine
- Postoperatively to cyclodialysis surgery
- Accommodative esotropia treatment—anticholinesterase agents.

Dosage and Preparation

Direct acting cholinergics

Generic name	Trade name	Concentration	Dosage
Pilocarpine HCl	Pilocar	1,2,4% ed	4–6 hrly
		4% gel	15 mm od
	Occusert	Pilo–20	20 mg/hr
		Pilo–40	40 mg/hr
Carbachol	Miostat	1.5,2,3% ed	6 hrly

Cholinesterase inhibitors

Generic name	Trade name	Concentration	Dosage	Remarks
Physostigmine	Eserine	0.25,0.5% ed	4–6 hrly	Reversible
		0.25% eo		
Echothiophate iodide	Phospholine iodide	0.06%,0.125% ed	12 hrly	irreversible
Isoflurophate		0.025% eo	0.25" 8–72 hrs	Irreversible

Accommodative esotropia without amblyopia or anisometropia these drugs have to be instilled in both eyes. Dosage is as follows:
- *Echothiophate:* 0.125 percent od for 2–3 weeks
- *Isoflurophate:* 0.25 percent eo at bedtime for 2 weeks, then once a week for 2 months.

Potential Side Effects

Ocular
- Miosis resulting in diminished night vision and constriction of visual fields

- Ciliary muscle contraction resulting in myopia, accommodative spasm, headache, forward lens movement and pupillary block glaucoma (Paradoxical increase in IOP)
- Activation of iritis (especially anticholinesterases), iris cyst formation and lacrimal punctual stenosis.
- Retinal tears and retinal detachment.

Systemic
- GI overactivity
- Cardiac irregularities
- Salivation
- Breathing difficulties.

Antidote: Overdosage can be treated with parenteral atropine sulfate. The dose is 0.05 mg/kg IV initially followed by maintenance with 0.02 to 0.05 mg/kg titrated.

Contraindications

These drugs are not to be used in inflammatory glaucoma and malignant glaucoma. Anticholinesterases are not to be used in narrow angle glaucoma.

Because the muscle tendon attachments are not well formed in infants, miotics are not very effective in the pediatric age group.

Prostaglandin Analogs

Mechanism of Action

They are analogs of F2-alpha prostamides and activate metalloproteinases to remodel the extracellular matrix of the uveoscleral pathway thereby facilitating outflow. The also enhance nocturnal ciliary muscle tone.

Dosage and Preparations

Generic name	Trade name	Concentration	Dosage
Latanoprost	Latoprost 9 PM	0.005%	At bedtime
Bimatoprost	Lumigan	0.03%	At bedtime
Travoprost	Travatan	0.004%	od/bd
Unoprostone	Rescula	0.15%	bd

Potential Side Effects

Local side effects include increased eyelash growth, increased iris pigmentation, periorbital skin changes and punctate keratitis. Sleep disturbances and sweating have been reported in some children.

When used in a group of pediatric patients, latanoprost was found effective in only a minority of cases, although the drug appears to be well tolerated for short-term use.

These newer class of medications are mainly used in adults due to its impressive potency in adults, once daily dosing, flat diurnal cycle effects and few side effects.

In summary, timolol gel once daily is the recommended first line glaucoma medication in pediatrics age group due to its low cost and once daily dosing.

A combination of timolol with dorzolamide (Dorzox T) is more efficacious than taking the concomitant medications. However, the combination does not have the advantage of sustained release and dorzolamide causes stinging which can deter pediatric compliance.

Brimonidine is contraindicated in young children due to the CNS side effects and sympathomimetics are ineffective. The newer agents, prostaglandin analogs seem promising in juvenile-onset open angle glaucoma but long-term studies have to be carried out.

ANTI-INFLAMMATORY DRUGS

Steroids

Mechanism of Action

Corticosteroids are anti-inflammatory drugs for inflammatory eye disease. The inflammatory action is by altered protein transcription in white blood cells (WBCs) results in reduced due to depicts corticosteroid anti-inflammatory activity Table 63.3.

Hydrocortisone	1
Prednisolone	4
Triamcinolone	5
Methylprednisolone	5
Betamethasone	25
Dexamethasone	25

Indications

Inflammatory and allergic conditions of the eye. In children the common inflammatory/allergic condition include:
- *Lids*: Blepharitis, chalazion
- *Conjunctiva and cornea* : Vernal conjunctivitis, phlyctenular keratoconjunctivitis
- *Uveitis*
- *Postoperative*: Cataract, squint

Systemic corticosteroids are used in the treatment of severe inflammatory conditions of the eye. Corticosteroid injections are used in intermediate and posterior uveitis and capillary hemangiomas.

Dosage and Preparations

Steroids can be administered topically as drops (solutions, suspension) and ointments. They can be given as periocular injections through subconjunctival, retrobulbar or intralesional routes. Systemic administration either oral or parenteral is also prescribed in certain conditions.

TABLE 63.3: Lists the various corticosteroid preparations

Generic name	Concentration	Preparation	Trade name
Betamethasone Sodium phosphate	0.1% 0.5 mg 4 mg/ml	ed/eo tab injection	Betnesol
Dexamethasone Sodium phosphate	0.1% 0.05% 0.5 mg 4 mg/ml	ed (soln) ed tab inj	Decadron Lodex Wymeson Decadron
Hydrocortisone acetate	1% 2.5%	ed (soln) eo	Allocort Hydrocortistab
Prednisolone acetate	0.12% 0.125% 1%	ed ed (suspension) "	Pred mild Ecopred Predace Predmet
Prednisolone sodium phosphate	0.125% 1%	ed (soln)	AK-Pred/Inflamase Inflamase Forte
Prednisolone	5,10,20 mg	tab	Wysolone
Methylprednisolone	40 mg/ml 1 gm/16 ml	Inj	Depomedrol Solumedrol
Medrysone	1%	ed (suspen.)	HMS/Flarex
Fluoromethalone acetate	0.1% 0.25%	ed (suspen.) eo ed (suspen)	FML/Flomon FML SOP FML forte.
Loteprednol etabonate	0.5%	ed (soln)	Lotepred/Loteflam
Rimexolone	1%	ed (suspen.)	Vexol
Triamcinolone	1 mg/4 mg 10/20 mg/ml 40 mg/ml	tab inj	Kenacort Cyanamid Ledercort

The topical preparations are dosed as 1 to 2 drops every 1 hour to once daily or less, depending on the severity of the inflammation. Ointments are usually used at night for inflammatory conditions of the eyelid.

Dosage, duration and type of systemic steroids use depend on the severity and type of ocular disease. The dose for periocular injections is 0.5 ml in adults. In children the dose can be adjusted according to the age of the child. Systemic administration of steroids needs to be done in consultation with a pediatrician.

Potential Side Effects

Severe undesirable side effects limit topical corticosteroids use. They are
- Ocular hypertension (within 3 to 6 weeks in steroid responsive individual)
- Steroid induced glaucoma

- Posterior subcapsular cataracts
- Reactivation of herpes infections
- Perforation in presence of corneal or scleral thinning
- Systemic effects like headache and hypotension are rare or not commonly complained by children until they are very severe.

Systemic steroids besides having the same side effects like topical can also cause.
- Gastrointestinal—Gastritis, peptic ulcer
- Metabolic worsening diabetes, increased appetite, weight gain, sodium
- Fluid retention
- Vascular—Hypertension, capillary fragility
- Skeletal—Osteoporosis, aseptic necrosis of the hip
- Infective—Exacerbations of infections
- Psychiatric—Sleep disturbance and mood problems.

Corticosteroid infections (e.g. Kenacort) have been known to cause ophthalmic artery occlusion during intralesional infection to treat capillary hemangioma. A case of CRAO in a 4-year-old child has also been reported.

Relative Potential Side Effects of Various Corticosteroids

The safety of most of the steroids has not been established in children. Among the newer steroids safety of FML has not been established in children less than two years. In view of the serious side effects caused by prolonged corticosteroid use, benefits should outweigh the risks of steroid treatment. These drugs should be used with caution in patients diabetes, hypertension, myopia > 5 D or Krukenberg spindle.

Betamethasone, dexamethasone, and prednisolone are potent corticosteroids with excellent intraocular penetration but high chances of causing IOP spikes. Medrysone has poor intraocular penetration and therefore used for lid inflammations.

The newer generation steroids like fluorometholone and loteprednol are powerful corticosteroids with fewer propensities to cause rise in IOP. These are indicated for short-term treatment and prophylaxis of severe ocular surface disease (VKC). Rimexolone is a derivative of prednisolone that is metabolized to its inactive form in the anterior chamber thus reducing the risk of increased IOP. The ocular hypertensive effect is dose dependent and is more profound than in adults. Although the newer steroids claim to have less effect on IOP, their anti-inflammatory effect is probably limited.

Precautions

- IOP checked if steroids are used for more than 10 days.
- Subjects on long-term steroids monitored closely and frequently for complications.
- Dosage should be titrated for effect from the smallest possible dose and tapered as soon as possible.
- To consider use of diluted topical corticosteroids (1:10) to produce sufficient anti-inflammatory activity but least side effect.

Nonsteroidal Anti-inflammatory Drugs (NSAIDs)

Mechanism of Action

They inhibit cyclooxygenase and lipooxygenase enzymes, which lead to inhibition of inflammatory products. They are unable to modulate inflammatory cytokines other than those generated by arachidonic acid metabolism.

They have synergistic activity with steroids.

Indications

- Maintain intraoperative mydriasis
- Postoperative inflammation
- Allergic and giant papillary conjunctivitis
- Episcleritis and scleritis (Chronic inflammation associated with JRA)
- Certain uveitis along with steroids
- Cystoid macular edema.

Dosage and Preparations

Topical

Generic name	Concentration	Trade name
Indomethacin	1% ed (Soln/Suspn)	Incicin
Flurbiprofen	0.03% ed (Soln)	Flur/ocuflur
Diclofenac	0.1% ed	Voveran
Ketorolac	0.5% ed	Acular/Doloket/Ketlur

They are instilled every 6 hourly. Systemic NSAIDs have an analgesic, antipyretic and anti-inflammatory effect.

Potential Side Effects

The safety and efficacy of these drugs have not been established in children. The greatest advantage these have over steroids is anti-inflammatory activity without affecting IOP. The topical formulations do cause local irritation and sometimes allergic reactions. They may increase risk of bleeding in ocular tissues post-procedures.

Oral NSAIDs are useful when tapering corticosteroids. These have to be used carefully as they cause serious systemic side effects.

Diclofenac 0.1 percent when used for various condition in 208 pediatric patients along with corticosteroids including neonates was found to be effective and safe. In another study of 90 cases of VKC, flurbiprofen was found to be less effective than betamethasone but a safer alternative.

ANTI-ALLERGY MEDICATIONS

Allergic ocular disease is one of the common problems seen in childhood. It might be mild as in allergic conjunctivitis or more severe as in vernal keratoconjunctivitis (VKC). Most of them are primarily type-I hypersensitivity reactions (IgE mediated) with type-IV hypersensitivity playing a varying degree of role. Histamine release is responsible for most of the signs, symptoms and sequelae. Current antiallergy medical therapy is aimed at altering mediator production, release or effect on end organ. Besides the anti-allergy groups of drugs mentioned in this section, topical steroids, NSAIDs and immunosuppressors are also being used.

Mast Cell Inhibitors

Mechanism of Action

They prevent calcium influx into the mast cells thus inhibiting degranulation.

Indications

These are used in allergic ocular disorders like vernal keratoconjunctivitis, giant papillary conjunctivitis, vernal keratitis and allergic keratoconjunctivitis.

Dosage and Preparations

Generic name	Concentration	Trade name	Dosage
Sodium cromoglycate	2 % ed	Cromal	qd
4 % ed	Cromal forte		
Lodoxamide	0.1 % ed	Alomide	qd
Ketotifen	0.025 % ed	Ketorid	td/bd
Nedocromil	2 % ed	Alocril	qd

Potential Side Effects

As there is minimal systemic absorption of the mast cell stabilizer, the toxicity is negligible. Local irritation is common after instillation but these are relatively safe drugs.

In various studies it was found that Lodoxamide and Nedocromil were more efficacious for the treatment of VKC in children. Lodoxamide can be used in children two years or older up to a maximum of 3 months.

Decongestants (Antihistaminics and Sympathomimetics)

Mechanism of Action

Antihistaminics are H_1 receptor antagonists that prevent vasodilatation caused by histamine release. Sympathomimetics are decongestants that cause vasoconstriction by acting on the alpha advenergic receptors.

Preparation and Dosage

These are available as combinations and occasionally along with astringents. Some of the common are listed below:

Generic name	Concentration	Trade name	Remarks
Phenylephrine HCl	0.12%	I-kul	Sympathomimetic
Naphazoline HCl Menthol-camphor	0.05%		
Naphazoline HCl	0.056%	Andre	Sympathomimetic
Chlorpheniramine maleate	0.01%		Antihistaminic
$ZnSO_4$, Boric acid, NaCl			
Oxymetazoline	0.25 mg/ml	Oxylin	Sympathomimetic
Naphazoline HCl	0.01%	Clearine	Sympathomimetic
Boric acid, glycerol			
Tetrahydrazoline HCl	0.05%	Visine AC	Sympathomimetic (NA)
Zn sulfate			
Naphazoline HCl	0.05%	Naphcon-A	Sympathomimetic
Antazoline	0.5%		Antihistaminic
Levocabastine HCl	0.05%	Livostin	H_1-antagonist
Emedastine difumarate	0.05%	Emadine	H_1-antagonist

Usual dosage is 1 to 2 drops 3 to 4 times daily.

Potential Side Effects

None of these drugs have been proven safe in children. While the adverse effect of somnolence is less likely with second generation as compared to first, none of them are completely free of CNS effects such as impaired concentration, dizziness, headache and insomnia. They should be used with caution in older children and avoided in those less than 6 years of age. These can precipitate angle closure glaucoma.

Dual Agents

Mechanism of Action

These provide mast cell stabilizing effect along with H_1-receptor binding.

Indication

These are used in treatment of allergic conjunctivitis.

Dosage and Preparation

Generic name	Concentration	Trade name	Dosage
Olopatadine	0.1%	Patanol	bd
Azelastine	0.05%	Optivar	bd
Ketotifen	0.025%	Ketorid	bd

Potential Side Effects

Besides causing local irritation, the systemic effects include headache, asthenia, pharyngitis and alteration in taste. The safety of azelastine has been established down to age 3 years.

ANTIBIOTICS

Antibiotics are routinely prescribed in ophthalmology for both treatment and prophylaxis. The eye is particularly suitable for local application of antibiotics, which can be administered by various routes. Systemic administration of antibiotics has the disadvantage of poor ocular penetration especially in an inflamed eye as well as toxic side effects of the drug to a larger extent. A number of antibiotics that cannot be safely used systemically due to their toxicity can be used locally for external or intraocular infections.

The lipoidal and the blood eye barrier pose significant obstacles in achieving optimum concentrations of the drug in anterior or posterior segment respectively. Drug penetration may be improved by frequent instillation, increasing viscosity of drug, a suitable vehicle, alteration of pH or increasing concentrations of the drug. Delivery of drug into vitreous cavity in severe infections like endophthalmitis can be achieved by intravitreal injections.

To prevent development of resistant organisms follow the following principles:
- Avoid chronic use of antibiotics
- Completely treat all clinical infections
- Use antibiotics only when indicated
- Limit antibiotic use to diagnosed infections
- Use newer antibiotics when there is resistant to traditional therapy.

The antibiotics are subdivided into various groups as follows:
- Beta-lactams
- Sulfonamides
- Aminoglycosides
- Macrolides
- Tetracyclines
- Chloremphenicol
- Fluoroquinolone.

Indications

Antibiotics are used in ophthalmology for the following conditions:

Prophylaxis
To prevent bacterial infection from occurring as in:
- Foreign bodies and corneal abrasion
- Pre-and postoperatively.

Treatment
To treat ocular infections. These may be:
- External infections like
  - Blepharitis, lid infections
  - Dacryocystitis and orbital infections

- Bacterial conjunctivitis
- The common organisms affecting this age group are Gram +ve particularly *Staphylococcus* and *Streptococcus*.
- Keratitis
    This is rare in children but can be seen after trauma, surgery or contract lens wear. The common pathogens are *Pseudomonas*, staphylococci, alpha-hemolytic streptococci as well as herpes simplex virus.
- Intraocular infections like
  - Deep keratitis and corneal ulcers
  - Endophthalmitis
    - Bacterial/fungal can be by direct microbial penetration or hematogenous spread.

Dosage

In mild infections one drop is instilled four times daily for 5–7 days. Ointments have a longer duration in the eye and preferred when the eye needs to be padded. Severe infections can be treated with increased frequency of instillation. These can be given as fortified drops, subconjunctival injections, intravitreal injections as well through the systemic route depending on the severity and site of infection. They are also combined with steroids to prevent detrimental effects of inflammation, which usually accompany any infective pathology.

Table 63.4 gives an overview of various antibiotics and their dosages via the different routes. These are adult doses and need to be given in lower doses in children according to their age.

Beta-lactams

Mechanism of Action

These groups of drugs are bactericidal and act by interfering with bacterial cell wall synthesis. They include:
- Penicillins
  - Natural penicillin
  - Semisynthetic penicillin
- Cephalosporins

These drugs are not available as eyedrops. They can be used for subconjunctival, intravitreal or systemic use. Some of them can be used as eyedrops when reconstituted from the injection form.

Preparations

Penicillin prep	Type	Effectivity
Penicillin G	Natural penicillin	Streptococcal, pneumococcal gonococcal infections
Methicillin	Semisynthetic	Endophthalmitis of penicillinase resistant org
Cloxacillin	Semisynthetic	*Staphylococcus, Pneumococcus Streptococcus*
Ampicillin Amoxycilllin	Semisynthetic	Gram +ve, Gram –ve organisms Ineffective for *Staphylococcus*

TABLE 63.4: Concentration and dosages of principal antibiotics

Generic name	Trade name	Topical	Sub-conjunctival	Intravitreal	Systemic	Remark
Amikacin	Amicin (100 mg, 250 mg and 500 mg per 2 ml)	10 – 15 mg/ml	25 – 50 mg	100–400 µg	10–15 mg/kg/day (Total max dose 15 g) 3 times/day	Modify dose in case of renal failure
Amoxycillin	Mox, novamox, Amoxil, Flemoxin	—	—	—	250–500 mg (thrice a day)	—
Ampicillin	Ampillin, Bacipen Roscillin	50 mg/ml	50 – 250 mg	500 µg	2.0 – 4.0 g/4 hr	
Bacitracin	Nebasulf	10,000 units/ml	10,000 units	—	—	
Cefazolin	Alcizon, Reflin Azolin	50 mg/ml	100 mg	2.25 mg	2 – 4 g/day (in 3 – 4 doses)	
Cefotaxime	Claforan	33 – 66 mg/ml	—	2.00 mg	1 – 2 g (bid)	—
Ceftazidime	Ceftidin	50 mg/ml	100 mg	2.25 mg	2 – 6 g/day (in 2 doses)	
Cephalexin	Cephaxin, Nufex	30 – 60 mg/ml	—	—	1 – 4 g/day (in 4 days)	On empty stomach
Cephaloridine		—	100 mg	250 µg	0.5 – 1.0 g/6 hr	
Cefoxitin		30 – 60 mg/ml	—	—	—	—
Chloramphenical	Chloromycetin	5 mg/ml	50 – 100 mg	1.0 – 2.0 mg	50 mg/kg/day	
Ciprofloxacin	Ciftan, Ciplox, Ciprobid, Supraflox Milflox (Milmet)	3 mg/ml	20 mg	100 – 200 µg	0.5 – 1.5 g/day (Oral)	
Clindamycin	Dalacin Calcap	5 – 10 mg/ml	15 – 50 mg	1.00 mg	900 – 1800 mg/day (2 – 3 divided doses)	

Contd...

Contd...

Generic name	Trade name	Topical	Sub-conjunctival	Intravitreal	Systemic	Remark
Cloxacilline	Klox	—	—	—	250 – 500 mg (thrice a day)	
Doxycycline	Doxy	—	—	—	100 – 200 mg (times/day)	
Erythromycin	Althrocin, E-mycin Eltocin, Erythrocin	50 mg/ml	100 mg	500 µg	250 – 500 mg (3 – 4 times/day)	Max 4 gm daily
Gentamicin	Garamycin	8 – 15 mg/ml	20 – 40 mg	100 – 400 µg	5.0 – 7.5 mg/kg/day	
Methicillin		—	150–200 mg	2.0 mg	2.0 mg – 4 hr	
Norfloxacin	Norbactin, Norbid Norflox, Normax	3 mg/ml	—	—	200 – 400 mg (bid) orally	
Ofloxacin	Tarivid, Zanocin	3 mg/ml	—	—	200 – 800 mg/day	Not recommended for children
Penicillin G	Penivoral, Pentids, Crystapen	100,000 units/ml	0.5 – 1.0 million	200 units	2.0 – 6.0 mega units/4 hr	
Sulfacetamide	Albucid	100 – 300 mg/ml	—	0.5 mg	4 – 8 g/day	
Tetracycline	Resteclin	0.5–1.0% (5–10 mg/ml)	2.5 – 5.0 mg	—	1 – 4 g/day (in 4 doses)	Antifungal action also
Tobramycin	Tobacin	3 mg/ml (8 – 16 mg/ml) 0.3%	20 mg	100 µg	3 – 5 mg/kg/day (2 – 3 doses)	
Vancomycin	Vancocin CP	5 – 50 mg/ml	25 mg	1.0 mg (up to 2.00 mg)	2 g/day (in 2 doses)	Solution remain stable for 21 days At 40 C or 250 C

Cephalosporins	Type	Effectivity
Cefazolin	1st generation	Good activity against Gram +ve
Cephaloridine		modest activity against Gram –ve
Cephalexin		Ineffective for enterococci
Cefuroxime	2nd generation	Gram +ve org esp staphylococcus and streptococcus
		More effective than 1st gen against gram –ve
Cefatoxime	3rd generation	Gram –ve organism only
Ceftazidime		

Cephalosporins are execellent adjuncts to aminoglycosides in the treatment of severe infectious keratitis and endophthalmitis. Ceftazidime with vancomycin or cefazolin with amikacin provide execellent broad spectrum coverage in cases of infective endophthalmitis.

Dosage and Routes of Administration

Dosage and routes of administration see Table 63.4.

Side Effects and Safety

Penicillins: The most common adverse reaction is that of hypersensitivity which might be mild to a very severe anaphylaxis. Hence, contraindicated in known cases of allergy to this group of drugs.

Cepholosporins: Hypersensitivity reactions, nephrotoxicity, pseudomemberanous colitis, vitamin K deficiency and pain after im injections are known.

SULFONAMIDES

Mechanism of Action

These are bacteriostatic agents, which inhibit bacterial folate synthetase.

Indications

Superficial ocular infections as in trachoma used to be treated with sulfonamides both systemic and topical. Newer antibiotics have now superceded them. The systemic preparations are also used in ocular toxoplasmosis in combination with pyrimethamine and trimethoprim.

Effectivity

These are effective against both Gram +ve and Gram –ve organisms.

Resistance

They are not very effective against *Staphylococcus, Neisseria* and *Pseudomonas* organisms.

Preparation and Dosage

The topical eye drops are available as 10 percent, 20 percent, and 30 percent of sulfacetamide (trade name Albucid). The systemic sulfonamides are sulfadiazine and sulfamethoxazole. Their doses in adult are as follows:
- Oral – 2–4 g day in 4 divided doses
- Parenteral – 100 mg/kg/day in 4 divided doses

Side Effects and Safety

They are cheap drugs but cause significant stinging after instillation. They are contraindicated in patients with allergy to sulpha drugs and are not to be used in infants less than 2 months. Severe fatalities like Steven Johnson' Syndrome, hepatic necrosis, and blood dyscrasias although rare can occur.

AMINOGLYCOSIDES

Mechanism of Action

Bactericidal agents, which result in abnormal protein production fatal to microbes.

Effectivity

They are broad spectrum antibiotics effective against Gram –ve bacilli and *Staphylococcus aureus.*

Resistance

Streptococcus and *Chlamydia* organisms are resistant to them.

Preparation and Dosage

The various aminoglycosides used topically are:

Gentamicin	0.3% soln/eo	Genticin
Tobramycin	0.3% soln/eo	Tobrex
Amikacin	0.3% soln	Amikin
Neomycin	0.17% ed	
	5 mg/g oint.	

Other drugs belonging to this group are netilmicin, kanamycin, framycetin and streptomycin.
For dosage refer to Table 63.4.

Side Effects and Safety

Corneal toxicity is seen with long-term use. They are epithelial and endothelial toxic drugs resulting in dryness of eyes, congestion and corneal ulcer. Subconjunctival injections of gentamicin commonly cause subconjunctival hemorrhage. Intravitreal or accidental injection into the eye results in ischemic infarct of retina. Amikacin has the least toxicity and is more effective against aminoglycoside resistance strains. Best used short-term. Neomycin commonly causes contact allergy.

Systemic administration can cause ototoxity, nephrotoxicity and neurotoxicity.

MACROLIDES

Mechanism of Action

These are bacteriostatic agents inhibiting protein synthesis in the bacterial cell.

Effectivity

These are effective against gram-posititive organisms and atypical microbes like *Mycoplasma, Chlamydia, Legionella* and certain mycobacteria. Intravitreal vancomycin has been recommended as initial therapy for exogenous endophthalmitis. Oral clindamycin is also recommended in treatment of ocular toxoplasmosis.

Preparation and Dosage

The various drugs belonging to this group are:
- Erythromycin
- Clindamycin
- Vancomycin
- Roxithromycin
- Azithromycin
- Clarithromycin.

For details of doses and preparations of commonly used macrolides refer to Table 63.4.

Side Effects and Safety

They are relatively safe when given topically but are used only in mild bacterial conjunctivitis. Systemic administration can cause GI disturbances.

TETRACYCLINES

Mechanism of Action

These are bacteriostatic agents acting by inhibiting protein synthesis in ribosomes.

Effectivity

Gram-positive organisms, gram-negative bacilli, anaerobes, *Mycoplasma, Actinomyces, Rickettsia, Chlamydia* and spirochaetes. Surface ocular infections respond well to tetracyclines. Topical tetracyclines along with 1 percent Silver nitrate is recommended in prophylaxis of ophthalmia neonatorum. Acute trachoma is also treated with both systemic and topical preparations. Systemic tetracyclines are indicated in adult inclusion conjunctivitis acquired from genital contact, phlyctenular conjunctivitis, ocular toxoplasmosis, Lyme's disease and ocular rosacea.

Resistance

These are resistant to *Proteus* and *Pseudomonas*.

Preparation

Some of the drugs belonging to this group are:
- Tetracycline
- Doxycycline
- Minocycline

See Table 63.4 for details.

Side Effects and Safety

Surface ocular infections caused by susceptible microorganism respond well to tetracycline although intraocular penetration is poor. Topical preparations are relatively safe. Systemic administration can cause GI disturbances, yellow discoloration of teeth, photosensitization, nephrotoxicity and benign intracranial hypertension. Not recommended for use systemically in children due to the side effects.

CHLORAMPHENICOL

Mechanism of Action

It is a bacteriostatic agent interfering with protein synthesis. Being lipophilic it has good intraocular penetration. It is one of the most commonly used topical antibiotic ointment.

Effectivity

It is a broadspectrum antibiotic against gram-positive, gram-negative organism and anaerobes.

Resistance

It is resistant to *Pseudomonas aeruginosa*.

Preparation and Dosage

See Table 63.4 for details.

Side Effects and Safety

The ointment can cause allergic reactions although it is relatively rare. Bone marrow hypoplasia including aplastic anemia and death has been reported following local application of chloramphenicol. In infants it can cause gray baby syndrome. Hence, it should not be used when less potentially dangerous agents would provide effective treatment.

FLUOROQUINOLONES

Mechanism of Action

They are bactericidal agents interfering with enzyme DNA gyrase required for bacterial DNA synthesis. They have good ocular penetration.

Effectivity

Broad spectrum antibiotic effective against gram-positive, gram-negative organism including *Pseudomonas, Haemophilus*.

Preparation

Generic name	Concentration	Trade name	Remarks
Norfloxacin	0.3% soln/eo	Norflox	Corneal epithelial toxicity
Ciprofloxacin	0.3% ed/eo	Ciplox	Resistant to *Streptococcus*
Ofloxacin	0.3% ed/eo	Oflox	More effective than ciprofloxacin
Pefloxacin	0.3% ed	Pflox	Inactive against anaerobes. Effective against *N. gonorrhoea*
Lomefloxacin	0.3% ed		Deep acting
Sparfloxacin	0.3% ed	Sparflox	Good penetration
Levofloxacin	0.5% ed		Good penetration. Safe in children
Gatifloxacin	0.3% ed	Gatiflox	Safe in children >1 yr
Moxifloxacin	0.5% ed	Mosi	Safe in children >1 yr

Dosage of topical eyedrops depends on severity of infections. Refer to Table 63.4 for other doses.

Side Effects and Safety

Fluoroquinolones are relatively safe for topical use in children, Safety is not established in infants below 1 year of age. They are expensive but extremely effective with good ocular penetration. Fourth generation fluoroquinolones are active against quinolone resistant strains of *S. aureus*.

ANTIVIRALS (TABLE 63.5)

Viral disease in pediatric patients is often systemic and frequently accompanied by significant ocular inflammation with risk of amblyopia. Immunocompromised children have complex courses with persistence and recurrence of the disease. Unlike bacteria, viruses use host cell machinery for its metabolism and can lie dormant in the host for a long period. Antivirals act on actively replicating viruses only and are toxic to the host cells to a variable extent. As yet no antiviral in available which inhibit viral entry into host cells. Difficulty in diagnosis during incubation and latent period compound the problem.

TABLE 63.5: Antivirals

Generic name	Concentration	Trade name	Dose	Duration	Indication	Remarks
Idoxuridine (IDU)	0.1% ed 0.5 eo	Ridinox	1 hrly 2 hrly night 6 times	2 weeks	Superficial HSV Injn	Corneal toxicity
Vidarabine	3% eo 200 mg/ml	Ara – A	5 times 5–15 mg/kg. 8 hrly	2–3 weeks	HSV keratitis HSV encephalitis	Decreased host cell toxicity
Trifluridine (TFT)	1% ed	Viroptic	6 – 9 times	2 weeks	HSV keratitis Recurrent HSV Resistant HSV Deep infection	Less toxic than IDU or Ara - A
Acyclovir	3% eo 5% dermal cream 200 mg) 400 mg) Tablet 800 mg) 250 mg powder (IV)	Zovirax	5 times 200 – 800 mg 5 times 5 mg/kg 8 hrly (IV)	2 Weeks 10 days 7 – 10 days	HSV Herpes zoster Acute retinal necrosis Immunocompromised Recurrent and deep infections	Potent at anti-herpetic and selective to virus cells
Zidovudine	100 mg cap	Retrovir	200 mg 8 hrly Oral		HIV	Expensive bone marrow suppression

Contd...

Contd...

Generic name	Concentration	Trade name	Dose	Duration	Indication	Remarks
Foscarnet	24 mg /ml viral diluted to 12 mg ml with dextrose	Foscavir	60 mg/kg 8 hrly IV	2–3 weeks	CMV in AIDS acyclovir resist HSV and VZV	Nephrotoxic Administer diluted
Famciclovir	–	–	500–700 mg 8 hourly	1 week	HZV	Effective in 1000 doses
Ganciclovir	250 mg cap 500 mg powder	Cytovene	5 mg/Kg 12 hourly	2–3 weeks	CMV	Bone marrow toxicity
Valacyclovir	500 mg/ig (Oral)	Valtrex			HZV	Better Pani relief Oral availability Less dosing
Fomivirsen sodium		Vitravene	330 mcg intravitreal alternate week X 2 every 4 weeks		CMV in AIDS	
Cidofovir	75 mg/ml		5 mg/kg once weekly/ 2 weeks		CMV in AIDS	Nephrotoxic
Bromovinyl deoxyuridine	0.1% ed		8 times	8 – 10 days	HSV keratitis	Least toxicity

The common viral infections causing ocular diseases in childhood are:
- DNA viruses – Herpes simplex
  Herpes zoster
- RNA viruses – Measles
  Mumps
  Rubella

Mechanism of Action

In general, antivirals act by inhibiting viral DNA synthesis and thereby its replication. These agents are virustatic and cause various degree of host cell toxicity.

Preparations and Dosage

Preparation and dosage see to Table 63.5.

Side Effects and Safety

Host cell toxicity is present to a variable degree, acyclovir being least toxic and idoxuridine/trifluridine most when administered topically.

Local toxicity in the form of superficial punctate keratitis, punctual occlusion, and conjunctival congestion are seen. Safety of ganciclovir implant in children below 9 years is not established.

Oral acyclovir is highly effective for HSV epithelial keratitis, stromal keratitis, recurrence and HZV infections in immunocompromised pediatric patients, oral valacyclovir may be the preferred substitute of IV acyclovir due to better bioavailability in children although it has been studied only in adults.

Bone marrow suppression and nephrotoxicity are seen with systemically administered antivirals. Therefore renal function and blood cell counts must be monitored.

ANTIFUNGALS

Fungi do not invade the cornea except when it is compromised by injury, or immunosuppression fungal infections are commoner in tropics due to favorable climate. Infections with yeast fungi usually follow alterations in host defenses. While filamentous fungi infect normal eyes after injury from vegetable matter.

Various antifungals are:

Polyenes

Mechanism of Action

These bind to ergosterol, after cell membrane permeability and disrupt the fungal cell.

Preparation and Dosage

Generic name	Concentration	Trade name	Dose	Effectivity
Nystatin	100000 units/g ointment (Oral/IV)	Nystatin	2 hourly	Fungistatic superficial infections
Amphotericin B	0.075–3% 0.8–1 mg 5 mg	Fungizone	1 hourly topical SC 24–48 hr Intravitreal intravenous	Deep mycosis
Natamycin	5% (Suspension)	Natacyn	5 times/day	Superficial infections initial drug of choice

Side Effects and Safety

These drugs in general are insoluble, cause irritation and are unstable. Natamycin is well tolerated but can cause local irritation and punctate ketatitis. Amphoterin B has poor ocular penetration and can cause anaphylaxis, nausea, vomiting and nephrotoxicity when given systemically.

Imidazole Derivatives

Mechanism of Action

They inhibit ergosterol synthesis, and cause fungal cell inhibition

Preparations and Dosage

Generic name	Concentration	Trade name	Dose	Remarks
Clotrimazole	1% ed 5–10 mg 60 mg/kg 1 day	Mycocid	1 hourly subconj oral	Fungistatic effective for *Aspergillus*
Miconazole	1% ed 5–10 mg 10–40 mg	Micogel	2 hourly subconj intravitreal	Highly effective for *Candida* (Broad Spectrum)
Econazole	1% ointment	Ecanol	4–6 times	Poor penetration sup infections
Ketaconazole	2% ointment 200 mg tab	Fungicide	200 mg 800 mg od	Highly effective deep infections
Fluconazole	0.3% eyedrop 50–200 mg cap 100 mg	Forcan	4 hourly 200–600 mg/day Intravitreal	Excellent Ocular penetration broad-spectrum
Intraconazole	100 mg cap 0.01 mg	Sporanox	50–400 mg/day Intravitreal	Not effective against *Fusarium*

Side Effects and Safety

Topical imidazoles cause local irritation to a variable degree. Fluconazole, ketoconazole and miconazole cause the least and are well tolerated when systemically administered they can cause GI disturbances and hepatotoxicity.

Fluorinated Pyrimidines—Flucytosine

Mechanism of Action

It blocks fungal thymidine synthesis.

Preparation and Dosage

Generic name	Concentration	Dose	Remarks
Flucytosine	1–1.5% ed	1 hrly	Used as an adjunct to
	250/500 mg cap	50–150 mg/kg/d	other antifungals

Side Effects and Safety

Topical preparations can cause local irritation and systemic use can cause GI disturbances.

CONCLUSION

Many of the medications commonly used in children do not have pediatric dosing labeling presenting a dilemma while treating these patients. Studies on this age group are difficult due to inadequate sample size and objective measurements of signs and symptoms being problematic. It is advisable that physicians analyse risk benefit profile while prescribing in children, establish an appropriate dosage while monitoring the patient closely for local and systemic side effects.

BIBLIOGRAPHY

1. Alm A, Stjernschantz J. Effects on intraocular pressure and side effects of 0.005 percent latanoprost applied once daily, evening or morning. A comparison with timolol. Scandinavian Latanoprost Study Group. Ophthalmology 1995;102:1743-52.
2. Bielory L. Ocular allergy guidelines: A practical treatment algorithm. Drugs 2002;62:1611-34.
3. Bill A. Uveoscleral drainage of aqueous humor: physiology and pharmacology. Prog Chin Biol Res 1989;312:417-27.
4. Bito LZ, Racz P, Ruzsony MR, et al. The Prostaglandin analogue, PhXA41, significantly reduces daytime and night time intraocular pressure (IOP) by itself, and in timolol-treated glaucomatous eyes [ARVO abstract]. Invest Ophthalmol Vis Sci 1994;35(Suppl):2178.
5. Bowman RJ, Cope J, Nischal KK. Ocular and systemic side effects of bromonidine 0.2 percent eye drops (Alphagan) in children. Eye 2004;18:24-6.
6. Camras CB. Comparison of latanoprost and timolol in patients with ocular hypertension and glaucoma: A six month masked,

multicenter trial in the United States. The United States Latanoprost Study Group. Ophthalmology 1996;103:138-47.
7. Carlsen JO, Zabriskie NA, Kwon YH, et al. Apparent central nervous system. Depression in infants after the use of topical brimonidine. Am J Ophthalmol 1999;128:255-6.
8. Controlled evaluation of loteprednol etabonate and prednisolone acetate in the treatment of acute anterior uveitis. Loteprednol Etabonate US Uveitis. Loteprednol Etabonate US Uveitis Study Group. Am J Ophthalmol 1999;127:537-44.
9. Egbert JE, Schwartz GS, Walsh AW. Diagnosis and treatment of an ophthalmic artery occlusion during an intralesional injection of corticosteroid into an eyelid capillary hemangioma. Am J Ophthalmol 1996;121:638-42.
10. Enyedi LB, Freedman SF, Uckley EG. The effectiveness of latanoprost for the treatment of pediatric glaucoma. J AAPOS 1999;3(1):33-9.
11. Enyedi LB, Freedman SF. Latanoprost for the treatment of pediatric glaucoma. Surv Ophthalmol 2002;47:1:S129-32.
12. Enyedi LB, Freedman SF. Safety and efficacy of brimonidine in children with glaucoma. J AAPOS 2001;5(5):281-4.
13. Fan DS, NgJS, Lam DS. A prospective study on ocular hypertensive and anti-inflammatory response to different dosages of fluorometholone in children. Ophthalmology 2001;108:1973-7.
14. Fitzgerald DA, Hanson RM, West C, Martin F, Brown J, Kilham HA. Seizures associated with 1 percent cyclopentolate eyedrops. J Paediatr Child Health 1990;26(2):106-7.
15. Foster CS, Alter G, DeBarge LR, et al. Efficacy and safety of rimexolone 1 percent ophthalmic suspension vs 1 percent prednisolone acetate in the treatment of uveitis. Am J Ophthalmol 1996;122:171-82.
16. Gerinec A, Kostolna B. Diclof 0.1 percent eyedrops in pediatric ophthalmology. Cesk Slov Oftalmol 2001;57(3):200-3.
17. Katzung, B, et al. Basic and Clinical Pharmacology, 8th edn. San Francisco, Lange Medical Books/McGraw-Hill 2001.pp.134-5.
18. Pucci N, Novembre E, Cianferoni A, Lombardi E, Bernardini R, Caputo R, et al. Efficacy and safety of cyclosporine eyedrops in vernal keratoconjunctivitis. Ann Allergy Asthma Immunol 2002;89:298-303.
19. Ruttum MS, Abrams GW, Harris GJ, Ellis MK. Bilateral retinal embolization associated with intralesional corticosteroid injection for capillary hemangioma of infancy. J Pediatr Ophthalmol Strabismus 1993;30:4-7.
20. Shorr N, Seiff SR. Central retinal artery occlusion associated with periocular corticosteroid injection for juvenile hemangioma. Ophthalmic Surg 1986;17:229-31.
21. Sud RN, Greval RS, Bajwa RS. Topical flurbiprofen therapy in vernal keratoconjunctivitis. Indian J Med Sci 1995;49(9):205-9.
22. Terasa MM, David Wallace, Sandra Johnson. Ophthalmic medications in pediatric patients. Comprehensive update 2005; 6(2):85-1001.
23. Textbook of Ocular Therapeutics Ashok Garg, 2001.
24. Verin PH, Dicker ID, Mortemousque B. Nedocromil sodium eye drops are more effective than sodium cromoglycate eyedrops for the long-term management of vernal keratoconjunctivitis. Clin Exp Allergy 1999;29(4): 529-36.

Management of Uveitis in Children

Gagandeep Singh Brar, SPS Grewal (India)

Inflammation of the uveal tract when presenting in children and adolescents younger than 16 years of age is termed as pediatric uveitis although some studies advocate using 18 years as the cut-off age.[1] The incidence of uveitis in children has been reported to be less than that of adults and 2.2-10.6 percent of the total number of uveitis patients belong to the pediatric age group.[2-6] Wide variation in the incidence as well as varying prevalence within the same population over time has been reported.

There are some basic differences between childhood uveitis and adult uveal inflammation. Systemic associations of the uveitis are not as common in children as in adults and ANA positive oligoarticular juvenile idiopathic arthritis (JIA) presents as the most common systemic disorder.[7,8] Also, the uveitis is mostly asymptomatic in the early stages in children and they may be presenting to the ophthalmologist at a very late stage. Thirdly, the mainstay of management of uveitis in adults, namely corticosteroids, may not be safe in growing children with permanent adverse effects so steroid sparing agents may have to be employed more frequently for controlling the inflammation. Complications of uveitis are also more common in children because of the chronic and relentless course of the disease in many cases coupled with delayed presentation. Results of surgical intervention in this age group have also been poorer when compared to adults and visual outcomes are less encouraging. Lastly, many children may be at a stage of visual immaturity and attendant amblyopia may further compromise visual rehabilitation.

As with adult uveitis, marked variability has been observed in the patterns of uveitis in children when studied over time and has been attributed to geographical variations, racial and genetic differences, recognition of newer clinical entities, better diagnostic capabilities and better control of infections. In children, in almost one-fourth of all cases, no cause can be ascertained and these are termed as idiopathic uveitis. As already stated, JIA associated uveitis is the most common form of anterior uveitis and toxoplasmosis the most common posterior uveitic entity. Other common entities in children include pars planitis, Behçet's disease and Fuchs' heterochromic uveitis. In one study, anterior uveitis accounted for 30-40 percent, posterior uveitis for 40-50 percent, intermediate uveitis for 10-20 percent, and diffuse uveitis for 5-10 percent of childhood uveitis.[9]

JUVENILE IDIOPATHIC ARTHRITIS ASSOCIATED UVEITIS

In children, JIA has been reported as the accompanying systemic manifestation in 81 percent of children with uveitis[7] and in 95 percent of children with anterior uveitis.[10] More recently, JIA was found to be the associated systemic manifestation in 41.5 percent of 130 children with uveitis.[8] This change has in part been brought about by better recognition of other diseases associated with uveitis in childhood which may strongly resemble JIA. Chronic anterior uveitis may also occur associated with other systemic diseases, such as inflammatory bowel disease and sarcoidosis, and as an isolated phenomenon. Sarcoidosis of childhood frequently manifests in the joints, skin, and eyes and rarely in the lungs.[11] Posterior segment manifestations in the form of retinal vasculitis, peripheral multifocal choroiditis, or choroidal granuloma may help to differentiate this entity from JIA associated uveitis.

Screening guidelines for JIA associated uveitis vary and are mainly based on the perceived risk of developing uveitis: risk factors include the pattern of initial joint disease, the patients' sex, ANA status, and age at onset.

Diagnosis

The uveitis is chronic, non-granulomatous and bilateral in about three-fourths of all cases. Children with pauciarticular involvement are at more risk for developing uveitis than those with polyarticular or 'systemic' JIA. Hypoyon is rare although the intraocular inflammation may be severe. The JIA associated uveitis is a 'white uveitis'; the eye is rarely congested even when the inflammation is severe. Girls seem to have a more indolent course than boys and need more careful follow-up. Antinuclear antibody (ANA) positivity may precede uveitis. Seronegativity for rheumatoid factor is the rule. Some cases may be HLA B27 positive and the uveitis may be similar to ankylosing spondylitis associated anterior uveitis. Filiform synechiae with a 'festooned pupil' are common in long standing cases (Figs 64.1A and B). In chronic cases, complicated cataract develops in more than 50 percent cases, band-shaped keratopathy in almost 40 percent and secondary glaucoma in 15–20 percent.

Management

Topical corticosteroids are the mainstay of therapy. They are titrated according to anterior chamber cellular reaction although chronic flare may persist despite therapy and should not be aggressively treated. Some children may require depot steroid injections for control of inflammation. A short course of systemic steroids may be necessary in older children but they should be used with caution as they retard normal growth of the child. Systemic immunosuppression has also been found to be useful in severe cases but an internist and pediatrician co-management is mandatory when using systemic therapies in these

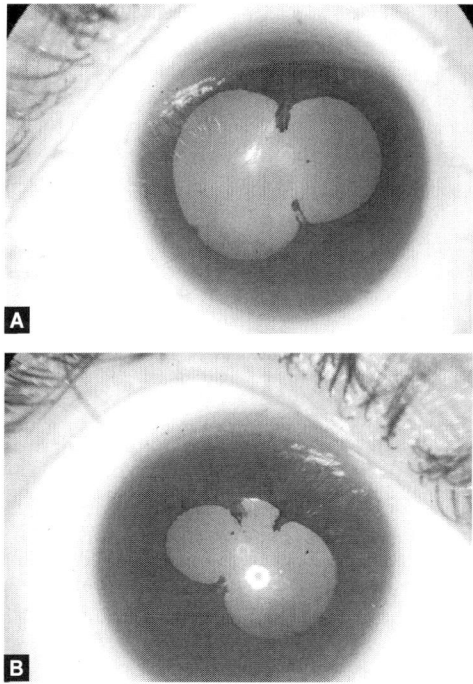

Figs 64.1A and B: Filiform synechiae OU in a 16-year-old child with juvenile rheumatoid associated uveitis

children. Surgical intervention is warranted for management of cataract, glaucoma and severe band-shaped keratopathy. Ideally, inflammation should be controlled prior to surgery. The control of inflammation implies a lack of anterior chamber cellular reaction. At times, in younger children, surgery may be planned despite some inflammatory reaction persisting in order to take care of risk of amblyopia. In some cases with cyclitic membranes, hypotony and low grade inflammation, surgery and removal of these membranes may actually help to control the inflammation and its sequelae. The two surgical techniques of use today for managing complicated cataracts in JIA associated uveitis are phacoaspiration with or without intraocular lens implantation and lensectomy with anterior vitrectomy. The largest series of cataract surgery in JRA patients reports surgical results in 162 eyes, 61 of which underwent needling and aspiration and the rest underwent lensectomy with anterior vitrectomy.[7] Phthisis bulbi was seen in 25 percent of eyes undergoing needling and aspiration versus only 3 percent eyes after lensectomy. Visual acuity of 20/60 or better was achieved in 56 percent of cases undergoing lensectomy versus 21 percent with needling and aspiration. However, improvement in microsurgical techniques have also improved the results of extracapsular surgical techniques and Foster et al reported 6 eyes undergoing extracapsular cataract extraction and 4 eyes achieved 20/40 or better and no eye went into phthisis over a follow-up period of up to 7 years.[12]

Glaucoma in JIA associated uveitis may be related to inflammation or may be caused by papillary block due to posterior synechiae. Pupillary block may be relieved by an iridectomy which may have to be surgical as laser iridotomies frequently close. Medical management is difficult and many cases require surgical management in the form of trabeculectomy with antimitotic agents or implantation of glaucoma drainage devices. Cyclocryotherapy or cyclophotocoagulation should be reserved as a last resort in eyes with poor visual prognosis.

For band-shaped keratopathy, chemical chelation with 0.37M EDTA is done after debridement of epithelium. This improves corneal clarity in majority of cases with severe involvement.

FUCHS HETEROCHROMIC UVEITIS

Although described by Lawrence in 1843, the syndrome is named after Ernst Fuchs who first analyzed 38 patients and reported features of a 'new' condition in 1906.[13] Although the typical patient is a young adult who presents with visual symptoms and heterochromia, rarely children under 16 years of age may be affected. The uveitis is nonprogressive, mild, and in general nonresponsive to corticosteroid therapy. The diagnosis is usually made on the basis of small, white, diffusely scattered keratic precipitates; minimal cells and flare; lack of posterior synechias; and atrophic changes in the iris. In the full blown case, cataract is invariably present and is most often posterior subcapsular in location (Figs 64.2A to D). Glaucoma remains perhaps the main sight threatening component of this syndrome and may be seen in 6.3–59 percent of cases.[14]

Management

The inflammatory component usually does not need any treatment as it is mild and does not respond very well to steroids. Complicated cataract is frequently seen, typically posterior subcapsular in morphology, and usually occurs in patients after 40 years of age. It has been managed using different techniques including lens aspiration and intracapsular cataract extraction (ICCE) and extracapsular cataract extraction. The 1990s brought the increasing use of intraocular lenses (IOLs) in patients with FHU. A general consensus has evolved on the good prognosis of posterior chamber IOL (PC IOL) implantation in these patients. However, most studies used manual ECCE and reported postoperative complications such as hyphema, glaucoma, and intractable uveitis. Recently, good results have been reported after phacoemulsification and foldable intraocular lens implantation in FHU.[15]

Management of glaucoma poses the same challenges as in any other form of uveitic glaucoma. Control of inflammation may be required in cases with glaucoma. Surgery for management of glaucoma may be required in a majority of patients with equivocal results.

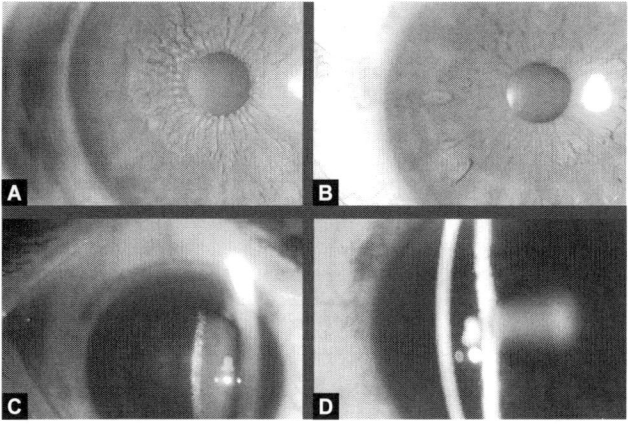

Figs 64.2A to D: A 15-year-old female patient was diagnosed as a case of Fuchs' heterochromic cyclitis on the basis of iris heterochromia, Koeppe nodules, Stellate keratic precipitates and posterior subcapsular cataract

INTERMEDIATE UVEITIS

Intermediate uveitis (IU) is a chronic intraocular inflammation, mainly affecting the anterior vitreous and the pars plana. The disease predominantly affects patients under the age of 40 years and forms approximately 8–22 percent[16] of all uveitis in the general uveitic population. The percentage of IU increases in the uveitis population aged less than 16 years.[7,8,17] The visual prognosis in adults is usually favorable.[16] The visual outcome of IU in children is not known. The ocular inflammation in children is frequently discovered late in the disease process, and the child might already be presenting with advanced signs and complications.[18-21] The etiology of IU in adults is considered to be an idiopathic autoimmune disease, and was occasionally associated with sarcoidosis, multiple sclerosis (MS), or infectious diseases.[22] In the pediatric population, the causes and prognosis of IU have not yet been systemically studied. Remission of the disease has been reported, but the incidence of remissions reported was low.[19]

The International Uveitis Study Group has used the term 'Intermediate uveitis' to classify cases with intraocular inflammation restricted to the peripheral retina and adjoining vitreous. Pars planitis refers to a specific form of intermediate uveitis in which white fluffy collection termed as 'snowbanking' is present over the ora serrata and pars plana. Intermediate uveitis is most often idiopathic.

Diagnosis

Patients usually present with a symptom of floaters and occasionally blurring of vision. On examination, anterior chamber reaction is mild to moderate with fine keratic precipitates and usually an absence of posterior synechiae. The main site of inflammation is the pars plana area and peripheral retina and hence anterior

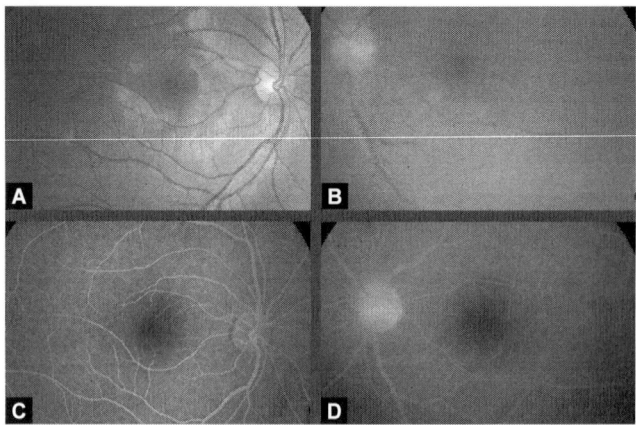

Figs 64.3A to D: A 13-year-old girl presented with 6/24 vision in the left eye. Examination showed evidence of pars planitis in the left eye with vitritis, pars plana snowbanking and disk hyperemia. FFA showed left disk leakage

vitreous cells are seen. More than half of all cases develop cystoid macular edema resulting in visual impairment. A specific problem noted in the pediatric age group is development of optic disc edema (Figs 64.3A to D).

Management

Many cases with mild involvement and without macular edema do not require any treatment. Since the etiology of IU is not very well defined, treatment is mainly symptomatic. In some previous studies, the young patients were less frequently systemically treated than adults.[23] One should consider the presence of CME as an indication for treatment and periocular corticosteroid injections are the mainstay of management of CME. A short course of oral steroids may be necessary in cases with severe anterior vitreous inflammation. Since CME is the major cause of visual loss or impairment of IU in children, early detection and treatment of CME are crucial for the prevention of visual loss.

BEHÇET'S DISEASE

Behçet's disease (BD) is a multisystem inflammatory disorder dominated clinically by recurrent oral and genital ulceration, uveitis, and erythema nodosum. It is characterized by a chronic course, with exacerbations and remissions. Behçet's disease is most frequently seen in adults, although a childhood-onset has been reported. About 2–3 percent of all affected individuals have childhood-onset.[24] Onset of this disease in children as young as 2 years of age has been reported, but most children develop clinical features after 6–7 years of age.[25] The cause remains unknown, although an autoimmune reaction triggered by an infectious agent in a genetically predisposed individual has been suggested.

Behçet's disease is a vasculitis, affecting vessels of different types, sizes, and localizations. Since the etiology of Behçet's disease is unknown, treatment tends to be empirical and is usually comprised of systemic corticosteroids and immunosuppressants.

The International uveitis Study Group Criteria for diagnosis of Behçet's disease are:[26]

Recurrent oral ulceration	Minor aphthous, major aphthous or herpetiform ulceration observed by physician or patient, which recurred at least 3 times in one 12-month period
Plus 2 of:	
Recurrent genital ulceration	Aphthous ulceration or scarring, observed by physician or patient
Eye lesions	Anterior uveitis, posterior uveitis, or cells in vitreous on slit lamp examination; or retinal vasculitis observed by ophthalmologist
Skin lesions	Erythema nodosum observed by physician or patient, pseudofolliculitis or papulo-pustular lesions; or acneiform nodules observed by physician in postadolescent patients not on corticosteroid treatment
Positive pathergy test	Read by physician at 24–48 hrs, performed with oblique insertion of a 20-gauge or smaller needle under sterile conditions

Ocular manifestations include panuveitis, anterior uveitis, posterior uveitis, bilateral disc edema, and retinal vasculitis (Figs 64.4A and B). Ocular involvement is usually bilateral, although severity of disease may differ between eyes. Ocular disease is the most common cause of significant morbidity in Behçet's disease, since it may lead to visual loss in about five years if not treated.

Management

The treatment of BD is symptomatic and empirical, but generally specific to the clinical features of each patient. The acute anterior inflammation may respond well to topical steroids initially. However, posterior segment involvement requires systemic therapy and steroids are usually not effective. Many patients will require immunosuppressive agents in the form of azathioprine, methotrexate or cyclophosphamide which must be prescribed in conjunction with internist or pediatrician.

TOXOPLASMOSIS

Toxoplasmosis is caused by infestation in humans by a protozoan parasite *Toxoplasma gondii* for whom cat is the definitive host and other animals including human beings are the intermediate hosts.

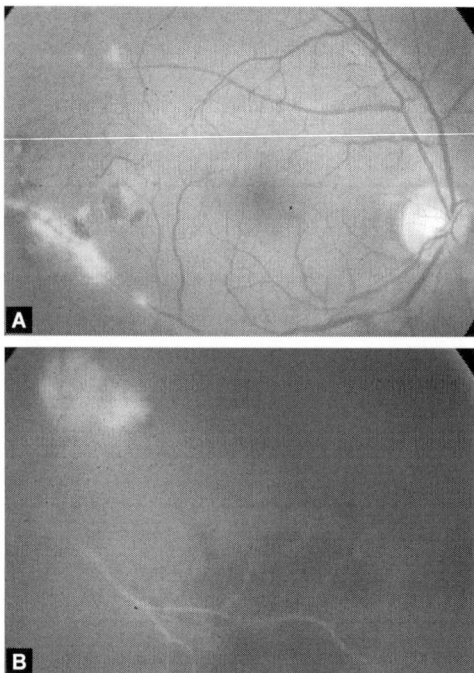

Figs 64.4A and B: A 14-year-old child presented with poor vision in both eyes. His BCVA was 6/9 in right eye and 6/60 in the left. He had dense vitritis in the left eye and evidence of vasculitis in both eyes. He gave history of recurrent orogenital ulcerations. He was diagnosed as a case of Behçets disease and was treated with oral corticosteroids and immunosuppressive agents

While undercooked meat and food contaminated with oocysts from cat feces remain the major sources of infection, contaminated water may be an important additional source in some settings. In most cases, infection is acquired transplacentally when a pregnant mother gets infested.

Clinical Features

If the mother acquires infection in the first or second trimester, the child is either still born or there may be spontaneous abortion or the child may be born with brain damage. In children with inactive disease at birth, most cases are subclinical with chorioretinal scars (Figs 64.5A and B). Reactivation of disease from these scars occurs between the ages of 10–35 years and manifests as a focal necrotizing retinitis with severe overlying vitritis giving a 'headlight-in-fog' appearance. The active lesion is usually adjacent to an old chorioretinal scar in the posterior pole area.[27,28] Spillover mild anterior segment inflammation may also be present. The choroid and retinal vessels may be indirectly involved. The course may be complicated by development of cystoid macular edema, macular pucker, tractional retinal detachment, rhegmatogenous retinal detachment and choroidal and retinal neovascularization.

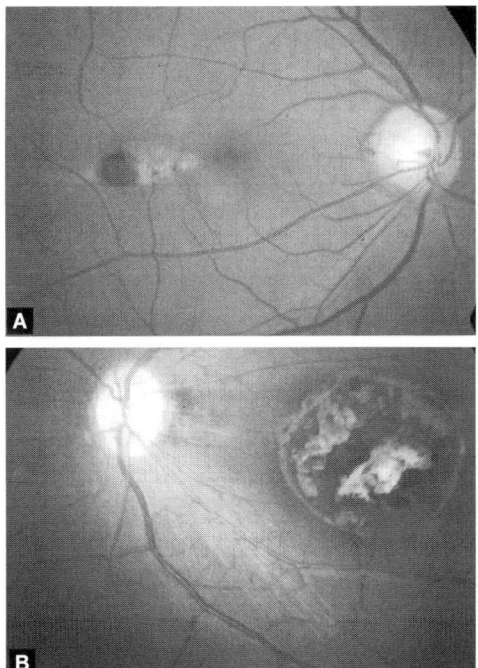

Figs 64.5A and B: A 15-year-old child presented with poor vision in both eyes. His BCVA was 6/6 in right eye and CF 1 meter in the left. Fundus examination showed bilateral toxoplasmosis scars

Management

Not all lesions require treatment; only vision-threatening lesions in the form of those close to fovea, papillomacular bundle and rarely the optic nerve head require to be treated. Treatment is in the form of steroids to control the inflammation and antimicrobials. Steroids may be used orally and topically. Antimicrobials in the form of clindamycin 300 mg QID, sulphadiazine 2 gm loading followed by 1 gm QID, or pyrimethamine 75–150 mg loading followed by 25 mg daily, are given for a period of 3-4 weeks. Clindamycin use can cause pseudomembranous colitis and one should be careful when using the drug. Patients on pyrimethamine need follow up for thrombocytopenia and leukopenia.

TOXOCARIASIS

This disease is an infestation with a roundworm found in dogs and cats (*Toxocara canis* and *Toxocara cati*). Young children in close contact with pets or ingesting contaminated food or soil are at risk. The eggs of the worm are ingested which develop into larva which in turn migrate to the lungs, liver, brain or eyes. Ocular toxocariasis is characterized by a chronic endophthalmitis-like picture or a granuloma formation in the posterior pole or retinal periphery (Fig. 64.6). The complications could be in the form of cyclitic membranes, macular drag or retinal detachment. Management

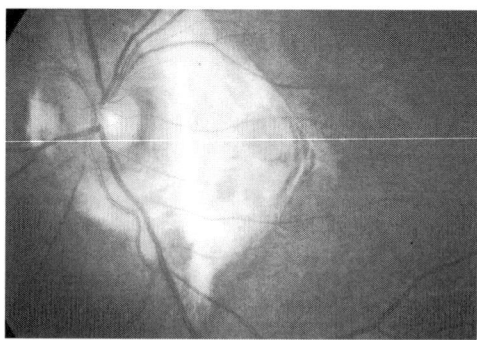

Fig. 64.6: A 6-year-old child presented with esotropia in the left eye. Fundus showed a white dense toxocara granuloma scar in the left eye

is restricted to surgical intervention in the form of pars plana vitrectomy for the complications.[29,30]

SUMMARY

Uveitis in children, although less common than in adults, is fairly frequently seen and assumes great importance because of the higher number of complications observed and a poorer visual outcome. The major proportion of cases are either idiopathic or associated with juvenile idiopathic arthritis. Other entities commonly seen are pars planitis, toxoplasmosis and Fuchs heterochromic uveitis. In some regions, Behçet's disease may also assume significant proportions. The management of uveitis in children is particularly challenging as the use of aggressive systemic medications may interfere with the growth of the child. The fact that some of these children are in the amblyopic age group further complicates the issue. However, useful vision may be salvaged in a majority of these cases with judicious management.

REFERENCES

1. BenEzra D, Cohen E, Maftzir G. Uveitis in children and adolescents. Br J Ophthalmol 2005;89:444-8.
2. David M. Endogenous uveitis in children; associated band-shaped keratopathy and rheumatoid arthritis. Arch Ophthalmol 1953;50:443-54.
3. Perkins ES. Patterns of uveitis in children. Br J Ophthalmol 1966;50:169-85.
4. Kimura SJ, Hogan MJ, Thygeson P. Uveitis in children. Arch Ophthalmol 1954;51:80-8.
5. Blegvad O. Iridocyclitis and diseases of the joints in children. Acta Ophthalmol 1941;19:219-36.
6. Kimura SJ, Hogan MJ. Uveitis in children: analysis of 274 cases. Trans Am Ophthalmol Soc 1964;62:173-92.
7. Kanski JJ, Shun-Shin A. Systematic uveitis syndromes in childhood; an analysis of 340 cases. Ophthalmology 1984;91:1247-52.
8. Tugal-Tutkun I, Harvlikova K, Power WJ, et al. Changing patterns in uveitis of childhood. Ophthalmology 1996;103:375-83.

9. Cunningham ET Jr. Uveitis in children. Ocul Immunol Inflamm 2000;8:251-61.
10. O'Brien JM, Albert DM. Therapeutic approaches for ophthalmic problems in juvenile arthritis. Rheumatol Dis Clin N Amer 1989;15:413-22.
11. Fink CW, Cimaz R. Early onset sarcoidosis: not a benign disease. J Rheumatol 1977;24:174-7.
12. Foster CS, Fong LP, Singh G. Cataract surgery and intraocular lens implantation in patients with uveitis. Ophthalmology 1989; 96:281-7.
13. Fuchs E. Über Komplicationen der Heterochromie. Z Augenheilkd 1906;15:191-212.
14. Jones NP. Fuchs' Heterochromic Uveitis. An Update. Surv Ophthalmol 1993;37:253-72.
15. Ram J, Kaushik S, Brar GS, Gupta A, Gupta A. Phacoemulsification in patients with Fuchs' heterochromic uveitis. J Cataract Refract Surg 2002;28:1372-8.
16. AT Vitale, M Zierhut, CS Foster. Intermediate uveitis. In: CS Foster, AT Vitale (Eds). Diagnosis and treatment of uveitis. Philadelphia: WB Saunders 2001.pp.844-57.
17. Boer de JH, Wulffraat N, Rothova A. Causes of blindness in uveitis of childhood. Br J Ophthalmol 2003;87:879-84.
18. Smith RE, Godfrey WA, Kimura SJ. Complications of chronic cyclitis. Am J Ophthalmol 1976;82:277-82.
19. Hogan MJ, Kimura SJ, O' Connor GR. Peripheral retinitis and chronic cyclitis in children. Trans Ophthalmol Soc UK 1965;85:39-52.
20. Aaberg TM. The enigma of pars planitis. Am J Ophthalmol 1987;103:828-30.
21. Giles CL. Pediatric intermediate uveitis. J Pediatr Ophthalmol Strabismus 1989;26:136-9.
22. Nussenblatt RB, Whitcup SM, Palestine AG. Intermediate uveitis. In: L Craven (Ed). Uveitis, fundamentals, and clinical practice. St Louis: Mosby 1996.pp.279-88.
23. Guest S, Funkhouser E, Lightman S. Pars planitis a comparison of childhood onset and adult onset disease. Clin experiment Ophthalmol 2001;29:81-4.
24. Saylan T, Mat C, Fresko I, Melikoglu M. Behçet's disease in the Middle East. Clin Dermatol 1999;17:209-23.
25. Kari JA, Shah V, Dillon MJ. Behçet's disease in UK children: clinical features and treatment including thalidomide. Rheumatology 2001;40:933-8.
26. International Study Group for Behçet's Disease. Criteria for diagnosis of Behçet's disease. Lancet 1990;335:1078-80.
27. Holland GN, O'Connor GR, Belfort Jr R, Remington JS. Toxoplasmosis. In: JS Pepose, GN Holland, KR Wilhelmus, (Eds). Ocular infection and immunity, St Louis: Mosby-Year Book, Inc. 1996.pp.1183-1223.
28. Hogan MJ, Kimura SJ, O'Connor GR. Ocular toxoplasmosis. Arch Ophthalmol 1964;72:592-600.
29. Werner JC, Ross RD, Green WR, Watts JC. Pars plana vitrectomy and subretinal surgery for ocular toxocariasis. Arch Ophthalmol 1999;117:532-4.
30. Belmont JB, Irvine A, Benson W, O'Connor GR. Vitrectomy in ocular toxocariasis. Arch Ophthalmol 1982;100:1912-5.

Management of Anticoagulation Therapy in Elective Ophthalmic Procedures

Purendra Bhasin, Prateek Gujar, Priyamvada Bhasin, Prachi Tomar (India)

Cardiovascular diseases are the leading cause of death for both men and women around the world. The number of patients on antithrombotic medications, such as warfarin, clopidogrel and ticlopidine is on a rise. Medical conditions, such as atrial fibrillation and valvular heart disease, require the regular use of anticoagulants (e.g. Warfarin), whilst antiplatelet therapy is used in high-risk populations to reduce vascular events.[1,2]

Many of the patients encountered by an ophthalmic surgeon have been placed on anticlotting drugs by another physician. The challenge for the ophthalmic surgeon treating a patient who is on anticoagulant therapy revolves around the complex, delicate calibration of weighing the risk of poorly controlled bleeding vs the risk of a thromboembolic event. In other words, the ophthalmologist must balance the potential loss of eyesight against the potential loss of life.

Antithrombotic medications are routinely discontinued preoperatively due to a perceived increased risk of severe bleeding intra and postoperatively. However, this practice is generally not based on published evidence and the potential risks to the patient may be poorly understood. Nonetheless, the risk of perioperative bleeding in patients on anticoagulants is dependant on multiple factors including age of the patient, other systemic diseases, the type of surgery as well as the international normalized ratio (INR).[3-5] The primary issues to consider in these patients are the purpose of the anticoagulation, the level of risk for both ocular bleeding and systemic thrombosis, and the type of surgery being performed.

IDENTIFYING THE PATIENTS AT RISK

It is important to identify patients at risk of thrombotic complications on altering the antithrombotic therapy. The very basic question that one should ask is—"Why the patient is on anticoagulants?" Patients on antithrombotics may be placed in two broad overlapping groups: those with significant cardiovascular risk factors where these drugs play a significant cardioprotective and antithrombotic role, and those taking them to keep the circulation "healthy".

Patients belonging to the former group, like those having deep venous thrombosis, atrial fibrillation, valvular disease, and post-coronary stents, are at increased risk of thrombogenic events. The current guidelines recommends dual antiplatelet therapy after coronary stenting especially with drug eluting stents, as early antiplatelet discontinuation may increase the risk of stent thrombosis.[6]

Another important consideration in such patients is the phenomenon of rebound hypercoagulability. Although disputed by many authorities, there is an evidence to suggest that the risk of thromboembolism is increased on abrupt cessation of warfarin by a combination of this phenomenon and the prothrombotic effect of surgery.[6,7]

In addition to the underlying systemic condition requiring anticoagulation, the thrombotic risk also depend on the duration of disruption of antithrombotic therapy and the use of bridging therapy.[8-12]

RISK OF BLEEDING COMPLICATIONS

Though more common than thrombosis, bleeding is often more of a nuisance for patients and surgeons than a serious life-altering event. Many types of ophthalmic surgeries are considered as lower risk for bleeding, especially those with smaller incisions, and procedures of short duration.

Cataract Surgery

Most of the patients undergoing cataract surgery are elderly and a significant minority are on anticoagulants.[13] Studies have shown that the use of aspirin, clopidogrel and warfarin in the perioperative period in patients undergoing cataract surgery does not appear to be associated with an increased risk of significant bleeding complications.[13-18]

Katz et al have reported that the rate of thrombotic complications are much higher on interruption of anticoagulants than the rate of bleeding complications on continued use during cataract surgery.[13]

Study by Kumar et al on patients undergoing cataract surgery found a greater incidence of subconjunctival hemorrhage in patients who were receiving either clopidogrel or warfarin compared to aspirin or no antithrombotic drugs, although there were no sight-threatening bleeding complications.[19]

Vitreo-retinal Surgery

Although more invasive than cataract surgery, vitreo-retina surgery also appears to be safe in patients taking aspirin.[20] In a retrospective study on 54 patients who underwent 57 vitreoretinal surgical procedures while on warfarin anticoagulation therapy found that there were no intraoperative hemorrhagic complications and only four postoperative hemorrhages, all of them resolved spontaneously.[21]

Glaucoma Surgery

Patients using warfarin appears to be at a risk of developing clinically significant hyphema during trabeculectomy. Glaucoma surgery appears to be safe in patients using aspirin.[22]

Lacrimal Surgery

Lacrimal surgery can be associated with significant blood loss.[23] Poor visibility during the procedure due to bleeding can lead to poor surgical outcome. Good hemostasis is desirable not only during surgery, but also to prevent bleeding in the immediate postoperative period.

A study investigating oculoplastic surgery in anticoagulated patients has concluded that the incidence of serious hemorrhagic complication is low.[24]

MODIFYING ANTITHROMBOTIC THERAPY DURING OPHTHALMIC SURGERY

Patients who fall in "high-risk category", like those using dual antiplatelet therapy (aspirin+ clopidogrel) for an acute coronary syndrome or after recent stent implantation deserves special consideration. A thorough evaluation, collaboration with the internist or cardiologist is indispensable and highly recommended in such cases. Elective ophthalmic surgery should be delayed if it has been less than a month since the thrombotic episode. In cases, where discontinuing antithrombotics is warranted, they may be stopped before surgery with oversight from the cardiologist or internist.

Warfarin (Coumadin): This is a complex drug to manage, as after discontinuation, it takes several days for the antithrombotic effect to recede and, when resumed, several days to become re-established. In general, warfarin is stopped about four to five days prior to elective surgery. If discontinued, close monitoring is mandatory, using the international normalized ratio (INR). Bridging therapy with low molecular weight heparin should be instituted in patients at a moderate to high-risk of thrombotic complications.[15]

Intravenous heparin: It is to be discontinued about 12 hours before surgery.[13]

Platelet inhibitors: Aspirin, a nonreversible platelet inhibitor, is usually stopped about 7 to 10 days before surgery, although studies have shown that stopping aspirin 48 hours before coronary bypass surgery is just as effective as seven days.[25]

Thienopyridine agents: Commonly prescribed after coronary artery stent placement, these agents should only be stopped following advice from a cardiologist or prescribing physician. It is recommended to start aspirin therapy, if possible, if thienopyridine derivatives, such as clopidogrel and ticlopidine, are discontinued, and restarting the former drugs as soon as possible.[13]

Enoxaparin sodium: Discontinue 12 to 24 hours before surgery with monitoring of the Platelet levels before surgery since enoxaparin can cause thrombocytopenia.[13]

INTRAOPERATIVE CONSIDERATIONS TO REDUCE BLEEDING IN PATIENTS USING ANTICOAGULATION THERAPY

- Topical anesthesia/sub-tenon's anesthesia is preferable as compared to retrobulbar anesthesia.
- Meticulous surgical technique and a good understanding of local anatomy to reduce surgical trauma.
- Local infiltration with adrenaline is a tried and tested method of achieving local hemostasis and is especially useful in cutaneous, oculoplastic, and lacrimal surgery, and a dilution of 1:80,000 to 1:200,000 is effective when infiltrated about 10 minutes before surgery.[26]
- Radiofrequency cutting diathermy to reduce bleeding at the operative site.

In summary, various types of ophthalmic surgery appear to be safe in anticoagulated patients. Aspirin does not appear to be associated with an increased risk of significant bleeding in patients undergoing any type of ophthalmic surgery or infiltration of local anesthesia. Also no evidence of excessive thromboembolism on its discontinuation has been identified. To reduce oozing at the operative site, aspirin may be discontinued in the perioperative period in patients without significant cardiovascular risk factors.

Patients using warfarin are to be dealt more cautiously in the perioperative period, in close discussion with a cardiologist and/or clinical hematologist. The risk of significant bleeding in patients using warfarin and undergoing ophthalmic surgery appears to be relatively low when the INR is within the therapeutic range, as compared to the probability of thromboembolism on its interruption. Thus, reducing the warfarin dose preoperatively to bring down the INR to the lower limit of the therapeutic range is a safer alternative to disrupting it and exposing the patient to a risk of thromboembolism. When the discontinuation of warfarin is considered essential, it should be for the minimal possible time with low molecular weight heparin 'bridging; cover during the period of discontinuation. There is also insufficient evidence to make precise recommendations about the newer antiplatelet drugs like clopidogrel.

REFERENCES

1. Kitchin AH, Milnes JS. Longitudinal survey of ischaemic heart disease in a randomly selected sample of the older population. Br Heart J 1997;39:889-93.
2. Secondary prevention in non-rheumatic atrial fibrillation after transient ischaemic attack or minor stroke. EAFT (European Atrial Fibrillation Trial) Study Group. Lancet 1993;342:1255-62.
3. Schulman S, Beyth RJ, Kearon C, Levine MN. American College of Chest Physicians. Hemorrhagic complications of anticoagulant

and thrombolytic treatment: American College of Chest Physicians Evidence-Based Clinical Practice Guidelines (8th Edition). Chest 2008;133(6 Suppl):257S-98.
4. Palareti G, Cosmi B. Bleeding with anticoagulation therapy—who is at risk, and how best to identify such patients. Thromb Haemost 2009;102(2):268-78.
5. Hughes M, Lip GY. Guideline Development Group for the NICE national clinical guideline for management of atrial fibrillation in primary and secondary care. Risk factors for anticoagulation-related bleeding complications in patients with atrial fibrillation: a systematic review. QJM 2007;100(10):599-6.
6. Grines CL, Bonow RO, Casey DE Jr, Gardner TJ, Lockhart PB, Moliterno DJ, O'Gara P, Whitlow P. American Heart Association; American College of Cardiology; Society for Cardiovascular Angiography and Interventions; American College of Surgeons; American Dental Association; American College of Physicians. Prevention of premature discontinuation of dual antiplatelet therapy in patients with coronary artery stents: A science advisory from the American Heart Association, American College of Cardiology, Society for Cardiovascular Angiography and Interventions, American College of Surgeons, and American Dental Association, with representation from the American College of Physicians. J Am Coll Cardiol 2007;49:734-9.
7. Palareti G, Legnani C, Poller L, Thomson J. Warfarin withdrawal. Pharmacokinetic-pharmacodynamic considerations and evidence for "rebound" hypercoagulability after stopping anticoagulants. Clin Pharmacokinet 1996;30:300-13.
8. Lip GY, Lowe GD. Fibrin D-dimer: a useful clinical marker of thrombogenesis? Clin Sci (Lond) 1995;89:205-14.
9. Carrel TP, Klingenmann W, Mohacsi PJ, Berdat P, Althaus U. Perioperative bleeding and thromboembolic risk during non cardiac surgery in patients with mechanical prosthetic heart valves: an institutional review. J Heart Valve Dis 1999;8:392-8.
10. Katholi RE, Nolan SP, McGuire LB. Living with prosthetic heart valves. Subsequent noncardiac operations and the risk of thromboembolism or hemorrhage. Am Heart J 1976;92:162-7.
11. Katholi RE, Nolan SP, McGuire LB. The management of anticoagulation during noncardiac operations in patients with prosthetic heart valves. A prospective study. Am Heart J 1978;96:163-5.
12. Tinmouth AH, Morrow BH, Cruickshank MK, Moore PM, Kovacs MJ. Dalteparin as periprocedure anticoagulation for patients on warfarin and at high risk of thrombosis. Ann Pharmacother 2001;35:669-74.
13. Katz J, Feldman MA, Bass EB, Lubomski LH, Tielsch JM, Petty BG, et al. Risks and benefits of anticoagulant and antiplatelet medication use before cataract surgery. Ophthalmology 2003;110:1784-8.
14. Dunn AS, Turpie AG. Perioperative management of patients receiving oral anticoagulants: A systematic review. Arch Intern Med 2003;163:901-8.
15. Douketis JD, Berger PB, Dunn AS, Jaffer AK, Spyropoulos AC, Becker RC, Ansell J. The perioperative management of antithrombotic therapy: American College of Chest Physicians Evidence-Based Clinical Practice Guidelines 8th Edn. Chest 2008;133(6 Suppl):299S-339S.

16. Kallio H, Paloheimo M, Maunuksela EL. Haemorrhage and risk factors associated with retrobulbar/peribulbar block: a prospective study in 1383 patients. Br J Anaesth 2000;85:708-11.
17. Carter K, Miller KM. Phacoemulsification and lens implantation in patients treated with aspirin or warfarin. J Cataract Refract Surg 1998;24:1361-4.
18. Shuler JD, Paschal JF, Holland GN. Antiplatelet therapy and cataract surgery. J Cataract Refract Surg 1992;18:567-71.
19. Kumar N, Jivan S, Thomas P, et al. Sub-Tenon's anesthesia with aspirin, warfarin, and clopidogrel. J Cataract Refract Surg 2006; 32:1022-102.
20. Narendran N, Williamson TH. The effects of aspirin and warfarin therapy on haemorrhage in vitreoretinal surgery. Acta Ophthalmol Scand 2003;81:38-40.
21. Dayani PN, Grand MG. Maintenance of warfarin anticoagulation for patients undergoing vitreoretinal surgery. Arch Ophthalmol 2006;124:1558-65.
22. Cobb CJ, Chakrabarti S, Chadha V, Sanders R. The effect of aspirin and warfarin therapy in trabeculectomy. Eye 2007;21:598-603.
23. Hannah IT, Powrle S, Rose GE. Open lacrimal surgery: A comparison of admission outcome and complications after planned day case or inpatient management. Br J Ophthalmol 1998;82:392-6.
24. Custer PL, Trinkaus KM. Hemorrhagic complications of oculoplastic surgery. Ophthal Plast Reconstr Surg 2002;18:409-15.
25. Matsuzaki K, Okabe H, Kajihara N, Haraguchi N, Nagano I, Tatewaki H, et al. A prospective study on the timing of discontinuation of aspirin before coronary artery bypass grafting. Nippon Kyobu Geka Gakkai Zasshi 1997;45:1710-4.
26. Rasgon BM, Cruz RM, Hilsinger RL, Jr., Korol HW, Callan E, Wolgat RA, et al. Infiltration of epinephrine in tonsillectomy: A randomized, prospective, doubleblind study. Laryngoscope 1991;101:114-8.

Ocular Pharmacology of Intravitreal Dexamethasone Sustained Release Implant

Priyamvada Bhasin, Amit Basia, Purendra Bhasin (India)

INTRODUCTION

Corticosteroids have been the mainstay for treatment for various noninfectious inflammatory diseases. They can be administered systemically or locally by topical, periocular, or intravitreal routes. Persistent inflammation and cystoid macular edema (CME) secondary to ocular inflammation are often vision-threatening and pose a significant therapeutic challenge. However, significant ocular and systemic side effects limit their use. In an effort to avoid the damage to ocular structures that can ensue with recurrent episodes of ocular inflammation, the side effects associated with systemic steroids, and the need for repeated administration of both topical and locally injected corticosteroids, sustained-release intraocular corticosteroid implants have been developed. These novel implants provide long-term, slow release of steroids to the eye providing sustained control of intraocular inflammation. The Ozurdex (Ozurdex; Allergan, Inc, Irvine, CA, USA) dexamethasone drug delivery system (DDS) is a biodegradable intravitreal implant that delivers sustained release of 700 μg preservative-free dexamethasone to the retina and vitreous.

It is approved by the United States Food and Drug Administration as a first-line therapy for the treatment of macular edema following branch or central retinal vein occlusion, as well as for noninfectious posterior uveitis.[1-3] The results of its use in uveitis in clinical practice and animal models for controlling inflammation and improving CME and visual acuity have been encouraging.[4,5]

MECHANISM OF ACTION

The anti-inflammatory effects of corticosteroids are mediated by the cytosolic glucocorticoid receptors which increase expression of anti-inflammatory proteins.[6] Glucocorticoids can also inhibit the release of proinflammatory cytokines both systemically and in the eye.

Dexamethasone is a widely used corticosteroid for the treatment of systemic inflammatory conditions. Dexamethasone is five times more potent than triamcinolone acetonide, which is commonly used for periocular injections (Kenalog) and intravitreal injections (Triesence). Due to hydrophilicity, it allows for higher vitreous concentration than triamcinolone acetonide. The drawback with dexamethasone formulation is that it is required in higher concentrations to cross the cellular junctions at the ocular surface and through the blood–retinal barrier which can cause significant toxicity.[7] Dexamethasone has a shorter half-life in comparison with other corticosteroids.[8] This brief half-life precludes the use of dexamethasone injections as a long-term treatment for ocular inflammation. These shortcomings have been addressed with the development of a biodegradable dexamethasone drug delivery system (Ozurdex, Allergan, Inc, Irvine, CA). These polymers have been used to create nanoparticles and microparticles for systemic drug delivery that can be targeted to specific human tissues such as the heart, or have novel peptide coatings which can be directed towards human malignancies such as intracranial tumors.[9] Having a biodegradable implant as a platform for drug delivery is ideal, particularly for ocular tissues, given the small size of the organ and significant risk in placing and removing permanent implants as with FA implant. The sustained-release dexamethasone drug delivery system is made of a solid biodegradable polymer composed of a polylactic acid-co-glycolic acid (PLGA) matrix.[10] The PLGA polymer matrix dissolves completely *in vivo* into its components, lactic acid and glycolic acid. These products are in turn converted to carbon dioxide and water which can be easily eliminated by ocular tissue.[11,12] The biodegradable matrix is saturated with 0.7 mg of dexamethasone. As the polymer dissolves, dexamethasone is slowly released into its target tissues, the vitreous and retina. The implant was not only developed to be biodegradable but was also designed to be administered as an office-based procedure.

CHEMICAL FORMULA

The chemical name for dexamethasone is pregna-1,4-diene-3,20-dione, 9-fluoro-11,17,21-trihydroxy-16-methyl-, (11β,16α)-. Its structural formula is:

MW 392.47; molecular formula: $C_{22}H_{29}FO_5$

Dexamethasone occurs as a white to cream-colored crystalline powder having not more than a slight odor, and is practically insoluble in water and very soluble in alcohol. The PLGA matrix slowly degrades to lactic acid and glycolic acid.

Storage: Store at 15°–30°C (59°–86°F).

TECHNIQUE

The intravitreal injection procedure should be carried out under controlled aseptic conditions which include the use of sterile gloves, a sterile drape, and a sterile eyelid speculum (or equivalent). Adequate anesthesia and a broad-spectrum microbicide applied to the periocular skin, eyelid and ocular surface are recommended to be given prior to the injection.

Remove the foil pouch from the carton and examine for damage. Then, open the foil pouch over a sterile field and gently drop the applicator on a sterile tray. Carefully remove the cap from the applicator. Hold the applicator in one hand and pull the safety tab straight off the applicator. Do not twist or flex the tab. The long axis of the applicator should be held parallel to the limbus, and the sclera should be engaged at an oblique angle with the bevel of the needle up (away from the sclera) to create a shelved scleral path. The tip of the needle is advanced within the sclera for about 1 mm (parallel to the limbus), then re-directed toward the center of the eye and advanced until penetration of the sclera is completed and the vitreous cavity is entered. The needle should not be advanced past the point where the sleeve touches the conjunctiva. Slowly depress the actuator button until an audible click is noted. Before withdrawing the applicator from the eye, make sure that the actuator button is fully depressed and has locked flush with the applicator surface. Remove the needle in the same direction as used to enter the vitreous. Following the intravitreal injection, patients should be monitored for elevation in intraocular pressure and for endophthalmitis. Monitoring may consist of a check for perfusion of the optic nerve head immediately after the injection, tonometry within 30 minutes following the injection, and biomicroscopy between two and seven days following the injection. Patients should be instructed to report any symptoms suggestive of endophthalmitis without delay.

Each applicator can only be used for the treatment of a single eye. If the contralateral eye requires treatment, a new applicator must be used, and the sterile field, syringe, gloves, drapes, and eyelid speculum should be changed before administered to the other eye.

PHARMACOKINETICS

Chang-Lin et al by using mass spectrometry and expression of the dexamethasone-sensitive gene cytochrome *P450A38 (CYP3A8)*, which is a marker of dexamethasone biological activity in the retina in monkeys determined the pharmacokinetics and pharmacodynamics of the sustained-release dexamethasone drug delivery system.[11] The peak concentration of dexamethasone in the retina reached 1110 ± 284 ng and 213 ± 49 ng/ml in the vitreous at 2 months (day 60). There was minimal systemic absorption with a peak concentration of 1.11 ng/ml in the serum at 2 months. Following the first 2 months there was a steady decline in steroid concentration from 2 to 3 months, after which a second steady state was achieved and maintained until 6 months. The *CYP3A8* expression increased more than three-fold in implanted eyes and was sustained for 6 months. This study confirmed what was noted in clinical trials: the dexamethasone implant has persistent effects on target tissue up to 6 months after implantation. In addition, it was noted that the initial burst release of dexamethasone from the implant upon administration reaches an initial steady state at therapeutic concentration, which is then followed by decline to a second steady state with lower sustained release of dexamethasone. These results also confirmed the low risk of systemic absorption of medication. The high concentrations of corticosteroid exert immunologic effects, such as T-cell apoptosis accounting for prolonged immunosuppression.[13,14] The concentrations of DEX in the retina during the first 2 months was sufficient to induce this effect suggesting that it may benefit patients with retinal diseases, such as uveitis, in which T cells play a central role in pathogenesis. By binding to cytoplasmic glucocorticoid receptors, corticosteroids in high doses increase the activation of anti-inflammatory genes, whereas at low concentrations they have a role in the suppression of activated inflammatory genes. Therefore, a drug-release profile that consists of an initial phase of high concentration of DEX, followed by a second phase of lower concentration, may continue to contribute to the anti-inflammatory action of DEX for the duration of the implant.

Pharmacokinetics in Vitrectomized and Non-vitrectomized Eye

In another study Chang-Lin et al confirmed that vitreoretinal pharmacokinetic profiles were similar between nonvitrectomized and vitrectomized eyes in rabbit model maintained for at least 31 days.[12]

INDICATIONS

1. Macular edema secondary to retinal vein occlusion, Irvine-Gass syndrome, Diabetes, Persistent inflammation
   A. *Early clinical trial:* Initial clinical studies were performed to evaluate the safety and efficacy of the dexamethasone implant in patients with persistent macular edema. Subsequent studies would be performed to evaluate use in posterior uveitis. Kuppermann et al performed a multicenter, Phase II trial enrolling patients with persistent macular edema for 90 days or more despite laser and medical treatment.[2] The underlying cause could be diabetic retinopathy, retinal vein occlusion, postoperative complications such as Irvine-Gass syndrome, or uveitis. The patients were randomized to observation, treatment with surgically implanted dexamethasone implant of two different concentrations, 0.35 mg and 0.7 mg in a 1:1:1 ratio. A significantly greater proportion of patients who received either dexamethasone implant achieved ten or more letters of visual improvement 90 days after implantation

(24% in 0.35 mg group and 35% in the 0.7 mg group) than control eyes (13%). In addition, patients receiving the higher concentration implant had a greater rate of visual improvement (35% in 0.7 mg implant vs 24% in 0.35 mg implant). These results were similar in all patients despite the etiology of their macular edema. Eleven percent of patients treated with the dexamethasone implant had an increase in IOP of 10 mm Hg or higher compared to the control group (2%). None of these patients required laser or surgical intervention for IOP control and were managed successfully with medication. Finally, there was no significant difference in the number of reported cataracts among the different study groups. The authors concluded that the dexamethasone implant was well tolerated and had a satisfactory safety profile. Further subset analysis was performed examining effectiveness of treatment with the dexamethasone implant in patients with macular edema from Irvine–Gass syndrome and uveitis.[3] This analysis confirmed that patients with persistent macular edema from these entities had a significant improvement in BCVA at 90 days with the dexamethasone implant. It was found that 41.7 percent of patients in the 0.35 mg group and 53.8 percent of patients in the 0.7 mg group had a ten letter or more improvement in BCVA (observation was 14.3%). Furthermore, a 15-letter improvement in BCVA was achieved in 53.8 percent of patients receiving the 0.7 mg dexamethasone implant. These findings were supported by a decrease in fluorescein leakage in treated patients compared to control patients. The adverse effects in this subgroup analysis of IOP increase and cataract formation were equivalent to the adverse events in the overall study.

B. *Ozurdex Geneva Study Group:* The findings of this earlier study were confirmed with a multicenter, randomized, controlled clinical trial (Ozurdex Geneva Study Group) comparing 0.35 mg and 0.7 mg dexamethasone implant with sham in eyes with macular edema associated with retinal vein occlusion.[1] The greatest response was seen at day 60 in the 0.7 mg implant group with 29 percent of patients achieving 15-letter improvement. Significant adverse events were eye pain, ocular hypertension, and anterior chamber cellular reaction. There was no statistically significant increase in cataract formation in the treated group. Sixteen percent of implanted eyes had an increase in IOP that was greater than 15 mm Hg. Most of these episodes of ocular hypertension were transient and there was no difference in IOP elevation between sham and treatment groups at 180 days. They concluded that the dexamethasone implant is a therapeutic alternative for patients with vision loss due to retinal vascular occlusion-induced macular edema. This study led to FDA approval of the dexamethasone implant for the treatment of macular edema associated with retinal vein occlusion.

C. *Treatment of diabetic macular edema in vitrectomized eyes—ozurdex champlain study group:* Boyer et al in a prospective, multicenter, open-label, 26-week study evaluated the safety and efficacy of dexamethasone intravitreal implant 0.7 mg in the treatment of diabetic macular edema in vitrectomized eyes.[15] Author reported that the mean (95% confidence interval) change from baseline central retinal thickness was greatest at 8th week. The mean (95% CI) increase in best corrected visual acuity from baseline (54.5 letters) was 6.0 letters (3.9, 8.1 letters) at 8th week (P-0.001) and 3.0 letters (0.1, 6.0 letters) at 26th week (P = 0.046). At 8th week, 30.4 percent of patients had gained 10 letters in best-corrected visual acuity. Conjunctival hemorrhage, conjunctival hyperemia, eye pain, and increased intraocular pressure were the most common adverse events. Treatment with dexamethasone intravitreal implant led to statistically and clinically significant improvements in both vision and vascular leakage from diabetic macular edema in difficult-to-treat vitrectomized eyes and had an acceptable safety profile.
2. Posterior segment non-infectious uveitis
    A. *Preclinical studies: animal models:* A nonbiodegradable dexamethasone implant containing 5 mg of dexamethasone was first developed by Cheng et al for the treatment of experimental uveitis by inducing two episodes of severe panuveitis separated by 2 weeks in rabbit eyes.[16] The implants were explanted at 99 days and found to have 30 percent of the drug remaining. Electroretinography (ERG) performed showed significant depression in untreated eyes compared to treated eyes. In addition, clinical findings noted significantly less inflammation in treated eyes when graded by two masked observers. The authors concluded that intravitreal implantation of a sustained-release dexamethasone device provided effective suppression of severe ocular inflammation for more than 3 months and allowed for prevention of ocular complications from recurrent inflammatory episodes in animal models. This study provided the initial support for the use of dexamethasone as a treatment for posterior uveitis.
    B. *Dexamethasone intravitreal implant for the treatment of uveitis: clinical trials:* Lowder et al evaluated the efficacy of two doses of dexamethasone (DEX) intravitreal implant in patients diagnosed with noninfectious intermediate or posterior uveitis.[17] A total of 229 patients were randomized in 1:1:1 ratio to receive sham procedure or treatment with dexamethasone implant (either 0.35 mg or 0.7 mg). The proportion of patients with vitreous haze score of 0 at 8th week was 47 percent, 36 percent, and 12 percent for the 0.7 mg dexamethasone implant, the 0.35 mg implant, and the sham group, respectively. Response peaked at 8th week but was maintained for up to 26th week. BCVA was significantly improved by 2 to 6-fold greater in the dexam-

ethasone treated eyes than the sham group throughout the study period. Less than 10 percent of eyes had an IOP of 25 mm Hg or greater. Twenty-three percent of eyes in the 0.7 mg DEX implant group required IOP-lowering medications. Most patients were either observed or treated with 1 IOP-lowering topical medication. No eyes required surgical or laser therapy for elevated IOP. Cataract formation was not statistically significant in comparison groups. The authors concluded that a single dose of the DEX implant was well tolerated in patients with noninfectious posterior uveitis with significant improvement in intraocular inflammation and visual acuity at 26th week follow-up. The 0.7 mg DEX implant demonstrated greater efficacy than the 0.35 mg implant with a similar safety profile.
3. Hypotony.

CONTRAINDICATIONS

- Ocular or periocular infections
- Advanced glaucoma
- Aphakic eyes with rupture of the posterior lens capsule
- ACIOL and rupture of the posterior lens capsule
- Hypersensitivity.

ADVERSE EFFECTS

Intravitreal injection–related effects—endophthalmitis, eye inflammation, increased intraocular pressure, and retinal detachments.
- Steroid–related effects—posterior subcapsular cataracts, increased intraocular pressure, glaucoma, and may enhance the establishment of secondary ocular infections due to bacteria, fungi, or viruses.
  Corticosteroids should be used cautiously in patients with a history of ocular herpes simplex.
- Risk of implant migration—patients in whom the posterior capsule of the lens is absent or has a tear are at risk of implant migration into the anterior chamber.
- Implant misplacement.
- Device dislocation with or without corneal edema.
- Hypotony of the eye (associated with vitreous leakage due to injection).

REFERENCES

1. Haller JA, Bandello F, Belfort R Jr, et al. Ozurdex® Geneva Study Group Randomized, sham-controlled trial of dexamethasone intravitreal implant in patients with macular edema due to retinal vein occlusion. Ophthalmology 2010;117:1134-46.
2. Kupperman BD, Blumenkranz MS, Haller JA, et al. Randomized controlled study of an intravitreous dexamethasone drug delivery system in patients with persistent macular edema. Arch Ophthalmol 2007;125:309-17.

3. Williams GA, Haller JA, Kuppermann BD, et al. Dexamethasone posterior-segment drug delivery system in the treatment of macular edema resulting from uveitis or Irvine-Gass syndrome. Am J Ophthalmol 2009;147:1048-54.
4. Myung JS, Aaker GD, Kiss S. Treatment of noninfectious posterior uveitis with dexamethasone intravitreal implant. Clin Ophthalmol 2010;4:1423-6.
5. Ghosn CR, Li Y, Orilla WC, Lin T, Wheeler L, Burke JA, et al. Treatment of experimental anterior and intermediate uveitis by a dexamethasone intravitreal implant. Invest Ophthalmol Vis Sci 2011;52(6):2917-23.
6. Taylor SR, Isa H, Joshi L, Lightman S. New developments in corticosteroid therapy for uveitis. Ophthalmologica 2010;224 (Suppl)1:46-53.
7. Sivaprasad S, McCluskey P, Lightman S. Intravitreal steroids in the management of macular oedema. Acta Ophthalmol Scand 2006;84(6):722-33.
8. Edelman JL. Differentiating intraocular glucocorticoids.Ophthalmologica 2010;224 (Suppl)1:25-30.
9. Sawyer AJ, Saucier-Sawyer JK, Booth CJ, et al. Convection-enhanced delivery of camptothecin-loaded polymer nanoparticles for treatment of intracranial tumors. Drug Deliv Transl Res 2011;1(1):34-42.
10. London NJ, Chiang A, Haller JA. The dexamethasone drug delivery system: indications and evidence. Adv Ther 2011;28(5):351-66.
11. Chang-Lin JE, Attar M, Acheampong AA, et al. Pharmacokinetics and pharmacodynamics of a sustained-release dexamethasone intravitreal implant. Invest Ophthalmol Vis Sci 2011;52:80-6.
12. Chang-Lin JE, Burke JA, Peng Q, et al. Pharmacokinetics of a sustained release dexamethasone intravitreal implant in vitrectomized and nonvitrectomized eyes. Invest Ophthalmol Vis Sci 2011;52(7):4605-9.
13. Leussink VI, Jung S, Merschdorf U, Toyka KV, Gold R. High-dose methylprednisolone therapy in multiple sclerosis induces apoptosis in peripheral blood leukocytes. Arch Neurol 2001;58(1):91-7.
14. Migita K, Eguchi K, Kawabe Y, et al. Apoptosis induction in human peripheral blood T lymphocytes by high-dose steroid therapy. Transplantation 1997;63(4):583-7.
15. Boyer DS, Faber D, Gupta S, Patel SS, Tabandeh H, Li XY, et al. Dexamethasone intravitreal implant for treatment of diabetic macular edema in vitrectomized patients. Retina 2011;31:915-23.
16. Cheng CK, Berger AS, Pearson PA, Ashton P, Jaffe GJ. Intravitreal sustained-release dexamethasone device in the treatment of experimental uveitis. Invest Ophthalmol Vis Sci 1995;36(2):442-53.
17. Lowder C, Belfort R Jr, Lightman S, et al. Dexamethasone intravitreal implant for noninfectious intermediate or posterior uveitis. Arch Ophthalmol 2011;129(5):545-53.

Nanotechnology in Ophthalmology

NR Biswas, Harivenkatesh N, KP Biswas, Alok K Ravi, Madhurjya Gogoi (India)

INTRODUCTION

Nanotechnology is a field of science comprising the body of theories and techniques that allow the production and manipulation of minute objects that measure a little as one billionth of a meter; the nanometer (1 nanometer = 10^{-9} meter). Although research in this field dates back to Richard P Feynman's work in 1959, the term *nanotechnology* was first coined by K Eric Drexler in 1986 in the book *Engines of Creation*.

Nanotechnology involves research and technology development at the atomic, molecular, or intracellular levels in the critical dimension range of approximately 1-100 nanometers. Nanoparticles have relatively high surface are: volume ratio. Nanotechnology research and development includes control at the nanoscale and integration of nanoscale structures into larger material components and systems. Within these larger scale assemblies, the control and construction of their structures and components remains at the nanometer scale.

Of relevance to medicine is *Nanomedicine*, which may be defined as the monitoring, repair, construction and control of human biological systems at the molecular level, using engineered nanodevices and nanostructures. The goal is to deliver the potential benefit of discoveries in the laboratory to society.

The power of nanotechnology can be encapsulated in an apparently simple and minute device. Packed with miniature chemical processors, computing, and robotics, it will produce a wide-range of items quickly, cleanly, and inexpensively, building products directly from blueprints. The enabling technologies include optics, nanolithography, mechanochemistry and 3D prototyping.

Although nanotechnology is in the research stage as of now, it is likely to arrive into the clinics in near future. It is being extensively pursued for research on aging, cancer, neurodegenerative disorders, ophthalmology, drug development and drug delivery systems.

MEDICINE AND NANOTECHNOLOGY

Nanotechnology is highly interdisciplinary and features a close collaboration between life scientists, physical scientists, chemists and engineers. Medicine attempts to make the best use of the body's natural healing powers and homeostatic mechanisms. The underlying principle is that, all else being equal, those interventions are best that intervene least. The promise of nanotechnology in medicine lies in the potential to achieve this by target specific and controlled delivery of intervention measures at the cellular level. Nanosystems have significantly different biological properties from large-sized systems (e.g. implants) that could be used effectively to overcome problems in drug and gene therapy using programmable and controllable microscale robots. This will hopefully unlock the indefinite extension of human health and the expansion of human abilities.

Medical Nanodevice/Nanomachines

The typical medical nanodevice will probably be a micron-scale robot assembled from nanoscale parts ranging from 1-100 nm and might be fitted together to make a working machine measuring perhaps 0.5-3 microns (1 micron = 10^{-6} meter) in diameter. Three microns is about the maximum size for blood borne medical nanorobots, the limiting factor being capillary passage. These nanomachines can be used to measure various biological parameters like oxygen tension, blood pressure, intraocular pressure, pH, temperature and oxidative status of a cell, etc.

Carbon will likely be the principal element comprising the bulk of a medical nanorobot, probably in the form of diamond or diamondoid/fullerene nanocomposites—largely because of the tremendous strength and chemical inertness of diamond. Other elements such as hydrogen, sulfur, oxygen, nitrogen, fluorine, silicon, etc. will be used for special purposes.

Properties

The medical nanodevice should be visualized as two spaces: its interior and its exterior. The exterior will be exposed to the diverse chemical brew that makes up our human biochemistry. But the interior of the nanorobot may be a highly controlled environment into which external liquids would not normally intrude, except in specific instance.

The ideal model of the medical nanodevice will consist of an injection of a few cubic centimeters of micron-sized nanorobots. The circulating nanorobots will be designed to accomplish a specific task, and would remain absolutely inactive outside of the target volume. Even once inside the target treatment volume, nanorobots would still remain inactive until the physician tells them to begin the active treatment, or the precise antigenic signature of the target tissue is detected.

Nanorobots will communicate their positions, operational status, and the outcome of treatment using encoded acoustic messaging for internal communications as well as for communication with the physician, who will retain complete control. It may not be necessary to image the nanodevices directly, and procedures such as biopsy should be rarely needed. They will have a high level of redundancy to ensure effectiveness and safety. *In vivo* medical nanodevices could metabolize local glucose and oxygen for energy, or use externally supplied acoustic power. Their exfusion from the body will occur via the usual excretory channels or other scavenger systems. The only physical change to be seen in the patient will hopefully be his recovery.

Question of Immune Response

Many medical nanorobots will have only temporary residence in the body, and the issue of nanodevice biocompatibility is in principle similar to the biocompatibility of medical implants generally. It is not expected to be a major problem. The design of the exteriors will be critical to minimize bioactivity and opsonization. Passive diamond is one such design.

Nanotechnology and Genetics

Of great importance is the use of nanotechnology in genetics. DNA is a unique material for nanotechnology since it is possible to use base sequences to encode instructions for assembly in a predetermined fashion at the nanometer scale. This emerging field of DNA-nanotechnology is now exploring DNA-programmed processes for the assembly of organic compounds, biomolecules, and inorganic materials. Bioconjugated nanoparticles have been evaluated for biosensing and bioimaging, such as cell staining, DNA detection and separation, rapid single bacterium detection, and biotechnological application in DNA protection.

Pegylated compacted DNA nanoparticles have been investigated for gene therapy applications in eye, lung and brain. Nanoparticles can also be used to deliver the genes effectively into the stem cells.

Nanotechnology in Drug Development and Drug Delivery Systems

Nanosystems comprising nanoparticles and nanodevices such as nanobiosensors and nanobiochips, are being developed for targeted drug therapy. Among these nanomaterials, carbon nanotubes (CNT) have emerged as an efficient and safe tool for transporting and translocating therapeutic molecules such as bioactive peptides, proteins, nucleic acids and drugs.

Nanoparticles that contain the specific drug can be dispersed either in a polymer matrix (nanosphere) or encapsulated in a polymer (nanocapsule) as shown in Figure 67.1.

Many polymerizable surfactants have been synthesized with all possible combination of the various types (anionic, cationic, zwitterionic or non-ionic group) and of classical polymerizable groups (acrylate, methacrylate, acrylamide, vinyl, allyl, diallyl, etc.). The polymerizable group can be located at different parts of the surfactant molecule most often near the polar head or at the end of hydrophobic tail, or even in the counterion (Fig. 67.2).

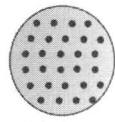
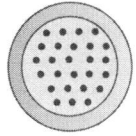

Fig. 67.1: Schematic representation of nanosphere (left) and nanocapsule (right). Black dots in the figure represent the drug molecules

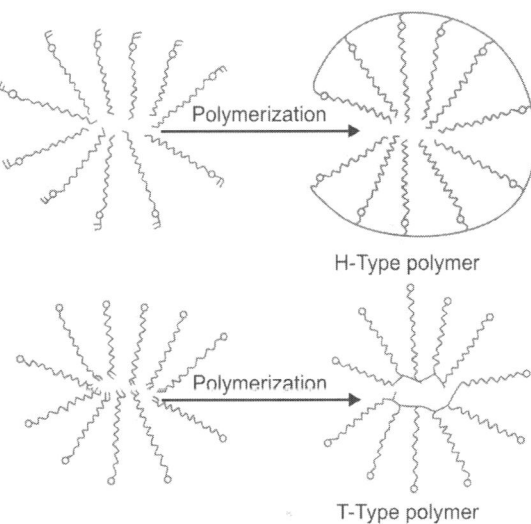

Fig. 67.2: Schematic structure of a polymeric micelle. Water insoluble drug can be loaded in the core of the micelle

Another important parameter, which synergies the release kinetics of the drug in different pH solutions, is the swelling behavior of the polymer. The ability to ionize/deionize at different pH is the salient feature of some copolymers. The pores of the particles are controlled by overall -COOH content and the ionization of –COOH groups. At acidic pH, the carboxylic groups exhibit inter-chain hydrogen bonding creating a tighter overall network and hence the pore size becomes smaller. Consequently due to small pore size, the release of drug from the micelles is quite slow. At alkaline pH, -COOH groups become ionized and due to repulsion among the ionized –COO groups swelling take place. As a result of swelling, pore size of the polymer increases and the drug release becomes faster (Fig. 67.3).

Liposomal based drug delivery systems are gaining wider therapeutic uses. In fact liposomes were the first nanoparticles to be used therapeutically as lipid emulsion for parenteral administration. Liposomes are small artificially prepared vesicles that contain a lipid bilayer prepared from nontoxic phospholipids and cholesterol. Liposomes show promising results when used as

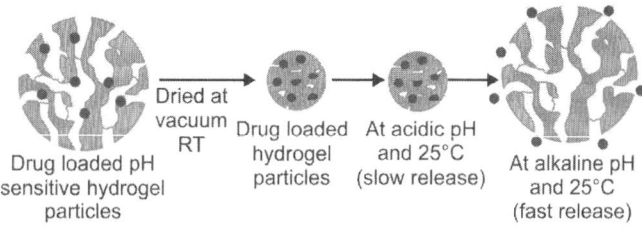

Fig. 67.3: Schematic representation of drug release from polymer at different pH

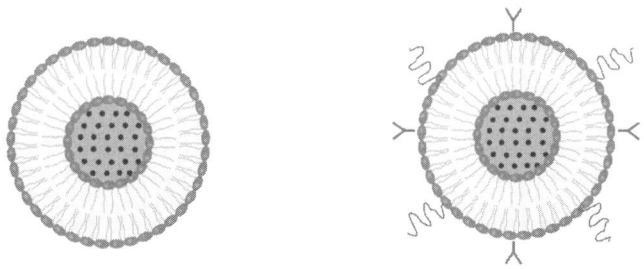

Fig. 67.4: Schematic diagram of liposomal drug delivery system (left) and immunoliposomal drug delivery system (right). Black dots represent the drug; red Y represents the antibody and violet curved structure represents polyethylene glycol (PEG)

drug delivery systems. Liposomes can be pegylated and conjugated with antibodies for selective targeting of cells (Fig. 67.4). Neosomes are similar to liposomes but contain non-ionic surfactant vesicles rather than phospholipids.

Dendrimers are artificially synthesized highly branched polymers with nono-scale scaffolding that can be precisely controlled (Fig. 67.5). These dendrimers have been investigated as the carriers for controlled targeted drug delivery. Drugs explored for delivery through dendrimers include anti-cancer drugs, pilocarpine and vascular endothelial growth factor (VEGF) inhibitors.

NANOTECHNOLOGY IN OPHTHALMOLOGY

Nanotechnology has been applied in ophthalmologic research for diagnosis and treatment including optimized drug delivery. Some examples of nanotechnology applications in ophthalmology are summarized below.

Nanoceria Particles for Ocular Diseases Associated with Free Radical Damage

Nanoceria particles (cerium oxide nanoparticles) act as free radical scavengers that can scavenge ROS (reactive oxygen species). They have been shown to prevent light induced photoreceptor damage

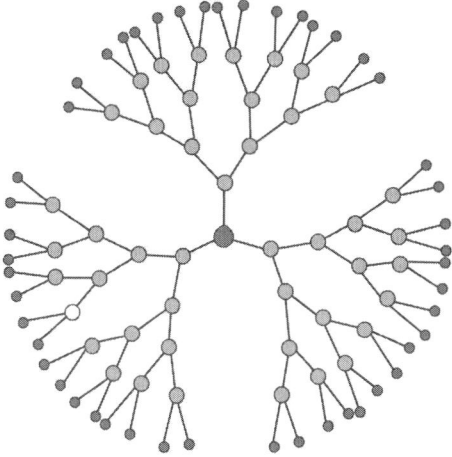

Fig. 67.5: Schematic structure of a dendrimer

in rodent models when injected intravitreally. This may pave way for treatment of ocular conditions associated with oxidative damage like age-related macular degeneration (AMD), retinitis pigmentosa and diabetic retinopathy.

Nanosensors for Continuous IOP Monitoring

Nanosensors that can measure intraocular pressure (IOP) have been embedded in contact lens (Fig. 67.6), intraocular lens, intrascleral and intraimplants. These devices have been investigated for continuous noninvasive/minimally invasive measurement of intraocular pressure that can revolutionize glaucoma management in the future.

Nanotechnology and Theragnostics

The process in which individualized diagnosis for a particular patient is coupled to specific targeted therapy is known as theragnostics.

The oxidative stress seen in conditions like retinopathy of prematurity activates antioxidant response element (ARE) in the DNA of retinal pigment epithelial cells. A biosensor DNA/gene tethered to magnetic nanoparticles has been injected subretinally in diabetic rats and it was found that these biosensor nanoparticles detected the activation of ARE in the retinal pigment epithelium of diabetic rats. These antioxidant biosensor nanoparticles can identify the potential candidates for therapy at an earlier stage. Neonates with retinopathy of prematurity may be identified earlier using these sensors and appropriate therapy like laser photocoagulation can be initiated before the onset of severe disease. Simultaneously therapeutic genes that encode for antioxidants like catalase or superoxide dismutase can be coupled to the biosensors (theragnostics approach). In conditions like

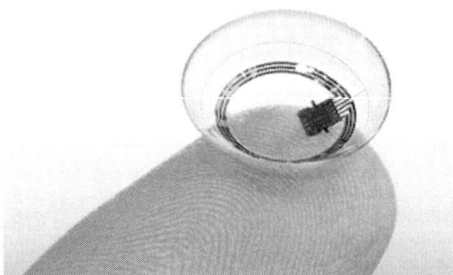

Fig. 67.6: Scientist holding a nanosensor embedded contact lens in the pulp of his finger

oxidative stress, these genes will be taken up by retinal pigment epithelial cells to enable self treatment.

Nanotechnology and Ocular Gene Therapy

Compacted DNA nanoparticles can act as carriers/vehicles for gene therapy. These nanoparticles cross the cell surface and ultimately enter the nucleus in a short time span. These DNA nanoparticles when delivered to the target tissue result in good transfection rates and are being investigated for treatment of some ocular conditions like retinopathy of prematurity.

Nanoparticles for Ophthalmic Drug Delivery

The main objective of employing nanoparticles as a carrier for ophthalmic drug delivery is to enhance drug permeation and provide sustained drug release and hence prolonged therapeutic activity.

Dendrimers have been investigated as vehicles for controlled delivery of some drugs like pilocarpine, gatifloxacin, VEGF (Vascular Endothelial Growth Factor) inhibitors into the eye. In rabbit eye, dentrimer-gatifloxacin complex was found to cross the ocular barriers effectively and attain excellent gatifloxacin concentrations in aqueous and vitreous humor, cornea and conjunctiva.

Microemulsions are dispersions of oil and water that require the presence of surfactant to stabilize them (Fig. 67.7). When applied topically to the eye, these microemulsions have good corneal permeability and achieve sustained drug release in aqueous humor thereby decreasing the frequency of drug administration. In rabbit eye, pilocarpine microemulsion was shown to produce sustained miosis resulting in sustained ocular hypotensive effect. Pilocarpine microemulsions can be given twice daily instead of giving 6th hourly conventional preparations.

Polymeric nanoparticle suspensions made from inert polymer resins can be used as carriers for delivering certain drugs in order

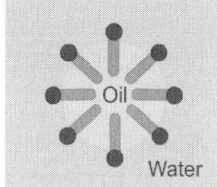 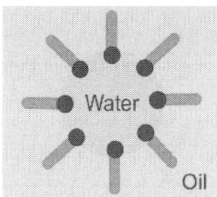

Fig. 67.7: Schematic representation of microemulsions—oil in water microemulsion (left) and water in oil microemulsion (right). Orange colored rods represent lipophilic component and violet dots represent hydrophilic component

to increase bioavailability and prolong drug release. Flurbiprofen, a non-steroidal anti-inflammatory drug (NSAID) has been loaded in polymeric nanosuspensions prepared from Eudragit RS 100® and RL 100® polymer resins and has been found to prevent miosis and inflammatory edema induced by surgical traumas, such as cataract extraction.

Albumin nanoparticles are non-toxic to retina, non-antigenic and are biodegradable. Albumin nanoparticles have been studied as vehicles for delivering certain drugs like ganciclovir and oligonucleotides in treatment of CMV (cytomegalovirus) retinitis.

Nanoparticles made from chitosan, a natural polymer (Fig. 67.8) are being studied as vehicles for certain drugs used in treatment of ocular diseases.

Liposomes show promising results as ocular drug delivery systems. Liposomes get adsorbed to the corneal surface and transfer the drug to corneal epithelium resulting in enhanced corneal penetration. In rabbit cornea, positively charged unilamellar liposomes were shown to enhance the corneal flux of penicillin G. Liposomal preparations of acetazolamide, pilocarpine and oligonucleotides have been investigated in various studies. Intravenous administration of liposomal verteporfin has been approved for photodynamic therapy of age-related macular degeneration.

Immunoliposomes of some antiviral drugs like ganciclovir and iododeoxyuridine have been investigated. These immunoliposomes are conjugated to herpes simplex virus (HSV) glycoprotein D monoclonal antibodies and selectively target the viral cells.

Neosomes have been successfully studied as vehicles for cyclopentolate. Studies have reported increased ocular bioavailability of timolol when entrapped with vehicles like neosomes and discomes (modified neosomes).

It has been reported that ocular bioavailability and corneal penetration of poorly water soluble drugs like dexamethasone, acetazolamide and cyclosporin can be increased by using cyclodextrins as drug carriers.

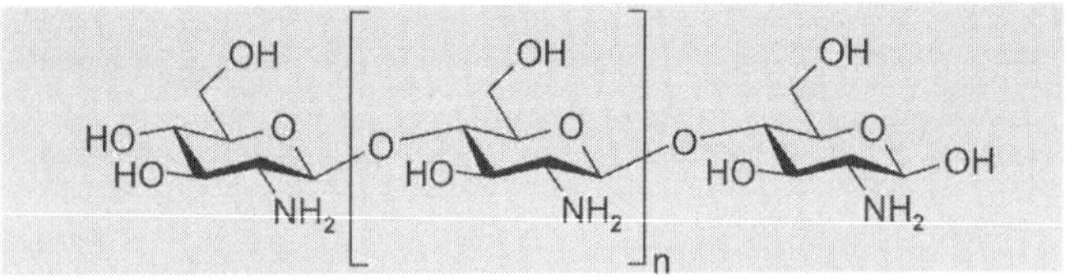

Fig. 67.8: Chemical structure of chitosan

Ocular Drug Delivery Using Nanobubble

Anti-VEGF medications like ranibizumab and bevacizumab target Vascular Endothelial Growth Factor and retard the growth of abnormal retinal blood vessels in patients suffering from age-related macular degeneration. They are given as intravitreal injections. Research is underway for development of a more efficient method to deliver anti-VEGF drugs by using microscopic particles known as nanobubbles.

Drug-loaded nanobubbles increase the transit time of the drug in the retina and are selectively activated using ultrasound. The nanobubbles are mixed with fluorescent dyes that make them visible to imaging and can be guided and released when they are in place. The biodegradable nanobubbles prevent the medication from disbursing before reaching the target area and maintain higher drug concentration for longer duration.

Nanofibers for Glaucoma

The trabecular meshwork is responsible for drainage of aqueous humor and thereby maintaining a constant intraocular pressure (IOP). Any problem or blockage in trabecular meshwork impairs the aqueous drainage leading to elevated intraocular pressure and glaucoma. By using woven miniature nanofibers, scientists are creating artificial trabecular meshwork complex for treatment of glaucoma.

OCULAR DISTRIBUTION OF NANOPARTICLES

The fate of nanoparticles in the body depends on the physicochemical properties of the nanoparticles. Properties such as pH, surfactant, and stabilizers influence the mucoadhesion properties to the ocular membrane and thereby modify the precorneal retention of the nanoparticles. It has been shown that the molecular weight of the polymer influences the residence time of nanoparticles in the precorneal area. As the molecular weight increases, the polymer becomes poorly retained, whereas low molecular weight polymers are retained for a longer time. Experimental data on the disposition of polyhexylcyanoacrylate nanoparticles in tears, the aqueous humor, cornea and conjunctiva of albino rabbits clearly showed adhesion of nanoparticles to adsorbing tissue.

FUTURE OF NANOTECHNOLOGY

Nanoparticles appear to offer several advantages in the area of ophthalmic drug delivery. Particularly attractive are their bioadhesive properties which, if optimized, may overcome major shortcomings of current ophthalmic preparations like inadequate retention time in the precorneal site. Another important feature is the versatility of nanoparticles as a drug carrier. Many different types of compounds can be incorporated or adsorbed to nanoparticles, and depending on the composition, nanoparticles with different release characteristic can be designed. Furthermore, nanoparticles are easy to manufacture and form a stable, yet biodegradable product. Biodegradability suggests that nanoparticles will have low toxicity.

Despite promising results of nanoparticle ophthalmic drug delivery systems, there is a need for further studies to elucidate the pharmacodynamic and pharmacokinetic fate of nanoparticle ophthalmic products, the safety of long-term use of this new type of ophthalmic dosage form, and also the aspects of the industrial product development.

Regenerative nanomedicine is an upcoming branch of nanomedicine which aims at repairing or replacing damaged tissues by using nanoparticles of gene transcription factors and other molecular modulators for *in vivo* reprogramming of the damaged cells. Nanotechnology will provide better and effective treatment modalities for various ocular diseases in the near future.

BIBLIOGRAPHY

1. Araujo J, Gonzalez E, Egea MA, Garcia ML, Souto EB. Nanomedicines for ocular NSAIDs: safety on drug delivery. Nanomedicine 2009;5(4):394-401.
2. Cattaneo AG, Gornati R, Sabbioni E, Chiriva-Internati M, Cobos E, Jenkins MR, et al. Nanotechnology and human health: risks and benefits. J Appl Toxicol 2010;30(8):730-44.
3. Cai X, Conley S, Naash M. Nanoparticle applications in ocular gene therapy. Vision Res 2008;48(3):319-24.
4. Das S, Bellare JR, Banerjee R. Protein based nanoparticles as platforms for aspirin delivery for ophthalmologic applications. Colloids Surf B Biointerfaces 2012;93:161-8.
5. de la Fuente M, Ravina M, Paolicelli P, Sanchez A, Seijo B, Alonso MJ. Chitosan-based nanostructures: a delivery platform for ocular therapeutics. Adv Drug Deliv Rev 2010;62(1):100-17.
6. Diebold Y, Calonge M. Applications of nanoparticles in ophthalmology. Prog Retin Eye Res 2010;29(6):596-609.
7. Gupta HL, Gupta P, Gupta R. Nanotechnology in ophthalmology. Indian J Ophthalmol [Epub ahead of print] [cited 2012 Sep 14]. Available from: http://www.ijo.in/preprintarticle.asp? id=97557
8. Jain KK. Nanomedicine: application of nanobiotechnology in medical practice. Med Princ Pract 2008;17(2):89-101.
9. Jain KK. Role of nanobiotechnology in the development of personalized medicine. Nanomedicine (Lond) 2009;4(3):249-52.
10. Jo DH, Kim JH, Yu YS, Lee TG. Antiangiogenic effect of silicate nanoparticle on retinal neovascularization induced by vascular endothelial growth factor. Nanomedicine 2012;8(5):784-91.

11. Jo DH, Lee TG, Kim JH. Nanotechnology and nanotoxicology in retinopathy. Int J Mol Sci 2011;12(11):8288-301.
12. Kalishwaralal K, Barathmanikanth S, Pandian SR, Deepak V, Gurunathan S. Silver nano—a trove for retinal therapies. J Control Release 2010;145(2):76-90.
13. Kanwar JR, Mohan RR, Kanwar RK, Roy K, Bawa R. Applications of aptamers in nanodelivery systems in cancer, eye and inflammatory diseases. Nanomedicine (Lond) 2010;5(9):1435-45.
14. Kanwar JR, Sun X, Punj V, Sriramoju B, Mohan RR, Zhou SF, et al. Nanoparticles in the treatment and diagnosis of neurological disorders: untamed dragon with fire power to heal. Nanomedicine 2012;8(4):399-414.
15. Kim JH, Kim KW, Kim MH, Yu YS. Intravenously administered gold nanoparticles pass through the blood-retinal barrier depending on the particle size, and induce no retinal toxicity. Nanotechnology 2009;20(50):505101.
16. Leary JF. Nanotechnology: what is it and why is small so big? Can J Ophthalmol 2010;45(5):449-56.
17. Lin TT, He YJ. [The ophthalmic applications of nanotechnology]. Zhonghua Yan Ke Za Zhi 2007;43(11):1048-52.
18. Liu S, Jones L, Gu FX. Nanomaterials for ocular drug delivery. Macromol Biosci 2012;12(5):608-20.
19. Nagarwal RC, Kant S, Singh PN, Maiti P, Pandit JK. Polymeric nanoparticulate system: a potential approach for ocular drug delivery. J Control Release 2009;136(1):2-13.
20. Nguyen P, Meyyappan M, Yiu SC. Applications of nanobiotechnology in ophthalmology—Part I. Ophthalmic Res 2010; 44(1): 1-16.
21. Orosz KE, Gupta S, Hassink M, Abdel-Rahman M, Moldovan L, Davidorf FH, et al. Delivery of antiangiogenic and antioxidant drugs of ophthalmic interest through a nanoporous inorganic filter. Mol Vis 2004;10:555-65.
22. Pignatello R, Bucolo C, Ferrara P, Maltese A, Puleo A, Puglisi G. Eudragit RS100 nanosuspensions for the ophthalmic controlled delivery of ibuprofen. Eur J Pharm Sci 2002;16(1-2):53-61.
23. Raghava S, Goel G, Kompella UB. Ophthalmic Applications of Nanotechnology. In: Tombran-Tink J, Barnstable JC, editors. Ocular Transporters in Ophthalmic Diseases and Drug Delivery: Humana Press; 2008. pp. 415-35.
24. Sahoo SK, Dilnawaz F, Krishnakumar S. Nanotechnology in ocular drug delivery. Drug Discov Today 2008;13(3-4):144-51.
25. Vandervoort J, Ludwig A. Ocular drug delivery: nanomedicine applications. Nanomedicine (Lond) 2007;2(1):11-21.
26. Zarbin MA, Montemagno C, Leary JF, Ritch R. Nanotechnology in ophthalmology. Can J Ophthalmol 2010;45(5):457-76.
27. Zarbin MA, Montemagno C, Leary JF, Ritch R. Nanomedicine in ophthalmology: the new frontier. Am J Ophthalmol 2010;150(2): 144-62 e2.
28. Zarbin MA, Montemagno C, Leary JF, Ritch R. Regenerative nanomedicine and the treatment of degenerative retinal diseases. Wiley Interdiscip Rev Nanomed Nanobiotechnol 2012;4(1):113-37.
29. Zuo L, Wei W, Morris M, Wei J, Gorbounov M, Wei C. New technology and clinical applications of nanomedicine. Med Clin North Am 2007;91(5):845-62.

Photochemical Therapy for Corneal Infections

Ammar M Al Mahmood, Ashley Behrens (Saudi Arabia)

INTRODUCTION

Photochemical therapy (PCT) stands for the application of photosensible compounds followed by exposure to a suitable source of light to achieve specific therapeutic goals. The most known procedures in the field of ophthalmology are corneal collagen cross-linking (CXL) and photodynamic therapy (PDT). More recently, another type of corneal PCT has been proposed for the treatment of microbial keratitis. We will call this application "photochemical treatment for corneal infections (PCTCI)" in the flow of the article. The principles of PCTCI are somewhat similar to CXL, which is growing in popularity for the treatment of keratoconus.

Researchers are optimistic about PCTCI as it holds a promise as a future antimicrobial therapy through the course of corneal infections.[1,2] In the following chapter we will describe the mechanism of action, preliminary *in vitro* and *in vivo* studies and early clinical results of this potential new treatment modality for a broad spectrum of infectious keratitis. Similarly, we will discuss other findings published in the literature that may result contradictory for the indications proposed initially. The goal is to stress the importance of a methodology that is still in process of development.

ANTIMICROBIAL EFFECTS OF PCTCI

In the 1960s, it was established that riboflavin, could inactivate the RNA of tobacco mosaic virus after exposure to either visible or UV-light source.[3] Since then, it has been revealed that this phenomenon can be used to inactivate a wide range of viruses, bacteria, and parasites in different clinical settings.

In the cornea, the benefits of PCTCI may have two possible mechanisms which may operate in synergy. Firstly, the pathogens implicated in corneal melting are known to effect this by enzymatic digestion of the corneal tissue. Since CXL has been reported to increase tissue resistance to enzymatic digestion,[4] the improvement in symptoms can be attributed to the greater resistance of corneal tissue to enzyme activity. Secondly, the phenomenon of cell damage after CXL may include not only keratocytes but also pathogens, thus arresting the infectious process. Riboflavin byproducts generated after UV light exposure seem to be competitive to nucleotides present in both DNA and RNA, generating disruption of DNA/RNA material and cell death. (reference Gambro) Via this second and important mechanism, any bacteria, virus, fungus or parasite, regardless of the type, should be equally affected and damaged by these byproducts. Therefore, the theoretical "sterilization" of the cornea may be feasible and eradication of infection warranted in the exposed area.

Antibacterial Effect Trials

The antibacterial effectiveness of CXL has been demonstrated *in vitro* against some common pathogens, selected from a panel of clinical ocular isolates obtained from patients with severe bacterial keratitis.[5] Tested organisms included *Pseudomonas aeruginosa* (PA), *Staphylococcus aureus* (SA), *Staphylococcus epidermidis* (SE), methicillin-resistant *S. aureus* (MRSA), multidrug-resistant PA, drug-resistant *Streptococcus pneumoniae*, and *Candida albicans*. A modified disk-diffusion system using Kirby-Bauer disks was utilized, and the mean growth inhibition zone in square millimeters was measured in the area of UV-A exposure to riboflavin). Treatment was found effective against SA, SE, PA, MRSA, multidrug-resistant PA, and drug-resistant *Streptococcus pneumoniae*, but ineffective on *Candida albicans*. Schrier et al[6] tested UV light alone, and the combination of riboflavin and UV light on SA, MRSA, and PA. All plates exposed to the combination of riboflavin and UVA light showed bacterial death. Makdoumi et al[7] evaluated the antibacterial efficacy of riboflavin/Ultraviolet A UVA on three bacterial strains: SA, SE and PA. Extensive eradication of bacteria with combination treatment with potent reduction in bacterial number was reported in all studies.

Other reports have looked on the effects of PCTCI *in vivo*. Animal studies in New Zealand white rabbits have shown improvement in models of *Staphylococcus aureus* induced keratitis after PCTCI. In a study by Khan et al[8] they demonstrated significant clinical improvement after established bacterial keratitis in the rabbit model compared to controls, in as soon as 24 hours after treatment (Figs 68.1A to C).

Makdoumi et al[9] reported the results of seven eyes with infectious keratitis (four culture-positive) associated with melting that underwent PCTCI. All but one eye showed symptomatic improvement, with re-epithelialization occurring in all eyes at 1–6 months follow-up. A recent study by the same authors investigated the role of PCTCI as a primary therapy in 16 eyes with infectious keratitis and found that inflammation improved and epithelium healed in all eyes, although two eyes required additional antibiotics and one required amniotic membrane.[10] Iseli et al[11] evaluated the efficacy of CXL for treating infectious melting keratitis. Five patients with infectious keratitis associated with corneal melting were treated with CXL. CXL was performed when the infection did not respond to systemic and topical antibiotic therapy. Follow-up after cross-linking ranged from 1 to 9 months. In all cases, the progression of corneal melting was halted after CXL treatment. Emergency keratoplasty was not necessary in any of the 5 cases

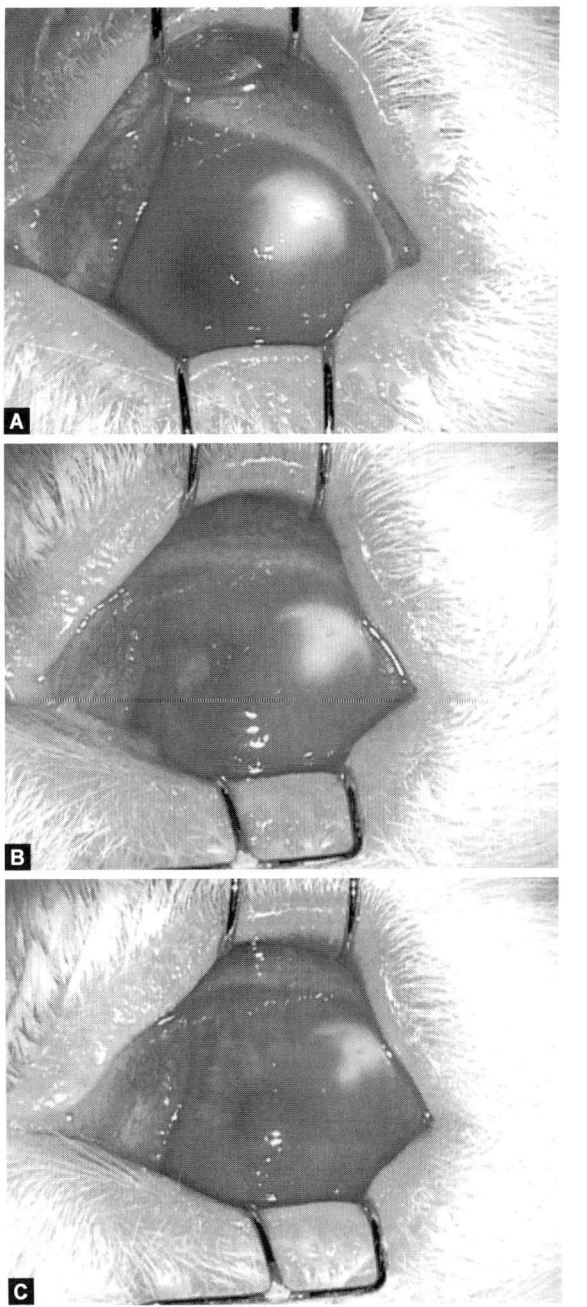

Figs 68.1A to C: Experimental model of *Staphylococcus aureus* in New Zealand white rabbits. The photos show clinical progression after PCTCI applied on day 0. (A) Day 0 (prior PCTCI application); (B) 24 hours after PCTCI application, no other antimicrobial applied. Note reduction in both infiltrate and edema; (C) 48 hours after PCTCI application, no further antimicrobial therapy applied. Note much less infiltrate and details of the iris observed after edema clearance in one area of the cornea

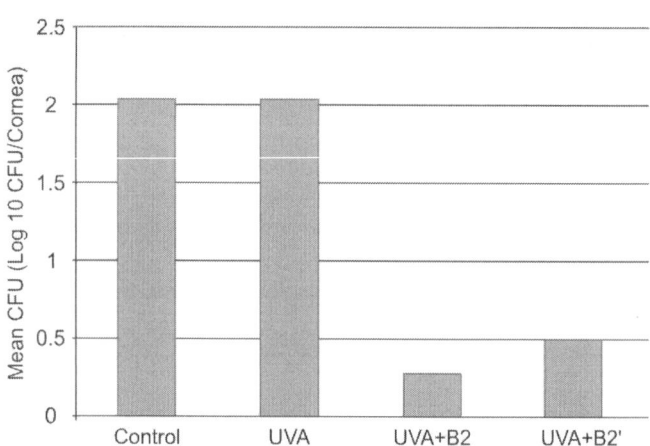

Fig. 68.2: Colony forming units obtained from the corneal samples exposed to treatment vs. controls. Control: No treatment. UVA: Exposure to UV-A light only. UVA + B2: Exposure to riboflavin solution + UV-A light. UVA + B2': Exposure to UV-A light and preactivated riboflavin solution

presented. Kymionis et al[12] reported keratitis with corneal melt due to microbiologically proven atypical mycobacteria that was treated simultaneously with combined flap amputation, phototherapeutic keratectomy, and CXL, which resulted in a favorable visual outcome without further surgical intervention.

CXL has also been beneficial in treating a patient with *Escherichia coli* keratitis,[13] leading to complete healing of corneal ulceration, regression of edema, and disappearance of painful symptoms.

A significant improvement of visual acuity was recorded in the treatment of 2 cases of bullous keratopathy combined with corneal ulcer.[14]

Antiamoebic Effect

del Buey et al[15] evaluated *in vitro* amoebicidal effects of riboflavin/UVA collagen CXL. Two different strains of *Acanthamoeba* species were tested identically. In all cases, cysts and trophozoites were detected 24 hours after treatment at a radial distance from the center of the seeding point more than 5 mm, indicating that the amoebae were viable. The treatment was considered ineffective for *Acanthamoeba* isolates. Same conclusion was reached in another study by Kashiwabuchi.[16] Similar results were reached when riboflavin/UVA CXL was applied to rabbit eyes.[17] However, Camacho et al (unpublished data) were able to demonstrate lysis of *Acanthamoeba* cysts after PCTCI + Brolene in cultures isolated from a patient with keratitis who was a contact lens wearer (Figs 68.3A to D).

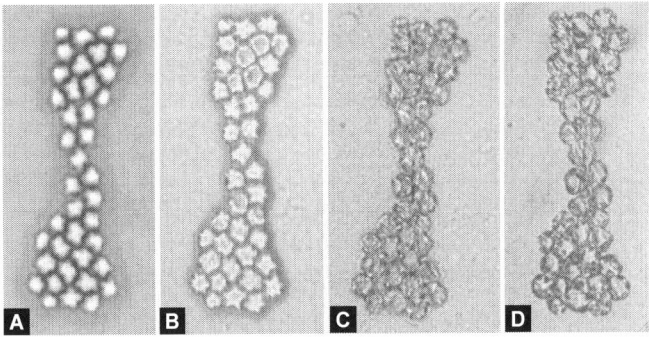

Figs 68.3A to D: Time-lapse photography 4 hours after exposure to PCTCI treatment + Brolene *in vitro* in an *Escherichia coli* enriched media. (A) Prior exposure; (B) One hour after exposure, cysts start to show some structural changes; (C) 3 hours after exposure, cyst skeleton looks disorganized and cyst content seems to start disintegrating; (D) 4 hours after exposure, disorganization and disruption of the walls of *Acanthamoeba* cysts at the endpoint. In the Brolene only group, cysts remained intact (100 X)

Clinical results did not seem to be in agreement with its preceding *in vitro* studies. Few case reports were enthusiastic of PCTCI antiamoebic effect for clinically established infections in some patients. Khan et al[18] reported the first 3 cases of *Acanthamoeba* keratitis, unresponsive to medical treatment, that were successfully treated with adjunctive therapy using PCTCI. Garduño-Vieyra et al[19] also reported excellent outcome in a patient with *Acanthamoeba* keratitis three weeks following PCTCI treatment. These facts may corroborate the lack of direct correlation between *in vitro* sensitivity tests and clinical efficacy, which is not uncommon in clinical practice.

Antiviral Effect

In 1960, it was found that riboflavin exposed to UV light can inactivate the RNA of some viruses.[3] More recently, more studies suggest that this is feasible using a similar principle.[20,21]

Antifungal Effect

Sauer et al[22] evaluated the antimicrobial properties of riboflavin/UVA, with or without previous treatment with amphotericin B, on three groups of fungi selected from severe cases of keratomycosis: *Candida albicans*, *Fusarium* species and *Aspergillus fumigatus*. They were tested by using Kirby-Bauer disks and measurement of mean growth inhibition zone according to sensitivity tests proposed originally by Martins et al[5] Amphotericin with PCTCI was effective in increasing the growth inhibition zone of *Candida albicans*, *Aspergillus fumigatus* and *Fusarium* species, which ultimately represents more efficacy than either treatment alone. In an earlier study riboflavin/UVA was ineffective on *Candida albicans*.[5] Galperin et al[23] evaluated the efficacy of riboflavin/UVA CXL as a simple therapy in *Fusarium* keratitis in rabbits. The study found that treatment was effective in decreasing the intensity and severity of infections, but this treatment alone is not a suitable cure for fungal keratitis. They proposed a combined treatment of PCTCI with standard antifungals as a better approach to treat these cases.

Despite these promising results, studies are limited in terms of case numbers, and further investigations are needed before PCTCI can be incorporated into routine clinical practice for the treatment of infectious keratitis.

MICROBIAL KERATITIS FOLLOWING CXL

CXL using riboflavin–UVA is a minimally invasive method but traditionally requires epithelial removal for surgery and corneal stroma exposure for 30 minutes of irradiation. The epithelial defect usually takes from 2-5 days to heal completely. The compromised corneal epithelial integrity caused by the surgical procedure, along with possibly reduced immunity status caused by depletion of defensive cells by the treatment itself are probably predisposing factor to develop keratitis.

Bacterial Keratitis

Pérez-Santonja et al[24] reported the first case of keratitis following CXL. In his case, *Staphylococcus epidermidis* was isolated two days following uneventful procedure. The patient was treated successfully with ofloxacin 0.3 percent and topical fortified tobramycin. Final examination revealed a mild residual haze in the mid-peripheral cornea. Pollhammer et al[25] reported a case of bacterial *Escherichia coli* keratitis three days after corneal CXL for keratoconus (KC). The case was successfully treated with fortified tobramycin and cephazolin eye drops for several weeks leading to permanent reduction of the visual acuity. Zamora et al[26] reported a case of polymicrobial keratitis caused by *Streptococcus salivarius*, *Streptococcus oralis*, and coagulase-negative *Staphylococcus* species three days after CXL for KC. The patient was successfully treated with fortified cephalotin 5 percent and gentamicin 0.9 percent. Patient ended with residual central corneal stromal haze and subepithelial scar in ring-like configuration. In this case the triggering factor was removing the bandage contact lens and cleaning it by mouth before reapplying it in the eye. *Pseudomonas aeruginosa* has been reported by Sharma et al[27] one day after CXL. Following treatment, the infiltrates decreased in size and the hypopyon gradually disappeared, leaving a leucomatous corneal opacification.

Amoebic Keratitis

Rama et al[28] reported *Acanthamoeba* keratitis resulting in perforation 5 days following CXL for KC. The patient was unaware that he was wearing a bandage contact lens and repeatedly rinsed his face and eyelids with tap water. A large therapeutic keratoplasty was performed.

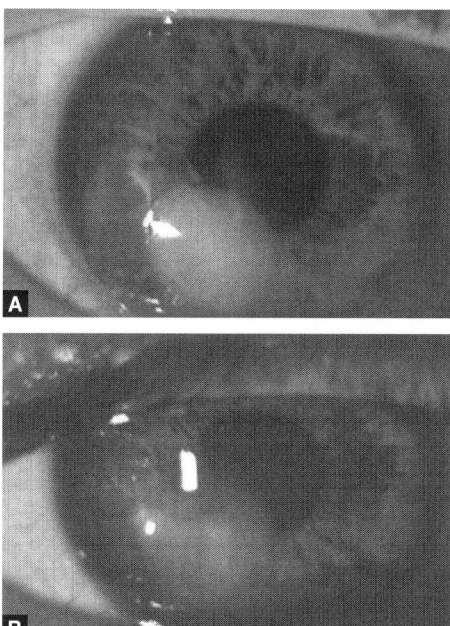

Figs 68.4A and B: Culture-proven *Acanthamoeba* keratitis. (A) Prior PCTCI treatment after two-month therapy with Brolene, PHMB and chlorhexidine with no improvement; (B) Two-month after two PCTCI applications, epithelial defect healed and BCVA is 20/25

Viral Keratitis

Ultraviolet A light was suggested as a potent stimulus to trigger reactivation of latent herpes simplex virus infections. Kymionis et al[29] reported a case of herpes keratitis with iritis five days following CXL. Diagnosis was confirmed with analysis of tear samples by polymerase chain reaction. Oral steroids and acyclovir were employed in the treatment. No evidence of herpetic disease recurrence was noted. This patient ended with mild paracentral corneal subepithelial opacity. Yuksel et al[30] reported a case of herpetic keratitis in a patient without a prior history of herpetic eye disease or cold sores. The diagnosis was confirmed with polymerase chain reaction analysis of the corneal swab for herpes simplex. He suggested that herpetic keratitis can be induced by CXL even in patients with no history of previous herpetic eye disease.

Fungal Keratitis

A single case report of *Fusarium solani* keratitis three weeks following corneal cross-linking was reported.[31] Following treatment with topical antifungal medications, the patient ended with large central leucoma with poor visual acuity.

Microbial keratitis following CXL is a potential source of permanent visual loss. It is important to mention that these patients may be locally immunosuppressed due to the effects of the procedure itself. We believe that broad-spectrum antibiotic therapy should be initiated after CXL until complete re-epithelialization is achieved, in order to prevent the occurrence of these infections. Once these infectious processes are in place, diagnosis and proper treatment are essential for a favorable outcome. Techniques adjustment to avoid epithelium debridement and therefore the need for a bandage contact lens may eliminate risk factors for infection.

MICROBIAL KERATITIS FOLLOWING OTHER PDT APPROACHES

Photodynamic therapy with a photosensitizer can produce microvascular thrombosis, leading to selective occlusion of neovascular vessels. Among several photosensitizers, verteporfin has been widely used to treat many chorioretinal diseases.[32,33] Currently it has been proven to be safe and effective in the treatment of corneal neovascularization in humans as well as animal models.[34-36]

There is very minimal in the literature on occurrence of microbial keratitis following PDT. A case of recurrent of herpes simplex keratitis three days after verteporfin PDT for corneal neovascularization was reported.[37]

ANTIMICROBIAL EFFECT OF OTHER PDT APPROACHES

Antibacterial Effect

In the 1990s, it was observed that there was a fundamental difference in susceptibility to PDT between gram-positive and gram-negative bacteria. It was found that, in general, neutral or anionic photosensitizers molecules are efficiently bound to and photodynamically inactivate gram-positive bacteria, whereas they are bound only to the outer membrane of gram-negative bacterial cells, but do not inactivate them after illumination.[38] The high susceptibility of gram-positive species is explained by their physiology, as their cytoplasmic membrane is surrounded by a relatively porous layer of peptidoglycan and lipoteichoic acid that allows photosensitizers to cross.[38] The cell envelope of gram-negative bacteria consists of an inner cytoplasmic membrane and an outer membrane that are separated by the peptidoglycan-containing periplasm. The outer membrane forms a physical and functional barrier between the cell and its environment. There are two basic mechanisms that have been proposed to account for the lethal damage caused to bacteria by PDT: (i) DNA damage and (ii) damage to the cytoplasmic membrane, allowing leakage of cellular contents or inactivation of membrane transport systems and enzymes.[39]

Several bacteria were inactivated successfully *in vitro*. These include: *Staphylococcus* bacteriophages,[40] *Bacillus* Spores,[41] *Escherichia coli*,[42] *Staphylococcus aureus*,[42] *Mycobacterium bovis*,[43] *Mycobacterium marinum* infection[44] and MRSA.[45] Non-tuberculous mycobacterial were tested both *in vitro* and *in vivo*.[46] PDT was found effective against *Mycobacterium fortuitum*.

Antiamoebic Effect

Ferro et al[47] reported the effect of PDT with a tetracationic Zn(II)-phthalocyanine (RLR068) on *Acanthamoeba*. After incubation with 5 mmol/l of RLP068, followed by exposure to light for 20 min at a fluence rate of 50 mW/cm^2, the cysts lost their excystment ability up to day 10 and were clearly damaged when observed under an interference contrast microscope.

Chen et al[48] evaluate the effectiveness of Hypocrellins B PDT on *Acanthamoeba* trophozoites and cysts, and its cytotoxic potential on the corneal epithelial cells and stromal cells *in vitro*. Hypocrellins B PDT had amoebacidal properties and showed a better effectiveness on the trophozoites than the cysts. On the other hand, Hypocrellins B PDT demonstrated cytotoxicity on the corneal epithelial and stromal cells.

Antiviral Effect

Experimental keratitis produced in rabbits by infection with herpesvirus isolated from a human periorbital lesion was treated with proflavine and light. The herpetic keratitis could be rapidly resolved by the dye-light treatment, whereas improvement was not seen in untreated rabbits.[49] Another experimental model of primary ocular infection with herpesvirus, we found that proflavine and light had a significant effect in suppressing herpetic disease of the cornea and that the effect was similar to that-produced with idoxuridine given four times daily.[50]

O'Day et al[51] used the photodynamic inactivation technique with proflavine as the photoactive dye to treat herpetic epithelial keratitis in a preliminary study of patients who had idoxuridine toxicity or resistance. A comparative study with idoxuridine in treating dendritic ulcerations of the cornea showed a good therapeutic effect. But the investigation was suspended when adverse reactions, consisting of a generalized epithelial keratitis and an anterior uveitis, possibly of phototoxic origin, developed in a few patients receiving treatment.

Myers et al[52] evaluated photodynamic inactivation in recurrent infections with herpes simplex virus. Neutral red (a heterotricyclic dye) and light was evaluated in a placebo-controlled study of 170 episodes of recurrent infection with herpes simplex virus in 96 patients. The technique inactivated herpes simplex virus *in vitro*. However, no beneficial effect, either on the rate of resolution of herpetic lesions or on the interval to subsequent recurrences, was observed in treated patients.

Antifungal Effect

Candida albicans has been inactivated by the photosensitizers Photofrin (Porfirmer sodium), Rose Bengal, and Al(III)-tetrasulphonted phthalocyanine. It is most efficiently destroyed by cationic photosensitizer, including, Methylene blue, when efflux pumps of *C. albicans* are blocked.[53,54] No *in vivo* studies related to treatment of fugal keratitis with PDT are available.

CONCLUSION

Microbial keratitis is a source of potential failure following CXL leading to devastating visual outcomes. On the other hand, PCTCI is emerging as an answer for resistant cases of microbial keratitis. It is important to understand the pathophysiology of these new therapeutic modalities for the eye, to prevent corneal infections in the case of CXL, and to potentially treat infections in case of PCTCI. Wise selection of patients is important in achieving good results. Further clinical trials are required to set guidelines for a more effective treatment using these exciting novel treatment strategies.

REFERENCES

1. Hamblin MR, Hasan T. Photodynamic therapy: a new antimicrobial approach to infectious disease? Photochem Photobiol Sci 2004;3(5):436-50. Epub 2004 Feb 12.
2. Huang L, Dai T, Hamblin MR. Antimicrobial photodynamic inactivation and photodynamic therapy for infections. Methods Mol Biol 2010;635:155-73.
3. Tsugita A, Okada Y, Uehara K. Photosensitized inactivation of ribonucleic acids in the presence of riboflavin. Biochim Biophys Acta 1965;103:360-63.
4. Spoerl E, Wollensak G, Seiler T. Increased resistance of crosslinked cornea against enzymatic digestion. Curr Eye Res 2004;29:35-40.
5. Martins SA, Combs JC, Noguera G, Camacho W, Wittmann P, Walther R, Cano M, Dick J, Behrens A. Antimicrobial efficacy of riboflavin/UVA combination (365 nm) *in vitro* for bacterial and fungal isolates: a potential new treatment for infectious keratitis. Invest Ophthalmol Vis Sci 2008;49(8):3402-8. Epub 2008 Apr 11.
6. Schrier A, Greebel G, Attia H, et al. *In vitro* antimicrobial efficacy of riboflavin and ultraviolet light on *Staphylococcus aureus*, methicillin-resistant *Staphylococcus aureus*, and *Pseudomonas aeruginosa*. J Refract Surg 2009;25: S799-S802.
7. Makdoumi K, Bäckman A, Mortensen J, Crafoord S. Evaluation of antibacterial efficacy of photo-activated riboflavin using ultraviolet light (UVA). Graefes Arch Clin Exp Ophthalmol 2010; 248:207-12.
8. Khan YA, Martins SA, Camacho W, Castro-Combs J, Wittmann P, Walther R, Dick J, Behrens A. Riboflavin/UVA Combined Treatment in a Rabbit *Staphylococcus aureus* Keratitis Model: A New Approach for Corneal Infections. Invest Ophthalmol Vis Sci 2008;49:E-Abstract 5535.
9. Makdoumi K, Mortensen J, Crafoord S. Infectious keratitis treated with corneal crosslinking. Cornea 2010;29:1353-8.

10. Makdoumi K, Mortensen J, Sorkhabi O, Malmvall BE, Crafoord S. UVA-riboflavin photochemical therapy of bacterial keratitis: a pilot study. Graefes Arch Clin Exp Ophthalmol 2012;250(1):95-102. Epub 2011 Aug 27.
11. Iseli HP, Thiel AM, Hafezi F, et al. Ultraviolet A/riboflavin corneal cross-linking for infectious keratitis associated with corneal melts. Cornea 2008;27(5): 590-4.
12. Kymionis GD, Kankariya VP, Kontadakis GA. Combined treatment with flap amputation, phototherapeutic keratectomy, and collagen crosslinking in severe intractable post-LASIK atypical mycobacterial infection with corneal melt. J Cataract Refract Surg 2012;38(4):713-5. Epub 2012 Feb 23.
13. Micelli Ferrari T, Leozappa M, Lorusso M, Epifani E, Micelli Ferrari L. *Escherichia coli* keratitis treated with ultraviolet A/riboflavin corneal cross-linking: a case report. Eur J Ophthalmol 2009;19(2):295-7.
14. Kozobolis V, Labiris G, Gkika M, Sideroudi H, Kaloghianni E, Papadopoulou D, Toufexis G. UV-A Collagen Cross-Linking Treatment of Bullous Keratopathy Combined With Corneal Ulcer. Cornea 2010;29(2):235-8.
15. del Buey MA, Cristóbal JA, Casas P, Goñi P, Clavel A, Mínguez E, Lanchares E, García A, Calvo B. Evaluation of *in vitro* efficacy of combined riboflavin and ultraviolet a for *Acanthamoeba* isolates. Am J Ophthalmol 2012;153(3):399-404. Epub 2011 Oct 11.
16. Kashiwabuchi RT, Carvalho FR, Khan YA, de Freitas D, Foronda AS, Hirai FE, Campos MS, McDonnell PJ. Assessing efficacy of combined riboflavin and UV-A light (365 nm) treatment of *Acanthamoeba* trophozoites. Invest Ophthalmol Vis Sci 2011;52(13):9333-8. Print 2011.
17. Berra M, Galperín G, Boscaro G, Zarate J, Tau J, Chiaradia P, Berra A. Treatment of *Acanthamoeba* Keratitis by Corneal Cross-linking. Cornea 2012 Aug 27. [Epub ahead of print].
18. Khan YA, Kashiwabuchi RT, Martins SA, Castro-Combs JM, Kalyani S, Stanley P, Flikier D, Behrens A. Riboflavin and ultraviolet light a therapy as an adjuvant treatment for medically refractive *Acanthamoeba* keratitis: report of 3 cases. Ophthalmology 2011; 118(2):324-31. Epub 2010 Sep 29.
19. Garduño-Vieyra L, Gonzalez-Sanchez CR, Hernandez-Da Mota SE. Ultraviolet-a light and riboflavin therapy for *Acanthamoeba* keratitis: a case report. Case Report Ophthalmol 2011;2(2):291-5. Epub 2011 Aug 31.
20. Vanlandingham DL, Keil SD, Horne KM, Pyles R, Goodrich RP, Higgs S. Photochemical inactivation of chikungunya virus in plasma and platelets using the Mirasol pathogen reduction technology system. Transfusion. 2012 May 25. doi:10.1111/j.1537-2995.2012.03717.x. [Epub ahead of print]
21. Ruane PH, Edrich R, Gampp D, Keil SD, Leonard RL, Goodrich RP. Photochemical inactivation of selected viruses and bacteria in platelet concentrates using riboflavin and light. Transfusion 2004;44(6):877-85.
22. Sauer A, Letscher-Bru V, Speeg-Schatz C, Touboul D, Colin J, Candolfi E, Bourcier T. *In vitro* efficacy of antifungal treatment using riboflavin/UV-A (365 nm) combination and amphotericin B. Invest Ophthalmol Vis Sci 2010;51(8):3950-3. Epub 2010 Mar 24.

23. Galperin G, Berra M, Tau J, Boscaro G, Zarate J, Berra A. Treatment of fungal keratitis from *Fusarium* infection by corneal cross-linking. Cornea 2012;31(2):176-80.
24. Pe´rez-Santonja JJ, Artola A, Javaloy J, Alio´ JL, Abad JL. Microbial keratitis after corneal collagen crosslinking. J Cataract Refract Surg 2009;35:1138-40.
25. Pollhammer M, Cursiefen C. Bacterial keratitis early after corneal crosslinking with riboflavin and ultraviolet-A. J Cataract Refract Surg 2009;35:588-9.
26. Zamora KV, Males JJ. Polymicrobial keratitis after a collagen cross-linking procedure with postoperative use of a contact lens: a case report. Cornea 2009;28:474-6.
27. Sharma N, Maharana P, Singh G, Titiyal JS. *Pseudomonas* keratitis after collagen crosslinking for keratoconus: case report and review of literature. J Cataract Refract Surg 2010;36(3):517-20.
28. Rama P, DiMatteo F, Matuska S, Paganoni G, Spinelli A. *Acanthamoeba* keratitis with perforation after corneal crosslinking and bandage contact lens use. J Cataract Refract Surg 2009;35:788-91.
29. Kymionis GD, Portaliou DM, Bouzoukis DI, Suh LH, Pallikaris AI, Markomanolakis M, Yoo SH. Herpetic keratitis with iritis after corneal crosslinking with riboflavin and ultraviolet A for keratoconus. J Cataract Refract Surg 2007;33:1982-4.
30. Yuksel N, Bilgihan K, Hondur AM. Herpetic keratitis after corneal collagen cross-linking with riboflavin and ultraviolet-A for progressive keratoconus. Int Ophthalmol 2011;31(6):513-5. Epub 2011 Dec 3.
31. Garcia-Delpech S, Díaz-Llopis M, Udaondo P, Salom D. *Fusarium* keratitis 3 weeks after healed corneal cross-linking. J Refract Surg 2010;26(12):994-5. doi: 10.3928/1081597X-20100804-02. Epub 2010 Aug 16.
32. Blinder KJ, Bradley S, Bressler NM, et al. Treatment of Age-related Macular Degeneration with Photodynamic Therapy study group; Verteporfin in Photodynamic Therapy study group. Effect of lesion size, visual acuity, and lesion composition on visual acuity change with and without verteporfin therapy for choroidal neovascularization secondary to age-related macular degeneration: TAP and VIP report no. 1. Am J Ophthalmol 2003; 136:407-18.
33. Blinder KJ, Blumenkranz MS, Bressler NM, et al. Verteporfin therapy of subfoveal choroidal neovascularization in pathologic myopia: 2-year results of a randomized clinical trial—VIP report no. 3. Ophthalmology 2003;110:667-73.
34. Yoon KC, Ahn KY, Lee SE, et al. Experimental inhibition of corneal neovascularization by photodynamic therapy with verteporfin. Curr Eye Res 2006;31:215-24.
35. Fossarello M, Peiretti E, Zucca I, et al. Photodynamic therapy of corneal neovascularization with verteporfin. Cornea 2003;22:485-8.
36. Yoon KC, You IC, Kang IS, et al. Photodynamic therapy with verteporfin for corneal neovascularization. Am J Ophthalmol 2007;144:390-95.
37. Yoon KC, Im SK, Park HY. Recurrent herpes simplex keratitis after verteporfin photodynamic therapy for corneal neovascularization. Cornea 2010;29(4):465-7.

38. Malik Z, Ladan H, Nitzan Y. Photodynamic inactivation of Gram-negative bacteria: problems and possible solutions. J Photochem Photobiol B 1992;14:262-6.
39. Hamblin MR, Hasan T. Photodynamic therapy: a new antimicrobial approach to infectious disease? Photochem Photobiol Sci 2004;3(5):436-50. Epub 2004 Feb 12.
40. Schultz EW, Krueger AP. Inactivation of *Staphylococcus* bacteriophage by methylene blue. Proc Soc Exp Biol Med 1928;26:100-1.
41. Demidova TN, Hamblin MR. Photodynamic inactivation of *Bacillus* spores mediated by phenothiazinium dyes. Appl Environ Microbiol 2005;71:6918-25.
42. Phoenix DA, Sayed Z, Hussain S, Harris F, Wainwright M. The phototoxicity of phenothiazinium derivatives against *Escherichia coli* and *Staphylococcus aureus*. FEMS Immunol Med Microbiol 2003;39(1):17-22.
43. O'Riordan K, Sharlin DS, Gross J, et al. Photoinactivation of mycobacterial *in vitro* and in a new murine model of localized *Mycobacterium bovis* BCG-induced granulomatous infection. Antimicrob Agents Chemother 2006;50:1828-34.
44. Wiegell SR, Kongshoj B, Wulf HC. *Mycobacterium marinum* infection cured by photodynamic therapy. Arch Dermatol 2006; 142:1241-2.
45. Tang HM, Hamblin MR, Yow CM. A comparative *in vitro* photoinactivation study of clinical isolates of multidrug-resistant pathogens. J Infect Chemother 2007;13(2):87-91. Epub 2007 May 8.
46. Shih MH, Huang FC. Effects of photodynamic therapy on rapidly growing nontuberculous mycobacteria keratitis. Invest Ophthalmol Vis Sci 2011;52(1):223-9. Print 2011 Jan.
47. Ferro S, Coppellotti O, Roncucci G, Ben Amor T, Jori G. Photosensitized inactivation of *Acanthamoeba* palestinensis in the cystic stage. J Appl Microbiol 2006;101(1):206-12.
48. Chen Z, Xuguang S, Zhiqun W, Ran L. *In vitro* amoebacidal activity of photodynamic therapy on *Acanthamoeba*. Br J Ophthalmol 2008;92(9):1283-6.
49. Conard Moore, Craig Wallis, Joseph L. Melnick, and Michael D. Kuns Photodynamic Treatment of Herpes Keratitis Infect Immun 1972;5(2):169-71.
50. Jeffrey D Lanier, John P Whitcher, Chandler R Dawson, Jang O. Oh Proflavine and Light in the Treatment of Experimental Herpetic Ocular Infections. Antimicrob Agents Chemother 1974;6(5):613-9.
51. O'Day DM, Jones BR, Poirier R, Pilley S, Chisholm I, Steele A, Rice NS. Proflavine photodynamic viral inactivation in herpes simplex keratitis. Am J Ophthalmol 1975;79(6):941-8.
52. Myers MG, Oxman MN, Clark JE, Arndt KA. Photodynamic inactivation in recurrent infections with herpes simplex virus. J Infect Dis 1976;133 Suppl:A145-50.
53. Bliss JM, Bigelow CE, Foster TH, Haidaris CG. Susceptibility of *Candida* species to photodynamic effects of photofrin. Antimicrob Agents Chemother 2004;48: 2000-6.
54. Lazarova G. Effect of glutathione on rose bengal photosensitized yeast damage. Microbios 1993;75: 39-43.

Recent and Future Drugs in Ophthalmology

Roberto Bellucci, Carlo Bellucci (Italy)

INTRODUCTION

The current status of ocular pharmacology and therapeutics is satisfying as for many aspects. We can prevent and treat many diseases, obtaining full restoration of both anatomy and function in most eyes. We reduced postoperative endophthalmitis rate to a minimum by intraocular application of antibiotics, and found drugs to improve macular degeneration. We can preserve vision in glaucoma by hypotensive medications, and shorten the course of uveitis eventually restoring vision. However, the percentage of patients is still high, requiring better care than that available either to heal from currently untreatable diseases or to shorten the healing process of treatable diseases. For these reasons the research in experimental and clinical therapeutics in ophthalmology is very active, and any update will face a huge amount of new material.

RECENT AND EMERGING DRUGS

Every area of ophthalmic diseases is interested in new drugs/treatment modalities. However, research on antibiotics is somewhat pausing at the moment, as we are still satisfied with existing drugs. Currently, the main interest is in anti-VEGF drugs, in glaucoma medications, in anti-inflammatory agents, and in agents for vitreous liquefaction. As anti-VEGF drugs are:

Future Drugs for Glaucoma Treatment

Glaucoma is an optic nerve disease where therapy aims at reducing intraocular pressure (IOP), that is considered to be the main risk factor. There are several categories of antiglaucoma drugs: Alpha-adrenergic agonists (e.g. brimonidine), beta-adrenergic blockers (e.g. timolol), carbonic anidrase inhibitors (e.g. dorzolamide), cholinergic agonists (e.g. pilocarpine), and prostaglandin analogs (e.g. latanoprost).

At the moment, there is only one beta-blocker under investigation, but acting in a different way than existing beta-blockers. The company Sylentis is proposing an agent capable of interfering with RNA potentially reducing IOP through knockdown of beta-adrenergic receptors. The name of the compound is SYL 040012, and is currently in phase II investigational trial.[1]

A few prostaglandin-analog drugs are under investigations from different companies, but so far the research for a better and safer drug that those currently available was not successful. One of these new drugs, taprenepag, is being developed by the very Pfizer company that commercializes latanoprost.[2]

The importance of melatonin analogs is enphasized by Crooke (Crooke). Melatonin is a hormone incretvd in the blood mainly by the pineal gland, allowing the entrainment of circadian rhythm of several biological functions. Melatonin and its analogs reduce IOP in animals and humans, also exerting neuroprotective activity and, therefore, proposing as a candidate for glaucoma treatment.[3]

Other novel compounds evaluated in clinical trials include an actin polymerization inhibitor, Ras homolog associated protein kinase inhibitors, adenosine receptor agonists, cannabinoid receptor agonists, and a serotonin receptor agonist.[1] However, the initial data about penetration and efficacy indicate that these compounds still need refinement to compare favorably with existing drugs. Therefore, in the near future glaucoma therapy may take advantage from new methods of delivery existing drugs rather than from new drugs.

Emerging Drugs for Uveitis

After 60 years, corticosteroids remain the milestone for the treatment of uveitis. New drugs in this field are new formulations of steroids, designed for intraocular use. Both Retisert (Bausch & Lomb, Rochester, NY, USA) and Ozurdex (Allergan, Irvine, CA, USA) are steroid implants designed for intravitreal use, that have been extensively studied and that are available in most of the world. Their efficacy has been proven several times, however with the side effects of cataract formation and of IOP rise. In addition, the risks of intravitreal injections must be considered.[4]

Other drugs used in uveitis therapy are antimetabolites (methotrexate, azathioprine, and mycophenolate mofetil), T-cell inhibitors (cyclosporine, tacrolimus, and sirolimus), alkylating agents (cyclophosphamide and chlorambucyl). While these drugs are well known and probably familiar to most ophthalmologists, biologic agents have been introduced more recently and warrant some discussion.

Biologic agents are a class of drugs that have been designed following better understanding of the immune system. In inflammatory disease, and in uveitis as well, a key role is played by tumor necrosis factor alpha (TNF-α), a proinflammatory cytokine. TNF-α inhibitors are a class of compounds that show anti-inflammatory properties. Infliximab and adalimumab are monoclonal antibodies available for systemic usage, that have been found more active than cyclosporine in the treatment of Bechet's disease.[5-8] Adalimumab is fully humanized, then probably more tolerated. It has been used in children to control anterior uveitis associated or not to juvenile rheumatoid arthritis. Another TNF-α inhibitor, etanercept, seems to be less active on ocular inflammation.[9]

Other drugs used in uveitis are cytokine receptor antibodies, already used for systemic diseases like tumors, multiple sclerosis, and immune disorders. Rituximab is a chimeric monoclonal antibody against CD20, a B cell marker, which result in depletion of B cells.[4] Rituximab has been used successfully to treat Wegener's granulomatosis,[10] and retinal vasculitis associate with Bechet's disease.[11]

Vitreous and Ocriplasmin

Ocriplasmin (also known as microplasmin) is the truncated form of human plasmin with retained protease activity (Fig. 69.1). It is a recombinant protein, developed because the isolation of plasmin from patients' blood requires a considerable amount of time and is therefore impractical. The rationale of ocriplasmin use in ophthalmology is the achievement of vitreous detachment from the retina and/or vitreous liquefaction, to facilitate the subsequent vitreoretinal surgery.

Ocriplasmin was first employed in experimental setting about 15 years ago,[12] and it was thoroughly studied thereafter,[13-18] but only recently its use reached the clinical level. The first study published in 2009 enrolled sixty patients, and pointed out some advantages and some disadvantages of the treatment.[19] The intravitreal optimal dosage of 125 mg was set following a second study published in 2010,[20] and confirmed subsequently.[19] In addition, it was demonstrated the advantage of repeating injections, that led to a higher percentage of eyes with detached vitreous.[21]

Recently, the results of a multicenter controlled trial enrolling 652 eyes have been published.

A number of 464 patients with vitreomacular adhesion received 125 mg of ocriplasmin, and 188 patients received placebo.[22] Following the injection, the vitreomacular adhesion

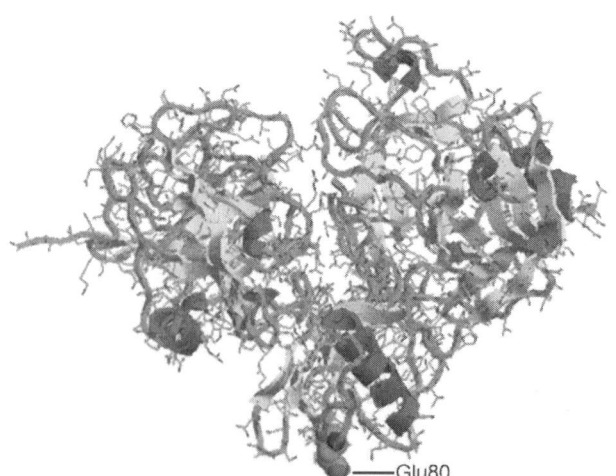

Fig. 69.1: Proposed structure for microplasmin-glu80

resolved in 26.5 percent of ocriplasmin eyes, and in 10.1 percent of placebo eyes. Total posterior vitreous detachment was found in 13.4 percent of ocriplasmin eyes, and in 3.7 percent of the placebo eyes. The most important finding of this study was the nonsurgical resolution of the macular hole in 40.6 percent of ocriplasmin eyes, and in 10.6 percent of the placebo eyes. All the differences were highly significant at statistical analysis. However, minor adverse events were also more frequent with ocriplasmin (68.4 vs 53.5%), while serious adverse events were similar in the two groups. According to these results, ocriplasmin appears to be the most important new drug of this period, a potent toll once available for clinical use. The possibility to completely avoid surgery is of great interest for all the patients with vitreomacular disease, and especially those with high myopia.

NEW DRUG DELIVERY IN OPHTHALMOLOGY

There is no doubt that drug delivery is going to change in the near future, and that new methods especially related with nanotechnology and nanoparticles will become popular. These modalities will in turn change the way we are treating ophthalmic diseases, proposing new strategies with current treated morbidities, and enlarging the area of treatable morbidities, gradually transitioning from simple eye-drop applications to more complex yet quicker procedures. As a consequence, a part of the new drugs will be studied not only (or not at all) as aqueous solutions, but they will be designed for different administration routes. Anti-VEGF drugs are probably among the first and best examples of this approach. Intravitreal injections, that were anecdotical only 10 years ago, are now popular all over the world. This chapter will focus on some aspects of drug delivery, and on a few drugs that appear promising for large clinical application in the near future.

Ophthalmic drug delivery must overcome the natural defences of the eye, also known as "barriers". Anatomical barriers include the different layers of the cornea, sclera and retina, as well as the blood/aqueous barrier and the blood/retinal barrier. Functional barriers are those related with flow removal of therapeutic agents by tear film, by lymphatic clearance, by blood flow.[23] In addition, many drugs bind to melanin and may therefore be less bio-available inside the eye.[24-27] Finally, drug clearance and degradation after penetration takes place as usually, and even at higher rate for selected ocular structures.

Traditionally, drug delivery has been based on several routes of administration. Ophthalmic routes include eye drops application, subconjunctival and sub-Tenon injections, retrobulbar and juxtascleral injections, and intracameral and intravitreal injections. General routes include oral and parenteral administration, still used when the ratio between local activity and general toxicity and local activity is high. The drug visudyne is one excellent example of the parenteral administration route.

A few methods have recently being developed to increase drug penetration and availability inside the eye. The most accepted methods include: facilitating penetration through the identification of drug carriers or through iontophoresis; designing of specific drug formulations to take advantage of these processes; new drug preparation in colloidal forms like nanoparticles, liposomes and so on; new formulations like bioadhesive gels and fibrin sealant-based approach.[23]

BIOLOGICAL TRANSPORTERS AND PRODRUGS

Ocular bioavailability of current preparations depends on drug solubility and lipophilicity, however a transporter-targeted structure of the compound would be a better approach. Biological transporters are membrane-bound proteins that play an important role in active transportation of nutrients across biological membranes. They are present in various tissues of the human eye, some facilitating drug penetration (influx transporters), others promoting drug removal (efflux transporters). Influx transporters play a specific role when prodrugs are specifically designed to bind them and to form a substrate that easily penetrates biologic membranes being less affected by the efflux pump. Valacyclovir is one of the best examples of this approach, but several other prodrugs are available in ophthalmology. The NSAID agent nepafenac has little intrinsic activity, but as a prodrug of amfenac it penetrates the cornea at a high rate, to be metabolized to the more potent amfenac inside the eye.[28] Prodrugs developed with the purpose of targeting the influx transporters can significantly enhance the absorption of poorly permeating parent drugs, thus allowing either the increase of activity or the reduction of concentration. In addition, physicochemical properties of the drug such as solubility, stability and other properties of the parent drug can be improved.[23]

Amino acid and peptide transporters are the influx transporters of most interest in ophthalmology. They transport various amino acids and nutrients into ocular tissues, and therefore may have a definite role in ocular drug delivery if the drug is formulated to bind them. In addition, the drug may be designed as a prodrug to increase both ocular absorption and bioavailability after the required change in chemical structure that takes place in ocular tissues.

A recent example of prodrug employment in ocular therapeutics is Hexadecyloxypropyl-cyclic Cidofovir (HDP-cCDV). HDP-CDV is a prodrug for cidofovir (CDV), an antiviral agent especially useful against human cytomegalovirus resistant to Ganciclovir. Like Ganciclovir, Cidofovir can be injected into the vitreous cavity of affected eyes, but the necessity of repeated injections threatens the advantages of the drug, as hemorrhages and infection can happen following the injection. For this reason HDP-CDV has been developed. Once injected into the vitreous cavity, the prodrug form a depot within the vitreous, from which it can migrate into the retina where the prodrug HDP-cCDV is converted into the active form through phospholipase C cleavage of HDP and hydrolysis of the cCDV to CDV.[29] However, the HDP-cCDV may also be hydrolyzed to HDP-CDV within the vitreous, and assume the form of micelles, that are then transported into the retinal cells to be further metabolized to release the active drug. The paper of Wang demonstrated success in obtaining a new, active and long-lasting drug against cytomegalovirus, however indicating how complex the matter is when intraocular pharmacokinetics is studied at the molecular level.[29]

COLLOIDAL CARRIERS AND NANOPARTICLES

The combination of various molecules of the drug to form a supramolecular structure to increase efficacy has been widely studied in ophthalmology,[30] still its diffusion as a therapeutic tool remains low. These colloidal carrier preparations include micelles, liposomes, nanoparticles, micro- and macroemulsions and so on. They offer controlled and sustained release of the drug at the targeted site, prolonged activity with reduced number of administration, capability to pass ocular barriers, reduced removal from the activity site.[31] The interest in ophthalmology is to treat chronic conditions like glaucoma, uveitis, retinal edema, intraocular tumors, macular degeneration, and may be used to treat previously untreated conditions like retinitis pigmentosa or Stargardt's disease.[32]

The identification of the most effective delivery system for each ocular disease, pathology and drug is a difficult task that depends in part on the molecular properties of the drug, both chemical and physical.

Micelles

Micelles are self-assembling nanosized colloidal particles with a hydrophobic core and a hydrophilic shell. They are used as pharmaceutical carriers for drugs that are insoluble in water, and are especially useful for corneal penetration. Being more nature-driven that artificially obtained, their stability may depend on their polarity (Fig. 69.2).

Emulsions

Emulsions of oil in water are already used in ophthalmology, but an entire new category of well-tolerated emulsifiers like polysorbate-80 is becoming available. As aseptic processing has also improved recently, more emulsions will probably be studied in the near future.

Ion-activated Gel

Conventional eye drops bioavailability is poor due to the short contact time with the cornea. Ion-activated *in situ* gelling systems interact with cations present in the tear fluid, forming a gel on the ocular surface that results in prolonged contact time.[33] In an animal experiment employing miotic drugs, this delivery system increased by 2.5 times the area under the curve reporting miosis versus time, as compared with the aqueous solution.[34]

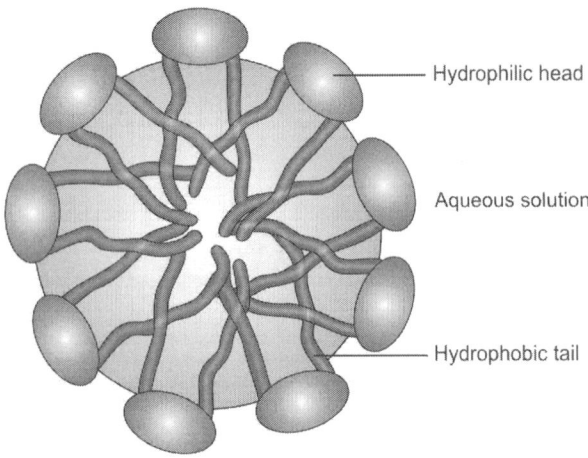

Fig. 69.2: Scheme of a micelle, with the hydrophobic parts of the molecules inside

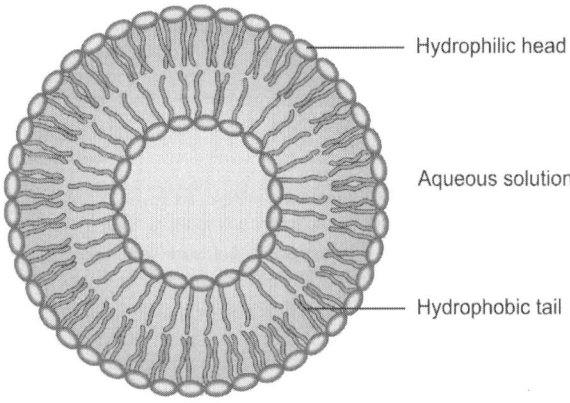

Fig. 69.3: Scheme of a liposome, with a cavity inside that can host drugs

Liposomes

Liposomes are vesicles consisting of one or more concentric phospholipid bilayers alternating aqueous or lipophilic compartments, with diameter ranging from 80 nm–10 μm (Fig. 69.3). They are biodegradable, allow sustained drug release and tend to remain at the site of administration.[35] Hydrophilic compounds can be encapsulated in the inner aqueous cavity, and lipophilic compounds can be incorporated in the membrane. Liposomes can also protect drug molecules from enzymes present on the corneal surface, thus increasing drug penetration up to 15 folds.[36] Liposomes have been extensively used in experimental settings to deliver cyclosporine, both as eyedrops and as subconjunctival injection.[37,38] Despite the claimed advantages, liposomal encapsulation is nor widely used in ophthalmology, maybe because of the high manufacturing cost.[37]

Liposomes can also be injected directly into the eye. Following intracameral injection they can be found in all the ocular tissues of the anterior and posterior segment, suggesting optimal penetration both into the retina and into the corneal epithelium.[35] To increase liposome stability in the vitreous, pegylation has been advocated, that is the conjugation of poly (ethylene glycol), but with some resulting toxicity in investigational studies.[39] At the moment, the most promising application of liposomes in ophthalmology is as a carrier for nucleic acid-based drugs for retinal therapy.

Nanoparticles

Nanoparticles are small solid colloid particles, usually artificially obtained, consisting of a polymer base (polymeric nanoparticles), a lipid base (solid lipid nanoparticles) or a peptide base (peptide nanoparticles) that encapsulate or condense with the drug of interest.[35] Their size varies from 1–1000 nm, therefore being much smaller than liposomes, and they are actually the smallest particles available (Figs 69.4A to D). Compared with micron-grade particles, nanoparticles have strong mobility because of their small size and can enter cells easily to accumulate at the lesion site.[40] In addition, nanoparticles are more stable under different temperature, pH and osmolarity conditions.[35]

They have been used also for gene therapy,[41-43] to alleviate oxidative stress for the retina, and to deliver growth factor to cells.[44]

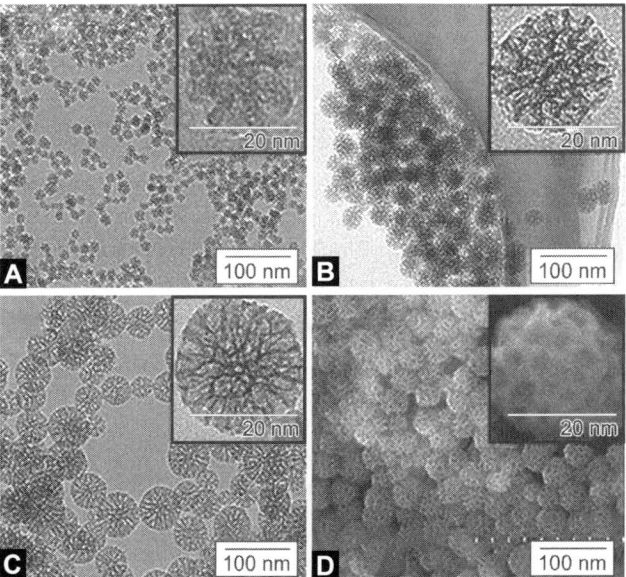

Figs 69.4A to D: Various types of nanoparticles

Recently, core-shell nanospheres loaded with ciprofloxacin were incorporated into a conventional, transparent contact lens to provide sustained and effective bactericidal activity up to 72 hours.[45]

The diffusion of nanoparticles within the ocular structures is size-depending. Following periocular administration, small 20 nm particles could cross the sclera, but were rapidly removed by blood flow, while 200 nm nanoparticles remained longer in the injection site, but could not cross the sclera.[46,47] For this reason nanoparticles are especially considered for intravitreal injection, with demonstrated retinal penetration with limited or no damage.[48] Implantable polymeric microspheres are usually based on two compounds: Chitosan (CH) and its oligomer CHO, and hyaluronan (HY).

Chitosan is a copolymer produced by removing an acetate moiety from chitin through hydration in concentrated alkali (Fig. 69.5). It is soluble in most diluted acids, and as a natural product shows good biocompatibility. It is not toxic for the human body, showing some positive properties.[49] Drugs carried by chitosan nanoparticles are released as chitosan is degraded and corroded, leading to a clear sustained-release effect. Tested drugs include a variety of agents, but timolol is one of the most interesting because its delivery through nanoparticles may manifold prolong its activity.[50] At the moment, several modifications of chitosan nanoparticles are under investigation, with the purpose of improving drug penetration and accuracy.

Hyaluronan is well known to ophthalmologists. It has been demonstrated that HY can be used to prepare nanoparticles, and that HY nanoparticles remain in tissues longer than CH nanoparticles.[51]

Dendrimers

Dendrimers are monodispersed symmetric macromolecules that host a central core with at least two functional groups, surrounded by a large number of active end groups.[52] They are globe or ellipsoid-shaped, resembling spheres with countless cavities that can host macromolecular therapeutic agents (Fig. 69.6). The diameter of dendrimers used in ophthalmology ranges from 1.5–100 nm. The surface functional groups determine dendrimer's physical properties, usually enhancing the solubility of poorly water soluble drugs by electrostatic interaction or covalent conjugation.[53]

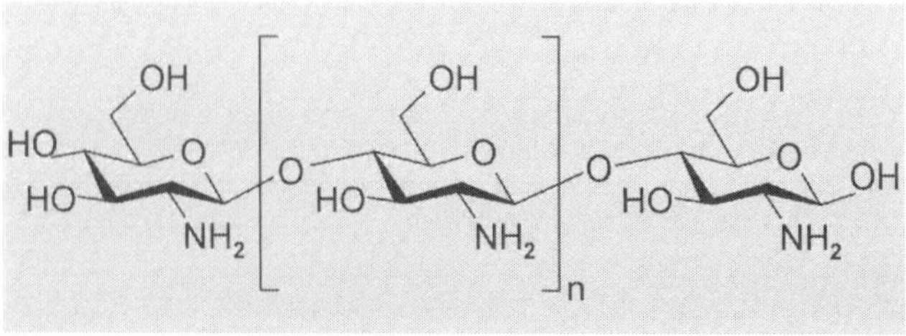

Fig. 69.5: Structure of chitosan

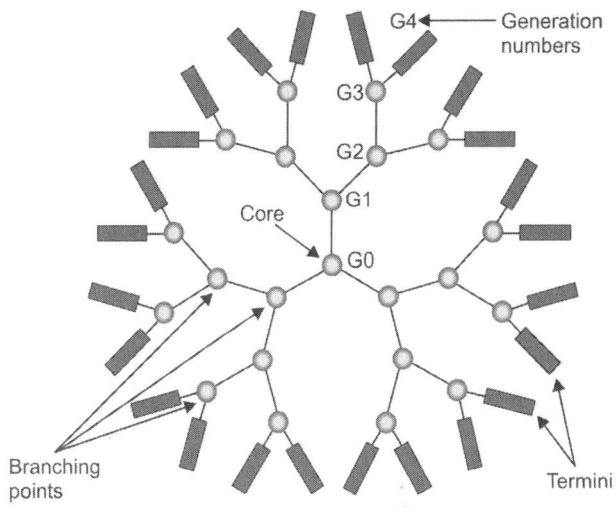

Fig. 69.6: Structure of dendrimers

Dendrimers are being extensively studied both for ocular therapy and for reconstructing pieces of ocular tissues, namely the cornea.[54]

Polyplexes

Polyplexes are complexes of cationic polymers and nucleic acid such as plasmid DNA. These particles are small (<8 nm) but have high vector capacity, and they are stable in nuclease-rich environment.[32] They have been used to deliver siRNA to decrease conjunctival inflammation and fibrosis.[55]

Vision Regeneration

Probably the most exciting application of nanoparticles is the attempt to restore vision in retinitis pigmentosa. Greenbaum and associates used proteoliposomes as vehicles to deliver photoactive transmembrane structures to mammalian cells.[56,57] By placing photosystem reaction centers close to voltage-gated ion channels, the light induced charge separation potential they generate can trigger a change in the membrane potential, thus generating a vision sensation. A series of studies are being carried out in this area, that may open the way to prostetic electrochemical vision.

CONCLUSION

Although the studies are promising, the clinical application of nanovectors in ophthalmology must face the difficulties related with particles penetration into the ocular structures. The ocular barriers required to protect the eye and maintain its function tend to block penetration of nanoparticles, suggesting different administration routes, namely intraocular injection.

In addition, targeting diseases like retinitis pigmentosa means facing the fate of nanoparticles inside the eye, sometimes desiring their disappearance sometimes looking for them to remain forever in the injection site. Following intravitreal injection of nanoparticles, and because of the negative charge of vitreal hyaluronan, positively charged molecules tend to aggregate within the vitreous humor, a problem partially solved through PEGylation.[58] However, internal limiting membrane limits retinal absorption, and high periocular concentrations of nanoparticles is required to reach the retina. To avoid removal by conjunctival and periocular vessels, a fibrin sealant containing the drug has been developed and successfully studied to deliver antibiotics, antitumoral agents, and insulin.[23]

Despite all these inconveniences, and although manufacturing cost and safety issues have not been properly addressed, nanotechnology and nanoparticles will play an increasing role in ocular therapeutics in the near future. While nanovectors are being studied for drug delivery, the development and selection of those capable of crossing the ocular barriers has not yet started.

REFERENCES

1. Chen J, Runyan S, Robinson R. Novel ocular antihypertensive compounds in clinical trials. Clin Ophthalmol 2011;5:667-77.
2. Shachar RA, Raber S, Courtney R, et al. Dose-escalating, double-masked, vehicle controlled trial of the IOP reducing effect of the EP agonist PF-04217329. Invest Ophthalmol Vis Sci 2010;51: ARVO abstract 175.
3. Crooke A, Colligris B, Pintor J. Update in glaucoma medicinal chemistry: Emerging evidence for the importance of melatonin analogues. Curr Med Chem 2012;19:3508-22.
4. Larson T, Nussenblatt RB, Sen HN. Emerging drugs for uveitis. Expert Opin Emerg Drugs 2011;16:309-22.
5. Ohno S, Nakamura S, Hori S, Shimakawa M, Kawashima H, Mochizuki M, et al. Efficacy, safety, and pharmacokinetics of multiple administration of infliximab in Behçet's disease with refractory uveoretinitis. J Rheumatol 2004;31:1362-8.
6. Yamada Y, Sugita S, Tanaka H, Kamoi K, Kawaguchi T, Mochizuki M. Comparison of infliximab versus ciclosporin during the initial 6-month treatment period in Behçet's. disease. Br J Ophthalmol 2010;94:284-8.
7. Jap A, Chee SP. Immunosuppressive therapy for ocular diseases. Curr Opin Ophthalmol. 2008;19:535-40.
8. Mushtaq B, Saeed T, Situnayake RD, Murray PI. Adalimumab for sight-threatening uveitis in Behçet's disease. Eye. 2007;21:824-5.
9. Tynjala P, Lindahl P, Honkanen V, Lahdenne P, Kotaniemi K. Infliximab and etanercept in the treatment of chronic uveitis associated with refractory juvenile idiopathic arthritis. Ann Rheum Dis. 2007;66:548-50.
10. Taylor SR, Salama AD, Joshi L, Pusey CD, Lightman SL. Rituximab is effective in the treatment of refractory ophthalmic Wegener's granulomatosis. Arthritis Rheum 2009;60:1540-47.
11. Sadreddini S, Noshad H, Molaeefard M, Noshad R. Treatment of retinal vasculitis in Behçet's disease with rituximab. Mod Rheumatol. 2008;18:306-8.

12. Sebag J. Pharmacological vitrelysis. Retina 1998;18:1-3.
13. Gandorfer A, Ulbig M, Kampik A. Plasmin-assisted vitrectomy eliminates cortical vitreous remnants. Eye 2002;16:95-7.
14. Gandorfer A, Rohleder M, Sethi C, et al. Posterior vitreous detachment induced by microplasmin. Invest Ophthalmol Vis Sci 2004;45:641-7.
15. Gandorfer A, Kampik A. Intrasurgical plasmin enzyme in diabetic macular edema. Am J Ophthalmol 2005;139:949.
16. Sakuma T, Tanaka M, Mizota A, et al. Safety of *in vivo* pharmacological vitreolysis with recombinant microplasmin in rabbit eyes. Invest Ophthalmol Vis Sci 2005;46:3295-9.
17. De Smet MD, Valmaggia C, Zarranz-Ventura J, Willekens B. Microplasmin: *in vivo* characterization of its activity in porcine vitreous. Invest Ophthalmol Vis Sci 2009;50:814-9.
18. Gandorfer A. Enzymatic vitreous disruption. Eye 2008;22:1273-7.
19. De Smet MD, Gandorfer A, Stalmans P, et al. Microplasmin intravitreal administration in patients with vitreomacular traction scheduled for vitrectomy: the MIVI I trial. Ophthalmology 2009;116:1349-55.
20. Benz MS, Packo KH, Gonzalez V, et al. A placebo-controlled trial of microplasmin intravitreous injection to facilitate posterior vitreous detachment before vitrectomy. Ophthalmology 2010; 117:791-7.
21. Stalmans P, Delaey C, de Smet MD, et al. Intravitreal injection of microplasmin for treatment of vitreomacular adhesion: Results of a prospective, randomized, sham-controlled phase II trial (the MIVI-IIT trial). Retina 2010;30:1122-7.
22. Stalmans P, Benz MS, Gandorfer A, et al. Enzymatic vitreolysis with ocriplasmin for vitreomacular traction and macular holes. N Engl J Med 2012;367:606-15.
23. Gaudana R, Ananthula HK, Parenky A, Mitra AK. Ocular drug delivery. AAPS J 2010;12:348-60.
24. Schoenwald RD, Tandon V, Wurster DE, Barfknecht CF. Significance of melanin binding and metabolism in the activity of 5-acetoxyacetylimino-4-methyl-delta2–1, 3, 4,-thiadiazolin e-2-sulfonamide. Eur J Pharm Biopharm 1998;46:39-50.
25. Larsson BS. Interaction between chemicals and melanin. Pigment Cell Res 1993;6:127–33.
26. Leblanc B, Jezequel S, Davies T, Hanton G, Taradach C. Binding of drugs to eye melanin is not predictive of ocular toxicity. Regul Toxicol Pharmacol 1998;28:124–32.
27. Pitkanen L, Ranta VP, Moilanen H, Urtti A. Binding of betaxolol, metoprolol and oligonucleotides to synthetic and bovine ocular melanin, and prediction of drug binding to melanin in human choroid-retinal pigment epithelium. Pharm Res 2007;24:2063-70.
28. Bucci FA Jr, Waterbury LD. Pharmacokinetics and pharmacodynamics of nepafenac, amfenac, ketorolac, and bromfenac. J Cataract Refract Surg 2008;34:1226.
29. Wang H, Chhablani J, Freeman WR, et al. Intraocular safety and pharmacokinetics of hexadecycloxypropyl-Cidofovir (HDP-CDV) as a long-lasting intravitreal antiviral drug. Invest Ophthalmol Vis Sci 2011;52:9391-6.
30. Gaudana R, Jwala J, Boddu SH, Mitra AK. Recent perspectives in ocular drug delivery. Pharm Res 2009;26:1197-1216.

31. Mainardes RM, Urban MC, Cinto PO, et al. Colloidal carriers for ophthalmic drug delivery. Curr Drug Targets 2005;6:363-71.
32. Zarbin MA, Montemagno C, Leary JF, Ritch R. Nanomedicine in ophthalmology: The new frontier. Am J Ophthalmol 2010;150: 144-62.
33. Rupenthal ID, Green CR, Alany RG. Comparison of ion-activated *in situ* gelling systems for ocular drug delivery. Part 1: physicochemical characterization and *in vitro* release. Int J Pharm 2011;411:69-77.
34. Rupenthal ID, Green CR, Alany RG. Comparison of ion-activated *in situ* gelling systems for ocular drug delivery. Part 2: Precorneal retention and *in vivo* pharmacodynamics study. Int J Pharm 2011;411:78-85.
35. Khar RK, Jaun GK, Warsi MH, et al. Nano-vectors for the ocular delivery of nucleic acid-based therapeutics. Indian J Pharm Sci 2010;72:675-88.
36. Masuda I, Matsuo T, Yasuda T, Matsuo N. Gene transfer with liposomes to the intraocular tissues by different routes of administration. Invest Ophthalmol Visual Sci 1996;37:1914–20.
37. Yavuz B, Pehlivan SB, Unlu N. An overview on dry eye treatment: Approaches for cyclosporin A delivery. Scientific World J. 2012: ID 1948;8:1-11.
38. Mosallaei N, Banaee T, Farzadnia M, et al. Safety evaluation of nanoliposomes containing cyclosporine A after ocular administration. Curr Eye Res 2012;37:453-6.
39. Bochot A, Couvreur P, Fattal E. Intravitreal administration of antisense oligonucleotides: Potential of liposomal delivery. Prog Retin Eye Res 2000;19:131-47.
40. Singh R, Lillard J Jr. Nanoparticle-based targeted drug delivery. Exp Mol Pathol 2009;86:215-23.
41. Naik R, Mukhopadhyay A, Ganguli M. Gene delivery to the retina: Focus on non-viral approaches. Drug Dis Today 2009;14:306-15.
42. Liu X, Rasmussen CA, Gabelt BT, Brandt CR, Kaufman PL. Gene Therapy Targeting Glaucoma: Where Are We? Surv Ophthalmol 2009;54:472-86.
43. Conley SM, Naash MI. Nanoparticles for retinal gene therapy. Prog Retin Eye Res 2010;29:376-97.
44. Chen Y, Moiseyev G, Takahashi Y, Ma JX. RPE65 gene delivery restores isomerohydrolase activity and prevents early cone loss in Rpe65-/- mice. Invest Ophthalmol Visual Sci 2006;47:1177-84.
45. Garwhal R, Shady SF, Ellis EJ, et al. Sustained ocular delivery of ciprofloxacin using nanospheres and conventional contact lens materials. Invest Ophthalmol Vis Sci 2012;53:1341-52.
46. Amrite AC, Kompella UB. Size-dependent disposition of nanoparticles and microparticles following subconjunctival administration. J Pharm Pharmacol 2005;57:1555-63.
47. Amrite AC, Edelhauser HF, Singh SR, Kompella UB. Effect of circulation on the disposition and ocular tissue distribution of 20 nm nanoparticles after periocular administration. Mol Vis 2008;14:150-60.
48. Jani PD, Singh N, Jenkins C, Raghava S, Mo Y, Amin S, et al. Nanoparticles sustain expression of Flt intraceptors in the cornea and inhibit injury-induced corneal angiogenesis. Invest Ophthalmol Vis Sci 2007;48:2030–36.
49. Wang JJ, Zeng ZW, Xiao RZ, et al. Recent advances in chitosan nanoparticles as drug carriers. Intern J Nanomed 2011:6:765-73.

50. Fulgencio GO, Viana FA, Ribeiro RR, et al. New mucoadhesive chitosan film for ophthalmic drug delivery of timolol maleate: *In vivo* evaluation. J Ocular Pharmacol Ther 2012;28:350-58.
51. Fuente M, Seijo B, Maria JA. Novel hyaluronic acid-chitosan nanoparticles for ocular gene therapy. Invest Ophthalmol Vis Sci 2008;49:2016-24.
52. Sahoo SK, Labhasetwar V. Nanotech approaches to druf delivery and imaging. Drug Discov Today 2003;8:1112-20.
53. Tomalia DA, Baker H, Dewald J, Hall M, Kallos G, Martin S, et al. A new class of polymers: Starburst-dendritic macromolecules. Polym J 1985;17:117-32.
54. Shaunak S, Thomas S, Gianasi E, Godwin A, Jones E, Teo I, et al. Polyvalent dendrimer glucosamine conjugates prevent scar tissue formation. Nat Biotechnol 2004;22:977-84.
55. Kim B, Tang Q, Biswas PS, Xu J, Schiffelers RM, Xie FY, et al. Inhibition of ocular angiogenesis by siRNA targeting vascular endothelial growth factor pathway genes: Therapeutic strategy for herpetic stromal keratitis. Am J Pathol 2004;165:2177-85.
56. Pennisi CP, Jensen PE, Zachar V, et al. Incorporation of photosyntetic reaction centers in the membrane of human cells: toward a new tool for optical control of cell activity. Cell Mol Bioeng 2009;2:156-65.
57. Kuritz T, Lee G, Owens ET, et al. Molecular photovoltaics and the photoactivation of mammalian cells. IEEE Trans Nanobioscience 2008;7:164-71.
58. Cheruvu NP, Amrite AC, Kompella UB. Effect of diabetes on transscleral delivery of celecoxib. Pharm Res 2009;26:404-14.

INDEX

Page numbers followed by f refer to figure and t refer to table

A

Abacavir 198, 215, 216
Abdominal pain 367, 455
Abnormal
    conjugate gaze 482
    oculography 479
    retinal pigmentation 531
Abnormalities of hypothalmic-pituitary adrenal axis 448
Absent pupil light reflex 485, 487
Absorbable gelatin film 335, 510
Absorption 940
Abuse of topical ocular anesthetics 460
Acanthamoeba 69
Acantholysis 525
Accommodative
    paralysis 473-489
    spasm 482
Acetaminophen 170
Acetate
    ointment 158, 494
    solution 158, 494
    suspension 158, 494
Acetazolamide 500
Acetic acid 435
Acetone 423
Acetylcholine 499
Acetylcysteine 336
Acetylsalicylic acid 170, 172
Acid-fast bacilli 68
Acquired immunodeficiency syndrome 391
Actinomyces israelii 68
Activation of
    infections 169
    tuberculosis 617
Acute
    and chronic hepatitis C infection 211
    angle closure glaucoma 387, 948
    CSC 686
    hydrops 387
    multifocal placoid pigment epitheliopathy 829
    postoperative endophthalmitis 847, 853
    retinal necrosis 407, 519
    trachoma 126
Acyclovir 196, 199, 203, 497, 546
Addison's disease 533
Adefovir 197, 212, 213
Adenovirus 69, 193
Adjustable pump 86
Adrenaline 340, 505
Adrenals Cushing's disease 533
Advantages of
    hyaluronic acid in ophthalmic viscomicrosurgery 321
    ICG 822
    intracameral injection of lidocaine 304
Age-related
    eye disease study 642
    macular degeneration 191, 362, 512, 514, 635, 641, 702, 816, 883, 917, 991
Agranulocytosis 455
Air in anterior chamber 878
Alanine 20, 53
Albumin 20, 637
Alcoholic rub-in hand disinfectant 423
Aldose reductase inhibitors 512
Alkali burns 523
Alkaptonuria 539
Allergic
    conjunctivitis 285
        and blepharitis 157
    disease 730
    disorders 615
    ocular disease 725
    reactions of lid and conjunctiva 308
Allergy 476, 777
    and idiosyncratic reactions 458
Allylamines 227, 239
Alopecia 186, 454
Alpha
    chymotrypsin 328, 464, 509
    linoleic acid 839
Alteration of lacrimation 457
Alternate day therapy 616
Alternations in lipid metabolism 450
Amantadine 197, 222, 223
Amaurosis fugax 532
Amblyopia 942
Amides 303
Amikacin 117, 121, 149-151, 406, 854
    solution 492

Amino acid 20, 26, 52, 53
  composition of human tear lysozyme 20t
Aminocaproic acid 435
Aminoglycosides 103, 116, 541, 582, 849, 961
Aminopenicillins 106
Amoebic keratitis 1012
Amoxicillin 107, 493
Amphotericin B 227-229, 443, 498, 652
  for intraocular injection 657t
Ampicillin 106, 107, 150, 151, 493
Amprenavir 198
Amylase 29
Amyloidosis 535
Anaerobic streptococcus 67
Anatomy of orbital cavity 4f
Anemia and opportunistic infections 186
Anesthesia trends in ophthalmology 899
Angioneurotic edema 459, 478
Aniridia 527, 537
Anisocoria 473, 475, 483, 484, 532, 538
Ankyloblepharon 527
Ankylosing spondylitis 526
Anorexia 454
Antazoline 503
  phosphate 548
Anterior
  blepharitis 775f
  chamber angle in cross-section 47f
  ischemic optic neuropathy 168
  membrane dystrophies 387
  segment
    ischemia 619
    OCT of IOL 865f
    OCT of scleral flap 865f
  stromal edema 461
Antiallergy
  medication 281, 953
  therapy 280, 502, 547
Antiangiogenic drugs 689
Antiarthritic drugs 473
Antibacterial therapy 97
Antibiotic
  cyclosporin 758
  prophylaxis 607
  therapy 492
Anticataract therapy 511
Anticoagulation therapy 985
Antifungal 476, 967
  drugs 226
  regime for keratomycosis 655t
  spectrum 229, 242
  therapy 225, 498, 546

Antiglaucoma therapy 499, 548
Antihistamine 288, 475, 503
  eyedrops 719
Anti-inflammatory
  drugs 543, 950
  therapy 155
Antileprosy drugs 477
Antimalarial drugs 472
Antimetabolites 457, 502, 757
Antimicrobial
  combination therapy 100
  peptides 103, 147
  spectrum 114, 119, 124, 127, 134, 141, 145
  therapy 99
Antineoplastic drugs 479
Antinuclear antibody 972
Antioxidant 434, 512
  therapy 511
Antiplatelet trialists collaboration 886
Antiprostaglandin therapy 295
Antiproteinases 24
Antipyrine 548
Antiretroviral drugs in ophthalmic infections 516
Antisense oligonucleotide 197
Antiseptic solutions 460
Antithyroid drugs 487
Antituberculosis drugs 478
Antiviral therapy 193, 496, 545
Aortic arch syndrome 533
Aplastic anemia 440
Applanation tonometry 354
Apraclonidine 500
Aqueous
  humor 16
    composition 48
    dynamics 38
    formation 42, 44
  outflow system 46f
Arachidonic acid metabolites and inflammation 172
Arcus senilis 532
Arginine 20, 53
Argon laser photocoagulation 691
Arrhythmia 453, 455
Arteriosclerosis 532
Artificial tear
  and lubricants 506
  inserts 64
  solutions 370, 373
Asbestos disk filters 418
Ascorbate 52, 638
Ascorbic acid 640, 640f
Aspartic acid 20
Aspergillus
  flavus 71, 657
  fumigatus 71, 1011
Aspirin 172, 544

Astemizole 294
Asthenia 367, 453, 454
Asthma 454, 455, 524
Astringent ophthalmic solution 431, 567
Ataxia 453, 454
    telangiectasia 526
Atazanavir 198, 219
Atomic radiation 524
Atopic keratoconjunctivitis 280, 281, 282f, 285, 296
Atovaquone 405, 518
Atrophy 474, 477, 479, 488, 533
Atropine 344, 345
    sulfate 345, 349, 506, 942
Atypical mycobacteria 68
Autoclave sterilization 417t
Autologous serum tears 837
Automated lamellar keratoplasty 631
Average blood volume 940
Awareness of ocular surface disease 740
Azathioprine 186, 188, 496, 758
Azelastine 547
    hydrochloride 287, 502
Azithromycin 102, 130, 130f, 132, 151, 494, 542, 589, 906f, 962
    in ophthalmology 905
Azole derivatives 232
Aztreonam 112

B

Bacillocid 425
Bacillus
    anthracis 68
    cereus 68
    subtilis 68, 115
Bacitracin 102, 115, 151, 541, 542, 584
    zinc 542
Back pain 367
Bacterial
    cell membrane 116
    conjunctivitis 573, 596
    DNA 136
    keratitis 574, 596, 1012
    ulcers 152t
Bacteroides fragilis 105, 110, 611
Balanced salt solution 803, 894, 931
Balofloxacin 142
Band keratopathy 534, 535
Basic structure of fluoroquinolones 138f
Basis of tetracyclines 593f

Behçet's disease 187, 188, 190, 756-758, 976, 977
Benoxinate 308, 505
    HCl 308
Benzalkonium chloride 373, 434, 466, 577
Benzodiazepines 483
Benzoic acid 227
Benzyl penicillin 105, 493
Besifloxacin 140, 142, 151, 542, 579
Best corrected visual acuity 674
Beta-adrenergic blockers 453
Beta-lactam antibiotics 104, 585
Betamethasone 158, 494, 495, 543-545
Betapropiolactone 423
Betaxolol 500
Bevacizumab 884
Bicarbonate 28
Biguanides 421
Bilateral
    corneal deposits 491
    toxoplasmosis scars 979f
Bilirubin 638
Bimatoprost 501
Bioflavonoids 641
Biopsy of conjunctiva 32
Birdshot chorioretinopathy 188, 758, 828
Birth trauma 387
Bitot's spot on conjunctiva 535
Blastomyces dermatidis 237
Bleb-associated endophthalmitis 854
Blepharitis 201, 525, 775
    exacerbates dry eyes and allergy 735
Blepharoclonus 484, 489
Blepharoconjunctivitis 476, 478, 490
Blepharospasm 335, 482-484
Blindness 536
Blond fundus 535
Blood
    agar 70
    aqueous barrier 38
    dyscrasia 455
Blue
    sclera 525, 536
    vision 483
Boceprevir 197, 214
Boeck's sarcoid uveitis 618
Bone marrow depression 455
Boric acid 433, 435, 567
Borrelia burgdorferi 105
Bradycardia 453, 458
Brain heart infusion broth 70
Branch vein occlusion 533
Breakthrough retinitis 404

Breast
  carcinoma 537
  neoplasm 539
Brimonidine 500, 502
Brinzolamide 501
Bromfenac 172, 182, 544
Bromovinyl deoxyuridine 202, 497, 546
Brompheniramine 294
Bronchiectasis 537
Bronchogenic carcinoma 537
Bronchospasm 454
Brow
  growth 479
  loss 475, 479
Brown violet lid discoloration 485
BSS
  containing 508
  plus 327
  solution containing 327
Bullous pemphigoid 470, 757
Bupivacaine 306
Butacaine 308, 313, 505
  solution 505
Butoconazole 227

C

Calcium
  deposits in conjunctiva and cornea 535
  deposits in cornea, sclera 490
Calcofluor stain 70
Campylobacter jejuni 133
Canal of Schlemm 45
Candida
  albicans 393, 530, 856, 1008, 1011, 1016
  endophthalmitis 237
  keratomycosis 232
Capsular opacity 183
Carbapenems 102, 113
Carbenicillin 107, 150, 151
Carbolic acid 337
Carbon nanotubes 998
Carbonic anhydrase inhibitors 454, 500, 769, 946
Carboxymethyl cellulose 371, 372, 506, 833, 834
  sodium 434
Carboxypenicillin 106, 493
Cardiac
  arrest 453
  glycosides 482
Cardiovascular symptoms of toxicity 300
Carotenoids 638, 639
Carteolol 500
Caspofungin 227, 241, 242

Cataract 444, 487, 488, 490, 523-525, 528-531, 533-537, 617
  snowflake 533
  surgery 313, 324, 383, 606, 983
Catecholamines 26
Cecocentral scotomas 487
Cecropins 148
Cefaclor 493
Cefadroxil 109, 493
Cefamandole 493
Cefazolin 109, 150, 151, 493, 854
Cefdinir 110
Cefixime 110, 493
Cefonicid 493
Cefoperazone 110, 151, 493
Ceforanide 493
Cefotaxime 110, 151, 493
Cefotetan 493, 854
Cefotiam 493
Cefoxitin 112, 493
Cefpirome 112
Cefpodoxime 110
Cefsulodin 493
Ceftazidime 110, 112, 149-151, 493, 849, 854
Ceftibuten 110
Ceftizoxime 110, 112, 493
Ceftriaxone 110, 112, 151, 493
Centbucridine 301, 306, 308, 310
  solution 505
Central
  foveal thickness 918
  nervous system 38, 453, 458, 944
  retinal
    artery occlusion 880
    vein occlusion 639
  scotomas 483, 485, 488, 535
  serous
    chorioretinopathy 685, 827
  retinopathy 449
Cephalexin 109, 112, 493
Cephaloridine 109, 493
Cephalosporins 102, 108, 111, 854
Cephalosporium 69, 108
  acremonium 108
Cephalothin 109, 493
Cephapirin 493
Cepholosporins 960
Cephradine 109, 493
Cerebral ischemia 453
Ceruloplasmin 22, 637
Cetrimide 423
Cetrizine 294
Cetylpyridinium chloride 434
Cetylthonium chloride 434
Chain-breaking antioxidants 638

Chemical
  composition of
    aqueous humor 49
    tear fluid 18
  disinfection systems 515
  injury 387
  structure of
    aminoglycosides 118f
    azathioprine and
      methotrexate 188f
    azithromycin 591f
    azoles 232f
    benoxinate 308f
    betamethasone 159f
    bupivacaine 306f
    butacaine 313f
    chloramphenicol 127f
    chloroprocaine 303f
    clindamycin 135f
    cocaine 310f
    cyclophosphamide 186f
    cyclosporin A 189f
    dibucaine 312f
    diclofenac 182f
    difluprednate 165f
    dimethocaine 312f
    flucytosine 231f
    fluorometholone 163f
    flurbiprofen 177f
    hydrocortisone 158f
    ketorolac 178f
    lidocaine 304f
    linezolid 134f
    maraviroc 221f
    mepivacaine 305f
    metronidazole and
      tinidazole 144f
    mupirocin 148f
    nalidixic acid 576f
    phenocaine 311f
    piperocaine 312f
    polyenes 228f
    prednisolone 159f
    prilocaine 305f
    procaine 302f
    proparacaine 309f
    quinupristin/dalfopristin
      137f
    raltegravir 222f
    rimexolone 161f
    telithromycin 133f
    terbinafine 239f
    tetracaine 303f
    tetracycline 124f, 924f
    tigecycline 127f
    triamcinolone 159f
    vancomycin 115f
    verteporfin 362f
Chemosis 534, 539
Cherry red spot 536
  of macula 532
Chicken pox 204
Chlamydia
  psittaci 68
  trachomatis 68, 101, 145
Chlamydial disease 126
Chlamydophila pneumoniae 133
Chlorambucil 186, 496
Chloramphenicol 102, 127, 149-
    151, 492, 541, 544,
    545, 587, 609, 854
Chlorhexidine 414, 421
Chloride 27
Chlorobutanol 434
Chloroprocaine 302, 504
Chlorpheniramine 294
Chlorpromazine 472
Chlortetracycline 125, 492, 493
Chocolate agar 70
Cholinesterase inhibitors 948
Chondroitin sulfate 323
  solution 323
Chorioretinal scars 532
Chorioretinitis 477, 525, 527-531
Choroidal
  and retinal metastasis 537,
    539
  hemangioma 526
  metastasis 539
  neovascular membranes 883
  neovascularization 191, 687,
    702, 816, 917
  tuberculosis 396
Choroiditis 527, 530, 828
Chronic
  CSC 686
  follicular conjunctivitis 441
  hepatitis B infection 211
  myelogenous leukemia 211
  open angle glaucoma 948
  postoperative endophthalmitis
    853
Chrysarobin 485
Cicatricial pemphigoid 525
Ciclopirox olamine 227
Cidofovir 197, 206, 209, 497, 546
Ciliary
  body
    epithelial microcysts 449
    microcysts 487
  flush 489
Ciprofloxacillin 406
Ciprofloxacin 139, 142, 149-151,
    494, 542, 854
  solution 492
Citrate 52
Clarithromycin 102, 130, 130f, 132,
    150, 151, 406, 494, 962

Classification of
    antibacterial drugs 102
    antioxidants 637
    antiviral drugs 196
    cephalosporins 108
    endophthalmitis 847*t*
    quinolones 138
Clavulanic acid 108
Clear corneal incision 783*f*
Clemastine 294
Clinafloxacin 542
Clindamycin 103, 135, 149-151, 405, 493, 518, 854, 962
Clofazimine 406
Clonidine 500
Clostridia
    tetani 68
    welchii 68
Clostridium
    botulinum 510
    difficile 135, 144
Clotrimazole 227, 234, 235, 498, 546, 652
Cloxacillin 106, 107, 493
Coagulation and cell growth inhibitors 50
Cocaine 308, 310
    hydrochloride 341
    solution 505
Coloboma 536
    of lower lids 536
Color
    Doppler scanography 36
    vision
        defect 449, 474-487
        impairment 534
        tests 439
Comma-shaped conjunctival vessels 532
Complement targeted therapies 840
Complementary test 687
Complete
    blood count 757
    hemogram 400
Complications of
    contact lens solutions 465
    intravenous fluorescein 466
    steroids 443
    topical
        antimicrobial agents 440
        ocular anesthetic agents 457
    human tears and plasma 17*t*
Compound sodium lactate solution 327
Computer vision syndrome 431
Concentrated cold sterilizer 424

Congenital
    cataract 528, 537
        surgery 316
    glaucoma 387, 526, 527, 537
    microphthalmos 527
Congestive angle-closure glaucoma 40
Conjunctival
    allergen challenge 716, 717, 719
    allergy 475
    chemosis 461, 530
    closure during strabismus surgery 813
    depigmentation 488
    edema 480, 481
    hemorrhage 191, 529
    hyperemia 478, 527
    keratinization and scarring 202
    photosensitivity 476
    telangiectasia 526
    vessel
        blanching 523
        dilation 532
Conjunctivitis 366, 524-531, 535, 538
Constipation 454
Contact
    allergy 778*f*
    blepharodermatitis 202
    dermatitis of eyelids 157
    dermatoconjunctivitis 441
    lens 63, 354
        care products 514, 559
        fitting 313
        intolerance 485, 490
Contraindications of antibiotic-steroid combination 166
Convulsion 454
Copper
    and silver wire appearance of retinal vessels 532
    corneal ring 536
Corneal
    abrasions and trauma 341
    barrier 56
    blindness 523
    clouding 201
    collagen shield 75
    concentrations of azithromycinhthalmol 907*f*
    deposits 474, 481, 486
    edema 308, 489, 527, 528, 895
    epithelial
        damage 524
        debridement 313

erosion 524, 525
folds 533
graft
    reactions 157
    rejection 387, 617
hyperpigmentation 484
infections 1007
iritis 524
neovascularization 736, 810*f*
opacities 477, 485, 525
pannus 529
perforation 523, 525, 527, 529
peripheral edema 475
polychromatic crystals 477
recurrent erosion 533
refractive surgery 631
scarring 525
shields 63
stromal edema 202
surgery 317
transplant surgery 318, 320
ulcer 480, 525, 529
    and pannus 524
    perforation 847
vortex whorls 477

Cortical
blindness 191, 179, 480, 486, 488, 759
cataract 534
Corticosteroid
antibiotic combinations 495
in infective corneal diseases 615
mydriasis 618
Corynebacterium 71
difficile enterocolitis 405
xerosis 71
Cotrimoxazole 103, 146, 147, 494
Cotton
pledgets 63
wool
    exudates 533, 534
    spot 392, 393, 395*f*
Craniofacial syndromes 536
Cromolyn sodium 284, 502, 547
Cryptococcus
infections 530
neoforman 393
Crystalline
lens proteins 50
penicillin 105
Crystalluria 455
Crystals in conjunctiva and cornea 531
Curvularia lunare 69
Cutaneous hypersensitivity reactions 392, 397
CVS accident 453

Cyanoacrylate tissue adhesive 337, 509, 811
Cyclooxygenase inhibitors 512
Cyclopenthiazide 511
Cyclopentolate 344, 345, 349, 943
    HCl 347, 506
Cyclophosphamide 186, 496, 757
Cycloplegic
mydriatics 343, 344*t*, 506
refraction 942, 943
Cycloserine 102, 478
Cyclosporin 191, 759
    A 188, 496
Cysticercosis 530
Cysticerus cellulosae 69
Cystoid macular edema 175, 535, 620, 744, 745, 762, 895, 988
Cytarabine 497, 545
Cytokine-targeted therapies 840
Cytomegalovirus 193, 196, 205, 208, 209
infection 399, 516
retinitis 392, 393

D

Dacryoadenitis 528
Dacryocystitis 528, 530, 656
Dacryocystorhinostomy 321
Dalbavancin 102
Dapirazole 500
Daptomycin 102
Dark pigmentation of sclera 539
Darunavir 198, 220
Daunorubicin 502
Decrease in vision 191, 473, 479
Decreased
corneal sensation 480
dark adaptation 480, 485
depth perception 483
epithelial mitosis and migration 308
pupil
    light reflex 486, 490
    reflex and convergence 483
vision 481, 487, 489, 535
visual acuity 473, 475, 477, 478
Degeneration of rod outer segment 535
Delavirdine 198, 217, 398, 516
Delayed
epithelial healing 201, 202
wound healing 169, 444, 474, 487
Dematiaceous fungi 69, 71
Demecarium 499

Demeclocycline 125
Demodex folliculorum 777
Dendrimer 84, 1028
 formation 84*f*
Dendritic keratitis 528
Deposition of scales in
 conjunctival sac 525
Depression 453
Dermatitis 444
Dermatomyositis 526
Descemet membrane 3
Desloratadine 293, 503
Detection of
 corneal epithelial defects 354
 penetration of globe 354
Dexamethasone 158, 165, 494, 495,
 543, 544
 phosphate 841
 sodium 544
Dexchlorpheniramine 294
Diabetes mellitus 533
Diabetic
 hyperglycemia 457
 neuropathy 639
 retinopathy 512, 568, 642, 746,
 916
Diarrhea 455
Dibucaine 308, 311
 solution 505
Dichlorphenamide 501
Diclofenac 172, 496, 767
 sodium 180, 543
Dicloxacillin 106, 107, 149
Didanosine 198, 216, 398, 516
Diffuse
 choroiditis 529
 lamellar keratitis 629
 subretinal fibrosis syndrome
 190
Difluprednate 164
Digital subtraction 823
Dilated
 fundoscopy 400
 retinal
 veins 531
 vessels 531, 533
Dimethocaine 308, 311
 solution 505
Dioxahexane 424
Diphenhydramine 294
Diphtheria 529
Dipivefrine 500
Diplococcus pneumoniae 67
Diplopia 473-478, 483-485, 487,
 489, 490, 526, 533,
 535, 536, 538
 and extraocular muscle
 paralysis 474

Disinfection
 hydrogen peroxide soft lenses
 563
 nonhydrogen peroxide soft
 lenses 563
Disinfective and antiseptic agents
 in ophthalmology
 569
Dislocated crystalline lenses 806
Disodium cromoglycate 285, 502,
 547
DNA viruses 69, 193
Docosahexaenoic acid 839
Docosanol 196
Doripenem 113
Dorzolamide 501
Dosage of cotrimoxazole 146
Doxycycline 125, 493
Dracunculus medinensis 144
Drug
 active against
 cytomegalovirus 197, 205
 hepatitis virus 211
 herpes simplex virus 196
 human
 immunodeficiency
 virus 197
 influenza virus 197, 222
 respiratory syncytial virus
 197
 delivery system 55, 988
 induced
 ocular cicatricial
 pemphigus 471*f*
 Stevens-Johnson
 syndrome 472*f*
 resistant *Streptococcus*
 pneumoniae 1008
Dry
 cornea 535
 eye 169, 202, 369, 473-475,
 479-486, 490, 534,
 537, 539, 730
 and photophobia 525
 and punctate keratitis 477
 disease 839
 syndrome 377
 heat 410
Dryness of mucous membrane 480
Durasite drug delivery system 907
Dyspnea 454
Dystrophy 387

E

Eales' disease 188, 758
Ecchymosis 451
Echinocandins 227, 241, 654

Echinococcus granulosus 69
Echothiophate 499
Econazole 227, 235, 498, 546
Ectropion 525
Edema 476, 718, 719, 721
Efavirenz 198, 217
Eicosapentaenoic acid 839
EIS solution containing 328
Elasticity 316
Electrolytes 51
    and hydrogen ions 27
Electroretinography 81, 313, 439
Elephantiasis of lids 529
Emedastine 292, 504
Emedastine difumarate 288, 289, 547
Emerging drugs for uveitis 1021
Emphysema 537
Emtricitabine 198, 215, 216
Encephalotrigeminal angiomatosis 526
Endocarditis 533, 538
Endogenous endophthalmitis 855
Endolaser photocoagulation 803*f*
Endophthalmitis 529, 656, 880
    vitrectomy study 847, 670
Endothelial
    dystrophies 387, 462
    toxicity 458
Enfuvirtide 198
Enoxaparin sodium 985
Entecavir 197, 212, 214
Enteric bacilli 71
Enterococcus
    faecalis 136, 909
    faecium 136
Enzymatic cleaners 515, 562
Enzyme 28
    lactic dehydrogenase 53
Ephedrine 504, 547
Epidemic keratoconjunctivitis 528
Epidermolysis bullosa 525
Epinephrine 291, 340, 500, 505
Episcleritis 157, 162, 175, 526, 527, 535, 536, 623
Epithelial
    desquamation 308
    keratopathy 202
    toxicity 457
Epstein-Barr virus 193
Ertapenem 113
Erythema 459, 478, 524, 525, 718, 719, 721
    multiforme 369, 454
    of lids 524
Erythromycin 102, 129, 130*f*, 131, 151, 493, 541, 588, 854, 906*f*, 962
    ointment 492

Escherichia coli 101, 583, 1010
Essential fatty acids 839
Ethacrynic acid 485
Ethambutol 406, 518
Ethionamide 478
Ethoxazolamide 501
Ethylene
    diaminetetra-acetic acid 507
    oxide 418
Ethylenediaminetetra acetate 336, 434
Etidocaine 306
Etravirine 198, 217
Evaluation of corneal abrasions 313
Ewing's tumors 618
Except bacitracin 102
Excessive sweating 459
Excimer Laser PRK and LASIK surgery 313
Exophthalmos 169, 439, 474, 484, 487, 488, 490, 526, 531, 533-536, 538, 617
Exposure keratitis 534, 536
External ophthalmoplegia 537, 539
Extracapsular cataract
    extraction 782
    surgery 316
Extraocular
    irrigating solution 327, 508
        containing 328
    muscle
        myalgia and palsy 528, 538
        palsy 526, 528, 535, 538
        paralysis 474, 476, 478, 479, 481, 483, 487
        paresis 473, 478, 490
Eye
    hypotony 764
    pain 366
Eyelash 479
    loss 480, 483, 486
Eyelid
    infiltration 313
    integrity 833, 840
    margins 833

F

Facial
    deformity syndromes 536
    nerve block 313
Facilitates capsulorrhexis 318
Famciclovir 196, 199, 205, 497
Femoral head ischemia necrosis 617
Fenamates 169, 171
Fenoprofen 179, 544

Fever 454, 457
Fexofenadine 294
Fibrin glue 860
    seals conjunctiva 864f
Fick's diffusion equation 871
Fifth generation cephalosporins 111
Filamentous fungi 225
Filter paper strips 63
Filtering surgery for glaucoma 324, 383
First generation
    cephalosporins 109
    drugs 545
Fitting of rigid contact lenses 354
Flashing colored lights 484
Flashing lights 477, 478, 486
Flavonoids 638, 641
Flickering vision 478
Flu syndrome 367
Fluconazole 227, 233, 236, 498, 546, 653
Flucytosine 227, 231, 498, 547
Fluid retention 452
Fluorescein
    angiography 355, 439, 687
    dye
        disappearance test 35
        test 353f
    sodium 351, 512
    stain of dendritic ulcer 445f
    strips 355, 513
        for applanation tonometry 352f
        for dry eye disorder 352f
        for evaluation of conjunctival injuries and infections 352f
Fluorexon 351, 356, 513
Fluorinated pyrimidine 231, 547, 969
Fluorometholone 103, 136, 138, 162, 495, 452, 543, 545, 575, 964
    acetate 495
    suspension 159
Flurbiprofen 172, 176, 495, 543
Flurometholone 545
Focal
    keratitis 387
    spots 825
Follicular conjunctivitis 528
Fomivirsen 197, 209, 546
    sodium 407, 519
Forced duction testing 313
Forceps injury 387
Foreign body sensation 183
Formaldehyde 427
Fosamprenavir 198

Foscarnet 197, 206, 399, 403, 497, 516
    sodium 208, 546
Fosfomycin 102, 115
Fourth generation
    cephalosporins 110
    fluoroquinolones 611
Fractionated purified silicone oil 330, 509
Framycetin 123, 151, 541
    solution 492
Fuchs heterochromic
    cyclitis 975f
    uveitis 974
Functions of aqueous humor 54
Fundus
    autofluorescence imaging 687
    contact lens biomicroscopy 313
Fungal
    diseases 166
    infections 407
    keratitis 1013
Fusarium solani 1013
Fusidic acid 103, 136
Fusidium coccineum 136
Future
    of nanotechnology 1005
    viscoelastics 326

G

Galactosemia 536
Ganciclovir 197, 205, 206, 399, 497, 516, 546
    implant 401
        design 402f
    intravitreal lmplant 207
    resistance 402
Gastrointestinal
    disturbances 943
    drugs 486
Gatifloxacin 140, 142, 151, 494, 542, 854
    ophthalmic solution 577
    solution 492
Gemifloxacin 142, 494, 542
    solution 492
Gentamicin 117, 120, 149-151, 543, 545, 609, 854
    solution 492
    sulfate 541
German measles 527
Giant
    papillary conjunctivitis 176, 281, 283f, 285, 623
    retinal tear 803f
    tears 802
Giardia lamblia 144

Giemsa stain 70
GIT
  disorders 451
  disturbances 186, 758
Glare sensitivity 490
Glaucoma 169, 439, 474, 487, 527, 533, 535, 537, 618, 639, 895
  filtration surgery 320
  retinopathy 523
  surgery 318, 617, 984
Glaucomatocyclic crisis 534
Glucocorticoids inhibiting drugs 690
Glucose 25, 52
  imbalance 453
Glutamate 53
Glutamic acid 20
Glutaraldehyde 420, 424, 427
Glutathione peroxidase 637
Glycerine 435, 501
  solution 389, 510
Glycopeptide antibiotics 113
Glycosuria 455
Glycylcycline 102, 126
Gold salts 473
Goldman's and other contact lenses 426
Gonioscopy 313
Gonorrhea 529
Gram stain 70
Gramicidin 542
Gram-negative bacteria 71
Gram-positive bacteria 71
Gray corneal opacities 485
Green
  angiography 822
  vision 487
Griseofulvin 227

H

Haemophilus
  aegyptius 67
  ducreyi 133
  influenzae 67, 133, 575, 578, 590, 609, 855, 906
Halogenated benzamidozole 405
Hamameli's
  ophthalmic solution 433
  water 567
Hamycin 227
Hansel stain 70
Harada's disease 617
Hard
  exudates 532
    and microaneurysm 533
  lenses 559-561
Hay fever conjunctivitis 281

Headache 367, 453-455
Heart block 453, 458
Helicobacter pylori 777
Hemangioma 157
Hematuria 455
Hemianopia 478-482, 488, 490
Hemolytic anemia 455
Hemorrhage 537, 759
Hemorrhagic cystitis 186
Hepatitis
  B virus 196
  C virus 196
Hepatotoxicity 189, 759
Herpes
  simplex 395, 528
    virus 193, 194, 196
  zoster 528
    infection 204
    keratitis 157
    ophthalmicus 168, 392, 395, 396f, 405, 518
    virus 196
Herpetic chorioretinitis 528
Hexachlorophene 485
High
  molecular fluorescein 355
  polyunsaturated fatty acid 643
  viscosity methylcellulose 378
Histamine 26
Histidine 20, 53
Histoplasma capsulatum 69, 237, 393
Histoplasmosis 530
HIV-related retinopathy 391, 392
Homatropine 344-346, 506, 943
Homolateral congenital glaucoma 526
Homonymous hemianopia 532
Hot air oven 411, 416
HSV keratitis 204
Human
  fibrin glues 812
  immunodeficiency virus 193, 196, 391
  papovavirus 69
  tear
    electrolytes 27t
    lysozyme 21
Hyalectin 322, 508
Hyalophora cecropia 148
Hyaluronic acid 317, 377, 836
Hyaluronidase 329, 465, 509
Hydatid cyst 530
Hydrochloric acid 435
Hydrocortisone 158, 494, 495, 543, 545
Hydrodissection 786f
Hydrogel contact lens 57
Hydrogen peroxide 337, 427

Hydroxazine 294
Hydroxyamphetamine 342, 505
Hydroxyethyl cellulose 434, 506
Hydroxymethyl progesterone 160
Hydroxypropyl
    guar galactomannan 841
    methylcellulose 434, 506, 834
Hyperemia 524
Hyperpigmentation 477, 479, 485
Hypersecretion of tears 33
Hypersensitivity of drug 166
Hypertension 300, 455, 532
Hypertensive retinopathy 533
Hypertrichosis 488, 525, 759
Hyperuricemia 189, 758, 759
Hypofluorescence of fluorescein 459
Hypokalemic alkalosis 452
Hypoparathyroidism 534
Hypopyon 322, 487
Hyposecretion of tears 30
Hypotension 453, 458

I

Iatrogenic inflammation of eye 156
Ibuprofen 179, 544
Ichthyosis 525
Identification of neoplasms 126
Idiopathic
    polypoidal choroidal
        vasculopathy 825, 827f
    sclerosing orbital
        inflammation 190
Idoxuridine 196, 198, 200, 443, 496
Imidazole 227, 232
Imipenem 113, 149, 150
Immunoglobulin 22, 50
    A 22
    D 24
    E 24
    G 23
    M 23
Immunoliposomal drug delivery system 1000f
Immunosuppressive
    agents in ophthalmology 184, 496
    drugs 756
Impaired
    conjugate gaze 534
    dark adaptations 490
    vision 484-489
Impairment of vision 482
Impression cytology mapping 15f, 370f
Inadvertent intra-arterial
    injections 468
Increased
    intracranial pressure 449
    intraocular pressure 183
Indications of
    combination therapy 100
    topical antibiotic steroid
        combinations 166
Indinavir 198, 399, 497, 516, 546
Individual drugs 120
Indocyanine 822
    green 351, 358, 513, 790, 822, 823, 828
        angiography 687, 702, 822
        dye 790, 824f
Indoles 169, 179
Indomethacin 172, 179, 543, 767
Indoxuridine 545
Infantile capillary hemangioma 913
Infection and ulceration 444
Infectious
    endophthalmitis 892t
    epithelial keratitis 204
    mononucleosis 528
Inflammatory
    diseases 763
    eye diseases 639
Infliximab 190
Influenza 528, 538
Infrared radiation 524
Infusion 548
Inhibition of
    epithelial wound healing 442
    post-translational processing 211
    transcription 211
    translation 211
    viral
        maturation and release 211
        penetration 211
Inhibits human cytomegalovirus 407
Injection of gas 878
Inner mucin layer 6
Innovative strategies for ocular
        surface diseases 730
Insomnia 453
Instillation of vasoconstrictor 719
Integrase inhibitor 222
Interferons 211, 497
Intermediate uveitis 975
International task force 842
Interstitial
    keratitis 157
    pneumonitis 758
Intracameral
    antibiotics 612
    injections 97
Intracapsular cataract extraction 974

Intraocular
  antibiotics 848
  foreign body 617
  gas 870
    geometry 871
    injection 876
    kinetics 871
  inflammation 387, 463
  irrigating solutions 326, 508
  lenses 419, 806, 974
  pressure 40, 463, 895
    monitoring 439
  surgery 387
  tumors 827
Intrastromal hemorrhage 461
Intravenous
  dosage 516
  fluorescein 355, 513
Intraventricular hemorrhage 915
Intravitreal
  amphotericin B 656
  antiangiogenic drugs 708
  antibiotic injections 150*t*
  devices 401
  implant 206
  injection 617
    of ganciclovir 400
  medication 769
Intravitreous triamcinolone-associated endophthalmitis 856
Intubation dacryocystography 35
IOL implantation 168, 313, 316, 318, 324
  and phacoemulsification 383
Ionizing radiation 410, 418
Iontophoresis 77
Iridocyclitis 526, 527, 536
Iris and ciliary body cysts 531
Iritis 308, 322, 473, 477-482, 487, 524, 527-535, 538
Irreversible bullous keratopathy 461
Irrigating solutions 326, 508
Ischemic iritis 533
Isofluorophate 499
Isoleucine 20, 53
Isoniazid 478
Isopropyl alcohol 420
Isosorbide 501
Isotretinoin 490
Itching 721
Itraconazole 227, 233, 237, 498, 546, 653

J

Jaundice 186
Jerky pursuit 482, 484

Jones test 354
Juvenile idiopathic arthritis 971, 972

K

Kanamycin 123, 150, 151, 493
Kaposi's sarcoma 211, 222, 392, 397
Keratitis 474, 478, 479, 485, 488, 523-531, 534, 538
  medicamentosa 442
  sicca and band keratopathy 527
Keratoconjunctivitis 485
  sicca 32, 369, 930
Keratoconus 524
  and dry eyes 524
Keratomalacia 535
Keratomycosis 651
Keratoplasty 324, 383
Ketoconazole 227, 234, 236, 498, 546, 653
Ketolides 102, 133
Ketoprofen 179, 544
Ketorolac tromethamine 177, 573
Ketotifen 503
  fumarate 286, 547
Kinyoun's method 70
Klebsiella pneumoniae 837, 856
Koeppe nodules 975*f*

L

Lacrimal
  dilation and irrigation 313
  duct stenosis 525
  gland
    lesions 530
    swelling 527
  surgery 984
  testing 354
Lacrimation disorder 366
Lactate 26, 52
  dehydrogenase 28
Lactophenol cotton blue mount 70
Levocysteine 336
Lamivudine 197, 214-216, 398, 516
Laser
  assisted
    in situ keratomileusis 625, 631
    subepithelial keratectomy 631
  photocoagulation 705
LASIK surgery 383, 520
Laws of refraction 797
Lens
  dislocation 536
  opacities 880

Lenticular opacity 491
Leprosy 529
Lethal toxicity 458
Lethargy 453
Leucine 20, 53
Leukemias 531
Leukocytic and platelet aberrations 451
Leukokoria 530
Leukopenia 455
Levocabastine 547
Levocetrizine 293, 503, 547
Levofloxacin 139, 142, 151, 494, 542, 580
    solution 492
Lid
    blue discoloration 486
    bullae 525
    edema 201, 473, 477, 479-482, 486, 528, 529, 534, 538, 539
    infections 527
    inflammation 478, 485
    lesions 526
    margins scars and loss 538
    paralysis 529
    photosensitivity 489
    redness 485
    retraction and lag 534
    scarring and burn 523
    scrubs 63, 430, 566
    thrush 530
    twitch sign 536
    vesicles 527
Lidocaine 303, 308, 504
    HCl 309
        solution 505
Limbal dendritis 528
Lincomycin 149, 150
Lincosamide 103, 135
Linezolid 103
Lipemia retinalis 533
Lipid keratopathy 532
Liposomal drug delivery system 1000f
Liposomes 81, 297, 760, 1026
Liquid perfluorocarbons 435
Lissamine green 351, 358, 513
Listeria monocytogenes 68, 101, 134
Liver
    disease 534
    function tests 400
Loa loa 69
Lobucavir 497, 546
Local
    anesthetic agents 299, 307, 504
    injectable anesthetics 300, 313

Lodoxamide 285, 502
    tromethamine 547
Lomefloxacin 142, 149-151, 494, 542, 610
    solution 492
Lopinavir 198, 219
Loratadine 294
Loss of
    eyelashes 191
    red reflex 766f
Lotemax 841
Loteprednate 545
Loteprednol etabonate 160, 164, 495, 543
Low
    density lipoprotein 817
    molecular weight components 330
Lowe's syndrome 537
Löwenstein-Jensen media 70
Lung neoplasm 539
Lyme's disease 962
Lymphogranuloma venereum 529
Lymphoma 531, 538
    of orbit 397
Lysine 20, 53
Lysosomal enzymes 28, 30
Lysozyme 20, 30
    assay 32

M

Macrolides 102, 128, 588, 962
Macular
    degeneration 477, 481, 487
    edema 168, 191, 474, 476-478, 481, 488
    hole surgery 878
    photocoagulation study 816
    scarring and optic neuritis 530
Maintenance
    of intraoperative mydriasis 174
    therapy 400
Major causes of corneal edema 387
Malaria 538
Malignant exophthalmos 168
Management of
    cystoid macular edema 762
    dry eye 833
    endophthalmitis 847
    iatrogenic inflammation of eye 615
    myopic choroidal neovascularization 674
    post- refractive keratitis 625
    uveitis in children 971

Marfan's syndrome 536
Marginal corneal ulcer 526
Marked mydriasis 480
Mast cell inhibitors 547, 954
Measles 193
Medrysone 543
Meibomian gland
    dysfunction 840
    plugging 777*f*
Melena 454
Membrane bound
    devices 57
    inserts 64
Membranous conjunctivitis 529
Mepivacaine 305
Meropenem 113
Metastatic endophthalmitis 539
Methacycline 493
Methazolamide 501
Methemoglobinemia 458
Methicillin 106, 107, 149-151, 493
    resistant *Staphylococcus aureus* 111
Methionine 20, 53
Methotrexate 186-188, 496
Methylcellulose 324, 371, 373, 434, 506, 507
Metronidazole 144, 494
Mezlocillin 107
Micafungin 241, 242
Miconazole 227, 234, 235, 498, 546, 652
Microbial antibiotic resistance 672
Microfilarial invasion of ocular tissues 531
Microlides 541
Microperimetry 688
Microphthalmos 528, 536
Micropsia 486
Microvascular damage 763
Middle aqueous layer 5, 12
Mikulicz's syndrome 369
Mild
    adverse reactions 467
    keratitis and iritis 538
    papilledema 537
    retinopathy 537
Minimum
    bactericidal concentration 938
    inhibitory concentration 937
Minocycline 125, 493
Minor surgery of conjunctiva 313
Miosis 474, 482, 484, 485, 489, 490
Mitogen activated protein kinase 925
Mitomycin C 502
Moderate iritis 524
Modes of corticosteroid delivery 167

Modified Schirmer test 31*f*
Moist heat 410, 416
Molecular structure of
    aztreonam 112*f*
    carbapenems 113*f*
    cephalosporins 108*f*
    flavonoid 642*f*
    macrolides 130*f*
Molluscum contagiosum 69, 392
Monobactams 102, 112
Mooren's ulcer 189, 759
Moraxella catarrhalis 133
Moxalactam 110, 112
Moxifloxacin 140, 142, 151, 494, 542, 545
    ophthalmic solution 578
    solution 492
Mucoadhesive polymers 88
Multifocal choroiditis 829
Multiple
    evanescent white dot syndrome 830
    myelomas 531
    pupils 536
Multiplication of virus 195*f*
Multipurpose solution 515
Mumps 193, 528
Mupirocin 103, 147
Muscular dystrophy disorders 537, 539
Myasthenia 453
    gravis 536
Myasthenic block 473, 487-489
Mycobacterium
    avium 132, 141
        complex 132
        intracellulare 393, 406
    bovis 1015
    fortuitum 1015
    leprae 68, 132
    marinum infection 1015
    tuberculosis 68, 134, 406, 518
Mycoplasma pneumoniae 125, 133, 440
Mydriasis 169, 473-487, 489
Myesthenic block and toxic amblyopia 449
Myopathy 451
Myopia 473, 485, 486, 536
Myopic subfoveal choroidal neovascularization 674

N

Naepaine 308, 311
    solution 505
Nafcillin 106, 107
Naftifine 227, 240

Nanofibers for glaucoma 1004
Nanoparticles 1002, 1027
Naphazoline 291, 547
    HCl 291, 503
Naproxen 179, 544
Narrowed optic foramina 490
Nasolacrimal duct 656
Natamycin 227, 228, 230, 498
Nature of allergic disease 727
Necrotic keratopathy 539
Necrotizing retinitis 395f, 396f
Neisseria
    gonorrhea 101, 573, 590
    meningitides 101
    sicca 101
Nelfinavir 198, 498, 546
Neomycin 117, 122, 151, 541, 542, 544, 545
    solution 492
    sulfate 542, 544
Neovascular
    age-related macular degeneration 190
    glaucoma 191
    myopic maculopathy and retinopathy of prematurity 911
Neovascularization of nerve head 533
Nephrotic syndrome 537
Netilmicin 122, 150, 151, 493
Neuraminidase inhibitors 197
Neurofibromatosis 526
Neuromuscular
    blockade 120
    drugs 489
Neutrophil count 400
Nevirapine 198, 217, 398, 516
Niemann-Pick disease 536
Night blindness 481, 483, 484, 534, 539
Nitrofurantoin 103
Nitroimidazoles 103, 143
Nodular scleritis 538
Nonexpansile concentration 872, 876
Nonfatal
    hemorrhagic stroke 886
    ischemic stroke 886
    myocardial infarction 886
Non-nucleoside reverse transcriptase inhibitors 198, 216, 398, 516
Nonopportunistic infections 391, 394
Nonpigmented epithelial cells 38

Nonsteroidal
    antiestrogens 488
    anti-inflammatory
        agents 543
        drugs 155, 169, 474, 619, 623, 767, 935, 953, 1003
Nonsurgical contusion injury 387
Norfloxacin 142, 150, 151, 494, 542
    solution 492
Normal
    ciliary epithelium 39f
    microbial flora of eye 70
    tear drainage 15
Ntravenous heparin 984
Nucleoside reverse transcriptase inhibitors 196f, 198, 216, 398, 516
Nystagmus 473-490, 525-527, 534-536, 538
Nystatin 227, 228, 230, 498

O

Occlusive vascular diseases 532
Ocular
    allergic diseases 727
    allergy 730
    defense system 3
    and immunity 380
    disposition of ophthalmic formulations 74f
    distribution of nanoparticles 1004
    drug toxicity 438
    gene therapy 1002
    hypertension 951
    hypotensive lipids 501
    inflammation 619
    iontophoresis 841
    irritation 485
    manifestations of
        AIDS cytomegalovirus retinitis 394f
        HIV infections in children 397
        systemic diseases 523
    pain 481
    palsy 531, 532, 538
    pemphigoid 618
    pseudotumor 481
    rosacea 126, 928
    syphilis 407, 518
    tuberculosis 166
    uses of
        cephalosporins 111
        fluoroquinolones 142
        tetracyclines 126

Oculogyric crisis 477, 479, 482-484, 489
Ocusert system 57
Ofloxacin 139, 142, 149-151, 494, 542, 611
  solution 492
Olopatadine 502, 547
  hydrochloride 286
Onchocerca volvulus 69
Onchocerciasis 531
Open-angle glaucoma 40
Ophthalmic
  decongestants 291*t*
  diagnostic tear test strips 431
  dyes 351, 512
  gel 206
  nonsteroidal anti-inflammatory drugs 744
  surgery 984
  viscosurgical devices 315, 508
Ophthalmoscopy 439
Opportunistic infections 189, 759
  of eye 391, 393
Optic
  atrophy 473, 476, 477, 481, 484, 485, 490, 527, 528, 531, 533, 534, 536
  nerve
    amyloid 535
    diseases 765
    glioma 526
    pathology 439
  neuritis 439, 474-484, 487-489, 491, 525, 527-529, 533-535, 537, 538
  neuropathy 491
Optical coherence tomography 688, 767
Oral
  antihistamine 283, 293, 294*t*
  fluorescein 513
  ganciclovir 206, 400
  pseudoephedrine 292
Orbital
  cellulitis 655
  edema 529
  hemorrhage 532
Orbital
  infiltration 531
  mass 537
  metastasis frequent 537, 539
  myositis 618
  pain 479
  pseudotumor 168
  puffiness 534
Ornidazole 144
Orogenital ulcer 978*f*
Oscillopsia 484

Oseltamivir 197, 223
Osmotic
  flow model of aqueous production 42*f*
  pressure 17
  pump 58, 86
Osteoporosis 451, 617
Other
  ocular drug delivery systems 86
  lipid layer 5
Oval shaped cornea and corneal opacity 531
Oxacillin 106, 107, 149, 150, 854
Oxazolidinones 103, 134
Oxiconazole 227
Oxygen 52
  induced retinopathy 912
Oxymetazoline 291, 547
  HCl 292, 504
Oxyphenbutazone 172, 544
Oxytetracycline 125, 493, 541, 542, 545
Ozurdex Geneva study group 992

P

Painful eye movements 530
Painless lid swelling 531
Palivizumab 197
Palpebral conjunctivitis 530
Palpitation 453, 455
Pancreatic diseases 534
Pancreatitis 451
Panuveitis 162
Papillary conjunctivitis 201
Papilledema 169, 474-476, 479, 484, 485, 487-490, 530-538
  and optic neuritis 480, 485
  and retinal hemorrhage 473, 475
Papillitis 168, 528, 531, 533, 539
Para-aminophenols 169, 171
Parabulbar local anesthesia 60*f*
Paracentral scotomas 480
Paradoxical lid retraction 536
Paresthesia of extremities 454
Pars
  plana
    cysts 531
    vitrectomy 770, 791
  planitis 187
Partial ophthalmoplegia 526
Partially reversible renal toxicity 189, 759
Pefloxacin 142, 149-151, 494, 542
  solution 492
Pegaptanib 191, 883

Pemphigoid lupus erythematosis 369
Pemphigus 470
Penciclovir 196, 199, 205
Penetrating trauma surgery 317
Penetration
　of foreign body 387
　tracking 938
Penicillin 102, 104, 107, 854, 960
　G 105, 107, 149, 151
　V 106, 107
Penicillinase resistant penicillins 106
Pentoxyphylline 512
Peptic
　ulcer diseases 534
　ulceration 617
Perennial allergic conjunctivitis 280
Perfluorocarbon liquids in vitreoretinal surgery 795
Perfluoro-N-octane 795
Perfluoro-phenanthrene 795, 802
Perfluoro-tributylamine 795
Periarteritis nodosa 538
Peribulbar anesthesia 313
Periocular steroids 446
Periorbital edema 479, 480, 524, 530
Peripheral
　disease 400
　retinal lesions 764
　ulcerative keratitis 538
　vasodilation 300, 458
Persistent epithelial defects 126
Phacoemulsification 313, 316, 318
Pharmacologic therapy for ocular inflammation 746
Pheniramine maleate 503, 547, 548
Phenocaine 310
　solution 505
Phenols 423
Phenoxymethyl 493
　penicillin 106
Phenylacetates 169
Phenylacetic acid 171, 180
Phenylalanine 20, 53
Phenylalkanoic acids 169, 171, 176
Phenylbutazone 172, 544
Phenylephrine 290, 291, 341, 348, 505, 542, 547, 548
　and cyclopentolate 348
　and tropicamide 349
　HCl 291, 503, 548
　hydrochloride 941
　with tropicamide 348
Phenylmercuric
　acetate 434
　nitrate 434

Phlyctenular
　conjunctivitis 529
　disease 930
　keratoconjuctivitis 157
Phosgene stimulation 488
Phosphate and
　ciprofloxacin 544
　framycetin 544
　gentamicin 544
　lomefloxacin 544
　ofloxacin 544
　sparfloxacin 544
　tobramycin 544
Phosphate solution 494
Phosphonoformic acid 208
Phosphoric acid 435
Photochemical therapy 1007
Photodynamic therapy 674, 688, 691, 706, 816, 817, 820, 1007
Photophobia 201, 367, 473-481, 484-489, 534
Photorefractive keratectomy 520, 748
Photosensitivity 454, 476, 478, 479, 481, 485, 486
Phthirus pubis 69
Physical
　defense system of eye 4f
　properties of
　　gases 870
　　tears 16
Physiological protection of eye 6f
Physostigmine 499
Picorna virus 193
Pigment epithelium detachments 706
Pigmentary
　glaucoma 485
　retinitis 525
　retinopathy 490, 537, 539
Piperacillin 107, 151
Piperocaine 308, 311
　solution 505
Piroxicam 179, 544
Plastic surgery 321, 324
　for congenital ptosis surgery 317
Platelet
　count 400
　inhibitors 984
Pneumatic
　displacement of submacular hemorrhage 878
　retinopexy 876-878
Pneumocystis
　carinii 393, 394
　　choroiditis 394, 407, 519
　jiroveci 135, 146, 147
　　pneumonia 146

Pneumonia 539
Polyacrylamide 325
Polyaminopropyl biguanide 434
Polyarteritis nodosa 369, 756, 757
Polychromatic cataract 539
Polydimethyl siloxane 509
Polyene 227, 546, 652, 967
    antibiotics 227
Polyethylene glycol 835
Polyhexamethyl biguanide 654
Polyhexanide 421
Polymethylmethacrylate 52
Polymixin B 116, 544
    sulfate 542, 544
Polymorphonuclear 171
Polyoxythylene 388
Polypeptide 541
    antibiotics 102
Polyplexes 1029
Polypoidal choroidal vasculopathy 689
Polyuria 455
Polyvinyl
    alcohol 370, 401, 434, 506, 835
    base solutions 372, 506
    pyrrolidone 373, 434, 507
    polymer base tear solution 373, 507
Porfirmer sodium 1016
Posaconazole 233, 239
Posterior
    chamber intraocular lens 860
    mucin layer 13
    segment surgery 317
    subcapsular cataract 169, 474, 488, 524, 952
    uveitis 168
Post-LASIK infectious keratitis 626f
Postoperative intraocular pressure management 879
Postprocedure
    ocular therapeutic module 520
    therapeutic
        medications 632
        modulation 521
Post-traumatic endophthalmitis 855
Potassium
    bicarbonate 435
    borate 435
    chloride 435
    imbalance 453
Povidone iodine 414, 422, 510, 654
Preclusion of sequential testing 459
Prednisolone 158, 494, 543, 545
Preoperative
    mydriasis 943
    ocular therapeutics 520

Preparation of
    gas 877
    intravitreal antibiotic injections 664t
Preservative free saline solutions 564
Prilocaine 304
Primary prophylaxis of CMV end organ disease 400
Procaine 301, 504
Progression of glaucoma 450f
Proliferative
    diabetic retinopathy 191, 805
    vitreoretinopathy 804, 805f, 806f, 875
Promethazine 294
Prominent choroidal vessels 535
Proparacaine 308, 309, 443
    solution 505
Propionibacterium acnes 853
Proptosis 531, 538
Propylene glycol 434, 836
Protease inhibitors 198, 218, 399
Proteins 19, 49, 101
Prulifloxacin 142
Pruritis 454
Pseudallescheria boydii 657
Pseudogaze palsy 536
Pseudomembranes 528, 529
Pseudomonas
    aeruginosa 64, 67, 101, 110, 578, 609, 837, 849, 963, 1012
    cepacia 67, 848
    corneal ulcers 592
Pseudoretinitis 527
Pseudotumor cerebri 449, 475, 479, 480, 485, 487-490, 617, 619
Ptosis 169, 201, 449, 473, 475, 476, 480-484, 489, 531, 535-539
Pulmonary
    edema 457
    interstitial fibrosis 186, 757
Pulse therapy 617
Punctate
    epithelial keratitis 308
    keratitis 461, 475, 477, 485, 487, 489, 529
    marginal keratitis 442
Purulent conjunctivitis 529
Pyrazinamide 406, 518
Pyrazolones 169, 171
Pyridoxine 518
Pyrilamine 294
    maleate 503, 548
Pyrimethamine 103, 146, 405, 518
Pyrimidines 652

Q

Quaternary ammonium compounds 427
Quinidine 481
Quinupristin-dalfopristin 102

R

Radiation injury 387
Raised intraocular pressure 880
Reactivation of herpes infections 952
Recent
   advances in
      antiretroviral drug therapy 407, 519
      immunosuppressive therapy 296, 759
      multipurpose soft lens care systems 515
Red
   dyschromatopsia 489
   green color vision defect 474, 481, 482
Reduced
   tear secretion 480
   vision 480-485
   visual acuity 480, 490
Reduction of postoperative inflammation 174
Refraction of light 797*f*
Refractive
   index 797
   keratotomy 168
Reiter's syndrome 526
Renal
   calculi 455
   colic 455
   toxicity and testicular atrophy 186, 757
   transplantation 537, 539
Repository injection 616
Resident flora 71
Respiratory
   distress syndrome 915
   failure 454
   syncytial virus 196*f*, 214
Retapamulin 103, 136
Retinal
   angiography 354
   angioma 526
   angiomatous proliferation 702
   cyst 530
   detachment 525, 526, 530, 536, 617
   surgery 324
   dysfunction 490
   edema 476, 537
   and exudates 531, 532
   and hemorrhage 487, 531
   and papilledema 527
   hemorrhage 191, 439, 449, 473-479, 481-486, 488, 490, 526, 527, 533, 534, 538, 539, 759
   microvasculopathy 222
   periphlebitis 528
   perivasculitis 535
   pigment
      epitheliopathy and macular edema 439
      epithelium 38, 642, 685, 816
      epithelium disturbances 191, 475, 480, 488, 759
   reattachment surgery 320
   traction 765
   vascular
      dilatation 537
      occlusion 488
      spasm 482
      tumor 190
   vasculitis 188, 528, 758
   vasodilation 481
   vasospasm 488
   vein occlusion 483
   venous congestion 533
   vessel
      dilation 529, 532
      tortuosity 533
Retinitis 523, 527, 530
Retinopathy 538
   of prematurity 191, 915, 941
Retrobulbar
   anesthesia 313
   neuritis 168, 478, 487-489, 535
   route 56, 59
Reversible inflammation 727
Rewetting solutions 514, 515, 560
Rheumatoid arthritis 527, 757
Rhinosporidium seeberi 69
Ribavirin 197, 212, 214
Rifabutin 406
Rifampicin 406
Rigid gas permeable lenses 561
Rimantadine 197, 222, 223
Rimexolone 159, 161, 543
Ritonavir 198, 399, 497, 516, 546
RNA viruses 69, 193
Rose
   bengal staining test 357
   petal aqueous infusion 292, 504
Roth's spots 529, 533, 538, 539
Routes of aqueous outflow 45
Roxithromycin 102, 129, 130*f*, 132, 493, 541, 962

Rubella 193, 527
Rubeosis iridis 533

S

Saboroud's medium 70
Salicylates 169, 171
Salicylic acid 227
Saquinavir 198, 220, 399, 497, 516, 546
Sarcoid lid nodule 527
Sarcoidosis 369, 470
Scanning laser ophthalmoscopes 822
Schiotz tonometer 426
Schirmer
    tear test sterile strips 432
    test 31, 459
Scintillating scotomas 476
Scintillography 36
Scleral
    barrier 56
    fixated IOL 860
    icterus 534
Scleritis 157, 162, 168, 175, 473, 476, 480, 527, 529, 536, 636
Scleroderma 369, 538
Scleromalacia perforans 190
Scopolamine 344, 345, 347, 506
Scotomas 475, 477, 478, 482-484, 488-490
Seasonal
    allergic conjunctivitis 282f
    iritis 524
Secnidazole 144
Second generation
    cephalosporins 109
    drugs 546
Secondary glaucoma 529, 531, 534
Seidel's sign 354
Selecting optimal ophthalmic antibiotic 595
Selenium 638, 641
Septic retinitis 530, 539
Septicemia 529
Serous
    detachment of neurosensory retina 697f
    retinopathy 474
Serpiginous choroiditis 188, 758, 829, 829f
Serratia marcescens 101, 574, 777
Severe
    anterior uveitis 168
    dry eye 480

membranous conjunctivitis 470
ocular
    rheumatoid disease 190
    surface disease 952
skin burns 523
Sexual dysfunction 454, 455
Shimmering lights 476
Sickle cell disease 532
Sildenafil 490
Silicone oil 509
Silver sulfadiazine 243, 498, 547, 654
Silvery skin scales 525
Sisomicin 122, 151, 541
Sjögren's syndrome 369, 470, 931f
Skin necrosis 469
Slow epithelial healing 308
Small optic disc 490
Sno test strips 432
Snowy vision 482
Sodium
    acetate 435
    benzoate 434
    bicarbonate 435
    bisulfite 434
    chloride 435
    cromoglycate 284
    hyaluronate 317, 319f, 323, 508
    hypochlorite 414, 427, 420
    metabisulfite 434
    phosphate 158, 544
        ointment 494
        solution 494
    propionate 434
    retention 452
    salicylate 511
    sulfacetamide 542, 545
    thiosulfate 434
Soft
    contact lens
        products 514
        therapy 376
    lenses 57, 563-565
Solution containing combination 508
Sorbic acid 434
Sparfloxacin 142, 149, 151, 494, 542, 611
Spectinomycin 103, 123
Spiramycin 132, 493
Spirochetal infection 126
Spirohydantoin 511
Squamous cell carcinoma of conjunctiva 397
Squint surgery 383
Staphylococcal blepharitis 778f

1056 Ocular Therapeutics

Staphylococcus
   aureus 67, 71, 101, 104, 111, 116, 127, 136, 147, 573, 578, 606, 611, 625, 628, 776, 777, 847, 849, 1008, 1009*f*, 1015
   epidermidis 67, 71, 98, 101, 111, 573, 611, 1008, 1012
   saprophyticus 67
Star maculopathy 532
Stasis retinopathy 533
Stavudine 197, 216, 398, 516
Sterile technique 415
Sterilization 790
   methods 415
      in ocular surgery 415*t*
Steroid-induced
   cataract 447*f*
   dendritic keratitis 445*f*
   fungal keratitis 446*f*
   glaucoma 447*f*-448*f*
Stevens-Johnson syndrome 397, 440, 458, 470
Stimulation of tears 377
Strabismus 486, 487, 489, 490, 526, 527, 530, 531, 536, 617
   oscillopsia 483
   surgery 317, 321, 324
Streptococcus
   faecalis 101
   pneumoniae 67, 101, 114, 141, 573, 574, 578, 590, 611, 849, 909, 1008
   pyogenes 67, 136, 147
   salivarius 1012
   viridans 611, 837
Streptogramins 102, 136
Streptomyces
   aureofaciens 924
   erythreus 128
   fradiae 122
   griseus 123
   natalenses 230
   nodosus 229
   noursei 230
   roseosporus 116
   venezuelae 127, 609
Streptomycin 118, 123
Structure of
   6-aminopenicillanic acid 105*f*
   bacteria 102*f*
   bromfenac 183*f*
   chitosan 1028*f*
   chlorambucil 187*f*
   dendrimer 1001*f*, 1029*f*
   fungal cell 226*f*
   indomethacin 181*f*
   loteprednol 164*f*
   nepafenac 184*f*
   retapamulin 137*f*
   suprofen 180*f*
   virus 194*f*
Subconjunctival
   antibiotics 612
   hemorrhage 449, 475, 476, 478, 479, 485, 531, 535
   route 56, 59
Subepithelial corneal
   opacities 490
   whorl opacities 480
Subluxated IOL 863*f*
Subretinal
   fish eggs 880
   hemorrhage 367
Sub-Tenon's plane relationship 58*f*
Sulbactam 108
Sulfacetamide 592
   solution 492
Sulfadiazine 146
Sulfamethoxazole 146
   trimethoprim 103
Sulfasoxazole
   diolamine 541
   solution 492
Sulfonamides 103, 145, 147, 443, 485, 493, 960
Sulfonyl ureas 512
Sulphacetamide 541, 545
Sulphadiazine 405, 518
Superficial
   foreign body removal 313
   lipid layer 11
   punctate
      epithelial keratopathy 204
      keratitis 157, 201, 477
      keratopathy 201
Superoxide dismutase 637
Suprofen 172, 179, 496, 504, 543
Surface keratopathy 459
Surfactant cleaning solutions 515, 562, 565
Surgery for giant retinal tears 803*f*
Surgical techniques of glued IOL 860
Suture removal 313
Sutured scleral fixated intraocular lenses 860
Sutureless lamellar keratoplasty 813
Sweating 455
Symblepharon 523, 525, 527
Sympathetic ophthalmia 168, 757
Syphilitic uveitis 396
Systemic
   antibiotics 850
      in ophthalmology 493
   disease 833, 840
   hypertension 189, 759

lupus erythematosus 527
nonsteroidal anti-
inflammatory agents
621*t*
steroids 168, 447
therapy 511, 616, 737
uses of
fluoroquinolones 142
tetracyclines 125

T

Tachycardia 300, 455
Taenia solium 69
Tazobactam 108
TB granuloma of choroid 392
T-cell-targeted therapies 840
Tear
albumin 19
drainage system 10*f*
film layers 6*f*, 12*f*
globulin assay 32, 33*f*
osmolarity 32
test strips 567
Telaprevir 197, 213
Telavancin 102, 114
Telbivudine 197
Telithromycin 102
Tenofovir 197, 198, 212, 213, 216
Tenon's capsule 58, 335
Terbinafine 227, 239, 499, 547
Terfenadine 294
Tetracaine 302, 308, 309, 504
solution 505
Tetracycline 102, 123, 125, 151, 541, 593, 962
ointment 492
Tetrahydrozine HCl 291
Tetrahydrozoline 291, 503, 547, 548
Tetramethylglutaric acid 511
Thalassemia 532, 538
Thayer-Martin medium 70
Thermal circulation 45
Thiazides 486
Thickened corneal nerves 526
Thioglycolate broth 70
Thioridazine 490
Thiourea 434
Third
generation cephalosporins 110
nerve palsy sparing pupil 533
Three layers of precorneal tear film 6*f*
Threonine 20, 53
Thrombocytopenia 186, 455, 532, 757, 758

Thygeson's superficial punctate keratitis 202
Ticarcillin 107, 151
Tinidazole 144
Tinnitus 454
Tipranavir 198, 220
Tobramycin 118, 121, 149-151, 541, 545, 854
solution 492
Tolosa-Hunt syndrome 619
Topical
anesthesia 632
antibiotic 609, 632
anticataract therapy 568
anti-inflammatory therapy 494
azithromycin eyedrop 905
brimonidine 500
burning sensation 204
fluorometholone 632
fluoroquinolones 143, 610
glycerine solution 388
immune therapy 380, 383, 510, 559
immunosuppressors 283, 296, 504
levocabastine 503
mast cell
inhibitors 283, 502
stabilizers 283
NACl
ointment 388
solution 388
nonsteroidal anti-
inflammatory
agents 621*t*
drugs 495
solution 157
containing 354
steroid 283, 295, 444, 504
antibiotic combinations 165, 544
tetracycline 126
vitamin A 839
Tortuous vessels 532
Toxemia of pregnancy 532
Toxic
amblyopia 474-484, 487
anterior segment syndrome 891, 892*f*
endothelial cell destruction syndrome 893
impaired vision 486
miosis 481
Toxocara canis 69, 979
Toxoplasma
gondii 69, 132, 393, 394, 405, 517, 977
infection 394, 405, 517

Toxoplasmosis 126, 530, 619, 977
Trachoma 470
Transcorneal iontophoresis 78, 79*f*
Transient
    flora 71
    vision disturbances 366
Transpupillary thermotherapy 706
Trans-scleral iontophoresis 78
Traumatic inflammation of eye 157, 162
Treatment of
    bacterial endophthalmitis 153*t*, 668*t*
    central serous choroidopathy 685
    cytomegalovirus retinopathy 80
    dacryocystitis 656
    diabetic macular edema 993
    drug resistant HSV keratitis 211
    fungal keratitis 651
    hairy cell leukemia 211
    ocular surface diseases 926
    retinal angiomatous proliferation 702
    vernal keratoconjunctivitis 285
Treponema pallidum 68, 105, 141
Triamcinolone 158
    acetonide 494, 543
Triazoles 227, 232
Trichiasis 523, 525
Trichinosis 530
Trichomonas vaginalis 144
Trifluorothymidine 201
Trifluridine 197, 199, 201, 497, 545
Trimethoprim 103, 146, 492
    polymyxin b sulphate 609
    sulfamethoxazole 146
    sulfate 542
Tripelennamine 294
Triprolidine 294
Tropicamide 344, 345, 347, 506, 943
Trypsin 20
Tryptophane 20
Tuberculosis 529
Tumoral diseases 764
Tunnel vision 490
Turner's syndrome 531
Two-chamber pump 86
Tyrosine 53

U

Ulcer 479
Ulcerative colitis 535
Ultraviolet radiation 523
Uncontrolled leukopenia 758
Unique ocular drug delivery systems 73, 75
Unrolling giant retinal tear 878
Urea powder 501
Uric acid 638
    crystals 536
Urinary frequency 455
Urokinase 329, 509
Urticaria 454
Use of
    antibiotics in irrigating solutions for intraocular surgery 149
    beta-adrenergic blockers in ocular vascular diseases 911
    corticosteroids in
        alkali burns of cornea and conjunctiva 616
        pseudophakic bullous keratopathy 616
    echinocandins 243
    macrolides 133
    methylcellulose 324
    nonsteroidal anti-inflammatory drugs in inflammation 619
    tissue adhesives in ophthalmology 810
Uveitis 175, 387, 525-531, 538, 617, 622, 942, 950
Uveoscleral
    aqueous outflow pathway 48*f*
    outflow pathways 47

V

Vaccinia 527
    virus 193
Vacuolation theory 45
Valacyclovir 196, 199, 205, 498, 546
Valganciclovir 197, 206, 208
Valine 20, 53
Vancomycin 102, 114, 149-151, 493, 543, 594, 849, 854, 962
    resistant *Staphylococcus aureus* 116
Vapor pressure 801, 801*f*
Variable color vision 477
Varicella zoster
    infection 204
    virus 193, 194, 196*f*, 407, 519
Vascular
    dilation 478
    endothelial growth factor 185, 676, 883, 911, 915

Ventricular arrhythmias 458
Vernal
    conjunctivitis 157, 281
    keratoconjunctivitis 280, 282*f*, 295, 954
Verteporfin 362, 363, 817
Vertical gaze palsy 484
Vesicular rashes 528
Viagra 490
Vidarabine 196, 198, 201, 496, 545
Vigabatrin 490
Vinca alkaloids 480
Viral
    disease of eyelids 395
    keratitis 1013
    protein synthesis 196
    resistance 200
Viruses 69
Visceral perforation 451
Viscoelasticity 316
Viscosity 316, 800, 800*f*
Viscosurgical devices 436
Vision regeneration 1029
Visual
    acuity 438
    evoked potential 439
    field
        constriction 478, 480, 488
        defects 487, 489, 490
        hemianopia 478
        scotoma 474
    hallucinations 191, 473, 474, 475, 477-479, 480, 481, 483-490, 759
Vitamin
    A deficiency 535
    B deficiency 535
    C 638, 640
        deficiency 535
    D 490
    E 638
        therapy 511
Vitrectomy 324, 852
    and posterior segment surgery 383
Vitreo-retinal surgery 174, 983
Vitreous
    cyst 530
    floaters 487
    fluorophotometry 354
    haziness 529
    hemorrhage 367, 530, 532, 533
    humor 16
    opacity 527, 535
    surgery 617
Vitritis 528, 530, 531, 538
Vogt-Koyanagi-Harada disease 168, 190, 525, 830
von Hippel's disease 526

W

Walls of orbit 4*f*
Wegener's granulomatosis 757
White
    blood cells 950
    snow vision 483
    vision 478
Wilms' tumor 537
Wilson's disease 536
Wright stain 70
Wuchereria bancrofti 69
Wyburn syndrome 526

X

Xalcom 501
Xanthophylls 638
Xenopus laevis 148
Xeroderma pigmentosum 526
Xerophthalmia 534, 535, 539
Xerosis of cornea and conjunctiva 535

Y

Yeast fungi 225
Yellow
    sclera 477
    vision 486

Z

Zalcitabine 198, 216, 398, 516
Zanamavir 197, 223
Zero order kinetics 56
Zidovudine 197, 215, 216, 398, 497, 516, 546
Ziehl-Neelsen's stain 70
Zinc 638
    sulfate 431, 548
Zone-Quick test 432, 433
Zonular cataract 535